Volume 2

Fluid, Electrolyte, and Acid–Base Disorders

Volume 2

Fluid, Electrolyte, and Acid–Base Disorders

Edited by

Allen I. Arieff, M.D.

Professor of Medicine
University of California San Francisco
Chief, Clinical Nephrology
Veterans Administration Medical Center
San Francisco, California

and

Ralph A. DeFronzo, M.D.

Associate Professor of Medicine
Yale University School of Medicine
Section of Nephrology
New Haven, Connecticut

CHURCHILL LIVINGSTONE
NEW YORK, EDINBURGH, LONDON, AND MELBOURNE 1985

Acquisitions editor: *Lewis Reines*
Sponsoring editor: *Lynne Herndon*
Copy editor: *Peggy Brigg*
Production editor: *Fred L. Kantrowitz*
Production supervisor: *Sharon D. Tuder*
Compositor: *The Kingsport Press*
Printer/Binder: *The Murray Printing Co.*

Distributed in the United Kingdom by Churchill Livingstone, Robert Stevenson House, 1–3 Baxter's Place, Leith Walk, Edinburgh EH1 3AF and by associated companies, branches and representatives throughout the world.

First published 1985

Printed in USA

ISBN 0–443–08190–5

7 6 5 4 3 2 1

Library of Congress Cataloging in Publication Data
Main entry under title:

Fluid, electrolyte, and acid-base disorders.

Includes bibliographies and index.
1. Body fluid disorders. 2. Water-electrolyte imbalances. 3. Acid-base imbalances. 4. Water-electrolyte balance (Physiology) I. Arieff, Allen I. (Allen Ives), 1938 II. DeFronzo, Ralph A. [DNLM: 1. Acid-Base Balance. 2. Acid-Base Imbalance. 3. Water-Electrolyte Balance. 4. Water-Electrolyte Imbalance. WD 220 F6438]
RC630.F56 1985 616.3'9 84–11392
ISBN 0–443–08190–5 (v. 1)

To my loving and supportive family—my parents, Alex and Betty, and my children, Allison and Adrienne

Allen I. Arieff

I would like to dedicate this book to my father. His devotion to hard work and perfection has set the standards that have guided me throughout my life. He may have been a poor man, but he possessed a richness of heart that is unmatched in today's society.

Ralph A. DeFronzo

Contributors

Sheldon Adler, M.D.
Professor of Medicine; Head, Renal and Electrolyte Unit; Assistant Chief of Medicine, University of Pittsburgh School of Medicine, Montefiore Hospital, Pittsburgh, Pennsylvania

Zalman S. Agus, M.D.
Associate Professor of Medicine; Chief, Renal-Electrolyte Section, Department of Medicine, University of Pennsylvania School of Medicine, Philadelphia, Pennsylvania

Robert Alvis, M.D.
Assistant Professor, Department of Medicine, Temple University School of Medicine, Philadelphia, Pennsylvania

Allen I. Arieff, M.D.
Professor of Medicine, University of California San Francisco; Chief, Clinical Nephrology, Veterans Administration Medical Center, San Francisco, California

Robert A. Bear, M.D., F.R.C.P.(C)
Associate Professor of Medicine, Department of Medicine, University of Toronto, Toronto, Ontario

Bruce E. Berger, M.D.
Clinical Assistant Professor, Department of Medicine, University of North Carolina, Chapel Hill, North Carolina

Margaret Johnson Bia, M.D.
Associate Professor of Medicine, Section of Nephrology, Yale University School of Medicine, New Haven, Connecticut

Edward G. Biglieri, M.D.
Professor of Medicine, Department of Medicine, University of California San Francisco; Chief of Endocrine Service, San Francisco General Hospital, San Francisco, California

Stanley A. Blumenthal, M.D.
Professor of Medicine, State University of New York, Upstate Medical Center; Department of Medicine, Veterans Administration Medical Center, Syracuse, New York

Barry M. Brenner, M.D.
Samuel A. Levine Professor of Medicine, Harvard Medical School; Director, Renal Division and Laboratory of Kidney and Electrolyte Physiology, Brigham and Women's Hospital, Boston, Massachusetts

Hugh J. Carroll, M.D.
Professor of Medicine; Director, Electrolyte-Hypertension Division, State University of New York, Downstate Medical Center, Brooklyn, New York

Jack W. Coburn, M.D.
Professor of Medicine, Department of Medicine, UCLA School of Medicine; Medical Investigator, Veterans Administration Medical Center, West Los Angeles, California

Malcolm Cox, M.D.
Associate Professor, Department of Medicine, University of Pennsylvania School of Medicine; Chief, Renal Section, Philadelphia Veterans Administration Medical Center, Philadelphia, Pennsylvania

Ralph A. DeFronzo, M.D.
Associate Professor of Medicine, Yale University School of Medicine, Section of Nephrology, New Haven, Connecticut

John Dobbins, M.D.
Associate Professor, Division of Gastroenterology, Department of Medicine, Yale University School of Medicine, New Haven, Connecticut

Gary Dubois, M.D.
Clinical Instructor, Department of Medicine, University of Oklahoma; Staff Physician, Veterans Administration Medical Center, Oklahoma City, Oklahoma

Leon G. Fine, M.D.
Professor of Medicine; Chief, Division of Nephrology, Center for the Health Sciences, UCLA School of Medicine, Los Angeles, California

Walter Flamenbaum, M.D.
Professor of Medicine, Mt. Sinai School of Medicine; Chief, Division of Nephrology and Hypertension, Beth Israel Medical Center, New York, New York

Donald S. Fraley, M.D.
Associate Professor of Medicine, Assistant Head of Renal-Electrolyte Unit, Director of Medical Intensive Care Unit, University of Pittsburgh School of Medicine, Montefiore Hospital, Pittsburgh, Pennsylvania

Richard Friedman, M.D.
Division of Nephrology and Hypertension, Beth Israel Medical Center, New York, New York

Michael Geheb, M.D.
Assistant Professor and Assistant Chairman, Department of Medicine, Wayne State University School of Medicine, Detroit, Michigan

Stanley Goldfarb, M.D.
Associate Professor of Medicine, Renal-Electrolyte Section, Department of Medicine, University of Pennsylvania School of Medicine, Philadelphia, Pennsylvania

Marc B. Goldstein, M.B., F.R.C.P.(C)
Professor of Medicine; Coordinator, Division of Nephrology, University of Toronto, Toronto, Ontario

David A. Goodkin, M.D.
Instructor in Medicine, Temple University Health Sciences Center, Philadelphia, Pennsylvania

Mitchell L. Halperin, M.D., F.R.C.P.(C)
Professor of Medicine, Department of Medicine, Saint Michael's Hospital, University of Toronto, Toronto, Ontario

Rosemary E. Hernandez, M.D.
Nephrology Fellow, Department of Medicine, University of California San Francisco, San Francisco, California

Henry N. Hulter, M.D.
Adjunct Lecturer, Division of Nephrology, Department of Medicine, University of San Francisco, San Francisco, California

Khursheed N. Jeejeebhoy, M.B., Ph.D, F.R.C.P.(C)
Professor, Department of Medicine, University of Toronto; Chief of Gastroenterology, Gastroenterology Division, Toronto General Hospital, Toronto, Ontario

Edward R. Jones, M.D.
Assistant Professor of Medicine, Temple University Health Sciences Center, Philadelphia, Pennsylvania

Robert G. Josse, M.D., F.R.C.P.(C), F.A.C.P.
Assistant Professor of Medicine, Department of Medicine, Saint Michael's Hospital, University of Toronto, Toronto, Ontario

Adrian I. Katz, M.D.
Professor of Medicine, Department of Medicine, University of Chicago, Pritzker School of Medicine, Chicago, Illinois

Alan S. Kliger, M.D.
Associate Clinical Professor, Renal Division, Department of Medicine, Yale University School of Medicine, New Haven, Connecticut

Kiyoshi Kurokawa, M.D.
Professor of Medicine, Department of Medicine, UCLA School of Medicine; Chief, Nephrology Section, Veterans Administration Wadsworth Medical Center, Los Angeles, California

Ira Kurtz, M.D.
Fellow in Nephrology, University of California San Francisco, San Francisco, California

Neil A. Kurtzman, M.D.
Chief, Section of Nephrology, Department of Medicine, University of Illinois Hospital; Professor of Medicine and Physiology, University of Illinois College of Medicine at Chicago; Consultant, West Side Veterans Administration Hospital, Chicago, Illinois

Melvin E. Laski, M.D.
Department of Nephrology, University of Illinois Hospital; Staff Nephrologist, West Side Veterans Administration Hospital, Chicago, Illinois

William E. Lattanzi, M.D.
Professor of Clinical Pediatrics, Yale University School of Medicine; Chairman, Department of Pediatrics, Hospital of Saint Raphael, New Haven, Connecticut

Kai Lau, M.D.
Director of Nephrology Division, Michael Reese Hospital; Associate Professor of Medicine, University of Chicago, Chicago, Illinois

David B.N. Lee, M.D.
Associate Professor of Medicine, Department of Medicine, UCLA School of Medicine; Chief, Nephrology Division, Veterans Administration Sepulveda Hospital, Sepulveda, California

Barton S. Levine, M.D.
Assistant Professor of Medicine, Department of Medicine, UCLA School of Medicine; Assistant Chief, Nephrology Section, Veterans Administration Wadsworth Medical Center, Los Angeles, California

David Z. Levine, M.D.
Professor of Medicine, Department of Medicine, University of Ottawa; Chief, Renal Service, Ottawa General Hospital, Ottawa, Canada

Marshall D. Lindheimer, M.D.
Professor of Medicine and Obstetrics & Gynecology, Departments of Medicine and Obstetrics and Gynecology, University of Chicago, Pritzker School of Medicine; Head, Medical High Risk Clinic, Chicago Lying in Hospital, Chicago, Illinois

Shaul G. Massry, M.D.
Professor of Medicine and Chief, Division of Nephrology, Department of Medicine, University of Southern California, School of Medicine, Los Angeles, California

R. Curtis Morris, M.D.
Professor of Medicine and Pediatrics, Department of Medicine, University of California San Francisco; Director of the General Clinical Research Center, San Francisco, California

Arnold M. Moses, M.D.
Professor of Medicine, State University of New York, Upstate Medical Center; Department of Medicine, Veterans Administration Medical Center, Syracuse, New York

Robert G. Narins, M.D.
Professor of Medicine; Head, Section of Nephrology, Department of Medicine, Temple University School of Medicine, Philadelphia, Pennsylvania

Edward P. Nord, M.D.
Assistant Professor of Medicine, Division of Nephrology, Center for the Health Sciences, UCLA School of Medicine, Los Angeles, California

Man S. Oh, M.D.
Associate Professor of Medicine, Co-Director, Electrolyte-Hypertension Division, State University of New York, Downstate Medical Center, Brooklyn, New York

Kent H. Raymond, M.D.
Renal Division, Department of Medicine, University of Texas Health Sciences Center, San Antonio, Texas

H. John Reineck, M.D.
Associate Professor of Medicine, Department of Medicine, University of Texas Health Sciences Center, San Antonio, Texas

John W. Rowe, M.D.
Associate Professor of Medicine and Director, Division on Ageing, Harvard Medical School; Director, Geriatric Research Education Clinical Center, West Roxbury Veteran's Administration Medical Center; Chief, Division of Gerontology, Department of Medicine and Thorndike Laboratory, Beth Israel and Brigham and Women's Hospital, Boston, Massachusetts

Morris Schambelan, M.D.
Professor of Medicine, Department of Medicine, University of California San Francisco, San Francisco, California

Anthony Sebastian, M.D.
Associate Professor, Department of Medicine; Associate Director of the General Clinical Research Center, University of California San Francisco, San Francisco, California

Robert J. Shay, M.D.
Instructor in Medicine, Temple University Health Sciences Center, Philadelphia, Pennsylvania

Norman J. Siegel, M.D.
Professor of Pediatrics and Medicine; Director, Section of Pediatric Nephrology; Vice Chairman, Department of Pediatrics, Yale University School of Medicine, New Haven, Connecticut

Irwin Singer, M.D.
Professor of Medicine, University of Pennsylvania School of Medicine; Director of Clinical Research, Renal-Electrolyte Section, Hospital of The University of Pennsylvania; Philadelphia Veterans Administration Medical Center, Philadelphia, Pennsylvania

Karl L. Skorecki, M.D.
Instructor in Medicine, Harvard Medical School; Associate Physician, Brigham and Women's Hospital, Boston, Massachusetts

J. Douglas Smith, M.D.
Assistant Professor of Medicine, Division of Nephrology, Yale New Haven Hospital, New Haven, Connecticut

Jay H. Stein, M.D.
Professor and Chairman, Department of Medicine; Director, Division of Renal Diseases, The University of Texas Health Sciences Center, San Antonio, Texas

David H.P. Streeten, M.B. D. Phil
Professor of Medicine, State University of New York, Upstate Medical Center, Syracuse, New York

Raymond Townsend, M.D.
Instructor in Medicine, Temple University Health Sciences Center, Philadelphia, Pennsylvania

David G. Warnock, M.D.
Associate Professor of Medicine, University of California San Francisco; Chief, Nephrology Section, Department of Medicine, Veterans Administration Medical Center, San Francisco, California

Foreword

The study of the volume and composition of body fluids was one of the earliest examples of clinical research growing from an emerging laboratory capability. The ability to measure electrolytes and pH in body fluids initially led to a better definition of clinical states of disordered volume, tonicity, and acid-base regulation. As a result, more basic questions were progressively posed about physiology and pathophysiology. As the questions have become more basic, so have the techniques for answering them. In place of the original balance and clearance studies, we now have micropuncture, microperfusion, and isolated membrane preparations as model systems. We are able to define hormonal regulation of body fluid homeostasis at the level of receptors and postreceptor events. The mechanisms controlling cellular production, processing, and secretion of these hormones are also being elucidated. The importance of the concept that abnormalities of function elicit predictable compensatory responses has been recognized. Knowledge of normal compensatory responses in terms of mechanism, time, and extent has helped, for example, to clarify the pathophysiology of uremia, to predict the effects of altered tonicity and its treatment on cell volume and function, and to define simple versus mixed acid-base disturbances.

Understanding basic pathophysiology has permitted the design and monitoring of sophisticated therapeutic programs. It has also facilitated improved pharmacologic approaches to the regulation of volume, tonicity, and composition of body fluids. In a field where basic observations and clinical application proceed as rapidly as this one, a new text that interprets the state of the art for the practicing physician is always welcome.

This book, which is sophisticated enough to serve the nephrologist, is broad and informative enough to be part of the library of a general internist. It provides an excellent overview of normal acid-base, electrolyte, and water physiology. The basic understanding of these processes is essential for what follows, which is the diagnostic and therapeutic approach to clinical disorders founded on a firm knowledge of pathophysiology and pharmacology. Discussions of basic physiology are followed by general chapters on pathophysiology, covering, for example, abnormalities of volume regulation, abnormalities of tonicity, and abnormalities of acid-base regulation. Normal and abnormal metabolism of potassium, calcium, magnesium, and phosphorus are handled in individual chapters. After reviewing the effects of diuretics on the previously described physiology, the text then shifts to a group of disease states and deals with the broad spectrum of fluid, electrolyte, and acid-base problems as they occur in, for example, uremia, pulmonary disease, and gastrointestinal disease. There are additional chapters that should be especially helpful and are not always presented in a text of this sort; for example, special considerations in the pediatric age group and in the geriatric age group. This book has a distinguished group of authors presenting coverage of a dynamic subject. Though it is directed primarily at nephrologists and internists, it will almost certainly be of value to all of those interested in the field of fluid, electrolyte, and acid-base disorders.

Samuel O. Thier, M.D.

Preface

Fluid, electrolyte, and acid-base disturbances are among the commonest disorders encountered in clinical medicine. In addition to internal medicine and pediatrics, the practitioners of neurology, general surgery, gynecology, obstetrics, and the various other subspecialties will encounter fluid, electrolyte, and acid-base abnormalities as a part of their everyday practice. Among the subspecialties of internal medicine, the nephrologist traditionally has been assumed to be the reigning authority in matters pertaining to fluid, electrolyte, and acid-base metabolism. Nonetheless, it is important that all general internists, particularly those with subspecialities in endocrinology/metabolism, gastroenterology, cardiology, pulmonary disease and oncology, have a firm working knowledge of the disorders of water, electrolyte, and acid-base since they must deal with these problems on a day to day basis.

Each book should have a "raison d'être" and in the case of this work that reason is the rapid growth in knowledge relating to water, electrolyte, and acid-base physiology and pathophysiology. The book has been conveniently divided into three sections, each of which may prove useful in different circumstances. In section I, entitled "Normal Water and Acid-Base Regulation," the biochemistry, physiology and clinical correlates of the regulation of intracellular and extracellular volume, tonicity and pH as well as the content and concentration of sodium, potassium, chloride, calcium, magnesium, and phosphorous are discussed. The editors have deliberately sought out opposing viewpoints in an attempt to present a balanced overview of a variety of topics (e.g., see the discussion of fluid volume regulation presented in chapter 1 as opposed to chapter 3). The first section should be useful to all of those who seek to explore the normal regulatory processes. It is hoped that this will lead to an increased understanding of pathophysiology of common fluid, electrolyte, and acid-base disturbances.

Section II deals with specific pathologic states. The fluid, electrolyte, and acid-base abnormalities associated with acute and chronic renal failure, gastrointestinal diseases, pituitary and adrenal disease and diabetes, particularly diabetic comas, are exhaustively described. There is now a worldwide dialysis population which exceeds 100,000, and specific emphasis is placed on the complications relating to the dialysis (hemodialysis, peritoneal dialysis, and chronic ambulatory peritoneal dialysis) population. Among the major problems confronting many patients with end-stage renal failure are renal osteodystrophy and various central nervous system disorders, such as impaired mental function, uremic encephalopathy, and dialysis dementia. The current state of knowledge about these disorders is addressed. In recent years our understanding of the effects of pregnancy on water and electrolyte metabolism, as well as on renal function, has undergone significant changes. More and more women with impaired renal function are becoming pregnant, and the therapeutic implications of this are discussed.

In section III, entitled "Special Considerations," we discuss a variety of unrelated, yet clinically important topics, which are commonly associated with disturbances in water, electrolyte, and acid-base metabolism. Drugs have become pervasive in our practice of medicine. Many commonly prescribed medications have profound effects on the composition of all body fluids. This is particularly true of the diuretics. Their uses, as well as abuses, are discussed in detail. Total parenteral nutrition has become an increasingly popular therapeutic tool. The different types of therapy, as well as side effects, are explored. The special problems of fluid, electrolyte, and acid-base abnormalities presented by both the very old and very young are not well appreciated. These important areas are explored in depth. Lastly, it is important that the physician be able to recognize the clinical manifestations associated with disturbances in water, electrolyte, and acid-base metabolism. Therefore, a detailed discussion of the signs and symptoms resulting from these disorders has been included.

It is our hope that we and our many outstanding contributors have compiled a useful and enduring work. We thank these contributors, for this is, in fact, their book.

Allen I. Arieff, M.D.
Ralph A. DeFronzo, M.D.

Contents

Volume 1

Section I: Normal Water and Acid-Base Regulation

1. Regulation of Extra- and Intracellular Fluid Composition and Content 1
   Man S. Oh, Hugh J. Carroll
2. Sodium Metabolism and Maintenance of Extracellular Fluid Volume 39
   Kent H. Raymond, H. John Reineck, Jay H. Stein
3. Edema Forming States: Congestive Heart Failure, Liver Disease and Nephrotic Syndrome 77
   Karl L. Skorecki, Barry M. Brenner
4. Disorders of Thirst and Renal Water Excretion 119
   Malcolm Cox, Michael Geheb, Irwin Singer
5. Hypo- and Hyperosmolar States: Diagnostic Approaches 185
   Robert Alvis, Michael Geheb, Malcolm Cox
6. Acid-Base Regulation: Cellular and Whole Body 221
   Sheldon Adler, Donald S. Fraley
7. Metabolic Acid-Base Disorders: Pathophysiology, Classification, and Treatment 269

   Part I: Definitions 269
   Part II: Metabolic Acidosis 281
   Part III: Metabolic Alkalosis 335

   Robert G. Narins, Jr., Edward R. Jones, Raymond Townsend, David A. Goodkin, Robert J. Shay
8. Acid-Base Disturbances in Pulmonary Medicine 385
   Melvin E. Laski, Neil A. Kurtzman
9. Clinical Disorders of Potassium Metabolism 413
   J. Douglas Smith, Margaret Johnson Bia, Ralph A. DeFronzo
10. Calcium Metabolism: Normal and Abnormal 511
    Zalman S. Agus, Stanley Goldfarb
11. Magnesium Metabolism: Normal and Abnormal 575
    Kai Lau

12. Physiology of Phosphorus Metabolism and Pathophysiology of Hypophosphatemia and Hyperphosphatemia 625
Kiyoshi Kurokawa, Barton S. Levine, David B.N. Lee, Shaul G. Massry

Index

Volume 2

Section II: Specific Pathologic States

13. Acute Renal Failure 661
Walter Flamenbaum, Richard Friedman

14. Chronic Renal Failure 683
Leon G. Fine, Edward P. Nord

15. Renal Osteodystrophy 729
Jack W. Coburn

16. Complications of Dialysis: Hemodialysis, Peritoneal Dialysis, CAPD 777
Alan S. Kliger

17. Gastrointestinal Disorders 827
John Dobbins

18. Acid-Base and Electrolyte Disorders Associated with Endocrine Disease: Pituitary and Thyroid 851
Arnold M. Moses, Stanley A. Blumenthal, David H.P. Streeten

19. Acid-Base and Electrolyte Disorders Associated with Adrenal Disease 893
Anthony Sebastian, Morris Schambelan, Henry N. Hulter, Ira Kurtz, Rosemary E. Hernandez, Edward G. Biglieri, R. Curtis Morris

20. Diabetic Comas 933
Mitchell L. Halperin, Marc B. Goldstein, Robert A. Bear, Robert G. Josse

21. Effects of Water, Acid-Base, and Electrolyte Disorders on the Central Nervous System 969
Allen I. Arieff

22. Fluid and Electrolyte Metabolism in Normal and Abnormal Pregnancy 1041
Marshall D. Lindheimer, Adrian I. Katz

Section III: Special Considerations

23. Clinical Manifestations of Electrolyte Disorders 1087
Gary D. Dubois, Allen I. Arieff

24. Drugs and Water Metabolism 1145
Arnold M. Moses, Stanley A. Blumenthal, David H.P. Streeten

25. Sites of Action and Clinical Uses of Diuretics 1159
Bruce E. Berger, David G. Warnock

26. Total Parenteral Nutrition 1191
Khursheed N. Jeejeebhoy, Mitchell L. Halperin, David Z. Levine

27. Fluid and Electrolyte Therapy in Children 1211
Norman J. Siegel, William E. Lattanzi

28. Aging and Renal Function 1231
John W. Rowe

Index

SECTION II

Specific Pathologic States

13

Acute Renal Failure

Walter Flamenbaum
Richard Friedman

Acute renal failure (ARF) is a syndrome that may be functionally defined as a rapid and progressive decrease in renal function with an acute onset and a limited course.[1] Acute renal failure has been variously termed acute tubular necrosis, implying a histopathologic diagnosis, and by terms suggesting a pathophysiologic mechanism, such as vasomotor nephropathy. To avoid either histopathologic or pathophysiologic inferences, we will use the term acute renal failure. This definition of acute renal failure is broad enough to include renal diseases other than those associated with this diagnosis. The generality of this term, acute renal failure, requires a clinical approach in establishing its diagnosis by excluding other processes resulting in abrupt changes in renal function.[2]

The alterations in renal function characteristic of acute renal failure include a decrease in glomerular filtration rate, as well as associated changes in tubular function.[3-7] Azotemia, the accumulation of nitrogenous wastes manifested by rises in blood urea nitrogen (BUN) and creatinine concentrations, along with changes in other body fluid constituents, is the hallmark of this decline in glomerular filtration rate. The abnormalities in fluid and electrolyte homeostasis, most typically an inability to normally conserve salt and water, are due to the associated abnormality in tubular function. A quantitative description of alterations in urine volume, usually a 24-hour urine volume of <400 ml as being oliguric, was previously included within the descriptive definition of acute renal failure. Recent clinical studies have virtually eliminated urine volume as part of the definition of acute renal failure, since acute renal failure may occur without oliguria.[7-9] While it may be proposed that oliguric and nonoliguric acute renal failure differ in terms of either pathogenesis or pathophysiology, it is easier to accept the differences in the clinical course of these two forms of acute renal failure. Nonoliguric acute renal failure is characterized by a lower morbidity and mortality, diminished need for therapy with dialytic techniques, and, in general, a more benign course.

Just as a static definition of acute renal failure (such as acute tubular necrosis) or an inflexible requirement for diagnosis (such as oliguria) is no longer reasonable, an inflexible clinical approach cannot be used, since acute renal failure varies depending on when clinical intervention is occurring during the course of the syndrome. For this purpose, acute renal failure may be subdivided into the initiation, maintenance, and recovery phases.[10-12] Each of these subdivisions of the temporal course of acute renal failure has important clinical implications, since therapy relative to the phase of acute renal failure varies. The initiation phase of acute renal failure is the interval between the etiologic event and the first clinical manifestations of acute renal failure. Included within this phase is the clinical description of "incipient" acute renal failure, during which therapy may prevent acute renal failure, convert oliguric to nonoliguric acute renal failure, or modify the clinical course of acute renal failure. Once acute renal failure is established the patient enters the maintenance phase and treatment is directed at the fluid, electrolyte, acid base, and nutritional consequences of the disease. The maintenance phase of acute renal failure covers the interval of progressive azotemia until the onset of the recovery phase, which is characterized by a gradual and progressive return in renal function. Initially during the recovery phase, patients demonstrate increasing urine volume, most marked in patients who have been oliguric, followed by a slower return in tubular function. The recovery phase concludes when renal function reaches its new plateau and may last as long as 12 to 18 months. It will be extremely useful to keep these phases in mind when considering each of the physiologic consequences of acute renal failure.

CLINICAL ACUTE RENAL FAILURE: A REVIEW

In this and subsequent sections the primary data base used for discussion will be clinically derived. The information available from experimental models or nonclinical situations cannot be excluded, since these form the basis for clinical advances and a more complete understanding of clinical events. The next section of this chapter deals with a detailed review of the physiologic consequences of acute renal failure, whereas the current section provides the reader with a basis for placing those observations and comments in perspective.

Acute Renal Failure: A Diagnosis of Exclusion

The definition of acute renal failure as noted requires that other processes be excluded before the clinician reaches the conclusion that a patient has acute renal failure.[2,7] In general, a complete history and physical examination, a urinalysis, and generally available biochemical determinations of urine and plasma composition, along with appropriate radiographic studies, permit one to delineate the cause of any observed reduction in renal function.[2,13] The various subsets of disease entities that must be considered when evaluating a patient with a sudden onset of deteriorating renal function are listed in Table 13–1.

Prerenal azotemia is the commonest clinical disorder resulting in a sudden deterioration in renal function. The etiology of prerenal azotemia may be subdivided into those associated with true hypovolemia, such as external fluid losses due to hemorrhage or vomiting, or fluid sequestration, as occurs in patients developing large third-space accumulations or those events associated with an ineffective circulating blood volume (e.g., cardiogenic shock, hypoalbuminemia due to nephrosis or cirrhosis, or vascular pooling due to sepsis or anaphylaxis). Regardless of the etiology, renal hypoperfusion occurs, resulting in azotemia, and appropriate physiologic responses of salt and water conservation through stimula-

Table 13–1. Diagnosis by Exclusion of ARF: Entities to Be Considered

Prerenal azotemia
True hypovolemia
Ineffective circulating volume
Renal parenchymal diseases
Nephritis
Nephrosis
Disorders of calcium or urate homeostasis
Obstructive uropathy
Intrinsic
Extrinsic
Renovascular disease
Arterial
Venous

tion of the renin–angiotensin–aldosterone axis, release of antidiuretic hormone, and other homeostatic mechanisms. Although there are no specific changes in urine sediment, the urine composition is characterized by decreased sodium concentration and increased specific gravity or other indices of water conservation. The ability of the kidney to respond appropriately to hyperperfusion with conservation of salt and water clearly indicates intact tubular function. A prompt diagnosis is important, since these observed changes are functional and revert with treatment. Alternatively, failure to correct the hemodynamic alterations responsible for prerenal azotemia may result in acute renal failure.

Renal parenchymal diseases are perhaps the second most common category of non-ARF-associated acute changes in renal function. While any renal parenchymal disease may result in this pattern of clinical change, they may be subdivided into renal diseases associated with nephritis, nephrotic syndrome, or disorders of calcium or urage homeostasis. Diagnosis of these processes is important, since specific therapy may be required to restore renal function to normal and to prevent their progression to chronic renal failure. Many patients with renal parenchymal diseases may undergo an acute decrease in renal function due to a superimposed process, such as dehydration, infection, hypertension, or urinary tract obstruction. The superimposed process mimicking acute renal failure may be reversed by appropriate therapy, only to find that the patient has a specific renal parenchymal disease resulting in reduced renal function. The diagnosis of renal parenchymal disease may require specific procedures related to that process, including renal biopsy. Last, the disorders of calcium or urate homeostasis are also important, since they represent preventable causes of renal disease. For example, uric acid nephropathy, which may be observed in patients with myeloproliferative disorders undergoing chemotherapy, can be prevented or minimized through hydration, urinary alkinization, and the use of allopurinol.

Obstructive uropathy and renovascular disease may also result in a sudden change of renal function suggestive of acute renal failure. The diagnosis of obstructive uropathy is usually suggested by the history and physical examination and is an important correctable cause of sudden renal failure. Obstruction may result in renal failure, with or without oligoanuria, when there is bladder outlet obstruction, bilateral ureteral obstruction, unilateral obstruction in a solitary kidney, or an obstructive component superimposed on preexisting renal disease. The anuria that may occur in patients with obstructive uropathy may also be suggestive of renal cortical necrosis or fulminant glomerulonephritis. Alternatively, urine flow in obstructed patients may consist of a sequential pattern of ologoanuria and polyuria, due to a "ball-valve"-like obstruction. The etiology of obstruction includes any event resulting in intrinsic or extrinsic compression of the urinary system. Extrinsic causes of obstruction include tumor (either local or metastatic) and extensive retroperitoneal disease. Renal calculi, blood clots, benign prostatic hypertrophy, and papillary necrosis or necrotizing papillitis are examples of intrinsic causes of obstruction. Radiographic procedures are usually required to establish the site of obstruction. These studies include procedures ranging from a plain x-ray film of the abdomen (KUB) or ultrasound examination, a computed tomography (CT) scan (with or without contrast media enhancement), intravenous pyelography, or retrograde ureteral catheterization.

In order for renovascular disease to result in severe changes in renal function both arteries or both veins must be involved, save for those patients with a single kidney or preexisting renal disease. Both embolic and thrombotic renal arterial disease have been reported to result in acute decreases in renal function. Renal arterial emboli may occur in patients after major vascular surgery or arteriography, when they are most frequently composed of cholesterol or atheromatous plaque material, or from the heart in patients with myocardial infarcts, bacterial endocarditis, atrial fibrillation, or intramural cardiac tumors. Arterial and venous thrombotic events are less common causes of renal failure. Acute renal vein thrombosis usually presents with flank pain, tender, enlarged kidneys, and a urinalysis demonstrating proteinuria and hematuria. Acute renal vein thrombosis has been observed in patients with nephrotic syndrome, sickle cell disease, renal cell carcinoma, or in patients having vena caval or renal vein compression due to tumor or fibrosis. Arterial thrombotic phenomena are most often observed in patients subjected to trauma or having hyperviscocity, such as may occur in patients with polycythemia vera. Although the diagnosis of arterial or venous occlusive disease may be suggested by history, confirmation is usually made with arteriography or venography.

A brief consideration of the etiologies of acute renal failure is in order, since the specific diagnosis may be suggested by the patient's history or physical examination.[2,9,14–16] As indicated in Table 13–2, the etiologies of acute renal failure may be subdivided into those related to ischemic episodes, to nephrotoxic events, or to pigment nephropathy. It is not uncommon for patients with acute renal failure to have multiple etiologies, although the clinician is usually able to delineate the most probable cause in any given patient. Ischemic acute renal failure occurs in patients with a reduced extracellular fluid volume due to hemorrhage, fluid and electrolyte losses resulting from diuretics, diarrhea, sequestration of fluid into a third space, plasma losses associated with large body surface area burns, or in association with placenta previa or abruptio placenta. Renal ischemia also occurs with a normal extracellular fluid volume in patients with cardiogenic shock, cerebral infarction, renal artery clamping, sepsis, or intravascular hemolysis. While acute renal failure associated with renal hypoperfusion and an ischemic episode has been the most common form of this process, increased use of potentially nephrotoxic agents has resulted in an increased incidence of nephrotoxic acute renal failure. The causes of nephrotoxic acute renal failure are diverse, although aminoglycoside antibiotics, radiocontrast agents, and nonsteroidal antiinflammatory agents account for most cases of nephrotoxic acute renal failure. Of recent clinical import has been the acute renal failure associated with the use of a heavy metal complex, cis-platinum, a cancer therapeutic agent. Pigment nephropathy appears to combine elements of both ischemic and nephrotoxic acute renal failure, since it occurs frequently in patients with hypotension or volume depletion but requires circulating levels of myoglobin or hemoglobin.

Table 13–2. Etiologies of Acute Renal Failure

Ischemic
Reduced extracellular fluid volume
"Normal" extracellular fluid volume
Nephrotoxic
Antibiotics
Radiocontrast agents
Nonsteroidal antiinflammatory drugs
Heavy metals
Pigment nephropathy
Myoglobinuric
Hemoglobinuric/methemoglobinemic
Mixed

In summary, the diagnosis of acute renal failure is made by excluding other causes of acute decreases in renal function. This can usually be accomplished without any invasive diagnostic procedures.[1,2,5,7] The urine sediment (Table 13–3) of patients with acute renal failure demonstrates coarse granular casts that are pigmented in patients who have hemoglobinuria or myoglobinuria, renal tubular epithelial cells, usually present as "muddy brown" casts, a minimal amount of proteinuria, and occasional white or red blood cells. Patients with prerenal azotemia have a benign urine sediment, demonstrating occasional hyaline casts or fine granular casts, and an absence of proteinuria, hematuria, or pyuria. The urine of patients with obstructive uropathy may be remarkable for its absence of findings or for crystalluria in the sediment, which may reflect the etiology of the obstruction when it is due to stone disease. Patients with glomerulone-

Table 13–3. Alterations in Urine Sediment and Composition

	Prerenal Azotemia	Obstructive Uropathy	Renovascular Disease	Renal Parenchymal Disease	Acute Renal Failure
Sediment	"Benign," occasional hyaline or pine granular casts	Negative or crystalluria or pyuria and renal papilla	Arterial: hematuria venous: proteinuria	Glomerulonephritis: RBC casts interstitial nephritis: pyuria, proteinuria, eosinophiluria	Muddy brown renal tubular epithelial cell casts, WBCs, RBCs
Composition	*Sodium conservation*				
	FE_{Na+} ↓, < 1%		Variable		↑, > 1%
	U_{Na+} ↓, < 20 mEq/liter		Variable		↑, > 40 mEq/liter
	RFI ↓, < 1		Variable		↑, > 1
	Water conservation				
	Sp.Gr. ↑, > 1.2		Variable		↑, > 1.015
	U_{osm} ↑, > 450 mOsm		Variable		↑, > 400 mOsm
	U/P_{osm} ↑, > 1.2		Variable		↑, > 1.1
	U/P_{cr} ↑, > 25		Variable		↑, > 20

Abbreviations: FE_{Na+} = Parachonal excretion of sodium; U_{Na+} = random urine sodium concentration; RFI = renal failure index (U_{Na}/U_{Pc_r}); SpGr = specific gravity; U_{osm} = urine osmolality; U/P_{osm} = ratio of urine to plasma osmotality; U/P_{c_r} = ratio of urine to plasma creatinine concentration.

phritis or vasculitis may have urine sediments containing red blood casts, whereas patients with interstitial nephritis may demonstrate pyuria and variable proteinuria with or without eosinophiluria. Additional readily available studies point toward the differences in tubular function characteristic of acute acute renal failure and prerenal azotemia.

Salt and water conservation are intact and normally responsive in patients with prerenal azotemia, whereas in patients with acute renal failure they are remarkably abnormal (Table 13–3).[1,2] Typically patients with prerenal azotemia will conserve sodium and have a urine sodium concentration on a random specimen of <20 mEq/liter, or a fractional sodium excretion of less than 1 percent. Conservation of water in prerenal azotemia results in increased urine to plasma creatinine concentration ratios, enhanced urine osomolality, or increased urine specific gravity. In contrast, patients with acute renal failure usually have a high urine sodium concentration, typically >40 mEq/liter or one-third of the concurrent plasma sodium concentration, on a random urine specimen, and a fractional excretion of sodium in excess of 1 percent. A parallel decrease in water conservation results in urine osomolality approaching plasma tonicity and decreased urine: plasma creatinine concentration ratio to a value of <20. Because of the gray zones due to biologic variability and sampling errors due to non-steady-state conditions, the renal failure index, a derivative of the fractional excretion of sodium, has been used to increase the specificity and accuracy of urinary indices as a diagnostic criterion.[7] The renal failure index is obtained when the urine sodium concentration (an estimate of sodium conservation) is divided by the urine: plasma creatinine concentration ratio (an index of overall water conservation). A renal failure index of >1 is highly suggestive of acute renal failure in appropriate circumstances, whereas a value of <1 is typically associated with prerenal azotemia.

The change in urinary indices between initiation and maintenance phases of acute renal failure is due to quantitative rather than qualitative differences. Early in the initiation phase, when patients may be considered to have incipient acute renal failure,[17] sodium conservation is better maintained and there is less diminution in water conservation, resulting in a tendency toward lower urine sodium concentrations and higher urine osmolalities. During the maintenance phase there is a trend toward increased urine sodium concentration and decreases in water conservation, with the most severe abnormalities occurring in those patients with oliguric acute renal failure. During the recovery phase there is continued isosthenuria and a reversal of the urine sodium : potassium concentration ratio, suggesting a return toward normal of sodium conservation, which precedes recovery of urine concentrating ability.

Radiographic procedures are more useful in establishing diagnosis in renal diseases other than acute renal failure. The usefulness of radiographic procedures in helping establish the diagnosis of obstructive uropathy and renovascular abnormalities of either the arterial or venous system resulting in a sudden decline in renal function is obvious. More recently, observations by Fry and Catell[18] have suggested that prior radiocontrast procedures may help confirm the diagnosis of acute renal failure. These workers observed a persistent but diminished nephrogram phase well after the administration of radiocontrast material in patients with acute renal failure. It was their observation that the nephrogram phase could persist for periods of up to 96 hours after a radiocontrast agent had been administered.

Table 13–4. Pathogenetic Mechanisms Proposed to Account for the Major Pathophysiologic Events in Acute Renal Failure

Renal hemodynamic alterations
Enhanced vasoconstriction (renin–angiotensin system)
Diminished vasodilation (prostaglandins)
Glomerular structural changes
Endothelial cell swelling
Perturbed glomerular dynamics
1. Decreased glomerular capillary surface area, and/or
2. Decreased hydraulic conductivity
Intraglomerular coagulation
Abnormalities in renal tubules
Obstruction of renal tubules
Extrinsic (interstitial edema)
Intrinsic (cast formation)
Acute tubular necrosis

Although we would not suggest that a radiocontrast agent be administered to patients suspected of having acute renal failure in order to confirm the diagnosis, it is worthwhile obtaining a KUB in anyone being evaluated for acute renal failure who has recently (within the last 4 to 5 days) had a radiocontrast study. The presence of a persistent nephrogram would be consistent with acute renal failure; however, failure to observe one does not exclude the diagnosis.

Pathophysiology of Acute Renal Failure

The failure of research efforts to decide on a single responsible pathogenetic mechanism (Table 13–4) for the pathophysiology of acute renal failure is not surprising in view of the diversity of pathophysiologic events that must be accounted for by such a single mechanism. These include a marked reduction in glomerular filtration rate (out of proportion to the modest changes in renal blood flow) and tubular dysfunction, ranging from tubular necrosis to sustained viability of tubular epithelial cells, despite marked abnormalities in salt and water conservation. Regardless of the severity of the resultant renal disease there is the potential for recovery from rather marked renal insufficiency. It has become apparent that acute renal failure is a multifactorial disease, resulting from the interplay of multiple pathogenetic events.[2,6,12,14,15,19,20] Thus, while each of the proposed pathogenetic mechanisms may be discussed singly, they should be viewed as acting in concert, with varying intensities at varying times during the course of acute renal failure.

The most extensively studied pathophysiologic mechanism for acute renal failure concerns renal hemodynamic alterations, consisting of reduced total renal blood flow and a redistribution of intrarenal blood flow with outer cortical ischemia. Reduced renal blood flow has been consistently observed, especially early in the course of acute renal failure. A variety of mechanisms have been proposed to account for these renal hemodynamic alterations, including activation of the renin–angiotensin system or deficiencies in prostaglandin synthesis/release. It has been suggested that the renin–angiotensin system is activated through the mechanism of tubuloglomerular feedback, which proposes an interrelationship between alterations in tubular function, resulting from ischemia or nephrotoxins, and control of glomerular filtration rate.[21] Either an ischemic or nephrotoxic initiating event reduces the proximal tubular reabsorption of glomerular filtrate, changing the composition of tubular fluid in distal nephron segments in general, and within the macula densa segment in particular. According to this theory, through an unknown mechanism the macula densa segment recognizes this tubular fluid alteration, and there is enhanced synthesis and release of renin, resulting in increased generation of angiotensin II and decreased renal afferent arterial blood flow and glomerular filtration rate. Alternatively, decreased prostaglandin synthesis, a major renal vasodilator, may result in a vasoconstrictor excess—with or without enhanced renin–angiotensin system activity. This would be associated with similar changes in renal blood flow and glomerular filtration rate. Alterations in renal hemodynamics are most prominent during the initiation phase of acute renal failure, and may return toward normal in the latter phases of acute renal failure.[22] It has been demonstrated that pharmacologic agents may return renal blood flow to normal without an associated improvement in renal function.

Given that the hallmark of acute renal failure is a reduction in glomerular filtration rate, it has been proposed that alterations in glomerular structure and/or function may account for the physiologic abnormalities of acute renal failure. There are two major theories that center around changes in glomerular structure or function in acute renal failure. An early theory suggested that ischemic or nephrotoxic insults induced metabolic change in capillary endothelial cells, resulting in cell swelling and occlusion of glomerular capillary blood flow, decreased renal blood flow, decreased glomerular filtration rate and azotemia.[23] Studies in experimental acute renal failure demonstrating increased endothelial cell size, and their reversibility with osmotic agents, have not been reproducible. In addition, studies of clinical acute renal failure do not support changes in endothelial cell size, a requisite for this theory. Recently it has been proposed that alterations in glomerular dynamics account for the decrease in glomerular filtration rate observed in acute renal failure.[24] The surface area of the glomerulus available for filtration and the filtration characteristics of the glomerular structure are determinants of glomerular permeability. Decreases in either surface area or the hydraulic conductivity of the glomerular structure result in decreased glomerular filtration rate. Experiments are unable to distinguish clearly between changes in surface area, which may be the result of enhanced synthesis of vasoconstrictors, and changes in hydraulic conductivity. While studies of experimental acute renal failure have demonstrated changes consistent with this thesis, histopathologic analyses of clinical acute renal failure have failed to confirm any consistent glomerular ultrastructural changes. More recently it has been suggested that activation of the coagulation system may, through occlusion of glomerular capillaries or fibrin deposition along glomerular endothelial cell surfaces, result in reductions in glomerular filtration rate.[25] Regardless of the precise mechanism resulting in changes in glomerular function, these abnormalities appear to be operative only early in the course of acute renal failure (i.e., during the initiation phase), and no single change appears to be universally present.

Abnormalities in tubular function have long been a favorite mechanism proposed as being responsible for the pathophysiology of acute renal failure. Either renal tubule obstruction, due to external compression from interstitial edema, or intratubular obstruction due to the accumulation of necrotic cellular debris could result in a decrease in glomerular filtration rate through increases in intratubular pressure. In order for this mechanism to be operative, a consistent demonstration of increased intratubular pressure of sufficient magnitude to offset effective glomerular capillary pressure must be demonstrated. This has not uniformally been the case in animal models of experimental acute renal failure, suggesting that tubular obstruction does not have a consistent role in the pathogenesis of acute renal failure. Alternatively, tubular epithelial cell necrosis, permitting the transtubular leakage of a normally formed glomerular filtrate to return to the systemic circulation via renal lymphatics, may account for the observed decrease in glomerular filtration rate. Until recently the sole evidence supporting this theory has been the inconsistent histologic observation of necrotic tubular epithelial cells and an inconsistent demonstration that intratubularly injected radioactive inulin is not quantitatively recoverable in models of experimental acute renal failure. Myers and colleagues, however, have adapted studies using dextran particles of various sizes that may be used to determine the sieving characteristics of the glomerular membrane, in order to analyze the role of tubular fluid leak in human acute renal failure.[26-28] These workers chose patients with acute renal failure secondary to cardiovascular surgery because of their availability and their reproducible clinical course. These studies demonstrated alterations in the clearance of various-sized dextran particles consistent with tubular fluid leak during the maintenance phase of acute renal failure and, less consistently and of lesser magnitude, during the recovery phase of acute renal failure. Relying on these elegant and interesting experiments, it may be proposed that (*1*) tubular fluid leak plays a significant role during the maintenance phase of acute renal failure, and (*2*) the healing occurring during the recovery phase is associated with the dimunition of tubular leak. However, at best tubular fluid leak can only account for a proportion of the reduced glomerular filtration rate observed in acute renal failure, and additional pathophysiologic mechanisms are required to be operative simultaneously to account for the remaining changes.

Parallel observations suggesting the participation of multiple mechanisms during the course of acute renal failure are available from recent studies of experimental acute renal failure due to cis-platinum.[29,30] During the maintenance phase of acute renal failure in rats receiving cis-platinum intraperitoneally, evidence was obtained indicating a role for tubular fluid leak and intratubular obstruction. However, these two mechanisms alone could not account for the entire reduction in glomerular filtration rate, suggesting that other mechanisms, such as alterations in glomerular dynamics or renal hemodynamics, must be operative as well. Were one to try and place all these clinical and experimental studies into perspective, the only logical conclusion would be that various mechanisms are operative at different times in the course of acute renal failure, and that the magnitude of their contribution to the reduction in renal function is dependent on the etiology of the acute renal failure as well as the particular phase during which they are studied. Reductions in renal blood flow and intrarenal blood flow distribution play a significant role in the initiation of acute renal failure, particularly that resulting from ischemic events. Tubular abnormalities, resulting either from tubular fluid leak or from intratubular obstruction, most markedly in patients developing acute renal failure subsequent to the administration of nephrotoxic agents, play a very important role, but not to the exclusion of renal hemodynamic or glomerular abnormalities. Regardless of the initiating event—either nephrotoxic or ischemic—an altered pattern is observed during the maintenance phase of acute renal failure, which is characterized by a major role for tubular obstruction and tubular fluid leak, and a minor role for renal hemodynamic or glomerular abnormalities. Subsequently, during the recovery phase of acute renal failure, return of tubular integrity, as noted initially from an increased urine volume and subsequently improved quality of the urine formed, would appear to result from the return of tubular epithelial cells back toward normal.

Therapy

The remainder of this chapter concentrates on the consequences of acute renal failure and their treatment, particularly during the maintenance and recovery phases. However, any discussion of the topic would be incomplete without consideration of those efforts that can prevent acute renal failure from occurring or the treatment of acute renal failure during the initiation phase, when the etiologic event may still be active. While there are no specific therapeutic maneuvers that act as a prophylaxis against the development of acute renal failure, it is generally accepted that maintenance of adequate hydration and volume status diminish the risk of developing acute renal failure, regardless of the initiating event.[17,31] Avoiding, wherein possible, the use of potentially nephrotoxic agents especially during a period of volume depletion may also be accepted as a general rule. There are, however, only limited circumstances under which the clinician may anticipate acute renal failure. For example, the clinician who recognizes that the major objective of dehydration before urography is to enhance the quality of the resulting pyelogram phase will be better prepared to regulate the conditions under which radiocontrast material is given. Even when oral hydration is to be avoided, parenteral hydration may diminish if not prevent associated renal dysfunction in patients receiving radiocontrast material for arteriograms, venograms, or enhanced CT scans.

While no specific drugs are known to prevent the development of acute renal failure, duiretics have been used to manage and treat acute renal failure in its initiation phase. Although the use of such agents remains somewhat controversial, there is sufficient evidence to indicate that when appropriately used there is minimal risk of renal damage, and the potential benefits are great. Mannitol and the "loop" diuretics, furosemide or ethacrynic acid, have received the greatest attention.[32] Their use may be considered from two points of view: enhanced removal of potential nephrotoxins and modification of the incidence, if not the course, of acute renal failure. Increasing urine flow will increase the excretion of any nephrotoxic agent filtered at the glomerulus. In this regard, mannitol would appear to be more efficacious, since the concurrent administration of loop diuretics with certain antibiotics may enhance the nephrotoxicity of the antibiotic. Mannitol may be used to promote the excretion of myoglobin, hemoglobin and acid hematin, radiocontrast materials, and uric acid. Despite the plethora of studies available, data concerning the ability of diuretic agents to prevent the development of acute renal failure are inconclusive. Whereas a similar statement could be made concerning the ability of diuretics in general and furosemide in particular to convert acute renal failure from its oliguric form, which carries a higher degree of morbidity and mortality, to the nonoliguric form, recent evidence would suggest that a more affirmative statement is in order. Anderson and colleagues have demonstrated that the systematic administration of furosemide to patients having acute renal failure will result in a more benign course in those responding with an increase in urine volume and maintenance if not development of nonoliguric acute renal failure. It is therefore our general rule to administer furosemide unless there is a clear-cut contraindication to its use in a given patient.

PHYSIOLOGIC ABNORMALITIES IN ACUTE RENAL FAILURE

The kidney has a central role in the homeostasis of fluid and electrolyte balance and adaptations to acid–base changes. The physiologic consequences of changes in renal function must be considered relative to both the degree and duration of alterated renal function. Physiologic consequences of acute renal failure can be anticipated to be of a differing magnitude and severity depending on when in the course of acute renal failure they are clinically apparent.[2,3,6,10-12,14] The following discussion of the major physiologic abnormalities developing in patients with acute renal failure considers both the specific phase during which the abnormality occurs, as well as whether that abnormality is associated with oliguric or nonoliguric acute renal failure.[8,9,21]

Dialytic therapy, with peritoneal dialysis or hemodialysis, has become relatively available over the past two decades. Hemodialysis and peritoneal dialysis are not without associated risks, although with appropriate use their benefit well outweighs these risks (33). The subsequent discussion does not cover the use of dialysis to treat the metabolic and physiologic consequences of acute renal failure. Rather, we have chosen to concentrate our efforts on a review of alterations in salt and water homeostasis, abnormalities in potassium balance, acid–base changes, and perturbations in calcium–phosphorus homeostasis. We would also be remiss in failing to consider the role of nutrition in patients with acute renal failure, despite the lack of general consensus concerning the efficacy of parenteral nutrition in these patients.

Sodium Chloride and Water

INITIATION PHASE

Given the very nature of the initiation phase (i.e., it precedes clinical recognition of renal disease), abnormalities of salt and water balance are important due to the influence of dehydration on the development of acute renal failure, as well as the potential therapeutic effects of diuretics in preventing or modifying the subsequent course of acute renal failure. If patients developing acute renal failure are nonoliguric during the initiation phase, the inability to conserve sodium and water may contribute to clinically significant dehydration and the severity of the ensuing renal failure. Given the influence of volume loss and dehydration on renal blood flow and renal function, it may be assumed that patients with sustained salt and water losses during the initiation phase may be more likely to develop oliguric acute renal failure, although little evidence is available to support this conclusion.[15,16]

When the initiation phase is characterized by oliguria, with a marked decrease in both urine volume and sodium excretion, retention of salt and water may occur, resulting in volume overload, congestive heart failure, and hypertension. If there is a significant time interval between reduced urine output and the clinical recognition of renal insufficiency, and standard fluid replacement therapy is continued, volume overload and its attendant problems could occur.

Not infrequently, patients undergo a variety of therapeutic interventions during the initiation phase in an attempt to prevent the occurrence of acute renal failure. Several of these maneuvers, such as a fluid challenge with normal saline, the infusion of large amounts of mannitol, or the administration of large doses of furosemide, can also drastically affect the patient's salt and water balance.[32] This may occur either by rapidly causing the formation of large amounts of urine in a previously oliguric patient, or by precipitating fluid overload in a nonoliguric patient who fails to respond to these maneuvers. These therapeutic endeavors, which have an appropriate and reasonable objective, contribute to the difficulties in maintaining salt and water balance during the maintenance phase.[7,32]

MAINTENANCE PHASE

In general, glomerular filtration rate is reduced to approximately 10 percent of normal in patients with acute renal failure.[2,32] Despite comparable reductions in glomerular filtration rate, patients with nonoliguric acute renal failure have a relatively well-maintained urine volume.[7-9] This is in contrast to patients with either nonoliguric acute renal failure or a marked decrease in glomerular filtration rate due to prerenal factors. Despite the reduced glomerular filtration rate, maintenance of urine volume results in considerably fewer difficulties in management of salt and water problems in patients with nonoliguric acute renal failure. Because of the tubular dysfunction characteristic of acute renal failure, characterized by an inability to conserve salt and water normally, these patients may undergo inordinantly large volume losses.[3-5,12,21] Even though urine sodium concentrations are lower in nonoliguric than in oliguric patients, the concentrations are still higher than values encountered in patients with prerenal azotemia.[7-9] On occasion, as recently reported by Diamond and Yoburn,[34] the urine sodium concentration may be low enough to be consistent with prerenal azotemia, although other parameters suggest the diagnosis of acute renal failure. It is therefore important to maintain the extracellular fluid volume status of patients with nonoliguric acute renal failure by replacing their urinary losses. This approach avoids both dehydration and other cardiovascular consequences due to volume depletion. In patients with oliguric acute renal failure, water and sodium chloride losses are limited by the extent to which they can be eliminated by the skin and lungs and in the small amount of urine excreted. In order to maintain fluid balance and prevent the complications associated with an expanded extracellular fluid volume, such as congestive heart failure or hypertension, greater care must be exercised to balance the intake of sodium chloride and water with the measured or inferred losses.

In an afebrile resting adult, fluid losses via the skin and lungs, referred to as insensible losses, amount to ~0..5 to 0.6 ml/kg body weight/hr. These insensible loses are increased by approximately 13 percent for each degree Centigrade (7 percent for each degree Fahrenheit) in a febrile patient.[14,32,35] To these insensible losses must be added any volume losses resulting from urine output, as well as measured fluid losses due to vomiting, diarrhea, or gastrointestinal drainage. The endogenous production of water that results from the oxidation of proteins, fats, and carbohydrates offsets these fluid losses.[36] In the absence of carbohydrate supplementation, a 70-kg man will metabolize ~1 g of protein/kg body wt and ~2 g of fat/kg of body wt in a 24-hour interval. As a result of these metabolic events, endogenous water production is ~560 ml/24 hr. Carbohydrate is usually supplemented, and the addition of 100 g of carbohydrate/day results in a 50 percent reduction in protein metabolism. This reduces endogenous water production by 15 to 20 percent and results in a net water production of ~460 ml/24 hr. Given the above rate of insensible fluid loss, assuming no other measurable fluid losses and estimating endogenous water production as noted, it may be calculated that additional fluid therapy in a 70-kg man should approximate 400 ml/24 hr in order to maintain fluid losses. Since there are always other measurable fluid losses (e.g., urine volume, GI losses), this approach will usually result in a persistent slightly negative water balance. In view of this, an alternative method of assessing fluid balance is the frequent and accurate monitoring of body weight. In a patient not receiving supplemental nutrition, a daily weight loss of ~0.2 to 0.4 kg is consistent with the above scheme of fluid replacement and minimizes the risk of developing fluid overload. In general, since fluid deficits can easily be replaced, whereas fluid removal in patients with acute renal failure is a complex event, it is more appropriate to err on the conservative side and possibly end up with a fluid deficit rather than risk the problems associated with excessive volume expansion.[2]

Even though for the purposes of the present discussion the problems related to sodium chloride balance are addressed separately, it must be appreciated that sodium chloride and water homeostasis are inseparable.[3] They are treated concordantly during the maintenance phase of acute renal failure. From a philosophic point of view, it is best to approach all patients with acute renal failure as having a limited means of excreting sodium chloride, and with the concept that sodium chloride excretion correlates with volume homeostasis.

Simple approximations can be made, therefore, using urine volume as an index of salt and water handling.[8,32] Typically, the urine sodium concentration in patients with acute renal failure is 40 to 60 mEq/liter. Patients with oliguric acute renal failure have a daily urine volume of 400 ml, resulting in a net sodium excretion of 20 mEq/day, which is the equivalent of a dietary sodium intake of 500 mg.[35] While patients with nonoliguric acute renal failure may have a correspondingly larger sodium excretion, they also tend to have a lower urine sodium concentrations, hence similar limitations in sodium excretion. The overzealous use of sodium chloride, in either diet or parenteral solutions, may rapidly lead to volume expansion, congestive heart failure, and hypertension.

In addition to the disturbance in total body sodium content, manifested as volume depletion or edema formation, disturbances in serum sodium concentration are frequently encountered. Hyponatremia is commonly due to a failure to consider both endogenous water production and exogenous fluid administration in determining optimum fluid balance. This results in the accumulation of a relative excess of water as compared with sodium, as well as dilutional hyponatremia.[37] Hypernatremia is less commonly encountered and is often due to the administration of excessive sodium, frequently in the form of sodium bicarbonate administered to correct the systemic acidosis observed in acute renal failure. These abnormalities in serum sodium concentration can best be treated by carefully regulating the amount of fluid intake relative to sodium chloride intake, although not infrequently a prolonged interval may be required to normalize the serum sodium concentration.

RECOVERY PHASE

During the recovery phase of acute renal failure there is a progressive, often stepwise, increase in urine volume. While this quantitative increase in urine volume is often reassuring, it must be recognized that the quality of the urine formed is extremely poor. The diuresis that characterizes the recovery phase is most clearly observed in patients with oliguric acute renal failure. In patients with nonoliguric acute renal failure there may be little change in urine volume, and clinicians must rely on improved biochemical parameters as heralding improved renal function. During the recovery phase, urine volume may reach proportions considered frankly polyuric. Multiple factors, other than an increase in the number of filtering nephron units, contribute to the increased urine volume noted during the recovery phase, including: (*1*) prior overhydration and volume expansion during the maintenance phase of acute renal failure; (*2*) osmotic diuresis secondary to the excretion of retained solutes, such as urea; and (*3*) a continued inability to conserve salt and water as the renal tubule recovers from its prior damage. Neither the increased urine volume in patients with oliguric acute renal failure nor the continued maintenance of urine volume in patients with nonoliguric acute renal failure should be interpreted to mean that attention to sodium chloride and water homeostasis can be forgotten. Inadequate fluid and electrolyte therapy can lead to significant volume depletion and associated problems attributable to continued impairment of salt and water homeostasis.[6]

Potassium Homeostasis

Potassium homeostasis is extremely important in patients with acute renal failure and hyperkalemia is a leading cause of death in these patients.[38] The ratio of intracellular to extracellular potassium concentration is the critical determinant of neuromuscular function. Given that ordinarily only 2 percent of total body potassium is extracellular, it is evident that relatively small changes in extracellular potassium concentration have a marked effect on this ratio, and subsequently on neuromuscular transmission.[14] Even though serum potassium concentrations cannot be used as an estimate of total body potassium content, they do represent an approximation of potential potassium toxicity in this circumstance. The major clinically significant disorder in potassium concentration is hyperkalemia and the associated changes in cardiac electrical events.[39]

INITIATION PHASE

In patients in whom acute renal failure develops, increases in extracellular or serum potassium concentration are due to an inability to excrete a normal potassium load. Potassium intake may be derived from either exogenous or endogenous sources. The exogenous component of potassium balance may be controlled by means of strict potassium restriction, with particular emphasis on dietary potassium content, or the potassium contained in therapeutic sources (e.g., K-penicillin). The endogenous sources of potassium that must be excreted by the kidney are more difficult to control. A principal endogenous source of potassium is from protein catabolism; it usually occurs in association with an altered nutritional status, fever, sepsis, or other catabolic states. In addition, intravascular hemolysis or the absorption of blood released into the gastrointestinal tract leads to an increase in endogenous potassium load.

In patients having a urine volume of ≥ 1 liter/day, hyperkalemia tends to be less of a clinical problem. The ability of these patients to maintain potassium homeostasis and a normal serum potassium concentration in spite of severe acidemia may be attributed to several factors. Patients who are nonoliguric, even during the initiation phase, may have a greater proportion of remaining functioning nephrons; these nephrons may excrete a higher than normal load of potassium per nephron unit in order to compensate for nephron units that are no longer functioning. There is also a component of potassium excretion in distal nephron segments that depends on urine flow, related to maintaining the electrochemical gradient for potassium secretion, which in patients with maintained urine volumes favors net potassium secretion.[40] In contrast, patients with oliguria are less able to maintain a normal serum potassium concentration, and hyperkalemia may rapidly become a significant problem.

Additional factors determining the potential severity of hyperkalemia in the initiation phase of acute renal failure are related to excessive releases of endogenous potassium. For example, patients developing myoglobinuric acute renal failure due to rhabdomyolysis may rapidly show increases in serum potassium concentration. Tissue damage generally results in the release of a large amount of intracellular potassium from damaged cells into the circulation. Whether this leads to hyperkalemia due to the kidney's inability to excrete this potassium is unclear.[41]

MAINTENANCE

Parallel changes in serum potassium concentration occur during the maintenance phase in patients with oliguric and nonoliguric acute renal failure, although hyperkalemia continues to occur more frequently and tends to be more severe in patients with lower urine volumes. The most threatening consequence of hyperkalemia is the associated cardiac toxicity.[42] The earliest alterations noted on the electrocardiogram consist of peaking of the T waves, followed by broadening of the QRS complex, prolongation of the P-R interval, and disappearance of the P wave. Subsequently there may be even further widening of the QRS complex resulting in a sine-wave appearance, which may rapidly be followed by ventricular fibrillation. When serious hyperkalemia develops, as evidenced by electrocardiographic abnormalities or a serum potassium concentration in excess of 6.5 mEg/liter, several modes of therapy are available to offset cardiotoxicity and/or normalize serum potassium concentration. The emergency treatment of choice for hyperkalemia with life-threatening electrocardiographic changes is the IV administration of calcium, usually as a 10 percent calcium gluconate solution, as a rapid infusion over 1 to 5 minutes. Although calcium neither diminishes serum potassium concentration nor enhances its excretion from the body, it protects the myocardium from hyperkalemic arrhythmias by resetting the threshold potential for excitable cardiac neuromuscular tissue. Infusions of sodium bicarbonate or a glucose-insulin-containing solution may be used in the emergency situation to bring about a rapid lowering of serum potassium concentrations. Sodium bicarbonate, probably through an increase in serum pH, promotes the entrance of potassium into cells, thereby reducing serum potassium concentration. An additional method of promoting the entrance of potassium to cells is the IV administration of glucose (25 to 50 g as a 50 percent solution) along with 5 to 10 units of regular insulin, or 1 unit of regular insulin per 5 g glucose. Alternatively, a continued infusion of a solution containing 400 ml of 5 percent dextrose in water, 100 ml of 50 percent dextrose in water, 2 ampules of calcium gluconate, and 15 units regular insulin infused at a rate of 30 ml/hr and adjusted to maintain serum potassium concentration at a safe level may be used as long as the patient can tolerate the additional fluid volume represented by this mixture. While none of the above therapeutic maneuvers results in the net removal of potassium from the body, they are effective since they serve either to stabilize the electrophysiologic response to hyperkalemia or to redistribute potassium from extracellular fluid into an intracellular location.

Having resolved the emergency hyperkalemic problems, and usually concurrent with this emergency treatment, efforts must be made to remove potassium and thus diminish total body potassium. Kayexalate, a cation exchange resin acting in the large intestine, exchanges sodium for potassium with the subsequent excretion of potassium in the stool. Each gram of Kayexalate removes ~1 mEq of potassium and simultaneously results in the absorption of 1 mEq of sodium. Kayexalate may be administered either orally or by retention enema in doses of 40 to 100 g mixed with 70 percent sorbitol in order to prevent constipation. Unlike insulin or $NaHCO_3$, an effect of Kayexalate on serum potassium will not be observed for several hours. Potassium removal may also be accomplished using peritoneal dialysis or hemodialysis. While hemodialysis is more efficient in the removal of potassium and results in a larger amount of potassium being removed in a shorter period of time, peritoneal dialysis does represent a safe and adequate alternative. From a practical point of view, most hyperkalemic patients can be treated by eliminating exogenous sources of potassium intake, minimizing endogenous sources of potassium release, and promoting potassium removal with Kayexalate. Dialytic techniques are most often needed in those patients who are severely oliguric, hypercatabolic, and have marked and difficult to control sources of potassium release.[43]

RECOVERY PHASE

During the recovery phase of acute renal failure, most patients have a normal serum potassium concentration. Occasional patients with marked or persistent polyuria during the recovery phase may excrete large amounts of potassium, leading to hypokalemia. For this reason, potassium losses in the urine should be monitored during the recovery phase, and on occasion small amounts of potassium supplementation may be required in order to remain serum potassium concentration at ~3.5 mEq/liter. With progressive stabilization and normalization of urine volume and diminution of acidemia, potassium homeostasis returns toward normal, and prolonged potassium therapy is usually not required.

Calcium, Phosphate, Parathyroid Hormone

Although considerable controversy remains as to the specific mechanisms involved, it is evident that an elevation of parathyroid hormone is one of the first hormonal changes observed in patients with acute renal failure.[44,44a] This secondary hyperparathyroidism is usually associated with hypocalcemia and hyperphosphatemia. The increased levels of parathyroid hormone (PTH), as well as the concomitant changes in calcium and phosphorus, tend to persist throughout the initiation phase and maintenance phase of acute renal failure. During the recovery phase of acute renal failure these parameters begin to return toward normal.

INITIATION PHASE

During the initiation phase of acute renal failure, multiple factors are responsible for the development of secondary hyperparathyroidism, of which hypocalcemia is very important. Hyperphosphatemia, a biochemical abnormality characteristic of patients with acute renal failure, is a contributory factor in the genesis of hypocalcemia subsequent hyperparathyroidism in this clinical situation. Under circumstances of normal renal function approximately 70 percent of the phosphate ingested is excreted by the kidneys. In order to maintain phosphate balance, the kidney must excrete 10 to 15 percent of the filtered load of phosphate. However, in patients with incipient renal failure as well as during the remainder of the initiation phase of acute renal failure there is a progressive decrease in the number of functioning nephron units, and the amount of phosphate excreted by the remaining functioning nephron units must increase in order to keep a normal serum phosphate concentration. This adaptation, referred to as the intact nephron hypothesis, occurs through the interrelationship of calcium, phosphate, and parathyroid hormone.[45,46]

According to the intact nephron hypothesis, during the course of progressive renal failure, as the number of available functioning nephron units decreases, slight, often clinically undetectable increases in serum phosphate concentration occur. This retention of phosphate due to a decrease in excretion leads to a decrease in blood levels of ionized calcium, probably through the binding and subsequent deposit of calcium phosphate in various body tissues. As a result of the ensuing hypocalcemia, parathyroid hormone (PTH) secretion is stimulated; the enhanced secretion of PTH returns serum phosphate concentration levels to normal by decreasing the tubular reabsorption of phosphate by the kidney. This renal action of PTH normalizes the serum concentrations of both phosphate and calcium. Serum PTH concentrations must remain elevated, however, in order to maintain serum phosphate concentration at near-normal levels.[47,48] In addition, this cycle of increased serum phosphate concentration and enhancement of PTH secretion continues with each decrement in glomerular filtration rate. Indeed, this mechanism functions well enough to maintain a relatively normal serum phosphate concentration until the glomerular filtration rate has decreased to less than 25 percent of normal, or to a value below ~25 ml/min. Below this level of renal function there are insufficient remaining functioning nephron units to maintain serum phosphate concentration at a normal level, due to an inability to obtain any further increases in phosphate excretion per nephron unit.

Another factor contributing to the hypocalcemia observed in patients with acute renal failure is the skeletal resistance to the calcium-mobilizing effects of PTH.[49] It has been observed that in patients with moderate to advanced renal failure hypocalcemia persists despite high levels of circulating immunoreactive PTH. In fact, the finding that infusions of PTH lead to blunted changes in serum calcium concentration, regardless of the level of serum phosphate concentration, has led to the postulate that this is an important factor in the pathogenesis of secondry hyperparathyroidism in patients with renal failure.[49-51]

Derangements in vitamin D metabolism are also a contributing factor to the developments of hyperparathyroidism in patients with renal disease. Renal parenchyma participates in the formation of $1,25(OH)_2$ D from 25(OH) D. Therefore, any decrease in the amount of functioning renal parenchyma will also cause a decrease in the formation of the active form of vitamin D (see also Chap. 15). Furthermore, the effect of PTH in increasing absorption of calcium in the presence of hypocalcemia is modulated by its effect of increasing production of $1,25(OH)_2$ D. If the active form of vitamin D is not produced in adequate amounts, as would be expected to occur in patients with chronic renal failure, the secretion of PTH will continue and increase to higher levels due to a failure to enhance gastrointestinal calcium absorption. It has also been suggested that diminished production of $1,25(OH)_2$ D or perhaps other active metabolites of vitamin D, during acute renal failure may be the factor that renders the skeleton less responsive to the actions of PTH. In addition, a low level of the liver metabolite of vitamin E, 25(OH) D, has been observed in patients with acute renal failure.[52] The diminution of 25(OH) D and the decreased generation of $1,25(OH)_2$ D results in decreases in calcium absorption from the gastrointestinal tract, persistent hypocalcemia, secondary hyperparathyroidism, as well as skeletal resistence to parathyroid hormone, all of which contribute to the hypocalcemia observed in patients with acute renal failure.[51,53]

MAINTENANCE PHASE

Once acute renal failure is established, the abnormalities in calcium and between calcium and phosphate become more stable and persist throughout the maintenance phase. In spite of persistent hyperphosphotemia and hypocalcemia, the abnormalities may actually be less profound and easier to control than during the early initiating phase of acute renal failure.

RECOVERY PHASE

During the recovery phase of acute renal failure there is slow resolution of the secondary hyperparathyroidism as renal function returns toward normal. During this phase, abnormalities in serum calcium and phosphate concentrations, PTH synthesis and release, and vitamin D metabolism all return toward normal. Hypercalcemia has also been observed in a small number of patients recovering from acute renal failure. In general, hypercalcemia has only been observed in some patients who have had profound hypocalcemia, hence, an increased stimulus for PTH synthesis and release. From a clinical point of view, this usually occurs in patients with myoglobinuric-induced acute renal failure resulting from rhabdomyolysis.[2,32] This form of acute renal failure is commonly associated with drug or alcohol overdose and is characterized by severe myolysis and deterioration of renal function. This form of acute renal failure may be characterized by marked elevation of muscle enzymes and a more profound hyperphosphatemia, hyperuricemia, and hypocalcemia. In the diuretic phase of acute renal failure secondary to myolysis some patients have been observed to have a marked hypercalcemia that subsequently resolves. The resulting hypercalcemia has been postulated to be due in part to the resolution of soft tissue calcifications formed during the oliguric phase of this disorder.[54] There are, however, a number of other factors contributing to the hypercalcemia observed in these clinical circumstances. Llach and colleagues[55] have demonstrated an association between the profound hypocalcemia observed during the oliguric phase of myoglobinuric-induced acute renal failure and low levels of $1,25(OH)_2$ D. Subsequently, during the polyuric phase, hypercalcemia was associated with a rise in this active vitamin D metabolite to supernormal levels. This increase in $1,25(OH)_2$ D probably contributes to the hypercalcemia by increasing gastrointestinal calcium absorption, as well as bone and soft tissue reabsorption of calcium salts.

Metabolic Acidosis

The kidney represents the primary route for the excretion of nonvolatile acids. Consequently, patients with acute renal failure usually develop metabolic acidosis. The severity and extent of the metabolic acidosis is greater when it occurs in patients in a hypercatabolic state due to sepsis or cardiogenic shock or who have considerable tissue necrosis.[56]

INITIATION PHASE

The potential acid–base disturbances occurring in patients entering the initiation phase of acute renal failure are multiple, and consist of abnormalities in acid–base homeostasis which precede the development of acute renal failure, as well as any superimposed due to the development of a progressive renal insufficiency. Excluding a consideration of preexisting acid–base abnormalities, there are several factors that determine both the severity and type (i.e., "nonanion gap" versus "anion gap") of metabolic acidosis that develops. In the normally functioning kidney acid–base homeostasis is maintained by conservation of filtered bicarbonate, through reclamation of bicarbonate contained in glomerular filtrate, and the excretion of the normal daily load of acid produced by metabolism. During the excretion of this acid load, which is ~1 mEq/kg body wt/day, additional bicarbonate is generated in distal nephron segments as this acid is excreted.[56] In general, patients developing acute renal failure have a diminished ability to excrete an acid load due to the marked decrease in glomerular filtration rate rather than having abnormal tubular function resulting in bicarbonate wasting due to a failure of bicarbonate reclamation. Uremic acidosis is the most common form of metabolic acidosis, and is characterized by a measurable anion gap due to failure of filtration and excretion of the unmeasured anions of metabolic acids, such as sulfate and phosphate. This is consistent with relatively well-maintained tubular function in the face of a progressive decrease in glomerular function. On occasion, however, during the early phases of acute renal failure there may be more marked abnormalities in tubular function than glomerular filtration rate. When this occurs, patients may have a "non-anion gap" acidosis due to the associated hyperchloremia, which results from the increased reabsorption of chloride resulting from the decreased availability of reabsorbable bicarbonate. In this instance, there is decreased filtered bicarbonate as plasma bicarbonate is titrated against systemic acids, resulting in the necessity for sodium to be reabsorbed with an available anion, which would be chloride.[56] Usually, with continued declining glomerular filtration rate, the pattern will evolve toward the more usual form of uremic acidosis.

In order to excrete metabolic acids ammonia must be available as a major urine buffer. As glomerular filtration rate declines and phosphate retention occurs, there is enhanced renal ammonia synthesis and ammonium excretion, which would counter the fall in phosphate excretion, and result in maintenance of net renal acid excretion. With renal insufficiency, the biosynthesis of ammonia cannot be substantially increased, and there is an inability to excrete the acid load represented by phosphate retention. In this context, renal ammonium excretion may be looked at as an index of remaining functional renal mass. As functional renal mass decreases, due to renal metabolic disturbances, the total amount of ammonia synthesized limits acid excretion, becoming an important factor in the subsequent development of uremic acidosis.[57]

MAINTENANCE PHASE

During the maintenance phase of acute renal failure most patients have an established anion gap uremic acidosis that is relatively mild and, in the absence of active catabolic events, is nonprogressive. Serum bicarbonate concentrations of 12 to 18 mEq/liter with arterial pH values >7.30 are the general rule. A metabolic acidosis of this modest degree usually does not require any specific treatment. However, patients with acute renal failure who are catabolic develop a more flagrant form of acidosis and may rapidly become symptomatic. They are more succeptible to the hemodynamic consequences of metabolic acidosis, including depressed myocardial contractility, decreased venous capacitance due to venoconstriction, and diminished pulmonary function. These patients may require specific therapy for their metabolic acidosis, which must be cautiously approached, since the administration of sodium bicarbonate may result in volume-related problems. To minimize the risk of volume overload due to the sodium bicarbonate solution, therapy should be restricted to that amount of base necessary to maintain a serum bicarbonate concentration at ~20 mEq/liter. In a recent study, it has been demonstrated that acidemic persons tolerate sodium bicarbonate better than sodium chloride, with a lesser degree of resultant edema and weight gain.[58]

Sodium bicarbonate therapy may result in alterations other than normalization of serum acid–base status. Alkalinization may reduce the ionized calcium concentration. In patients with acute renal failure who are already hyperphosphatemic and hypocalcemic, this reduction in ionized calcium concentration may cause enhanced neuromuscular excitability and even tetany. Therefore, additional caution is required in the use of alkaline therapy.

RECOVERY PHASE

During the recovery phase of acute renal failure there is continued return of glomerular filtration rate, tubular function, and overall renal metabolic function toward normal. As result, acid–base disturbances are minimized. However, in those patients with a persistent catabolic state these difficulties may persist and require specific therapy.

Nutrition

Disturbances in nutritional status represent one of the major problems encountered in patients with acute renal failure. At the very least, patients with acute renal failure are anorectic and unable to sustain normal nutrition, and acute renal failure represents a catabolic state in which loss of lean body mass may occur.[32] The state of catabolism may be extremely severe and may become a major determinant of survival in patients with acute renal failure after surgery or trauma, or in those instances associated with sepsis or burns. Major problems arise in providing these patients with adequate caloric intake, since administration of protein may be curtailed due to the patient's azotemia; oral administration of nonprotein nutrients is limited due to the anorexia, nausea, and vomiting associated with acute renal failure. In addition to these problems with enteral nutrition, additional difficulties arise with parenteral administration of nutrients due to the associated fluid volume difficulties that may occur. Given the self-limited course of acute renal failure and the associated decreases in glomerular filtration rate, these patients usually do not develop hypomagnesemia, and little is known concerning deficiencies of trace elements.

Controversy persists concerning the precise role of enteral or parenteral nutrition in the management of patients with acute renal failure. It has been firmly suggested by Abel and co-workers[59,60] that parenteral nutrition, consisting of hypertonic glucose and essential amino acids, improves patient survival and diminishes associated morbidity. That patients with acute renal failure complicated by gastrointestinal disease have a higher morbidity and mortality has been demonstrated. However, conflicting experimental results are available.[61] Toback[62] has obtained evidence suggesting that infusions of glucose or glucose combined with both essential and nonessential amino acids diminish the levels of renal insufficiency in rats in whom acute renal failure is induced with mercuric chloride. A similar study using amino acids in rats with acute renal failure was not confirmatory.

INITIATING PHASE

During the early phases of acute renal failure the patient's state of catabolism may be the greatest, due to associated clinical events. It is, therefore, during this time that adequate nutrition is of the utmost importance. The provision of sufficient calories to offset the catabolic events may take many forms. Calories may be provided in the form of glucose, since the administration of 100 g of carbohydrates per day has been shown in healthy persons to reduce endogenous protein breakdown during periods of starvation. In patients with acute renal failure the administration of glucose has two major consequences: reduction of protein catabolism and prevention of associated starvation ketosis. Both might exacerbate the underlying metabolic acidosis. Without protein sparing, endogenous protein catabolism results in enhanced protein synthesis, which requires amino acids. Amino acids may not be readily available for this protein synthesis, since their normal dietary intake is curtailed. Therefore, during a maintained catabolic period, the provision of insufficient calories necessitates the use of available amino acids as a source of nutrition. The breakdown of endogenous protein thus enhances the overall depletion of the body's protein mass. Administration of glucose, along with essential, and occasionally nonessential, amino acids, permits sparing of the body's amino acid pool from use as a substrate for metabolism in addition to promoting maintenance of a normal lean body mass.[63]

MAINTENANCE PHASE

Given that most studies have been performed in patients with well-established acute renal failure, additional information is available concerning the use of amino acids during this phase. During the maintenance phase it has been demonstrated that the addition of amino acids to glucose infusions in patients with acute renal failure leads to a clinically improved state, with a decrease in associated nausea and vomiting, as well as a decrease in the rate of rise in BUN concentration and an improvement in wound healing. While a detailed discussion of the role of parenteral nutrition in patients with acute renal failure is beyond the scope of the present chapter, it may be stated that at the clinical extremes of acute renal failure (i.e., in patients with either extremely mild acute renal failure or extremely severe forms of acute renal failure), mortality is little influenced by hyperalimentation. There are a relatively large number of patients having acute renal failure of intermediate severity in whom hyperalimentation may play a beneficial role in allowing them to tolerate their renal insufficiency, possibly shorten the duration of their renal insufficiency, and even contribute to diminished overall morbidity and mortality. In those patients with acute renal failure who require dialysis hyperalimentation has an additional important role. Hemodialysis is associated with significant loss of amino acids, ~2 to 3 g/hr of treatment, although protein losses do not occur. In contrast, patients undergoing peritoneal dialysis have sustained losses of both amino acids (~30 g/48 hr of treatment) and protein (20 to 40 g/48 hr of treatment). These losses must be taken into consideration when evaluating the state of nutrition of patients with acute renal failure and their nutritional requirements.[62]

RECOVERY PHASE

Unless a patient has a consistent catabolic state during the recovery phase there would appear to be no role for enteral or parenteral nutrition as a specific therapeutic modality. Certainly given the catabolism that occurs during the earlier phases of acute renal failure, nutritional therapy should be individualized on the basis of the preceding disturbances in nutritional status. Thus, a patient who has been subjected to trauma or surgery, with or without associated sepsis, may have sustained a decrease in lean body mass that will require more specific therapy during the recovery phase.

CONCLUSION

The physiologic consequences of acute renal failure are for the most part preventable or treatable. In the absence of prolonged oliguria, a protracted duration of reduced glomerular filtration rate, or associated catabolic problems many patients may proceed through acute renal failure requiring little or no dialysis. Clearly the physiologic consequences should contribute minimally to the mortality and moderately to the morbidity of acute renal failure. In support of this, most reviews clearly point to nonrenal causes of death in patients with acute renal failure, such as infection or gastrointestinal hemorrhage. While the "uremic milieu" including the alterations discussed in this chapter may contribute to these events, it is not surprising that many physicians consider these deaths as occurring in patients with renal insufficiency rather than from renal failure.

Acute renal failure is encountered relatively frequently in clinical medicine and has been the focus of ongoing clinical and experimental evaluations for many years. Yet there has not been a remarkable diminution in morbidity and mortality. Certainly some of this apparent lack of progress may be ascribed to the changing pattern of the patients being treated with acute renal failure. Older, sicker and more difficult to manage patients are being frequently encountered, resulting in greater morbidity and mortality.

REFERENCES

1. Levinsky NG: Pathophysiology of acute renal failure. N Engl J Med 296:1433, 1977
2. Gross M, Gehr M, Flamenbaum W: Acute renal failure. p. 505. In Flamenbaum W, Hamburger RJ (eds): Nephrology: An Approach to the Patient with Renal Disease. JB Lippincott, Philadelphia, 1982
3. Swann RC, Merrill, JP: The clinical course of acute renal failure. Medicine (Baltimore) 32:215, 1953
4. Eliahou HE, Bata A: The diagnosis of acute renal failure. Nephron 2:287, 1965
5. Espinel CH: The FE_{Na} test: Use in the differential diagnosis of acute renal failure. JAMA 236:579, 1976
6. Maxwell MA, Kleeman CR (eds): Franklin SS; Maxwell MA: Acute renal failure. p. 745. In Clinical Disorders of Fluid and Electrolyte Metabolism, 2nd ed. McGraw-Hill, New York, 1980
7. Miller TJ, Anderson RJ, Linas SL, et al: Urinary diagnostic indices in acute renal failure: A prospective study. Ann Intern Med 89:47, 1978
8. Anderson RJ, Linas SL, Berns AS, et al: Nonoliguric acute renal failure. N Engl J Med 296:1134, 1977
9. Anderson RJ, Schrier RW: Clinical spectrum of oliguric and nonoliguric acute renal failure, p. 1. In Brenner BM, Stein JH (eds): Acute Renal Failure. Churchill Livingstone, New York, 1980
10. Bull GM, Joekes AM, Lowe KG: Renal function studies in acute tubular necrosis. Clin Sci 9:379, 1950
11. Brun C, Munck O: Pathophysiology of the kidney in shock and in acute renal failure. Prog Surg 4:1, 1964
12. Flamenbaum W: Pathophysiology of acute renal failure, p. 795. In Kurtzman NA, Martinez-Maldonado M (eds): Pathophysiology of the Kidney. Charles C Thomas, Illinois, 1977
13. Bash CP, Rudnick MR, Narins RG: Diagnostic approaches to acute renal failure. p. 17. In BM Brenner, JH Stein (eds): Acute Renal Failure. Churchill Livingstone, New York, 1980
14. Finn WF: Acute renal failure. p. 167. In Earley L, Gottschalk C (eds): Diseases of the Kidney. 3rd ed. Little, Brown, Boston, 1979
15. Levinsky NG, Alexander EA, Venkatachalamm MA: Acute renal failure, p 1181. In Brenner B, Rector F (eds): The Kidney. 2nd ed. WB Saunders, Philadelphia, 1981
16. Brenner BM, Stein JH: Acute Renal Failure. Churchill Livingstone, New York, 1980
17. Luke RG, Briggs JD, Allison MEM, et al: Factors determining response to mannitol in acute renal failure. Am J Med Sci 259:168, 1970
18. Fry JK, Catell WR: The nephrographic pattern during excretion urography. Br Med Bull 28:227, 1972
19. Stein JH, Lifschitz MD, Barnes LD: Current concepts on the pathophysiology of acute renal failure. Am J Physiol 243:F171, 1978

20. Hostetter TH, Wilkes BM, Brenner BM: Mechanisms of impaired glomerular filtration in acute renal failure. p. 52. In Brenner BM, Stein JH (eds): Acute Renal Failure. Churchill Livingstone, New York, 1980
21. Thurau K, Boylan J: Acute renal success: The unexpected logic of oliguria and acute renal failure. Am J Med 61:308, 1976
22. Hollenberg NK, Adams DF, Oken DE, et al: Acute renal failure due to nephrotoxins: Renal hemodynamic and angiographic studies in man. N Engl J Med 282:1329, 1970
23. Flores J, Dibona DR, Beck CH, et al: Role of cell swelling in ischemic renal damage and the protective effect of hypertonic solute. J Clin Invest 51:118, 1972
24. Daugharty TM, Ueki IF, Mercer PF, et al: Dynamics of glomerular ultrafiltration in the rat. V. Response to ischemic injury. J Clin Invest 53:105, 1974
25. Mandal HD, Haygood CC, Bell RC, et al: Effect of acute and chronic splenectomy on experimental acute renal failure. J Lab Clin Med 92:698, 1978
26. Myers BD, Chui F, Hilberman M, et al: Transtubular leakage of glomerular filtrate in human acute renal failure. Am J Physiol 6:F319, 1979
27. Myers BD, Carrie BJ, Yee RR, et al: Pathophysiology of hemodynamically mediated acute renal failure in man. Kidney Int 18:415, 1980
28. Myers BD, Hilberman M, Spencer RJ, et al: Glomerular and tubular function in nonoliguric acute renal failure. Am J Med 72:642, 1982
29. Sarifstein R, Miller P, Dickman S, et al: Cisplatin nephrotoxicity in rats: Defect in papillary hypertonicity. Am J Physiol 10:F175, 1981
30. Chopra S, Kaufman JS, Jones TW, et al: Cis-diamminedichloroplatinum induced acute renal failure in the rat. Kidney Int 21:54, 1982
31. Barry KG, Cohen A, Knochel JP, et al: Mannitol infusion. II: The prevention of acute functional renal failure during resection of an aneurysm of the abdominal aorta. N Engl J Med 264:967, 1961
32. Gehr M, Gross M, Schmitt G, et al: Treatment of acute renal failure. p. 341. In Cowley RA, Trump BF (eds): Pathophysiology of Shock, Anoxia and Ischemia. Williams & Wilkins, Baltimore, 1982
33. Schmitt GW, Bach C: Peritoneal dialysis and hemodialysis. p. 561. In Flamenbaum W, Hamburger RJ (eds): Nephrology. An Approach to the Patient with Renal Disease. JB Lippincott, Philadelphia, 1982
34. Diamond JR, Yoburn DC: Nonoliguric acute renal failure associated with a low fractional excretion of sodium. Ann Intern Med 96:597, 1982
35. Gambos EA: Acute renal failure. Principles of management. NY State J Med 73:1055, 1973
36. Lawson LJ, Blaney JD, Dawson-Edwards P, et al: Dietary management of acute oliguric renal failure. Br Med J 3:292, 1962
37. Bluemle LW Jr; Potter HP, Elkinton Jr. Changes in body composition in acute renal failure. J Clin Invest 35:1094, 1956
38. Levinsky NG: Management of emergencies. VI. Hyperkalemia. N Engl J Med 274:1076, 1966
39. Levine HD: Electrolyte imbalance and the EKG. Mod Concepts Cardiovasc Dis 23:246, 1953
40. Stanton B, Giebisch G: Mechanism of urinary potassium excretion. Mineral Electrolyte Metab 5:100, 1981
41. Grossman RA, Hamilton RW, Morse BM, et al: Nontraumatic rhabdomyolysis and acute renal failure. N Engl J Med 291:807, 1974
42. Finch CA, Marchand JF: Cardiac arrest by the action of potassium. Am J Med Sci 206:507, 1943
43. Cohen JJ, Gennari FJ, Harrington JT: Disorders of potassium balance, p. 908. In Brenner BM, Rector FC Jr (eds): The Kidney. 2nd ed. WB Saunders, Philadelphia, 1981
44. David DS: Calcium metabolism in renal failure. Am J Med 58:48, 1975
44a. Cooper JD, Lazarowitz VC, Arieff AI: Neurodiagnostic abnormalities in patients with acute renal failure: Evidence for neurotoxicity of parathyroid hormone. J Clin Invest 61:1448, 1978
45. Bricker NS, Avioli LV, Reiss E, et al: Calcium, phosphorus and bone in disease and transplantation. Arch Intern Med 123:543, 1969
46. Bricker NS: On the meaning of the intact

nephron hypothesis. Am J Med 46:1, 1969
47. Massry SG, Ritz E: The pathogenesis of secondary hyperparathyroidism of renal failure. Is there a controversy? Arch Intern Med 138:853, 1978
48. Slatopolsky E, Caglar S, Pennell JP, et al: On the pathogenesis of hyperparathyroidism in chronic experimental renal insufficiency in the dog. J Clin Invest 50:492, 1971
49. Massry SG, Arieff AI, Coburn JW, et al: Divalent ion metabolism in patients with acute renal failure: Studies on the mechanism of hypocalcemia. Kidney Int 5:437, 1974
50. Massry SG, Coburn JW, Lee DBN: Skeletal resistance to parathyroid hormone in renal failure. Studies in 105 human subjects. Ann Intern Med 78:357, 1973
51. Arnaud CD: Hyperparathyroidism and renal failure. Kidney Int 4:89, 1973
52. Pietrek J, Kokot F, Kuska J: Serum 25-hydroxyvitamin D and parathyroid hormone in patients with acute renal failure. Kidney Int 13:178, 1978
53. Massry SG, Broutbar N, Goldstein DA: Calcium, phosphorus and magnesium. p. 179. In Flamenbaum W, Hamburger RJ (eds): Nephrology. An Approach to the Patient with Renal Disease. JB Lippincott, Philadelphia, 1982
54. Akman M, Goldstein DA, Telfer N, et al: Resolution of muscle calcification in rhabdomyolysis and acute renal failure. Ann Intern Med 89:928, 1978
55. Llach F, Felsenfeld AJ, Haussler MR: The pathophysiology of altered calcium metabolism in rhambdomyolysis induced acute renal failure. Interactions of parathyroid hormone, 25-hydroxycholecalciferol, and 1,25 dihydroxycholecalciferol. N Engl J Med 305:117, 1981
56. Narins RG: The renal acidoses. p. 30. In Brenner BM, Stein JH (eds): Acid–Base and Potassium Homeostasis. Churchill-Livingstone, New York, 1978
57. Cogan MG, Rector FC, Jr, Seldin DW: Acid–base disorders. p. 841. In Brenner BM, Rector FC Jr (eds). The Kidney. 2nd ed. WB Saunders, Philadelphia, 1981
58. Husted FC, Nolph KD, Maher JF: $NaHCO_3$ and NaCl tolerance in chronic renal failure. J Clin Invest 56:414, 1975
59. Abel RM, Beck CH Jr, Abbott WM, et al: Improved survival from acute renal failure after treatment with intravenous essential L-amino acids and glucose. Results of a prospective double-blind study. N Engl J Med 288:695, 1973
60. Abel RM, Shih VE, Abott W, et al: Amino acid metabolism in acute renal failure: Influence of intravenous essential L-amino acid hyperalimentation therapy. Ann Surg 180:350, 1974
61. Leonard CD, Luke RG, Siegel RR: Parenteral essential amino acids in acute renal failure. Urology 6:154, 1975
62. Toback FG: Amino acid enhancement of renal regeneration after acute tubular necrosis. Kidney Int 12:193, 1977
63. Toback FG: Amino acid treatment of acute renal failure. p. 202. In Brenner BM, Stein JH (eds): Acute Renal Failure. Churchill Livingstone, New York, 1980

14

Chronic Renal Failure

Leon G. Fine
Edward P. Nord

GENERAL CHARACTERISTICS OF HOMEOSTATIC SYSTEMS IN UREMIA

During the course of chronic renal disease, stresses are placed on numerous homeostatic systems in which the kidney serves as the principal excretory component. Not only are the various organ systems of the body required to function in a milieu that is no longer normal, but the kidneys themselves undergo significant adaptations in function that appear to be geared to maintaining the composition of the body fluids in as normal a state as possible for as long as possible. It is only when these systems ultimately fail that the uremic syndrome manifests clinically. When this stage is reached, only replacement of renal function by means of dialysis or transplantation can maintain life.

This chapter deals with the perturbations of composition of the body fluids and the nature of the adaptations in renal function that occur before the advent of terminal renal failure. It will become evident that the ability of the diseased kidney to maintain the composition of the body fluids in a state close to normality, even when the total nephron population is reduced by as much as 90 percent, is due to an intricate array of renal and extrarenal adaptations. Elucidation of the mechanisms of these adaptations remains a major challenge for the future.

Potential Consequences of Nephron Loss

ACCUMULATION OF SUBSTANCES NORMALLY EXCRETED BY GLOMERULAR FILTRATION

A persistent fall in glomerular filtration rate could be due either to a decrease in the rates at which all nephrons filter or to complete ablation of some nephrons, leaving others intact. The net effect of both situations is to reduce the "filtered load" of all substances that normally enter the tubular fluid via glomerular filtration. Certain solutes, including creatinine and urea, are excreted almost exclusively by this process. (Both substances are transported to some extent by the tubular epithelium and are thus not ideal markers of glomerular filtration; creatinine appears to be secreted by the renal tubule, especially in proteinuric states,[1] whereas urea reabsorption by the proximal tubule is enhanced under conditions of extracellular fluid volume contraction associated with low urine flow rates.[2]) A reduction in glomerular filtration rate (GFR) leads to a decrease in filtered load, that is, GFR × plasma concentration. This leads to a fall in the excretory rate of substances eliminated largely by glomerular filtration with a consequent rise in the concentration of these solutes in the body fluids. The result of the elevated plasma concentration is a secondary rise in the filtered load so that the excretory rate returns to its previous level. At this point a new steady state is established in which the rate of entry of creatinine or urea into the extracellular fluid is exactly balanced by an equal rate of excretion. However, this is achieved at the expense of an increased concentration of the solute in the extracellular fluid. Initially the rise in serum concentrations of urea and creatinine may be imperceptible, and even with a reduction in glomerular filtration rate of 50 percent may remain within the normal range. For instance, if a patient starts with a serum creatinine concentration of 0.6 mg/dl and filtration rate falls by 50 percent, a rate of creatinine excretion equal to the original rate can be attained with a serum creatinine concentration of 1.2 mg/dl.

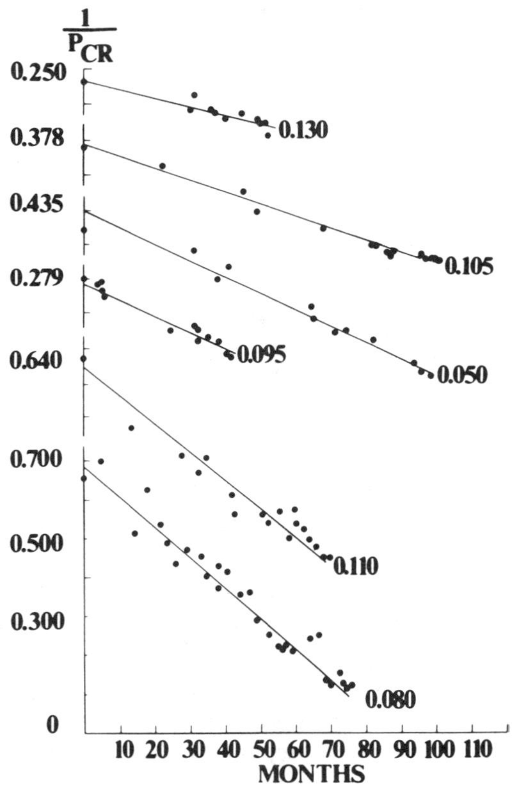

Fig. 14–1. Rate of loss of renal function measured as the linear change in the reciprocal of serum creatinine concentration with time. Data from six patients are shown: two with glomerulonephritis, two with interstitial nephritis, and two with medullary cystic disease. (From Mitch WE, Buffington GA, Lemann J, et al: A simple method of estimating progression of chronic renal failure, Lancet 2:1326, 1976.)

This relationship between serum creatinine concentration and glomerular filtration rate has been exploited to predict the course of chronic renal failure.[3] If the reciprocal of the serum creatinine concentration is plotted as a function of time in patients with chronic renal failure of diverse etiologies, a linear relationship is observed (Fig. 14–1). As long as the rate of creatinine acquisition remains constant, this relationship is valuable in predicting when renal function will be inadequate to support life. Furthermore, if a deviation from linearity is observed, the likelihood of a superimposed acute process unrelated to the intrinsic disease must be considered.

ACCUMULATION OF SUBSTANCES NORMALLY EXCRETED BY TUBULAR SECRETION

Organic anions, organic bases, uric acid, ammonia, and potassium are eliminated largely by tubular secretion. Uric acid and potassium are handled both by tubular reabsorption and by secretion, whereas organic anions such as lactate and hippurate are transported from the peritubular surface of the nephron into the tubular lumen. Ammonia is synthesized within the tubular epithelial cells and as such represents a different form of secretion. Nevertheless all these solutes share common fates as the nephron population decreases. The rate of excretion of a solute as a function of glomerular filtration rate can be expressed as the ratio of its clearance to the clearance of creatinine or inulin, that is, fractional excretion ($C_{solute}/C_{creatinine}$). As glomerular filtration rate falls, this ratio rises dramatically and C_{PAH}/GFR, C_{NH4}/GFR, and C_{urate}/GFR[4] have all been shown to increase. In essence this increased clearance ratio indicates an adaptation in tubular function, which serves to prevent a rise in the extracellular fluid (ECF) concentrations of these substances.

The effectiveness of each adaptation in maintaining serum concentrations within normal limits varies from solute to solute (Fig. 14–2), and the reasons for the differences are not apparent. Serum potassium concentration remains within normal limits until the glomerular filtration rate falls to approximately 10 percent of normal.[5,6] In contrast, serum levels of urate,[7-11] ammonia,[12-16] and phosphate[17-20] rise earlier in the course of renal failure. For these substances, despite significant adaptations in each of the surviving nephrons, the net amount excreted depends on the number of functioning nephrons. For instance, the values for ammonia excretion/GFR may be supranormal in uremia, yet total excretion may be decreased if the amount of surviving renal tissue is sufficiently small.

ACCUMULATION OF SUBSTANCES HANDLED BY FILTRATION AND TUBULAR REABSORPTION

In normal subjects 99 percent of the filtered load of sodium and 90 percent of filtered phosphorus are reclaimed by the renal tubules. In advanced renal failure tubular reabsorption of sodium may be depressed to 70 percent of the filtered load and phosphorus to 50 percent or more. Despite these similarities in tubular adaptation, serum phosphorus begins to rise when glomerular filtration rate falls to 25 to 30 percent of normal values,[20] whereas serum Na concentration is maintained within normal limits even down to a glomerular filtration rate of ≤10 ml/min.[21,22] The reason for the earlier rise in serum phosphorus is not immediately apparent. For instance, at a glomerular filtration rate of 25 ml/min and a serum phosphorus concentration of 4.5 mg/dl, the filtered load is 1620 mg/day. Daily gastrointestinal absorption of phosphorus from a normal diet is ~800 mg; thus a fractional excretion of 50 percent would be adequate to maintain phosphate balance at a glomerular filtration rate of 25 ml/min, obviating a rise in serum phosphorus concentration. Despite the fact that this fractional excretion rate can be attained, serum phosphorus concentration rises.

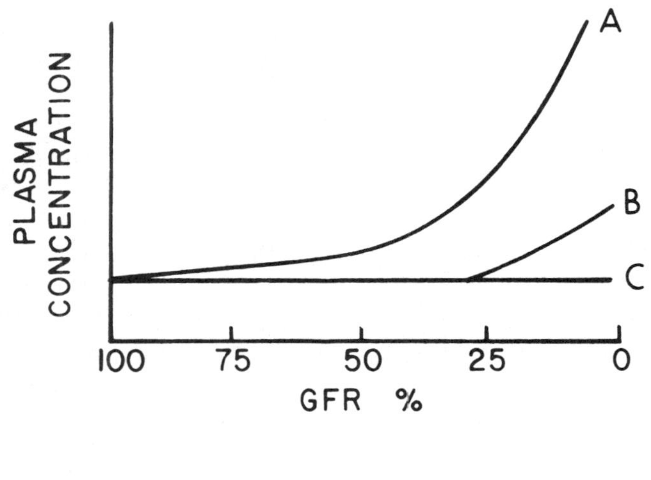

Fig. 14–2. Patterns of adaptation for different solutes in chronic progressive renal disease. Curve A shows no regulation of plasma contraction of the solute, which rises progressively as *glomerular filtration rate* (GFR) falls. Curve B shows that this rise occurs only when GFR approaches 25 percent of normal. Curve C represents perfect regulation of solute concentration. (From Bricker NS, Fine LG: The renal response to progressive nephron loss. p. 1058. In Brenner BM, Rector FC Jr (eds): The Kidney. WB Saunders, Philadelphia, 1981.)

The Concept of Balance and Its Maintenance in Uremia

"Balance" implies that the rate of elimination of a solute from the body exactly equals the rate at which it is ingested. For solutes that are not ingested as such (e.g., creatinine), the same concept would apply, except that the rate of excretion would equal the rate of accumulation within the body fluids from endogenous production.

The ability to maintain balance permits constancy of the composition of the body fluids to be maintained. If excretory rate falls below the acquisition rate, net positive balance results. If the total excretory mass of the kidney falls, balance can only be maintained if the surviving units (nephrons) increase their individual contributions to the total excretory rate. The theoretical requirements for this process to occur are discussed in the section on homeostasis in chronic renal failure.

At the outset it should be appreciated that although we are accustomed to measuring balance in human subjects and experimental animals over 24-hour periods, the ingestion of solutes actually occurs over shorter periods of time, that is, during meals. Thus the extracellular fluid is normally subjected to one or more acute changes in solute content during the day. Presumably each perturbation of the steady state acts as a signal that sets into motion one or more regulatory processes, the ultimate purpose of which, is to return the extracellular fluid to its original condition. If a change in the solute composition or total content of extracellular fluid is very small, it may not result in any adjustments. It is probable that some threshold must be exceeded in order to activate the regulatory process and that some fluctuations in concentration or content normally do occur. The extent of these fluctuations becomes an indirect measure of the sensitivity of the system.

When a number of different substances are added simultaneously to the extracellular fluid, balance requirements dictate that there must be a means of discriminating between one solute and another, that is, homeostasis requires independent regulation of each solute. Thus if sodium intake happens to coincide with a low-potassium intake on one day and the pattern is reversed on the following day due to normal dietary variation, excretion of each ion by the kidney must be regulated totally independently.

Biologic Control Systems: Do They Exist for All Solutes?

The precision with which the body fluids are regulated has led to the proposal that separate biologic control systems exist that oversee the excretion of each solute. A "system" is something having more than one component part. For most excretory processes, the kidney is the end organ or effector component. A key question is whether a given perturbation of extracellular fluid composition ultimately leads to activation of the end organ via a sensor and one or more mediators (and possibly an integrator to set the priorities for a variety of incoming signals) or whether the perturbation activates the renal response by directly altering cellular function within the kidney.

EXTRARENAL CONTROL

The control of extracellular volume represents, par excellence, an example of an extrarenal control system.[4] Such a system is conceived of as having volume sensors located somewhere in the thorax. Activation of the sensing mechanism leads to an alteration in one or more meditors, including neurogenic impulses to the kidney, a change in cardiac output, mean arterial pressure (MAP), and hormones (including catecholamines, vasopressin, natriuretic factors, dopamine, angiotensin, and aldosterone). Whether alterations of these hemodynamic, humoral, and neurogenic phenomena are concomitants of changes in extracellular fluid volume or whether they actually mediate the excretory response is the subject of ongoing investigation. It is clear that, in a multifactorial system, deletion of one or more of these factors is unlikely to abolish the appropriate excretory response. It is also entirely predictable that a system as critical to survival as the control of volume would have such built-in safety mechanisms.

With so many parallel changes taking place, it has been proposed that there is an integrator element that handle this diversity of information.[23] On the other hand, the need to postulate the existence of an integrator falls away if many of these humoral and neurogenic changes are not mediators of sodium excretion per se, but rather exist to defend cardiovascular and hemodynamic stability.

Finally, the end organ (the kidney) is activated to adjust its excretion of sodium and water so as to restore volume toward normal. Despite the obvious primacy of the kidney as the excretory organ in health, in advanced uremia other excretory routes may be recruited. A good example is the enhanced excretion of potassium by the colon in uremia.[24]

INTRINSIC RENAL CONTROL

An alternative explanation for solute homeostasis is that the elements of the kidney respond directly to alterations in content and composition of the body fluids. Even the control of extracellular volume may be explained in this way. If, for instance, subtle changes in perfusion pressure, filtration dynamics, or renal interstitial pressure were to alter changes in overall extracellular fluid volume, such events could mediate natriuresis or sodium retention.[25]

Potassium homeostasis may well be regulated entirely by the kidney despite the acknowledged regulatory role of adrenocortical hormones in modulating this process. For instance, very small elevations of serum potassium concentration (i.e., <0.5 mEq/liter) are associated with increases in renal potassium excretion.[26] Since an increase in serum potassium may elevate cellular potassium levels in the distal and collecting tubule by altering the flux across the peritubular membrane,[27] this could alter potassium excretion directly. Indeed, in the isolated perfused kidney the potassium concentration of the perfusate is directly correlated with fractional potassium excretion. In this system, no extrarenal influences are present.[28]

Many excretory processes are regulated by events initiated outside the kidney. Hormones, by definition, are substances that are released at one site and act on an effector cell different from that which produced the hormone. The fact that the kidney has target cells with receptors responsive to a variety of hormones indicates that these messengers must play at least some important roles in regulating excretion. Indeed the critical role of parathyroid hormone in modulating phosphorus excretion is indisputable, and the role of aldosterone in altering the renal handling of both sodium and potassium is well documented. For other hormones, precise roles in excretory processes are yet to be delineated (prostaglandins, kinins, catecholamines, and dopamine), whereas in certain cases the circumstantial evidence implicating the role of a hormone (e.g., natriuretic hormone) has preceded the isolation and purification of such a substance(s).

It is clear that biologic control is based on multifactorial processes, and in many cases there are more missing pieces than those that have found a place in the puzzle. Extracellular fluid volume control has been extensively investigated; nevertheless, a specific sensing element has not been identified, the signal to such a putative sensor has not been defined, and the hormonal and neurogenic mediators remain poorly understood.

Homeostasis in Chronic Renal Failure

The uncertainties in defining the homeostatic processes make it mandatory to define the process of homeostasis in uremia in its simplest possible terms. Only two elements are required: (1) a signal, and (2) an effector. When renal mass is reduced by disease, constancy of the extracellular fluid could be achieved if (1) the signal for excretion is enhanced, or (2) the response of the end organ to a normal signal is enhanced.

These possibilities are illustrated in Figure 14–3. The "signal" refers to the message imparted to the kidney indicating the extent to which the extracellular fluid composition has been perturbed. Addition of a solute to the extracellular fluid can result in either a rise in its concentration or, if water is added to the extracellular fluid in isotonic proportions, a change in total content without a change in concentration. Regardless of which of these two possibilities occurs, a signal is generated that triggers an increase in renal excretion of the solute. This signal may be extrinsic to the kidney or may occur within the kidney itself, according to one of three theoretical patterns.

AUGMENTED SIGNAL FOR EXCRETION

One way in which a reduced functioning renal mass can achieve a normal rate of excretion is to receive an excretory signal that is exaggerated. This increased signal would trigger an augmented secretion per nephron so that the steady-state level would be restored within the normal period of time. An example of this situation is seen when an acute potassium load is administered to uremic dogs.[29-31] Possibly because of altered extrarenal potassium disposal, serum potassium rises to a higher concentration than is observed when the same load is given to a normal animal and the direct effect on renal potassium excretion would be consequently exaggerated.

PROLONGED SIGNAL FOR EXCRETION

Another means whereby a reduced nephron population can dispose of an acute load of a solute is if the duration of the signal is increased, that is, the signal persists for a longer period of time even if the magnitude of the change in extracellular fluid concentration or content is the same as normal. This prolonged signal ultimately permits the reduced number of functioning nephrons to accomplish the same net excretion. Acute potassium loading also illustrates this example. In normal dogs the oral administration of 100 mEq of KCl leads to an elevation in serum potassium of

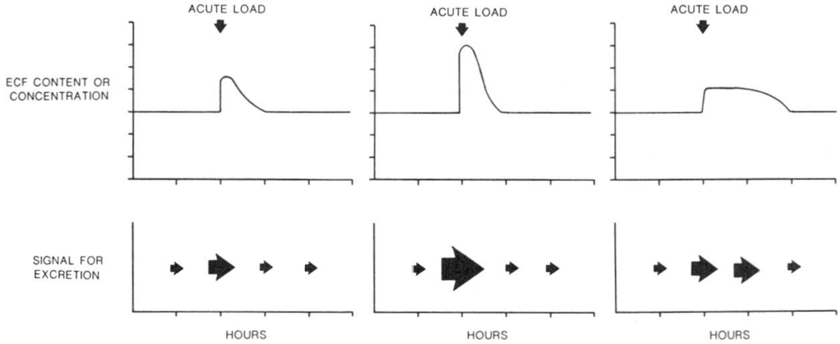

Fig. 14–3. Effect of an acute solute load in uremia. (Left) An example showing a normal signal for renal excretion, triggered by a rise in the extracellular fluid content or concentration of a solute. (Middle) Demonstration of how an exaggerated signal to diseased kidneys can be generated by a greater change in extracellular fluid (ECF) content or concentration. (Right) Normal signal magnitude, but of extended duration. Both methods of restoring the ECF toward normal have been demonstrated in uremia.

1 to 1.5 mEq/liter, but this elevation returns to baseline between 5 and 6 hours. In contrast, uremic dogs with remnant kidneys receiving the same load show serum potassium concentrations elevated ~1.5 mEq/liter above baseline even after 5 hours.[29] Since potassium excretion is directly related to serum potassium concentration, it is evident that the stimulus to potassium excretion is both an increase in the magnitude of the early signal (as in the augmented signal for excretion) and prolongation of a signal that may be normal in magnitude at a later point in time.

ENHANCED END-ORGAN RESPONSE

The final mechanism by which a diseased kidney can achieve a normal excretory rate despite the existence of a reduced number of functioning nephrons is to alter its response to an excretory signal. Even if the signal is normal in magnitude and duration, an enhanced end-organ response will achieve a greater rate of excretion. An example of this is the enhanced response to parathyroid hormone in uremia,[32,33] which is reflected by a greater than normal phosphaturia in response to a given amount of the hormone. Although this area has not been extensively explored, it is possible that the enhanced excretory rate per nephron of a number of substances regulated by extrarenal factors is achieved by this mechanism.

SPECIFIC ADAPTATIONS

Renal Blood Flow and Glomerular Filtration

RENAL HEMODYNAMIC AND GLOMERULAR RESPONSES TO NONGLOMERULAR DISEASE

Although chronic glomerulonephritis constitutes the most common form of chronic renal disease in humans, nonglomerular injury may also lead to chronic renal failure. This latter category includes uninephrectomy, subtotal nephrectomy (either by surgical excision of part of the kidneys or by ligation of branches of one renal artery with contralateral, i.e., a "remnant" kidney), and chronic interstitial diseases such as pyelonephritis.

Renal Blood Flow

Alterations in the intrarenal distribution of blood flow may be important in determining the total glomerular filtration rate of the diseased kidney, since the single-nephron glomerular filtration rate of the juxtamedullary nephrons is greater than that of the superficial nephrons.[34] Increases in the single-nephron glomerbular filtration rate of both superficial and deep nephrons occur in response to a reduction in renal mass.[35,36] The single-nephron glomerular filtration rate of superficial nephrons increases within less than 24 hours of uninephrectomy.[37] When studied at a later point in time (approximately 1 week), superficial single-nephron glomerular filtration rate may increase fourfold, whereas juxtamedullary nephron single-nephron glomerular filtration rate only increases by a factor of 2 in the remnant kidney.[35,36] After 2 to 4 weeks, it appears that single-nephron glomerular filtration rate increases proportionately in both nephron populations. Despite these observations, consistent changes in intrarenal blood flow distribution have not been demonstrable, even at an early phase of the disease. Carriere et al.[38] showed that marked reduction in nephron mass leads to obvious vasodilatation in the remnant kidney, affecting all regions of the cortex equally. On the other hand, Kaufman et al.[39] were able to show redistribution to the inner cortical region, which varied directly with the extent of ablation of renal mass. In view of the critical dependence of single-nephron glomerular filtration rate on plasma flow rate, it seems likely that early increases in superficial single-nephron glomerular filtration rate are related to changes in plasma flow through the superficial cortex. It is also possible that limitations in the techniques of measuring blood flow distribution have made it difficult to demonstrate such changes with any degree of consistancy.

Glomerular Filtration

An increase in single-nephron glomerular filtration rate, varying from two- to fourfold, has been a consistent observation in the remnant kidney.[35,36,40-43] Deen et al.[42] attempted to elucidate the major determinants of single-nephron glomerular filtration rate that lead to this increase in the uninephrectomized rat. These workers demonstrated that the ultrafiltration coefficient (K_f) of the uninephrectomized kidney is unchanged at 2 to 4 weeks, but that the ultrafiltration pressure was elevated due to an increase in single-nephron plasma flow and mean transcapillary hydraulic pressure difference. Similar findings, but of greater magnitude, have been described by Hostetter et al.[43] in Wistar rats with solitary remnant kidneys. Of interest is the fact that filtration pressure disequilibrium occurs in the remnant kidney (i.e., filtration continues along the entire length of the glomerular capillaries), making it possible to calculate the ultrafiltration coefficient (K_f). Although Hostetter et al. could not demonstrate a difference in K_f compared with normal values, Finn et al.[44] found an increase in the K_f of uninephrectomized Sprague-Dawley rats.

The ultrafiltration coefficient, K_f, is the product of the hydraulic conductivity of the glomerular capillary wall and the total surface area of the glomerular capillaries. Since an increase in the glomerular volume observed in the remnant kidney[45] could be due to an increase in the number or size of the cells within the glomerulus, morphometric analysis is required to delineate changes in capillary surface area. Such studies were performed by Olivetti et al.[46] and Shea et al.,[47] who demonstrated an increase in capillary surface area in uninephrectomized and 5/6 nephrectomized rats studied at 2 to 21 weeks. Since measured values of K_f appear to be unchanged, yet surface area is increased, it is possible that the hydraulic conductivity of the glomerular capillary wall may actually be decreased in this disease model. It is not clear, however, whether the increase in the glomerular volume is due to increased pressure within the glomerulus (i.e., a distention phenomenon reproduced when glomeruli are fixed during perfusion) or to a real increase in size due to compensatory hypertrophy. Measurements of glomerular capillary surface area using an in vivo antibody technique failed to show an increase in surface area up to 22 days after uninephrectomy,[48] but, since the relationship between surface area and antigenic sites may be altered in the hyperfiltering glomeruli, these studies do not clarify the issue further.

The changes in single-nephron glomerular filtration rate observed in the remnant kidney are also seen in experimental chronic pyelonephritis.[49,50] This finding suggests that, when the renal insult does not reside in the glomerulus, the unaffected nephrons respond by increasing their filtration rates. In the remnant kidney, this affects all surviving nephrons, whereas in pyelonephritis there is a patchy distribution of hyperfiltering nephrons that have been spared from the destructive interstitial disease. However, the nephron-to-nephron variation in single-nephron glomerular filtration rate from within the same kidney does not appear to be greater than the variation found in the normal kidney.

RENAL HEMODYNAMIC AND GLOMERULAR RESPONSES TO CHRONIC GLOMERULAR DISEASE

Glomerular function has been studied in two models of chronic glomerular disease: immune-complex (IC) nephritis and antiglomerular basement membrane (anti-GBM) antibody disease.[51-58]

During the early phase of immune-complex nephritis (heterologous phase), single-nephron glomerular filtration rate and total-kidney glomerular filtration rate are reduced.[51,58]

Heterogeneity of single-nephron glomerular filtration rate values is also increased. Ichikawa et al.[58] have shown that the reduction is due to a fall in single-nephron plasma flow and to a decrease in K_f. Transcapillary hydraulic pressure is increased, but not sufficiently to counteract the influences of the other determinants of filtration.[58] Allison et al.[52] demonstrated that, in the latter stage of IC disease (autologous phase), the mean single-nephron glomerular filtration rate remains depressed with an increased dispersion of values within the same kidney (Fig. 14–4). Some nephrons have markedly reduced filtration rates and some have supernormal values. Glomerular capillary pressure (PGC), estimated by the stopflow technique, varies directly with the single-nephron glomerular filtration rate.[52] A more recent study, by Ichikawa et al.,[58] demonstrated that the observed heterogeneity of single-nephron glomerular filtration rate values in autologous immune-complex nephritis is due to differences in single-nephron plasma flow and, to a lesser extent, to a decrease in K_f.[58]

In antiglomerular basement membrane nephritis, mean single-nephron glomerular filtration rate is similarly decreased with an increased internephron variation. K_f is also reduced, and the mean hydraulic pressure difference increased, as is observed in immune-complex nephritis.[52,55] In puromycin-induced nephritis, a "minimal-change" lesion, there is a reduction in K_f as well as a fall in plasma flow.[59]

It is evident from these observations that a fall in the ultrafiltration coefficient appears to be a critical determinant of the reduction in glomerular filtration rate in models of glomerular disease. Once again it is not clear

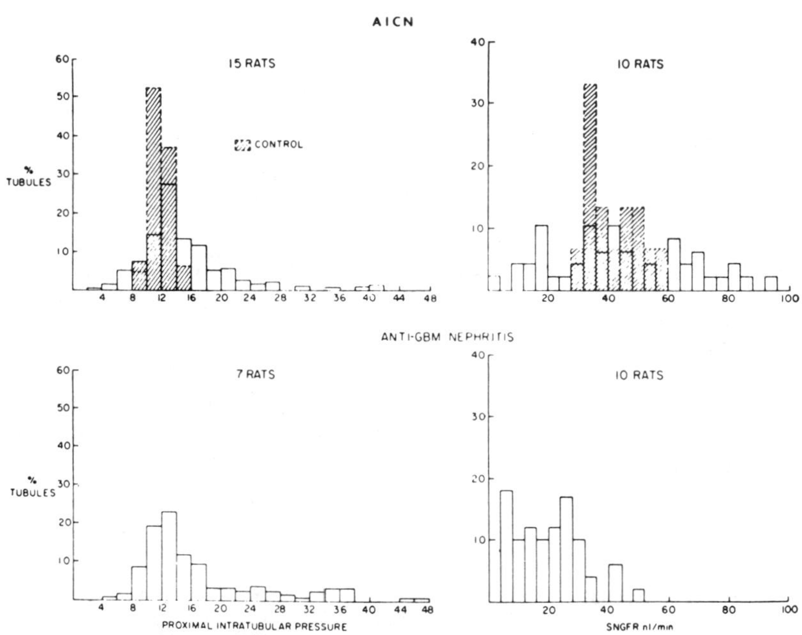

Fig. 14–4. Frequency histograms depicting distributions of proximal intratubular pressure and single nephron glomerular filtration rates (SNGFR) in rats with autologous immune complex nephritis (AICN), rats with antiglomerular basement membrane nephritis, and controls. (From Allison MEM, Wilson CB, Gottschalk CW: Pathophysiology of experimental glomerulonephritis in rats, J Clin Invest 53:1402, 1974. By permission of the American Society for Clinical Investigation.)

whether this reduction represents an intrinsic change in glomerular capillary hydraulic conductivity or an obliteration or collapse of capillary loops within the glomerulus. The latter may well be the more likely possibility in light of the finding that volume expansion can decrease the heterogeneity of single-nephron glomerular filtration rate values and reverse the patchy appearance of the kidney surface.[60] In puromycin-induced nephrosis, an angiotensin antagonist, saralasin, reverses the fall in renal plasma flow and K_f, suggesting that an increase in vasoconstrictor substances or a decrease in vasodilator substances plays an important role in the pathophysiology of this experimental disorder.[61] Indeed, inhibition of prostaglandin synthesis with a resulting obliteration of their vasodilatory effects leads to a pattern of glomerular function remarkably similar to that observed in puromycin nephrosis, that is, a decrease in K_f and single-nephron plasma flow.[62]

CHANGES IN GLOMERULAR STRUCTURE AND PERMEABILITY TO MACROMOLECULES

The elevation in the glomerular filtration rate of the surviving glomeruli, which follows reduction of a renal mass, provides a means of achieving augmented excretion of substances removed largely by glomerular filtration. A disconcerting observation, which has recently received renewed attention, is that removal of 75 percent or more of the renal mass leads to progressive uremia, hypertension, and proteinuria, even though the remaining renal tissue was intact at the time of the initial reduction in renal mass.[43]

In adult rats subjected to 5/6 nephrectomy, an increase in glomerular size is associated with vacuolization of epithelial cells and fusion of foot processes. Within 6 months, enlargement of the mesangial region and finally sclerosis of glomeruli occur. Similar observations were made in rats subjected to unilateral nephrectomy and contralateral segmental infarction of the kidney.[63] Recent studies by Olson et al.[65] demonstrated abnormalities of partial renal ablation as early as 1 week. These workers further showed that the severity of injury was proportional to the extent of reduction of renal mass.

This progressive glomerulosclerosis is associated with massive proteinuria, which has been shown, by analysis of fractional dextran clearances, to be associated with an enhanced passage of molecules of radius >38 A and a defect in the ability of the glomerulus to restrict the passage of negatively charged macromolecules[64] (Fig. 14–5). In rats with severe reductions of renal mass, the changes in permselectivity to macromolecules are coincident with structural alterations of the capillary wall and mesangial accumulation of fibrin. Low-protein feeding, which prevents the hemodynamic changes in the remnant glomeruli, reduces these structural changes.[66]

PROGRESSIVE NATURE OF RENAL DISEASE AND ITS POTENTIAL REVERSAL

It is clearly important to understand the mechanisms underlying the progressive glomerular sclerosis in the remnant kidney, since they may provide insight into the progressive nature of many renal diseases. There does not appear to be an immunologic basis for the lesion, although some deposition of immunoglobins has been detected by immunofluorescence.[64] Significant immune-complex or antiglomerular basement membrane antibody deposition are absent. Reversal of systemic hypertension does not prevent the lesion but does appear to attenuate its severity.[64]

In a provocative study, Hostetter and colleagues[43] have examined whether reversal of the single-nephron hyperfiltration of the remnant kidney can prevent the progression of the lesion. By restricting dietary protein intake, these workers prevented the doubling of single-nephron glomerular filtration rate seen in rats on a normal diet, and there was an impressive attenuation of both the proteinuria and the histologic lesion[43] (Fig. 14–6). These findings led these investigators to pro-

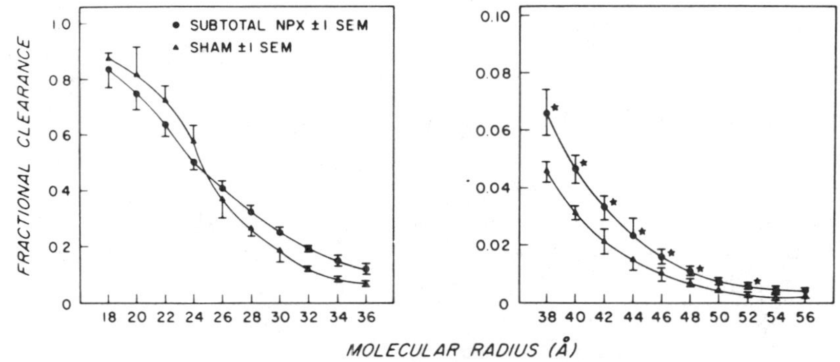

Fig. 14–5. Fractional clearance of neutral dextran molecules plotted as a function of effective molecular radii for sham-operated rats and rats subjected to subtotal nephrectomy of ~ 1 and ⅚ of renal mass. (Left) Data for molecules ranging 18 to 36 A in radius. (Right) Data for molecular radius of 38 to 56 A on an expanded scale for fractional clearance. Asterisks (*) denote statistically significant differences versus sham. (From Hostetter TH, Brenner BM: Glomerular adaptations to renal injury. p. 19. In Brenner BM, Stein JH (eds): Chronic Renal Failure, Churchill Livingstone, New York, 1981.)

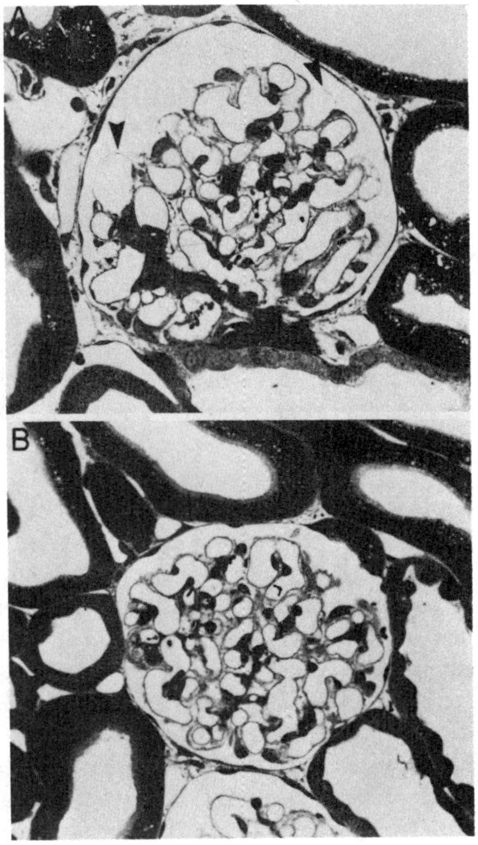

Fig. 14–6. Light micrographs of glomeruli from rats with 1 and ⅚ of their renal mass removed 1 week before study. (Top) Sequential increases in the mesangium and blebs (arrowheads) in the epithelial cells. These animals were on a normal protein intake. (Bottom) Glomerulus from rats subjected to the same surgical procedure, but maintained on a low-protein diet. The glomerulus is normal. (From Hostetter TH, Olson JL, Rennke HG, et al: Hyperfiltration in remnant nephrons: A potentially adverse response to renal ablation. Am J Physiol 241:F85, 1981.)

pose that hyperfiltration per se could be the cause of the progressive nature of renal failure in this model and in other diseases such as diabetes mellitus. Recent studies by Brenner and co-workers[67] suggest that long-term protein restriction can prevent the development of renal failure in this experimental model.

The mechanism of the glomerular sclerosis is unclear. The increased movement of filtrate across the capillary wall could lead to proteinuria via an increased convective flux of macromolecules. Altered barrier function of the glomerular capillary would enhance this effect, and the transglomerular movement of protein could ultimately damage some component of the glomerulus.[65,66] Ferritin deposition, for instance, is greatly increased in the mesangial region in the remnant glomeruli and, if long-term protein deposition occurs in this region, it may well initiate the sequence of events that ultimately leads to glomerular sclerosis.

GLOMERULAR FUNCTION IN HUMAN RENAL DISEASE

It is obviously difficult to obtain a detailed analysis of the dynamics of glomerular ultrafiltration in humans, but the available information does provide clues to the nature of the altered glomerular function. In human glomerulonephritis, filtration fraction (GFR/renal plasma flow) is decreased.[68,69] This suggests a fall in K_f which, together with a reduction in renal plasma flow, would lead to a fall in single-nephron glomerular filtration rate.[70]

The progressive nature of a variety of clinical disorders of renal function is also evident, especially when a period of hyperfiltration can be demonstrated.[71] Patients with diabetic glomerulosclerosis subjected to unilateral nephrectomy show rapid progression of glomerulopathy, whereas unilateral renal artery stenosis appears to protect the kidney from the diabetic lesion. After bilateral cortical necrosis, there is a period of recovery of glomerular filtration rate (presumably due to hyperfiltration in the surviving glomeruli), followed by a progressive downhill course of renal failure.[72] The glomerulosclerosis of reflux nephropathy is also progressive,[73] even if the reflux, the urinary tract infection, and the hypertension are corrected. Presumably the initial insult, if it destroys a sufficient number of nephrons, can lead to a perpetuation of the disease mediated by hyperfiltration in the surviving glomeruli.

CLINICAL EVALUATION OF GLOMERULAR FILTRATION RATE IN UREMIA

The observation that the fall in glomerular filtration rate that occurs in a variety of renal diseases is linearly related to the reciprocal of serum creatinine concentration has provided an important means of predicting the course of renal failure. This relationship holds despite the existence of a significant extrarenal clearance of creatinine (as will be seen in the section on nitrogen metabolism). The slope of the reciprocal of serum creatinine concentration ($1/S_{Cr}$) varies from patient to patient, but usually does not deviate from linearity as long as the nature of the disease process remains the same[3] (Fig. 14–1). Indeed, it is a deviation from this linearity that should raise suspicion of a superimposed insult, such as volume contraction, heart failure, obstruction (including unilateral obstruction, since the presence of advanced disease limits compensatory increases in the function of the contralateral kidney), superimposed acute glomerulitis, and administration of nephrotoxins, including contrast media.

Creatinine clearance becomes an unreliable index of true glomerular filtration rate (as measured by inulin clearance) as the latter falls below 20 to 25 ml/min. This is apparently due to tubular creatinine secretion, which is especially marked in heavy proteinuric states.[1] The mean of the creatinine and the urea clearance are a reasonable estimate of the true glomerular filtration rate. In practice, however, it is rarely of importance to know the precise glomerular filtration rate and, if serum creatinine concentration is related to a given creatinine clearance at some point in the course of the disease, it can be assumed that a doubling of serum creatinine concentration reflects a halving of glomerular filtration rate.

Compensatory Renal Hypertrophy

Enlargement of the surviving nephrons is an almost universal concomitant of loss of functioning renal mass. An increase in both cell number (hyperplasia) and in cell size (hypertrophy) occurs, with the latter process predominating.[74] Hypertrophy is generally defined as an increase in the RNA:DNA, protein:DNA, or protein:cell ratios, whereas in hyperplasia these ratios are unchanged. The term "compensatory hypertrophy" includes all of these processes.

Much emphasis has been placed on compensatory increases in glomerular and tubular function, but the relationships between such changes and increases in cell size are less clearly delineated. It is obvious that a functional alteration that occurs within minutes to hours is unlikely to be secondary to an increase in cell size. On the other hand, more chronic changes in tubular function, for instance, could be solely related to an increase in cell size. Thus, an adaptation of a specific transport process could be induced by a selective increase in that particular process, or it could be accomplished by a more global change in which all cell functions are increased symmetrically in parallel with an increase in the size of the cell and its constituent organelles and membranes.

THE NATURE OF RENAL COMPENSATORY HYPERTROPHY

Hypertrophy and Hyperplasia

Loss of nephrons results in a rapid increase in the mass of the remaining renal tissue. An increase in dry weight has been observed within 24 to 36 hours,[75-77] and in certain species, such as the rabbit, this increase may occur within hours.[78] After uninephrectomy, the remaining kidney can grow to up to 90 percent of the original combined two-kidney mass or increase in size at more than twice the expected growth rate of normal animals of the same size and age.[79] Within 1 to 2 weeks, kidney weight is increased by 40 percent above control levels in the rat.

Within minutes of the removal of one kidney, ^{14}C-choline incorporation into phospholipids increases by nearly 40 percent.[80] This phenomenon is observed first in the papilla and later in the outer medulla and cortex. The activity of choline kinase, a key enzyme in membrane biosynthesis, is increased within 6 hours after uninephrectomy. DNA synthesis is marginally increased, and an increase in RNA and protein content occurs within 24 hours.[81] Over the ensuing 24 to 48 hours, the rate of protein synthesis diminishes, but increases again around the fourth day and may exceed the prenephrectomy control value by some 30 percent.[82,83] The RNA:DNA ratio thus increases (due to an increase in ribosomal RNA) to a greater extent than does renal mass during the first 2 days after nephrectomy. Thereafter, the ratio remains constant as renal mass continues to increase.[84-87]

Cyclic nucleotide metabolism during compensatory hypertrophy has recently been investigated.[88,89] Cyclic guanosine monophosphate (cGMP) has been shown to be 200 to 300 percent above basal levels with parallel changes in insoluble guanylate cyclase activity. In contrast, cyclic adenosine monophosphate (cAMP) levels remain constant. Although it is tempting to postulate that a change in the cGMP:cAMP ratio plays a key role in initiating or modulating hypertrophy, additional information is required to evaluate this concept.

New Nephron Formation?

In adult animals, no increase in the number of nephron units has been observed on the basis of glomerular counts.[90-92] In neonatal rats, however, the total glomerular count was found by one group of investigators to rise by nearly 50 percent of the original number after removal of one kidney. This occurred only if the surgery was performed before the age of 50 days.[93] There are no data to indicate whether this process occurs in humans. Furthermore, the observation has not been confirmed using improved methods for glomerular counting, even in weanling rats.[94] Thus, new nephron formation probably does not contribute to the increase in renal mass seen clinically in compensatory hypertrophy.

Sites of Hypertrophy in the Nephron

Most evidence points to the fact that the entire nephron is involved in the process of hypertrophy. Glomerular size (and presumably capillary surface area) is increased, as are length and internal and external diameters of the tubules. Increases in tubular dimensions and in protein content per unit length have been demonstrated in proximal, convoluted, and straight tubules as well as in the loops of Henle and the collecting tubule[45,95,96,97] (Fig. 14–7).

When kidneys suffer patchy involvement by disease, as in glomerulonephritis, or by toxins such as potassium dichromate and mercuric chloride, compensatory growth may occur only in the intact or minimally involved nephrons, which leads to a marked variation from one nephron to another.

STIMULI FOR HYPERTROPHY

Loss of Renal Mass Versus Loss of Renal Function

Diversion of ureteral urine from one kidney into the peritoneal cavity effectively reduces renal excretory function by 50 percent without

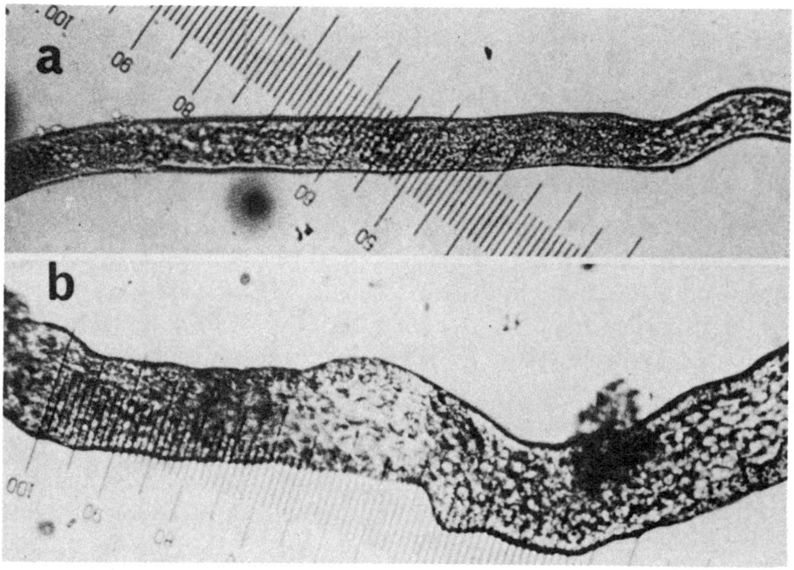

Fig. 14–7. Nonperfused proximal straight tubules from a normal rabbit (top) and from a rabbit that had undergone 1 and ¾ nephrectomy 3 months previously (bottom). A significant increase in tubular diameter due to an increase in the volume of tubular cells is seen. (From Fine LG, Trizna W, Bourgoignie JJ, et al: Functional profile of the isolated uremic nephron. Role of compensatory hypertrophy in the control of fluid reabsorption by the proximal straight tubule. J Clin Invest 61:1508, 1978. By permission of the American Society for Clinical Investigation.)

altering total renal mass. Under these circumstances, no increase in renal mass was observed in the contralateral kidney, even after 4 days.[98] Parabiotic experiments in rats have shown that cross-circulation from rats with bilateral ureteral ligation does not lead to compensatory hypertrophy, whereas a similar procedure using uninephrectomized rats does lead to an increase in size.[99] These observations would suggest that it is loss of mass rather than loss of function that is the primary stimulus for hypertrophy. The issue, however, is far from being resolved, since other experiments have shown an increase in size and in RNA:DNA ratio after unilateral ureteral ligation and unilateral ureterocaval anastomosis.[100,101] It is of interest that, if vascular parabiosis between a uninephrectomized rat and a normal rat is attempted within 48 hours, the renal hypertrophy is reversed. The hypertrophy can be restimulated in the same animal by subsequent nephrectomy.[102]

Conditioning Factors

Several factors are known to influence the ability of surviving renal tissue to hypertrophy in response to the loss of kidney mass. The most important of these factors is age.[74] Both in human beings and in experimental animals, compensatory growth is greatest in the young, with both hyperplasia and hypertrophy contributing to growth. With advancing age, hyperplasia becomes less and less prominent and ultimately ceases entirely. Compensatory hypertrophy thus becomes progressively more limited. Starvation and water deprivation retard compensatory growth, whereas a high-protein diet appears to increase the degree of compensatory growth after uninephrectomy.[103-105] Numerous hormones have been implicated in the process of compensatory hypertrophy. Hypothyroidism impairs the compensatory hypertrophy response.[106-108] When growth hormone is removed by hypophysectomizing animals subjected to experimental reduction of renal mass, profound inhibition of hypertrophy occurs. However, there may well be additional undefined pituitary growth factors that have not been excluded by these studies.

A pituitary factor that specifically enhances the rate of growth of renal cells has recently been partially purified.[113] This renotropic factor is different from other known pituitary tropic hormones, but its precise chemical structure has not yet been determined. The occurrence of compensatory renal hypertrophy in mice with congenital deficiency of growth hormone, thyrotropin, and prolactin, suggests that none of these known pituitary hormones is required for the process.[114] On the other hand, adrenocorticotropic hormone (ACTH) administration for 1 week has been found to enhance significantly the rate of compensatory hypertrophy, even in hypothyroid animals.[111] This effect may be mediated by an increase in plasma testosterone levels. Androgens lead to both an increase in the size and in the amino acid incorporation of the kidney undergoing hypertrophy. However, exogenous testerone administration has been shown to enhance renal hypertrophy only in female rats.[115]

Humoral Regulation of Renal Hypertrophy

A large body of experimental evidence has been accumulated that suggests the existence of circulating humoral factors that induce renal hypertrophy.[116] In 1958, Braun-Menendez[117] was the first to propose the existence of such a humoral regulator, which he called renotropin. Since then, numerous parabiotic experiments have been performed, unfortunately, with inconsistent results. The results of these studies have recently been summarized.[116] In vivo infusions of sera from uni- or bilaterally nephrectomized animals have been employed in an attempt to demonstrate the existence of a humoral factor that stimulates hypertrophy, but these experiments have not provided consistent results. While various explanations for negative results can always be found, such negative experiments, if sufficiently varied in nature, should be carefully considered before the existence of a renotropin is accepted.[118-121]

In vitro assays have also provided some evidence for the existence of renotropin. These studies include a variety of experiments using either plasma, serum or dialyzed serum obtained from either uninephrectomized rats or hamsters. Evidence of renotropin activity was provided by measurements of mitotic index and radioactive labeling of DNA. The studies of Preuss and Goldin[122] have consistently shown that plasma from uninephrectomized rats augments incorporation of ^{3}H-thymidine into DNA and ^{14}C-uridine into RNA and that this effect is specific for the renal cortex. This organ specificity may relate to the existence of an activator in the kidney itself. Dicker and Morris[123] found that plasma from uninephrectomized rats promoted an increase in renal cortical dry weight and protein content. Most studies have shown that renotropic activity is maximal at about 24 hours postnephrectomy. Urine reinfusion studies have also demonstrated the existence of a factor that stimulates renal growth and that is not dialyzable. When half the urine volume of rats was reinfused continuously over 7 days (effectively halving the excretory function of the kidneys, while maintaining renal mass intact), significant bilateral hypertrophy was noted.[124] The recent isolation and partial purification of a pituitary factor that enhances kidney growth[113] has been alluded to above.

CONTROL OF GROWTH OF KIDNEY EPITHELIAL CELLS IN CULTURE

Important insights into the control of kidney cell growth have recently been provided by studies of kidney cell growth in vitro. The ease with which the constituents of the culture medium can be manipulated makes this an ideal system for determining the roles of specific growth factors. This area has been well summarized by Holley.[125] The list of potential growth-controlling factors includes such varied compounds as polypeptide growth factors, corticosteroids, prostaglandins, cholera toxin, cyclic nucleotides, lithium ions, vasopressin, common nutrients, proteolytic enzymes, lectins and phorbol esters. Thus, the mechanisms controlling cell growth are very complex indeed.

THE PRIMARY EVENT IN COMPENSATORY HYPERTROPHY: A REEVALUATION OF THE WORK HYPOTHESIS

The work hypothesis as an explanation for renal hypertrophy holds that the increase in renal size is secondary to an increase in renal work. Thus, it was thought that the hypertrophy induced by a high-protein diet was caused by an increased generation of urea and the need to excrete more urea. It is now quite clear, however, that increased excretion of urea does not constitute a tubular work load since it is excreted largely by glomerular filtration. Attention has also been focused on a possible role of increased tubular reabsorption of sodium as the primary stimulus to hypertrophy. This has largely depended on the observation that the filtered load of sodium per nephron is increased in the subtotally nephrectomized animal and that reclamation of this increased load is accomplished by an increase in tubular reabsorption. Since feeding with a high-salt diet does not lead to hypertrophy per se, it has been argued that hypertrophy cannot be due to excess work.[126] It should be appreciated, however, that the increase in sodium excretion (which accompanies ingestion of a high-salt diet) actually reflects a decrease in tubular reabsorption (as long as the filtered load remains constant), since it is reabsorption rather than excretion that reflects tubular work. (A high-salt diet could result in an increase in tubular sodium reabsorption only if it led to an increase in glomerular filtration rate secondary to volume expansion.) An important argument against the work hypothesis is provided by studies using diversion of ureteral urine back into the extracellular fluid (ureteroperitoneostomy). This maneuver increases single-nephron glomerular filtration rate and tubular reabsorption of sodium, but does not lead to hypertrophy of the kidneys.[98] Another situation in which Tubular reabsorption of sodium and hypertrophy are dissociated is in an animal maintained on a low-potassium diet. Here, renal hypertrophy can occur in the absence of an increase in TR_{Na}.[127] In contrast to these important dissociations, we have observed that proximal tubular hypertrophy is associated with an increase in tubular reabsorption of sodium in a model of renal failure with an increased single-nephron glomerular filtration rate, but that no such hypertrophy is associated with a model of experimental glomerular disease, in which tubular reabsorption is decreased in parallel with a fall in single-nephron glomerular filtration rate.[128] Thus, although the work hypothesis has fallen from favor, it may require reevaluation in light of improved methods for measuring growth and transport function in the same nephron segment. The known difficulties of measuring TR_{Na} with any accuracy in vivo makes the interpretation of whole animal studies particularly difficult.

ADAPTATIONS IN HOMEOSTASIS FOR SPECIFIC SOLUTES IN RENAL FAILURE

Sodium Homeostasis in Chronic Renal Failure

VOLUME AND COMPOSITION OF BODY FLUID SPACES IN RENAL FAILURE

Extracellular Fluid Space

It has commonly been assumed that the adaptations that occur in the surviving nephrons of diseased kidneys serve to maintain the constant composition of the extracellular fluid compartment until renal function approaches 10 to 15 percent of normal. From a clinical standpoint, this is a reasonable generalization since, in the absence of overt congestive heart failure or severe hypoalbuminemia, total body sodium content does not appear to be altered. More careful measurements, however, indicate that body fluid spaces may indeed be altered in uremia. An important problem that relates to all measurements of body composition in uremia is that lean body mass tends to be decreased.[129] Since body water is distributed within this mass and not within body fat, the nutritional status of the patient is of critical importance if fluid spaces are expressed per unit of body weight. A loss of body fat would increase body water in relationship to body weight and such an increase would not be reflective of a true increase in total body water. These problems of interpretation have recently been summarized by Mitch and Wilcox,[130] who concluded that total body water may be increased in patients with chronic renal failure if nutrition is poor, but returns to normal if nutritional defects are corrected.

Measurements of extracellular fluid volume are notoriously vulnerable to the shortcomings of the methods of measurement. The most important flaw in these methods is that the injected tracers (e.g., bromide, sulfate, and thiocyanate) are probably not exclusively confined to the extracellular space, so that movement of the tracer out of the extracellular space may be altered by uremia. An example is the possibility of increased movement of bromide into cells and its increased loss in gastrointestinal secretions in chronic renal failure.[131] Despite these reservations, inulin, bromide, and sulfate spaces are increased in a significant number of chronically uremic patients.[130] Total body sodium and exchangeable sodium is also increased, but the extent to which this is contributed to by a rise in intracellular sodium is unclear. Direct measurements of blood and plasma volumes using dye dilution (Evans blue), radioiodinated serum albumin, and ^{51}Cr-labeled red cells, indicate that these vol-

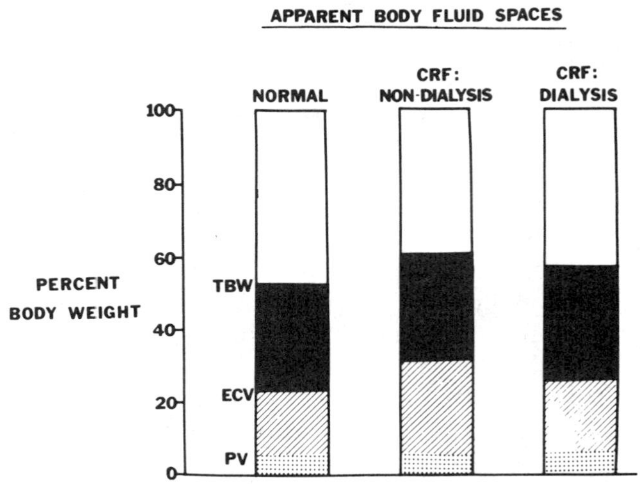

Fig. 14–8. Distribution of body water as a percentage of body weight in normal subjects and in patients with chronic renal failure not receiving dialysis and in those receiving dialysis. Mean values for total body water (TBW), extracellular fluid volume (ECFV), and plasma volume (PV) are shown. The increased fraction of body weight is represented by water in patients with chronic renal failure. Of those patients not on dialysis, intracellular fluid volume (dark shaded area) remains normal, yet there is an increase in ECFV due to an increase in PV and interstitial fluid volume (cross-hatched area). These apparent abnormalities are diminished in patients receiving regular dialysis. (From Mitch WE, Wilcox CS: Disorders of body fluids, sodium and potassium in chronic renal failure. Am J Med 72:536, 1982.)

umes are also increased in uremia. Thus, as indicated in Figure 14–8, there is an increase in extracellular fluid volume because of an increase in plasma volume and interstitial volume, while intracellular volume remains normal. However, a caveat is appropriate, since it should be noted that there is great variability in the results obtained by different workers, and in many instances extracellular fluid volume may be normal.

Intracellular Fluid Space

Although the volume of the intracellular space in uremic patients (as derived from the difference between total body water and extracellular fluid volume) is the same as in normal subjects, the ionic composition of this compartment appears to be deranged, particularly in patients with advanced renal failure. The first observations in this direction were made by Welt and co-workers[132–134] who demonstrated that the potassium content of erythrocytes of certain uremic patients was increased while the sodium content was decreased. This was shown to be due to a decrease in ouabain-sensitive Na–K-ATPase activity and could be reduced in normal erythrocytes by uremic plasma. Subsequent studies extended these findings to leukocytes and muscle, suggesting the existence of a humoral inhibitor of the Na–K pump with widespread effects.[135–138] In the skeletal muscle of uremic patients, this is reflected by a fall in transmembrane potential difference (E_m), but only if creatinine clearance is reduced below 6 ml/min. After approximately 2 months of hemodialysis, both the E_m and the intracellular electrolyte derangements can be reversed.[138]

RENAL TUBULAR HANDLING OF SODIUM IN UREMIA

Observations in Human Subjects

The fact that the total extracellular fluid volume remains normal, or slightly increased, and serum sodium concentration is maintained within normal limits well into the course of chronic renal failure (i.e., until the glomerular filtration rate approaches 7 to 10 ml/min) attests to the existence of an effective adaptation of the excretory function of the diseased kidney. A progressive and predictable increase in the fractional excretion of sodium accompanies the fall in glomerular filtration rate so that sodium balance is maintained[139-141] (Fig. 14–9). This statement applies, however, to a more restricted range of salt intake in uremic patients than it does in normal subjects leading to the concept of a "floor" and "ceiling" for salt intake. In essence, balance for sodium can be maintained as long as salt intake is neither too low nor too high. If intake is restricted or exaggerated, volume depletion or overload may ensue. The acceptable range of intake varies from patient to patient.[4]

Despite the long-recognized fact that uremic patients are subject to an "obligatory" sodium loss of 20 to 30 mEq/day leading to negative sodium balance if intake is abruptly reduced,[142] this salt-losing tendency has been shown by Danovitch et al. to be adaptive in nature, in that slow weaning from salt over a period of weeks to months can lead to the maintenance of balance on sodium intakes as low as 5 mEq/day[143] (Fig. 14–10). While this gradual reduction of intake has limited clinical application, it does demonstrate that the observed inability of uremic patients to lower their urinary sodium concentrations to very low levels is not a function of the disease process per se, but rather a characteristic imposed upon them by the requirement to maintain sodium balance.

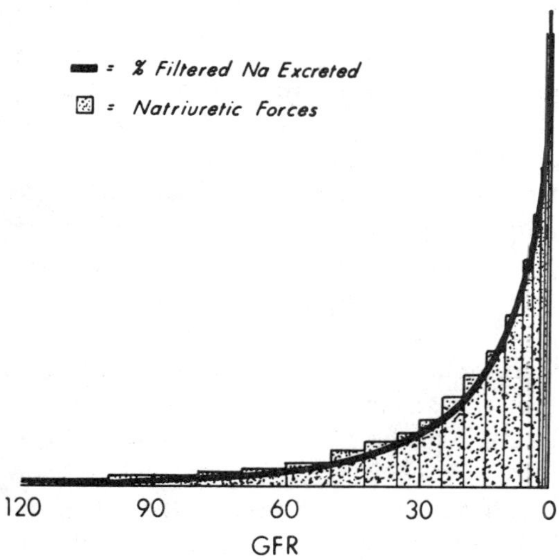

Fig. 14–9. Hyperbolic curve depicting the rise in the percentage of filtered sodium excreted with decreasing glomerular filtration rate (GFR) during the course of chronic progressive renal disease on any given salt intake. Vertical bars depict the theoretical parallel increments in the total natriuretic forces effecting the progressive increase in fractional sodium excretion. (From Bricker NS, Fine LG: p. 799. In Maxwell MH, Kleeman CR (eds): Clinical Disorders of Fluid and Electrolyte Metabolism. McGraw-Hill, New York, 1980. © 1980, McGraw-Hill. Used with the permission of the McGraw-Hill Book Company.)

In uremic man, fractional excretion of sodium ranges from 1 to 25 percent and varies with sodium intake.[140] Furthermore, acute volume expansion leads to an exaggerated natriuresis compared with normal persons. This progressive increase in excretory function per functioning nephron has been referred to as the magnification phenomenon.[144] When a normal person increases salt intake from 3.5 to 7 g/day, FE_{Na} increases by only 0.25 percent to restore balance. In a patient with a glomerular filtration rate of 2 ml/min, a comparable dietary increase requires a change in FE_{Na} that is 60 times greater, that is, FE_{Na} increases from approximately 15 percent to 20 percent. Since serum sodium concentration and extracellular fluid volume do not change perceptibly with these small increments in intake, filtered load of sodium is essentially unaltered, and the changes are all effected by alterations in tubular reabsorption.

Observations in Experimental Animals

Balance studies in animals with experimentally induced chronic renal failure have essentially shown the same adaptations as described above. Animal models have, however, permitted study of the process of adaptation at the

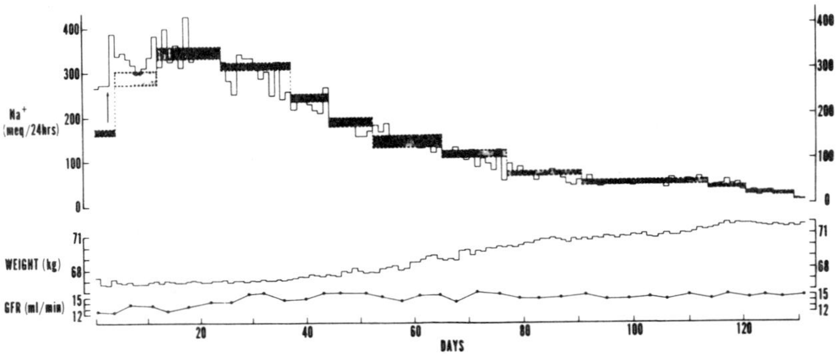

Fig. 14–10. Reduction of sodium intake over a period of 130 days in a patient with polycystic renal disease. Na^+ (mEq/24 hr) refers to daily urinary sodium excretion (solid lines) and daily dietary sodium intake (interrupted lines). The shaded areas represent the range of dietary sodium intake. This patient was able to reduce urinary sodium excretion to 5.4 mEq/day. (Reprinted by permission of the New England Journal of Medicine, from Danovitch GM, Bourgiognie JJ, Bricker NS: Reversibility of the "salt-losing" tendency of chronic renal failure. N Engl J Med 296:15, 1977.)

level of the individual nephrons.[145–153] Since the observations made in nonglomerular diseases differ from those in the glomerulopathies, these will be treated separately.

NONGLOMERULAR DISEASE. This category includes models of bacterial pyelonephritis, interstitial nephritis, and partial ablation of renal mass (subtotal nephrectomy). This latter model has been of particular value in that the subtotally nephrectomized animal, that is, the remnant kidney model, can be studied first in the presence and then in the absence of a contralateral intact kidney.[145,154–158] In the first instance, the animal is not uremic (azotemic), whereas in the latter instance it is. Since the same surviving nephrons can be examined under both circumstances, the influence of uremia on nephron adaptations can be separated from changes that are inherent in the remnant kidney per se. In these disease models, serum sodium concentration is either normal or decreased. However, since the single-nephron glomerular filtration rate and filtered load of sodium are markedly increased, the absolute reabsorptive rate is increased. Distal delivery of sodium is thus increased as well.

It is of interest that both the single-nephron glomerular filtration rate and the rate of reabsorption of sodium by the proximal tubule are independent of sodium intake (and excretion), suggesting that the main function of the proximal tubule is reclamation of filtrate rather than regulation of excretory rate. The increased rate of reabsorption by the proximal tubule in renal failure is accompanied by an increase in the size of the tubule. This is reflected by an increase in lumen volume, tubule length, and the size of the proximal tubular cells.[98] Since it is of importance to know whether the increased reabsorptive rate is determined by peritubular "physical" factors (i.e., hydrostatic and oncotic pressures in the peritubular capillaries) or by intrinsic alterations in the function of the proximal tubule, studies have been performed on proximal tubules isolated from remnant kidneys and perfused in vitro.[45,128] These tubules demonstrate a "memory" effect in that the increased fluid reabsorptive rate, J_v, per unit length persists in the in vitro situation (Fig. 14–11). This has been demonstrated in the late convoluted and the straight portions of the superficial proximal tubule and is associated with an increase in cellular volume per unit length and in pro-

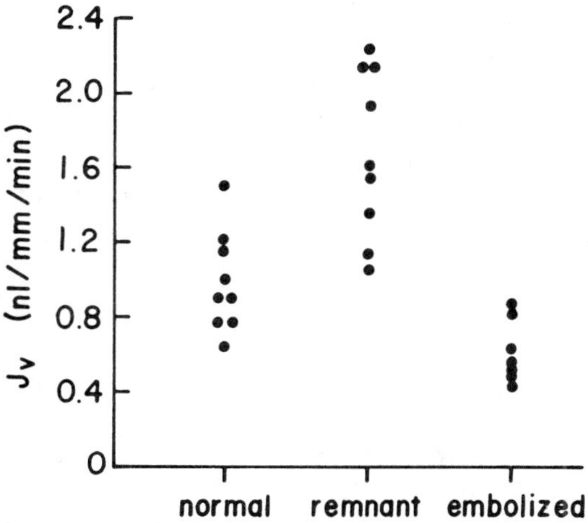

Fig. 14–11. Fluid reabsorption J_v of proximal convoluted tubules from remnant kidneys and embolized kidneys perfused in vitro. The remnant kidneys have elevated single-nephron glomerular filtration rate (SNGFR), while the kidneys in which glomeruli were embolized with microspheres have a decreased GFR. The rate of fluid reabsorption in vitro parallels the in vivo SNGFR. (From Trizna W, Yanagawa N, Bar-Khayim Y, et al: Functional profile of the isolated uremic nephron. Evidence of proximal tubular "memory" in experimental renal disease. J Clin Invest 68:760, 1981. By permission of the American Society for Clinical Investigation.)

tein content per unit length. On the other hand, in a disease in which single-nephron glomerular filtration rate is uniformly decreased by embolizing the glomeruli with microspheres, J_v is decreased, while tubule size remains unchanged.[128] This parallelism between single-nephron glomerular filtration rate and proximal tubular reabsorption suggests an important link between these processes and one that is programmed into the function of the proximal tubular cells. This same glomerulotubular balance has been observed in vivo in pyelonephritic kidneys.[159]

Distal nephron function has been less extensively studied, as has the pattern of function of the juxtamedullary nephrons. Distal tubular reabsorption of sodium is increased in the remnant kidney[158] and is also accompanied by an increase in the size of the nephron. While quantitatively slightly different, the adaptations described above apply equally to the deeper nephrons.[35] A problem inherent in determining reabsorptive rates in uremic nephrons is the fact that almost all nephron segments show flow dependence, that is, transport rates increase in parallel with delivery rates to the segment. Whenever single-nephron glomerular filtration rate is increased, the rate of delivery into each segment is increased. In the remnant kidney, the relationship between sodium reabsorption and sodium delivery appears to be the same as normal. On the other hand, in the terminal collecting tubule, but the absolute reabsorptive rate for water is increased when related to delivery, it is only 30 percent of the normal rate in absolute terms.[35] No sodium reabsorption occurs in this segment in the remnant kidney, whereas 40 percent of the delivered load is reabsorbed under normal circumstances. It is not possible from such studies to determine whether reabsorption is actually decreased or whether admixture of fluid from superficial and deep nephrons contributes to this apparent inhibition of sodium reabsorption. Under conditions of volume expansion in normal rats, differences in superficial and juxtamedullary handling of sodium have been described, and it is possible that the same applies to the remnant kidney.

GLOMERULAR DISEASE. Overall renal handling of sodium in animals with chronic glomerulonephritis is similar to that described in nonglomerular disease, that is, fractional sodium excretion is increased. At the level of the individual nephron, the situation is vastly different. In all forms of chronic experimental glomerular disease, there is a wide dispersion of single-nephron glomerular filtration rate values among various nephrons within the same kidney. Since fluid and solute delivery rates differ from nephron to nephron, a number of investigators have examined whether fractional reabsorption in the proximal tubule is the same in all nephrons. Allison et al.[52] found uniformity of glomerulotubular balance in nephrons of kidneys with both autologous immune-complex nephritis (AICN) and nephrotoxic serum nephritis. Similar findings were described by Ichikawa et al.[58] for both disorders. These workers were able to delineate the factors that determine glomerular ultrafiltration and those which determine peritubular capillary uptake of fluid. They suggest that the close coupling between single-nephron glomerular filtration rate and proximal reabsorption in individual nephrons is due to the functional response of the glomeruli to heterogeneous injury. In those glomeruli with the greatest fall in single-nephron glomerular filtration rate, single-nephron plasma flow and the ultrafiltration coefficient were also depressed, resulting in a lowering of peritubular reabsorption and the maintenance of a uniform pattern of glomerulo-tubular balance. A reverse situation applies to glomeruli with higher single-nephron glomerular filtration rate values. While these studies highlight the role of peritubular factors, other important factors (alluded to above) should not be overlooked. These factors include the memory effect in altering the intrinsic reabsorptive rate of the tubule and the flow dependence of proximal tubular reabsorption. This latter phenomenon is possibly dependent on the concentrations of substances cotransported with sodium in the proximal tubule, for example, glucose, amino acids, and organic ions. At higher flow rates, the concentrations of these substances are maintained at higher levels within the luminal fluid, thereby enhancing gradient-dependent uptake across the luminal membrane, coupled to sodium. The net effect would be an increase in the reabsorption of Na^+ and water along the length of the tubule. The physical effects of tubular distention and altered diffusion barriers cannot be excluded as contributing factors.

MEDIATORS OF SODIUM EXCRETION IN UREMIA. It is probable that the regulators of tubular sodium reabsorption in uremia are the same as those operating in health. Despite a large body of experimental work in this area, there is relatively little definitive information on the nature of the key elements in this system. In health the principal mediators of sodium excretion are (1) aldosterone, (2) "physical" factors or intrarenal hemodynamic alterations, (3) redistribution of filtration between different nephron subpopulations, and (4) other humoral natriuretic or autinatriuretic substances, including natriuretic factor, prostaglandins, catecholamines, bradykinin, and dopamine.

Aldosterone probably plays a role in altering the capacity of nephrons to reabsorb sodium in uremia[160-163] but does not seem to be a critical regulator of sodium balance. Sodium homeostasis is maintained in adrenalectomized uremic animals receiving a fixed maintenance dose of a mineralocorticoid. Supramaximal doses of aldosterone given to animals with intact adrenal glands also maintaines sodium balance.[145] The role of aldosterone appears to be more important in the maintenance of potassium homeostasis.

Adaptations in glomerular filtration rate and redistribution between nephron subpopulations appears to have no influence on the ability of an experimental animal to maintain sodium balance. Neither experimental increments nor decrements perturb sodium balance[145]; the fact that a wide range of single-nephron glomerular filtration rates exists in the same glomerulonephritic kidney despite the maintenance of perfect sodium balance suggests that other influences are at play.

Of the various humoral factors controlling sodium excretion in uremia, much attention has been directed to a humoral inhibitor of sodium transport, termed the natriuretic factor.[164-173] The precise nature of this substance(s) remains to be elucidated.

Urinary prostaglandin excretion is elevated in uremia, but it appears that the prostaglandins may have a more important role in modulating blood flow and glomerular filtration than in regulating sodium balance in experimental uremia.[174] The roles of other vasoactive agents have not been systematically evaluated in uremia.

Potassium Homeostasis in Chronic Renal Failure

OBSERVATIONS IN EXPERIMENTAL ANIMALS. Fractional excretion of potassium is increased dramatically in animals with chronic renal failure and may exceed 100 percent of the filtered load. Since close to 90 percent of filtered potassium is reabsorbed in nephron segments proximal to the distal and collecting tubules in rats with remnant kidneys, secretion by the latter nephron segments must be the source of urinary potassium.

The rapidity with which an animal with a reduced nephron population can increase renal potassium excretion per nephron is remarkable. Within 24 hours of removal of the contralateral kidney in a dog with one intact and one partially nephrectomized (remnant) kidney, the remnant kidney increases potassium excretion fourfold.[175] This excretion, however, is accompanied by an increase in serum potassium concentration. In light of the close correlation observed between serum potassium and renal potassium excretion,[26] and considering the fact that changes in potassium concentration of the perfusate can alter fractional potassium excretion by the isolated perfused kidney,[28] it is probable that this early adaptation is related to moderate hyperkalemia. After 7 days, however, when serum potassium has returned to its normal level, FE_K reaches levels of 150 percent. Since neither adrenalectomy plus DOCA nor the administration of large doses of 9α-fluorohydrocortisone attenuated this response, the adaptation appears to be governed by a mineralocorticoid-independent mechanism.[175] It is not clear whether some mineralocorticoid is required in a permissive role or whether glucocorticoids such as dexamethasone are more effective in this regard. A similar pattern of potassium adaptation has been observed in the subtotally nephrectomized rat.[176] The nephron site for this adaptation appears to be at a point beyond the superficial distal convoluted tubule, that is, in the collecting tubule. In vivo micropuncture studies have shown that whereas 45 percent of filtered potassium entered the surface collecting tubules in both normal and uremic rats, the FE_K was 7 percent and 60 percent, respectively, in the two groups, indicating an adaptation at a distal nephron site.[176] Analogous to the situation for sodium excretion, it is possible that an altered deep nephron contribution to final urinary potassium excretion underlies this difference, but data from normal rats suggest that this is not the case. It appears, therefore, that augmented potassium secretion by the collecting tubule is responsible for the adaptation.

Fine et al.[177] studied isolated cortical collecting tubules obtained from rabbits with remnant kidneys. On a normal potassium diet, potassium secretion per millimeter of tubule was twice as great as that observed in normal cortical collecting tubules. This could be augmented even further (up to six times normal) by doubling dietary potassium intake and could be reduced to normal levels by restricting dietary potassium in proportion to the reduction in nephron mass (Fig. 14–12). These findings are indicative of a true adaptation in that they parallel the requirements to maintain potassium balance. The cellular mechanisms underlying these changes are not clear. Neither hypertrophy, serum aldosterone levels, nor transtubular potential difference could account for the adaptation.[177] The Na–K-ATPase specific activity in outer medullary and cortical microsomes increases in the remnant kidney.[178] These changes also occur in adrenalectomized animals. When dietary potassium was reduced, the increase in Na–K-ATPase specific activity was obviated. It is likely that these changes are paralleled by the increase in the basolateral membrane sur-

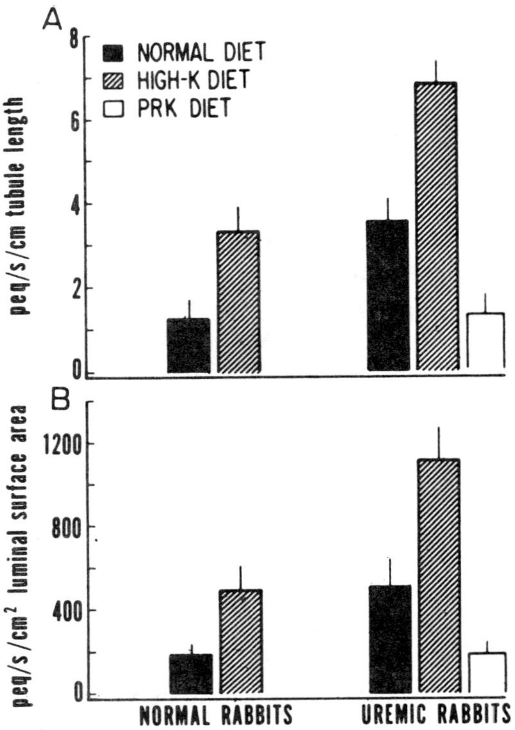

Fig. 14–12. Net potassium secretion, J_K, by isolated perfused cortical collecting tubules of normal and uremic rabbits maintained on normal, high, and proportional reduced PRK (i.e., in proportion to the reduction in GFR) potassium diets. (Top) Secretion per unit length of tubule. (Bottom) Data expressed per unit luminal surface area. In both normal and uremic rabbits, high-potassium diets induce an increased rate of transport. The true adaptive nature of the large increase in the uremic tubules is shown by the return to normal values when dietary potassium was restricted. (From Fine LG, Yanagawa N, Schultze RG, et al: Functional profile of the isolated uremic nephron. Potassium adaptation in the rabbit collecting tubule. J Clin Invest 64:1033, 1979. By permission of the American Society for Clinical Investigation.)

face area, which has been observed when dietary potassium intake is increased in normal animals.[179,180] Under all circumstances in which whole-kidney or single-tubule Na–K-ATPase activity has been shown to increase, the magnitude of the potassium loading has been considerable. It is possible that the changes represent epiphenomena, which are not necessarily related to changes in potassium transport. Indeed, when dietary potassium was increased modestly, the increment in Na–K-ATPase in the cortical collecting tubules was not observed.[177]

In uremia, it is not only the kidney, but also the colon that contributes to potassium excretion. Potassium loading in normal rats or induction of chronic renal insufficiency increases Na–K-ATPase activity and potassium secretion by the colon.[181] Extrarenal disposal of potassium in uremia does not appear to be specifically regulated by insulin or glucagon, but these hormones undoubtedly do contribute to cellular uptake of potassium as they do in normals.

Although chronic regulation of potassium excretion is maintained, the disposal of acute potassium loads in uremic animals is less adequate and may be associated with hyperkalemia, which is more severe and more prolonged than is observed in normal animals receiving the same potassium load.[29] Since potassium uptake under normal circumstances is in the form of a series of acute dietary loads, it is possible that the extent and prolongation of the hyperkalemia are directly responsible for the ability of the diseased kidney to maintain potassium balance when viewed over a prolonged period.

OBSERVATIONS IN PATIENTS. It is reasonable to assume that the mechanisms of the adaptation described herein are applicable to patients with renal failure. Serum potassium concentration is maintained within normal limits until the glomerular filtration rate approaches 10 percent of normal, so that hyperkalemia becomes a problem only when renal failure is far advanced. Comparable to the situation described for sodium homeostasis, the flexibility of potassium excretion is probably more restricted than in normal subjects. This is reflected by the commonly observed advent of hyperkalemia in patients on spironolactone, or in patients who develop constipation secondary to oral phosphate-binding compounds. A similarly increased tendency to develop hyperkalemia occurs under conditions of acute illness with hypercatabolism and metabolic acidosis, administration of beta-blocking agents which may decrease cellular uptake of potassium, and depolarizing muscle relaxants such as succinyl choline.

There are a number of specific conditions in which hyperkalemia occurs out of proportion to the reduction of glomerular filtration rate. Patients with mild renal failure due to sickle cell disease and systemic lupus erythematosus have been reported to develop hyperkalemia of early onset. Similarly, patients with hyperchloremic acidosis, normal urine pH, and hypoaldosteronism often present with hyperkalemia.[182] Most such patients are diabetics with renal function in the range of 30 to 50 percent of normal. Recently, the syndrome of hyperkalemia with distal renal tubular acidosis has been highlighted in patients with obstructive uropathy.[183] These patients are unable to lower urine pH below 5.5 during acidosis, and their baseline FE_K is lower than that seen in patients with other forms of renal disease and comparable loads of glomerular filtration rate.

Renal Concentrating and Diluting Mechanisms in Uremia

A normal person on a standard diet excretes ~450 mOsm of solute/day. A uremic patient must excrete the same amount of solute on a comparable diet. Urine volume in both will equal ~1.5 liters/day or 1 ml/min, with a urinary osmolality of 300 mOsm/kg of water. The difference between normal and uremic persons in terms of tubular resorption of filtered water, however, is quite remarkable. In the normal individual on an average water intake, less than 1 percent of the filtered water will be excreted. In contrast, the uremic patient with a glomerular filtration rate of 2 ml/min drinking the same amount of water must excrete more than 50 percent of the filtered water in order to produce an equal rate of urine flow. In both subjects, water balance may be maintained with precision but, as with the limitations in the excretion of sodium, the range of water excretion becomes increasingly narrowed in the patient with renal disease as glomerular filtration rate falls.

A normal person may excrete 450 mOsm/day of solute in a volume of water varying from ~375 ml to >20 liters. In the uremic patient with a glomerular filtration rate of 2 ml/min, urine volume can be varied only from ~1300 to 1850 ml/day, and urinary osmolality will vary from ~266 to 350 mOsm/kg. The restriction in the lower limits of urinary osmolality occurs despite the fact that free water clearance (CH_2O) per nephron (which reflects diluting ability) is well maintained, even in far-advanced uremia.[184-186] In a normal person the maximal value for the $CH_2O/$:GFR ratio is ~12 ml/100 ml H_2O glomerular filtration rate, and at glomerular filtration rate of 170 l/day, almost 21 liters of free water can be generated. In the uremic patient with a glomerular filtration rate of 2 ml/min (or 2880 ml/day), the same rate of generation of free water per 100 ml glomerular filtration rate will provide only 350 ml/24 hr. Thus the addition of this quantity of water to the 1.5 liter urine required to excrete the solute load in an isomotic solution will have only minimal effects on total urine volume.

A restriction on the upper limit of urinary osmolality occurs despite supramaximal doses of vasopressin and is due to a combination of nephron loss and impaired concentrating ability in the residual nephrons. Solute-free water resorption is ~6 ml/100 ml of glomerular filtration rate in normal subjects. It is much lower, and occasionally even negative, in advanced uremia.[187] However, even if 6 ml/100 ml of glomerular filtration rate of solute free water could be removed from the final urine, a uremic subject with a glomerular filtration rate of 2 ml/min could conserve only 175 ml/day of water from the ~1.5 liters of water required to excrete the daily solute load as an isosmotic solution.

The high rate of urine flow per nephron influences the inability of the diseased kidney to attain high urinary osmolalities, but this cannot be the sole explanation.[188] Thus there is a true concentrating defect in uremia, the mechanism of which has long been an intriguing but poorly understood phenomenon. A number of explanations have been proposed. Anatomic alteration could interfere with the concentrating mechanism[189]; indeed, in some patients with interstitial lesions and cystic diseases of the kidney, a concentrating defect appears to occur early in the course of the disease.[186] The urinary concentrating defect occurs in all forms of chronic glomerular disease, however, and the presence of a concentrating defect does not differentiate between patients with glomerular and those with nonglomerular disease.[190] A cogent argument against the thesis that the medullary anatomic alterations are the major cause of the impaired concentrating ability of the diseased kidney is the fact that maximal urinary concentration is only minimally reduced in the presence of a normal contralateral kidney and in the absence of uremia.[191,192] This same phenomenon has been observed in human subjects with unilateral renal disease.[193]

An increase in blood flow through the medullary circulation in uremia has also been thought to play a role in the concentrating defect by dissipating the interstitial solute concentration gradient required for the normal operation of the countercurrent multiplication system. An additional possibility is that the transport of chloride and sodium by the ascending limbs of the loops of Henle might be impaired or inhibited in advanced uremia. This type of transport defect, however, would not explain why diluting ability, which also depends on sodium chloride transport in the loop, is preserved.

An abnormality in the intrarenal recycling of urea has been demonstrated in the pyelonephritic rat.[194] In normal rats the delivery of urea of the early distal tubule is significantly greater than the amount emerging from the proximal tubule. No such increase, however, was observed in the pyelonephritic animals. Analysis of tissue slices in these animals demonstrated the absence of a corticopapillary concentration gradient both for total solute and for urea. Failure to recycle urea and to sustain a high medullary interstitial solute concentration must, according to current interpretations of the concentrating mechanisms, inevitably lead to a concentrating defect. These results, however, do not exclude the possibility that other factors are operative in the concentrating defect of experimental pyelonephritis in the rat or in spontaneously occurring chronic renal disease in humans.

It appears that there is also an acquired impaired responsiveness of the collecting tubule to vasopressin in the uremic state.[196,197] In this regard, studies on isolated collecting tubules from uremic rabbits have demonstrated a blunted water permeability and adenylate cyclase response to vasopressin stimulation.[96] Impairment of water resorption by the collecting tubule would also lead to a failure of urea to reach maximal concentrations within the lumen of the medullary collecting tubule and could contribute to or explain the defect in the recycling of urea.

Although it is commonly stated that uremic patients produce urine of a fixed osmolality that is isosmotic with plasma, a significant number of patients have urine that is persistently hypotonic. This hypostheuria is vasopressin resistant, but the urine may be diluted even further in response to a water load.

In the uremic patient, the restricted range of water excretion that accompanies advancement of renal disease requires that the range of water intake be restricted as well. Forced fluids and excessive fluid restriction are both inappropriate. Because diurnal variations in urine flow (normally urine flow is less during the night than the day) are altered or reversed in uremia, the hourly rate of urine formation at night may be equal to or greater than that during the waking hours; nocturia is thus a consistent symptom in patients with renal failure. In 4 hours of sleep, with a urine flow rate of 1 ml/min, 240 ml of urine will enter the bladder. The abrupt subsidence of nocturia is therefore an ominous sign in patients with chronic renal failure.

Nitrogen Metabolism in Uremia

UREA

The fact that urea is the main end product of protein metabolism and that this small molecule is eliminated from the body largely by the kidney makes the impact of reduced renal function on nitrogen balance an important one. An increase in protein intake leads to an increase in urea appearance, since the rate of enzymatic synthesis is proportional to substrate concentration. Although some of the synthesized urea is degraded to ammonia and carbon dioxide by intestinal bacteria, this is not considered quantitatively important.

In normal subjects an influx of urea into body water would be excreted rapidly, whereas in renal failure the urea accumulates more readily and elevates the BUN level. Thus, whereas urea excretion rate can be used as an index of urea appearance in normal persons, urea appearance in uremia must take into account changes in the urea pool (i.e., urea accumulation). The value of determining urea appearance is the ability to detect changes in protein intake in a uremic patient and to predict the rise in BUN if protein intake and urea clearance are known. A major problem is obviously the accurate determination of urea nitrogen (UN) accumulation, but a rough estimate would be 60 percent body weight × BUN (mg/dl). The rate of accumulation in grams per day can thus be determined. (The nitrogen excreted as non-urea compounds (e.g., creatinine, uric acid, protein) has been estimated to be ~2.5 g/day and is of little practical importance.)

For a normal person in a steady state, the following obtains:

$$\text{Nitrogen intake/day} = \text{nitrogen excretion/day} = (U_{UN}\ V) + 2.5 \text{ g N/day}$$

Where U_{UN} is the urinary urea nitrogen concentration and V is the urine flow rate. Since

$$\text{Urea clearance} = U_{UN} \cdot V/\text{BUN}$$

$$\text{BUN} = (N_{intake} - 2.5 \text{ g})/\text{urea clearance (liters/day)}$$

or

$$N_{intake}\ (\text{g/day}) = (\text{BUN} \times \text{urea clearance}) + 2.5 \text{ g/day}$$

Mitch has pointed out how a doubling of protein intake from 40 to 80 g/day in a patient with a urea clearance of 6 ml/min would elevate BUN from 45 to 120 mg/dl, assuming no change in the size of the body urea pool.[198] If BUN rises to a greater extent than predicted by the formula, it would imply that the numerator (i.e., the intake) is greater than the value being used in the calculation. This may be due to an increase in dietary intake or to a gastrointestinal bleed with its concomitant acute nitrogen load.

It is now well established that urea per se is not an important source of nitrogen for protein synthesis in patients with renal failure and that there is no significant recycling of urea. Thus, the urea that is retained as a result of the falling glomerular filtration rate accumulates in the body fluids and may be responsible for at least some of the symptoms of uremia. Infusions of urea into stable hemodialysis patients have led to lassitude, fatigue, nausea, vomiting, bleeding, and headache, but not to mental obtundation or asterixis. Urea may also decompose spontaneously to produce cyanate and ammonia, the former being a potential inhibitor of many enzymes via a process of carbamylation. Whether this in fact occurs in the clinical setting is not clear.

CREATININE

Creatinine arises from endogenous synthesis, from amino acids and from preformed dietary creatine. Although it is evident that both dietary creatine and dietary creatinine affect the level of serum creatinine and probably explain the daily fluctuations that occur in creatinine excretion, dietary intake of these substances is quantitatively of little importance. Since muscle contains more than 90 percent of creatinine, the size of the creatinine pool is a measure of total muscle mass.

In chronic renal failure, creatinine appearance (excretion plus accumulation) falls progressively as renal function diminishes. This has been thought to be due to a nonrenal route of elimination, possibly degradation by the gastrointestinal flora. This was confirmed by Mitch and Walser, who found evidence of the recycling of creatinine to creatine and degradation to noncreatinine products.[199] Although this extrarenal clearance amounts to less than 2 percent of total creatinine clearance when renal function is intact, this value may approach 50 percent in patients with severe reductions of glomerular filtration rate.

In the steady state:

$$\text{Creatinine excretion} = \text{production} - \text{catabolism}$$

In patients with chronic renal failure, production of creatinine is the same as in age- and sex-matched normal subjects. Thus production minus catabolism, which equals excretion, can be substituted in the clearance formula:

$$C_{Cr} = (U_{Cr}\ V)/P_{Cr}$$

$$C_{Cr} = (Cr_{production} - Cr_{catabolism})/P_{Cr}$$

Since production and catabolism are regarded as being constant and equal, creatinine clearance will be linearly related to reciprocal of plasma creatinine:

$$C_{Cr} \alpha 1/P_{Cr}$$

The reciprocal of P_{Cr} declines linearly with time as renal disease progresses and is an easy way to predict the time course of renal failure.

URIC ACID

Renal clearance of uric acid falls in chronic renal failure, but fractional excretion (C_{UA}/C_{Cr}) is increased, possibly as an adaptive phenomenon.[10] Despite the reduced rate of excretion, serum uric acid does not reach very high levels in uremia. This is because uric acid production falls as a result of decreased meat intake and because uric acid is degraded by gastrointestinal bacteria.

Divalent Ion Metabolism in Uremia

PHOSPHORUS

A significant amount of information is available on phosphate homeostasis in uremia largely because of the existence of an easily defined modulator of renal phosphorus excretion, that is, parathyroid hormone. In a variety of renal diseases, serum phosphorus concentration remains normal until the glomerular filtrations rate falls to 20 to 30 percent of normal (Fig. 14–13), at which point there is a progressive rise in serum phosphorus concentration as the renal failure progresses.[200] Exaggerated fluctuations in serum phosphorus levels following meals[201] may be an important factor in the pathogenesis of secondary hyperparathyroidism in uremia. Why the rise in serum phosphorus occurs early in the course of renal failure compared with the rise in other ions such as potassium, is not clear.

In advanced renal failure gastrointestinal absorption of phosphorus is diminished[202,203] and it is possible that this serves a protective role. Dietary intake of phosphorus also tends to be lower in uremics who consume 1000 to 1500 mg/day compared with a normal intake of 1500 to 2000 mg/day in the United States.[204] Low-protein diets contain even less phosphorus, and coincident abnormalities in vitamin D metabolism may cause phosphorus absorption to fall significantly.[204] Phosphate retention is thought to be an important pathogenetic factor in the genesis of secondary hyperparathyroidism.[205-210] Bricker and coworkers have argued that renal retention of phosphorus leads to a transient fall in serum-ionized calcium concentration, which in turn

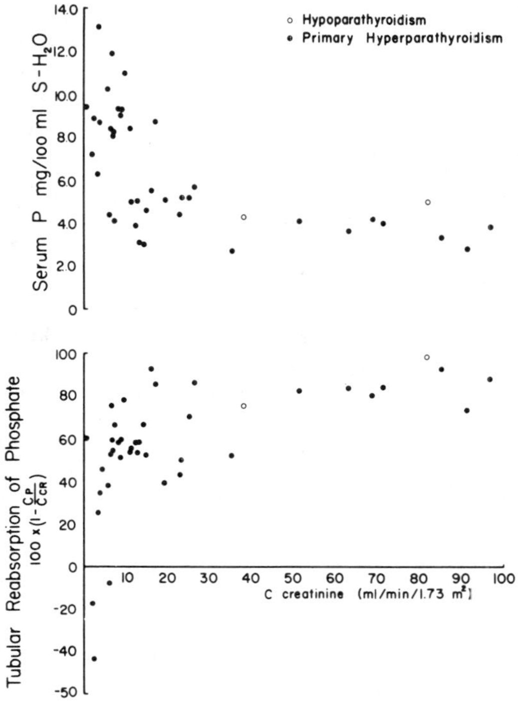

Fig. 14–13. Relationship between the extent of renal failure and serum phosphorus concentration (top) and tubular reabsorption of phosphorus (bottom). No change is observed until glomerular filtration rate (GFR) approaches 20 percent of normal, at which point serum phosphorus concentration rises and tubular reabsorption of phosphorus decreases with advancing renal failure. (From Kleeman CR, Better O, Massry SG, et al: Divalent ion metabolism and osteodystrophy in chronic renal failure. Yale J Biol Med 40:1, 1967.)

acts as the definitive stimulus to increased parathyroid hormone secretion. Elevated parathyroid hormone levels promote an increase in phosphate excretion by the nephrons of the diseased kidney so that serum phosphorus is returned to its original level, but at the expense of a higher circulating level of parathyroid hormone and its attendant bone disease. This forms the basis of the "trade-off hypothesis" which highlights the undesirable effects of certain homeostatic processes in uremia.[4] The hyperparathyroidism can be partially prevented by short-term[208,210] or long-term[211] dietary restriction of phosphorus.

Other factors that play an equally important role in the development of secondary hyperthyroidism are alterations in vitamin D metabolism, skeletal resistance to parathyroid hormone, and altered metabolism of parathyroid hormone. The administration of 25-hydroxycholecalciferol to dogs maintained on a diet reduced in phosphorus content in proportion to the reduction in glomerular filtration rate maintained serum-immunoreactive parathyroid hormone levels within normal limits over a period of 2 years.[211]

The mechanism of the progressive increase in the fractional excretion of phosphorus by the diseased kidney has been the subject of controversy for some time. While it is evident that parathyroid hormone plays an important role,[205-211] there is convincing evidence that other mechanisms, independent of parathyroid hormone, contribute to this phenomenon as well.[214-220] In essence these studies demonstrate under a variety of different experimental circumstances that fractional excretion of phosphorus may be increased even in the absence of parathyroid hormone.

In addition to an intrinsic alteration in tubular handling of phosphate in uremia, there appears to be an altered sensitivity of the renal tubules to parathyroid hormone, at least in terms of its phosphaturic effect. In rats this is increased,[221] while in humans and dogs the response has been shown to be dependent on ambient parathyroid hormone levels. Humans with secondary hyperparathyroidism show a blunted response to parathyroid hormone[214] (Fig. 14–14). Uremic dogs maintained in a euparathyroid state by phosphate restriction show increased parathyroid hormone sensitivity. However, in the hyperparathyroid state, sensitivity to the hormone is normal or decreased.[212,213]

The site of these tubular adaptations is predominantly in the proximal tubule.[222] Filtered load is increased when single-nephron glomerular filtration rate and serum phosphorus are elevated. Although fractional reabsorption by the proximal tubule is decreased, the absolute rate of reabsorption by the hypertrophied

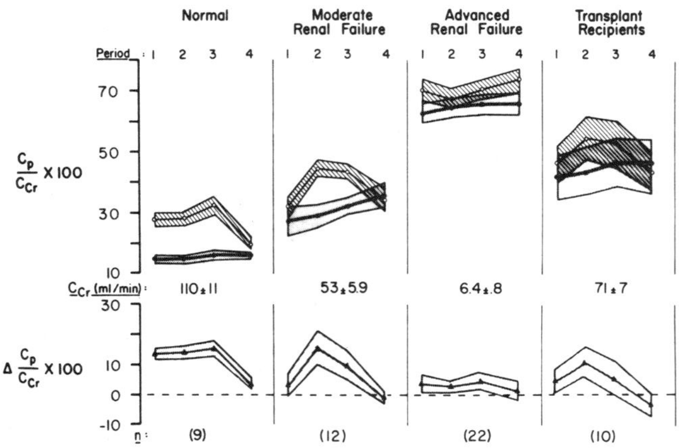

Fig. 14–14. Fractional phosphate excretion ($C_p/C_{Cr} \times 100$) on the control day (solid circles and shaded areas) and on the day of infusion of parathyroid extract (open circles and cross-hatched areas) to normal subjects and patients with varying degrees of renal failure (top). Change in fractional phosphate excretion produced by the infusion of parathyroid extract (bottom). Periods shown are at 4-hour intervals from 8 AM to 8 PM. Period 4 is an overnight period from 8 PM to 8 AM. The endogenous creatinine clearance C_{Cr} of each group is shown. It is evident that the phosphaturic response to exogenous parathyroid hormone is progressively blunted as renal failure progresses and that this is increased toward normal in transplant recipients. (From Massry SE, Coburn JW, Lee DBN, et al: Skeletal resistance to parathyroid hormone in renal failure. Study in 105 human subjects. Ann Intern Med 78:357, 1973.)

proximal tubule of the remnant kidney is actually increased.

Recent studies in the isolated perfused proximal tubule of the rabbit remnant kidney by Yanagawa et al.[223,224] have elucidated the nature of some of the discrepancies generated from in vivo observations (Fig. 14–15). It is apparent that the intrinsic rate of phosphate reabsorption (in the absence of parathyroid hormone) is conditioned by the in vivo parathyroid hormone status and by dietary phosphate intake. On the other hand, tubular sensitivity to parathyroid hormone is decreased in hyperparathyroid animals and increased in euparathyroid animals. An explanation for these differences based on down- or upregulation of parathyroid hormone receptors or receptor accuracy has been proposed.[225] In essence it appears as if the level of dietary phosphorus intake, circulating parathyroid hormone levels, and the degree of hypertrophy of the proximal tubule interact to determine the rate at which the filtered load of phosphorus is reclaimed by the proximal tubule.

A more detailed description of normal and abnormal phosphorus metabolism will be found in Chapter 12.

CALCIUM

Total serum calcium levels are commonly decreased in patients with chronic renal failure, particularly when creatinine clearance falls below 20 ml/min. Although total serum calcium values below 7.5 mg/dl are uncommon,[226] there is a concomitant increase in the complexed fraction of serum calcium due to the retention of a variety of organic anions. If this fraction is significantly elevated, ionized calcium may be subnormal. It is the ionized calcium (measured with an ion-sensitive electrode) that is the most physiologically relevant component of serum calcium. Protein-bound calcium remains within the normal range.

In mild renal failure, fractional excretion of calcium is lower than that seen in normal subjects,[227] the reason for which is unclear. In more advanced renal failure (i.e., creatinine clearance <20 ml/min), fractional excretion is increased and approaches 10 to 20 percent of the filtered load.

Occasionally hypercalcemia is observed that may be due to ingestion of calcium-containing antacids, vitamin D administration, thiazide diuretics, hyperparathyroidism, high-calcium

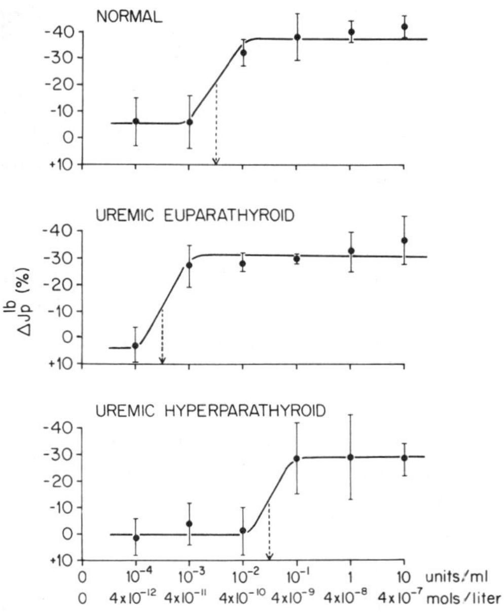

Fig. 14–15. Dose–response curve of phosphate flux $J_p$lb from lumen to peritubular surface of isolated perfused proximal tubules of normal and uremic rabbits. Tubules from euparathyroid uremic animals demonstrate a left shift (i.e., increased sensitivity), versus right shift of hyperparathyroid uremic animals (i.e., decreased sensitivity) in the dose–response curve. (Reprinted with permission from Kidney International. Yanagawa N, Rissenson RA, Edwards B, et al: Functional profile of the isolated uremic nephron. The intrinsic adaptation of phosphate transport in the rabbit proximal tubule. Kidney Int 23:674, 1983.)

dialysate, or hypophosphatemia. In certain cases hypercalcemia may appear from months to years after dialysis has been instituted. This has been ascribed to an increase in skeletal sensitivity to parathyroid hormone in patients with high circulating levels of the hormone. The fact that parathyroid hormone levels are not suppressed by the elevated calcium concentration is attributed to an increase in the mass of parathyroid hormone-secreting tissue rather than to true autonomy of the gland.[228]

See Chapter 15 for a more detailed description of renal osteodystrophy and other abnormalities of calcium metabolism accompaning the uremic state.

MAGNESIUM

Fractional excretion of magnesium increases with the progression of renal failure.[227] Nevertheless, there is a tendency for hypermagnesuria to develop, probably because gastrointestinal absorption of magnesium proceeds normally.[203] Serum magnesium usually rises when glomerular filtration rate falls below 30 ml/min.

A more detailed description of normal and abnormal magnesium metabolism will be found in Chapter 11.

Acid–Base Disturbances in Chronic Renal Failure

PATHOGENESIS OF ACIDOSIS

There is little evidence to suggest that serum pH, [HCO_3], or $PaCO_2$ decreases until glomerular filtration rate drops below 50 percent of control.[228] Thereafter, the pattern of metabolic acidosis that evolves may initially be of either the hyperchloremic or anion-gap variety. Since acid production by metabolism is not increased throughout the course of chronic renal insufficiency,[229] except when complicated by a superimposed catabolic event, such as sepsis, the development of a positive H^+ ion balance must reflect the inability of the kidney to completely dispose of protons.[230] The acidosis remains well-compensated until the glomerular filtration rate drops below 5 to 10 ml/min, that is, rarely does serum [HCO_3^-] drop below 12 to 15 mEq/liter, despite the net addition of protons to the body each day.

It is well established that metabolic acidosis of the hyperchloremic or non-anion gap variety may occur early in the course of chronic renal insufficiency. As renal function deteriorates (GFR <20 ml/min), the more common manifestations of an anion-gap metabolic acidosis become evident. The hyperchloremic or anion-gap form of acidosis has been reported to be more commonly associated with disease processes involving the renal interstitium,[231,232] but it is not clear that this is always the case. The pattern of the acidosis resembles proximal renal tubular acidosis in that patients lose HCO_3^- in the urine when plasma $[HCO_3^-]$ is raised to normal levels, yet maintain their ability to acidify the urine to < pH 5.4 when plasma $[HCO_3^-]$ is permitted to equilibrate of its own accord.[231,232] These patients often manifest an associated hyperkalemia.[233]

In a retrospective study, Widner and coworkers used data from ambulatory patients with graded degrees of uncomplicated renal failure to define the quantitative relationship between serum acid–base and electrolyte composition and the serum creatinine level.[234] Their findings indicate that a pattern of acid–base disturbance evolves in a consistent fashion as renal function deteriorates. With moderate renal insufficiency (serum creatinine 2 to 4 mg/dl), the serum total CO_2 (tCO_2) is reduced from a normal value of 28 to 22 mEq/liter. This fall in tCO_2 occurs uniformly in patients with primary glomerular and tubulointerstitial disease and is entirely offset by an increase in serum chloride concentration, the anion gap remaining within normal limits. As renal insufficiency becomes more severe (serum creatinine 4 to 14 mg/dl), further decrements in the serum tCO_2 occur in proportion to the increment in serum creatinine and are associated with a reciprocal increase in the anion gap, while serum chloride level remains unchanged at its previously elevated level.[234] This study suggests that the serum anion profile changes in a predictable manner throughout the course of chronic renal insufficiency independent of the nature of the underlying nephropathy.

Anion-gap metabolic acidosis is a uniform finding in advanced renal insufficiency (serum creatinine < 4 mg/dl) and is an expression of the inability of the surviving nephrons to excrete the daily acid load.[229] Another finding is retention of sulfuric acid, phosphoric acid, and incompletely oxidized organic acids,[235] which cannot be excreted by the kidney. The anion-gap increment reflects the anions of the accumulated acids. The plasma chloride level is normal or even elevated,[234] while the plasma $[HCO_3^-]$ level decreases. During the early compensatory phase of renal metabolic acidosis, there is a secondary lowering of the $Paco_2$ with a slight decrement in plasma pH. The respiratory response to chronic metabolic acidosis of renal origin is identical to that for other causes of metabolic acidosis at comparable degrees of severity.[236]

The relatively mild and nonprogressive nature of the acidosis is a characteristic feature of renal metabolic acidosis. As a rule, plasma $[HCO_3^-]$ rarely drops below 12 to 18 mEq/liter, and arterial pH is maintained at $\geq$ 7.3, despite the net accumulation in the extracellular fluid of $\leq$ 20 mEq/day of acid.[229] The nonprogressive nature of the acidosis has been attributed to the enormous buffering capacity of a nonextracellular buffer, namely bone.[237] Large calcium carbonate stores exist in the skeleton that provide this buffering capacity. The skeletal carbonate content has been estimated to be ~35,000 mEq,[229] thus contributing 20 mEq/day of HCO_3 to the bicarbonate buffer system. In support of the hypothesis that bone plays a crucial role as a cellular buffer is the observation that negative calcium balance is associated with positive H^+ ion balance.[237] The continued titration of bone carbonate may have a trade-off effect in that H^+ buffering by the skeleton may be attended by bone decalcification,[236,238] an important component of uremic bone disease.

RENAL CONTRIBUTION TO THE GENERATION OF METABOLIC ACIDOSIS

Throughout the course of chronic renal insufficiency it is the rule that urine pH seldom drops below 5.0 to 5.5. The amount of bicarbonate present in the urine at this pH is trivial, so that chronic bicarbonate wasting is an unlikely explanation for the metabolic acidosis. This does not imply that renal bicarbonate handling is intact in chronic renal insufficiency. Since neither acid production nor bicarbonate wasting appears to be a ready explanation for positive proton balance, the key to the pathogenesis of metabolic acidosis resides in the inability of the kidney to dispose of protons in the form of ammonium and/or titratable acids.

Ammonium Excretion

In the animal model of chronic renal insufficiency, the spontaneous rate of ammonium excretion every 24 hours increases by almost 100 percent compared with the control value,[239] despite a diminution in the total number of functioning nephrons. Thus, in response to a decrement in the nephron population, there is an adaptive increase in ammonium production per residual nephron. As the process of nephron destruction progresses, the adaptive increase in ammonium excretion per nephron fails to keep pace with daily body acid production, and ammonium excretion falls progressively. This reduction in ammonium excretion appears to be the most important factor in the pathogenesis of the metabolic acidosis of chronic renal insufficiency.

Factors that influence ammonia production may play an important role in determining the maximal ability of the kidney to excrete ammonium. Welborne and co-workers[240] studied patients with chronic renal insufficiency and demonstrated that the availability of glutamine, the major precursor for NH_3 production, is not a limiting factor. Since glutamine enters the renal tubular cell via both the luminal and antiluminal surface, it is feasible that glutamate entry into the cell may be a limiting factor. In a preliminary study, Windus et al.[241] observed that glutamate transport by brush-border membrane vesicles and basolateral membrane vesicles prepared from renal cortex of dogs rendered uremic were no different from normal values. These workers concluded that an adaptation resulting in changes in uptake of L-glutamine across either the luminal or the antiluminal membrane does not underly the increased ammonia production per nephron seen in chronic renal insufficiency. Of interest are the recent observations of Tizianello et al.,[242] who studied renal metabolism of amino acids and ammonia in subjects with intact renal function and in patients with chronic renal insufficiency. Ammonia production when corrected for glomerular filtration rate was increased fourfold in patients with renal insufficiency, yet glutamine extraction by the kidney was reduced. Their results suggest that in renal insufficiency most of the ammonia produced (approximately 65 percent) must derive from substrates other than glutamine and propose a role for precursors made available by protein and peptide degeneration within the kidney.

Phosphate Excretion

Since phosphate balance is well maintained until renal function drops below 25 to 30 ml/min, urinary phosphate as a component of titratable acid does not decline. Thus, short of severe dietary phosphate restriction, availability of this buffer cannot be incriminated as a likely cause for the evolving metabolic acidosis. With glomerular filtration rate values <10 ml/min, the number of surviving intact nephrons becomes the limiting factor for tubular phosphate availability.[243] It is important to note that under normal circumstances, acid retention consequent to a fall in phosphate excretion will be offset by an increase in ammoniagenesis. Since in advanced renal disease ammonia synthesis is near maximal, any fall in urinary phosphate buffer capacity would be poorly tolerated.

Bicarbonate Reclamation

Evidence for diminished bicarbonate reabsorptive capacity in patients with chronic renal insufficiency was first demonstrated by

Schwartz et al.[231] The serum bicarbonate of acidotic patients in stable renal failure was normalized and allowed to fall spontaneously. In contrast with normal persons, patients with renal disease continued to waste bicarbonate in the urine, despite serum [HCO_3^-] levels < 20 mEq/liter. Only when the serum [HCO_3^-] was restored to its previous level of 10 to 15 mEq/hr did maximal urinary acidification occur. A crucial link between bicarbonate wasting and volume status was elucidated by the studies of Slatopolsky et al.[244] Bicarbonate loading, as described by Schwartz and coworkers,[231] is usually associated with volume expansion, which in turn inhibits proximal tubular sodium reabsorption. Under conditions of minimal volume expansion there is a decrease in bicarbonate reabsorption both per unit glomerular filtration rate and in absolute terms in uremic patients.[245] This response is exaggerated in volume-loaded uremic patients. In summary, the threshold for bicarbonate excretion in the urine may be lowered in uremic patients, and this can be exaggerated by expansion of extracellular fluid volume. There is conflicting evidence on this point, with some workers describing an increase (rather than a decrease) in the threshold for bicarbonate reabsorption.[246]

The role of parathyroid hormone in inhibiting proximal tubular bicarbonate reabsorption is well documented and is probably independent of volume status. Muldowney and associates[247] have documented reduced bicarbonate resorption in states of secondary hyperparathyroidism, including chronic renal insufficiency which improves after parathyroidectomy or when parathyroid hormone secretion is diminished by calcium infusion. Interestingly, in states of primary hyperparathyroidism HCO_3^- wasting and acidosis are not consistent features, so that the role of parathyroid hormone in the acidosis of uremia remains uncertain.

Quantitation of bicarbonate reclamation in uremia dictates that the transport of H^+ ion per residual nephron must be increased. Studies on the nature of the adaptive response performed in an animal model of chronic renal insufficiency have supported this contention. Cohn et al.,[248] using isolated microvillar membrane vesicles prepared from the viable portion of uremic dog kidney, observed a twofold increment in the activity of the Na^+–H^+ antiporter. In a similar study on uremic rabbits, an increase in the maximum rate of Na-H antiport has been demonstrated under conditions in which a pH gradient exists across the membrane.[249]

CONSERVATIVE MANAGEMENT OF CHRONIC RENAL FAILURE

The term "conservative" applies to aspects of the management of patients with renal failure that do not include dialysis or transplantation. Essentially such management implies the substitution of adjusted dietary intake for the increased ability of the kidney to maintain homeostasis. Where the diseased kidney is able to maintain the constancy of the composition of the body fluids by its intrinsic adaptations, no such dietary intervention is required. This fact is often not appreciated. Indiscriminate dietary restrictions serve no purpose and may in fact lead to the adverse effects of solute deprivation (e.g., sodium, phosphate).

The goals of conservative management are (1) to detect and reverse any potentially reversible causes of renal failure, (2) to prevent the advent of alterations in the volume and content of the body fluids or to correct these if they have already developed, and (3) to prevent further loss of renal function where possible.

Factors Causing Reversible Deterioration of Renal Function

Table 14–1 lists the factors that should be considered in this context. Perhaps the most important cause of deterioration of renal func-

Table 14–1. Reversible Causes of Renal Failure

- Prerenal causes
  - Dehydration, volume depletion
  - Edema-forming states with decreased effective arterial blood volume (e.g., cardiac failure, nephrosis, liver failure)
- Intrinsic disorders or renal function
  - Acute glomerular disease (e.g., glomerulonephritis)
  - Alterations in renal blood flow (e.g., nonsteroidal anti-inflammatory agents)
  - Interstitial nephritis and papillary necrosis (e.g., analgesics)
  - Chronic infection (e.g., recurrent pyelonephritis)
  - Chronic electrolyte disturbances (e.g., persistent hypercalcemia or hypokalemia)
- Obstruction to urine flow
  - Uretero–pelvi–calyceal system
  - Bladder

tion (i.e., a rising BUN and serum creatinine concentration) is diuretic-induced volume contraction. Obstruction is often associated with infection, but the latter rarely occurs in the absence of an abnormality in the collecting system. Since intravenous pyelography relies on adequate filtration of the dye molecules to achieve adequate contrast, it is of no value in patients with low levels of glomerular filtration rate. Fortunately, ultrasound (sonography) has proved an effective and valuable method of revealing kidney size, pelvicalyceal or ureteral dilation or the presence of renal cysts or tumors.

Where renal function is adequate for visualization of the kidney by intravenous pyelography, the hazards of contrast media-induced deterioration of renal function should be borne in mind, especially in diabetic patients. Adequate hydration before and during the procedure appears to be protective in this regard.

Nutritional Requirements

Chronically uremic patients tend to demonstrate evidence of wasting, which is often identified only when specific measurements are carried out.[250] Table 14–2 lists the routine parameters that should be documented at regular intervals.

Table 14–2. Parameters for Routine Nutritional Assessment of Patients with Acute or Chronic Renal Failure

- Nutrient intake
  - Intake of total energy, protein, carbohydrate, fat, minerals, vitamins, and water
- Anthropometry
  - Height
  - Weight, percentage relative body weight and weight change as percent of usual weight
  - Triceps and subscapular skinfold thickness (actual measurements and percentages of the standard values)
  - Percent body fat
  - Mid-upper arm muscle circumference (actual measurements and percentages of standard values)
- Biochemical and other laboratory studies
  - Serum total protein, albumin, transferrin (transferrin concentrations may be estimated by [0.8 × total iron binding capacity] − 43)
  - Urea nitrogen appearance (UNA)
  - SUN/serum creatinine ratio (nondialyzed patients)
  - Creatinine height index (nondialyzed patients)
  - Serum sodium, potassium, chloride, bicarbonate
  - Serum calcium, phosphorus, and magnesium
  - Creatinine and urea clearance, daily urine volume
  - Fasting blood glucose, serum triglycerides, cholesterol, and high-density lipoproteins
  - Skin tests
  - Lymphocyte count
  - Radiographic skeletal survey

Reproduced with permission from Kopple JD: Nutritional therapy in kidney failure. Nutr Rev 39:193, 1981.

Protein intake: Although a variety of optimal regimens have been proposed, most require dietary supplements that are not generally available (e.g., ketoanalogues of essential amino acids) and use formulas of little practical value in the day-to-day management of patients. As a general rule, if BUN is maintained at <90 mg/dl, uremic symptoms are minimized. Protein is restricted only when the glomerular filtration rate falls <25 ml/min and initially should be moderate (~1 g/kg·day) to prevent wasting. When the glomerular filtration rate falls to ≤10 ml/min, a diet containing 0.5 to 0.6 g protein/kg·day (of which 50 percent is of high biologic value) should be instituted. Protein losses in the urine should be replaced gram for gram.

When dialysis is instituted, protein intake can be liberalized to ≥1 g/kg·day, especially in patients on chronic peritoneal dialysis in whom protein losses may be significant.

Caloric intake: The decrease in body fat that characterizes most uremic patients suggests that energy intake may often be inadequate. Approximately 35 kcal/kg·day is required. If serum triglycerides are elevated, 35 percent of the calories should be in the form of carbohydrate and 55 percent as fat with a polyunsaturated : saturated ratio of 2.

Vitamins: Pyridoxine, ascorbic acid, and folic acid should be routinely provided. The value of prophylactic use of vitamin D in the form of 1,25-dihydroxycholecalciferol has not been established and is used only when biochemical, radiologic, or biopsy evidence of secondary hyperparathyroidism is obtained. The starting dose is 0.25 to 0.5 μg/day. Because of the rapidity with which hypercalcemia may supervene, serum phosphorus should first be controlled to prevent any danger of metastatic calcification.

Calcium and phosphorus: An intake of 1200 mg of calcium, 1200 mg of phosphorus, and 300 mg of magnesium per day will maintain balance for all these minerals. Aluminum hydroxide is given when serum phosphorus concentration starts to rise.

Sodium and potassium: The only indicators for restriction of sodium are hypertension or an associated edema-forming state. Otherwise, a normal sodium intake can be tolerated until the glomerular filtration rate falls to 10 to 15 percent of normal. Normal dietary variations can be tolerated, but excessive restriction or loading will lead to profound volume depletion or overload because of the restricted flexibility of the sodium control system in uremia. Potassium homeostasis is likewise well preserved, and dietary restriction is warranted only if overt hyperkalemia supervenes.

Acid–Base: The metabolic acidosis of uremia is generally well tolerated. Alkali supplements in the form of calcium carbonate (which acts as a convenient source of calcium) may be instituted when serum bicarbonate concentration falls to <18 mEq/liter. Sodium bicarbonate ingestion may lead to an unacceptable level of sodium intake. Shol's solution (Na citrate–citric acid) provides 1 mEq bicarbonate per milliliter solution. The bicarbonate threshold may be lowered in patients with chronic renal failure, making it difficult to attain normal plasma bicarbonate levels. Arterial blood pH should thus be maintained above 7.35 and serum bicarbonate at ~18 mEq/liter.

Prevention of Progression in Chronic Renal Failure in Humans

A significant body of information is accumulating, largely from studies on animals with experimental uremia, suggesting that the progressive downhill course commonly observed in patients with most forms of chronic renal failure may not be as inevitable as previously thought. Although the literature of 1940–1950 provided reasonably solid evidence that the severity of renal failure in experimental animals could be attenuated by low-protein diets,[251] lack of a sound physiologic basis for such approaches led to gradual abandonment of dietary regulation as an important therapeutic modality in patients.

Two provocative and potentially important avenues of treatment—phosphate restriction and protein restriction—have proved effective in experimental animals with uremia, and in both, reasonably plausible explanations for the therapeutic effects have been provided.

Phosphorus restriction has proved effective in prolonging the survival of rats with remnant kidneys and chronic glomerulonephritis.[252] Deposition of calcium phosphate in the renal interstitium is prevented, and the histologic manifestations of the progressive disease are limited. Although it was supposed that secondary hyperparathyroidism was responsible for the destructive process in the kidney, selective parathyroidectomy was not effective in preventing the progressive renal failure. Patient studies have provided equally promising results, with significant prolongation of renal function being achieved by dietary phosphate restriction,[253] but these results are far from consistent.[254]

Another area that has essentially received renewed attention is the role of dietary protein intake on the progression of renal failure. Brenner and colleagues have provided a convincing scientific basis for the observed protective effect of low-protein diets in different forms of renal disease by showing that hemodynamically mediated renal injury can be abolished or markedly attenuated by dietary protein restriction in certain experimental animals.[256] Early reports suggest a similar protective effect in human renal disease,[256] but controlled studies on large patient populations are still lacking. Thus, while dietary manipulation may indeed prove to be the first consistent method of altering the course of chronic renal failure, it remains to be seen whether the management of human renal disease will benefit from this approach.

REFERENCES

1. Carrie BJ,Golbetz HV, Michaels AS, et al: Creatinine: An inadequate filtration marker in glomerular diseases. Am J Med 69:177, 1980
2. Shannon JA: The renal reabsorption and excretion of urea under conditions of extreme diuresis. Am J Physiol 123:182, 1938
3. Mitch WE, Buffington GA, Lemann J, et al: A simple method of estimating progression of chronic renal failure. Lancet 2:1326, 1976
4. Bricker NS, Fine LG: The renal response to progressive nephron loss. p. 1056. In Brenner BM, Rector FC Jr (eds) The Kidney. WB Saunders, Philadelphia, 1981
5. Berlyne GM: Exchangeable potassium and renal potassium handling in advanced chronic renal failure. Nephron 8:264, 1971
6. Kopple JD, Coburn JW: Metabolic studies of low protein diets in uremics. I. Nitrogen and potassium. Medicine (Baltimore) 52:583, 1973
7. Brochner-Mortensen K: Uric acid in blood and urine in Bright's disease. Acta Med Scand 96:438, 1938
8. Steele TH, Rieselbach RE: The contribution of residual nephrons within the chronically diseased kidney to urate homeostasis in man. Am J Med 43:876, 1967
9. Danovitch GM, Weinberger J, Berlyne GM: Uric acid in advanced renal failure. Clin Sci 43:331, 1972
10. Danovitch GM: Uric acid transport in renal failure, a review. Nephron 9:291, 1972
11. Rieselbach ER, Steele TH: Influence of the kidney upon urate homeostasis in health and disease. Am J Med 56:665, 1974
12. Schoolworth AC, Sandler RS, Hoffman S, et al: Effects of nephron reduction and dietary protein content on renal ammoniagenesis in the rat. Kidney Int 7:397, 1975
13. Elkington JR: Hydrogen ion turnover in health and in renal disease. Ann Intern Med 57:660, 1957
14. Dorhout Mees EJ, Machado M, Slatopolsky E, et al: The functional adaptation of the diseased kidney. III. Ammonium excretion. J Clin Invest 45:289, 1966
15. Simpson DF: Control of hydrogen homeostasis and renal acidosis. Medicine (Baltimore) 50:503, 1971
16. Welbourne T, Weber M, Bank N: The effect of glutamine administration on urinary ammonium excretion in normal subjects and in patients with renal disease. J Clin Invest 51:1852, 1972
17. Goldman R, Bassett S: Phosphorus excretion in renal failure. J Clin Invest 33:1623, 1954
18. Slatopolsky E, Robson AM, Elkan I, et al: Control of phosphate excretion in uremic man. J Clin Invest 47:1865, 1968
19. Massry SG, Friedler RM, Coburn JW: Excretion of phosphate and calcium. Physiology of their renal handling and relation to clinical medicine. Arch Intern Med 131:828, 1973
20. Kleeman CR, Better O, Massry SG, et al: Divalent ion metabolism and osteodystrophy in chronic renal failure. Yale J Biol Med 40:1, 1967
21. Platt R: Sodium and potassium excretion in chronic renal failure. Clin Sci 9:367, 1950
22. Slatopolsky E, Elkan IO, Weerts C, et al: Studies on the characteristics of the control

system governing sodium excretion in uremic man. J Clin Invest 47:521, 1968

23. Bricker NS: Extracellular fluid volume regulation: On the evidence for a biologic control system. P. 19. In M Epstein (ed) The Kidney in Liver Disease. Elsevier, New York, 1978
24. Hayes CP Jr, McLeod MI, Robinson R: An extrarenal mechanism for the maintenance of potassium balance in severe chronic renal failure. Trans Assoc Am Physicians 80:207, 1967
25. Seely JF, Levy M: Control of extracellular fluid volume. P. 371. In Brenner BM, Rector FC Jr (eds): The Kidney. WB Saunders, 1981
26. Young DB: Relationship between plasma potassium concentration and renal potassium excretion. Am J Physiol 242:F599, 1982
27. Giebisch G: Some reflections on the mechanism of renal tubular potassium transport. Yale J Biol Med 48:315, 1975
28. Silva P, Ross BD, Charney AN, et al: Potassium transport by the isolated perfused kidney. J Clin Invest 56:862, 1975
29. Bourgoignie JJ, Kaplan M, Pincus J, et al: Renal handling of potassium in dogs with chronic renal insufficiency. Kidney Int 20:482, 1981
30. Kahn J, Kaji DM, Nicolis G, et al: Factors related to potassium transport in chronic stable renal disease in man. Clin Sci Mol Med 54:661, 1978
31. Schon DA, Silva P, Hayslett JP: Mechanism of potassium excretion in renal insufficiency. Am J Physiol 227:1323, 1974
32. Yanagawa N, Nissenson RA, Edwards B, et al: Functional profile of the isolated uremic nephron. The intrinsic adaptation of phosphate transport in the rabbit proximal tubule. Kidney Int 23:674, 1983
33. Purkerson ML, Rolf DB, Yates J, et al: Factors that influence urinary phosphate excretion in rats with reduced renal mass. Evidence for increased sensitivity to parathyroid hormone. Mineral Electrolyte Metab 4:258, 1980
34. Jamison RL: Micropuncture study of superficial and juxtamedullary nephrons in the rat. Am J Physiol 218:46, 1970
35. Buerkert J, Martin D, Prasad J, et al: Response of deep nephrons and the terminal collecting duct to a reduction in renal mass. Am J Physiol 236:F454, 1979
36. Pennell JP, Bourgoignie JJ: Adaptive changes of juxtamedullary glomerular filtration in the remnant kidney. Pfluegers Arch 389:131, 1981
37. Diezi JP, Michoud A, Grandchamp A, et al: Effects of nephrectomy in renal salt and water transport in the remaining kidney. Kidney Int 10:450, 1976
38. Carriere S, Wong NLM, Dirks JH: Redistribution of renal blood flow in acute and chronic reduction of renal mass. Kidney Int 3:364, 1973
39. Kaufman JM, DiMeola HJ, Siegel NJ, et al: Compensatory adaptations of structure and function following progressive renal ablation. Kidney Int 6:10, 1974
40. Weber H, Lin K, Bricker NS: Effect of sodium intake on single nephron glomerular filtration rate and sodium reabsorption in experimental uremia. Kidney Int 8:14, 1975
41. Wen SF, Wong NLM, Evanson RL, et al: Micropuncture studies of sodium transport in the remnant kidney of the dog. The effect of graded volume expansion. J Clin Invest 52:386, 1973
42. Deen WM, Maddox DA, Robertson CR, et al: Dynamics of glomerular ultrafiltration in the rat. VII. Response to reduced renal mass. Am J Physiol 227:556, 1974
43. Hostetter TH, Olson JL, Rennke HG, et al: Hyperfiltration in remnant nephrons: A potentially adverse response to renal ablation. Am J Physiol 241:F85, 1981
44. Finn WF: Effect of unilateral nephrectomy on glomerular dynamics in Sprague-Dawley rats. Clin Res 28:445A, 1980
45. Fine LG, Trizna W, Bourgoignie JJ, et al: Functional profile of the isolated uremic nephron. Role of compensatory hypertrophy in the control of fluid reabsorption by the proximal straight tubule. J Clin Invest 61:1508, 1978
46. Olivetti G, Anversa P, Rigmonti N, et al: Morphometry of the renal corpuscle during normal postnatal growth and compensatory hypertrophy. J Cell Biol 75:573, 1977
47. Shea SM, Raskova J, Morrison AB: A stereological study of glomerular hypertrophy in the subtotally nephrectomized rat. Am J Pathol 90:201, 1978
48. Knutson DW, Chieu F, Benett CM, et al: Estimation of relative glomerular capillary

surface area in normal and hypertrophic rat kidneys. Kidney Int 14:437, 1978
49. Bank H, Aynedjian HS: Individual function in experimental pyelonephritis. I. Glomerular filtration rate and proximal tubular sodium, potassium and water reabsorption. J Lab Clin Med 68:713, 1966
50. Lubowitz H, Purkerson ML, Sugita M, et al: GFR per nephron and per kidney in chronically diseased (pyelonephritic) kidney of the rat. Am J Physiol 217:853, 1969
51. Rocha A, Marcondes M, Malnie G: Micropuncture study in rats with experimental glomerulonephritis. Kidney Int 3:14, 1973
52. Allison MEM, Wilson CB, Gottschalk CW: Pathophysiology of experimental glomerulonephritis in rats. J Clin Invest 53:1402, 1974
53. Lubowitz H, Mazumbar DC, Kawamura J, et al: Experimental glomerulonephritis in the rat: Structural and functional observations. Kidney Int 5:356, 1974
54. Lubowitz H, Mazumdarm DC, Kawamura J, et al: Experimental glomerulonephritis in the rat; structural and functional observations. Kidney Int 5:355, 1974
55. Maddox DA, Bennett CM, Deen WM, et al: Determinants of glomerular filtration in experimental glomerulonephritis in the rat. J Clin Invest 55:305, 1975
56. Blantz RC, Wilson CB: Acute effects of antiglomerular basement membrane antibody on the process of glomerular filtration in the rat. J Clin Invest 58:899, 1976
57. Blantz RC, Tucker BJ, Wilson CB: Acute effects of anti-glomerular basement membrane antibody on the process of glomerular filtration in the rat. Influence of dose and complement depletion. J Clin Invest 61:910, 1978
58. Ichikawa I, Hoyer JR, Seiler MW, et al: Mechanism of glomerulotubular balance in the setting of heterogeneous glomerular injury. Preservation of a dose functional linkage between individual nephrons and surrounding vasculature. J Clin Invest 69:175, 1982
59. Bohrer MP, Baylis C, Robertson CR, et al: Mechanisms of the puromycin-induced defects in the transglomerular passage of water and macromolecules. J Clin Invest 60:152, 1977
60. Bernard DB, Alexander GA, Couser WG, et al: Renal sodium retention during volume expansion in experimental nephrotic syndrome. Kidney Int 14:478, 1978
61. Ichikawa I, Hoyer JR, Seiler MW, et al: The physiological basis of altered GFR with glomerular injury induced by immune complex deposition. Clin Res 27:418A, 1979
62. Ichikawa I, Brenner BM: Local intrarenal vasoconstrictor-vasodilator interactions in mild partial ureteral obstruction. Am J Physiol 236:F131, 1979
63. Baylis C, Brenner BM: Modulation by prostaglandin synthesis inhibitors of the action of exogenous angiotensin II on glomerular ultrafiltration in the rat. Circ Res 43:889, 1978
64. Purkerson ML, Hoffsten PF, Klahr S: Pathogenesis of the glomerulopathy associated with renal infarction in rats. Kidney Int 9:407, 1976
65. Olson JL, Hostetter TH, Rennke HG, et al: Altered charge and size selective properties of the glomerular wall: A response to reduced renal mass. Kidney Int 16:857, 1979
66. Olson JL, Hostetter TH, Rennke HG, et al: Altered glomerular permeability and progressive sclerosis following extreme ablation of renal mass. Kidney Int 22:112, 1982
67. Meyer TW, Hostetter TH, Rennke HG, et al: Preservation of renal structure and function by long-term protein restriction in rats with reduced nephron mass. Abstr Am Soc Nephrol 15:125A, 1982
68. Bradley SE, Bradley GP, Tyson CJ, et al: Renal function in renal diseases. Am J Med 9:766, 1950
69. Earle D, Farber SJ, Alexander JD, et al: Renal function and electrolyte metabolism in acute glomerulonephritis. J Clin Invest 30:421, 1951
70. Baylis C, Brenner BM: The physiologic determinants of glomerular ultrafiltration. Rev Physiol Biochem Pharmacol 80:1, 1978
71. Hostetter TH, Rennke HG, Brenner BM: The case for intrarenal hypertension in the initiation and progression of diabetic and other glomerulonephritis. Am J Med 72:375, 1982
72. Kleinknecht D, Grunfeld JP, Comez PC, et al: Diagnostic procedures and long-term prognosis in bilateral renal cortical necrosis. Kidney Int 4:390, 1973

73. Torres VE, Velosa JA, Holley KE, et al: The progression of vesicoureteral reflux. Ann Intern Med 92:776, 1980
74. Malt RA: Compensatory growth of the kidney. N Engl J Med 280:1446, 1969
75. Halliburton IW, Thomson RY: Chemical aspects of compensatory renal hypertrophy. Cancer Res 25:1882, 1965
76. Johnson HA, Vera Roman JM: Compensatory renal enlargement: Hypertrophy versus hyperplasia. Am J Pathol 49:1, 1966
77. Coe FL, Korty PR: Protein synthesis during compensatory renal hypertrophy. Am J Physiol 213:1585, 1967
78. Fajers CM: On compensatory renal hypertrophy after unilateral nephrectomy. 2. Immediate effect of unilateral nephrectomy as judged by some renal function tests and karyometric studies in hydrated rabbits. Acta Pathol Microbiol Scand 41:34, 1957
79. Malt RA, Lemaitre DA: Accretion and turnover of RNA in renoprival kidney. Am J Physiol 214:1041, 1968
80. Toback FG, Smith PD, Lowenstein LM: Phospholipid metabolism in the initiation of renal compensatory growth after acute reduction of renal mass. J Clin Invest 54:91, 1974
81. Kurnick NB, Lindsay PA: Nucleic acids in compensatory renal hypertrophy. Lab Invest 18:700, 1968
82. Tomashefsky P, Tannenbaum M: Macromolecular metabolism in renal compensatory hypertrophy. I. Protein synthesis. Lab Invest 21:358, 1969
83. Tomashefsky P, Tannenbaum M: Macromolecular metabolism in renal compensatory hypertrophy. II. Protein turnover. Lab Invest 23:190, 1970
84. Toback FG, Lowenstein LM: Thymidine metabolism during normal and compensatory renal growth. Growth 38(1):35, 1974
85. Toback FG, Lowenstein LM: Uridine metabolism during normal and compensatory renal growth. Growth 38(1):17, 1974
86. Melvin WT, Kumar A, Malt RA: Conservation of ribosomal RNA during compensatory renal hypertrophy. A major mechanism in RNA accretion. J Cell Biol 69:548, 1976
87. Ouellette AJ: Messenger RNA in compensatory renal hypertrophy. Yale J Biol Med 51:413, 1978
88. Schlondorff D, Weber H: Cyclic nucleotide metabolism in compensatory renal hypertrophy and neonatal kidney growth. Proc Natl Acad Sci (USA) 73:524, 1976
89. Dicker SE, Greenbaum AL: Changes in renal cyclic nucleotide content as a possible trigger to the initiation of compensatory renal hypertrophy in rats. J Physiol (Lond) 271:505, 1977
90. Arakaki M: On the postnatal growth of the kidney with special reference to the number and size of the glomeruli. Am J Anat 36:399, 1926
91. MacKay EM, MacKay LC, Addis T: The degree of compensatory renal hypertrophy following unilateral nephrectomy. J Exp Med 56:255, 1932
92. Moore R: Number of glomeruli in kidney of adult rat unilaterally nephrectomized in early life. J Exp Med 50:709, 1929
93. Bonvalet JP, Champion M, Wanstok F, et al: Compensatory renal hypertrophy in young rats: Increase in the number of nephrons. Kidney Int 1:391, 1972
94. Kaufman JM, Hardy R, Hayslett JP: Age-dependent characteristics of compensatory renal growth. Kidney Int 8:21, 1975
95. Mandache E, Repciuc E: Microautoradiographic study of cell proliferation in compensatory renal growth. Morphol Embryol 21:71, 1975
96. Fine LG, Schlondorff D, Trizna W, et al: Functional profile of the isolated uremic nephron. Impaired water permeability and adenylate cyclase responsiveness of the cortical collecting tubule to vasopressin. J Clin Invest 61:1519, 1978
97. Hayslett JP, Kashgarian M, Epstein FH: Functional correlates of compensatory hypertrophy. J Clin Invest 47:774, 1968
98. Weinman EJ, Renquist K, Stroup R, et al: Increased tubular reabsorption of sodium in compensatory renal growth. Am J Physiol 224:565, 1973
99. Obertop H, Malt RA: Lost mass and excretion as stimuli to parabiotic compensatory renal hypertrophy. Am J Physiol 232:F405, 1977
100. Dicker SE, Shirley DG: Compensatory hypertrophy of the contralateral kidney after unilateral ureteral ligation. J Physiol (Lond) 220:199, 1972

101. Paulson DF, Fraley EE: Compensatory renal growth after unilateral ureteral obstruction. Kidney Int 4:22, 1973
102. Morris GC: Growth of rats' kidneys after unilateral ureterocaval anastomosis. J Physiol (Lond) 258:755, 1976
103. Konishi F: Renal hyperplasia in young and old rats fed high protein diet following unilateral nephrectomy. J Gerontol 17:151, 1962
104. Reiter RJ: Cellular proliferation and deoxyribonucleic acid synthesis in compensating kidneys of mice and effect of food and water restriction. Lab Invest 14:1636, 1965
105. Halliburton IW: Effect of unilateral nephrectomy and of diet on composition of kidney. P. 101. In Nowinski W, Goss RJ (eds): Compensatory Renal Hypertrophy. Academic Press, New York, 1969
106. Bradley SE, Coelho JB: Glomerular tubular dimensional readjustments during compensatory renal hypertrophy in the hypothyroid rat. Yale J Biol Med 57:327, 1978
107. Bradley SE, Coelho JB, Sealey JE, et al: Changes in glomerulotubular dimensions, single nephron filtration rates and renin–angiotensin system in hypothyroid rats. Life Sci 30:633, 1982
108. Stephan F, Reville P, de Laharpe F, et al: Impairment of renal compensatory hypertrophy by hypothyroidism in the rat. Life Sci 30:623, 1982
109. Astarabadi T: Some experimental evidence for dependence of kidney on pituitary gland. Acta Endocrinol (Suppl) 67:169, 1962
110. Reiter RJ, McCreight CE: Influence of adrenal glands on DNA synthesis in normal and compensatory kidneys. J Exp Zool 160:117, 1965
111. Ross J, Goldman JK: Compensatory renal hypertrophy in hypophysectomized rats. Endocrinology 87:620, 1970
112. Dicker SE, Greenbaum AL, Morris CA: Compensatory renal hypertrophy in hypophysectomized rats. J Physiol (Lond) 273:241, 1977
113. Nomura K, Puett D, Nicholson WE, et al: Partial purification and characterization of a renotropic fraction from avine pituitaries. Proc Natl Acad Sci (USA) 79:6675, 1982
114. Basinger GT, Gittes RF: Compensatory renal hypertrophy in male dwarf mice. Invest Urol 13(2):165, 1975
115. Schlondroff D, Trizna W, De Rosis E, et al: Effect of testerone on compensatory renal hypertrophy in the rat. Endocrinology 101:1670, 1977
116. Austin H III, Goldin H, Preuss HG: Humoral regulation of renal growth. Nephron 27:163, 1981
117. Braun-Menendez E: Evidence for renotropin as a causal factor in renal hypertension. Circulation 17:696, 1958
118. Van Vroonhoven TJ, Soler-Montesinos L, Malt RA: Humoral regulation of renal mass. Surgery 72:300, 1972
119. Ogden DA: Donor and recipient function 2 to 4 years after renal homotransplantation. A paired study of 28 cases. Ann Intern Med 67:998, 1967
120. Ogawa K, Nowinski WW: Mitosis stimulating factor in serum of unilaterally nephrectomized rats. Proc Soc Exp Biol Med 99:350, 1958
121. Lowenstein LM, Stern A: Serum factor in renal compensatory hyperplasia. Science 142:1479, 1963
122. Preuss HG, Goldin H: A renotropic system in rats. J Clin Invest 57:94, 1976
123. Dicker SE, Morris CA: Presence of a renotropic factor in plasma of unilaterally nephrectomized rats. J Physiol (Lond) 299:13, 1980
124. Harris RH, Best CF: Circulatory retention of urinary factors as a stimulus to renal growth. Kidney Int 12:305, 1977
125. Holley RW: Control of growth of kidney epithelial cells. p. 15. In Jiminez de Asna L (ed): Control Mechanisms in Animal Cells. Raven Press, 1980
126. Johnson HA, Knudsen KD: Renal efficiency and information theory. Nature 206:930, 1965
127. Epstein FH, Charney AN, Silva P: Factors influencing the increase on Na-K-ATPase in compensatory renal hypertrophy. Yale J Biol Med 51:365, 1978
128. Trizna W, Yanagawa N, Bar-Khayim Y, et al: Functional profile of the isolated uremic nephron. Evidence off proximal tubular "memory" in experimental renal disease. J Clin Invest 68:760, 1981

129. Coles GA: Body composition in chronic renal failure. Q J Med 41:25, 1972
130. Mitch WE, Wilcox CS: Disorders of body fluids, sodium and potassium in chronic renal failure. Am J Med 72:536, 1982
131. Bibrey GL, Carter NW, White MG, et al: Potassium deficiency in chronic renal failure. Kidney Int 4:423, 1973
132. Welt LG, Smith EKM, Dunn MJ, et al: Membrane transport defect: The sick cell. Trans Assoc Am Physicians 80:217, 1967
133. Cole CH, Balie JW, Welt LG: Induction of ouabain-sensitive ATPase defect by uremic plasma. Trans Assoc Am Physicians 31:213, 1968
134. Welt LG, Sachs JR, McManus TJ: An ion transport defect in erythrocytes from uremic patients. Trans Assoc Am Physicians 77:169, 1964
135. Patrick J, Jones NF, Bradford B, et al: Leukocyte potassium in uremia: Comparisons with erythrocyte potassium and total exchangeable potassium. Clin Sci 43:669, 1972
136. Patrick J, Jones NF: Cell sodium, potassium and water in uremia and the effects of regular dialysis in the leukocyte. Clin Sci Mol Med 46:583, 1974
137. Edmondson RPS, Hilton PJ, Jones NJ, et al: Leukocyte sodium transport in uremia. Clin Sci Mol Med 49:213, 1975
138. Cotton JR, Woodard T, Carter NW, et al: Resting skeletal muscle membrane potential as an index of uremic toxicity. J Clin Invest 63:501, 1979
139. Kleeman CR, Okun R, Heller RJ: The renal regulation of sodium and potassium in patients with chronic renal failure (CRF) and the effect of diuretics on the excretion of these ions. Ann NY Acad Sci 139:522, 1966
140. Slatopolsky E, Elkan IO, Weerts C, et al: Studies on the characteristics of the control system governing sodium excretion in uremic man. J Clin Invest 47:521, 1968
141. Kahn T, Mohammad G, Stein RM: Alterations in renal tubular sodium and water reabsorption in chronic renal disease in man. Kidney Int 2:164, 1972
142. Coleman AJ, Arias M, Carter NW, et al: The mechanism of salt wastage in chronic renal failure. J Clin Invest 45:1116, 1966
143. Danovitch GM, Bourgoignie JJ, Bricker NS: Reversibility of the "salt-losing" tendency of chronic renal failure. N Engl J Med 296:15, 1977
144. Bricker NS, Fine LG, Kaplan MA, Epstein M, et al: "Magnification phenomenon" in chronic renal disease. N Engl J Med 299:-1287, 1978
145. Schultze RG, Shapiro HS, Bricker NS: Studies on the control of sodium excretion in experimental uremia. J Clin Invest 48:869, 1969
146. Steinbeck AW: The plasma volume in glomerulonephritis. Clin Sci 12:327, 1953
147. Del Greco F, Simon NM, Roguska J, et al: Hemodynamic studies in chronic uremia. Circulation 40:87, 1969
148. Godon JP: Sodium and water retention in experimental glomerulonephritis. Kidney Int 2:271, 1972
149. Schacht R, Steele JM, Baldwin DS: Exaggerated natriuresis in glomerulonephritis. J Clin Invest 51:82a, 1972
150. Maddox D, Bennett C, Deen W, et al: Control of proximal tubule fluid reabsorption in experimental glomerulonephritis. J Clin Invest 55:1315, 1975
151. Bradley SE, Bradley GP, Tyson CJ, et al: Renal function in renal diseases. Am J Med 9:766, 1950
152. Earle DP, Farber SJ, Alexander, JD, et al: Renal function and electrolyte metabolism in acute glomerulonephritis. J Clin Invest 30:421, 1951
153. Farber SJ: Physiologic aspects of glomerulonephritis. J Chron Dis 5:87, 1957
154. Schmidt RW, Bourgoignie JJ, Bricker NS: On the adaptation in sodium excretion in chronic uremia: The effects of "proportional reduction" of sodium intake. J Clin Invest 53:1736, 1974
155. Bricker NS, Klahr S, Lubowitz H, et al: Renal function in chronic renal disease. Medicine (Baltimore) 44:263, 1965
156. Schultze RG, Weisser F, Bricker NS: The influence of uremia on fractional sodium reabsorption by the proximal tubule of rats. Kidney Int 2:59, 1972
157. Weber H, Lin KY, Bricker NS: Effect of sodium intake on single nephron glomerular filtration rate and sodium reabsorption in experimental uremia. Kidney Int 8:14, 1975
158. Wen SF, Wong NL, Evanson RL, et al: Micropuncture studies of sodium transport in

the remnant kidney. J Clin Invest 52:386, 1973
159. Bank N, Aynedjian HS: Individual nephron function in experimental bilateral pyelonephritis. II. Distal tubular sodium and water reabsorption and the concentrating defect. J Clin Med 68:728, 1966
160. Hayslett JP, Boyd JE, Epstein FH: Aldosterone production in chronic renal failure. Proc Soc Exp Biol Med 130:912, 1969
161. Cope CL, Person J: Aldosterone secretion in severe renal failure. Clin Sci 25:331, 1963
162. Schrier RW, Regal EM: Influence of aldosterone on sodium, water and potassium metabolism in chronic renal disease. Kidney Int 1:156, 1972
163. Berl T, Katz FH, Henrich WL, et al: Role of aldosterone in the control of sodium excretion in patients with chronic renal failure. Kidney Int 14:228, 1978
164. Bricker NS, Schmidt RW, Favre H, et al: On the biology of sodium excretion: The search for a natriuretic hormone. Yale J Biol Med 48:293, 1975
165. Bourgoignie JJ, Klahr S, Bricker NS: Inhibition of transepithelial sodium transport in the frog skin by a low molecular weight fraction of uremic serum. J Clin Invest 50:303, 1975
166. Bourgoignie JJ, Hwang KH, Espinel C, et al: A natriuretic factor in the serum of patients with chronic uremia. J Clin Invest 51:1514, 1972
167. Bourgoignie JJ, Hwang KH, Ipakchi E, et al: The presence of a natriuretic factor in urine of patients with chronic uremia. The absence of the factor in nephrotic uremic patients. J Clin Invest 53:1559, 1974
168. Kaplan MA, Bourgoignie JJ Rosecan J, et al: The effects of the natriuretic factor from uremic urine on sodium transport, water and electrolyte content, and pyruvate oxidation by the isolated toad bladder. J Clin Invest 53:1568, 1974
169. Favre H, Hwang KH, Schmidt RW, et al: An inhibitor of sodium transport in the urine of dogs with normal renal function. J Clin Invest 56:1302, 1975
170. Epstein M, Bricker NS, Bourgoignie JJ: Presence of a natriuretic factor in urine of normal men undergoing water immersion. Kidney Int 13:152, 1978
171. Licht A, Stein S, Bricker NS: Hormonal changes and transport adaptation in chronic renal failure: The possible role of a natriuretic hormone. Biochem Soc Trans (Lond) 6:13, 1978
172. Weber H, Bourgoignie JJ, Bricker NS: The effect of the natriuretic fraction from human serum on proximal tubular sodium reabsorption in the rat. Am J Physiol 226:419, 1974
173. Fine L, Bourgoigne JJ, Hwang KH, et al: On the influence of the natriuretic factor rom uremic patients on bioelectric properties and sodium transport of the isolated mammalian collecting tubule. J Clin Invest 58:590, 1976
174. Kirschenbaum MA, Serros ER: Effect of prostaglandin inhibition on glomerular filtration rate in normal and uremic rabbits. Prostaglandins 22:245, 1981
175. Schultze RG, Taggart DD, Shapiro H, et al: On the adaptation in potassium excretion associated with nephron reduction in the dog. J Clin Invest 50:1061,1971
176. Bank N, Aynedjian HS: A micropuncture study of potassium excretion by the remnant kidney. J Clin Invest 52:1480, 1973
177. Fine LG, Yanagawa N, Schultze RG, et al: Functional profile of the isolated uremic nephron. Potassium adaptation in the rabbit cortical collecting tubule. J Clin Invest 64:1033, 1979
178. Schon DA, Silva P, Hayslett JP: Mechanism of potassium excretion in renal insufficiency. Am J Physiol 227:1323, 1974
179. Kashgarian M, Taylor CR, Binder HJ, et al: Amplification of cell membrane surface in potassium adaptation. Lab Invest 581, 1980
180. Wade JB, O'Neil RG, Pryor JR, et al: Modulation of cell membrane area in renal collecting tubules by corticosteroid hormones. J Cell Biol 81:439, 1979
181. Bostle CP, Hayslett JP, Brudes HJ: Increased large intestinal secretion of potassium in renal insufficiency. Kidney Int 12:9, 1977
182. Cohen JJ, Gennari FJ, Harrington JJ: Disorders of potassium balance. p. 908. In Brenner BM, Rector FC Jr (eds): The Kidney. WB Saunders, Philadelphia, 1981
183. Battle DC, Arruda JAL, Kurtzman NA: Hyperkalemic distal renal tubular acidosis asso-

ciated with obstructive uropathy. N Engl J Med 304:373, 1981

184. Harrington JT, Cohen JJ: Clinical disorders of urine concentration and dilution. Arch Intern Med 131:810, 1973
185. Kleeman CR, Adams DA, Maxwell MH: An evaluation of maximal water diuresis in chronic renal disease. I. Normal solute intake. J Lab Clin Med 58:169, 1964
186. Martinez-Maldonado M, Yium JJ, Eknoyan G, et al: Adult polycystic kidney disease: Studies of the defect in urine concentration. Kidney Int 2:107, 1972
187. Dorhout Mees EJ: Relation between maximal urine concentration, maximal water reabsorption capacity, and mannitol clearance in patients with renal disease. Br Med J 1:1156, 1959
188. Bricker NS, Dewey RR, Lubowitz H, et al: Observations on the concentrating and diluting mechanisms of the diseased kidney. J Clin Invest 38:516, 1959
189. Finkelstein FO, Hayslett JP: Role of medullary structures in the functional adaptation of renal insufficiency. Kidney Int 6:419, 1974
190. Baldwin DS, Berman HJ, Heinemann HO, et al: The elaboration of osmotically concentrated urine in renal disease. J Clin Invest 34:800, 1955
191. Bricker NS, Kime SW Jr, Morrin PAF, et al: The influence of glomerular filtration rate, solute excretion and hydration on the concentrating mechanism of the experimentally diseased kidney in the dog. J Clin Invest 39:864, 1960
192. Lubowitz H, Purkerson ML, Bricker NS: Investigation of single nephrons in the chronically diseased (pyelonephritic) kidney of the rat using micropuncture techniques. Nephron 3:73, 1966
193. Bricker NS, Klahr S, Lubowitz H, et al: Renal function in chronic renal disease. Medicine (Baltimore) 44:263, 1965
194. Gilbert RM, Weber H, Turchin L, et al: A study of the intrarenal recycling of urea in the rat with chronic experimental pyelonephritis. J Clin Invest 58:1349, 1976
195. Holliday MA, Egan TJ, Morris CR, et al: Pitressin-resistant hyposthenuria in chronic renal disease. Am J Med 42:378, 1967
196. White AG, Kurtz M, Rubin G: Comparative renal responses to water and antidiuretic hormone in diabetes insipidus and in chronic renal disease. Am J Med 16:220, 1954
197. Tannen RL, Regal EM, Dunn MJ, et al: Vasopressin-resistant hyposthenuria in advanced chronic renal disease. N Engl J Med 280:1135, 1969
198. Mitch WE: Conservative management of chronic renal failure. P. 116. In Brenner BM, Stein JH (eds): Chronic Renal Failure. Churchill Livingstone, New York, 1981
199. Mitch WE, Walser M: A proposed mechanism for reduced creatinine excretion in severe chronic renal failure. Nephron 21:248, 1978
200. Goldman R, Bassett SH: Phosphorus excretion in renal failure. J Clin Invest 33:1623, 1954
201. Slatopolsky E, Rutherford WE, Hruska K, et al: How important is phosphate in the pathogenesis of renal osteodystrophy. Arch Intern Med 138:848, 1978
202. Stanbury SW, Lumb GA: Metabolic studies of renal osteodystrophy: I. Calcium phosphorus and hyperparathyroidism complicating chronic uremia and osteomalacia of the adult Fanconi syndrome. Medicine (Baltimore) 41:1, 1962
203. Kopple JD, Coburn JW: Metabolic studies of low protein diets in uremia. II. Calcium, phosphorus and magnesium. Medicine (Baltimore) 52:597, 1973
204. Coburn JW, Kurokawa K, Llach F: Altered divalent ion metabolism in renal disease and renal osteodystrophy. P. 1153. In Maxwell MH, Kleeman CR (eds): Clinical Disorders of Fluid and Electrolyte Metabolism. McGraw-Hill, New York, 1980
205. Reiss E, Canterbury JM, Kanter A: Circulating parathyroid hormone concentration in chronic renal insufficiency. Arch Intern Med 124:417, 1969
206. Arnaud CD: Hyperparathyroidism and renal failure. Kidney Int 4:89, 1973
207. Bricker NS, Slatopolsky E, Reiss E, et al: Calcium phosporus and bone in renal disease and transplantation. Arch Intern Med 123: 543, 1969
208. Slatopolsky E, Caglar S, Pennell JP, et al: On the pathogenesis of hyperparathyroidism in chronic renal disease. J Clin Invest 50:492, 1971
209. Slatopolsky E, Caglar S, Gradowska L, et

al: On the prevention of secondary hyperparathyroidism in experimental chronic renal disease using "proportional reduction" of dietary phosphorus intake. Kidney Int 2:147, 1972

210. Slatopolsky E, Bricker NS: The role of phosphorus restriction in the prevention of secondary hyperthyroidism in chronic renal disease. Kidney Int 2:141, 1973
211. Rutherford WE, Bordier P, Marie P, et al: Phosphate control and 25-hydroxycholecalciferol administration in preventing experimental renal osteodystrophy in the dog. J Clin Invest 60:332, 1977
212. Kaplan MA, Canterbury JM, Jaffe D, et al: Interpelations between phosphorus, calcium, parathyroid hormone and renal phosphate excretion response to an oral phosphorus load in normal and uremic dogs. Kidney Int 14:207, 1978
213. Kaplan MA, Canterbury JM, Gavellas G, et al: The calcemic and phosphaturic effect of parathyroid hormone in the normal and uremic dog. Metabolism 27:1785, 1978
214. Massry SG, Brautbar N: Renal handling of phosphate in renal failure. p. 307. In Massry SG, Fleisch H (eds): Renal Handling Phosphate. Plenum, New York, 1980
215. Popovitzer MM, Pinggera WF, Hutt MP, et al: Serum parathyroid hormone levels and renal handling of phosphorus in patients with chronic renal disease. J Clin Endocrinol Metab 35:213, 1972
216. Swensen RS, Weisinger JR, Rubberi JL, et al: Evidence that parathyroid hormone is not required for phosphate homeostasis in renal failure. Metabolism 24:197, 1975
217. Christensen MS, Brochner-Mortensen J, Tougaard L, et al: Minor influence of parathyroid hormone on fractional tubular reabsorption of phosphate in chronic renal failure. p. 131. In Massry SG, Ritz E (eds): Phosphate Metabolism. Plenum, New York, 1977
218. Fotino S: Phosphate excretion and chronic renal failure. Evidence for a mechanism other than circulatory parathyroid hormone. Clin Nephrol 8:499, 1977
219. Lorean N, Cosgus JP, Repreux C, et al: Renal calcitonic receptors and adenylate cyclase in rats immunized against tubular basement membrane. Kidney Int 12:184, 1977
220. Caverzasio J, Gloor HJ, Fleisch H, et al: Parathyroid hormone independent adaptation of the renal handling of phosphate in response to renal mass reduction. Kidney Int 21:471, 1982
221. Puckerson ML, Rolf DB, Yates J, et al: Factors that influence urinary phosphate excreted in rats with reduced renal mass. Evidence for increased sensitivity of parathyroid hormone. Mineral Electrolyte Metab 4:258, 1980
222. Bank N, Su W, Aynedjian HS: A micropuncture study of renal phosphate transplant in rats with chronic renal failure and secondary hyperparathyroidism. J Clin Invest 61:884, 1978
223. Yanagawa N, Nissenson RA, Edwards B, et al: Functional profile of the isolated uremic nephron. The intrinsic adaptation of phosphate transport in the rabbit proximal tubule. Kidney Int 23:674, 1983
224. Fine LG, Yanagawa N, Lang R: Adaptations of tubular handling of phosphate by the diseased kidney. Proc Eur Soc Ped Nephrol 16:34, 1982
225. Fine LG: Regulation of phosphate excretion by the diseased kidney: "Reabsorption sites" and hormone–receptor interactions." Mineral Electrolyte Metab 6:308, 1981
226. Coburn JW, Popovitzer MM, Massry SG: The physiochemical state and renal handling of divalent ions in chronic renal failure. Arch Intern Med 124:302, 1969
227. Popovitzer MM, Schainuck LI, Massry SG, et al: Divalent ion excretion in chronic kidney disease relation to degree of renal insufficiency. Clin Sci 38:297, 1970
228. Slatopolsky E, Rutherford WE, Hoffstein PE, et al: Non-suppressible secondary hyperparathyroidism in chronic progressive renal disease. Kidney Int 1:38, 1972
229. Goodman AD, Lemann JJ, Lennon EJ et al: Production, excretion and net balance of fixed acid in patients with renal acidosis. J Clin Invest 44:455, 1965
230. Schwartz WB, Relman AS: Acidosis in renal disease. N Engl J Med 256:1184, 1957
231. Schwartz WB, Hall PW III, Hays RM, et al: On the mechanism of acidosis in chronic renal failure. J Clin Invest 38:39, 1959
232. Wrong O, Davies HEF: The excretion of acid in renal disease. Q J Med 28:259, 1959

233. Lathem W: Hyperchloremic acidosis in chronic pyelonephritis. N Engl J Med 358:1031, 1958
234. Widmer B, Gerhardt RE, Harrington JT, et al: Serum electrolyte and acid base composition. The influence of graded degrees of chronic renal failure. Arch Intern Med 135:1099, 1979
235. Relman AS: The acidosis of renal disease. Am J Med 44:706, 1968
236. Albert MD, Dell RB, Winter RW: Quantitative displacement of acid–base equilibrium in metabolic acidosis. Ann Intern Med 66:312, 1967
237. Lemann JJ, Litzow JR, Lennon EJ: The effects of chronic acid loads in normal mass: Further evidence for the participation of bone mineral in the defense against chronic metabolic acidosis. J Clin Invest 45:1608, 1966
238. Litzow JR, Lemann J, Lennon EJ: The effect of treatment of acidosis on calcium balance in patients with chronic azotemic renal failure. J Clin Invest 46:280, 1967
239. Dorhout-Mees EJ, Hachado M, Slatopolsky E, et al: The functional adaptation of the diseased kidney. III. Ammonia excretion. J Clin Invest 45:289, 1966
240. Welbourne T, Weber M, Bank N: The effect of glutamine administration on urinary ammonium excretion in normal subjects and in patients with renal disease. J Clin Invest 51:1852, 1972
241. Windus D, Klahr S, Hammerman MR: Renal vesicle glutamine transport in health and chronic renal failure. Am Soc Nephrol 15:125A, 1982 (Abst).
242. Tizianello A, De Ferrari G, Garibotto G, et al: Renal metabolism of amino acids and ammonia in subjects with normal renal function and in patients with chronic renal insufficiency. J Clin Invest 65:1162, 1980
243. Bricker NS: On the pathogenesis of the uremic state: An exposition of the "trade-off hypothesis." N Engl J Med 286:1093, 1972
244. Purkerson MC, Lubowitz H, White RW, et al: On the influence of extracellular fluid volume expansion on bicarbonate reabsorption in the rat. J Clin Invest 68:1754, 1969
245. Slatopolsky E, Hoffsten P, Purkerson M, et al: On the influence of extracellular fluid volume expansion and of uremia on bicarbonate reabsorption in man. J Clin Invest 49:988, 1970
246. Arruda JAL, Nascimento L, Arevalo G, et al: Bicarbonate reabsorption in chronic renal failure in man and the rat. Pflügers Arch 376:193, 1978
247. Muldowney TP, Donahue JF, Carroll DV, et al: Parathyroid acidosis in uremia. Q J Med 41:321, 1972
248. Cohn DE, Hruska KA, Klahr S, et al: Increased Na^+–H^+ exchange in brush border vesicles from dogs with renal failure. (Renal Fluid Electrolyte Physiol 12.) Am J Physiol 263:F293, 1982
249. Hafezi A, Nord EP, Trizna W, Fine LG: A unique H^+-gradient-dependent increase in the J Max of the Na^+-H^+ antiporter in the luminal membrane of the remnant kidney proximal tubule. Abtr Am Soc Nephrol 16:108A, 1983
250. Kopple JD: Nutritional therapy in kidney failure. Nutr Rev 39:193, 1981
251. Addis T: Glomerular Nephritis: Diagnosis and Treatment. Macmillan, New York, 1948
252. Ibels LS, Alfrey AC, Hart L, et al: Preservation of functions in experimental renal disease by dietary restriction of phosphate. N Engl J Med 298:122, 1978
253. Maschio G, Oldrizzi L, Tessitore N, et al: Effects of dietary protein as phosphorus restriction on the progression of early renal failure. Kidney Int 22:371, 1982
254. Barrientos A, Arteaga J, Rodicio JL, et al: Role of the control of phosphate on the progression of chronic renal failure. Mineral Electrolyte Metab 7:127, 1982
255. Brenner BM, Meyer TW, Hostetter TH: Dietary protein intake and the progressive nature of kidney disease: The role of hemodynamically mediated glomerular injury in the pathogenesis of progressive glomerular sclerosis on aging, renal ablation and intrinsic renal disease. N Engl J Med 307:652, 1982
256. Giordano C: Protein restriction in chronic renal failure. Kidney Int 22:401, 1982

15

Renal Osteodystrophy

Jack W. Coburn

As the lives of patients with advanced renal failure are prolonged through conservative measures or by renal "replacement" with dialysis, renal osteodystrophy is observed with increased frequency. The term *renal osteodystrophy* is used in a global sense to include all the skeletal syndromes and alterations of divalent ion metabolism that arise as renal function decreases.

The kidneys are important in the regulation of the metabolism of calcium, phosphorus, and magnesium via the regulation of their urinary excretion and also through generation of the renal hormone, 1,25-dihydroxyvitamin D_3 ($1,25(OH)_2D_3$). The kidneys are both a target organ for the actions of parathyroid hormone (PTH) and are partly responsible for the degradation of parathyroid hormone (PTH). With failure of renal function, several homeostatic mechanisms are activated in an apparent attempt to adjust for the various disturbances of divalent ion metabolism. These homeostatic processes per se may have adverse effects: thus, increased PTH secretion, which occurs in renal insufficiency, can be a major pathogenic factor leading to altered bone structure and metabolism; moreover, excess PTH may contribute to other uremic symptoms. In addition, there is growing evidence that the renal retention of an element, aluminum, which normally enters the body in minute amounts and is excreted in the urine, can contribute to the bone disease in advanced renal failure.

Several forms of skeletal pathology occur with advanced renal failure. The type of bone disease may depend upon the actions of several pathogenic processes described in detail below, the presence of uremic toxicity, the age of the patient, the rate of skeletal turnover, the duration of renal insufficiency, differences in dietary intake, the type of pharmacologic intervention, the duration and adequacy of dialysis, and the purity of the water used for dialysate. The skeletal pathology varies from patient to patient; the most common form of pathology in uremic adults is osteitis fibrosa or fibroosteoclasia,[1,2] which arises due to the action of excess PTH. *Osteomalacia,* or impaired mineralization of bone, also occurs; osteomalacia is generally accompanied by a variable degree of osteitis fibrosa, and the term *mixed renal osteodystrophy* has been applied to this combination.[3] There are two forms of bone disease: "isolated" osteomalacia, with markedly impaired mineralization and little or no evidence of fibroosteoclasia, and a variety characterized by decreased mineralization but no increase in osteoid. The latter has been termed "aplastic" bone disease;[4] both have been attributed to aluminum accumulation.

SKELETAL PATHOLOGY IN RENAL OSTEODYSTROPHY

Osteitis Fibrosa (Fibroosteoclasia)

The bone with osteitis fibrosa exhibits increased numbers of both osteoclasts and osteoblasts and variable degrees of peritrabecular fibrosis. Osteoclast activation is mediated by the action of PTH, although this may occur secondary to an initial effect of PTH on osteoblasts.[5] The result is increased resorption of both mineral and matrix along the surfaces of trabecular bone and within the Haversian canals of cortical bone.[6] The increased resorption brings about increased bone formation through a "coupling" process that is not totally understood. Wide seams of newly synthesized collagen are laid down along the surfaces of trabecular bone and within earlier resorptive cavities or Howships lacunae. Thus, the excess unmineralized osteoid appears in osteitis fibrosa as a consequence of the rapid synthesis of matrix rather than arising due to impaired mineralization.

The presence of "woven" osteoid, with the layers of collagen arranged in haphazard, irregular directions, is another feature of osteitis fibrosa; this woven pattern contrasts with the orderly, lamellar arrangement of collagen fibrils deposited in normal bone. Woven osteoid is a nonspecific finding, and it occurs in other conditions with increased bone turnover, including Paget's disease, hyperthyroidism, and acromegaly. Another feature of woven bone is the deposition of calcium as amorphous calcium phosphate; this contrasts to the hydroxyapatite that is deposited in normal, lamellar bone. It has been suggested that a greater mass of woven than lamellar bone may be stimulated in an effort to achieve a similar degree of mechanical strength.[6] Also, it has been proposed that osteosclerosis, a common radiographic finding in the axial skeleton of patients with renal osteodystrophy, may represent increased mineralization with amorphous calcium phosphate as an attempt to maintain mechanical stability of woven bone.

Osteomalacia

The term *osteomalacia* is used to describe defective mineralization of bone, and various histologic criteria have been employed for this diagnosis.[7] Osteomalacia is commonly identified from the presence of wide osteoid seams, although widened osteoid seams do not, by themselves, indicate osteomalacia. Osteoid seams are widened in osteitis fibrosa because mineralization fails to keep pace with the enhanced matrix synthesis. Other "static" features of osteomalacia include increased numbers of osteoid lamellae or an increase in the trabecular surface covered with osteoid. The best method of identifying impaired mineralization involves the administration of tetracycline, which is incorporated into newly forming bone with its subsequent identification by its fluorescent characteristics.[8] Brief periods of treatment with tetracycline on two separate occasions, separated by a specific time interval, allow determination of bone formation rate. This offers a dynamic approach to the evaluation of bone, and such "double tetracycline labels" discloses delayed bone formation in osteomalacia.

In many uremic patients with osteomalacia, variable degrees of secondary hyperparathyroidism coexist and there are features of osteitis fibrosa, that is, peritrabecular fibrosis and increased resorption surface. Such a lesion has been classified as a "mixed" lesion, because of the features of both osteitis fibrosa and osteomalacia.[3,9]

A subset of patients with advanced renal failure have isolated or "pure" osteomalacia; these patients usually lack the features of secondary hyperparathyroidism.[10,11] The mineralized bone beneath the osteoid often shows resorption cavities, which may represent evidence of previous secondary hyperparathyroidism. Many of these patients have been treated with hemodialysis for a substantial period, and the pathogenesis of this vitamin D-refractory osteomalacia may be related to the accumulation of aluminum in bone.[12-14] Thus, this condition differs from both osteitis fibrosa and the mixed lesion characterized by both osteomalacia and osteitis fibrosa.

Another subgroup of renal failure patients has been identified with a bone biopsy lesion characterized by a varying reduction of bone volume, little or no separation of tetracycline labels, but no generalized increase in osteoid.[4] Because of the lack of bone formation, this group has been classified as "aplastic"; the biopsies show substantial uptake of aluminum along the surfaces which would normally exhibit new bone formation. Certain patients have shown this lesion on initial biopsy and then exhibit more typical osteomalacia on a subsequent biopsy.

PATHOPHYSIOLOGY OF ALTERED MINERAL HOMEOSTASIS

Normally, the kidneys play a vital role in mineral homeostasis. Thus, they act to maintain the external balance for calcium, phosphorous, and magnesium; they are the major organs which are physiologically responsible for the generation of 1,25-dihydroxyvitamin D_3, as well as 24,25-dihyroxyvitamin D_3. In addition, they are both target organs for parathyroid hormone (PTH), and they are partly responsible for the degradation of the intact PTH molecule and the clearance of fragments of PTH from the circulation. With the loss or reduction of these functions during renal insufficiency, it is not surprising that there is altered mineral homeostasis. Generally, these disturbances follow an orderly sequence, as there is progressive reduction in functioning nephron population; however, a preponderance of certain pathophysiologic processes can occur in certain renal diseases or syndromes. Thus, patients with Fanconi's syndrome may have long-standing hypophosphatemia due to long-standing excessive excretion of phosphate, and patients with the nephrotic syndrome have large urinary losses of 25-hydroxyvitamin D, which is excreted bound to the vitamin D-binding protein of plasma.[15]

Secondary Hyperparathyroidism

When the glomerular filtration rate (GFR) falls below 50 to 75 ml/min, an early and persistent feature is an elevated serum level of immunoreactive PTH (iPTH).[16,17] This increase in serum iPTH occurs partly because the secretion of PTH is increased, but the increment is magnified due to a reduced metabolic clearance of the PTH and its fragments. Many immunoassay procedures react primarily to the carboxyl (C) terminal fragments or mid-region terminal fragments of the PTH molecule. These fragments are normally cleared from the circulation entirely by glomerular filtration.[18] With progressive renal insufficiency, their metabolic clearance rate is greatly reduced, leading to a substantial increase in their blood levels. Thus, a moderately increased blood level of the mid-region fragments of PTH does not in itself indicate the presence of significant secondary hyperparathyroidism in a patient with end-stage renal disease.

Bone biopsies, done on patients with mild renal insufficiency, often show some evidence of increased PTH action.[1] As renal failure progresses and GFR falls below 30 ml/min, the degree of secondary hyperparathyroidism becomes more marked, and clear correlations have been noted between the elevated serum levels of iPTH and the morphologic features of hyperparathyroidism on bone biopsy, as is shown in Fig. 15–1.[19]

The major stimulus for increased PTH secretion is believed to be hypocalcemia, and several factors, including phosphate retention, an altered calcemic response to the action of parathyroid hormone, and abnormal vitamin D metabolism, are believed to contribute to the hypocalcemia.

In addition to the increased PTH secretion that arises as a consequence of hypocalcemia, parathyroid hypersecretion may also occur because of factors intrinsic to the parathyroid gland, such as the hyperplasia with an increase in cell mass and alterations in parathyroid cell function. In normal glands, the half-maximal

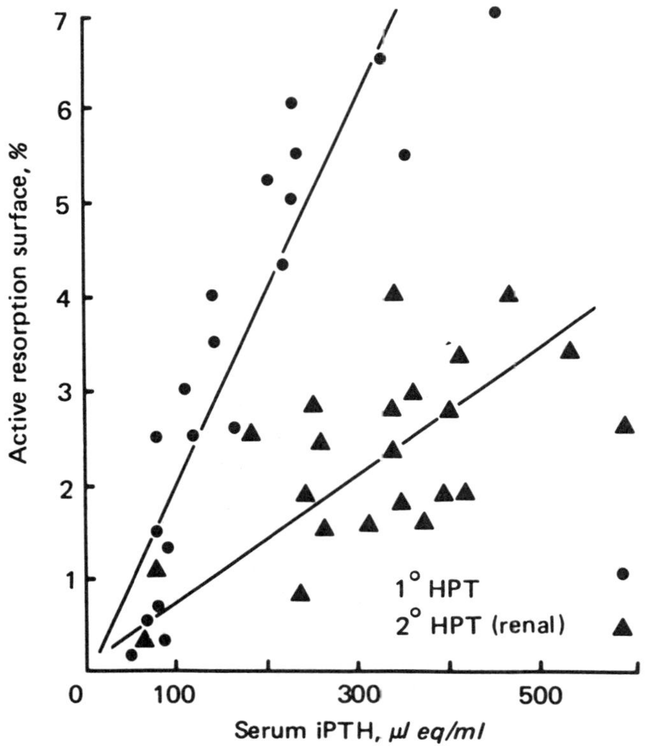

Fig. 15–1. Relation between bone biopsy features of active resorption surface on and the serum iPTH, measured with an antiserum now known to react against the mid-region of the carboxyl terminal of the PTH molecule. Data are given for patients with primary hyperparathyroidism (1° HPT) and those with secondary hyperparathyroidism due to advanced renal failure (2° HPT). The difference in the slopes most likely due to retention of inactive fragments of these iPTH fragments in the circulation of patients with renal failure. (From Bordier PJ, Arnaud C, Hawker C, et al: Relationship between serum immunoreactive parathyroid hormone, osteoclastic and asteocytic bone resorption and serum calcium in primary hyperparathyroidism and osteomalacia. In Frame B, Parfitt AN, Dunash HH (Eds): Clinical Aspects of Bone Disease, Excerpta Medica, Amsterdam, 1973.)

inhibition of PTH release, or the "set-point," occurs with an ionic calcium concentration above 1.03 m*M* (4.12 mg/dl). On the other hand, the set point was 1.03 m*M* or above in cell suspensions from 12 of the 14 hyperplastic parathyroid glands that showed suppression (Fig. 15–2). This shift of the set-point was common in the glands removed from patients with chronic renal failure,[20] while the maximal release of PTH per cell did not differ in glands from patients with secondary hyperparathyroidism compared to those from normal parathyroid glands.

The mechanism for this shift in set-point of PTH is not known; it has been shown that there is alteration of the activation constant for magnesium of the enzyme, adenylate cyclase, an important regulator of PTH secretion, in the cell membranes from parathyroid glands from patients with hyperplasia.[21] The addition of GTP to this incubation system largely restored activation of the adenylate cyclase to normal. These latter observations suggest that there are alterations in the characteristics of adenylate cyclase in parathyroid glands from patients with hyperplasia; this abnormality could contribute to altered control of PTH secretion under these circumstances. Other preliminary data suggest that the alteration of set-point is accompanied by changes in the intracellular calcium activity (Ca^{2+}) in response to alterations in extracellular calcium ion concentration.[22] Also, clinical observations that serum iPTH levels may not be reduced in dialysis patients unless the serum calcium exceeds 10.0 to 10.5 mg/dl is consistent with the in vivo occurrence of this shift in the set-point.[23]

Phosphate Retention

A substantial increase in plasma phosphorus level causes a reciprocal fall in plasma calcium, and the retention of phosphate due to a reduction in GFR early in the course

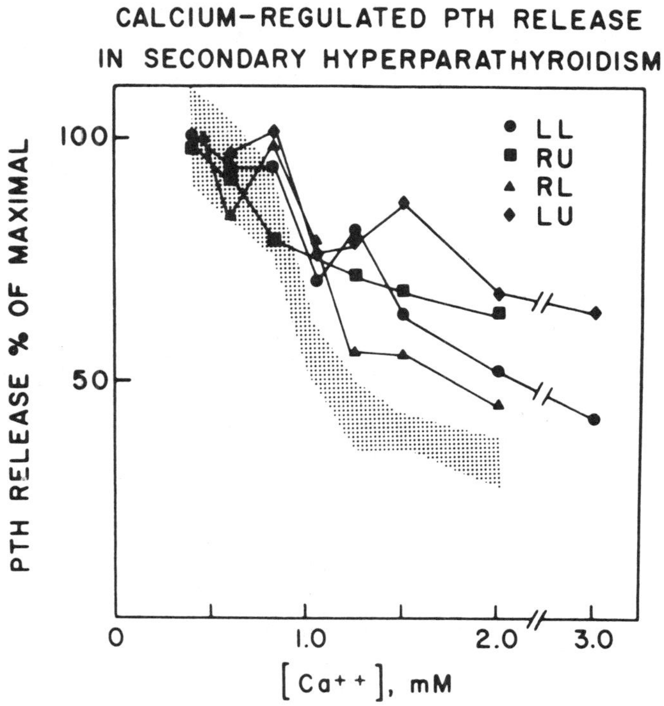

Fig. 15–2. The calcium-regulated release of PTH from suspensions of parathyroid cells obtained by parathyroid surgery in a patient with secondary hyperparathyroidism due to renal failure. Each symbol represents cells from a different parathyroid gland. The calcium-mediated change in PTH release from parathyroid cells from individuals those with normal parathyroid glands is indicated by the shaded area. (Reprinted from Brown EM: Setpoint for calcium its role in normal and abnormal parathyroid secretion. In Cohn D (Ed): Hormonal Control of Calcium Metabolism. Excerpta Medica, Amsterdam, 1982.)

of renal insufficiency was suggested to cause a fall in blood ionized calcium, which then increased the secretion of PTH. The increased PTH level would cause phosphaturia, which would then reduce serum phosphorus levels to normal and thereby restore the serum calcium to normal, but only with an increased serum iPTH level.

Slatopolsky and co-workers[24-26] have carried out studies showing the fundamental importance of phosphate intake in the pathogenesis of secondary hyperparathyroidism in dogs with experimental renal failure. They showed that feeding "uremic" dogs a diet containing an amount of phosphate that was restricted in exact proportion to the reduction in GFR largely prevented both the usual rise in serum iPTH and the development of bone lesions which on biopsy are characteristic of secondary hyperparathyroidism (Fig. 15–3). This observation contrasted to the substantial secondary hyperparathyroidism which developed in the azotemic dogs fed a constant, normal phosphate diet.[27]

The mechanism whereby phosphate retention stimulates PTH secretion remains uncertain. Thus, serum phosphorus levels have been normal or even slightly reduced in patients with mild-to-moderate renal insufficiency,[28-31] and it has been suggested that the postprandial levels of serum phosphorus may be elevated in patients with moderate renal insufficiency. However, controlled data indicate that in general even the postprandial levels of phosphate remain normal or subnormal.[28,32] Thus, the original theory, which suggested that phosphate retention increased the serum phosphorus level and thereby lowered ionized calcium level, may require revision. The possibility that phosphate retention may act through an effect on vitamin D metabolism is considered below under "Abnormalities of Vitamin D Metabolism."

When renal function decreases to below 25 percent of normal, overt and persistent hyperphosphatemia is common, and inverse correlations have been observed between serum phosphorus levels and the levels of serum Ca and iPTH in patients with advanced renal failure.[33]

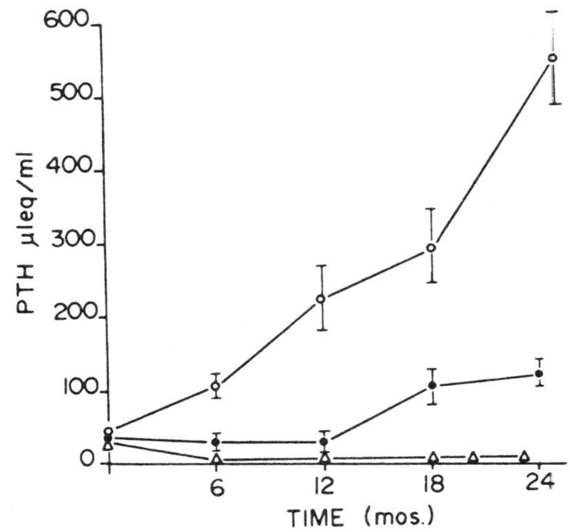

Fig. 15–3. Serial values of serum iPTH (mean ± SE) in dogs with chronic renal insufficiency. The dogs received either (1) a normal phosphate intake (○), (2) a dietary phosphate intake reduced in proportion to the reduction in glomerular filtration rate (●), or (3) a proportional reduction in dietary phosphate intake and 25(OH)-vitamin D_3, 30 μg twice weekly (△), for 2 years. (From Rutherford WE, Bordier P, Marie P, et al: Phosphate control and 25-hydroxycholecalcific administration in preventing experimental renal osteodystrophy in the dog. J Clin Invest 60:332, 1977. By permission of the American Society for Clinical Investigation.)

Resistance of Bone to the Calcemic Action of PTH

Another factor that contributes to hypocalcemia and secondary hyperparathyroidism in renal failure is skeletal resistance to the calcemic action of PTH; thus, greater PTH secretion may be needed to maintain the normal flux of calcium from bone into extracellular fluid. Otherwise, serum calcium would fall and further stimulate PTH secretion. Patients with either acute or advanced renal failure fail to exhibit a normal rise in serum Ca following the infusion of parathyroid extract.[34-36] Moreover, patients with mild renal insufficiency showed delayed recovery from hypocalcemia induced by the infusion of EDTA despite an adequate rise in serum iPTH level, as shown in Fig. 15–4.[31] Moreover, similar resistance to the skeletal response to PTH has been demonstrated in dogs with reduced renal function.[37-40] The factors responsible for skeletal resistance to the calcemic action of PTH have been reported to include decreased levels of $1,25(OH)_2D_3$,[38] and/or $24,25(OH)_2D_3$,[41] phosphate retention,[42] the presence of "uremic toxins,"[43] and alterations in the metabolism of PTH.[44] In some patients with advanced uremia, it is also possible that bone resorption may be maximal so that a further increase

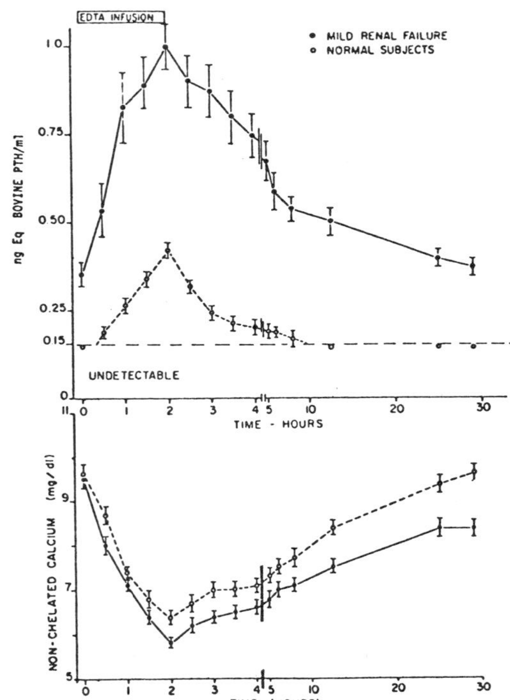

Fig. 15–4. Levels of serum iPTH and serum nonchelated calcium (both as mean ± SE) before, during and after the infusion of EDTA, given to reduced the nonchelated calcium levels. There was delayed recovery from hypocalcemia in the patients with mild renal insufficiency compared to observations data in normal subjects. (Serum iPTH levels below 0.15 mg/ml, below the horizontal interrupted line, could not be detected with high accuracy.) (From Llach F, Massry SG, Singer FR, et al: Skeletal resistance to endogenous parathyroid hormone in patients with early renal failure. A possible cause for secondary hyperparathyroidism. J Clin Endocrinol Metab 41:338, 1975.)

in PTH can cause little increase in its skeletal action.[45]

Abnormalities of Vitamin D Metabolism

The kidney is the organ responsible for the physiologic generation of circulating levels of $1,25(OH)_2D_3$, the active hormonal form of vitamin D. Recent in vitro observations, which show that cells from other tissues can produce $1,25(OH)_2D_3$ from an excess of radiolabeled $25(OH)D_3$,[46-48] are of uncertain physiologic significance. Only during pregnancy[49] and in the rare patient with sarcoidosis, uremia, and hypercalcemia[50] is there evidence for the extrarenal generation of $1,25(OH)_2D_3$ in physiologically important amounts. Normally, the blood levels of this renal hormone are maintained within relatively narrow limits. The generation of $1,25(OH)_2D_3$ from $25(OH)D_3$ is normally stimulated by a low-calcium diet, probably from the action of increased PTH, and by a reduction in phosphate intake or a fall in serum P level. This effect of phosphate restriction occurs independent of PTH.[51] Conversely, calcium loading or phosphate loading with hyperphosphatemia may reduce the generation of $1,25(OH)_2D_3$.[52,53] Physiologic events such as pregnancy, lactation, and growth are also associated with striking increments in the plasma levels of $1,25(OH)_2D_3$; moreover, $1,25(OH)_2D_3$ has a negative feedback effect to reduce its own generation.[54]

An effect of acidosis on the generation of $1,25(OH)_2D_3$ is less certain. The activity of $25(OH)D_3{}^{-1}$ alpha-hydroxylase, the enzyme responsible for generating $1,25(OH)_2D_3$, is inhibited by acidosis. However, it is less certain that acidosis produces this effect in vivo, particularly in the vitamin D-replete state.[55] However, others suggested that the effect of acidosis to raise serum phosphorus might block such an effect. In man, moderate acidosis has no effect on serum levels of $1,25(OH)_2D_3$.[57]

It has been suggested that an inability of the diseased kidney to produce $1,25(OH)_2D_3$ may play an important role in the pathogenesis of secondary hyperparathyroidism in patients with renal insufficiency.[58] In patients with advanced renal failure or end-stage renal disease, the intestinal absorption of calcium is impaired and the plasma levels of $1,25(OH)_2D$ are uniformly depressed.[59-61] Moreover, modest oral doses of $1,25(OH)_2D_3$ restore intestinal absorption of calcium to normal levels in such patients, as is shown in Fig. 15–5.[62]

Thus, vitamin D metabolism is abnormal in patients with advanced renal failure. How-

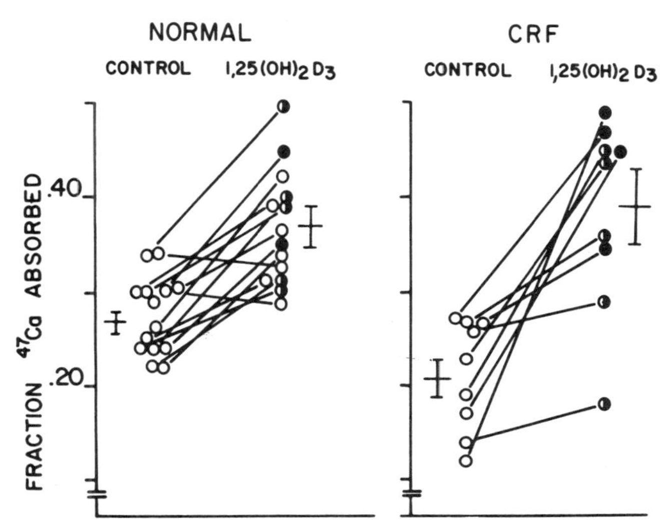

Fig. 15–5. Fraction of radiolabeled calcium absorbed (200 calcium mg carrier) in normal subjects and patients with advanced renal failure (CRF) studied both before and after receiving calcitriol ($1,25(OH)_2D_3$) for 7 to 10 days. The brackets encompass mean ± SE. (From Brickman AS, Coburn JW, Massry SG, Norman AW: 1-25-dihydroxy-vitamin D_3 in normal man and patients with renal failure. Ann Intern Med 80:161, 1974.)

ever, it is not clear at what time in the course of renal insufficiency there is a decrease of vitamin D activation. It is also not known how this contributes to the pathogenesis of hyperparathyroidism early in the course of renal insufficiency. Most patients with mild to moderate renal insufficiency (i.e., serum creatinine levels below 2.5 mg/dl or creatinine clearances above 50 ml/min) exhibit intestinal calcium absorption that cannot be distinguished from normal.[30,63] Preliminary data in adults with moderate insufficiency indicate that plasma levels of $1,25(OH)_2D$ may be normal,[64] although others have reported reduced levels.[65] Observations in children with moderate renal insufficiency, largely from tubulointerstitial disorders, revealed mean serum levels of $1,25(OH)_2D$ that are lower than normal.[28] Moreover, the findings of "normal" levels of $1,25(OH)_2D_3$ in early renal failure may not represent a normal response of renal tubular cells to high levels of PTH. Thus, increased serum levels of $1,25(OH)_2D_3$ are common in patients with high PTH levels due to primary hyperparathyroidism.[66]

The preliminary observations in both children and adults[67,68] indicate that many of the pathophysiologic features, including slightly reduced serum levels of $1,25(OH)_2D$ and high serum iPTH levels, can be returned to normal following the restriction of dietary phosphate intake. Such observations underscore the important link between dietary phosphate intake and alterations in vitamin D metabolism and suggest that the two are indeed inseparable. The observations that secondary hyperparathyroidism may persist and even progress in the case of normal or only slightly reduced serum levels of $1,25(OH)_2D_3$ raises the possibility that there may be an increased requirement for this sterol in the face of excess PTH activity.[23] The possibility exists that $1,25(OH)_2D_3$ may suppress PTH secretion by means of a direct effect on the parathyroid glands;[69,70] which is independent of hypercalcemia.

The kidney is also primarily responsible for the generation of 24,25-dihydroxyvitamin D_3 ($24,25(OH)_2D_3$),[71] a naturally occurring vitamin D sterol of uncertain physiologic role.[72] This sterol probably does not augment the intestinal absorption of calcium prior to its renal conversion to 1,24,25-trihydroxyvitamin D_3; however, the administration of $24,25(OH)_2D_3$ may have effects different from those of $1,25(OH)_2D_3$.[73,74] Presently, it remains uncertain whether reduced serum levels of $24,25(OH)_2D_3$ in uremic patients play any role in the pathogenesis of the bone disease.

FACTORS CAUSING OSTEOMALACIA (DEFECTIVE MINERALIZATION)

Several factors contribute to the pathogenesis of osteomalacia or defective mineralization in patients with advanced renal failure.

Abnormalities of Vitamin D

In occasional uremic patients, the plasma levels of 25(OH)D may be low;[75] this is probably evidence for coexisting nutritional deficiency of vitamin D in a patient who also has renal failure. Cases with reduced serum levels of 25(OH)D have been unusual in most studies of patients with advanced renal failure.[76-80] However, in a series of patients with both bone biopsies and vitamin D sterols, the presence of osteomalacia did correlate most closely with reduction in serum levels of 25(OH)D.[81]

Because of deranged vitamin D metabolism in advanced renal insufficiency, it is tempting to conclude that a deficiency of $1,25(OH)_2D_3$ is a major cause of osteomalacia. However, anephric patients, who cannot generate $1,25(OH)_2D_3$, do not invariably develop histologic features of osteomalacia.[82] The blood levels of $24,25(OH)_2D_3$ are also reduced or absent in anephric patients;[71] however, it is not certain whether this vitamin D sterol is needed for skeletal homeostasis.[72]

The role of the low serum $1,25(OH)_2D$ lev-

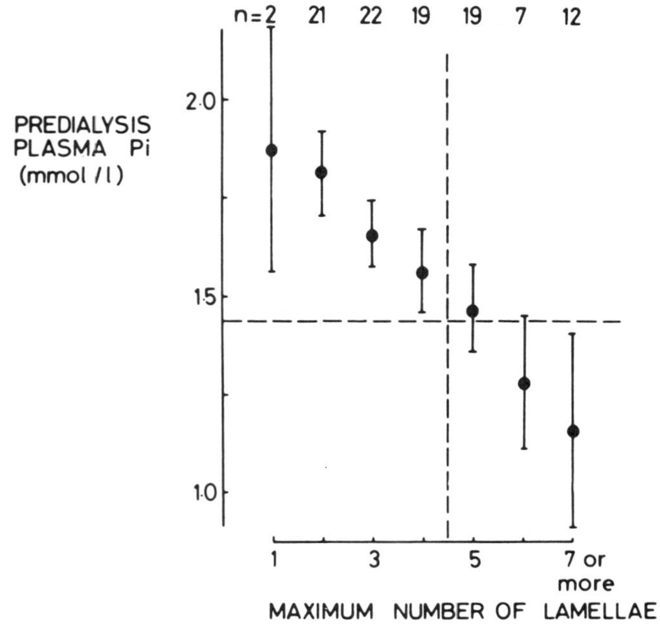

Fig. 15–6. Relation between the predialysis serum phosphorus level (1 mmol/liter = 3.1 mg/dl) and the maximum number of osteoid lamellae seen on bone biopsy. Values above 4.5 lamellae may indicate the presence of reduced mineralization of bone. (From Kanis JA, Adams NP, Earnshaw M, et al: Vitamin D, osteomalacia and chronic renal failure. In Norman AW, Schaefer K, Coburn JW, et al (Eds): Vitamin D, Biochemical, Chemical, and Clinical Aspects Related to Calcium Metabolism. de Gruyter, New York, 1977.)

els in causing osteomalacia in uremia is not known, in part, because it is uncertain how vitamin D produces mineralization of bone under normal circumstances. Thus, it is uncertain whether vitamin D and its metabolites have a direct effect on skeletal mineralization or whether they act to normalize mineralization merely by elevating the levels of the calcium and phosphorus in extracellular fluid which bathes the skeletal matrix. Observations that bone mineralization is normal in vitamin D-deficient animals when serum calcium and phosphorus levels are maintained normal by either dietary means or by the continuous infusions in calcium and phosphate,[83] certainly suggest that vitamin D sterols are not essential for normal mineralization.

PHOSPHATE DEPLETION

Case reports indicate an occasional role of phosphate depletion or hypophosphatemia in causing osteomalacia (Fig. 15–6). Thus, the intake of a low phosphate diet or the overzealous use of phosphate binders can cause phosphate depletion and hypophosphatemia, which is known to impair bone mineralization.[84,85] Such hypophosphatemia is probably the cause of osteomalacic bone disease in only a small number of uremic patients.

Treatment with certain drugs, including phenobarbital, diphenylhydantoin, or glutethimide, can occasionally be implicated in the pathogenesis of osteomalacia in patients with renal failure.[86] The number of cases of osteomalacia arising as a consequence of treatment with these drugs, which may cause osteomalacia by enhancing the degradation of 25(OH)D_3, must be relatively small.

Aluminum Accumulation

A growing body of evidence suggests that aluminum accumulation in bone may be a major factor in the development of osteomalacia in patients with end-stage renal disease (Figs. 15–7 and 15–8). Reports have shown a strong association between the use of untreated, aluminum-containing water for preparing dialysate and the prevalence of osteomalacia and encephalopathy.[87-89] Also, osteomalacic bone disease is less common following initiation of

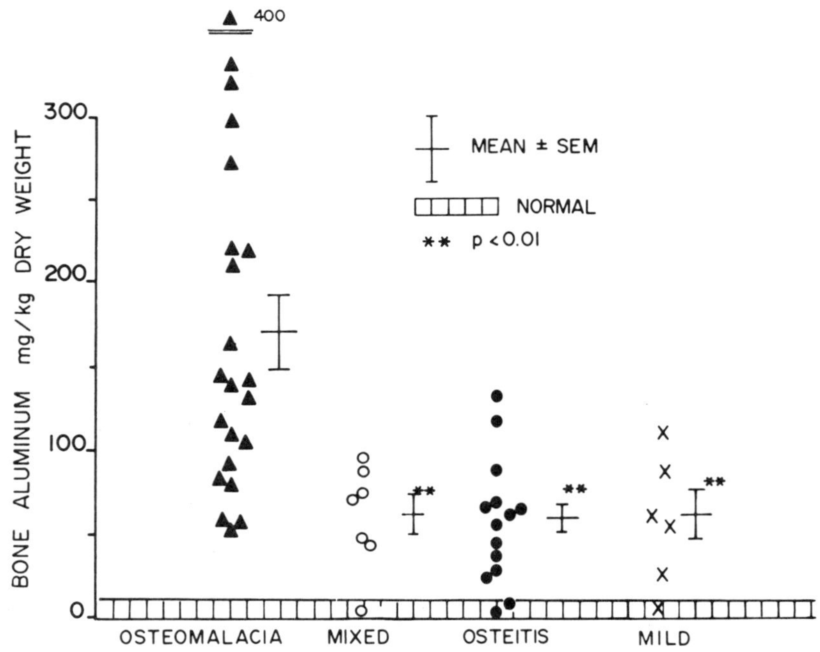

Fig. 15–7. The bone content of aluminum shown according to the type of bone histology in dialysis patients who underwent bone biopsy. The range of normal is indicated by the lower vertical hatched area. Some patients with "mild" disease were later reclassified as *aplastic.* The aluminum level in the patients with osteomalacia differed from that in each of the other groups. (From Hodsman AB, Sherrard DJ, Alfrey AG, et al: Bone aluminum and histomorphometric features of renal osteodystrophy. J Clin Endocrinol Metab 54:539, 1982.)

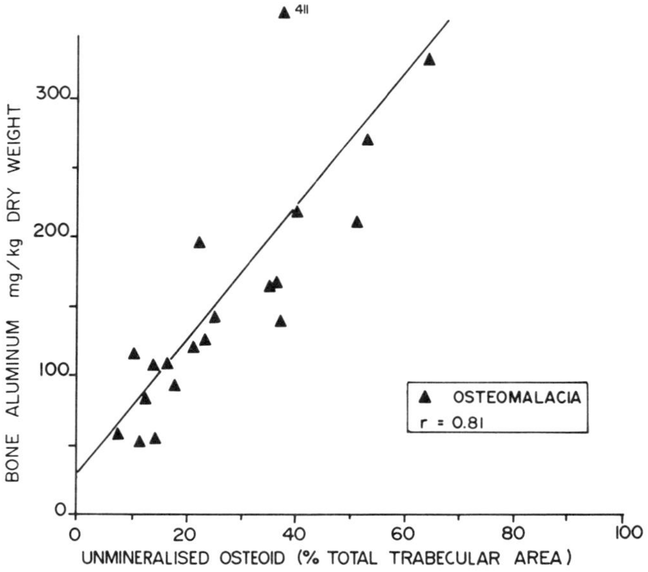

Fig. 15–8. Relation between bone aluminum content and the severity of osteomalacia, as indicated by the fraction of bone with unmineralized osteoid, in dialysis patients with "pure" osteomalacia. Each symbol represents a separate patient. (From Hodsman AB, Sherrard DJ, Alfrey AG, et al: Bone aluminum and histomorphometric features of renal osteodystrophy. J Clin Endocrinol Metab 54:539, 1982.)

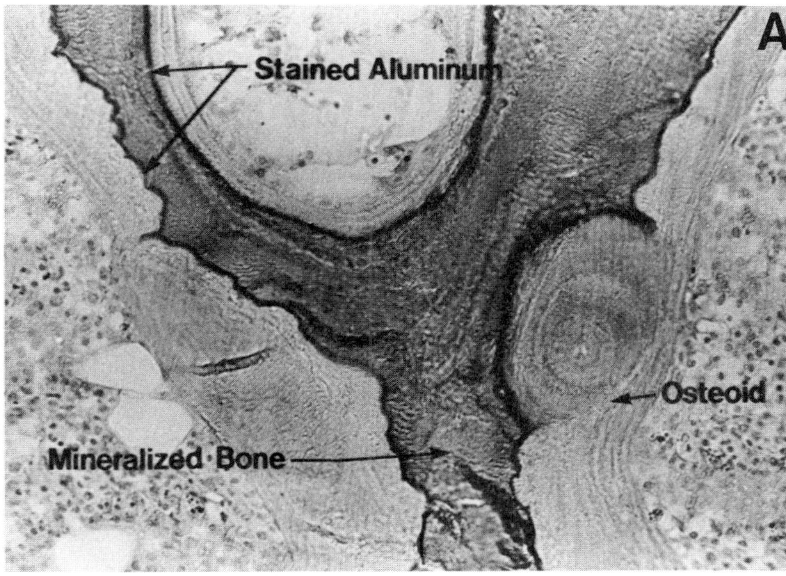

Fig. 15–9. Photomicrograph of trabecular bone in a hemodialysis with osteomalacia which is stained for aluminum with the aluminon stain. There is excess lamellar osteoid, and there is dense staining for aluminum, which can be seen as a bright red zone at the mineralization front. (× 270). (From Maloney NA,Ott S, Alfrey AC, et al: Histologic quantitation of aluminum in iliac bone from patients with renal failure. J Lab Clin Med 99:206, 1982.)

water purification,[89] providing compelling evidence that aluminum or some other contaminant of the water can increase the incidence of osteomalacia. Such epidemiologic observations of an association between osteomalacia and aluminum accumulation is strong, but they do not prove "cause and effect." Studies in experimental animals indicate that the parenteral administration of large quantities of aluminum can cause osteomalacia.[12,90-92] In addition, low-turnover osteomalacia has been described in patients with normal renal function who have received long-term infusions of total parenteral nutrition fluids, which inadvertently contained aluminum.[93] Histochemical techniques[94,95] and studies with the electron probe[13] indicate that aluminum in such cases is localized primarily along the mineralization front (Fig. 15–9). Moreover, the areas of bone showing an increased uptake of aluminum exhibit little or no uptake of tetracycline and no separation of the tetracycline label, providing a strong association between the local accumulation of aluminum and inhibition of bone formation.[96] Preliminary reports suggest that removal of aluminum through use of the chelating agent, desferrioxamine, may lead to improved bone mineralization,[97,98] providing further evidence for a important pathogenic role of aluminum.

Small amounts of aluminum can also enter the body via intestinal absorption during oral therapy with aluminum carbonate or aluminum hydroxide.[99,100] Since the kidney is the only organ capable of excreting the aluminum which does enter the body,[101] it is not surprising that aluminum can accumulate in patients with renal failure. Moreover, the occurrence of aluminum-associated osteomalacia disease in dialysis patients who have used water that was "appropriately treated" and in patients who have never undergone dialysis[102] indicate that pathogenic quantities of aluminum can enter through the enteric route.[100,103]

Another factor that has been implicated as contributing to development of aluminum associated or "pure" osteomalacia is a serum iPTH level that is lower than expected.[11,104] Moreover, total parathyroidectomy has been implicated as predisposing to this syndrome.[11,102,105] Other observations indicate that there is impaired release of PTH in response to hypocalcemia in dialysis patients with aluminum-associated osteomalacia.[57] The mechanisms whereby reduced parathyroid activity may either predispose to aluminum-associated osteomalacia or precipitate its appearance are not known. However, it is possible that the market reduction in bone turnover due to reduced plasma PTH levels may allow more aluminum to accumulate at the mineralization front, where it might impair bone formation even further. Conversely, it has been suggested that an excess of PTH may even be protective,[106] and there may be less aluminum accumulation at the mineralization front with high serum levels of parathyroid hormone and more rapid bone turnover.

Factors Contributing to Osteomalacia in Mixed Lesions

Bone biopsies in dialysis patients[4] indicate that aluminum accumulation is probably important in the pathogenesis of most cases of the "pure" osteomalacia that appear without the coexistence of significant hyperparathyroidism. However, the causes of the osteomalacic component of the mixed renal osteodystrophy may be different. Thus, evaluation of a large number of dialysis patients having bone biopsies suggests that the mean calcium-phosphate product in plasma was lower in patients with the mixed lesions with both osteitis fibrosa and osteomalacia than in patients with osteitis fibrosa alone.[4] It should be noted that even the Ca $\times$ P products observed were above normal, an observation raising the possibility that greater than normal levels of these minerals are needed to achieve normal bone mineralization in a usual patient with renal failure and secondary hyperparathyroidism.

Since there is a deficiency of $1,25(OH)_2D_3$ and $24,25(OH)_2D_3$, it is surprising that osteomalacia is not more common in patients with end-stage renal failure, and the search for the factor or factors which prevent the development of osteomalacia in uremic patients would be useful. With osteomalacia occurring due to other causes, including that which occurs from nutritional vitamin D-deficiency, that associated with mesenchymal tumors, and that developing with sex-linked hypophosphatemic rickets, *hypophosphatemia* is a prominent feature. On the other hand, serum phosphorus levels are elevated or normal in patients with end-stage renal disease. Thus, the absence of hypophosphatemia could be a factor which prevents the development of osteomalacia in uremic patients.

It has been suggested that fluoride may contribute to the genesis of osteomalacia.[107] However, interpretation of data that incriminate the use of fluoride-containing water in preparing dialysate must be tempered with knowledge that this water may have contained other potentially toxic agents, including aluminum. Purification of water supplies with the removal of the fluoride would also have removed aluminum and other trace compounds. Thus, such epidemiologic data do not prove that fluoride is the cause of abnormal bone formation in uremic patients.

Other factors in patients with advanced renal failure may contribute to impaired skeletal mineralization. Thus, acidosis and treatment with heparin may inhibit bone formation.[108] Alterations in collagen synthesis or crystal maturation may contribute to impaired mineralization and be an integral component of this skeletal abnormality.[109] Also, the bone of a uremic patient exhibits the accumulation of magnesium pyrophosphate[110] and the loss of carbonate,[111] alterations which may contribute to defective mineralization. Each of these pathophysiologic features, itself, might alter skeletal homeostasis, but there are no data to indicate that these factors are altered to any greater extent in the uremic patients who develop osteomalacia than in other uremic patients who lack this problem.

Thus, the assignment of a unified process to account for the development of osteomalacia as a component of the mixed renal osteodystrophy in some patients with end-stage uremia is impossible. Indeed, certain pathogenic factors, such as reduced serum levels of both $1,25(OH)_2D$ and $24,25(OH)_2D$ and the skeletal accumulation of aluminum, exist in most patients with far-advanced renal failure, and the factor or constellation of factors causing impaired mineralization remains uncertain.

CLINICAL MANIFESTATIONS

The symptoms and signs arising due to alterations in mineral metabolism and renal osteodystrophy are usually nonspecific and vague. Indeed, bone disease is usually not detected or recognized on the basis of symptoms and signs until the problem is very far advanced. Even when symptoms are marked, physical examination usually reveals little. Because of this, both the patient and his physician either ignore the symptoms or attribute them to the chronic illness associated with dialysis for end-stage renal failure. Certain laboratory and radiographic abnormalities generally appear long before there are any symptoms or signs. There are several specific syndromes and pathologic processes which are observed clinically; these will be considered followed by laboratory and radiographic features.

Bone Pain

Bone pain can be a common manifestation of metabolic bone disease in chronic renal failure. Despite the apparent "specificity" of this symptom, it is often vague and poorly localized. Bone pain is generally insidious in appearance and is often aggravated by weight bearing and sudden changes in position or posture. Positive physical findings are often absent.

Pain is most common in the lower back, hips, and legs, but it may occur in the peripheral skeleton and the joints of the ankles, knees, shoulders, and wrists. The pain is usually not aggravated by cold or damp weather, but it often disappears with rest or relaxation. Severe pain, particularly of the axial skeleton, is more common in patients with osteomalacia than in those with osteitis fibrosa or a mixed lesion. However, the presence or absence of bone pain is nonspecific regarding the prediction of a specific histologic type of bone lesion.

The sudden appearance of pain around the knee, ankle, or heel can suggest acute arthritis. Such pain is usually not relieved by massage or local heat; it is commonly perceived as deep-seated and not in the muscles or joints. Occasionally, pressure over the pelvis or ribs may elicit tenderness, but physical findings are more commonly absent. Evidence for an osseous origin of the pain include radiographic abnormalities,[112,113] typical features on scintiscan,[114] markedly elevated serum iPTH levels, and through exclusion of other causes, such as osteomyelitis.[115]

Since the separation of secondary hyperparathyroidism from aluminum-related osteomalacia is so important, consideration of the clinical features is also of great significance. The typical pain, itself, may provide a rough clue to the cause.

Features of Osteitis Fibrosa

When there is osteitis fibrosa or a mixed lesion, x-rays often reveal subperiosteal erosions, such as that shown in Figure 15–1 and 15–2. Serum iPTH levels are usually strikingly elevated, and the appearance of symptoms is often preceded by a slow progressive rise in serum alkaline phosphatase. The scintiscan of bone may reveal diffuse symmetrical increase in uptake of the diphosphonate in such patients (Fig. 15–3).

Features of Osteomalacia

When osteomalacia is the underlying process, the biochemical and roentgenographic features are less specific; thus, serum iPTH levels may be low, normal, or moderately elevated, and skeletal demineralization and spontaneous fractures may be the only clues to osteomalacia. Although pseudofractures or Looser's zones may be diagnostic of osteomalacia, they are unusual in uremic patients with osteomalacia. The scintiscan of bone may show a general decrease in uptake but with localized uptake at the site of fractures or pseudofractures at the ribs, pelvis, or spine.

In osteomalacia, pain may arise because of a spontaneous fracture, that is, low back pain from a vertebral crush fracture or pleuritic chest pain due to a rib fracture, and such fractures are more common with osteomalacia than osteitis fibrosa. However, a bone biopsy may provide the only means to confirm this diagnosis; this will disclose wide osteoid seams, increased areas of undecalcified osteoid matrix, and evidence for decreased apposition rate as measured by double tetracycline labeling. In cases of pure osteomalacia, bone biopsies also demonstrate a marked accumulation of aluminum, either by histochemical staining[94,95] or by direct biochemical measurement.[14] Other biochemical features often encountered in such patients include periodic episodes of hypercalcemia,[11,116] either occurring spontaneously or concomitant with the intake of small doses of vitamin D sterols or oral calcium salts. Although it has been stated that such patients may exhibit normal plasma alkaline phosphatase levels,[10] the levels can be elevated and such levels do not permit discrimination between pure osteomalacia, a "mixed" lesion or osteitis fibrosa.[11,14] The presence of radiographic features of osteitis fibrosa also does not exclude the presence of osteomalacia, since a delayed mineralization of previous radiographic erosions may occur due to concomitant presence of aluminum-associated osteomalacia;[117] thus, x-ray features of erosions may indicate an earlier pathologic process in such patients.

Muscle Weakness

Proximal myopathy can be particularly serious in patients with advanced renal failure. This muscle weakness affects the proximal muscles of the lower extremities more profoundly than those of the shoulder girdle. Symptoms appear insidiously, with the patient noting difficulty in climbing stairs or in rising from a sitting position without the aid of his arms. Gait abnormalities are common, and the patients may waddle with a typical "penguin" gait. When the upper extremities are involved, the patient may be unable to lift objects above his head or to comb his hair because of the weakness. These symptoms are often so insidious that they are overlooked by both the patient and the physician until there is marked disability.

Physical findings are usually absent, but the muscle weakness is often accompanied by varying degrees of pain, which is felt deep within the bone or around the joints. When the pain is present, it is aggravated by sudden motions of a limb, any effort against gravity, and by weight bearing. This proximal muscle weakness resembles that described in nutritional vitamin D deficiency.[118] The plasma levels of various muscle enzymes, including creatinine phosphokinase, aldolase, and the transaminases, are usually normal, and electromyographic features are nonspecific.

Biochemical abnormalities in the uremic patient with myopathy are variable; serum levels of calcium, phosphorus, and alkaline phosphatase are not distinctive; some patients have elevated serum iPTH levels, while the levels are normal in others. Also, the type of bone disease varies among patients with myopathy. Most of the patients with myopathy show osteomalacia, while occasional patients show striking osteitis fibrosa. Thus, proximal myopathy is more common in uremic patients with severe osteomalacia[11] than it is in those with osteitis fibrosa. Muscle biopsy may show Type 2 fiber atrophy, and features of neuropathy may coexist in many uremic patients.

Pathogenesis of Myopathy

The pathogenesis of proximal myopathy in uremic patients is uncertain; secondary hyperparathyroidism,[119] phosphate depletion,[85] abnormal vitamin D metabolism,[120] and uremic myopathy[121] have been incriminated in case reports. Some patients show striking improvement in muscular strength following treatment with $1,25(OH)_2D_3$ or $25(OH)_2D_3$,[122,123] and this suggests a role of altered vitamin D metabolism. Abnormalities of muscle function occur in vitamin D-deficient animals, which exhibit abnormal muscular relaxation[124] and reduced uptake of radiocalcium by the sarcoplasmic reticulum.[120] Some of these features can be corrected by the administration of vitamin D or $1,25(OH)_2D_3$ to animals with uremia or vitamin D-deficiency,[120,125] observations which support of a role of altered vitamin D metabolism in the pathogenesis of myopathy. However, the lack of demonstration of specific receptors for $1,25(OH)_2D_3$ within muscle is a problem in attributing a $1,25(OH)_2D_3$-deficiency as a cause of the myopathy.

It has been reported that 25(OH)D stimulates the phosphorylation of ADP in muscle, and a reduced action of 25(OH)D was proposed as a cause of uremic myopathy.[126] Myopathy can occur in uremic patients with normal serum levels of 25(OH)D.[11] The observation that the muscle from uremic animals exhibits impaired binding of 25(OH)D could explain why the action of 25(OH)D is altered in uremia despite the presence of normal serum levels.[127] It should be noted that many patients with myopathy show little or no response to treatment with a vitamin D sterol. Myopathy can occur from phosphate depletion and occur due to secondary hyperparathyroidism. Myopathy can also arise as a consequence of muscle ischemia.[121] The favorable response of certain patients with uremic myopathy to 25(OH)D or $1,25(OH)_2D_3$ suggests that in the absence of any contraindication, a therapeutic trial with a vitamin D sterol is warranted.

The occurrence of severe myopathy in patients with aluminum-associated osteomalacia indicates that proximal myopathy has a strong predilection to occur in the presence of osteomalacia. It is possible that inactivity and decreased muscle use secondary to the osteomalacia and bone pain are responsible for the myopathy. However, the presence of profound muscle weakness in the absence of bone pain in certain patients with aluminum-associated osteomalacia militates against this as the total explanation.

ACUTE JOINT SYNDROMES

Several syndromes with acute joint pain occur in patients with end-stage renal failure, and several are associated with renal osteodystrophy and altered mineral metabolism. They include: (1) pseudogout or articular chondrocalcinosis and (2) calcific periarthritis. These conditions must be distinguished from acute gouty arthritis, septic arthritis, and polyarticular arthritis of other causes, which occur in patients with end-stage renal failure.[115]

Pseudogout

Pseudogout is an acute monoarticular arthritis which resembles gout and usually affects the large joints, particularly the ankles and knees. X-rays typically show chondrocalcinosis and joint aspirate reveals positively birefringent, rhomboid crystals of calcium pyrophosphate. This condition appears to be more common in dialysis patients than in the general population;[128] its incidence increases with age, and there may be some relation to parathyroid hormone, in that there is greater frequency in patients with primary hyperparathyroidism.[129] Periarticular calcifications and marked hyperphosphatemia are usually lacking.

Calcific Periarthritis

Calcific periarthritis is characterized by attacks of acute arthritis, with periarticular warmth and redness, and often small joint effusions with synovial fluid lacking crystals under polarizing light.[74,130] X-rays usually disclose small periarticular calcifications, and often there is substantial hyperphosphatemia and other evidence of overt secondary hyperparathyroidism.[130,131] With appropriate reduction of hyperphosphatemia, the syndrome usually does not recur. Presumably, this syndrome arises from the deposition of hydroxyapatite crystals in periarticular tissues. This syndrome and pseudogout respond acutely to nonspecific antiinflammatory drugs.

MISCELLANEOUS MUSCULOSKELETAL SYNDROMES

There are several musculoskeletal syndromes which occur in patients with end-stage renal disease more frequently than in the general population;[115] these conditions, which are either linked to renal osteodystrophy or confused with it, include (1) spontaneous tendon rupture, (2) carpal tunnel syndrome, and (3) olecranon bursitis.

Spontaneous tendon rupture, occurring with only minimal stress, is seen in dialysis patients, particularly those with overt secondary hyperparathyroidism,[132–134] and this condition has also been noted in those with primary hyperparathyroidism.[135] It most commonly affects the quadriceps tendon, although the digits, that is, extensor digiturum longus, can also be involved. Immediate surgical repair is usually successful; subsequent therapy should include appropriate management of the secondary hyperparathyroidism.

Carpal tunnel syndrome is another condition that occurs commonly in patients with long-standing end-stage renal failure;[136] many of these patients exhibit either significant secondary hyperparathyroidism or have aluminum-related dialysis osteomalacia. The association may merely be coincidental and the responsible mechanism is totally unknown.

Olecranon bursitis or "dialysis elbow"[137] is a problem that may be related to pressure on the site during dialysis or the repeated heparin injections rather than be related to altered calcium metabolism.

EXTRASKELETAL CALCIFICATION

Although an association between extraskeletal calcification and uremia has been recognized for many years, this has only become a significant clinical problem with the widespread application of regular dialysis. On the basis of clinical, epidemiological, chemical and crystallographic characteristics, there seem to be three major distinct varieties: (1) visceral, (2) tumoral or periarticular, and (3) vascular. The chemical and crystallographic composition of visceral calcification differs from those noted with either vascular or periarticular calcification, and the x-ray diffraction patterns of visceral calcifications are consistent with amorphous or microcrystalline material.[138,139] This contrasts with the pattern showing carbonate-containing apatite with arterial and periarticular calcifications. Also, there are major peaks of whitlockite following the incineration of visceral calcification, in contrast to the apatite in the calcifications of the tumoral and vascular types. Pyrophosphate is a major constituent of visceral calcifications, while there are only small quantities of pyrophosphate in tumoral or vascular calcifications. The crystals of the apatitic type are more likely to induce inflammation than are the amorphous microcrystals characteristic of visceral calcification.[140]

Periarticular Calcifications

The major pathogenic factor contributing to the periarticular or tumoral type of deposition of calcium and phosphate is hyperphosphatemia, which increases the calcium-phosphate product in the extracellular fluid. Initially, there is believed to be precipitation of amorphous calcium phosphate, which is then spontaneously converted to hydroxyapatite. This type of calcification is associated with increased serum phosphorus levels,[130,131] an increase in Ca × P product and, in some series, higher serum iPTH levels than occur in a general population of dialysis patients.[131] Among the major clinical syndromes is calcific periarthritis, an acute joint syndrome described above. Also, large tumor masses can cause pain or limit the motion of an affected limb. These lesions often show prompt regression following reduction of serum phosphorus levels. A role of parathyroid hormone is not clear; thus, PTH may exert an effect to elevate the serum phosphorus level further, and the hyperphosphatemia may aggravate the extraskeletal calcifications. Such calcifications can clearly appear and be worsened following local tissue injury, and periarticular dystrophic calcification may be difficult to distinguish from that arising due to the renal failure.

Visceral Calcifications

In contrast to the associations noted between hyperphosphatemia and periarticular or tumoral calcifications, the occurrence of visceral calcifications has shown no relationship to hyperphosphatemia or the (Ca) × (PO_4) product in serum[141] or to the presence of clinical features of secondary hyperparathyroidism.[139] It has been suggested that alterations in pyrophosphate metabolism and/or magnesium homeostasis may play a role in leading to visceral calcifications.[140]

The tissues most commonly involved with

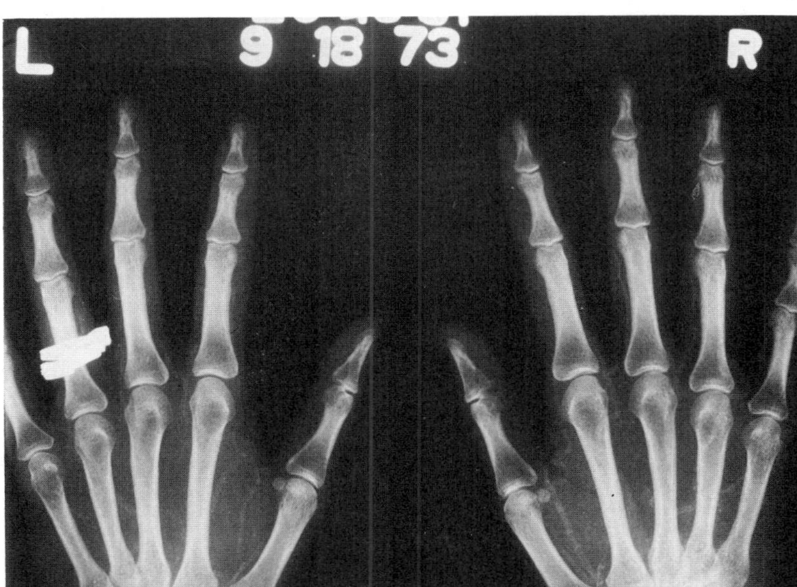

Fig. 15–10. Radiographs of the hands of a dialysis patient showing extensive calcification of the digital arteries.

visceral calcifications include the lungs, heart, and kidney; other organs affected include skeletal muscle, the stomach, and the dura.[142] Visceral calcifications involving the lungs or heart may have serious consequences. Thus, pulmonary calcifications can be associated with severe perfusion-ventilation abnormalities,[141] and cardiac calcifications may be associated with myocardial failure or abnormalities of the conduction system, with congestive heart failure or heart block as consequences.[143,144]

Vascular Calcifications

Two major types of vascular calcifications occur in patients with renal failure: (1) intimal calcifications in atherosclerotic lesions of the aorta and large arteries, and (2) medial calcifications, which involve the media of medium and large arteries. The medial calcifications are more characteristic of advanced renal failure; calcifications occur initially in the medial elastic fibers, the medial ground substance and the internal elastic lamella;[145] eventually, the entire media of the vessel can be involved.[146] Most patients are totally asymptomatic, and the vascular lumen usually remains patent. The pulses and the blood pressure may be difficult to detect or there may be falsely elevated blood pressure because of the rigidity of the vessels. Also, the surgical establishment of vascular access for dialysis may be difficult. Occasionally, these calcifications are associated with ischemia, and the syndrome of calciphylaxis, described below, is commonly associated with severe medial calcifications.[146]

Vascular calcifications, which can be best detected by a lateral radiograph of the ankle or an anteroposterior view of the foot, are observed with increasing incidence with age.[147] Also, their incidence increases both with the duration of dialysis[148] and with the time of follow-up in advanced renal failure without dialysis.[147] Whether there is a relationship between vascular calcifications and either hyperphosphatemia, an increase in (Ca) × (PO_4) product in serum, or high levels of serum iPTH is less certain. There are reports of regression of these lesions after parathyroidectomy[149,150] or following vitamin D treatment and control of hyperphosphatemia, with presumed reduction of serum iPTH levels.[151] However, there was no change in the vascular calcification either after parathyroidectomy or after successful renal transplant in other reports.[147,152]

Miscellaneous Calcifications

Calcifications commonly involve the eye, with either the bulbar conjunctivae and/or the corneal-scleral junction being involved. The latter is known as "band keratopathy." The conjunctiveal calcifications are believed to be hydroxyapatite crystals located beneath the epithelium.[153,154] Acute redness of the eyes, with a granular scratchy sensation, can occur in afflicted patients.[154] In all likelihood, the high local pH in the part of the eye exposed to the environment makes the lesions more prone to develop.

Calcifications can also involve the skin, where they may occur as macular plaques; usually these are clinically insignificant although they may be associated with pruritus. Children with end-stage renal failure usually have a lower incidence of soft tissue calcifications than is observed in adults.[6]

CALCIPHYLAXIS

Calciphylaxis is a rare syndrome with ischemic necrosis of the skin, muscles, and/or subcutaneous fat which develops in patients who have either advanced but stable renal failure, have been treated with dialysis, or who have been engrafted with a functioning kidney transplant.[146] Substantial vascular calcifications of the intimal type are usually present (Fig. 15–10).

Initial symptoms include Raynaud's phenomenon or muscle pain; there is the appearance of cutaneous lesions, with mottled discolorations and livedo reticularis. Ischemic lesions can involve the toes, ankles, and fingers,

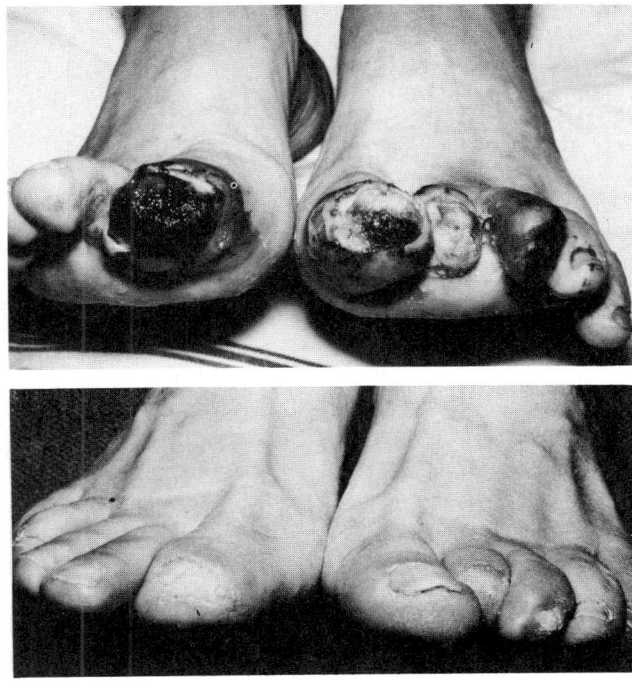

Fig. 15–11. Extensive ischemia and necrosis of the toes in a patient with calciphylaxis (above). The lesions progressed rapidly after successful renal transplantation. Subtotal parathyroidectomy was carried out, followed by prompt healing; the lower photograph was taken 3 months after parathyroid surgery.

but they may also involve the thighs and trunk (Fig. 15–11). Radiographs show extensive vascular calcifications of the medial type involving medium-sized arteries. Biopsy shows ischemic necrosis with fibrosis and intimal and medial calcification of the vessels; an inflammatory reaction is usually minimal. In patients with renal failure, there is usually hyperphosphatemia and serum Ca may be normal or slightly increased. In a successful transplant recipient, serum P may be normal or low but mild hypercalcemia is frequent. Skeletal radiographs often reveal subperiosteal resorption, and renal transplant recipients usually have had features of overt secondary hyperparathyroidism before renal transplantation.

The course of this syndrome may be rapidly progressive, with a patient dying from sepsis;[155] it is indolent and slowly progressive in others. A striking improvement has occurred in certain patients after subtotal parathyroidectomy;[146,149] this observation suggests that the high levels of PTH may play a pathogenic role in causing this problem. In other instances, a marked reduction of serum P to levels of 2.5 to 3.5 mg/dl is associated with gradual resolution of the ischemic lesions and calcifications; this has occurred in patients without evidence of hyperparathyroidism.[146]

The pathogenesis of this syndrome is unknown; it resembles the syndrome of calciphylaxis, induced in experimental animals by various maneuvers, including the induction of renal failure, oral phosphate loading, and treatment with glucocorticoids. The treatment of this syndrome in transplant recipients suggests that glucocorticoid plays a role in man. The condition seems less common than it was in the past, perhaps because of better prevention of hyperphosphatemia in end-stage renal disease.

The treatment of this condition remains difficult: if there is evidence of hyperparathyroidism (i.e., characteristic resorption on radiographs, markedly elevated iPTH levels, and bone biopsy evidence of osteitis fibrosa), parathyroid surgery should be considered, indeed, urgent surgery is at times needed. Vigorous procedures should be initiated to lower the levels of serum P.

OTHER FEATURES: PARATHYROID HORMONE AS A UREMIC TOXIN

A number of signs, symptoms, and biochemical features of uremia have been postulated to occur, at least in part, due to the high levels of parathyroid hormone noted in patients with advanced renal failure. Experimental studies have suggested that various neurobehavioral abnormalities, disturbances of the electroencephalogram, and peripheral nerve function[156] might be related to increased serum iPTH levels. Anemia could be related to the high iPTH levels for various reasons; thus, there is replacement of the marrow elements with peritrabecular fibrosis in some instances. Also, high levels of PTH can inhibit the proliferation of erythroid tissue in vitro,[152] and PTH also was shown to reduce the survival of red cells.[158] High concentrations of PTH may impair myocardial cell function in an in vitro system.[159] Other data have suggested that PTH could play a role in inducing altered carbohydrate tolerance and the hyperlipidemia of renal failure.[160] Additional observations are needed to critically test the theory that there is a role of PTH as a clinically important uremic toxin. Although there are many suggestive data, PTH has been shown only to alter the EEG and perhaps affect psychological testing in uremic subjects (see Chapter 21).

BIOCHEMICAL FEATURES OF RENAL OSTEODYSTROPHY

Alterations of Serum Phosphorus

Serum phosphorus levels are usually in the normal range or even slightly low in patients with early renal insufficiency; however, hyperphosphatemia is common when GFR decreases below 25 percent of normal. With marked renal insufficiency, changes in dietary phosphate intake can readily contribute to the degree of hyperphosphatemia. Some degree of dietary phosphate restriction is useful in these cases, and it is usually necessary to treat such patients with aluminum carbonate or aluminum phosphate gels to bind phosphate in the gastrointestinal tract. Thus, although hemodialysis can remove substantial phosphate, the continued use of aluminum-containing phosphate binders is required presently in 85 to 95 percent of patients undergoing treatment with dialysis.

Intestinal absorption of phosphorus is probably normal in most patients with renal failure.[161] Treatment with an active vitamin D sterol can enhance the absorption of phosphate as well as of calcium,[162] and hyperphosphatemia may become more marked. One thinks of parathyroid hormone as having an effect to reduce the serum phosphorus level because of its known phosphaturic action. However, this phosphaturic effect is quantitatively of little or no importance when renal function is markedly reduced. Thus, a patient with a GFR below 10 ml/min invariably has minimal tubular reabsorption of phosphate (i.e., the percentage tubular reabsorption of phosphorus approaches zero). Under such circumstances, PTH can cause no further phosphaturia, and any increase in bone resorption produced by PTH would enhance the release of both calcium and phosphate into extracellular fluid. Hyperphosphatemia can be aggravated by any acute catabolic stress, and, indeed, the hyperphosphatemia can be marked.

Occasionally, serum phosphorus levels are in the lower range of normal or subnormal in patients with advanced renal failure. In patients with mild renal insufficiency (i.e., GFR, 49–70 ml/min), the mean serum phosphorus levels are often lower than in controls.[28,30,31] A reduction in serum phosphatase may appear because of the overzealous use of phosphate binders or when the dietary phosphate intake is very low. Occasionally, the intestinal absorption of phosphate is below normal in uremic patients. Also, hypophosphatemia can occur during a time of tissue anabolism, that is, during the recovery from marked malnutrition or a catabolic illness.

Alterations of Serum Calcium

The mean level of serum calcium in a group of patients with advanced renal failure is lower than that seen in a control population; however, there is marked individual variation. The causes of hypocalcemia, which are reviewed above, are of considerable interest. Patients with end-stage renal failure often have a slight increase in the complexed fraction of plasma calcium, with more calcium complexed to citrate, phosphate, and other organic anions. Thus, there is a slightly lower blood level of ionized calcium for the total serum calcium concentration. Upon initiation of regular hemodialysis, serum calcium levels increase toward normal in most patients with end-stage renal disease. Occasionally, mild hypercalcemia occurs. In patients with advanced renal failure and marked secondary hyperparathyroidism ("tertiary" hyperparathyroidism), hypercalcemia may appear with excess intake of oral calcium or treatment with various vitamin D sterols; also, hypercalcemia is common in patients with aluminum-related osteomalacia.[11,116] Hypercalcemia can also arise in patients with renal failure due to independent causes unrelated to renal failure, that is, sarcoidosis, malignancy, etc.

During regular hemodialysis treatment, the use of dialysate with calcium levels of 3.0 to 3.5 mEq/L produces postdialysis serum calcium levels that are above normal.[163] By 48 to 72 hours, the serum calcium levels usually have decreased to normal. However, the continued use of a dialysate calcium level of 4.0 mEq/L leads to persistent hypercalcemia in some patients.[164]

Alterations of Serum Magnesium

Serum magnesium levels tend to increase as the GFR falls below 20 to 25 percent of normal, similar to the situation for serum phosphorus levels.[165] Acute hypermagnesemia can develop in uremic patients following an increase in the dietary intake of magnesium or ingestion of magnesium-containing antacids. When dialysate magnesium concentration is 0.5 to 0.8 mEq/L, serum magnesium often decreases to normal. Intestinal magnesium absorption is usually normal in uremic patients;[161] however, severe hypomagnesemia associated with hypocalcemia can develop in uremic patients with malabsorption or severe diarrhea.[166] Reduced secretion of parathyroid hormone and reduced skeletal responsiveness to the action of PTH[167] can contribute to the hypocalcemia which is often observed with severe magnesium depletion.

PLASMA ALKALINE PHOSPHATASE ACTIVITY

Total serum alkaline phosphatase activity reflects enzyme activities arising from hepatic, intestinal, and skeletal sources. Despite this nonspecific nature of total alkaline phosphatase, the finding of a slow, progressive increase in serum level in a patient with end-stage renal failure may be an important clue to the development of overt secondary hyperparathyroidism. Skeletal alkaline phosphatase arises largely from osteoblasts, and a correlation between the skeletal isoenzyme of alkaline phosphatase and bone biopsy findings of osteitis fibrosa has been reported.[168] In uremic patients with aluminum-associated osteomalacia, normal alkaline phosphatase activities have been reported,[10] although this has not been a universal finding.[11,14] With the measure of skeletal isoenzymes of alkaline phosphatase, a good correlation between the plasma activity of skeletal alkaline phosphatase and the response to treatment with an active vitamin D sterol was observed.[168] Other plasma markers of increased bone activity include plasma hydroxyproline,[169] and GLA-protein;[170] presently, these are not widely used.

Serum Immunoreactive Parathyroid Hormone

Serum levels of iPTH are almost invariably increased in patients with advanced renal failure. However, the degree of elevation above normal and the fraction of uremic patients showing markedly elevated levels vary widely with the antisera being used. With use of an antiserum which is directed toward the amino-terminus of the PTH molecule (N-terminal) and which primarily detects intact PTH, serum iPTH levels may be only mildly elevated in uremia.[171] On the other hand, measurements utilizing antisera directed toward the carboxyl, "C-terminal" fragments or the mid-region fragments, most of which are biologically inactive, reveal degrees of elevation that vary from modest to marked in uremic patients;[172] this occurs because these various fragments of PTH are cleared from the plasma largely by glomerular filtration.[18] With a number of assays, correlations between serum iPTH and bone biopsies have been reported.[19,172]

RADIOGRAPHIC FEATURES OF RENAL OSTEODYSTROPHY

Techniques of X-ray Radiography

The techniques commonly employed for bone radiographs often result in poor-quality films that are insensitive to the detection of metabolic bone disease. Thus, bone radiographs are often obtained to identify metastatic lesions or fractures rather than to detect the fine details of skeletal architecture. Use of precise and careful radiographic techniques can substantially improve the sensitivity and precision of skeletal radiographs for both detecting and identifying specific abnormalities of bone.[173]

Standard radiographic techniques and film are generally utilized for x-rays of the spine, pelvis, chest, and shoulder girdle, due to the energy of the x-rays and exposure time employed. Several techniques, however, can enhance both the sensitivity and accuracy of hand radiographs. Meema et al.[174] routinely utilize fine grain film (Kodak, Type M film); these films, which are hand-developed in the same manner as dental films, are then magnified six- to sevenfold with a hand lens. Direct magnification x-rays, enlarged 3.5- to 4-fold, are utilized by others,[173,175] but special equipment is required. Another technique is to utilize a fine grain film, such as mammography film, which can be developed with standard automatic processing; the films are then viewed with enlargement utilizing a hand lens.

There is disagreement about the sensitivity of these methods; those who use direct magnification techniques believe this method is more sensitive than is the visual magnification of standard mammography films with a hand lens. On the other hand, Meema et al.[176] have reported high sensitivity with enlargements of fine gain films utilizing a hand lens. The technique of xeroradiography[175] adds little to these techniques.

Using hand radiographs without magnification, Meema et al.[174] detected subperiosteal resorption in 8 percent of dialysis patients, while 29 percent displayed erosions after magnification with a hand lens. Using mammography film with no magnification, Carr et al.[173] detected superiosteal resorption in 6 percent of cases compared to 56 percent showing abnormalities with magnification films; also, intracortical striations were identified with increased frequency.

Radiographic Features of Osteitis Fibrosa

The most specific and consistent feature of secondary hyperparathyroidism on x-ray film is that of subperiosteal erosion. Hand radio-

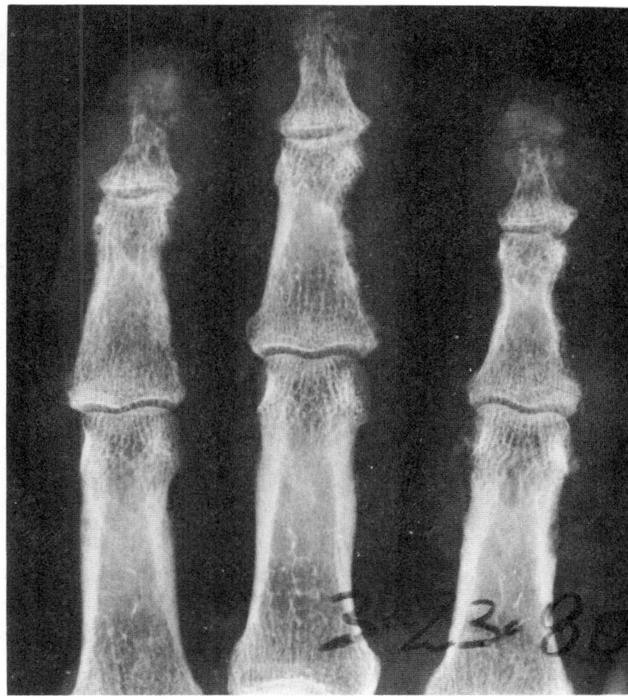

Fig. 15–12. Radiographs of the left hand of a dialysis patient with severe and symptomatic secondary hyperparathyroidism. There are marked subperiosteal erosions, which are evident on the radial surfaces of the 2nd and 3rd digits. Also, substantial resorption of the distal tuft and soft tissue calcification at the site of the tendon insertion are also shown.

graphs evaluated by one of the sensitive methods described above are the most sensitive for detecting these erosions (Fig. 5–12). There is some disagreement about the best site for evaluation; thus, Meema et al.[172] and Ritz et al.[113] emphasized the specificity of subperiosteal erosions on the radial surfaces of the phalanges of the first, second, and third digits. Thus, the presence of subperiosteal erosions correlated well with serum iPTH levels and with histologic features of osteitis fibrosa on bone biopsy. Sundaram et al.[173] reported that abnormalities of the terminal phalangeal tuft could be detected more frequently than erosions on the periosteal surfaces of the phalanges. They noted that "loss of the cortical margin of the tuft" was often accompanied by a fine fraying of the end of the phalanx. Ritz et al.[113] concluded that the abnormalities of the distal tuft, termed *acroosteolysis,* were less specific than were erosions; moreover, the abnormalities correlated less well with bone histologic features of osteitis fibrosa than did phalangeal subperiosteal erosions.

Subperiosteal erosions can be seen elsewhere, including the distal ends of clavicles (Fig. 5–13) and the surfaces of the ischium, pubis, and the long bones at the junction of the metaphysis and diaphysis. There may be problems in differential diagnosis; that is, intraarticular erosions of the humeral head may simulate the findings of erosive arthritis.[178] Other radiographic features of hyperparathyroidism include cortical striations, cystic abnormalities (brown tumors), and periosteal new bone formation.[179]

Correlations exist between the severity of subperiosteal erosions and the degree of osteitis fibrosa detected on bone biopsy. Thus, erosions are most common in patients with severe abnormalities on bone biopsy; the radiographs are often normal in patients with only mild to moderate histologic evidence of bone disease. A small fraction of patients who lack histologic features of osteitis fibrosa may exhibit superiosteal erosions. This may reflect the fact that changes in trabecular bone, with its higher apparent turnover, are revealed on

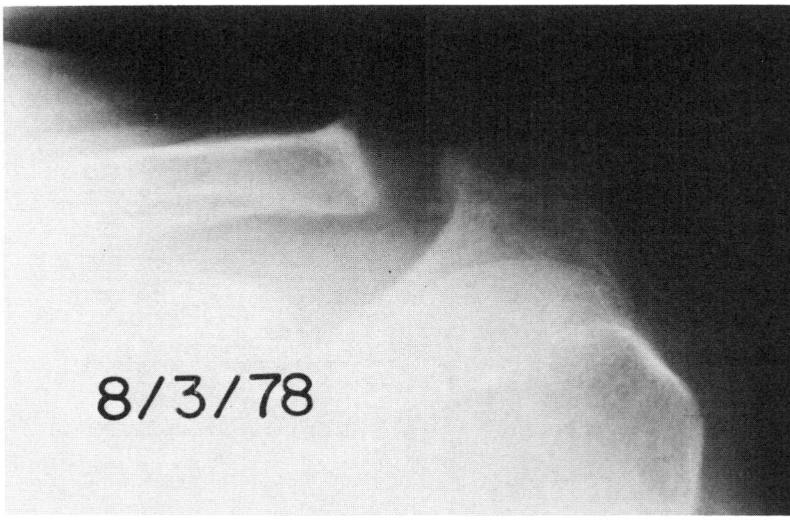

Fig. 15–13. Erosion of the distal end of the left clavicle of the dialysis patient with secondary hyperparathyroidism whose hands are shown in Fig. 15–12. One year earlier, radiographs had shown no abnormality of the clavicle. (Modified from Massry SG, Gordon A, Coburn JW, et al: Vascular calcification and peripheral necrosis in a renal transplant recipient: reversal of lesions following subtotal parathyroidectomy. Am J Med 49:416, 1970.)

bone biopsy, while the radiographic features of erosions reflect abnormalities of cortical bone, with its lesser overall change.

The radiographic abnormalities of the skull that occur with secondary hyperparathyroidism include: (1) a diffuse "ground glass" appearance, (2) a generalized mottled or granular appearance which probably represents areas of increased resorption alternating with sclerotic areas, (3) the presence of focal radiolucencies, and (4) areas with focal sclerosis.[112] Dental x-rays may reveal a loss of the lamina dura of the teeth; however, this finding is nonspecific. Deformities of the pelvis may slowly develop in patients with secondary hyperparathyroidism; these deformities occur due to the rapid remodeling of bone in a part of the skeleton involved with weight bearing.

In uremic children with secondary hyperparathyroidism, abnormalities of the growth zone are common. The distinction between secondary hyperparathyroidism occurring secondary to uremia from true "rickets" may be difficult; with the former there is no widening of the epiphyseal zone, and the metaphyseal lucent zone is very irregular and blends into subperiosteal erosions on the surface of the cortex.[180]

The effect of aluminum accumulation on the radiographic feature of secondary hyperparathyroidism is unclear; however, there are data suggesting that aluminum may prevent the healing of erosions in x-ray despite the significant decreases in serum iPTH and alkaline phosphatase.

Osteosclerosis, commonly observed in the spine or pelvis, is a radiographic feature that is common in those with end-stage renal failure. When it involves the spine, osteosclerosis may show a "rugger jersey" appearance. These features may correlate with other findings of osteitis fibrosa,[181] although an association between osteosclerosis and osteomalacia has also been reported.[182] The explanation for this is uncertain, and the presence of osteosclerosis in a patient with osteomalacia could represent a remnant of prior hyperparathyroidism. Others have noted no relationship between osteosclerosis and the type of skeletal pathology.[183]

Radiographic Features of Osteomalacia

Specific x-ray film features of osteomalacia are unusual in uremic patients, even when biopsy evidence of osteomalacia is profound. Thus, pseudofractures or Looser's zones, the characteristic features of osteomalacia, which appear as wide, straight radiolucent bands abutting upon the cortex of bone and usually perpendicular to or at an angle with the long axis of the bone, are not common in patients with renal failure. The pathogenesis of Looser's zones is unclear; at one time they were thought to represent an erosion around a nutrient artery. More recent views suggest that pseudofractures represent undisplaced, "stress" fractures, with resorption and slow healing around the edge of the fracture. A scintiscan of bone using technetium-labeled diphosphonate may be a more sensitive means for detecting pseudofractures. The other x-ray features of osteomalacia are nonspecific. Some degree of demineralization of the medullary bone and increased cortical striation are commonly seen. Generalized demineralization may be marked in patients with osteomalacia, but this finding is nonspecific. The syndrome, termed *dialysis osteopenia,* is indeterminant as to the nature of this skeletal disorder; such patients may have had some degree of osteomalacia. Fractures, particularly of the ribs, vertebral bodies, and the hips are more common in patients with pure osteomalacia than in uremic patients with osteitis fibrosa or a mixed renal osteodystrophy.[182]

Radiographic Features of Extraskeletal Calcification

Serial radiographs are the best means for detection and evaluation of extraskeletal calcifications, whether they are tumoral, periarticular, or vascular. Calcifications of the lungs may be detected by a scintiscan, using technetium-labeled diphosphonate, at a time when they cannot be seen on x-ray.[184,185] The clinical features of such calcifications, which are reviewed above, vary with their site and extent.

Measure of Bone Mass Using Radiographs

Various techniques, which utilize measurements on x-ray films, have been used to evaluate bone mass. The thickness of the cortex of metacarpal bones on hand radiographs and the ratios of cortical to total width also have been measured. Such measurements show a progressive decrease with time in the "bone mass" of patients with advanced renal disease. This loss of cortical bone mass has not correlated with either the type or extent of bone disease as assessed by iliac crest bone biopsy.[186] In a longitudinal study of patients treated with hemodialysis, there was a low-order correlation between the total dose of heparin given and the rate of fall in metacarpal cortical bone width in the male but not female patients. Other observations suggest that the rate of loss of cortical bone mass relates to the calcium concentration in dialysate.[187]

Other Techniques for Diagnosis

Scintiscans of bone, using ^{99}TcM-labeled diphosphonate, can detect and indicate the severity of skeletal disease in patients with renal osteodystrophy (Fig. 15–14). The degree of secondary hyperparathyroidism or osteitis fibrosa is usually manifested by a symmetrical increase in uptake of diphosphonate both by the axial skeleton and around epiphyseal areas of the long bones.[114] Others have noted increased uptake in osteomalacia, as well.[188] Scintiscans can also identify pseudofractures that are not visible on x-ray in patients with

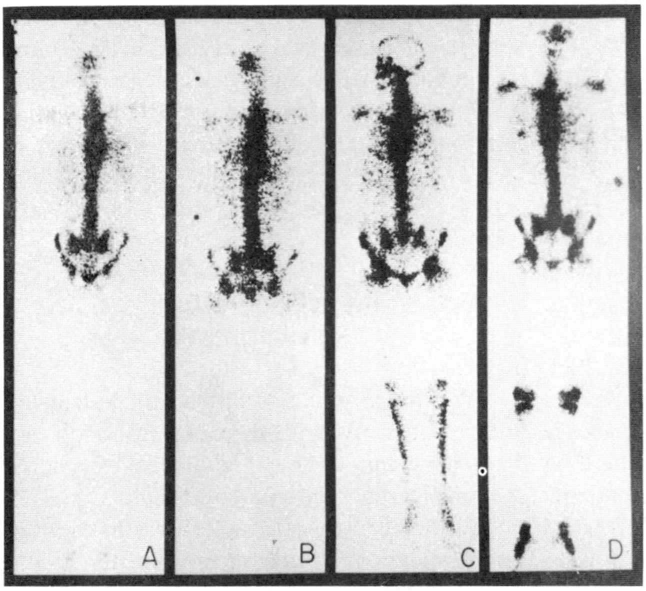

Fig. 15–14. Scintiscans of bone, obtained using the technetium-labelled bisphosphonate, EHDP, in (A) a normal subject and in patients with advanced renal failure (B, C, D) who have varying degrees of secondary hyperparathyroidism, graded as 1, 2, and 3, respectively. (From Olgaard K, Heerfordt J, Madsen S: Scintigraphic skeletal changes in uremic patients on regular hemodialysis. Nephron 17:325, 1976.)

osteomalacia as is shown in Fig. 15–15.[115] Also, the scintiscan can detect ectopic calcification, particularly in the lungs and other soft tissues.

MANAGEMENT OF RENAL OSTEODYSTROPHY

Control of Hyperphosphatemia

A major goal in managing patients with advanced renal failure is prevention of hyperphosphatemia. Thus, data indicating that phosphate retention plays a major role in the pathogenesis of renal osteodystrophy are strong. Moreover, hyperphosphatemia can contribute to the extraskeletal calcification observed in uremia. The serum phosphorus levels of patients undergoing hemodialysis exhibit a "saw tooth" pattern with an abrupt fall during each dialysis; under these conditions a predialysis serum phosphorus level of 4.0 to 5.5 mg/dl is preferred. Two procedures are needed to achieve such levels of serum phosphorus in most renal failure patients: (1) modest dietary phosphate restriction, with total phosphorus intake reduced to below 800 to 1000 mg/day, and (2) ingestion of aluminum-containing, phosphate binders. Thus, aluminum carbonate or aluminum hydroxide render phosphate nonabsorbable by binding it in the gut. The quantity of these phosphate-binders required varies from patient to patient; a small fraction of dialysis patients, e.g., less than 5 to 10 percent, can maintain normal serum phosphorus levels without the need for phosphate binders. The dosage of these compounds required to maintain the serum phosphorus needed varies from 4–6 capsules of aluminum hydroxide per day to as many as 30–40 capsules per day. Such variability depends on the intake of phosphate in the diet and the variation in intestinal absorption of phosphate in individual patients. Thus, most patients with advanced renal failure have normal phosphate absorption, while absorption of phosphate is impaired in other patients.

The suggested association between aluminum accumulation, dialysis encephalopathy,

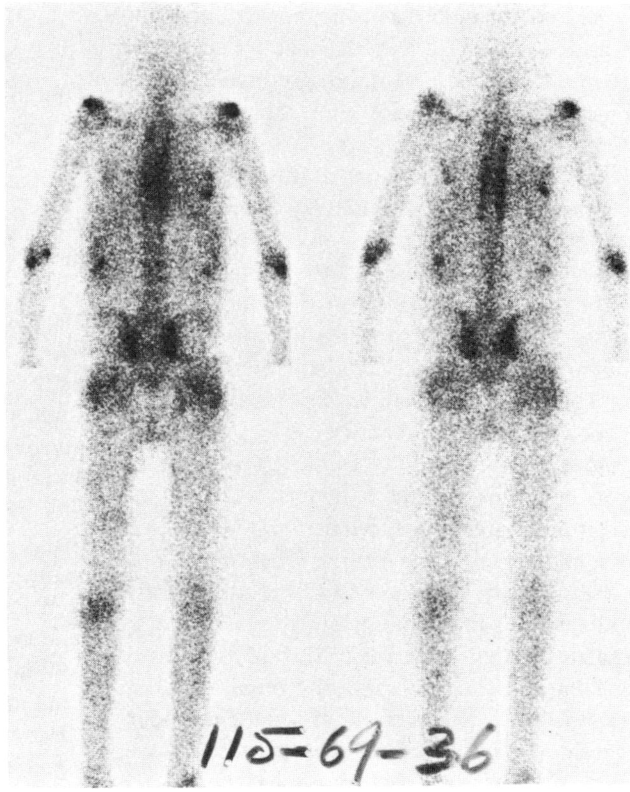

Fig. 15–15. A scintiscan of bone obtained using technetium-labeled EHDP, which shows increased uptake at the sites of bilateral rib fractures and moderate uptake at areas which increased uptake with secondary hyperparathyroidism. This patient had aluminum-related osteomalacia with little evidence of secondary hyperparathyroidism.

and vitamin D refractory osteomalacia has raised doubt about the safety of the long-term use of aluminum-containing phosphate binders in all patients. Epidemics of these syndromes have developed when aluminum was present in the water used for preparing dialysate. However, there are cases of aluminum accumulation that may have developed largely through intestinal absorption of the aluminum given in phosphate binders.[102] In considering the potential risks of aluminum-containing phosphate binders, it seems certain that a large fraction of patients with end-stage uremia will certainly develop severe secondary hyperparathyroidism or extraskeletal calcifications if hyperphosphatemia is allowed to occur. On the other hand, bone disease due to marked aluminum accumulation occurs in only a fraction of dialysis patients utilizing aluminum-free dialysate. Thus, the proper therapeutic choice of continuing to use aluminum-containing phosphate binders in most patients with renal failure seems obvious until phosphate-binding compounds are developed which do not contain aluminum. Alternatives to aluminum compounds that have been explored have included large doses of calcium carbonate.[189] The side effects have limited their use to those with known aluminum-related bone disease.

Adequate Calcium Intake

In patients with renal failure, calcium deficiency should be avoided by maintaining both the dietary intake of calcium at an adequate level and through use of appropriate concentrations of calcium in dialysate. Because of reduced ingestion of dairy products, dietary calcium intake is below normal in most patients with renal insufficiency.[30] It would seem best that dietary calcium intake should be increased. An increase in dietary calcium intake to 1500 mg/day or more can lead to a neutral or even positive balance for calcium in most patients with advanced renal failure and a dietary supplement providing 1.0 g/day of calcium has been recommended.[190,191]

There are practical, as well as theoretical, problems with the routine use of such oral calcium supplements. First, hypercalcemia can occur in uremic patients receiving oral calcium supplements, particularly when they also receive an active form of vitamin D. Thus, when an active vitamin D sterol is given, the efficiency of intestinal calcium absorption by dialysis patients is enhanced, but there is no mechanism for increasing the renal excretion of calcium. Moreover, such a patient undergoes dialysis utilizing a dialysate calcium level that often exceeds the diffusable level of calcium in blood. Thus, hypercalcemia can occur unless the bone accretion rate exceeds the rate of bone resorption. When the skeleton ceases to act as a "sump" for the deposition of calcium, hypercalcemia can occur during therapy with doses of $1{,}25(OH)_2D_3$ that do not increase the blood levels of $1{,}25(OH)_2D_3$ to normal. Thus, there is a theoretical reason why calcium supplementation should not be given to patients who are receiving an active vitamin D sterol. Presently, no controlled data are available to support or refute this possibility.

Dialysate calcium should be at a level that does not lead to a negative calcium balance during dialysis itself, and a dialysate calcium level of 3.0 to 3.25 mEq/liter is probably optimal. With dialysate calcium levels above 3.5 mEq/liter, there is no evidence for any beneficial effect on bone; moreover, there is the chance of persistent hypercalcemia with the possibility of related detrimental effects.

Control of Serum Magnesium

The kidney is the major route for the excretion of magnesium, and it is not surprising that hypermagnesemia often occurs in patients with renal failure following an increase in magnesium intake. This most commonly occurs following the ingestion of a laxative-containing magnesium (i.e., magnesium oxide, cascara sagrada, etc.) or a magnesium containing antacid. A dialysate magnesium level of 0.6–1.0 mg/dl (0.5–0.7 mEq/L) can cause predialysis serum magnesium levels that are only slightly above normal; also, significant hypomagnesemia is prevented during the postdialysis period. A dialysate magnesium of 1.5 mEq/liter produces moderate hypermagnesemia in dialysis patients. The suggestion that a high magnesium level in dialysate may suppress serum PTH levels[192] has not been substantiated by long-term observations.

When intestinal disorders that impair intestinal absorption of magnesium coexist, hypomagnesemia and magnesium depletion can develop in patients with renal insufficiency.[166] This may be associated with decreased secretion of PTH, reduced responsiveness of the skeleton to PTH and the development of hypocalcemia.

Vitamin D Sterols

1,25-DIHYDROXYVITAMIN D_3

Since the kidney is the only organ capable of generating 1,25-dihydroxyvitamin D_3 (calcitriol), the most active known, hormonal form of vitamin D, it seems logical that the use of this sterol should be considered in patients with renal failure.[58] Presently, there are no firm data on when treatment with an active vitamin D sterol should be initiated during the course of renal insufficiency. In three patients with moderate renal insufficiency (i.e., creatinine clearances of 32–51 ml/min), calcitriol treatment for 6 months at 1.0 μg/day led to a slight increase in serum Ca, a fall in serum iPTH, and improved the bone dis-

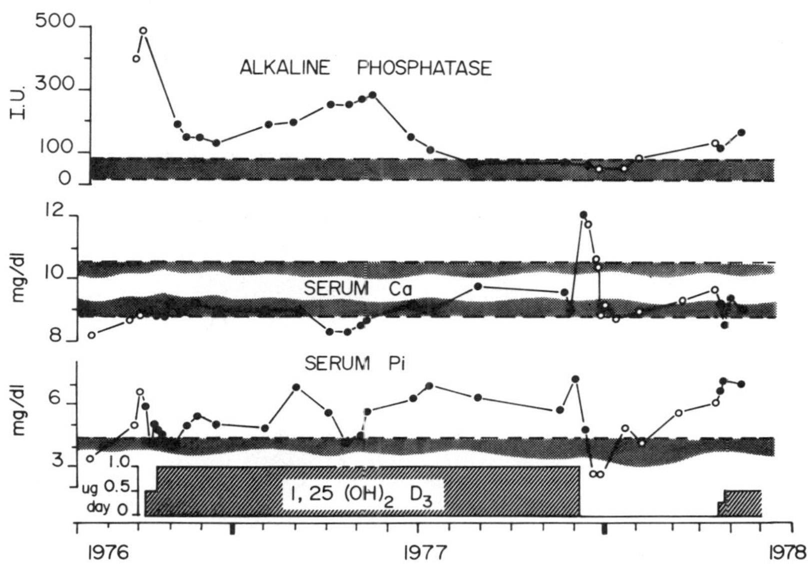

Fig. 15–16. Serial values of serum alkaline phosphatase, calcium, and phosphorus (Pi) in a dialysis patient with severe and symptomatic secondary hyperparathyroidism, who was treated with calcitriol ($1,25(OH)_2D_3$). (From Coburn JW, Brickman AS, Sherrard DJ, et al: Clinical efficacy of 1,25 di-hydroxy-vitamin D3 in renal osteodystrophy. In Norman AW, Schaefer K, Coburn JW, et al (eds): Vitamin D: Biochemical, Chemical and Clinical Aspects Related to Calcium Metabolism. Walter de Gowyter & Co., Berlin, 1977, pp 657–666)

ease. Urinary Ca excretion increased moderately in two of these patients and markedly in the third. Thus, calcitriol was safe and produced beneficial effects.[193] Other trials in patients with more advanced renal failure suggested that a reversible deterioration of renal function occurred during therapy with $1,25(OH)_2D_3$.[194] The mechanism for this change is uncertain; it is possible that the vitamin D sterol enhanced the absorption of both calcium and phosphorus, thereby aggravating hyperphosphatemia and contributing to an increased calcium content of the kidney. Together, these processes might cause more rapid deterioration of renal function. On the other hand, treatment with calcitriol might have a beneficial effect if PTH secretion was suppressed, particularly since PTH could be a factor contributing to the progressive decrease in renal function.

In patients with advanced renal insufficiency and those undergoing dialysis, the features of secondary hyperparathyroidism generally show improvement during treatment with calcitriol. Thus, features of secondary hyperparathyroidism, including the markedly elevated serum iPTH levels, increased alkaline phosphatase activity, radiographic findings of subperiosteal erosions, and bone biopsy features of osteitis fibrosa, generally show improvement during treatment with calcitriol (Fig. 15–16). Patients with secondary hyperparathyroidism and pretreatment hypercalcemia (serum Ca levels above 11.0 mg/dl) often exhibit rapid worsening of hypercalcemia, probably due to the marked parathyroid hyperplasia and also the right-ward shift in "set point," described above. In patients with skeletal lesions of both osteomalacia and osteitis fibrosa, that is, mixed renal osteodystrophy, there is improved mineralization and regression of osteitis fibrosa. Patients with osteomalacia associated with increased bone aluminum and little or no evidence of secondary hyperparathyroidism usually show little or no improvement during calcitriol therapy.[3,11,96]

Whether calcitriol or another active vitamin D sterol should be used as a prophylactic agent in patients with end-stage renal disease but no evidence of osteodystrophy is uncertain. Patients with only mild bone disease may be prone to the development of hypercalcemia.[195,196] When bone turnover is low with a limited rate of bone accretion, stimulation of intestinal absorption of calcium may cause hypercalcemia in a uremic patient with no ability to increase the renal excretion of calcium.

The dosage should be individualized when therapy with a vitamin D sterol is undertaken. Serum calcium levels, per se, have been suggested as a guide for adjusting the dosage. However, measurements of intestinal Ca absorption indicate there is substantial augmentation in all patients receiving calcitriol in doses of at least 0.5 μg/day.[62,197] Thus, the lack of an increase in serum calcium often indicates that there is increased net accretion of bone. Such patients often develop hypercalcemia after the serum alkaline phosphatase had decreased into the normal range (Fig. 15–16). For calcitriol, a dose of 0.5 to 0.75 μg/day may be optimal. Serial levels of alkaline phosphatase as well as Ca and P should be monitored; when alkaline phosphatase activity decreases to normal, the daily dose of calcitriol should be decreased by at least 0.25 μg/day.

Proximal myopathy, another common feature of symptomatic renal osteodystrophy, often shows substantial improvement during treatment with an active vitamin D sterol. Moreover, the myopathy may improve in patients who exhibit varying types of skeletal lesions, including osteitis fibrosa, osteodystrophy, and even pure osteomalacia.[11] It appears that there is little or no relationship between the improvement in proximal myopathy and changes in the various serum biochemical parameters, including calcium, phosphorus and iPTH.

Other Vitamin D Sterols

Several other vitamin D sterols, including vitamin D_2, dihydrotachisterol, and 25-hydroxycholecalciferol (calcifediol) have been utilized in uremic patients.[198,199] 1-alpha-hydroxyvitamin D_3 is extensively used in Europe; available data indicate that 1-alpha-hydroxyvitamin D_3 has actions similar to those of $1,25(OH)_2D_3$.[200,201] Dihydrotachisterol, when given in doses of 0.2 to 1.0 mg/day, can lead to improvement of the bone lesions of uremic secondary hyperparathyroidism.[202,203] Dihydroxytachisterol (DHT) is able to act in patients with end-stage renal disease because of the unique chemical structure of the A-ring of the sterol. Thus, the 3-hydroxyl group of the A-ring of DHT is rotated 180° so that it lies in a "pseudo-1-alpha-hydroxyl" position. This is why DHT can act without the necessity for renal 1-alpha-hydroxylation.

25-hydroxyvitamin D_3 (calcifediol) has been given to dialysis patients who have subsequently been studied with serial bone biopsies.[8] Dosages of calcifediol that increased the plasma 25(OH)D to values above normal often led to reversal of features of secondary hyperparathyroidism. In patients with mixed lesions, there was improved mineralization. The failure of these effects to occur until serum levels of 25(OH)D exceeded normal could indicate that $25(OH)D_3$ only exerts an action when it is given in pharmacologic quantities such that blood levels approach those seen with vitamin D toxicity.

Another sterol under evaluation as an investigational drug is $24,25(OH)_2D_3$. This sterol, which is generated largely in the kidney, is reduced in the serum of patients with advanced renal failure.[71,203] Short-term studies in patients with nutritional vitamin D deficiency suggest that 24,25-dihydroxyvitamin D_3 may have effects that are qualitatively dissimilar from those of $1,25(OH)_2D_3$ alone.[205]

Serum Ca levels fell slightly and alkaline phosphatase levels increased in dialysis patients given $24,25(OH)_2D_3$.[74] Moreover, certain uremic patients with aluminum associated osteomalacia showed improved mineralization of bone when given $24,25(OH)_2D_3$ compared to results with $1,25(OH)_2D_3$ alone.[206] Although such data suggest that $24,25(OH)_2D_3$ may exert actions different from those of $1,25(OH)_2D_3$, the results in experimental animals provide no evidence for a necessary action for this sterol.[72] Further physiologic or pharmacologic studies are needed to clarify any physiologic or pharmacologic role of $24,25(OH)_2D_3$.

PARENTERAL VITAMIN D STEROLS

Of considerable interest are the preliminary observations of the effects of parenteral calcitriol.[70] In this study, doses of $1,25(OH)_2D_3$, 0.50 to 4.0 μg were given intravenously thrice weekly during each dialysis procedure to hemodialysis patients; this treatment was associated with a substantial reduction in serum iPTH levels in all the dialysis patients evaluated. Moreover, an initial reduction in serum iPTH levels was observed before there was any detectable increase in serum calcium level. Upon discontinuing the calcitriol, serum iPTH levels increased toward pretreatment values. These observations may be consistent with a direct effect of the vitamin D sterol on the parathyroid glands to reduce the secretion of PTH by the parathyroid glands. The reason why similar suppressive effects of calcitriol have not been noted consistently following oral administration of the sterol is not readily apparent. Following its oral administration, the intestinal absorption of calcium could be stimulated to a greater degree than following its intravenous administration. If this were the only reason for the difference between oral and intravenous dosage, sterols such as 1-alpha-(OH)-vitamin D_3 or dihydrotachysterol would be expected to be superior to $1,25(OH)_2D$, since these two sterols must undergo 25-hydroxylation in the liver prior to their action. This has not proven to be the case. Another explanation might be the substantial elevation of serum levels of $1,25(OH)_2D$ that would be expected following the intravenous injection of the sterol in contrast to the rather modest increments observed following the oral administration of doses of 0.25 to 0.50 μg/day.[20]

PARATHYROID SURGERY

With the appropriate medical therapy described above, the degree of secondary hyperparathyroidism is usually reduced and improvement of osteitis fibrosa often occurs. However, surgical removal of hyperplastic parathyroid tissue may be indicated under certain circumstances. These include overt secondary hyperparathyroidism, characterized by a combination of radiographic features of bone erosions or bone biopsy features of osteitis fibrosa plus markedly elevated serum iPTH levels. Patients with such features may *require* parathyroid surgery under certain conditions which include: (1) persistent elevation of serum calcium to above 11.5 mg/dl; (2) an increase in serum (Ca) × (PO_4) product above 75 to 80 and progressive soft tissue calcification that persists despite vigorous efforts at phosphate restriction; (3) progressive skeletal lesions of secondary hyperparathyroidism, particularly when there are severe or debilitating symptoms and when a prompt clinical response to treatment is important; (4) intractable pruritus which is recalcitrant to standard medical therapy; and (5) the syndrome of calciphylaxis.

One important consideration is the availability of a surgeon who is highly experienced with parathyroid surgery. It is imperative that the four parathyroid glands be identified, since the existence of a single parathyroid adenoma in a patient with chronic renal failure is exceedingly uncommon. The favored surgical approach should either be (a) removal of 3½ to 3¾ glands, or (b) total parathyroidectomy with transplantation of parathyroid tissue to the forearm. During the postoperative period, marked hypocalcemia, hypophosphatemia, and hypomagnesemia can occur, with its severity depending on the extent of osteitis fibrosa noted preoperatively.[208] Preoperative treatment with calcitriol may aid in preventing or minimizing the hypocalcemia. During the postoperative period, severe tetanic seizures, which can cause fractures, may occur. Of interest, they usually occur during or immediately after hemodialysis. Therapy with supplemental calcium and an active vitamin D sterol may be needed for weeks or months. The decrease of the plasma alkaline phosphatase to normal may be an indication that such treatment can be reduced or even discontinued. It is imperative that there be efforts to prevent hyperphosphatemia after surgery to prevent recurrence of secondary hyperparathyroidism.

Management of Aluminum-associated Osteomalacia

Of all the syndromes of osteodystrophy encountered in patients with advanced renal failure, none has been so refractory to treatment as that of "dialysis osteomalacia," or "aluminum-related osteomalacia." Many patients had coexistent encephalopathy and these often died.[89] However, many such patients have suffered prolonged disability.[11] With institution of dialysis utilizing water free of aluminum, there has generally been little, if any change, in individual patients.[11] Early reports utilizing oral calcium carbonate instead of aluminum-containing compounds for phosphate binding,[189] have not been corroborated in large numbers of patients.

Preliminary and initial reports utilizing the chelating agent, desferrioxamine to treat bone disease associated with aluminum deposition have indicated substantial promise.[97,98] There seems to be little doubt that there is a substantial increase in aluminum removal during hemodialysis following the administration of this chelating agent. This contrasts to the rather ineffective removal of aluminum during regular hemodialysis, per se.[103] The reports on desferrioxamine therapy are preliminary but do suggest that chelation therapy may, indeed, hold substantial promise (Fig. 15–17). There have also been reports of rather substantial improvement of this syndrome following renal transplantation.[98]

ALTERED CALCIUM METABOLISM IN OTHER RENAL DISORDERS

Nephrotic Syndrome

Certain alterations of calcium metabolism, including hypocalcemia, hypocalciuria, and reduced intestinal absorption of calcium, have been described in patients with the nephrotic syndrome. The hypocalcemia exists in large part because of the decrease in serum albumin concentration with the consequent reduction in protein-bound calcium; however, several reports indicate that the ionized calcium activity, itself, can be reduced, particularly in patients with severe and long-standing nephrotic syndrome.[15,209,210]

Considerable data indicate that vitamin D metabolism is abnormal in patients with the nephrotic syndrome, and this abnormality probably accounts for most of the alterations in calcium metabolism that occur. The serum levels of 25(OH)D have been noted to be low.[15,211,212] Part of the reason may be that urinary excretion of 25(OH)D is markedly increased in these patients, due in part to concomitant increased urinary excretion of vitamin D-binding protein (a globulin with molecular weight of 59,000 daltons). Indeed, there was good correlation between the urinary excretion of 25(OH)D and the total protein excretion,[213] a reflection of the overall increased glomerular permeability in patients with the nephrotic syndrome. In some nephrotic patients, the serum levels of $1,25(OH)_2D$ have also been found to be low, presumably due to enhanced urinary losses of this sterol as well.[214] Thus, it seems likely that these altera-

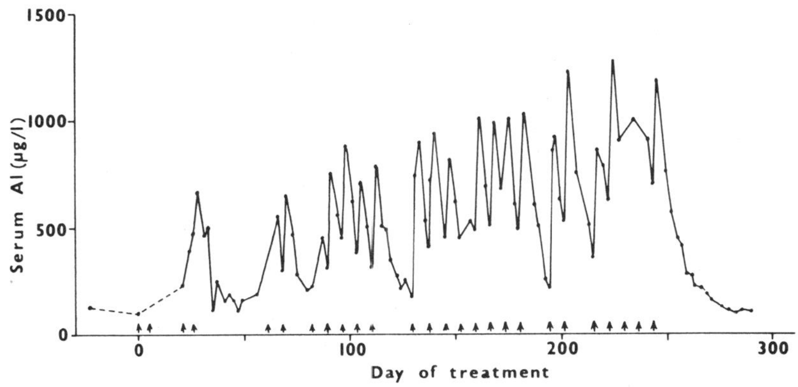

Fig. 15–17. Serial serum levels of aluminum in a patient with "dialysis encephalopathy" and symptoms of aluminum-related osteomalacia while the patient received intermittent injections of desferrioxamine, each of 6 g at the time of each arrow. There is substantial increments in serum Al after the desferrioxamine; during a 1-year period there was substantial improvement in both the neurologic and skeletal symptoms. (Modified from Ackrill P, Ralston AJ, Day JP, Hodge KC: Successful removal of aluminum from patient with dialysis encephalopathy. Lancet 2:692, 1980.)

tions in vitamin D metabolism account for most of the abnormalities in calcium metabolism noted. Reduced intestinal absorption of calcium has been noted in some patients,[15] and marked abnormalities of calcium homeostasis seem to be more prevalent in nephrotic children who have had the disease for a long period of time.[109,215] It should be noted that not all patients with the nephrotic syndrome exhibit reduced intestinal absorption of calcium;[216] this may be due to greater intake of vitamin D, more exposure to sunshine, or lower urinary losses of the vitamin D-binding protein.

The effects of these abnormalities on the skeleton have been variable. Rather substantial radiographic abnormalities of bone have been noted in children with the neprotic syndrome.[217] Date on bone biopsies in patients with the nephrotic syndrome have been variable. Evidence of osteomalacia and/or osteitis fibrosa have been observed in some adult patients;[218] on the other hand, normal bone biopsies have been reported in other studies of nephrotic adults.[219,220] Whether prophylactic vitamin D therapy should be given to all patients with the nephrotic syndrome is not apparent at present. The administration of vitamin D itself did result in an increase in serum 25(OH)D levels and the concentrations of $1,25(OH)_2D$ that were low returned to normal.[221]

Acute Renal Failure

Alterations of mineral metabolism and homeostasis are common in patients with acute renal failure (see Chapter 13). Because the pathogenetic factors are of recent onset and may be less complex than those existing in chronic renal failure, the abnormalities identified are of considerable interest. Hypocalcemia, hyperphosphatemia and elevated serum levels of iPTH have been noted early in the course of acute renal failure.[35,222,223] The hypocalcemia can be quite marked and persist well into the diuretic phase of acute renal failure. Because the hyperphosphatemia can be marked, it has been thought that the increase in serum phosphorus is the major factor responsible for hypocalcemia. However, various studies have shown no relation between serum calcium and phosphorus levels;[35] and hypocalcemia developed in patients with acute renal failure who had normal serum phosphorus levels.[224] There is good evidence for skeletal resistance to the calcemic action of parathyroid hormone in patients with acute renal failure.[35] In addition, animals with acute renal failure show a subnormal increase in serum calcium following a standardized infusion of PTH.[37] Moreover, the administration of $1,25(OH)_2D$ either alone or with $24,25(OH)_2D$ resulted in substantial improvement of the calcemic response to PTH,[37,38] an observation suggesting that vitamin D metabolism is abnormal in acute renal failure.

To date, the alterations of vitamin D metabolism in patients with acute renal failure have not been well defined. Pietrek et al[225] reported a fall in the plasma levels of 25(OH)D during the course of acute renal failure, with the rapid rate of decrease in its concentration most compatible with enhanced turnover of $25(OH)D_3$. These observations have not been confirmed, and Llach et al.[226] reported normal serum levels of 25(OH)D in patients with acute renal failure due to rhabdomyolysis. Plasma levels of $1,25(OH)_2D$ were subnormal in the patients with rhabdomyolysis; however, data on levels of vitamin D sterols in patients with acute renal failure due to other causes were not available for comparison. The possibility that the reduced levels of $1,25(OH)_2D$ may lead to altered interactions between serum calcium and PTH secretion in patients with acute renal failure is suggested by the observations of Madsen et al.[227] These workers reported that the parenteral administration of $1,25(OH)_2D$ caused a reduction in the high serum iPTH levels noted in patients who had acute renal failure. The patients were undergoing peritoneal dialysis with dialysate containing a low calcium concentration.

Marked hypocalcemia can occur in patients with acute renal failure, particularly when the acute renal failure occurs in association with rhabdomyolysis. This has been attributed to several factors, including the possible sequestration of calcium within the damaged muscle.[228-230] However, a recent study noted that hypocalcemia was no more common in patients with acute renal failure due to rhabdomyolysis than in acute renal failure arising from other causes.[224] During acute renal failure, both in experimental animals,[231] and in patients,[223] there is considerable evidence that the secondary hyperparathyroidism contributes to abnormalities of the EEG and perhaps to other central nervous system (CNS) abnormalities, as well.

During the diuretic phase of acute renal failure, serum phosphorus levels often decrease to normal or below. The factors accounting for the fall in serum phosphorus may include the osmotic diuresis occurring during recovery, the high serum iPTH levels causing phosphaturia, the presence of extracellular volume expansion, and the intracellular shift of phosphate occurring as the nutritional and metabolic state of the patient improves.

Hypercalcemia is occasionally noted during the diuretic phase and rarely even before the onset of diuresis in those with acute renal failure due to rhabdomyolysis.[224] The gret majority of these patients have had hypocalcemia early during the oliguric period. The mechanism for the hypercalcemia is probably multifactorial; it has been postulated to occur because of persistent and inappropriate secretion of PTH and the increased serum levels of $1,25(OH)_2D$;[226] it has also been attributed to the release of calcium from damaged muscle.[228,232] However, there are reports of cases with extensive tissue deposits of calcium who failed to develop hypercalcemia[232] and of patients with hypercalcemia and undetectable serum iPTH levels.[228] Occasionally the hypercalcemia can be marked and symptomatic. When treatment for hypercalcemia is needed, saline infusion and furosemide,[233] or calcitonin may be effective; if they are ineffective, a trial with mithramycin may be considered. Unless renal functional recovery is nearly complete, phosphate therapy should be used with great caution. Also, the potential deleterious effects of glucocorticoids in a patient recovering from acute renal failure should be carefully considered before initiating treatment with such an agent.

Mineral Metabolism Following Renal Transplantation

Many aspects of the altered mineral metabolism and bone disease present in patients with chronic renal failure are corrected following the transplantation of a well-functioning kidney. On the other hand, other new problems, such as aseptic necrosis of bone, develop with increased frequency. The high levels of serum iPTH often decrease toward normal[234,235] and there is recovery of the ability to generate $1,25(OH)_2D_3$ [236] after implanting of a normal functioning kidney. In addition, the functioning kidney contributes to the regulation and homeostasis of calcium and phosphate metabolism. The major factors causing continued alterations of mineral homeostasis following transplantation include the degree of function of the renal homograft, the degree of hyperplasia of the parathyroid glands, the levels of serum iPTH both before and after surgery, and the dosage of glucocorticoids taken by the patient. During the immediate posttransplant period, the renal handling of calcium, phosphate, and magnesium are affected by the degree of osmotic diuresis, the presence of extracellular volume expansion, and various hormonal factors, such as parathyroid hormone, which affects renal tubular reabsorption of calcium and phosphate. The major problems affecting mineral homeostasis identified in renal transplant recipients are hypercalcemia, hypophosphatemia, and asceptic necrosis of bone.

ALTERATIONS OF SERUM CALCIUM

When hypercalcemia appears, it makes its appearance weeks to months following renal transplantation; in one review hypercalcemia was noted in 28 percent of transplant recipients.[237] In general, such hypercalcemia has been attributed to the persistence of secondary hyperparathyroidism, and there has been the view that the function of the parathyroid glands can be autonomous in renal transplant recipients.[238] However, the parathyroid glands usually respond to appropriate physiologic stimuli.[239] With improved ability of the transplanted kidney to excrete phosphate and to generate $1,25(OH)_2D$ and the recovery of bone to show a more normal calcemic response to PTH, serum calcium levels usually rise with a fall in serum iPTH. Presumably, there will ultimately be involution of the hyperplastic glands in most cases.[240,241] In one series of transplant patients, elevated serum iPTH levels were present in 70 percent of normocalcemic patients, while the levels were elevated in all the hypercalcemic patients.[242] Continued secretion of PTH could occur due to the hyperplastic mass of "normally" functioning tissue, as has been shown to occur following transplantation of increased number of normal glands to normal rats.[243] Continued secretion of excess PTH might occur because of persistence of the shift of the "set point" described earlier, or be due to both factors. The magnitude of increment in serum iPTH occurring in response to an acute hypocalcemic stimulus has been shown to correlate closely to the magnitude of parathyroid hyperplasia.[239] Studies carried out in renal transplant recipients with persistent hypercalcemia indicate that substantial parathyroid hyperplasia can persist. Studies on the "set point" of these glands are not yet available to evaluate its possible contribution.

When hypercalcemia is encountered in a transplant recipient, other causes must be considered, and one factor that often occurs is hypophosphatemia with phosphate depletion.[240] The administration of phosphate led to improvement of the persistent hypercalcemia in certain cases.[240] Another factor that may contribute to the hypercalcemia is the rapid dissolution of extraskeletal calcifications;[244] This is probably not an important factor in patients who are well managed prior to the renal transplant.

Hypercalcemia, occurring during the early posttransplant period, has been associated with previous treatment with vitamin D_2 or D_3.[241,242] Presumably, this may occur because of the ability of the transplanted kidney to generate $1,25(OH)_2D_3$ and to the continued secretion of PTH to stimulate this conversion. Hypercalcemia is far more uncommon after the short-acting vitamin D sterols have been administered,[245] although an increase in serum calcium can also occur as the dosage of prednisone is reduced in transplant patients receiving $1,25(OH)_2D$.[246] Hypercalciuria is not common following renal transplantation,[247] although it can occur in patients who have persistent hypercalcemia. Under unusual circumstances, renal stones can develop in these patients.

Hypocalcemia can also occur during the posttransplant period. It can occur during a period of rapid skeletal remineralization[248] and hypocalcemia can occur due to hypomagnesemia which develops as a consequence of increased urinary magnesium losses.[249] An increase in the dosage of glucocorticoids, particularly during the early posttransplant period and before there is recovery of renal function, can cause a fall in serum calcium.[246]

ALTERATIONS IN SERUM PHOSPHORUS

A reduction in the serum phosphorus level is particularly common in renal transplant recipients, and serum phosphorus levels below 2.5 mg/dl during the first 6 months after transplant surgery have been reported in 60 to 70 percent of transplant recipients.[250,251] Several factors contribute to the hypophosphatemia, including: (1) reduced intestinal absorption due either to the antacids commonly ingested by these patients, an effect of glucocorticoids on the intestinal phosphate absorption or a primary intestinal abnormality in gut phosphate transport,[252,253] increased renal excretion of phosphate either due to excess PTH or a primary tubular defect; and (3) from the rapid remineralization of bone. Of these potential mechanisms, the continued renal loss of phosphate is probably the most common cause of long-lasting hypophosphatemia following renal transplantation. In patients with hypophosphatemia, the identification of the responsible mechanism involves the measurement of serum iPTH and renal phosphate handling (i.e., $TmPO_4/GFR$). In instances with low or undectable serum iPTH levels, the identification of renal phosphate wasting suggests a primary tubular defect.[250] When hypophosphatemia is associated with elevated serum iPTH levels and hypercalcemia coexists, parathyroid surgery may be indicated if there is no improvement following oral phosphate supplementation. Because of the tendency for the parathyroid glands to ultimately regress, this should be done with caution.[240]

The modest hypophosphatemia observed in transplant recipients is usually asymptomatic, and there are few sequelae when the serum phosphorus level is only slightly below 2.5 mg/dl. However, there have been unusual cases with marked phosphate depletion and osteomalacia has been described.[254] When serum phosphorus levels are very low, supplements of oral phosphate are clearly indicated.

ASEPTIC NECROSIS OF BONE

Aseptic necrosis of bone continues to be a major complication of renal transplantation,[255,256] occurring in 5 to 25 percent of those with successful renal transplants who received glucocorticoids for a period of several months to years.[237] Its pathogenesis is uncertain and probably multifactorial. Thus, there are data suggesting that the dosage of glucocorticoids plays a role,[257,258] while other groups have found no relationship between its incidence and the glucocorticoid dosage.[256,259,260] The mechanism whereby glucocorticoids may produce this effect is unclear; it may be related to the stimulation of increased numbers of fat cells with a subsequent increase in intraosseaous pressure.[261] It has been suggested that

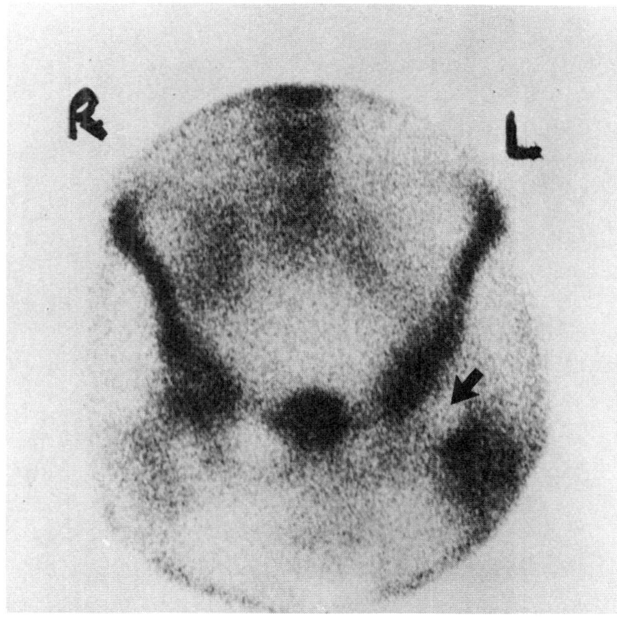

Fig. 15–18. Scintiscan showing early changes of aseptic necrosis of bone. Anterior view of the technetium diphosphate bone scan which demonstrates reduced uptake at the left femoral head (arrow); the changes are consistent with asceptic necrosis of the femoral head. (From Wright RS, Mehls O, Ritz E, Coburn JW: Musculoskeletal manifestations of chronic renal failure, dialysis, and transplantation. In Bacon P, Hadler N, Eds: Renal Manifestations in Rheumatic Disease. Butterworths, London, 1982.)

glucocorticoids may predispose to the development of multiple microfractures, which may cause impaired blood supply with subsequent bone necrosis;[262] others have challenged this view.[263]

Another risk factor for the development of aseptic necrosis is the degree of secondary hyperparathyroidism. Thus, aseptic necrosis has been reported in nontransplanted uremic patients with severe osteitis fibrosa.[264] Also, there are several reports indicating that aseptic necrosis had a higher incidence in transplanted patients showing evidence of hyperparathyroidism.[257,260,265] The finding of a very low incidence of aseptic necrosis in diabetic transplant recipients is of interest in that these patients had significantly lower serum iPTH levels than were observed in uremic patients without diabetes.[256]

Aseptic necrosis is recognized either by radiographs or from scintiscans of bone, with the latter technique more sensitive to detect earlier changes (Fig. 15–18). The early management should be conservative to allow time to ascertain whether spontaneous regression will occur. In more advanced cases, the surgical approach with hip replacement has often been successful.[266] With aseptic necrosis involving sites other than the hips, for example, the knees and shoulders, there is often spontaneous regression without the need for extensive surgical correction or reconstruction. It would seem that the application of more aggressive therapy of secondary hyperparathyroidism prior to renal transplantation might result in a lower incidence of this troublesome complication, although there are no prospective trials to evaluate this.

GROWTH IN CHILDREN

Following renal transplantation, there may be improved growth if the transplant is performed with a bone age less than 12 years, if there is normal or nearly normal function of the graft, and if the dosage of glucocorticoids can be maintained at the lowest possible dose.[267] Alternate day steroids have been suggested to aid in attaining normal growth,[268] but if the GFR falls below 50 ml/min, there is slowing of growth.

REFERENCES

1. Malluche HH, Ritz E, Lange HP: Bone histology in incipient and advanced renal failure. Kidney Int 9:355, 1976
2. Sherrard DJ, Baylink DJ, Wergedal JE, Maloney N: Quantitative histological studies on the pathologenesis of uremic bone disease. J Clin Endocrinol 39:119, 1974
3. Sherrard DJ, Coburn JW, Brickman AS, et al: Skeletal response to treatment with 1,25-dihydroxy-vitamin D in renal failure. Contrib Nephrol 18:92, 1980
4. Sherrard DJ, Ott S, Maloney N, et al: Uremic Osteodystrophy: Classification, cause and treatment. In Frame B, Potts JT, Eds: Proceedings of the Symposium on Clinical Disorders of Bone and Mineral Metabolism. Exerpta Medica, Amsterdam, 1984
5. Rodan G, Martin TJ: The role of osteoblasts in hormonal control of bone resorption: A hypothesis. Calcif Tiss Int 33:349, 1981
6. Ritz, E, Mehls O, Bommer, J, et al: Vascular calcification under maintenance hemodialysis. Klin Wochenschz 55:375, 1977
7. Frame B, Parfitt AM: Osteomalacia: Current concepts. Ann Intern Med 89:966, 1978
8. Frost HM, Griffith DL, Jee WSS, et al: histomorphometric changes in trabecular bone of renal failure patients treated with calcifediol. Metab Bone Dis Rel Res 2:285, 1981
9. Delling G, Luhmann H, Bulla M, et al: The action of $1,25(OH)_2D_3$ on turnover kinetic, remodelling surfaces and structure of trabecular bone in chronic renal failure. Contrib Nephrol 18:105, 1979
10. Alvarez-Ude F, Feest TG, Ward MK, et al: Hemodialysis bone disease: Correlation between clinical, histologic and other findings. Kidney Int 14:68, 1978
11. Hodsman AB, Sherrard DJ, Wong EGC, et al: Vitamin D-resistant osteomalacia in hemodialysis patients lacking secondary hyperparathyroidism. Ann Intern Med 94:629, 1981
12. Ellis HA, McCarthy JH, Herrington J: Bone aluminum in hemodialysed patients and in rats injected with aluminum chloride: Relationship to impaired bone mineralization. J Clin Pathol 32:832, 1979
13. Cournot-Witmer G, Zingraff J, Plachot JJ, et al: Aluminum localization in bone from hemodialyzed patients: Relationship to matrix mineralization. Kidney Int 20:376, 1981
14. Hodsman AB, Sherrard DJ, Alfrey AG, et al: Bone aluminum and histomorphometric features of renal osteodystrophy. J Clin Endocrinol Metab 54:539, 1982
15. Goldstein DA, Oda Y, Kurokawa K, Massry SG: Blood levels of 25-hydroxyvitamin D in nephrotic syndrome: Studies in 26 patients. Ann Intern Med 87:664, 1977
16. Reiss E, Canterbury JM: Genesis of hyperparathyroidism. Am J Med 50:679, 1971
17. Arnaud CD: Hyperparathyroidism and renal failure. Kidney Int 4:89, 1973
18. Hruska KA, Kopelman R, Rutherford WE, et al: Metabolism of immunoreactive parathyroid hormone in the dog: The role of the kidney and the effects of chronic renal disease. J Clin Invest 56:39, 1975
19. Bordier PJ, Arnaud C, Hawker C, et al: Relationship between serum immunoreactive parathyroid hormone, osteoclastic and osteocytic bone resorption and serum calcium in primary hyperparathyroidism and osteomalacia. p 222. In Frame B, Parfitt AN, Dunach HH, Eds: Clinical Aspects of Bone Disease. Exerpta Medica, Amsterdam, 1973
20. Brown EM: Set-point for calcium: Its role in normal and abnormal parathyroid secretion. p 35. In Cohn D, Ed: Hormonal Control of Calcium Metabolism. Excerpta Medica, Amsterdam, 1982
21. Bellorin-Font E, Martin KJ, Freitag JJ, et al: Altered adenylate cyclase kinetics in hyperfunctioning human parathyroid glands. J Clin Endocrinol Metab 52:499, 1981
22. Shoback DM, Brown EM: Direct determination of cytosolic calcium concentration in dispersed cells from neonatal and adult bovine and abnormal human parathyroid tissue. Calcif Tiss Int, in press.
23. Coburn JW, DiDomenico NC, Bryce GF, et al: Heterogeniety of secondary hyperparathyroidism in uremic patients on dialysis. Clin Res 30:539A, 1982
24. Slatopolsky E, Caglar S, Pennell JP, et al: On the pathogenesis of hyperparathyroidism in chronic experimental renal insufficiency in the dog. J Clin Invest 50:492, 1971
25. Slatopolsky E, Caglar S, Gradowska L, et al: On the prevention of secondary hyperparathyroidism in experimental chronic renal

disease using "proportional reduction" of dietary phosphorus intake. Kidney Int 2:147, 1972
26. Slatopolsky E, Bricker NS: The role of phosphorus restriction in the prevention of secondary hyperparathyroidism in chronic renal disease. Kidney Int 4:141, 1973
27. Rutherford WE, Bordier P, Marie P, et al: Phosphate control and 25-hydroxycholecalciferol administration in preventing experimental renal osteodystrophy in the dog. J Clin Invest 60:332, 1977
28. Portale AA, Booth BE, Tsai HC, Morris RC, Jr: Reduced plasma concentration of 1,25-dihydroxyvitamin D in children with moderate renal insufficiency. Kidney Int 21:627, 1982
29. Friis T, Hahnemann S, Weeke E: Serum calcium and serum phosphorus in uzaemia during administration of sodium phytate and aluminum hydroxide. Acta Med Scand 183:497, 1968
30. Coburn JW, Kopple MH, Brickman AS, Massry SG: Study of intestinal absorption of calcium in patients with renal failure. Kidney Int 3:264, 1973
31. Llach F, Massry SG, Singer FR, et al: Skeletal resistance to endogenous parathyroid hormone in patients with early renal failure. A possible cause for secondary hyperparathyroidism. J Clin Endocrinol Metab 41:338, 1975
32. Maschio G, Tessitore N, D'Angelo A, et al: Early dietary phosphorus restriction and calcium supplementation in the prevention of renal osteodystrophy. Am J Clin Nutr 33:1546, 1980
33. Fournier AE, Arnaud CD, Johnson WJ, et al: Etiology of hyperparathyroidism and bone disease during chronic hemodialysis. II. Factors affecting serum immunoreactive parathyroid hormone. J Clin Invest 50:559, 1971
34. Evanson, JM: The response to the infusion of parathyroid extract in hypocalcemic states. Clin Sci 31:63, 1966
35. Massry SG, Coburn JW, Lee DBN, et al: Skeletal resistance to parathyroid hormone in renal failure: Study in 105 human subjects. Ann Intern Med 78:357, 1973b
36. Massry SG, Arieff AI, Coburn JW, et al: Divalent ion metabolism in patients with acute renal failure: Studies on mechanism of hypocalcemia. Kidney Int 5:437, 1974
37. Kaplan MA, Canterbury JM, Gavellas G, et al: The calcemic and phosphaturic effects of parathyroid hormone in normal and uremic dogs. Metabolism 27:1785, 1978
38. Massry SG, Stein R, Garty J, et al: Skeletal resistance to the calcemic action of parathyroid hormone in uremia: Role of $1,25(OH)_2D_3$. Kidney Int 9:467, 1976
39. Massry SG, Dua S, Garty J, Friedler RM: Role of uremia in the skeletal resistance to the calcemic action of parathyroid hormone. Min Electrol Metab 1:172, 1978
40. Massry SG, Tuma S, Dua S, Goldstein DA: Reversal of skeletal resistance to parathyroid hormone in uremia by vitamin D metabolites. J Lab Clin Med 94:152, 1979
41. Somerville PJ, Kaye M: Resistance to parathyroid hormone in renal failure: Role of vitamin D metabolites. Kidney Int 14:245, 1978
42. Somerville PJ, Kaye M: Evidence that resistance to the calcemic action of parathyroid hormone in rats with acute uremia is caused by phosphate retention. Kidney Int 61:552, 1979
43. Wills MR, Jenkins MV: The effect of uraemic metabolites on parathyroid extract induced bone resorption in vitro. Clin Chim Acta 73:121, 1976
44. Jacob AI, Gavellas G, Canterbury J, Bourgoignie JJ: Calcemic and phosphaturic response to parathyroid hormone in normal and chronically uremic dogs. Kidney Int 22:21, 1982
45. Massry SG, Coburn JW, Lee, DBN, et al: Effect of the infusion of parathyroid extract on serum calcium in patients with renal failure. p. 578. In Frame B, Parfitt AM, Duncan H, Eds: Clinical Aspects of Metabolic Bone Disease. Amsterdam, Excerpta Medica, 1973
46. Weisman Y, Vargas A, Duckett G, et al: Synthesis of 1,25-dihydroxyvitamin D in the nephrectomized pregnant rat. Endocrinology 103:1992, 1978
47. Gray TK, Lester GE, Lorenc RS: Evidence for extra-renal 1 alpha-hydroxylation of 25-hydroxyvitamin D_3 in pregnancy. Science 204:1311, 1979
48. Howard GA, Turner RT, Sherrard DJ, et al: Human bone cells in culture metabolize

25-hydroxyvitamin D_3 to 1,25-dihydroxyvitamin D_3 and 24,25-dihydroxyvitamin D_3. J Biol Chem 256:7738, 1981

49. Kumar R, Cohen WR, Silva P, et al: Elevated 1,25-dihydroxyvitamin D plasma levels in normal human pregnancy and lactation. J Clin Invest 63:342, 1979
50. Barbour GL, Coburn JW, Slatopolsky E, et al: Extra-renal production of 1,25-dihydroxy-vitamin D in an anephric patient with sarcoidosis. N Engl J Med 305:440, 1981
51. Hughes MR, Haussler MR, Wergedal J, et al: Regulation of serum 1-alpha, 25-dihydroxyvitamin D_3 by calcium and phosphate in the rat. Science 190:158, 1975
52. Broadus AE, Magee JS, Mallette LE, et al: A detailed evaluation of oral phosphate therapy in selected patients with primary hyperparathyroidism. J Clin Endocrinol Metab 56:953, 1983
53. Van Den Berg CJ, Kumar R, Wilson DM, et al: Orthophosphate therapy decreases urinary calcium excretion and serum 1,25-dihydroxyvitamin D concentrations in idiopathic hypercalciuria. J Clin Endocrinol Metab 51:998, 1980
54. Horiuchi N, Suda T, Sasaki S: Direct involvement of vitamin D in the regulation of 25-hydroxycholecalciferol metabolism. FEBS Lett 43:353, 1974
55. Gafter U, Kraut JA, Lee DBN, et al: The effect of metabolic acidosis on intestinal absorption of calcium and phosphate. Am J Physiol (Gastrointest Liver Physiol) 239: G480, 1980
56. Bushinsky DA, Favus MJ, Sen PK, et al: Effects of chronic metabolic acidosis on serum $1,25(OH)_2D_3$ in the rat. Am J Physiol 243:F570, 1982
57. Kraut JA, Shinaberger JH, Singer FR, et al: Parathyroid gland responsiveness to acute hypocalcemia in dialysis osteomalacia. Kidney Int 3:725, 1983
58. Coburn JW, Hartenbower DL, Brickman AS: Advances in vitamin D metabolism as they pertain to chronic renal disease. Am J Clin Nutr 29:1283, 1976
59. Brumbaugh PF, Haussler DH, Bressler R, Haussler MR: Radioreceptor assay for 1 alpha, 25-hydroxy-vitamin D_3. Science 183: 1089, 1974
60. Eisman JA, Hamstra AJ, Kream BE, DeLuca HF: 1,25-dihydroxy-vitamin D in biological fluids: A simplified and sensitive assay. Science 193:1021, 1976
61. Shepard RM, Horst RL, Hamstra AJ, DeLuca HF: Determination of vitamin D and its metabolites in plasma from normal and anephric man. Biochem J 182:55, 1979
62. Brickman AS, Coburn JW, Massry SG, Norman AW: 1,25-dihydroxy-vitamin D_3 in normal man and patients with renal failure. Ann Intern Med 80:161, 1974
63. Malluche HH, Werner E, Ritz E: Intestinal absorption of calcium and whole body calcium retention in incipient and advance renal failure. Min Electrol Metab 1:263, 1978
64. Slatopolsky E, Gray R, Adams ND, et al: Low serum levels of $1,25(OH)_2D_3$ are not responsible for the development of secondary hyperparathyroidism in early renal failure (abstr). Kidney Int 12:733, 1978
65. Tessitore N, Lund B, Sorensen OH, et al: Vitamin D metabolites in patients with early renal failure: Effects of dietary phosphate restriction and calcium supplementation. Kidney Int 20:303A, 1981
66. Broadus AE, Horst RL, Lang R, et al: The importance of circulation 1,25-dihydroxyvitamin D in the pathogenesis of hypercalciuria and renal stone formation in primary hyperparathyroidism. N Engl J Med 302: 421, 1980
67. Llach F, Massry SG, Koffler A, et al: Secondary hyperparathyroidism in early renal failure: Role of phosphate retention. Clin Res 25:507A, 1977
68. Portale AA, Booth BE, Halloran BP, Morris RC, Jr: Effect of restriction and supplementation of dietary phosphate on plasma $1,25(OH)_2D$ and serum iPTH in children with moderate renal insufficiency. Kidney Int 23:108, 1983
69. Oldham SB, Smith R, Hartenbower DL, et al: The acute effects of 1,25-dihydroxycholecalciferol on serum immunoreactive parathyroid hormone in the dog. Endocrinology 104:248, 1979
70. Slatopolsky E, Weerts C, Thielan J, et al: Marked suppression of secondary hyperparathyroidism by intravenous $1,25(OH)_2D_3$ in uremic patients. Kidney Int 23:162, 1983
71. Horst RL, Littledike ET, Gray RW, Napoli JL: Impaired 24,25-dihydroxy-vitamin D

production in anephric human and pig. J Clin Invest 67:274, 1981

72. Tanaka Y, DeLuca HF: Biological activity of 24,24-Difluoro-25-hydroxyvitamin D_3. J Biol Chem 254:7163, 1979
73. Kanis JA, Cundy T, Bartlett M, et al: Is 24,25-dihydroxycholecalciferol a calcium regulating hormone in man? Br Med J 1:1382, 1978
74. Llach F, Brickman, AS, Singer FR, Coburn JW: 24,25-dihydroxy-cholecalciferol, a vitamin D sterol with qualitatively unique effects in uremic man. Metab Bone Dis Rel Res 2:11, 1979
75. Eastwood JB, Harris E, Stamp TCB, De Wardener HE: Vitamin D-deficiency in the osteomalacia of chronic renal failure. Lancet 2:1209, 1976
76. Bayard F, Bec P, Thon That E, Louvet JP: Plasma 25-hydroxycholecalciferol in chronic renal failure. Eur J Clin Invest 3:447, 1973
77. Offerman G, von Herrath D, Schaefer K: Serum 25-hydroxycholecalciferol in uremia. Nephron 13:169, 1974
78. Shen FU, Baylink DJ, Sherrard DJ, et al: Serum immunoreactive parathyroid hormone and 25-hydroxy-vitamin D in patients with uremic bone disease. J Clin Endocrinol Metab 40:1009, 1975
79. Christiansen C, Christensen MS, Melsen F, et al: Mineral metabolism in chronic renal failure with special reference to serum concentrations of $1,25(OH)_2D$ and $24,25(OH)_2D$. Clin Nephrol 15:18, 1981
80. Juttmann JR, Buurman CJ, DeKam E, et al: Serum concentrations of metabolites of vitamin D in patients with chronic renal failure (CRF). Consequences for the treatment with 1-alpha-hydroxy-derivatives. Clin Endocrinol 14:225, 1981
81. Mason RS, Lissner D, Wilkinson M, Posen S: Vitamin D metabolites and their relationship to azotaemic osteodystrophy. Clin Endocrinol 13:375, 1980
82. Bordier PJ, Tun-chot S, Eastwood JB, et al: Lack of histological evidence of vitamin D abnormality in the bones of anephric patients. Clin Sci 44:33, 1973
83. Underwood J, Weinstein R, DeLuca HF: Normal bone growth and mineralization in D-deficient rats with normal plasma calcium and phosphorus. Calcif Tiss Internat 35:704, 1983
84. Kanis JA, Adams ND, Earnshaw M, et al: Vitamin D, osteomalacia and chronic renal failure. In Norman AW, Schaefer K, Coburn JW, et al, Eds: Vitamin D, Biochemical, Chemical and Clinical Aspects Related to Calcium Metabolism. W de Gruyter, New York, 1977
85. Baker, LRI, Ackrill P, Cattel WR, et al: Iatrogenic osteomalacia and myopathy due to phosphate depletion. Br Med J 3:150, 1974
86. Pierides AM, Ellis HA, Ward M, et al: Barbiturate and anticonvulsant treatment in relation to osteomalacia with haemodialysis and renal transplantation. Br Med J 1:190, 1976
87. Ward MK, Feest TG, Ellis HA, et al: Osteomalacic dialysis osteodystrophy: Evidence for a water-borne aetiological agent, probably aluminum. Lancet 1:841, 1978
88. Parkinson IS, Feest TG, Ward MK, et al: Fracturing dialysis osteodystrophy and dialysis encephalopathy: An epidemiological survey. Lancet 1:406, 1979
89. Pierides AM, Edwards WG, Jr, Cullu UX, Jr, et al: Hemodialysis encephalopathy with osteomalacia fractures and muscle weakness. Kidney Int 18:115, 1980
90. Robertson JA, Felsenfeld AJ, Haygood CC, et al: An animal model of aluminum induced osteomalacia. In David DS, Ed: Calcium Metabolism in Renal Failure and Nephrolithesis. Williams & Wilkins, Baltimore, 1983
91. Chan Y, Alfrey AC, Posen S, et al: The effect of aluminum on normal and uremic rats: Tissue distribution, vitamin D metabolites and quantitative bone histology. Calcif Tiss Int 35:344, 1983
92. Goodman WG, Henry DA, Horst R, et al: Parenteral aluminum administration in the dog. II. Induction of osteomalacia and effect on vitamin D metabolism. Kidney Int 25:370, 1984.
93. Ott SM, Maloney NA, Klein GL, et al: Aluminum is associated with low bone formation in patients on chronic parenteral nutrition. Ann Intern Med 98:910, 1983
94. Buchanan MRC, Ihle BU, Dunn CM: Hemodialysis related osteomalacia. A staining method to demonstrate aluminum. J Clin Pathol 34:1352, 1981

95. Maloney NA, Ott S, Alfrey AC, et al: Histologic quantitation of aluminum in iliac bone from patients with renal failure. J Lab Clin Med 99:206, 1982
96. Ott SM, Maloney NA, Coburn JW, et al: The prevalence of aluminum in renal osteodystrophy and its relationship to response to calcitriol therapy. N Engl J Med 307:709, 1982
97. Ackrill P, Day JP, Garstang FM, et al: Treatment of fracturing renal osteodystrophy by desferroxamine. Proc EDTA 19:213, 1982
98. Ihle BU, Buchanan, MRC, Stevens B, et al: The efficacy of various treatment modalities on aluminum associated bone disease. Proc EDTA 19:195, 1982
99. Kaehny WD, Hegg AP, Alfrey AC: Gastrointestinal absorption of aluminum from aluminum-containing antacids. N Engl J Med 296:1389, 1977
100. Recker RR, Blotcky AJ, Leffler JA, Rack EP: Evidence for aluminum absorption from the gastrointestinal tract and bone deposition by aluminum carbonate ingestion with normal renal function. J Lab Clin Med 80:810, 1977
101. Kovalchik MT, Kaehny WD, Hegg AP: Aluminum kinetics during hemodialysis. J Lab Clin Med 92:712, 1978
102. Felsenfeld AJ, Gutman RA, Llach F, Harrelson JM: Osteomalacia in chronic renal failure: A syndrome previously reported only with maintenance dialysis. Am J Nephrol 2:147, 1982
103. Kaehny WD, Alfrey AC, Holman RE, Shorr WJ: Aluminum transfer during hemodialysis. Kidney Int 12:361, 1977
104. Felsenfeld AJ, Harrelson JM, Gutman RA, et al: Osteomalacia after parathyroidectomy in patients with uremia. Ann Intern Med 96:34, 1982
105. Teitelbaum SL, Bergfeld MA, Freitag J, et al: Do parathyroid hormone and 1,25-Dihydroxyvitamin D modulate bone formation in uremia? J Clin Endocrinol Metab 51:247, 1980
106. Ellis HA: Aluminum and osteomalacia after parathyroidectomy. Ann Intern Med 96:533, 1982
107. Siddiqui JY, Simpson W, Ellis HA, Kerr DN: Fluoride and bone disease in patients on regular haemodialysis. Proc EDTA 8:149, 1971
108. Griffith GC, Nichols G, Jr, Asher JD, Flanagant, B: Heparin osteoporosis. JAMA 221: 911, 1972
109. Avioli LV: Collagen metabolism, uremia and bone. Kidney Int 4:105, 1973
110. Alfrey AC, Solomons CC: Bone pyrophosphate in uremia and its association with extraosseous calcification. J Clin Invest 57:700, 1976
111. Pellegrino ED, Blitz RM: The composition of human bone in uremia. Medicine 44:397, 1965
112. Parfitt AM: Clinical and radiographic manifestations of renal osteodystrophy. In David DS, Ed: Calcium Metabolism in Renal Failure and Nephrolithiasis. Wiley, New York, 1977
113. Ritz E, Prager P, Krempien, et al: Skeletal x-ray findings and bone histology in patients on hemodialysis. Kidney Int 13:316, 1978
114. Olgaard K, Heerfordt, J, Madsen S: Scintigraphic skeletal changes in uremic patients on regular hemodialysis. Nephron 17:325, 1976
115. Wright RS, Mehls O, Ritz E, Coburn JW: Musculoskeletal manifestations of chronic renal failure, dialysis & transplantation. In Bacon P, Hadler N, Eds: Renal Manifestations in Rheumatic Disease. Butterworths, London, 1982
116. Boyce BF, Fell GS, Elder HY, et al: Hypercalcaemic osteomalacia due to aluminum toxicity. Lancet 2:1009, 1982
117. Shimada H, Nakamura M, Marumo F: Influence of aluminum on the effect of 1 alpha(OH)D_3 on renal osteodystrophy. Nephron 35:163, 1983
118. Smith R, Stern G: Myopathy, osteomalacia and hyperparathyroidism. Brain 90:593, 1967
119. Mallette LE, Patten BM, Engel WK: Neuromuscular disease in secondary hyperparathyroidism. Ann Intern Med 82:474, 1975
120. Matthews C, Heimberg K-W, Ritz F, et al: Effect of 1,25-dihydroxycholecalciferol in impaired calcium transport by the sarcoplasmic reticulum in experimental uremia. Kidney Int 11:227, 1977
121. Goodhue WW, Davis JN, Porro RS: Ischemic myopathy in uremic hyperparathyroidism. JAMA 221:911, 1972
122. Henderson RG, Russell RGG, Ledingham JGG, et al: Effects of 1,25-dihydroxycholecalciferol on calcium absorption, muscle

weakness, and bone disease in chronic renal failure. Lancet 1:379, 1974

123. Coburn JW, Brickman AS, Sherrard DJ, et al: Clinical efficacy of 1,25-dihydroxy-vitamin D_3 in renal osteodystrophy. In Norman AW, Schaefer K, Coburn JW, et al, Eds: Vitamin D: Biochemical, Chemical and Clinical Aspects Related to Calcium Metabolism. W de Gruyter, Berlin, 1977
124. Rodman JS, Baker T: Changes in the kinetics of muscle contraction in vitamin D-depleted rats. Kidney Int 13:189, 1978
125. Curry OB, Bastein JF, Francis MJO, Smith R: Calcium uptake by sacroplasmic reticulum of muscle from vitamin D-deficient rabbits. Nature 249:83, 1974
126. Birge SJ, Haddad JG: 25-hydroxycholecalciferol stimulation of muscle metabolism. J Clin Invest 56:1100, 1975
127. Harter HR, Birge SJ, Martin KJ, et al: Effects of vitamin D metabolites on protein catabolism of muscle from uremic rats. Kidney Int 23:465, 1983
128. Ellman MH, Brown NL, Katzenberg CA: Acute pseudogrout in chronic renal failure. Arch Intern Med 139:795, 1979
129. McCarty DJ, Silcox DC, Coe F, et al: Diseases associated with calcium pyrophosphate dihydrate crystal deposition. Am J Med 56:704, 1974
130. Mirahmadi KS, Coburn JW, Bluestone: Calcific periarthritis and hemodialysis. JAMA 223:548, 1973
131. Llach F, Pederson J: Acute joint syndrome and maintenance hemodialysis. Proc Clin Dial Transpl Forum 9:17, 1979
132. Lotem M, Robson MP, Rosenfeld JB: Spontaneous rupture of the quadriceps tendon in patients on chronic hemodialysis. Ann Rheumatic Dis 33:428, 1974
133. Morein G, Goldschmidt Z, Pauker M, et al: Spontaneous tendon ruptures in patients treated by chronic hemodialysis. Clin Orthopaed 124:209, 1977
134. Pierides AM, Ellis HA, Aljama P, Kerr DNS: Quadriceps tendon ruptures in uremia. Treatment with surgery and 1 alpha-hydroxy-cholecalciferol. Clin Nephrol 7:274, 1977
135. Preston ET: Avulsion of both quadriceps tendons in hyperparathyroidism. JAMA 221:406, 1972
136. Halter SK, DeLisa JA, Stolov WC, et al: Carpal tunnel syndrome in chronic renal dialysis patients. Arch Phys Med Rehabil 62:197, 1981
137. Cruz C, Shah SV: Dialysis elbow—olecrenon bursitis from long-term hemodialysis. JAMA 238:243, 1977
138. Contiguglia SR, Alfrey AC, Miller NL, et al: Nature of soft tissue calcification in uremia. Kidney Int 4:229, 1973
139. LeGeros RZ, Contiguglia SR, Alfrey AC: Pathological calcification associated with uremia. Two types of calcium phosphate deposits. Calcif Tiss Res 13:173, 1973
140. Alfrey AC: Extraosseous calcification in uremia. In Catto G, Coburn JW, Eds: Renal Osteodystrophy. M. Nijhoff, Amsterdam, in press
141. Conger JD, Hammond WS, Alfrey AC, et al: Pulmonary calcification in chronic dialysis patients. Ann Intern Med 83:330, 1975
142. Kuzela DC, Huffer WE, Conger JD, et al: Soft tissue calcification in chronic dialysis patients. Am J Pathol 86:403, 1977
143. Dreher W, Shelp W: Atrioventricular block in a long term dialysis patient. Reversal after parathyroidectomy. JAMA 234:954, 1975
144. Schwartz KV: Heart block in renal failure and hypercalcemia. JAMA 235:1550, 1976
145. Ibels LS, Alfrey AC, Huffer WE, et al: Arterial calcification and pathology in uremic patients undergoing dialysis. Am J Med 66:790, 1979
146. Gipstein RM, Coburn JW, Adams DA, et al: Calciphylaxis in man. Arch Intern Med 136:1273, 1976
147. Meema HE, Oreopoulos DG, deVeber GA: Arterial calcification in severe chronic renal disease and their relationship to dialysis treatment, renal transplant and parathyroidectomy. Radiology 121:315, 1976
148. Tatler GL, Gaillod RE, Varghese Z, et al: Evolution of bone disease over 10 years in 135 patients with terminal renal failure. Br Med J 4:315, 1973
149. Massry SG, Gordon A, Coburn JW, et al: Vascular calcification and peripheral necrosis in a renal transplant recipient: Reversal of lesions following subtotal parathyroidectomy. Am J Med 49:416, 1970
150. Griffiths HJ: Radiology of Renal Failure. Philadelphia, Saunders, 1976
151. Verberckmoes R, Bouillon R, Krempien B: Disappearance of vascular calcifications during treatment of renal osteodystrophy. Ann Intern Med 82:529, 1975

152. Katz AI, Hampers CH, Merrill JB: Secondary hyperparathyroidism and renal osteodystrophy in chronic renal failure. Metabolism 48:337, 1969
153. Llach F: Effects of renal failure and dialysis on divalent ion metabolism. In Brenner BM, Stein JH (eds): Contemporary Issues in Nephrology: Divalent Ion Homeostasis, Vol. 11. Churchill Livingstone, New York, 1983, pp. 291–318
154. Berlyne GM, Shaw AC: Red eyes in renal failure. Lancet 4:1967
155. Richardson JA, Herron G, Reitz R, Layzer R: Ischemic ulcerations of skin and necrosis of muscle in azotemic hyperparathyroidism. Ann Intern Med 71:126, 1969
156. Goldstein DA, Chui LA, Massry SG: Peripheral nerve calcium and motor nerve conduction velocity in acute renal failure. J Clin Invest 62:88, 1978
157. Meytes D, Bogin E, Ma A, et al: Effect of parathyroid hormone on erythropoiesis. J Clin Invest 67:1263, 1981
158. Bogin E, Massry SG, Levi J, et al: Effect of parathyroid hormone on somotic fragility of human red blood cells. J Clin Invest 69:1017, 1982
159. Bogin E, Massry SG, Harasy I: Effect of parathyroid hormone on rat heart cells. J Clin Invest 67:1215, 1981
160. Akmal M, Goldstein DA, Multani S, Massry SG: Parathyroid hormone (PTH) and glucose (G) intolerance in uremia. Proc Am Soc Nephrol 13:87A, 1980
161. Coburn JW, Hartenbower DL, Brickman AS, et al: Intestinal absorption of calcium, magnesium and phosphorus in chronic renal insufficiency. In David DS, Ed: Calcium Metabolism in Renal Failure and Nephrolithiasis. Wiley, New York, 1977
162. Brickman AS, Hartenbower DL, Norman AW, Coburn JW: Actions of 1 alpha-hydroxy- and 1,25-dihydroxy-vitamin D_3 on mineral metabolism in man. I. Effects on net absorption of phosphorus. Am J Clin Nutr 30:1064, 1977
163. Mirahmadi KS, Duffy BS, Shinaberger JH, et al: A controlled evaluation of clinical and metabolic effects of dialysate calcium levels during regular dialysis. Trans Am Soc Artif Intern Organs 17:118, 1971
164. Regan RJ, Peacock M, Rosen SM, et al: Effect of dialysate calcium concentration on bone disease in patients on hemodialysis. Kidney Int 10:246, 1976
165. Coburn JW, Popovtzer MM, Massry SG, Kleeman CR: The physiochemical state and renal handling of divalent ions in chronic renal failure. Arch Intern Med 124:302, 1969
166. Freitag J, Martin KJ, Hruska KA, et al: Impaired parathyroid hormone metabolism in patients with chronic renal failure. N Engl J Med 298:29, 1978
167. Estep, H, Shaw W, Watlington CO, et al: Hypocalcemia due to reversible hypomagnesemia and parathyroid hormone unresponsiveness. J Clin Endocrinol 29:842, 1969
168. Pierides AM, Skillen AW, Ellis HA: Serum alkaline phosphatase in azotemic and hemodialysis osteodystrophy. J Lab Clin Med 93:899, 1979
169. Hart W, Duursma, SA, Visser WJ, Njio LKF: The hydroxyproline content of plasma of patient with impaired renal function. Clin Nephrol 4:104, 1975
170. Price PA, Parthemore JG, Deftos LJ: New biochemical marker for bone metabolism. Measurement by radioimmunoassay of bone GLA protein in the plasma of normal subjects and patients with bone disease. J Clin Invest 66:878, 1980
171. Hawker CD, DiBella FP: Parathyroid hormone in chronic renal failure studies with two different parathyroid hormone immunoassays. Contrib Nephrol 20:2137, 1980
172. Hruska KA, Teitelbaum SL, Kopelman R, et al: The predictability of the histological features of uremic bone disease by non-invasive techniques. Metab Bone Dis Rel Res 1:39, 1978
173. Carr D, Davidson JK, McMillan M, Davidson M: Renal osteodystrophy: An underdiagnosed condition. Clin Radiol 31:55, 1980
174. Meema HE, Rabinovich S, Memma S, et al: Improved radiological diagnosis of azotemic osteodystrophy. Radiology 102:1, 1972
175. Sundaram M, Joyce PF, Shields JB, et al: Terminal phalangeal tufts: earliest site of renal osteodystrophy findings in hemodialysis patients. Am J Roentgenol 133:25, 1979
176. Memma HE, Memma S: Comparison of microradioscopic and morphometric findings in the proximal radius in thyrotoxicosis and in renal osteodystrophy. Invest Radiol 7:88, 1972
178. Bonavita JA, Dalinka MK: Shoulder ero-

sions in renal osteodystrophy. Skeletal Radiol 5:105, 1980
179. Meema HE, Oreopoulos DG, Rabinovich S, et al: Periosteal new bone formation (periosteal neostasis) in renal osteodystrophy. Radiology 110:513, 1974
180. Mehls O, Ritz E, Burkhard K, et al: Slipped epiphysis in renal osteodystrophy. Arch Dis Child 50:545, 1975
181. Zimmerman HB: Osteosclerosis in chronic renal disease. Report of 4 cases associated with secondary hyperparathyroidism. Am J Roentgenol 88:1152, 1962
182. Simpson W, Ellis HA, Kerr DNS, et al: Bone disease in long-term haemodialysis: the association of radiological with histologic abnormalities. Br J Radiol 49:105, 1976
183. Debman JW, Bates ML, Kopelman RC, Teitelbaum SL: Radiological pathological correlations in uremic bone disease. Radiology 125:653, 1977
184. Valentzas C, Meindok H, Oreopoulos DG, et al: Detection and pathogenesis of visceral calcification in dialysis patients with malignant disease. Can Med Assn J 1:45, 1978
185. Faubert PF, Shapiro WB, Porush JG, et al: Pulmonary calcification in hemodialysis patients detected by technetium-99M diphosphonate scanning. Kidney Int 18:95, 1980
186. Henderson RG, Russell RGG, Earnshaw MJ, et al: Loss of metacarpal and iliac bone in chronic renal failure: influence of haemodialysis, parathyroid activity, type of renal disease, physical activity and heparin consumption. Clin Sci 56:317, 1979
187. Bone JM, Davison AM, Robson JS: Role of dialysate calcium concentration in osteoporosis in patients on hemodialysis. Lancet 1:1047, 1972
188. deGraaf P, Schicht IM, Pauwels EKJ, et al: Bone scintigraphy in renal osteodystrophy. J Nucl Med 19:1289, 1978
189. Moriniere PH, Roussel A, Tahiri Y, et al: Substitution of aluminum hydroxide by high doses of calcium carbonate in patients on chronic haemodialysis: Disappearance of hyperaluminaemia and equal control of hyperparathyroidism. Proc EDTA 19:784, 1982
190. Clarkson EM, Eastwood JB, Koutsaimanis KG, DeWardner HE: Net intestinal absorption of calcium in patients with chronic renal failure. Kidney Int 3:258, 1973
191. Coburn JW, Slatopolsky E: Vitamin D, parathyroid hormone, and renal osteodystrophy. In Brenner BM, Rector F, Eds: The Kidney. Saunders, Philadelphia, 1981
192. Pletka P, Bernstein DS, Hampers CL, et al: Effect of magnesium on parathyroid hormone secretion during chronic hemodialysis. Lancet 2:462, 1971
193. Healy MD, Malluche HH, Goldstein DA, et al: Effects of long-term therapy with calcitriol in patients with moderate renal failure. Arch Intern Med 140:1030, 1980
194. Christiansen C, Rodbro P, Christensen MS, et al: Deterioration of renal function during treatment of chronic renal failure with 1,25-dihydroxycholecalciferol. Lancet, 2:700, 1978
195. Baker LRI, Muir JW, Cattell WR, et al: Use of 1,25$(OH)_2$-Vitamin D_3 in prevention of renal osteodystrophy: Preliminary observations. Contrib Nephrol 18:147, 1979
196. Binswanger U, Fischer JA, Iselin H, et al: 1,25-dihydroxycholecalciferol treatment of clinically asymptomatic renal osteodystrophy. Min Electrol Metab 2:103, 1979
197. Brickman AS, Coburn JW, Friedman GR, et al: Comparison of effects of 1 alpha-hydroxy-vitamin D_3 and 1,25-dihydroxy-vitamin D_3 in man. J Clin Invest 57:1540, 1976
198. Teitelbaum SL, Bone JM, Stein PM, et al: Calcifediol in chronic renal insufficiency: Skeletal response. JAMA 235:164, 1976
199. Recker R, Schoenfeld P, Letteri J, et al: The efficacy of calcifediol in renal osteodystrophy. Arch Intern Med 138:857, 1978
200. Kanis JA, Earnshaw M, Henderson RG, et al: Correlation of clinical, biochemical and skeletal responses to 1 alpha-hydroxyvitamin D_3 in renal bone disease. Clin Endocrinol 7(Suppl):45S, 1977
201. Madsen S, Olgaard K: 1-alpha-hydroxycholecalciferol treatment of adults with chronic renal failure. Acta Med Scand 200:1, 1976
202. Kaye M, Chatterjee H, Cohen GF, Sagar S: Arrest of hyperparthyroid bone disease with dihydrotachysterol in patients undergoing chronic hemodialysis. Ann Intern Med 73:225, 1970
203. Cordy PE, Mills DM: The early detection and treatment of renal osteodystrophy. Min Electrol Metab 5:311, 1981
204. Taylor CM, Mawer EB, Wallace JE, et al: The absence of 24,25-dihydroxychlecalciferol in anephric patients. Clin Sci Molec Med 55:541, 1978

205. Bordier PJ, Rasmussen H, Marie P, et al: Vitamin D metabolites and bone mineralization in man. J Clin Endocrinol Metab 46:284, 1976
206. Hodsman JW, Wong EGC, Sherrard DJ, et al: Preliminary trials with 24,25-dihydroxyvitamin D_3 in dialysis osteomalacia. Am J Med 74:407, 1983
207. Coburn JW, DiDomenico NC, Bryce GF, et al: Prospective, double blind trial with calcitriol in the prophylaxis bone disease in asymptomatic dialysis patients. In Norman AW, Schaefer K, Grigoleit HG, Herrath DV: Vitamin D: Chemical, Biochemical, and Clinical Endocrinology of Calcium Metabolism. W de Gruyter, Berlin, 1982
208. Felsenfeld AJ, Gutman RA, Llach F, et al: Postparathyroidectomy hypocalcemia as an accurate indicator of preparathyroidectomy bone histology in the uremic patient. Min Electrol Metab, in press.
209. Hooft C, Vermassen A, Van Belle M: On calcaemia and phosphataemia in the nephrotic syndrome. Comparative study of the period before and after the introduction of hormone therapy. Helv Paediat Acta 5:437, 1960
210. Lim P, Jacob E, Chio LF, Pwee HS: Serum ionized calcium in nephrotic syndrome. Q J Med 45:421, 1976
211. Schmidt-Gayk H, Schmitt W, Grawunder C, et al: 25-hydroxyvitamin D in nephrotic syndrome. Lancet 2:105, 1977
212. Barragry JM, France MW, Carter ND, et al: Vitamin D metabolism in nephrotic syndrome. Lancet 2:629, 1977
213. Sato KA, Gray RW, Lemann J, Jr: Urinary excretion of 25-hydroxyvitamin D in health and the nephrotic syndrome. J Lab Clin Med 99:325, 1982
214. Goldstein DA, Haldimann B, Sherman D, et al: Vitamin D metabolites and calcium metabolism in patients with nephrotic syndrome and normal renal function. J Clin Endocrinol Metab 52:116, 1981
215. Stickler GB, Rosevear JW, Ulrich JA: Renal tubular dysfunction complicating the nephrotic syndrome: The disturbance of calcium and phosphorus metabolism. Proc Mayo Clin 37:376, 1962
216. Mountokalakis TH, Virvidakis C, Singellakis P, et al: Intestinal calcium absorption in the nephrotic syndrome. Ann Intern Med 86: 746, 1977
217. Hooft C, Vermassen A: Metaphyseal decalcification of the bone in nephrosis, with reference to its origin. Ann Paediat (Basel) 191:129, 1958
218. Malluche HH, Goldstein DA, Massry SG: Osteomalacia and hyperparathyroid bone disease in patients with nephrotic syndrome. J Clin Invest 63:494, 1979
219. Korkor A, Schwartz J, Bergfeld M, et al: Absence of metabolic bone disease in adult patients with the nephrotic syndrome and normal renal function. J Clin Endocrinol Metab 56:496, 1983
220. Lim P, Jacob E, Tock EPC, Pwee HS: Calcium and phosphorus metabolism in nephrotic syndrome. Q J Med 46:327, 1977
221. Haldimann B, Trechsel U: Vitamin D replacement therapy in patients with the nephrotic syndrome. Min Electrol Metab 9:154, 1983
222. Kokot F, Kuska J: Der Einfluss der Hemodialyse auf die Parathormonkonzentration bei akuter nieren Insuffizienz. Z Gesamte Inn Med 29:416, 1974
223. Cooper JD, Lazarowitz VC, Arieff AI: Neurodiagnostic abnormalities in patients with acute renal failure. Evidence for neurotoxicity of parathyroid hormone. J Clin Invest 61:1448, 1978
224. Gabow PA, Kaehny WD, Kelleher SP: The spectrum of rhabdomyolysis. Medicine 61: 141, 1982
225. Pietrek J, Kokot F, Kuska J: Serum 25-hydroxyvitamin D and parathyroid hormone in patients with acute renal failure. Kidney Int 13:178, 1978
226. Llach, F, Felsenfeld AJ, Haussler MR: The pathophysiology of altered calcium metabolism in rhabdomyolysis-induced acute renal failure. Interactions of parathyroid hormone, 25-hydroxycholecalciferol and 1,25-dihydroxycholecalciferol. N Eng J Med, 305:117, 1981
227. Madsen S, Olgaard K, Ladefoged J: Suppressive effect of 1,25-dihydroxyvitamin D_3 on circulating parathyroid hormone in acute renal failure. J Clin Endocrinol Metab 53:823, 1981
228. deTorrente A, Berl T, Cohn PD, et al: Hypercalcemia of acute renal failure. Clinical

significance and pathogenesis. Am J Med 61:119, 1976

229. Meroney WH, Arney GK, Segar WE, Balch HH: The acute calcification of traumatized muscle with articular reference to acute post-traumatic renal insufficiency. J Clin Invest 36:825, 1957
230. Clark TG, Sumerling MD: Muscle necrosis and calcification in acute renal failure due to barbiturate intoxication. Br Med J 2:214, 1966
231. Arieff AI, Massry SG: Calcium metabolism of brain in acute renal failure. J Clin Invest 53:387, 1974
232. Akmal M, Goldstein DA, Telfer N, et al: Resolution of muscle calcification in rhabdomyolysis and acute renal failure. Ann Int Med 89:928, 1978
233. Suki WN, Yium JJ, von Minden M, et al: Acute treatment of hypercalcemia with furosemide. N Engl J Med 283:836, 1970
234. Christensen MS, Nielsen HE, Torring S: Hypercalcemia and parathyroid function after renal transplantation. Acta Med Scand 201:35, 1977
235. Gottlieb MN, Stephens MK, Lowrie EG, et al: Bone disease following renal transplantation. In David DS (Ed): Calcium Metabolism in Renal Failure and Nephrolithiasis. Wiley, New York, 1977, p 279
236. Piel CF, Roof BS, Avioli LV: Metabolism of tritiated 25-hydroxycholecalciferol in chronically uremic children before and after successful renal homotransplantation. J Clin Endocrinol Metab 37:944, 1973
237. Vincente F, Amend WJ, Jr: Mineral metabolism and skeletal disease after kidney transplantation. In Catto G, Coburn JW, Eds: Renal Osteodystrophy. M. Nijhoff, Amsterdam, 1984
238. McIntosh DA, Peterson EW, McPhaul JJ: Autonomy of parathyroid function after renal homotransplantation. Ann Intern Med 65:900, 1966
239. McCarron D, Mutheg RS, Lenfesty B, Bennet WM: parathyroid function in persistent hyperparathyroidism: Relationship to gland size. Kidney Int 22:662, 1982
240. Alfrey AC, Jenkins D, Groth CG, et al: Resolution of hyperparathyroidism after renal transplantation. N Engl J Med 279:1349, 1968
241. Schwartz GH, David DS, Riggio RR, et al: Hypercalcemia after renal transplantation. Am J Med 49:42, 1970
242. David DS, Sakai S, Brennen BL, et al: Hypercalcemia after renal transplantation. Am J Med 49:42, 1970
243. Gittes RF, Radde IC: Experimental model for hyperparathyroidism: effect of excessive numbers of transplanted isologous parathyroid glands. J Urol 95:595, 1966
244. Hornum I: Post-transplant hypercalcemia due to mobilization of metastatic calcifications. Acta Med Scand 189:199, 1971
245. Cundy T, Kanis JA, Fraher L, et al: The use of metabolites and analogues of vitamin D in prospective renal transplant recipients. Clin Nephrol 15:240, 1981
246. Wong EGC, Siemsen AW, Sugihara JG, Coburn JW: Interactions between treatment with $1,25(OH)_2D_3$ and glucocorticoids in uremic patients after kidney transplantation. Contrib Nephrol 18:152, 1980
247. Manra RS, Tambayah JA, Kinciad-Smith P: Calcium excretion in patients with renal allografts. Med J Austr 2:952, 1969
248. Pierides AM, Aljama P, Kerr DNS, et al: Effect of 1-alpha-hydroxycholecalciferol, 1,25-dihydroxycholecalciferol, 3 deoxy-1-alpha-hydroxycholecalciferol, 24,25-dihydroxycolecalciferol and successful renal transplantation on calcium absorption in hemodialysis patients. Nephron 20:203, 1978
249. Revusova V, Zvara V, Gratzlova J, et al: Magnesium deficit after renal transplantation with secondary posttransplantation hypocalcemia and hypophosphatemia. Urol Int 30:313, 1975
250. Olgaard K, Madsen S, Lund B, et al: Pathogenesis of hypophosphatemia in kidney necrograft recipients: A controlled trial. Adv Exp Med Biol 128:255, 1981
251. Herdman RC, Michael AF, Vernier RL, et al: Changes in phosphorous excretion and renal function after human renal homotransplantation. Nephron 5:170, 1968
252. Farrington K, Varghese Z, Newman SP: Dissociation of absorptions of calcium and phosphate after successful cadaveric renal transplantation. Med J 1:712, 1979
253. Walker FS, Peacock M, Marshall DH, et al: Factors influencing the intestinal absorption of calcium and phosphorus following

renal transplantation. Nephron 26:225, 1980
254. Moorhead JF, Ahmed KY, Varghese Z, et al: Hypophosphatemic osteomalacia after cadaveric renal transplantation. Lancet 1:694, 1974
255. Ibels LS, Alfrey AC, Huffer WE, Weil R: Aseptic necrosis of bone following renal transplantation. Experience in 194 transplant recipients and review of the literature. Medicine 57:25, 1978
256. Vincente F, Hattner R, Amend WJ, et al: Decreased secondary hyperparathyroidism in diabetic patients receiving hemodialysis. JAMA 245:930, 1981
257. Briggs WA, Hampers CL, Merrill JP, et al: Aseptic necrosis in the femur after renal transplantation. Ann Surg 175:282, 1972
258. Nielsen HE, Melsen R, Christensen MS: Aseptic necrosis of bone following renal transplantation. Acta Med Scand 202:27, 1978
259. Bewick M, Stewart PH, Rudge C, et al: Avascular necrosis of bone in patients undergoing renal allotransplantation. Clin Nephrol 5:66, 1976
260. Potter DE, Genant HK, Salvatierra O: Avascular necrosis of bone after renal transplantation. Am J Dis Child 132:1125, 1978
261. Zizic TM, Hungerford DS, Stevens MB: Ischemic bone necrosis in systemic lupus erythematosis. Medicine 59:134, 1980
262. Zinn WM (Ed): Idiopathic Ishemic Necrosis of the Femoral Head. G. Thieme Publishers, Stuttgart, 1971
263. Glimcher MJ, Kenzora JE: The biology of osteonecrosis of the human femoral head and its clinical implications. Clin Orthopaed Rel Res 104:273, 1979
264. Bailey GL, Griffiths HJL, Mocelin AJ, et al: Avascular necrosis of the femoral head in patients on chronic hemodialysis. Trans Am Soc Artif Intern Organs 18:401, 1972
265. Chatterjee, SN, Massry SG, Friedler RM, Singer FR, Berne TV: The high incidence of persistent secondary hyperparathyroidism after renal homotransplantation. Surg Gynecol Obstet 143:440, 1976
266. Springfield DS, Enneking WJ: Surgery for aseptic necrosis of the femoral head. Clin Ortho Related Resch 130:175, 1978
267. Pennisi A, Costin G, Phillips LS, et al: Linear growth in long-term renal allograft recipients. Clin Nephrol 8:415, 1977
268. Hoda Q, Hasinoff DJ, Arbus GS: Growth following renal transplantation in children and adolescents. Clin Nephrol 3:6, 1975

SELECTED READINGS

Ackrill P, Ralston AJ, Day JP, Hodge KC: Successful removal of aluminum from patient with dialysis encephalopathy. Lancet 2:692, 1980

Berlyne GM: Microcrystalline conjunctival calcification in renal failure: A useful clinical sign. Lancet 2:366, 1968

Coburn JW, Kurokawa K, Llach F: Altered divalent ion metabolism in renal disease and renal osteodystrophy. Clin Dis Fluid Electrolyte Metab 3:1153, 1980

Ellis HA: Aluminum induced osteomalacia in patients with chronic renal failure and in animals. Nieren- and Hochendruckkrankheit 12:198, 1983

Fine R: Treatment of end-stage renal disease in children. Pediatr Ann 10:45, 1981

Frost HM: The dynamics of human osteoid tissue. In Hioco DJ (Ed): L'Osteomalacie. Masson et Cie, Paris, 1967

Griswold W, Reinik V, Miendora SA, et al: Accumulation of aluminum in a non-dialysed uremic child receiving aluminum hydroxide. Pediatrics 71:56, 1983

Howard GA, Baylink DJ: Matrix formation and osteoid maturation in vitamin E-deficient rats were normocalcemic by dietary means. Min Electrol Metab 3:44, 1980

Kraut JA, Gordon EM, Ransom JC, et al: The effect of chronic metabolic acidosis on vitamin D metabolism in man. Kidney Int 24:644, 1983

Ritz E, Malluche HH, Krempien B, Mehls O: Bone histology in renal insufficiency. In David DS (Ed): Calcium Metabolism in Renal Failure and Nephrolithesis. Williams & Wilkins, Baltimore, 1983

Smith FW, Junor JR: Xeroradiography of the hand in patients with renal osteodystrophy. Br J Radiol 50:261, 1977

Wilson RE, Eastman RC, Pallotta J, Marynick SP: Abnormal regulation of parathyroid hormone release by calcium in secondary hyperparathyroidism due to chronic renal failure. J Clin Endocrinol Metab 54:172, 1982

16

Complications of Dialysis: Hemodialysis, Peritoneal Dialysis, CAPD

Alan S. Kliger

Acute and chronic renal failure cause many metabolic derangements, which, if untreated, lead to death. During the past 25 years dialysis therapy has been used widely to treat patients with renal failure. During these treatments, blood is exposed to dialysate solutions of glucose and electrolytes across a semipermeable membrane. Water and solutes move through the membrane according to their concentration and pressure gradients, providing a way to reestablish metabolic balance in patients with kidney failure. While development of this technology has proceeded in a largely empirical fashion, dialysis treatment now sustains the lives of more than 100,000 people in the world. There are two major forms of dialysis: hemodialysis and peritoneal dialysis. *Hemodialysis* treatments consist of the movement of blood out of the circulation into an artificial kidney. Dialysate solutions are placed on one side of an artificial semipermeable membrane; water, solutes, and uremic toxins that flow past the membrane on the opposite side diffuse down their concentration gradient into the dialysate, and the blood is then returned to the circulation. During *peritoneal dialysis,* dialysate solution placed into the peritoneal space exchanges water and solutes across the capillaries of the viscera, mesentery, and peritoneum, and is then removed and replaced with fresh solution. With either form of dialysis, patients with no renal function can remain relatively healthy for years.

The changes in water, electrolyte, and acid–base balance during dialysis treatment can be complex: patients with renal failure have many metabolic abnormalities, and dialysis may cause rapid shifts of fluids and electrolytes. This chapter considers the principles of water and solute flux during dialysis, then describes the complications of water, acid–base, and electrolyte balance that have been found in dialysis patients.

PRINCIPLES OF HEMODIALYSIS

When blood and a dialysate solution are apposed across a semipermeable membrane, water and solute may cross from one compartment into the other. The movement of these molecules is governed by the physical characteristics of the system and by concentration and pressure gradients across the membrane. These physical characteristics include the area and permeability of the membrane, tempera-

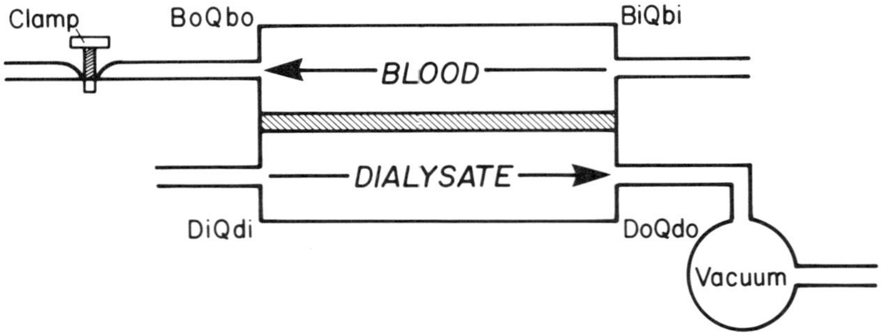

Fig. 16–1. Schematic representation of a hemodialysis device. Q_{bi}, Q_{bo}: blood flow rate entering and leaving the dialyzer, respectively; B_i, B_o: plasma solute concentration entering and leaving the dialyzer, respectively; Q_{di}, Q_{do}: dialysote flow rate entering and leaving the dialyzer, respectively; D_i, D_o: dialysote solute concentration entering and leaving the dialyzer, respectively.

ture, flow characteristics in the dialyzer, and solute size. During hemodialysis treatments, these principles are used to move water, metabolites, and some ions out of the blood, while substances in the dialysate move into the circulation. Figure 16–1 is a schematic representation of a hemodialyzer. Exchange of water and solute can be assessed by considering mass balance.

Solute Flux: Diffusive Transport

The net movement of a particular solute can be measured by considering the mass transfer of that molecule across the dialyzer (Fig. 16–1). The mass of a blood solute entering the dialyzer (M_{bi}) is equal to the product of blood concentration (C_{bi}) and blood flow rate entering the dialyzer (Q_{bi}) during that time period:

$$M_{bi} = C_{bi}Q_{bi} \tag{1}$$

Likewise, the mass of that plasma solute leaving the dialyzer (M_{bo}) may be expressed as

$$M_{bo} = C_{bo}Q_{bo} \tag{2}$$

This formulation presumes that blood is a simple solution of uniform solute concentration C_{bi}. In fact, blood is far from a uniform solution and contains many cells with solute concentrations differing from that of plasma. A consideration of plasma concentration and flow rates also would be inexact, since solutes and water may move from plasma to cells and vice versa. Although an oversimplification, this treatment is useful to describe solute flux.

Since the system conforms with laws of conservation of mass, the mass transfer of solute across the dialysis membrane per unit time (M) may be measured by

$$M = M_{bi} - M_{bo} \tag{3}$$

$$= C_{bi}Q_{bi} - C_{bo}Q_{bo} \tag{4}$$

Similarly, mass transfer also may be measured by changes in the dialysate compartment:

$$M = M_{do} - M_{di} \tag{5}$$

$$= C_{do}Q_{do} - C_{di}Q_{di} \tag{6}$$

M is dependent upon Q_{bi} and Q_{di} and is proportional to the concentration gradient of that solute across the membrane. When no solute is present in the initial dialysate, the transmembrane concentration gradient is determined by C_{bi}. A formula describing the relationship between mass transfer and this solute concentration gradient may be written

$$M = KC_{bi} \tag{7}$$

where K is a constant determined by solute molecular size and membrane characteristics, including area and permeability. Therefore,

$$K = \frac{M}{C_{bi}} \tag{8}$$

Combining (4), (6), and (8);

$$K = \frac{C_{bi}Q_{bi} - C_{bo}Q_{bo}}{C_{bi}} \tag{9}$$

$$K = \frac{C_{do}Q_{do} - C_{di}Q_{di}}{C_{bi}} \tag{10}$$

Since the initial dialysate contains no solute ($C_{di} = 0$),

$$K = \frac{C_{do}Q_{do}}{C_{bi}} \tag{11}$$

The term K is similar to the concept of *clearance* in renal physiology and indicates that the ratio of the mass of solute removed per unit time and the blood concentration of that solute is constant. The efficiency of solute removal during dialysis can be measured easily by the clearance K (ml/min) of that solute.

As in the kidney, the clearance rate is determined by the physical characteristics of the system and remains constant at any blood solute concentration. Therefore, during the dialysis treatment, as blood concentration of a solute falls, mass transfer of the solute into the dialysate fluid falls, but K remains constant. Clearance is a measure of dialysis efficiency, which is determined by the physical characteristics of the system.

When the solute studied is present in the dialysate, mass transfer is proportional to the concentration gradient of that solute:

$$M = D(C_{bi} - C_{di}) \tag{12}$$

where D is a constant analogous to K. D is called *dialysance* and defines more comprehensively the relationship between mass transfer and the transmembrane concentration gradient.

$$D = \frac{M}{C_{bi} - C_{di}} \tag{13}$$

or

$$D = \frac{C_{bi}Q_{bi} - C_{bo}Q_{bo}}{C_{bi} - C_{di}} \tag{14}$$

and

$$D = \frac{C_{do}Q_{do} - C_{di}Q_{di}}{C_{bi} - C_{di}} \tag{15}$$

Dialysance (D) is used to measure the solute flux of substances such as sodium, chloride, bicarbonate, calcium, magnesium, and potassium, which are present in blood and in dialysate mixtures. As noted by Gotch,[1] the relationship between clearance and dialysance, derived from equations (10) and (15) is

$$K = \frac{C_{bi} - C_{di}}{C_{bi}} \tag{16}$$

Thus, in the special case of dialysance where $C_{di} = 0$, clearance is equal to dialysance. When $C_{bi} = C_{di}$, $K = 0$, i.e., clearance ceases. D is independent of C_{bi} and C_{di}. Therefore the dialysance characterizes a dialyzer system and is not affected by whatever solute concentration(s) are present.

For practical purposes, clearance measurements are used to determine the efficiency of dialysis for solutes not present in the dialysate. Dialysance measurements are used to assess the efficiency of solute removal for solutes present in the dialysate and to compare the efficiencies of different dialysis systems.

Water Flux: Ultrafiltration

Water movement across the membrane is proportional to the hydrostatic and osmotic pressure differences across the membrane.[2]

$$Q_F = A(\Delta P - \Delta) \tag{17}$$

where

- Q_F = ultrafiltration rate, ml/min
- A = constant, determined by membrane hydraulic permeability and area
- ΔP = hydraulic pressure gradient across the membrane (mmHg)
- Δ = osmotic pressure gradient across the membrane (mmHg)

Most hemodialysis solutions contain glucose and are nearly isosmolar with blood. Therefore, no substantial osmotic pressure gradient is present across the membrane. Since a relatively large volume of fluid must be moved from the blood to the dialysate in most patients with end-stage renal failure, a hydrostatic pressure gradient is applied across the membrane. This is accomplished by placing a clamp resistance at the outflow side of the dialyzer blood path ("positive pressure") or applying a vacuum to the dialysate path ("negative pressure") (Fig. 16–1).

During standard hemodialysis, fluid is removed by sustaining a hydraulic pressure gradient across a cellulosic membrane of relatively low hydraulic permeability. A similar hydraulic pressure gradient can be established across the membrane when no dialysate is flowing through the dialyzer. This procedure is called pure *ultrafiltration* and can be used before standard hemodialysis (*sequential ultrafiltration*) for patients susceptible to develop hypotension or dialysis disequilibrium. Ultrafiltration also can be used independently to remove fluid rapidly from patients with severe fluid overload and congestive heart failure.

Noncellulosic membranes of high hydraulic permeability may be used. Such systems can increase Q_F by 20-fold. Under these conditions, most solute flux occurs by convection rather than diffusion, since the large bulk of water flow moves dissolved solutes with it across the membrane. During such treatments (*hemofiltration*) diluting fluids must be added to the blood compartment before (predilution) or after (postdilution) the blood flows by the membrane. A careful balance of ultrafiltration and diluting fluid must be maintained. The advantage of such systems is not only the ability to adjust Q_F, but also the increased mass transfer of blood solutes, especially those of higher molecular weights.

Convective Solute Movement

When water moves across the dialysis membrane during standard hemodialysis or during hemofiltration, dissolved solute moves with it ("solvent drag"). When cellulosic (cuprophan) membranes are used, Q_F is small, and relatively little total solute accompanies this bulk flow (convective movement). In contrast, noncellulosic membranes such as polyacrylonitrile (PAN) allow substantial convective flux. While diffusive transport is dependent upon the molecular size of the solute, convective transport may not have this dependency. Thus, mass transfer of middle size (500 to 5000 daltons) and larger molecules is substantially higher in hemofiltration than in hemodialysis. In this way hemofiltration is much closer than is hemodialysis to mass transfer across the glomerular capillary, and some have suggested that this design is therefore preferable to standard hemodialysis.[3]

During convective flux, the solute concentration is often lower in the ultrafiltrate than it is in the blood. This is caused by the physical characteristics of the membrane, which restrain the movement of solute through its pores. The extent of this resistance to convective solute movement can be defined by the sieving coefficient:

$$S = \frac{C_{uF}}{C_b} \qquad (18)$$

C_{uF} = concentration of solute in the ultrafiltrate

C_b = mean concentration of solute in the blood

$$C_b = \frac{C_{bi} + C_{bo}}{2} \qquad (19)$$

Combining (18) and (19), the sieving coefficient can be calculated:[1]

$$S = \frac{2C_{uF}}{C_{bi} + C_{bo}} \qquad (20)$$

PRINCIPLES OF PERITONEAL DIALYSIS

When a solution is introduced into the peritoneal space, solute movement occurs, primarily between the peritoneal capillaries and the dialysate.[4] The capillaries on the surface of the viscera, the mesenteric root, and the peritoneal membrane probably participate in this exchange to varying degrees, depending in part on the distance between the capillary and the peritoneal cavity.[5]

Mass balance considerations may be used to measure the effectiveness of solute diffusion:[6]

$$C = \frac{UV}{P} \tag{21}$$

where

C = clearance (in ml/min)
U = solute concentration in dialysis efflux
P = solute concentration in plasma
V = volume of dialysis efflux

Factors that may affect clearance include temperature, solute size, blood and dialysate flow rate, membrane area, and permeability. Peritoneal capillary blood flow is probably not a limiting factor to small solute clearance at high dialysate flow rates.[4] Vasodilators may enhance blood flow through previously nonperfused arterioles and capillaries,[7] increasing the effective surface area of the membrane available for dialysis exchange[8] and thereby increasing the rate of solute diffusion. Dialysate flow rate offers only a modest limitation to small solute clearance when the flow exceeds 30 ml/min.[4] The membrane itself offers little resistance to solute diffusion for solutes of molecular weight <30,000.[9,10] Stagnant fluid films within the peritoneum may impede solute diffusion,[4,5] and mixing the peritoneal fluid may enhance solute clearance.[11] Thus the relatively small number of peritoneal capillaries exchanging solute and unmixed fluid layers may be the main factors limiting small solute diffusion in peritoneal dialysis.[5]

In 1961 Boen[6] described the kinetics of peritoneal dialysis. When a solute diffuses from plasma to dialysate, its dialysate concentration rises at a rate proportional to the concentration gradient during diffusion. The rate of diffusion is highest at the start of each exchange, and declines with time as the dialysate concentration rises. The rate of diffusion is also inversely proportional to the molecular size of the solute: small molecules tend to equilibrate quickly, while large molecules equilibrate slowly (Fig. 16–2). Similar kinetics are found for molecules that diffuse from the dialysate into the blood, such as bicarbonate and glucose, although there is wide variability in the rates of glucose absorption from patient to patient. Peritoneal clearance also was found to increase as dialyzed volume increased to a maximum at 3.5 liters/hr (58 ml/min). However, only a modest increase in clearance was found when dialysate volume exceeded 2 liters/hr (~30 ml/min) for most molecules other than urea. Since many patients were uncomfortable with more than 2 liters in the peritoneal space, this is the volume used most frequently for peritoneal dialysis.

The term that best describes maximal mass transfer of solute across the peritoneal membrane, independent of the changing dialysate concentration, is *dialysance.* The dialysance of a solute describes the physical limitations to diffusion in a given system and is equal to the instantaneous clearance at the start of an exchange when the dialysate concentration of solute = 0.[12] During actual peritoneal dialysis, the minute-to-minute clearance falls from its dialysance value, as the dialysate concentration rises and the transmembrane driving gradient falls. To maximize mass transfer, the dialysate fluid should be drained and replaced frequently.

Based upon these considerations, intermittent peritoneal dialysis evolved, wherein 2 liters of dialysate was infused and drained every 30 to 60 minutes. Patients treated for 24 to 40 hours each week remained stable clinically, despite a weekly clearance of urea and other small molecules that was substantially less than weekly hemodialysis clearance rates.[13] When dialysate flow rates as high as 150 ml/min were achieved by automated cycling equipment,[14] urea clearance was equal to dialysance, 40 ml/min. Other ways to increase

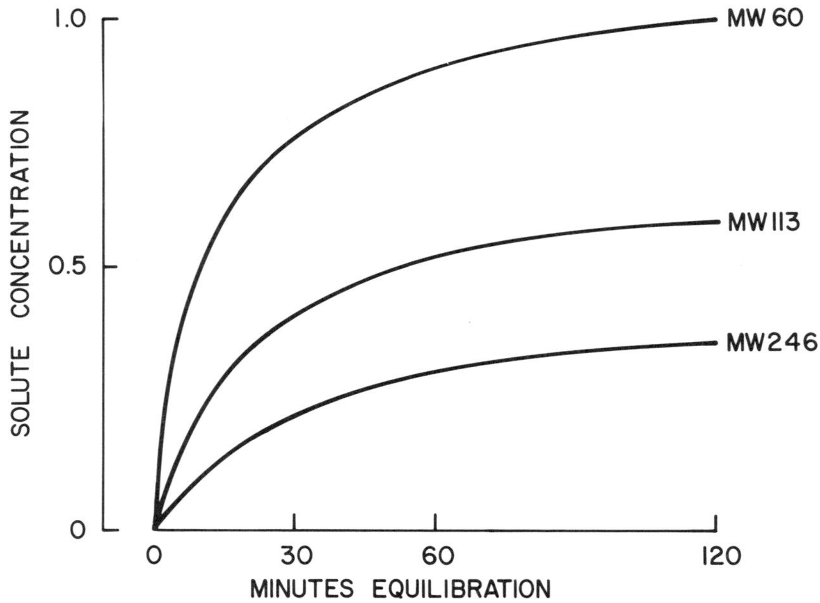

Fig. 16–2. Rates of equilibration of molecules during peritoneal dialysis according to their molecular weights (MW).

clearance rates were found, including vasodilators and hypertonic exchanges. Vasodilators increased clearances only modestly.[15–17] Hypertonic exchanges increase clearance[12,15,18] by at least two different mechanisms. Hypertonic dialysate causes ultrafiltration of water from the capillaries into the peritoneal space. Plasma solutes accompany this convective water movement,[18] and thus clearance is enhanced. However, enhanced clearance persists after isotonic fluid replaces hypertonic fluid in the peritoneum,[15] suggesting that membrane permeability per se may change with hypertonic fluid.[12]

Solute flux has two components: diffusion and convection. It is useful to consider separately the factors that affect each process. The rate of diffusion is determined by the permeability characteristics of the membrane, the membrane area, temperature, the size of the molecule, and the transmembrane concentration gradient. The diffusion rate is maximum in a given system the instant dialysis begins, when the concentration gradient is greatest. Diffusive movement per unit surface area under these conditions is the *mass transfer coefficient* (or dialysance), and the product of this value and the effective area of the peritoneal membrane is the mass transfer-area coefficient. Average mass transfer-area-coefficient values determined experimentally by Pyle et al.[19] are shown in Table 16–1.

Convective movement of solute occurs during ultrafiltration. While water and solutes move together, their respective mass transfer velocities may not be equal. An expression of the relative rates of solute and water movement during ultrafiltration is the sieving coefficient:[2]

$$S = \frac{C_F}{C_W} \tag{22}$$

S = sieving coefficient
C_F = solute concentration in dialysate efflux
C_W = solute concentration in plasma water

This value must be derived when there is no net diffusion of the solute and only convective solute movement is present. When diffusive transport is present,

Table 16–1

Solute	Molecular Weight	MTAC[a] (ml/min·1.73 m²) ± SD
Urea	60	17.7 ± 2.2
Creatinine	113	11.0 ± 3.0
Uric acid	158	9.3 ± 3.0
Glucose	180	9.2 ± 2.5
Insulin	5,500	5.9 ± 1.8
Dextran	70,000	2.0 ± 0.6
Total protein	340,000	0.047 ± 0.67

Adapted from Pyle WK, Moncrief JW, Popovich RP: Peritoneal transport evaluation in CAPD. p 35. In Moncrief JW, Popovich RP (eds): CAPD update. Masson, New York, 1981.
[a] MTAC = mass transfer-area coefficient.

$$S = \frac{\text{convective solute flux}}{C_W \cdot V_{uF}} \qquad (23)$$

where

V_{uF} = ultrafiltration volume

$$= \frac{\text{total solute flux} - \text{diffusive solute flux}}{C_W \cdot V_{uF}} \qquad (24)$$

$$\text{Total solute flux} = V_{Do} \cdot C_F \qquad (25)$$

where

V_{Do} = volume of dialysate efflux
C_F = solute concentration in dialysate efflux

The diffusive component of a small solute flux can be estimated at equilibrium as

$$V_{Di} \cdot C_W \qquad (26)$$

where

V_{Di} = volume of infused dialysate
C_W = solute concentration in plasma water

$$V_{uF} = V_{Do} - V_{Di} \qquad (27)$$

thus

$$S = \frac{V_{Do}C_F - V_{Di}C_W}{(V_{Do} - V_{Di})C_W} \qquad (28)$$

This determination of seiving coefficient presumes equilibrium conditions, which are not present during ordinary intermittent peritoneal dialysis. Nonetheless, estimates of the sieving coefficient during hypertonic peritoneal dialysis have been made.[20] The measured sieving coefficient for Na ranges from 0.12 to 0.78 (mean = 0.54) and for Cl from 0.29 to 1.0 (mean 0.78). Since $C_F < C_W$, patients may develop hypernatremia during such hypertonic peritoneal dialysis.

FLUID REMOVAL AND SODIUM BALANCE

Patients with end-stage renal failure usually are unable to excrete ingested salt and water normally, so dietary restriction and dialysis removal of water and sodium chloride are critical parts of dialysis therapy. An ultrafiltrate of plasma must be removed with each dialysis treatment. This is accomplished in two ways. During hemodialysis a transmembrane hydrostatic pressure is applied by increasing the pressure on the blood side ("positive pressure"), or a vacuum may be applied to the dialysate side of the membrane ("negative pressure"), or both may be employed (Fig. 16–1). This hydrostatic pressure difference induces water movement across the semipermeable membrane into the dialysate. During peritoneal dialysis, the dialysate solution has a higher tonicity than the plasma, and this osmotic pressure difference causes water to leave the vascular space and enter the dialysate.

Hemodialysis

The volume of ultrafiltration possible during hemodialysis depends upon the hydraulic permeability of the membrane, the transmembrane hydrostatic pressure, and the ability of the patient's cardiovascular system to sustain a rapid rate of fluid removal. Cuprophan membranes are modestly permeable, and under normal operating conditions with a 1.0-m^2 dialyzer and transmembrane pressures of 300 to 500 mm Hg, more than 1 liter/hr ultrafiltration can be performed. Noncellulosic membranes are 10 to 20 times more permeable than cuprophan and may be used for standard diffusive hemodialysis or convective hemofiltration.[2] Use of such membranes must be coupled with careful monitors of volume flux and reinfusion of a diluting fluid into the extracorporeal circuit. With this technology the major issue in fluid removal and sodium balance is the ability of patients to sustain large fluid losses over relatively short periods of time. Hypotension during hemodialysis is often the limiting factor in ultrafiltration.

Peritoneal Dialysis

Peritoneal dialysis solutions must be hypertonic to plasma in order to produce net ultrafiltration. To achieve hypertonicity, glucose has been added to the dialysate in concentrations of 5 to 70 g/liter. The glucose is absorbed at a variable rate into the plasma,[6] and water moves into the peritoneal space. When 1.5 percent dextrose (15 g/liter) solution is used, the maximum ultrafiltration rate is about 12 ml/min, and ~330 ml ultrafiltrate is present 140 minutes following infusion of 2 liters of dialysate.[19] When 4.25 percent (42.5 g/liter) dextrose is used, more than 1000 ml ultrafiltrate is present 4 hours following a 2-liter installation. After these times, the intraperitoneal fluid begins to be reabsorbed.

Several years ago, 7 percent dextrose dialysate solutions were available commercially and resulted in dramatic rates of ultrafiltration and glucose absorption. However, in many patients hypotension and death resulted from rapid volume depletion in some patients,[21] while in others severe hyperglycemia and hyperosmolarity developed.[22,23] Hemodynamic assessment showed decreased total blood volume and increased cardiac output in patients with severe heart failure treated with peritoneal dialysis.[24] Because of these complications the 7 percent dextrose dialysate is no longer available commercially, and great care must be taken when using the hypertonic 4.25 percent dextrose solutions that are available.

Hypernatremia is seen frequently among patients receiving aggressive intermittent hypertonic peritoneal dialysis.[20,23,25,26] The dialysate : plasma sodium concentration ratio is <1, particularly when 4.25 percent dextrose solution is used.[26] Thus ultrafiltrate is low in NaCl compared to the extracellular fluid, and hypernatremia results. This is thought to be caused by membrane sieving,[20,26] whereby extracellular fluid enters the peritoneal space through intercellular channels. Cell surface charges may interfere with the convective transport of charged ions, and some solute-free water is ultrafiltered. Alternately, some transcellular water movement may contribute to this hyponatric ultrafiltrate. To prevent hypernatremia, Nolph et al.[20] have suggested that, once the desired ultrafiltrate volume has been removed, all further ultrafiltrate be replaced with fluid having a sodium concentration equal to

$$S_{\mathrm{Na}} \cdot C_{\mathrm{Na}} \qquad (29)$$

where

S_{Na} = sieving coefficient for Na
C_{Na} = plasma Na concentration

Another alternative is to reduce the sodium concentration of the hypertonic peritoneal dialysis solutions to 110 mEq/liter.[27] This results in approximately isonatric extracellular fluid contraction. Alternatively, the plasma sodium concentration can be monitored frequently during the dialysis procedure, and appropriate amount of hypotonic fluid can be replaced intravenously.

Table 16–2. Hemodialysis Hypotension: Possible Causes

Intravascular volume depletion
Diffuse solute movement
Acetate in the dialysate
Hypoxemia
Osmolar shifts
Autonomic dysfunction

DIALYSIS HYPOTENSION

Nearly all hemodialysis patients at one time or another experience a sudden unpleasant feeling of nausea, dizziness, pallor, and abdominal cramps, which accompany a fall in the blood pressure during treatment. Patients and staff learn to respond quickly to these symptoms by decreasing the blood flow rate through the dialyzer, decreasing the transmembrane hydrostatic pressure difference, and infusing saline or other osmotic agents into the extracorporeal circuit. A delay in these remedial actions may result in vomiting, unconsciousness or seizures, and hypoperfusion of the heart or brain. The latter problem is of particular concern, since dialysis patients frequently have underlying coronary or cerebral vascular insufficiency. Approximately 25 percent of hemodialysis treatments are complicated by symptomatic hypotension,[28] and some patients experience the ordeal during nearly every treatment (see Table 16–2).

Role of Intravascular Volume and Cardiovascular Dynamics

Removal of fluid from the intravascular space at a rate exceeding movement of extra- and intracellular water into the circulation can cause hypotension. Early studies performed on patients receiving hemodialysis demonstrated rapid changes in the intravascular volume.[29] The first dialyzers required a large (800 to 1100 ml) extracorporeal circuit, and the machinery and tubing were primed with blood or other colloid. With such dialyzers there was an initial increase in the plasma volume, causing further vascular overload in an already volume-expanded patient. During subsequent hours of treatment, the plasma volume fell progressively, and many patients experienced symptomatic hypotension.

With the use of smaller saline primes the initial volume overload was minimized, but the problems with subsequent hypotension remained. delGreco et al.[30] showed that blood pressure was determined not only by the intravascular volume, but also by cardiac output and peripheral vascular resistance. These hemodynamic regulators vary with the intravascular volume.[30] In patients with circulatory congestion, total peripheral vascular resistance falls during dialysis, while cardiac output and cardiac index rise. In contrast, patients without circulatory congestion have increased peripheral vascular resistance and decreased cardiac output and cardiac index. The largest decline in cardiac output occurs during the first hour of dialysis,[31] when the blood volume and right atrial pressure are falling most quickly. During this time the saline prime (infused at the start of dialysis) rapidly moves out of the intravascular space and into the extracellular fluid. This intravascular volume depletion may cause hypotension in some patients. In one hemodynamic study the blood volume of patients who became hypotensive was 14 percent lower than the blood volume of patients with no fall in blood pressure.[32] When the dialysis coils were primed with dextran, which remains in the intravascular space, the blood volume did not fall during the first hour of dialysis. Patients with severe myocardial disease may be particularly susceptible to volume depletion and hypotension. Hemodynamic studies in such patients show a dialysis-induced fall in mean arterial pressure associated with decreased mean pulmonary artery and pulmonary capillary wedge pressures.[33] The heart responds appropriately to this decrease in venous return by increasing its rate and thereby increasing the cardiac output. However, the total peripheral resistance falls inappropriately. This failure of reflex vasoconstriction appears to be responsible for the resultant hypotension.

The major system that modulates intravascular volume in patients with functioning kidneys is the renin–angiotensin–aldosterone axis. Renin and aldosterone stimulate thirst[34] and therefore have a major impact on fluid balance even in patients with chronic renal failure. When thirsty patients drink large volumes of fluid between dialysis treatments, the ultrafiltration volume during dialysis must be high. Rapid hemodialysis ultrafiltration often results in hypotension. Most dialysis patients have high plasma levels of renin in relation to their exchangeable sodium, and these levels increase when a large volume of fluid is removed during dialysis.[35,36] In some patients this higher level of renin can induce postdialysis hypertension despite decreased intravascular volume. To reduce exchangeable sodium and thereby reduce renin-mediated thirst, and to prevent hypertension and interdialytic weight gains, a dialysate sodium concentration less than that of plasma was chosen in the original commercial dialysis solutions. Plasma sodium concentration declines during dialysis with these solutions, independent of the ultrafiltration rate. The possibility that falling plasma sodium may be a cause of dialysis hypotension will be considered below.

In 1976 Bergstrom et al.[37] speculated that dialysis-related hypotension may not be caused by volume changes alone. They performed *ultrafiltration* without diffusive dialysis by not circulating dialysate through the dialyzer. In this way, a high transmembrane hydrostatic pressure difference would force an ultrafiltrate of plasma to pass through the membrane into the "dialysate" side. This fluid was collected and its volume measured. Absence of circulating dialysate prevented diffusive movement of molecules across the membrane. During pure ultrafiltration, most patients tolerated high rates of fluid removal without developing hypotension, even though rates of fluid removal were equal to or greater than those that caused hypotension during standard dialysis. It therefore appeared that some factor(s) other than volume alone were responsible for dialysis-related hypotension. Hemodynamic studies of patients undergoing ultrafiltration followed by diffusive dialysis (*sequential ultrafiltration*) suggested that diffusion of solute during standard hemodialysis may in some way induce arterial vasodilatation and poor adaptation to falling intravascular volume.[38,39] During pure ultrafiltration, the pulmonary capillary wedge pressure and cardiac index fell. However, the peripheral vascular resistance increased, and as a result the blood pressure did not change. During diffusive dialysis, the cardiac index likewise fell, but the peripheral vascular resistance did not rise appropriately, and patients developed hypotension. Here again was evidence that diffusive dialysis in some way impaired reflex peripheral vasoconstriction, and hypotension resulted.

Hemofiltration, a process whereby a highly permeable membrane is used and most solute movement occurs by convection rather than diffusion, also can be used to remove a substantial volume of fluid without attendant hypotension. Here again, a major difference between the effect of this method and that of hemodialysis on the patient's hemodynamic response was observed. When patients were treated with acetate-containing hemodialysis, the total peripheral resistance fell, as did the blood pressure.[40] Treatment with acetate-containing hemofiltration caused a rise in the vascular resistance and a stable blood pressure.

These studies suggest that fluid removal is much better tolerated when not accompanied by diffusive hemodialysis. Substantial clinical experience with sequential ultrafiltration and hemofiltration has confirmed these findings. When patients have large interdialytic weight gain, or when dialysis hypotension occurs frequently, sequential ultrafiltration or hemofiltration can be used effectively to maintain fluid balance without inducing hypotension.

Role of Acetate

Acetate is substituted commonly for bicarbonate as the base for hemodialysis solutions. When high surface area dialyzers first were used with acetate dialysate solutions, the incidence of hypotension was quite high.[41] Hypotension and other symptoms of "dialysis disequilibrium," including nausea, vomiting, headache, tiredness, and dizziness were reduced when acetate was removed from the dialysate and bicarbonate was used. While many subsequent studies confirm a beneficial effect on the blood pressure when acetate is removed from the dialysate[42-47] others show no difference.[43,48-50] Here again, the reason for hypotension may be a failure of reflex vasocontriction. Acetate, particularly when used with a low sodium concentration in the dialysate, has been shown to decrease the systemic vascular resistance.[40,46,47] Despite increased cardiac output and heart rate, such patients dialyzed with acetate-containing baths developed hypotension.

Role of Hypoxemia

The use of acetate-based dialysis has been associated with a fall in the arterial Po_2. Since the hypoxia of other conditions such as acute pulmonary compromise may be associated with hypotension, it was reasoned that dialysis-related hypoxemia may play a role in the low blood pressures during dialysis. Possible causes of hypoxemia include pulmonary microemboli,[51] dialyzer membrane-induced leukostasis,[52] altered pulmonary function, which results from CO_2 loss across the membrane, or increased oxygen consumption.[53-69] Dolan et al.[54] found that the dead space fraction of tidal volume was slightly increased with acetate and bicarbonate dialysates, arguing against a major component of ventilation–perfusion mismatch as one might expect to see with pulmonary microemboli. Two studies argue against dialysis membrane-induced leukostasis as an important component of hypoxia. Brautbar et al.[70] performed sequential ultrafiltration dialysis and found that the peripheral white blood count fell during the initial ultrafiltration, but the arterial Po_2 remained unchanged. Later, during diffusive dialysis, the white blood count was not low, but the arterial Po_2 fell. A study of dialysis employing four different membrane materials also excludes leukostasis as a significant cause of hypoxia.[71] While hypoxia resulted in all cases, some membranes such as polyacrilonitrile did not result in a fall of white blood cell or platelet count. Thus altered pulmonary function is the best current explanation of dialysis-induced hypoxia. However, a simple decrease in ventilation will not explain the fall in arterial Po_2 in all cases. When patients on ventilators have their ventilation controlled during hemodialysis to prevent decreased minute ventilation, hypoxia still occurs.[72] A fall in the respiratory exchange ratio is probably responsible for the observed hypoxemia.[64]

Whatever the cause, hypoxemia during dialysis can be prevented by administration of oxygen. Several preliminary studies suggest that this maneuver may decrease the frequency of dialysis hypotension. When patients were studied in prospective double-blind protocols using compressed air or oxygen during hemodialysis,[65,73] the frequency of hypotension and other symptoms of dialysis disequilibrium decreased in the group receiving oxygen. The effects of oxygen administration on the pulmonary function of these patients were not recorded. Therefore it appears that, through some mechanism, the administration of oxygen to patients receiving acetate-based hemodialysis may decrease the frequency of hypotension.

Role of Changing Plasma Osmolarity

The widespread use of hyponatric dialysate to minimize interdialytic thirst, weight gain, and hypertension results in a decline of plasma osmolarity during hemodialysis treatments. As dialyzers of larger surface area and more efficient clearance characteristics were employed, the falling osmolarity occurred more quickly, and the frequency of hypotension rose. The possible role of falling osmolality with the accompanying shifts in the body's fluid compartments in dialysis-induced hypotension was investigated. In 1973 Port et al.[74] found that when the dialysate sodium concentration was adjusted during dialysis to maintain isosmolarity with the plasma, the incidence of electroencephalographic abnormalities and symptoms of disequilibrium fell dramatically. Subsequent studies[43,44,49,75–81] have confirmed a decreased incidence of symptomatic hypotension and disequilibrium when higher dialysate sodium concentrations are employed to minimize changes in plasma osmolarity. Boquin et al.[76] studied the effects of higher sodium concentration (140 mEq/liter) dialysate in patients receiving dialysis with large surface area membranes (2.5 m^2). While they found a clinically and statistically significant improvement in hypotension and cramps, they also noted that patients receiving higher sodium dialysis had higher interdialytic weight gains and a slightly higher incidence of hypertension. Therefore the choice of dialysate sodium concentration may need to be tailored to each patient, depending on the efficiency of the dialyzer used, history of hypotension or disequilibrium, cardiovascular stability, and ability to minimize interdialytic weight gain.

When glucose, mannitol, or both are infused during regular dialysis, there is an excellent correlation between the degree of change in serum osmolarity and the incidence of hypotension and disequilibrium.[82,83] Therefore it is clear that, independent of sodium concentration, osmolar shifts during dialysis play a major role in hypotension and disequilibrium. Bergstrom[78] found that sequential ultrafiltration-diffusive dialysis caused hypotension only when the low sodium rather than high sodium dialysate is employed. During sequential ultrafiltration, the serum osmolarity changes little in the first 1½ hours when compared with diffusive dialysis,[84] perhaps explaining the differing incidence of hypotension. Similarly, during high efficiency hemofiltration the serum osmolarity does not change as much as with diffusive dialysis.[85] Some have considered that hypoosmolarity and acetate dialysate may work together to cause hypotension. Wehle et al.[75] found that, while acetate had no effect on the blood pressure at high dialysate sodium concentration, it had a slightly additive deleterious effect at low sodium concentration. Raja et al.[43,86] prevented osmolar shifts during dialysis with a mannitol infusion and found that both acetate infusion and falling tonicity are important to blood pressure control.

The mechanisms whereby shifts in plasma osmolarity may induce hypotension have been studied in recent years. Aizawa et al.,[87] noting that the degree of fall in serum osmolarity correlated with the degree of hypotension, speculated that hypoosmolarity can affect circulating blood volume by an indirect effect of capillary refilling. When hyponatric dialysate is used, water leaves the intravascular space toward the dialysate and also leaves the intravascular space to enter cells.[79] In contrast, during hypernatric dialysis the same volume of fluid leaves the intravascular space to enter the dialysate, but more than half this loss is repleted by water movement out of cells into the extracellular space. Thus a falling serum osmolarity induces large fluid shifts out of the intravascular space, and hypotension may result.

Arguments have been made against a major role for osmolar shifts in dialysis hypotension. Shaldon et al.[88] observed that decreasing the dialysate flow rate and thereby decreasing the efficiency of diffusive transport reduced the incidence of hypotension despite the same osmolar shifts as with high dialysate flow rate. Furthermore, when Keshaviah et al.[46] performed isosmotic dialysis in dogs by adding sodium and urea to the dialysate in the same concentrations as in the plasma, the mean arterial pressure still fell early in dialysis. This was accompanied by falling systemic vascular resistance, a phenomenon reproduced by intravenous acetate but not by intravenous bicarbonate infusion. The authors concluded that acetate and not a fall in osmolarity was responsible for the early hypotension.

Role of Autonomic Dysfunction

Whatever is the underlying cause of dialysis-related hypotension, it is obvious that the effect is mediated through the autonomic nervous system. The autonomic nervous system, through its baroreceptors, catecholamine messengers, and cardiovascular effectors, regulates the blood pressure. When uremic dogs are volume depleted by pure ultrafiltration, heart rate and vascular resistance rise, and blood pressure is maintained.[89] When these same animals are volume depleted by diffusive dialysis, the peripheral resistance declines and the mean arterial pressure falls. Something happens during diffusive dialysis to interfere with the autonomic control mechanism, compensatory vasoconstriction fails, and hypotension develops. Since more than half the patients with chronic renal failure have a demonstrable impairment in autonomic nervous function even if they are asymptomatic,[90,91] this abnormality could be largely responsible for dialysis hypotension.

Kersh et al.[92] studied the integrity of the autonomic nervous system in patients with dialysis-induced hypotension and found that most were abnormal: hypotension was not accompanied by tachycardia, and the total systemic resistance fell. When these patients were given volume infusions, they had no response, but their blood pressure did rise when they received norepinephrine. Lilley et al.[93] found that patients suffering dialysis hypotension had higher mean arterial pressures before and after dialysis and higher plasma levels of dopamine β-hydroxylase than did nonhypotensive dialysis patients. Dopamine β-hydroxyalse is secreted into plasma on a mole-for-mole basis with epinephrine, but has a substantially longer biologic half-life than does epinephrine.[28] Its concentration can be used to assess effective sympathetic nervous system tone. When patients with dialysis hypotension were tested with amyl nitrite inhalation, a test of the entire baroreceptor reflex arc,[93] the R-R interval/MAP decrease was less than normal, suggesting a defect in the visceral afferent limb of the autonomic reflex arc. Lilley[93] speculated that hemodialysis hypotension may be neurogenic in origin and may result from a lesion in baroreceptors, cardiopulmonary receptors, or visceral afferent nerves.

Changes in sympathetic tone are mediated by circulating catecholamines, and some studies suggest that disordered norepinephrine control may play some role in dialysis hypotension. In 1978 Cannella et al.[94] studied patients with ultrafiltration and diffusive dialysis. During ultrafiltration, when the blood pressure remained constant, plasma norepinephrine levels rose. During diffusive dialysis, the blood pressure fell and norepinephrine levels did not rise. Cannella et al.[94] speculated that during diffusive dialysis, norepinephrine or another small molecule is removed, and hypotension results. Korchik et al.[95,96] found that, while norepinephrine is dialyzable with a substantial rate of clearance, plasma levels are not altered significantly by hemodialysis and respond to the upright posture with a normal increase. Corder et al.[97] confirmed these findings. Thus dialysance of norepinephrine plays no role in dialysis hypotension. During ultrafiltration dialysis, when the intravascular volume and the serum potassium concentration are falling, Henrich et al.[98] found that the heart rate did not increase and catecholamine levels fell. When isokalemic dialysis prevented a falling serum potassium, the heart rate increased appropriately and catecholamine levels remained elevated. However, later studies[83] found that isokalemic dialysis did not prevent hypotension, and that patients so treated demonstrated normal postural increases in norepinephrine levels. Changes in blood pressure could be dissociated from changes in plasma norepinephrine levels, discounting a major role for norepinephrine in dialysis hypotension. Finally, one study[99] of autonomic function in hypotensive and normotensive subjects failed to show a substantial difference between them, suggesting that autonomic dysfunction does not by itself induce hypotension.

In summary, it appears that dialysis hypotension is a common and complicated problem, with several possible causes. Rapid ultrafiltration or decreasing plasma osmolarity may result in rapid movement of fluid out of the intravascular space, causing volume contraction hypotension. Acetate, falling serum osmolarity, or some other molecule lost during diffusive dialysis may impair normal vasoconstriction, leading to a fall in mean arterial pressure. Hypoxia or defects in the autonomic reflex arc may predispose patients to hypotension, and any combination of these factors may be important in different patients. In addition to being unpleasant, intradialytic hypotension may be dangerous to the patient and may limit the amount of ultrafiltration that is possible. Therefore, a careful assessment of each patient who suffers frequent hypotension can improve the quality of life substantially. If interdialytic weight gain and blood pressure can be controlled, the dialysate sodium concentration should be raised to at least 140 mEq/liter, or to a level equal to the patient's serum sodium concentration. If large surface area hemodialyzers are used, or if dialysis disequilibrium commonly accompanies treatments, a trial of bicarbonate-based dialysate may be tried. For patients who develop hypoxia, low flow oxygen therapy may be useful. Finally, for many patients with frequent hypotension, or large intradialytic weight gains, sequential ultrafiltration followed by low dialysate flow isovolemic diffusive dialysis removes fluid effectively without hypotension. Should hemofiltration become more widely available, many hypertensive patients with dialysis hypotension might benefit by its use.

ACID–BASE BALANCE AND DIALYSIS

Chronic metabolic acidosis accompanies renal failure in virtually all patients who come to dialysis. Early in the course of kidney disease total plasma CO_2 is reduced significantly,[100] and this decline is offset by increased plasma chloride. The unmeasured anion concentration (the "anion gap"), representing fixed acids other than chloride, remains normal. As renal failure progresses, the total CO_2 declines further, Cl^- concentration remains stable, and the anion gap increases. A large fraction of this anion gap represents plasma sulfate,[101] which is increased manifold in chronic renal failure.[102] In patients with advanced renal failure this pattern is the same for primary glomerular diseases, interstitital diseases, or renal failure of unknown etiology. If these patients are given an acid load, total acid excretion is reduced,[103] and the patients appear to be in positive acid balance. When patients with chronic renal failure continue to eat an acid-producing diet, plasma pH and bicarbonate concentration remain stable at a reduced level,[104] even though their acid production rate is no different than that of healthy subjects on the same diet.[105] Therefore, some other buffer must accept protons chronically in patients with chronic renal failure. Lemann and Lennon[106] reviewed the evidence that much of this buffering takes place in the bones.

Bones as a Buffer

Patients with chronic renal failure frequently demonstrate skeletal demineralization. The adult skeleton contains ~35,000 mEq of potentially available base,[105,107] and demineralization can release alkali to buffer retained acid.[108] Patients with chronic renal failure have been shown to have a slow loss of total calcium[109,110] and a decline of bone calcium and carbonate in proportion to the duration of the renal disease.[111] Since calcium carbonate comprises 37 percent of bone carbonate, it may be the large buffer pool that titrates the daily retained acid load in these patients. Two lines of evidence support this hypothesis: studies of acid loads in normal animals and man,[112,113] and studies of bones and buffering capacity in azotemic animals and human subjects.[114,115] When normal human volunteers receive chronic oral acid loads, a positive acid balance develops buffered by intra- and extracellular buffers.[112] As acid retention continues, calcium losses suggest bone buffering, in a fashion similar to that of chronic renal failure patients. When the acid load is stopped, intra- and extracellular buffers are restored promptly, but some acid is not excreted, despite a return of serum bicarbonate to normal. In addition, the negative calcium balance is maintained for long periods after acid infusion is stopped. These findings suggest that bone mineral buffers the ingested acid, and the bones remain altered despite correction of acidemia. An analysis of bone from dogs with metabolic acidosis[113] demonstrates a 9.5 percent decline of calcium carbonate, an amount sufficient to account for buffering of the metabolic acid. Studies of vertebral bone from patients with chronic renal failure show decreased bone carbonate, which results from a carbonate–phosphate interchange within the apatite crystal.[114] The ability of bone to serve as a buffer may be dependent on presence of parathyroid hormone. Fraley and Adler[115] studied uremic animals with and without parathyroid glands. Animals with intact glands developed severe acidosis, but many survived, buffering 50 to 61 percent of the acid inside cells. All thyroparathyroidectomized animals died, buffering only 3 to 22 percent of the acid load intracellularly. When thyroparathyroidectomized animals were given exogenous parathyroid hormone, several of them survived. These workers suggested that bone is the target for parathyroid hormone-mediated increased cell buffering capacity.

The role of chronic acidosis in the genesis of uremic bone disease is unclear, but from the evidence discussed above it seems reasonable to expect that stopping the chronic acid load might result in less bony demineralization. When the chronic acidemia of renal tubular acidosis is corrected, the progression of bone disease is arrested.[107] Ten infants and children with classic renal tubular acidosis increased dramatically their mean height and rate of growth when chronic alkali therapy corrected their acidemia.[116] Finally, when patients with chronic renal failure and metabolic acidosis were treated with sodium bicarbonate, their calcium excretion fell, correcting their negative calcium balance.[110] These findings suggest that, when possible, chronic metabolic acidosis should be treated in patients with renal failure. For patients receiving chronic dialysis, maintenance of overall acid–base balance is possible if the diet is limited in acid-producing foods, and if the base concentration of the dialysate is sufficiently high to produce net alkali infusion with each dialysis.[117] When plasma bicarbonate falls below 15 mEq/liter, treatment with 1 to 2 mEq/kg/day sodium bicarbonate is probably indicated.[118] Shohls solution, a 1-mM solution of sodium citrate, may be better tolerated by some patients, and is as effective as sodium bicarbonate, since the citrate is metabolized to bicarbonate in the body.

Effects of Hemodialysis on the Acid–Base Balance

The earliest studies of 10 patients treated with hemodialysis showed changes in both the metabolic and respiratory control of acid–base balance.[119] As expected, dialysis with a bicarbonate-containing dialysate increased total serum base concentration, removed "anion gap"

Table 16–3. Effects of Hemodialysis on the Acid–Base Balance

Sustained respiratory alkalosis
Increased sensitivity to CO_2
CO_2 movement across the dialysis membrane
Hypoxemia
Bicarbonate and organic acid losses with acetate dialysate
Acetate or bicarbonate infusion

acids, and corrected hypochloremia. More surprising, respiratory alkalosis persisted unchanged throughout the dialysis, persisting to the end despite correction of metabolic acidosis.[119] Since that time, many investigators have sought to understand this persistent respiratory alkalosis (see Table 16–3).

Respiratory Alkalosis of Hemodialysis

Respiratory alkalosis, or a low P_{CO_2} at the end of dialysis has been confirmed widely with both bicarbonate- and acetate-containing hemodialysate baths[42,53-61,117,119-130] and with pure ultrafiltration where no dialysate bath is used.[131] Although some investigators have found that dialysis does not modify significantly the respiratory compensation of metabolic acidosis,[128] it has been known since 1917 that during rapid recovery from metabolic acidosis, many patients exhibit persistent hyperventilation and resulting respiratory alkalosis.[132] This phenomenon is seen in recovery from the acidosis of ammonium chloride administration, the acidemia of diarrhea, and diabetic ketoacidosis. While it may be no surprise that the same phenomenon is found following dialysis-induced rapid reversal of uremic acidemia, investigators have sought to understand its mechanism.

Cowie et al.[120] noted that, while plasma bicarbonate concentration rose by 11.2 mEq/liter following dialysis, cerebrospinal fluid bicarbonate concentration increased by only 1.5 mEq/liter. Since central nervous system pH may control the respiratory center, the resultant small change in cerebrospinal fluid pH (0.007) may be the reason for the relatively unchanged P_{CO_2} and the postdialysis alkalemia. However, studies in uremic goats do not support this hypothesis. Hamilton et al.[127] studied the ventilatory response to CO_2 after hemodialysis in acidemic uremic patients and in uremic goats. Both patients and animals demonstrated increased sensitivity to CO_2 within the first 30 minutes of dialysis, and the cerebrospinal fluid acid–base status in the goat could not explain the increased sensitivity to CO_2. When osmotic shifts during dialysis were minimized by adding urea to the dialysate, the increased sensitivity to CO_2 was eliminated. Hamilton and associates[127] concluded that when standard dialysis is performed on uremic patients, osmotic disequilibrium induces a transitory increased ventilatory response to CO_2, which results in respiratory alkalosis. Arguing against this hypothesis is a study showing no increased sensitivity to CO_2 immediately after hemodialysis in uremic[133] as well as in nonuremic patients.[134] When patients with normal renal function were hemodialyzed for schizophrenia, their P_{CO_2} values fell and respiratory alkalosis was present. Thus the mechanism for dialysis-induced respiratory alkalosis may be independent of both osmotic disequilibrium and the preexisting metabolic acidosis.

Several lines of evidence suggest that CO_2 moves across the dialyzing membrane, changing the P_{CO_2} by a mechanism other than hypo- or hyperventilation. In 1966 Henderson et al.[122] found that when 10 percent CO_2 is bubbled into a standard bicarbonate dialysate, the P_{CO_2} is higher in the bath, crosses the membrane, and enters the blood. Graziani et al.[125] speculated that the commonly observed postdialysis hypocapnia might be caused by CO_2 loss from the blood across the dialysis membrane, into the dialysis fluid. When CO_2 is added to the dialysate to prevent CO_2 loss[53] the arterial P_{CO_2} remains unchanged, suggesting that minute ventilation is controlled to maintain a constant P_{CO_2}. Recent measurements[54,59] have shown that the amount of CO_2 that crosses the dialysis membrane from blood to dialysate may be substantial, 3 mmol/min, or 30 ml/m^2/min. This represents one third of a patient's metabolic production of CO_2. However, since the prevention of CO_2 loss does not alter postdialysis hypocapnia, another explanation of the respiratory alkalosis must be found.[126] When high efficiency dialysis is performed using high (2.5 m^2) surface area membranes and acetate dialysate, the

P_{CO_2} falls substantially during the first part of the treatment, then rises to predialysis values at the termination of therapy.[42,61,129,130] Tolchin et al.[61] showed that this fall in P_{CO_2} was associated with a significant drop in minute ventilation volume, confirming a substantial dialyzer mass transfer of CO_2. The lower P_{CO_2} tends to raise the pH, offsetting the temporarily worsening metabolic acidosis found in such patients. While the intradialytic acid–base balance is affected by CO_2 movement across the dialysis membrane, the persistent respiratory alkalosis following dialysis remains unexplained.

Dialysis Hypoxemia

The arterial P_{O_2} falls during hemodialysis when acetate-containing dialysate is used.[45,53–69] While some evidence suggests that pulmonary artery microemboli[51] or dialyzer membrane-induced leukostasis[52] might be responsible in part for this hypoxia, altered pulmonary function, which results from CO_2 loss across the dialyzer and central control of respiratory alkalosis, is a major determinant of this finding. Sherlock et al.[55] found that both minute ventilation and the P_{O_2} fell during dialysis with acetate-based solutions. When CO_2 was bubbled into the dialysate to prevent CO_2 loss across the dialyzer, CO_2 output through the lungs (V_{CO_2}) increased, and the arterial P_{CO_2} remained unchanged. Although minute ventilation and the P_{O_2} remained depressed when CO_2 loss across the membrane was prevented, the hypoxemia was blunted.[57] Other investigators have confirmed an increased oxygen consumption during acetate-based dialysis,[54–56,60,62,68,69] causing a fall in the respiratory exchange ratio.[54,55,57,60,66,69] This alteration of alveolar gas content may be responsible for the observed hypoxia.[64] When bicarbonate bath is substituted for acetate, and CO_2 loss across the membrane is prevented by bubbling CO_2 into the dialysate, Aurigemma et al.[53] found that the P_{O_2} does not fall. While subsequent studies confirmed that the P_{O_2} does not fall[54,58,61] or falls only slightly[60,69] during bicarbonate-based dialysis, some studies showed the same degree of hypoxia with bicarbonate as with acetate-based dialysis.[63,66] Of particular note, oxygen consumption fell with bicarbonate bath, while it rose with acetate.[60] Thus, the respiratory quotient (V_{CO_2}/V_{O_2}) tends to fall more substantially with acetate dialysis, decreasing the P_{O_2}. However, the change in respiratory quotient is not the sole mechanism for hypoxia of acetate dialysis. In one study where the P_{O_2} fell, using both acetate and bicarbonate bath, the respiratory quotient fell only with the acetate bath.[66] In a sorbent regenerative acetate-based dialysis system, where CO_2 is lost across the membrane only early in the dialysis, the P_{O_2} fell early, but returned to baseline as CO_2 was regained across the membrane.[69]

These findings suggest that acetate induces an increase in oxygen consumption, which decreases the respiratory exchange ratio. When CO_2 is lost across the membrane, the respiratory exchange ratio may fall further. These acetate-induced changes may be responsible for the intradialytic hypoxia. When high surface area hemodialyzers are used,[61] the P_{CO_2} falls in association with a fall in minute ventilation and P_{O_2}. During such high-efficiency dialysis, loss of large amounts of CO_2 across the dialyzer induces hypoventilation to minimize the respiratory alkalosis, and this in turn causes the observed hypoxia. Thus, loss of CO_2 across the dialyzer and acetate-induced increased O_2 consumption both play a role in producing dialysis-related hypoxia. See Table 16–4.

Table 16–4. Dialysis Hypoxemia: Possible Causes

Pulmonary microemboli
Leukostasis
Acetate-induced increased oxygen consumption
CO_2 loss across the dialysis membrane

DIALYSIS-INDUCED CHANGES IN METABOLIC ACID–BASE BALANCE

During hemodialysis and hemofiltration, acids and bases move from dialysate to blood or blood to dialysate by diffusion or by convection (solute "drag" with water movement). Changes in overall acid–base balance depend upon the rate of movement of these substances across the membrane, the production rate of organic acids, and the ability of the body to metabolize dialysate base sources (acetate or lactate) to bicarbonate. In the most simple case, sodium bicarbonate is used as the dialysate base (Fig. 16–3).

Most patients with end-stage renal disease have a chronic metabolic acidosis, which depresses the plasma concentration of HCO_3^-. When the dialysate concentration of $NaHCO_3$ exceeds the plasma concentration, bicarbonate will diffuse from the dialysate into the blood. At the same time, organic acids such as pyruvate, acetoacetate, β-hydroxybutyrate, and citrate diffuse from the plasma into the dialysate. Since these organic anions can be metabolized to bicarbonate in muscle and liver cells, their loss is equivalent to base lost from the body. Net alkali balance may be expressed as

$$\text{net alkali} = \text{bicarbonate infusion} - \text{organic anion loss} \qquad (30)$$

The rate of bicarbonate infusion depends upon the concentration difference across the membrane, and the permeability and surface area of the membrane. Both cuprophan and noncellulose membranes offer little resistance to HCO_3 diffusion. The dialysate bicarbonate concentration falls as the bath P_{CO_2} falls. If CO_2 is bubbled into the dialysate, its P_{CO_2} is higher, the HCO_3 concentration remains stable in the bath, and CO_2 may diffuse across the membrane into the blood.[122] The result is a significant increase in the plasma HCO_3 concentration at the end of dialysis. During ultrafiltration of standard hemodialysis, HCO_3 moves into the dialysate according to the formula

$$\text{Convective } HCO_3 \text{ movement} = S_{HCO_3} \cdot V_{uF} \qquad (31)$$

where

S_{HCO_3} = sieving coefficient for bicarbonate
V_{uF} = ultrafiltration volume

For example, if the mean plasma HCO_3 concentration is 20 mEq/liter and 4 liters of ultrafiltrate are removed during dialysis, ~60 to 80 mEq HCO_3 will move from plasma to dialysate. While this loss may represent only 10 to 20 percent of the net HCO_3 gained during standard hemodialysis, bicarbonate loss increases substantially when the noncellulosic, highly permeable membranes are used for dialysis or hemofiltration. In these procedures, HCO_3 or other base equivalent such as acetate must be infused with diluting fluid to maintain the acid–base balance.

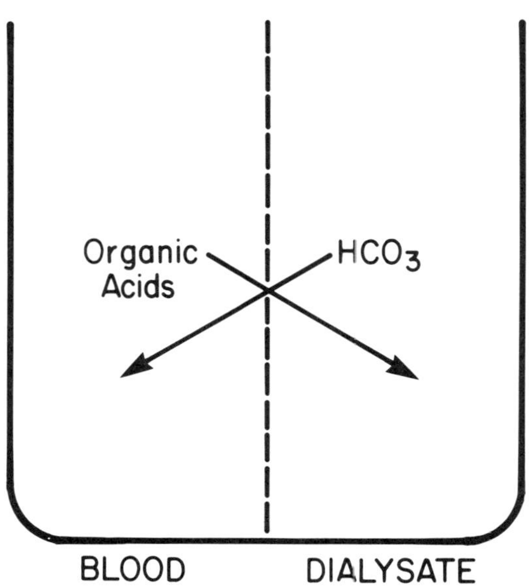

Fig. 16–3. Acid–base movement across a semipermeable membrane during dialysis with bicarbonate (HCO_3)-containing dialysate solutions.

Acetate in Hemodialysis

When the use of chronic hemodialysis grew during the early 1960s, centers were established to treat many patients simultaneously.

At that time, methods were sought to simplify the dialysis equipment and procedures, and to prepare large quantities of dialysate for hemodialysis centers. The preparation of dialysate containing bicarbonate was difficult, since delivery of bicarbonate and calcium to the same dialysate required an extra proportioning pump. A dialysate concentrate containing both HCO_3^- and Ca^{2+} would result in precipitation as calcium carbonate, so an alternative to HCO_3^- was sought in the preparation of commercial dialysate concentrates. Acetate was selected to substitute for bicarbonate in the dialysate.[135] Sodium acetate had been used previously for parenteral administration of alkali.[136] In the body it is converted to acetyl-CoA, which can then be oxidized in the Krebs cycle:

$$\text{Na acetate} \rightarrow \text{acetyl-CoA} \rightarrow \text{Na bicarbonate} + CO_2 + H_2O + 200 \text{ kcal/mol} \qquad (32)$$

Thus acetate, which diffuses across the dialysis membrane into the patient across the membrane, is converted mole for mole to bicarbonate in the muscle. It was recognized that dialysate containing acetate but no bicarbonate would result in a bidirectional movement of base according to the concentration gradients (see Fig. 16–4). In this early, relatively inefficient procedure with a Kiil dialyzer and blood flow of 150 ml/min, the bicarbonate lost from the blood into the dialysate was 90 mEq/hr.[135] If the dialysate acetate concentration is similar to bicarbonate, 32 mEq/liter, net base is lost during hemodialysis, and acidemia results.[137] A dialysate acetate concentration of 35 to 40 mEq/liter ensures that total acetate infused exceeds total bicarbonate lost from the blood, and a positive alkali balance results by the end of dialysis. This complicates formula (30) for net alkali gain during dialysis:[138]

$$\text{net alkali gain} = \text{acetate infusion} - (\text{bicarbonate loss} + \text{organic anion loss}) \qquad (33)$$

Early studies reported an initial decline in the serum bicarbonate concentration when acetate dialysate was used. This was followed by a steadily rising bicarbonate level.[66,123] Other studies showed only a rising bicarbonate level,[117,121,124,133] suggesting that infused acetate was converted rapidly to bicarbonate and was an excellent dialysate buffer as Mion et al.[135] had suggested. Intravenous infusion of acetate in uremic patients produced buffering similar to bicarbonate infusion, even in patients with severe liver disease.[139] This was not surprising, since Lindquist[140] had estimated that 300 mmol/hr of free acetate could be metabolized to bicarbonate in humans.[140] In subsequent studies, the mean utilization rate for acetate during hemodialysis was calculated to be 2.9 to 3.5 mmol/kg/hr, with a range of 2.8 to 4.4 mmol/kg/hr.[130,141] The rate of acetate infusion with early dialysis equipment did not reach these levels.

In 1975 Port and Easterling[142] studied patients treated with the new, highly efficient hemodialyzers with surface areas of 2.6 m². They found that acetate clearance and bicarbonate clearance were very high, only 10 percent less than urea clearance. The plasma acetate level rose with dialysis, reaching levels exceeding 9.5 mmol/liter in 17 percent of patients, and sometimes reached levels as high as 21.6 mmol/liter. The same group described patients who developed abdominal discomfort, chills, and hypotension during dialysis, each with strikingly elevated levels of acetate in the plasma ($>$15 mEq/liter) and a proportional fall in plasma bicarbonate.[143] While there was no correlation between these symptoms and postdialysis acetate levels,[142] this phenomenon was thought to represent acetate intolerance. Subsequent studies using acetate-containing dialysate and highly efficient dialyzers showed an initial fall, followed by a gradual rise in the plasma bicarbonate concentration.[42,129] Careful flux measurements showed that the rate of acetate infusion could exceed the maximum rate of acetate oxi-

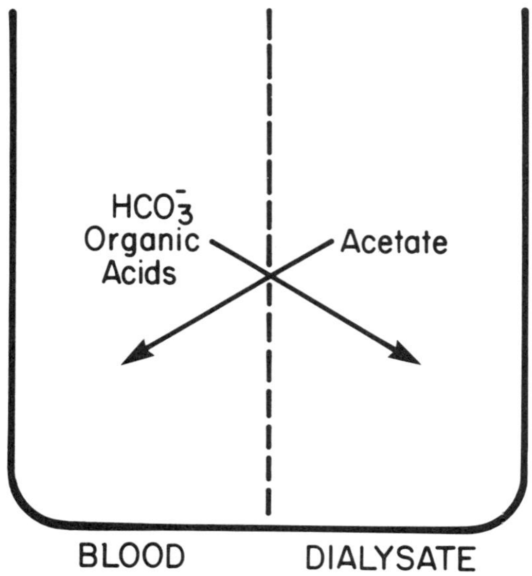

Fig. 16–4. Acid–base movement across a semipermeable membrane during dialysis with acetate-containing dialysate solutions.

dation to bicarbonate.[129,130,138,144] These high rates of acetate infusion were even found to increase the acetate utilization rate to as high as 7.2 mmol/min.[138] On the other hand, one reported patient had evidence for the presence of an inhibitor of acetate metabolism in the plasma or on cells, which reduced the ability of lymphocytes to metabolize acetate to bicarbonate by 65 percent.[145]

When the acetate infusion rate exceeds the ability of muscle to convert it to bicarbonate, alternate metabolic pathways may become prominent. These include conversion of acetate to cholesterol or to long-chain fatty acids.[146] As much as 9 percent of infused acetate could take such alternate pathways,[129,130] resulting in the conversion of ~70 mmol of acetate to cholesterol and fatty acids with each 4 hours of dialysis.[130]

It is possible that many symptoms commonly encountered during dialysis might be related to acetate infusion, including headaches, abdominal and muscle pain, chills, hypotension, nausea, vomiting, intolerance to ultrafiltration, and central nervous system symptoms. In the dog, acetate is a weak vasodilator and may cause a fall in systolic blood pressure. A direct depressant effect on the myocardium to decrease the force of contraction has also been proposed.[147] However, acetate infusion has also been shown to increase cardiac output, increase left ventricular *dP/dt,* increase coronary blood flow, and cause coronary vasodilatation.[148] In humans acetate dialysis has been variably reported to produce both a decrease in cardiac output[149] and an increase in cardiac index and heart rate.[39] In one study, repeated dialysis procedures with acetate resulted in improved cardiac performance.[47] Most importantly, acetate also produces a decrease in peripheral resistance,[39,149] even in the face of declining intravascular volume. Therefore, hypotension can result from a failure of reflex vasoconstriction or even vasodilatation whether or not acetate affects directly the myocardial contractility. One patient on acetate dialysis developed acute asthmatic attacks apparently related to the actate[150] (see Table 16–5).

If acetate is responsible, wholly or in part, for these troublesome symptoms during dialysis, substitution of bicarbonate for the acetate bath would result in substantial clinical improvement. Central delivery and individual proportioning hemodialysis equipment is now available, with separate infusions of calcium and bicarbonate, so that regular bicarbonate dialysis is technically feasible in large hemodialysis centers. Some studies do suggest that bicarbonate dialysis eliminates some of these symptoms,[42,48,151] while others find no difference between acetate and bicarbonate baths.[152]

Table 16–5. Acetate Dialysate: Possible Side Effects

Dialysis disequilibrium
Decreased myocardial contractility
Increased cholesterol and fatty acid production
Decreased peripheral vascular resistance and hypotension
Chronic retention of metabolic acids in bone buffers
Increased formation and loss of organic acids
Increased rate of oxygen consumption

When bicarbonate replaced acetate in the dialysate of 12 patients with recurrent hypotension, the blood pressure did not fall during the first hour of acetate hemodialysis.[153] Bicarbonate dialysis does not decrease the peripheral vascular resistance as does acetate,[149] possibly explaining the decreased incidence of hypotension.[154] When bicarbonate dialysate is recirculated at low flow rates through the dialyzer, and treatments are performed for 2 to 3 hours every other day, patients experience substantially fewer side effects,[155] perhaps as a consequence of better acid–base stability. As discussed earlier, many factors other than acetate may affect cardiac performance and cardiovascular stability. During chronic acetate dialysis, steady state is reached and H^+ balance equals zero. However, when these stable patients are converted to HCO_3 dialysis, 24 mEq of net alkali is retained per day,[156] suggesting that buffer depletion had occurred during acetate dialysis. Addition of bicarbonate removed H^+ from nonextracellular water buffers, presumably from bone. Although no evidence is available to suggest that correction of this chronic bone acid load will improve uremic bone disease, long-term studies in patients treated with bicarbonate-containing dialysate should answer this question.

Organic anion movement into the dialysate is an important determinant of overall acid–base homeostasis (Fig. 16–4) and may be equal to as much as 57 percent of net base gain during hemodialysis when acetate dialysate is used.[138] Plasma acetoacetate concentrations fall significantly during hemodialysis,[138] while lactate, citrate, and beta-hydroxybutyrate concentrations rise.[121,138,144] Pyruvate concentrations have been reported to rise[121] or fall.[138] Presumably, all of these organic acids diffuse into the dialysate, and movement of citrate and beta-hydroxybutyrate from cells into the plasma causes their rising concentrations. Vreman et al.[138] point out that factors altering plasma lactate concentration, such as hypotension or hypoxia, or conditions that increase the concentration of ketone bodies such as diabetes mellitus, fasting, or glucose in the dialysate may affect overall acid–base balance by inducing increased losses of organic anions into the dialysate.

In summary, the conflicting reports concerning the effects of acetate on the heart, and the many other factors that may affect the vascular system during dialysis make it difficult to reach firm conclusions concerning the use of acetate in hemodialysis. The use of high surface area hemodialyzers may result in acetate infusion rates that exceed the rate of metabolism and a higher incidence of intradialytic complications. Acetate may increase the formation and loss of organic anions, complicating the acid–base balance. A higher rate of oxygen consumption and increased CO_2 production may produce changes in the arterial Po_2 and respiratory dynamics, perhaps contributing to postdialysis respiratory alkalosis. Acetate-induced peripheral vasodilation may result in hypotension in those patients who cannot compensate adequately with an increased cardiac output. Finally, bicarbonate may correct the chronic acid load that is buffered in bones and may improve the course of uremic bone disease. It is clear that in some patients who experience frequent headaches, hypotension, abdominal or muscle pain, and chills, elimination of acetate from the dialysate and use of bicarbonate improves their lives substantially. Although some nephrologists believe that, were it technically feasible, all hemodialysis solutions should be bicarbonate-based, unresolved problems remain in the use of bicarbonate. If repletion of bone buffer is desirable, then a dialysate bicarbonate concentration somewhat higher than plasma is necessary. However, it should not be so high that metabolic alkalosis results. Furthermore, as bone buffer is repleted, the dialysate concentration of bicarbonate should be lowered. There is no clear way to know when the concentration should be decreased, or by how much. More information is needed before wholesale changes are made in the base content of hemodialysis.

EFFECTS OF PERITONEAL DIALYSIS ON THE ACID–BASE BALANCE

Metabolic Acid–Base Balance

Commercially prepared peritoneal dialysis solutions contain acetate or lactate to provide a stable source of alkali, and to allow addition of calcium and magnesium salts to the solution (see Table 16–6). Intermittent peritoneal dialysis for 30 to 36 hours gradually corrects the chronic metabolic acidosis of uremia, raising the serum bicarbonate concentration from 17.0 to 24.5 mEq/liter. When lactate is used as the dialysate base, it is absorbed rapidly and is metabolized by the Krebs cycle in the liver to glucose or CO_2.[157] When large amounts of lactate are absorbed, metabolic alkalosis may develop.[25] This complication is seen most frequently when hypertonic dialysate is used, and may result in part from a sieving effect on bicarbonate transport. The ultrafiltrate produced by hypertonic dialysate has a lower concentration of bicarbonate than does plasma. The loss of more water than bicarbonate may lead to a "contraction alkalosis."[23]

Since the liver is the main site of lactate metabolism, patients with disturbed hepatic function may be unable to convert lactate to bicarbonate.[158] In such patients the bicarbonate in the plasma moves across the membrane into the dialysis solution, decreasing the plasma bicarbonate concentration, and the metabolic acidosis actually may become worse.[157] Use of an acetate-based dialysis solution would obviate the problem. It should be noted that, while 71 percent of acetate infused during peritoneal dialysis is converted to bicarbonate, only 45 percent of infused lactate is converted to bicarbonate.[159] For this reason, the concentration of acetate should be lower than lactate for equivalent net alkali infusion. Acetate or lactate, together with the hyperosmotic glucose solutions of peritoneal dialysate, produce rapid dilation of the vascular bed,[160] thereby increasing the effective surface area of the dialysis membrane, and secondarily improve the efficiency of dialysis.

Peritoneal dialysate typically contains 3 mEq/liter of *titratable acids,* which may diffuse into the plasma to be buffered rapidly.[161] When this titratable acidity was reduced from 3.0 to 0.8 mEq/liter in two patients receiving intermittent peritoneal dialysis, the predialysis serum HCO_3 rose from 14.5 to 18 mEq/liter. This preliminary report suggests that the intradialytic acidemia may be improved by removing titratable acids from the dialysate solution.

Table 16–6. Effects of Peritoneal Dialysis on the Acid–Base Balance

Acetate or lactate infusion and conversion to bicarbonate
Titratable acid infusion
Respiratory alkalosis

Respiratory Alkalosis

Respiratory alkalosis may follow peritoneal dialysis.[25,123,157] One possible explanation of this finding is that two liters of fluid within the abdominal cavity might induce hyperventilation and lead to respiratory alkalosis. One study showed that, while the functional pulmonary residual capacity was reduced when 2 liters of dialysate was present in the peritoneum, pulmonary function studies were not affected.[162] No difference in vital capacity, FEV_1, or closing volume were detected before, during, or after peritoneal dialysis. Respiratory alkalosis may develop following peritoneal dialysis in a fashion similar to that observed in hemodialysis patients. It could result from rapid correction of metabolic acidosis, or from a direct effect of diffusion of some unknown molecule across the membrane.

Metabolic Alkalosis and Dialysis

Commercial dialysis fluids are designed to treat patients with chronic renal failure and metabolic acidosis. Therefore they contain bicarbonate, acetate, or lactate to correct this acid–base disturbance. However, the need sometimes arises to perform dialysis on patients with metabolic alkalosis. This situation usually arises when patients develop acute renal failure following severe vomiting or nasogastric suction. The usual treatment of metabolic alkalosis is to replete volume with NaCl and to treat accompanying hypokalemia with KCl. When renal function is impaired or alkalemia is severe, dilute hydrochloric acid can be infused[163] or acetazolamide can be given with KCl.[164] If severely alkalemic patients also have oliguric renal failure, these therapies may be unsuccessful or may induce volume overload. Since dialysis using standard dialysate could worsen the metabolic alkalosis, dialysis fluids containing no base,[165] low bicarbonate,[166] or low acetate[167] concentrations have been used successfully to correct volume overload, increase the chloride and hydrogen ion concentrations, and decrease the serum bicarbonate.

Dialysis and Lactic Acidosis

One of the most difficult acid–base disorders to treat is lactic acidosis. In this disorder, increased lactate production, decreased hepatic extraction of lactic acid or both[50,51a] may produce a severe "anion gap" metabolic acidosis and life-threatening acidemia (see Chapter 7). Underlying conditions that commonly lead to lactic acidosis are listed in Table 16–7. Therapy must be directed at two objectives: to eliminate specifically the source of lactic acid production and to correct the severe acidemia.[168] To correct the acidemia, large amounts of base are sometimes infused rapidly and continued for as long as lactate metabolism remains abnormal. The usual therapy is the intravenous infusion of large amounts of $NaHCO_3$. The primary complications resulting from the administration of such large amounts of base are the development of intravascular volume overload and hyperosmolarity. In addition, bicarbonate infusion may increase the rate of lactate production.[169–172,172a] For these reasons, treatments other than intravenous $NaHCO_3$ infusion may increase survival in patients with lactic acidosis. Recently, dichloroacetate has been shown to effectively reverse experimentally induced lactic acidosis,[172a] and may be efficacious in patients as well.[172b]

Table 16–7. Causes of Lactic Acidosis

Increased lactate production
Shock
Tissue hypoxia
Diabetes mellitus
Leukemia
Ethanol
Glycogen storage disease
Decreased lactate metabolism
Hepatocellular damage
Increased production and decreased metabolism
Phenformin

Adapted from Oliva PB: Lactic acidosis. Am J Med 48:209, 1970.

Peritoneal dialysis using an acetate base may have several benefits.[173,174] Excess fluid and sodium may be removed, allowing for more intravenous $NaHCO_3$ administration. The acetate will cross the dialysis membrane into the plasma, and muscle metabolism to bicarbonate will slowly add buffering capacity. A potential danger of acetate-based hemo- or peritoneal dialysis is the movement of bicarbonate from plasma to dialysate, worsening the metabolic acidosis until intravenous $NaHCO_3$ or acetate metabolism can correct its loss. Bicarbonate-based peritoneal dialysis can be performed successfully in patients with lactic acidosis.[175–178] It has the great advantage of allowing bicarbonate to infuse into the body without the complications of volume expansion or hypernatremia.[175] In addition, significant amounts of lactate can be removed,[175–177] although this per se will not correct the acidemia. As the metabolic acidosis corrects rapidly, the level of ionized calcium in the blood may fall. In addition, calcium and magnesium are not present in bicarbonate dialysate because it cannot be added easily to hypertonic bicarbonate dialysate without causing precipitation. During dialysis these

Table 16–8. Formula for the Preparation of 2 Liters Bicarbonate-Based Peritoneal Dialysate

	Na (mEq/liter)	Cl (mEq/liter)	HCO_3 (mEq/liter)	Glucose (g)
1 liter 0.9 NS	75	75	—	—
+ 60 ml $D_{50}W$	—	—	—	30
1 liter 0.45 NS	37.5	37.5	—	—
+ 50 mEq $NaHCO_3$	25	—	25	—
Final 2-liter solution (approximate)	137	112	25	1.5%

ions move out of the plasma into the dialysate and significant hypocalcemia and hypomagnesemia may result.[175] Therefore, serum levels of calcium and magnesium must be followed closely, and intravenous calcium gluconate and intramuscular magnesium sulfate should be administered when needed.[175] Table 16–8 shows how we prepare each 2 liters of peritoneal dialysate to treat lactic acidosis. A preliminary report[179] describes how hemoultrafiltration can be used with simultaneous infusion of isotonic $NaHCO_3$ to correct rapidly the severe acidemia of lactic acidosis.

POTASSIUM AND DIALYSIS

Potassium is the major intracellular cation. Overall potassium balance is accomplished when urinary and stool excretion balance daily oral intake. Less than 2 percent of total body potassium is located in the extracellular space, so that small changes in the transmembrane distribution of intra- to extracellular potassium can have dramatic effects on the plasma potassium concentration (see Chapter 9). Factors that influence potassium distribution include hydrogen ion balance and other determinants of the acid–base balance,[180] insulin, epinephrine, aldosterone, and the extracellular potassium concentration.[181] When renal function is normal, approximately 90 percent of ingested potassium is excreted by the kidneys and the remaining 10 percent by the gut. While urinary potassium remains the major source of potassium excretion in modest renal insufficiency, the end-stage kidney has an impaired ability to excrete an acute potassium load.[182] In renal failure the gut may play an increasing role in potassium homeostasis, excreting 35 to 50 percent of the ingested amount,[183,184] perhaps through an enhanced active transport process.[185]

Total exchangeable potassium, an index of the body's cell mass, has been reported to be normal[186,187] or decreased[188] in chronic renal failure. In one study, skeletal muscle potassium was reduced in patients with end-stage renal failure but returned to normal after 6 to 12 weeks of chronic hemodialysis treatment.[189] The potassium deficit may be caused by a decreased lean body mass in these chronically ill patients, or may be caused by chronic acidemia, dietary protein restriction, vomiting, diarrhea, or the use of kaliuretic agents often prescribed for these patients. In addition, patients with renal failure have been reported to have a reversible defect of the cell membrane, which impairs the cell's ability to maintain a high intra- to extracellular potassium gradient. Finally, as renal failure progresses, the kidney "adapts" by increasing its fractional potassium excretion, and thus maintaining overall potassium balance despite decreasing nephron mass.[190] It is not surprising, therefore, that increased extracellular concentration of potassium is not seen in patients with substantial renal disease (glomerular filtration rate = 10 ml/min) (see Chapter 9). Nonetheless, patients with end-stage renal failure are particularly prone to develop acute hyperkalemia if excessive amounts of potassium are ingested[191] if acute metabolic acidosis develops or if cell destruction suddenly increases the extracellular potassium pool. Such acute hyperkalemia may directly stimulate aldosterone production,[192,193] a mechanism of importance even when the diseased kidney is no longer able to increase substantially its potassium secretion. Aldosterone may enhance gut secretion of potassium[183,194] and probably plays an important role in extrarenal potassium homeostasis.[195] When potassium is infused into chronic hemodialysis patients, plasma aldosterone levels rise, and most of the potassium leaves the extracellular fluid and enters the cells.[196] Aldosterone levels may be increased by hemodialysis treatments, an effect that is enhanced by low sodium dialysate[197] and is reversed by a falling plasma potassium concentration.[98] The other potassium regulatory hormones, epinephrine[198] and insulin,[199] may be elevated in chronic renal failure and dialysis patients, and may participate in this transcellular regulation of infused potassium. As reviewed by Bia and DeFronzo,[200] these mechanisms of extrarenal potassium homeostasis are particularly important in patients with chronic renal failure. Further work is needed to determine whether these mechanisms are impaired in chronically uremic states.

When patients with end-stage renal failure are treated with chronic dialysis, overall potassium balance is maintained when

Oral K intake = dialysis K removal
+ gut K excretion + renal K excretion

While renal excretion is negligible in most dialysis patients, some continue a remarkable kaliuresis in a modest volume of urine. For such patients, dietary restriction of potassium may not be necessary, and indeed supplementary potassium and isokalemic dialysate solutions may be necessary to maintain the balance. Unfortunately, most patients do not have this luxury, and balance can be maintained only when substantially reduced dietary potassium intake is removed largely by dialysis. If this balance is not maintained, life-threatening hyperkalemia may result. This complication is still seen all too frequently among dialysis patients, usually as a result of dietary potassium "indiscretion."

Potassium Removal During Hemodialysis

The maximal amount of potassium a given hemodialyzer can remove per unit time is defined by its dialysance (D_d) when inflowing dialysate contains no potassium. The actual rate of clearance (K_d) for potassium when potassium is added to the dialysate can be described by Gotch's formula:[19]

$$K_d = \frac{C_{bi} - C_{di}}{C_{bi}} \qquad (33)$$

As dialysate potassium concentration is increased, the potassium clearance will decrease. Furthermore, as plasma potassium falls, the clearance rate declines, and when plasma potassium = dialysate potassium ($C_{bi} - C_{di} = 0$), the clearance of potassium ceases. This relationship points out two important characteristics of potassium removal during hemodialysis: first, it can be regulated substantially by altering the dialysate potassium concentration, and second, the system tends to self-regulate. At the start of dialysis, $C_{bi} - C_{di}$ is at its zenith, and the mass removal rate is maximal. As dialysis progresses and C_{bi} falls, the mass removal rate falls and reaches zero when $C_{bi} = C_{di}$. Thus, while the absolute rates of potassium movement vary and depend upon the initial plasma concentration and the dialyzer characteristics, the final plasma potassium concentration will approach the dialysate concentration if dialysis proceeds for an adequate length of time.

The above considerations presume that potassium behaves as a one-compartment model in the body, i.e., transcellular movement of potassium is so rapid that equilibration of intra- and extracellular spaces is virtually instantaneous. Several studies suggest that this is not true, since transcellular movement of potassium may be slower than dialysis clearance rates, and changing acid–base balance induced by dialysis may affect the distribution of potassium between intracellular and extracellular compartments. Decline of plasma potassium concentration during dialysis is followed by a rapid increase of potassium concentration 2 to 5 hours after dialysis.[201,202] This "rebound" probably represents delayed movement of potassium out of cells, suggesting at least two functional compartments for exchangeable potassium. In some hemodialysis patients, predialysis potassium concentration correlates with the H^+ concentration,[201] and correction of metabolic acidosis, coupled with glucose absorption and metabolism during dialysis, cause potassium to move into the cells. Thus the plasma potassium concentration might fall much more rapidly than predicted by the clearance formula, and hypokalemia may occur. This phenomenon was demonstrated dramatically in five patients with prolonged loss of potassium, marked metabolic acidosis, and moderate hypokalemia treated with hemodialysis.[203] Even though the dialysate contained 42 percent more potassium than predialysis serum, all five had a decline of serum potassium concentration on dialysis, and one developed hypokalemic quadriplegia and a near respiratory arrest. These reports emphasize that, although the kinetic model described by Gotch is useful to understand potassium movement in general, it must be considered with other factors in each patient in order to anticipate the effect of hemodialysis on overall potassium balance and the plasma potassium concentration.

Potassium Removal During Peritoneal Dialysis

When potassium-free dialysate is introduced into the peritoneal space, potassium moves rapidly down its concentration gradient into the dialysate. Boen[6] evaluated diffusive potassium movement by infusing 1.7 to 2.0 liters of fluid into the peritoneal space, and then removing small samples of dialysate at timed intervals. He found that the diffusion of potassium is nearly as rapid as the diffusion of urea. After 30 minutes, the dialysate: plasma concentration ratio for potassium was 0.55, and after 60 minutes, the concentration ratio was 0.77. Thus, when the initial serum concentration is 6.0 mEq/liter, a 2-liter peritoneal dialysis exchange of one hour removes 8 mEq of potassium. The rate of potassium diffusion was also found to be dependent upon the volume of infused dialysate in each exchange and was maximal when 3.5 liters was infused each hour. At that dialysate volume, the diffusional potassium clearance was 30 ml/min. When 2 liters was infused, a volume tolerated better by most patients, potassium clearance fell to 16 ml/min.

During intermittent peritoneal dialysis with potassium-free dialysate, the plasma potassium concentration falls rapidly during the initial exchanges, then gradually declines until it reaches 3.75 mEq/liter.[6] Thereafter the plasma potassium remains constant despite continued removal of potassium. The initial rapid fall reflects movement of potassium into cells as glucose is absorbed and metabolic acidosis begins to be corrected. Late in the dialysis, diffusion into the dialysate is balanced by efflux of potassium from the intra- to the extracellular compartment. When hypertonic dialysate is used, ultrafiltration occurs, and a convective component of potassium removal is seen.[204] After completion of dialysis, the plasma potassium concentration sometimes rises, perhaps related to cessation of glucose infusion.

Rapid changes in plasma potassium are sometimes undesirable, particularly in patients with metabolic acidosis or those taking digitalis. For this reason, potassium is added to the dialysate during intermittent peritoneal dialysis: 2 mEq/liter in patients with intermittent hyperkalemia and 3.5 to 4.0 mEq/liter for patients with normokalemia and for those taking digitalis. When continuous ambulatory peritoneal dialysis is performed, dialysate remains in the peritoneal space 24 hours a day, and the fluid is drained and replaced four to five times each day. When five 2-liter exchanges are performed daily, the serum potassium falls from a mean value of 5.1 mEq/liter at the start of dialysis to 4.0 mEq/liter by the eleventh week of treatment.[205] When 1.5 percent glucose solutions are used, the concentration ratio of drained fluid ranges from 0.76 to 1.01, with a mean value of 0.83, depending on cycle time.[206] This translates to a mass transfer of 7.9 mEq/2liters exchange. When 4.25 percent of glucose solution is used, the mean potassium concentration ratio rises to 0.88, and mass transfer is 10 mEq/2liters exchange; the greater potassium removal results from enhanced diffusion and increased convection of potassium across the membrane.

It is clear from this analysis that the weekly mass transfer of potassium during continuous ambulatory peritoneal dialysis is in the range of 250 mEq, while for intermittent peritoneal dialysis it is usually somewhat less. The constant removal of 35 to 45 mEq/day in continuous ambulatory peritoneal dialysis usually allows patients a normal diet, while intermittent potassium removal of intermittent peritoneal dialysis usually requires a potassium-restricted diet. Diabetic patients treated with continuous ambulatory peritoneal dialysis receive a constant intraperitoneal infusion of glucose. When a single morning dose of subcutaneous long-acting insulin is taken, a hyperglycemia-induced rise in serum potassium may occur toward the end of the day.[207] In such patients improved glucose and potassium control can be obtained by adding insulin to the dialysate, to provide continuous intraperitoneal absorption of insulin throughout the day.

Treatment of Acute Hyperkalemia in Patients with End-Stage Renal Failure

Acute hyperkalemia, serum K $\geq$ 7.0 to 8.0 mEq/liter, is a life-threatening emergency that causes weakness or paralysis, intestinal ileus, disordered cardiac conduction, and ventricular fibrillation or asystole. It may occur in acute or chronic renal failure, with the administration of large oral or parenteral doses of potassium, or when acidemia or tissue destruction enhance the movement of cellular potassium into the extracellular space (see Chapters 9 and 23). Therapy is designed to accomplish several steps:

1. Protect the cardiac conducting system against the effects of hyperkalemia.
2. Acutely shift potassium into cells.
3. Increase overall excretion of potassium.
4. Determine and prevent the underlying cause of the disturbance.

Increased extracellular calcium will decrease the incidence of ventricular arrhythmia; 14 mEq $CaCl_2$ (one standard ampul) should be injected intravenously as soon as the diagnosis is made. Potassium will shift into cells when metabolic acidosis is corrected; the standard therapy for hyperkalemia therefore includes intravenous infusion of $NaHCO_3$. However, patients with renal failure frequently are volume overloaded, and $NaHCO_3$ infusion may induce pulmonary edema. An assessment of the patient's volume status is important, therefore, before $NaHCO_3$ is administered.

A most useful technique to shift potassium into cells is the intravenous injection of glucose and insulin. Following the emergent injection of 100 ml of 50 percent dextrose solution with 10 units CZI insulin, a constant drip infusion can be employed to maintain the intracellular shift until more definitive therapy can eliminate the extra potassium from the body. Insulin can be infused at a rate of 1 to 2 U/hr in nondiabetic patients, and each unit should be accompanied by 2 to 5 g glucose. This can be accomplished by adding 40 units crystalline zinc ("regular") insulin to 1000 ml 10 percent dextrose, and infusing this solution at a rate of 25 ml/hr. Higher insulin infusion rates often are needed for diabetic patients. We have used this treatment in chronic hemodialysis patients who develop acute hyperkalemia immediately after surgery. At these times we wait at least 24 hours before starting dialysis, and we maintain the plasma potassium (and glucose) near normal levels by adjusting the rate of insulin (and glucose) infusion.

Potassium removal is accomplished in patients with renal failure by enhanced gut excretion of potassium or by dialysis. When oral or rectal instillation of the exchange resin sodium polystyrene sulfonate (Kayexalate) remains in contact with potassium-secreting cells of the colon for at least 30 minutes, 1 mEq of potassium is bound in each gram of resin, which is subsequently expelled. The resin is administered with sorbitol to produce an osmotic diarrhea and thereby enhance potassium excretion. The usual oral dose is 25 to 50 g resin with 50 ml of 70 percent sorbitol, or a 50-g Kayexalate enema with at least 30 minutes of retention. This treatment can be repeated as necessary and allows the removal of 50 to 100 mEq potassium within the first 2 hours.

Peritoneal dialysis is an inefficient way to remove potassium in a short time. Even when the plasma potassium concentration is 8 mEq/liter, the maximum mass transfer of this ion is 10 to 12 mEq/hr. In acidemic patients, peritoneal dialysis with bicarbonate-containing solutions may increase rapidly the plasma bicarbonate concentration and thereby lower the concentration of potassium. Resultant hyperglycemia and stimulation of insulin secretion may also contribute to the decline in plasma potassium concentration.

Hemodialysis with K-free dialysate can remove substantial amounts of potassium. Standard cellulosic membranes used at standard blood flow and dialysate flow rates may transfer up to 50 mEq/hr of potassium across the membrane.[1] Simultaneous correction of acidemia and glucose infusion usually result in a rapid fall of serum potassium, and the serum potassium concentration should be measured after 2 hours of dialysis. If the value has fallen to $\leq$6 mEq/liter, 2 mEq K/liter should be added to the dialysate.

The underlying source of potassium excess in patients with chronic renal failure (Table 16–9) is usually excessive dietary ingestion. In unusual cases exercise or seizure induced rhabdomyolysis, ischemic events such as myocardial infarction, or perhaps inadequate amounts or action of regulatory hormones such as aldosterone, insulin, or epinephrine may induce hyperkalemia. Malfunction of the epinephrine–potassium axis may occur or cause hyperkalemia when nonselective beta blockers are used to treat hypertension. Preliminary studies[208] suggest that propranolol (a beta-1 and beta-2 blocker) may result in higher plasma potassium levels after acute potassium infusion than when the beta-1 selective agent, metoprolol, is used.

TRACE ELEMENTS

Elements present in the body in micrograms per gram tissue amounts are defined as trace elements.[209] Several are important cofactors in enzymatic function and are either beneficial or essential in humans. Zinc, copper, and manganese are included in this group. Other elements are present in the environment and are potentially toxic to man. This latter group includes aluminum, lead, and mercury. Hemodialysis patients, exposed to large weekly volumes of fluid across a semipermeable membrane, may have altered metabolism of the essential trace element or increased expo-

Table 16–9. Causes of Hyperkalemia in Dialysis Patients

Excessive intake, "dietary indiscretion"
Metabolic acidosis
Endogenous potassium loading
Rhabdomyolysis
Hemolysis
Ischemic events
Regulatory hormone disturbance
Hyporeninemic hypoaldosteronism
Impaired epinephrine regulation: use of beta-2-blocking drugs

sure to the toxic ones. Atomic absorption spectrophotometry permits measurement of small concentrations of these substances and has been used to study these elements in dialysis patients.

Aluminum

Chronic dialysis patients have been found frequently to have high levels of aluminum in bones, muscles, other tissues, and blood. While this observation was made more than a decade ago,[210] it received little attention until clinical disorders of bone and neurologic function were associated with hyperaluminemia. Improved methods of measuring small quantities of aluminum using flameless atomic absorption[211] and careful epidemiologic studies[211-219] have shown clearly the toxicity of aluminum in the chronic dialysis population.

Dialysis patients are exposed to aluminum from two sources, oral phosphate binders and the water used to prepare the dialysate. Oral phosphate binders are prescribed for most hemodialysis patients to reduce the absorption of ingested phosphorus and thereby lower the serum phosphate concentration. This therapy is a cornerstone in the management of renal osteodystrophy and metastatic calcification, two common complications of renal failure. Calcium resins were used initially to bind phosphorus in the intestine, but much of the resin calcium was absorbed and hypercalcemia resulted. Aluminum-containing resins were substituted when it was presumed that virtually no aluminum would be absorbed by the intestine and the ingested aluminum would eventually be excreted in the feces. In 1970 Berlyne et al.[210] observed that more than one third of dialysis patients studied had increased levels of serum aluminum, including patients ingesting 45 g aluminum daily. However, they also noted three patients with abnormal serum aluminum who were not taking oral phosphate binders. These authors subsequently documented that the latter three patients were being dialyzed with high aluminum dialysate. Since then, the relative role of oral phosphate binders in the aluminum-associated abnormalities of dialysis patients has remained unclear. In 1972 Clarkson et al.[220] showed that dialysis patients taking aluminum hydroxide may absorb 87 to 478 mg of aluminum daily. While some aluminum is excreted in the urine, little if any is removed by dialysis, and patients are in positive aluminum balance. Since normal volunteers absorb only small amounts of aluminum from the intestine, some factor peculiar to dialysis patients may increase their aluminum absorption. Administration of parathyroid extract to rats before an aluminum-containing meal increases intestinal absorption of aluminum.[221] Since most dialysis patients have elevated levels of parathyroid hormone, enhanced intestinal absorption might result from the high parathyroid hormone levels. In 1979 Gorsky et al.[222] confirmed that as much as 25 percent of an ingested dose of aluminum may be absorbed. Furthermore, withdrawal of oral aluminum hydroxide resulted in a sustained fall of serum aluminum.[223] Nonetheless, elevated levels of serum aluminum are seen in patients ingesting no aluminum hydroxide,[210] and tissue aluminum levels may have no relationship to the intake of this phosphate binder.[217,224]

High serum and tissue concentrations of aluminum have been reported in patients dialyzed with high aluminum-containing dialysate. The importance of dialysate aluminum concentration was shown elegantly by Kaehny et al.,[225] who studied patients treated with low aluminum and high aluminum dialysate. Using a sensitive aluminum assay, this group found that small but significant amounts of aluminum are removed from the body when low aluminum dialysate is used. Of greater concern, a substantial increase of serum aluminum concentration is seen when patients receive dialysis with high aluminum-containing dialysate. They observed that plasma binding precludes almost any removal of aluminum during dialysis, and that significant amounts of aluminum can be transferred to plasma if the dialysate contains virtually any aluminum. This conclusion has been confirmed by Gorsky and Dietz,[226] who found no change in serum aluminum levels following dialysis with low aluminum dialysate.

DIALYSIS DEMENTIA

In 1972 Alfred et al.[227] reported five hemodialysis patients who developed a progressive neurologic disorder of unknown etiology (see Chapter 21). The first manifestations of this disease was slow, deliberate speech and stuttering, then dysnomia and dyspraxia of speech. Months later, tremulousness, myoclonus, asterixus, then dyspraxia of movement, memory impairment, personality changes and even psychosis were seen. Facial grimacing and focal seizures were common. The EEG was abnormal, showing multifocal bursts of slow waves, sometimes with spikes. A similar clinical syndrome was described in three hemodialyzed men in England, all of whom also had severe osteodystrophy and multiple spontaneous bone fractures.[218] All three were dialyzed with untreated tap water, while patients dialyzed with processed water did not develop the syndrome. The authors hypothesized that a toxic contaminant in untreated water might be responsible for the dementia and the bone fractures. These Denver investigators were impressed by the geographic localization of this disorder and studied intensively the brain, bone, and muscle tissue obtained at autopsy from affected persons. Four years later, they reported that muscle aluminum levels were 10 to 20 times higher in these patients than in nondialyzed controls, and that trabecular bone aluminum levels were 40 to 50 times higher than in controls.[211] Of most interest, they found that the aluminum levels of brain gray matter were significantly higher than either nondialyzed controls or uremic patients who did not have encephalopathy. While all affected patients had received aluminum-containing binders, the relative contribution of oral and dialysate aluminum was not established.

These reports stimulated worldwide interest in the potential toxicity of aluminum and several centers described apparent epidemics of dialysis dementia in well-circumscribed geographic locations. In a Columbia, South Carolina dialysis unit, 94 patients were treated in a 40-month period between 1974 and 1977.[214] Seven of these patients died with progressive encephalopathy, and 16 other patients had symptoms of this disorder. The dialysate for this center was prepared from untreated city tap water and it was noted that the water department added 0.7 to 6.0 grams of aluminum sulfate per gallon of water as a coagulant for colloidal material. The serum aluminum concentrations in these hemodialysis patients were 3 to 11 times higher than controls. In 1977 a water purification plant was installed, and the amount of prescribed aluminum-containing phosphate binders was decreased. Serum aluminum levels fell to near normal. Although several patients with previously established encephalopathy died, many others improved and no new cases of the disorder developed. Similar outbreaks of dementia associated with high dialysate aluminum concentrations were described from Trent[212] and Newcastle-upon-Tyne,[224] Chicago,[216] Scotland,[213] and Alma.[217] In Eindhoven[219] an outbreak of dialysis dementia was associated with contamination of the dialysate by an aluminum cathodic protection system in the boiler, which resulted in the dissolution of aluminum into the dialysate.

Other investigators have suggested the potential neurotoxicity of aluminum by systemic administration or direct injection into the central nervous system of laboratory animals.[228,229] Neurofibrillary degeneration in a pattern similar to that in Alzheimer's disease has been induced in cats and rabbits. Although these reports produced strong circumstantial evidence linking aluminum intoxication with dialysis dementia, a direct cause-and-effect relationship remains uncertain. While some investigators have found that brain gray matter aluminum concentration is higher in dialysis patients with encephalopathy than in those without neurologic disease,[211,214,219,224] other workers have not shown this association.[212,230] In subtle tests of intelligence, reasoning, memory, and manual dexterity, dialysis patients with high serum aluminum were not different than dialysis patients with normal serum aluminum.[231]

DIALYSIS OSTEOMALACIA

Renal osteodystrophy and other bone abnormalities that accompany chronic renal failure are found commonly among dialysis patients (see Chapter 15). Most affected individuals have osteitis fibrosa cystica, alone or in combination with osteomalacia. Only a small minority of patients have pure osteomalacia. This uncommon abnormality frequently causes pain, pathologic fractures, and proximal muscle weakness.[232] Two lines of evidence suggest that aluminum may play a role in some cases of osteomalacia.

First, many patients with dialysis dementia and exposure to aluminum also have osteomalacia.[212-214,210,233] A British survey of 18 dialysis centers showed a significant correlation between dialysate aluminum concentration and osteomalacia.[234] Histologic study[214] shows excess inactive osteoid covering large parts of the trabecular surfaces (Fig. 16–5). An identical osteomalacic lesion can be induced in rats by injecting aluminum chloride into the peritoneum.[235] Walker and colleagues[236] studied 40 hemodialysis patients with a high rate of bone fractures (38 percent) and osteomalacia (48 percent). They found that the patients with fractures had a significantly higher concentration of aluminum in their dialysate water and had been exposed to more total aluminum than the patients without fractures. Similarly, patients with osteomalacia had significantly higher water aluminum and total exposure to aluminum than those without osteomalacia.

Second, several investigators have found aluminum concentration in bones of patients with dialysis dementia and osteomalacia to be higher than in controls.[212,214,235] Bone aluminum is highest in patients treated with hemodialysis the longest,[215,237] and a clear relationship between bone aluminum and osteoid volume of bone has been shown.[238] The aluminum concentration of trabecular bone, the location of bone osteoid, may be 40 to 50 times higher than in nondialyzed controls.[211] Aluminum may remain in the bones after dialysis therapy is discontinued following successful renal transplantation.[235] Furthermore, osteomalacia may persist even after exposure to aluminum has been terminated. Dialysis patients with osteomalacia may have the same total bone aluminum content as dialysis patients without this bone lesion.[211,239] However, such patients localize their bone aluminum to the limit between the osteoid and calcified bone, while patients with osteitis fibrosa had no such localization.[239] The osteomalacia is not responsive to vitamin D.[239,240] When bone biopsies are stained using an aluminum method to localize areas of aluminum deposition, patients with osteomalacia have evidence of defective mineralization at a majority of sites with aluminum deposits.[241] Thus aluminum may induce severe osteomalacia by direct inhibition of the normal mineralization process.

Some authors have suggested that aluminum-induced osteomalacia is not an effect of aluminum on the bone, but rather an effect of chronic hypophosphatemia, which is sometimes seen with use of aluminum-containing antacids. A recent preliminary report[242] shows that strict phosphate control does not lead to osteomalacia, but may actually be associated with improved bone histomorphometry. The studies taken together suggest that excess aluminum may deposit between the osteoid and calcified bone, inhibit locally the mineralization process, and induce osteomalacia.

The most impressive finding in the aluminum story is that toxic effects on brain and bone are virtually eliminated when dialysate water is processed to remove solute impurities. The widespread use of deionized water and reverse osmosis in the preparation of dialysate has decreased the incidence of this disease. Nonaluminum oral phosphate binders such as magnesium hydroxide[243] can be used to elimi-

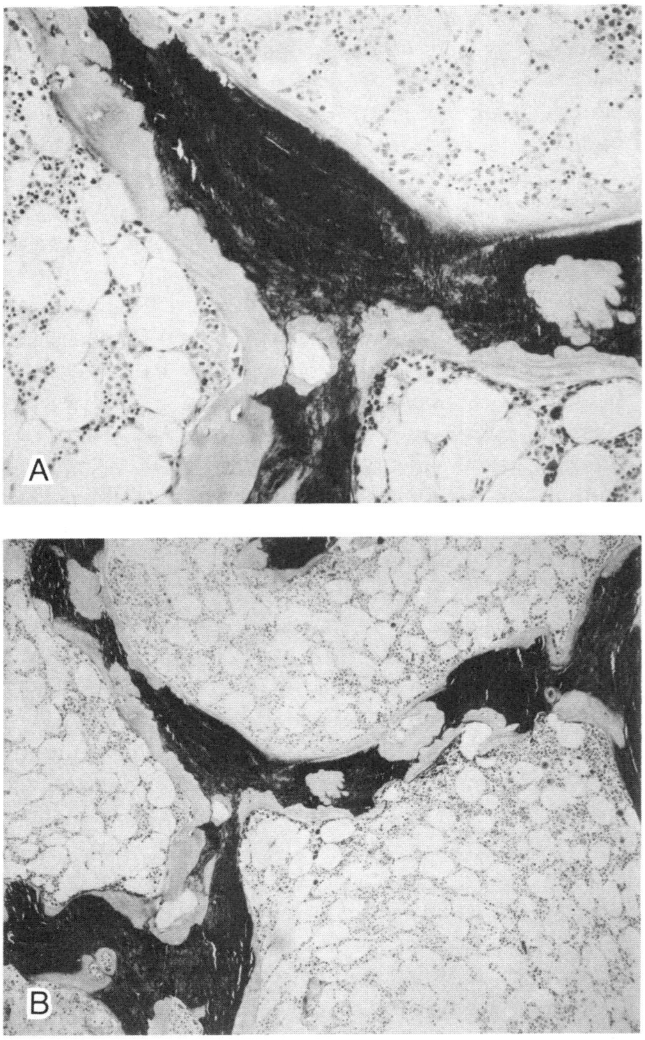

Fig. 16–5. Undecalcified sections of bone from a transileal biopsy in a patient with dialysis dementia and osteomalacia. Toluidine blue stain. (A) × 125 m. (B) × 300 m. Osteoid covers large surface areas of bone with few osteoblasts or osteoclasts visible. (Photographs courtesy of R. Baron.)

nate oral aluminum from the medical therapy. However, great care must be taken if magnesium is administered regularly because it is absorbed in the intestine and can lead to dangerous hypermagnesemia.[244] (See Chapter 23.)

Zinc

Zinc is a trace element that serves as an important cofactor for several enzymes, including alcohol dehydrogenase, alkaline phosphatase, and lactic acid dehydrogenase.[245] Dietary sources rich in zinc include animal proteins, particularly seafood and muscle meat.[239] Since the ingestion of these foods is often restricted in patients with renal failure, dietary zinc deficiency may be present. Even if ingested zinc is adequate, patients with chronic uremia may have a decreased intestinal absorption of this element. When plasma zinc levels were measured following an oral zinc load,[246] dialysis patients taking no supplementary vitamin D demonstrated reduced peak plasma zinc levels.

The plasma level of zinc has been shown to be decreased in patients on chronic hemodialysis.[245,247-250] Levels are low in uremic patients before they begin dialysis, and they may fall further once dialysis starts.[249] Despite low plasma zinc levels, tissue levels or intracellular zinc may be normal. For example, red blood cell zinc is normal in dialysis patients.[245] Therefore low plasma zinc does not necesarily mean zinc deficiency.[248] Serum and hair levels of zinc may be normal in pediatric dialysis patients.[251]

Zinc deficiency syndromes in patients with normal renal function result in clinical disorders similar to chronic renal insufficiency. For example, deficiencies of iron and zinc may result in a syndrome of anemia, hepatosplenomegaly, dwarfism, and hypogonadism.[252] Zinc supplementation in such patients is followed by increased growth and sexual maturation.[253] Since sexual dysfunction is a common characteristic of chronic renal failure, some authors have speculated that zinc deficiency might be responsible for this problem.[254,255] In a small controlled study[254] and a double-blind study[255] zinc or placebo was added to the dialysate of men receiving chronic hemodialysis. Zinc resulted in significant improvement in testicular function (testosterone levels and sperm counts) and subjective improvement in potency, libido, and frequency of intercourse. In two other studies 400 μg/liter zinc was added to the dialysate in the experimental group of a controlled[256] or double-blind crossover study.[257] While the serum zinc levels rose, no significant change could be detected in plasma testosterone or gonadotropin levels, and no change in sexual function was seen.

Disordered taste or smell, often accompanied by anorexia, is another problem that many dialysis patients experience. In 1971 a syndrome of idiopathic hypogeusia and hyposmia with low serum zinc was described[258] in people with normal renal function. These symptoms improved after oral zinc supplementation. Despite the fact that these same investigators did not confirm the efficacy of zinc in a double-blind study of more than 100 such patients,[259] several investigators have reported improved taste acuity and appetite in dialysis patients after zinc supplementation.[260-262] In one double-blind study of 22 chronic dialysis patients, taste threshold improved significantly in all patients supplemented with zinc acetate, while no correlation between zinc in plasma/tissue and taste/smell acuity was found.[263] Other uremic patients have impaired taste but normal plasma zinc.[264] Finally, in a group of 106 patients studied in double-blind fashion,[259] zinc sulfate did not improve hypogeusia.

Zinc deficiency has been associated with impaired cell-mediated immunity in humans[265] and rats.[266] Since delayed hypersensitivity is often abnormal in dialysis patients, Antoniou and colleagues[267] studied delayed hypersensitivity to mumps in 25 dialysis patients with a history of mumps infection. When zinc was added to the dialysate, 8 of 9 patients demonstrated a positive skin test. In the control group given no supplmentary zinc, 11 of 16 were positive. When 4 skin test-negative patients were then given dialysis with zinc supplements, 3 of 4 developed positive delayed hypersensitivity. The investigators speculated that protracted zinc deficiency may be a major cause of impaired cellular immunity in patients with chronic renal insufficiency. In vitro testing of lymphocyte blast transformation and granulocyte motility was performed by Briggs and colleagues[268] in zinc-treated and -untreated hemodialysis patients. They found that, while lymphocyte responses to several stimuli were no different in zinc-treated or -untreated patients, granulocyte motility was significantly greater. Granulocyte zinc concentration was significantly higher in treated than in untreated patients. The authors speculated that the state of zinc nutrition might affect granulocyte function, and may be important in patients experiencing recurrent or severe bacterial infections.

It is clear that some hemodialysis patients have decreased plasma zinc concentrations and may have low zinc concentration levels in some cells or tissues. Zinc supplementation for sexual dysfunction, disordered taste and smell, cell-mediated immunity, and granulocyte function has been found useful by some investigators but not by others. Such widespread discrepancies suggest a nonhomogeneous population, and it may be that certain subpopulations of hemodialysis patients will benefit from zinc treatment. Further studies of responsive and nonresponsive patients may elucidate the role of zinc in these many physiologic processes.

Copper

Nondialyzed, azotemic patients may have normal[250] or elevated[249] levels of copper in the plasma, and similarly hemodialysis patients may have increased[245,249,250] or normal[251] plasma copper. Red blood cell copper is normal.[245] These modest increases of plasma copper are not associated with known clinical abnormalities. In 1967 Lyle[269] wondered whether acute copper poisoning from contaminated dialysate might cause hemolytic anemia, which is sometimes seen in dialysis patients. He found that dialysate water prepared by a deionizer and passed through copper pipes had significantly elevated copper levels, particularly when the water stood in these pipes overnight. Copper appeared to diffuse across the dialyzer membrane, and episodes of pyrexia and transfusion requirements declined when the copper concentration was lowered. Plasma avidity for dialysate copper was later confirmed.[270] Several reports of fatal or life-threatening hemolysis accompanied by acidosis, methemoglobinemia, and hypoglycemia, with symptoms of chills, epigastric pain, vomiting, diarrhea, and headaches were traced to acute copper intoxication during hemodialysis.[271-274] This diagnosis was considered when the dialysate developed a green color. It was determined that when water used to prepare the dialysate was processed with a deionizer column that was at or near exhaustion, the water became acidic and readily ionized copper as it passed through a delivery system containing copper components. The copper then diffused across the dialyzing membrane into the plasma, inhibited red blood cell enzymes, and caused hemolysis and methemoglobinemia. Copper appears to enter the plasma following extraction from the cuprophan dialysis membrane.[271,275] More than 40 percent of the copper content of hemodialysis membranes is liberated during dialysis, resulting in progressive increases in serum copper and ceruloplasmin.[275] Copper-induced hemolysis has not recurred since copper was removed from the plumbing fixtures of all dialysis machines and care was taken to replace deionizer columns promptly to avoid acid water. Modern deionizer and reverse osmosis equipment removes virtually all copper from untreated water.[276] Although the dialysate concentrate may contain measurable amounts of copper, the concentration is so low as to be clinically unimportant. Patients treated with intermittent peritoneal dialysis have been reported to demonstrate rising serum copper levels during the dialysis for unclear reasons.[275]

Other Ions

Fluoride, 50 μM (1 ppm), is added to the municipal water supply in many areas. The effect of this ion on uremic bone disease is controversial. Reverse osmosis, a popular method to remove most solutes from water, removes fluoride only partially. Several case reports[277-280] describe increased serum and bone levels of fluoride when untreated fluoridated water was used to prepare the dialysate. Such patients had osteomalacia, with as much as a ninefold increase of osteoid formation in individuals treated with high fluoride (50 μM) compared to low fluoride (5 μM) water.[280] In one patient, an exhausted deionizer resulted in dialysate fluoride levels exceeding those in untreated water by severalfold.[281] The concomitant osteomalacia improved when fluoride was removed from the water. Two studies of small groups of patients comparing bone disease when fluoridated or nonfluoridated water was used suggested a higher incidence of excess osteoid formation with fluoridated water.[282,283] A strong argument against the importance of fluoride in osteomalacia was a prospective, double-blind study performed by Oreopoulos et al.[284] Deionized water was prepared for all patients and 50 μM fluoride was added back to the water in the experimental group, while no fluoride was added in the controls. There were no differences in osteitis fibrosa or osteomalacia between the two groups, although the osteoid index increased in all patients. One possible explanation of this discrepancy is that earlier studies showing an association between untreated water and osteomalacia may have been caused by a solute in tap water other than fluoride. Untreated water may contain high levels of aluminum, which may cause osteomalacia.

Another ion that should be removed from dialysate water is *sulfate*. Two patients dialyzed with high sulfate water (>200 mg/liter) developed nausea, vomiting and metabolic acidosis after each dialysis.[285] These symptoms were relieved completely when the sulfate level was reduced.

Many other trace metals may be toxic, although no specific toxic syndromes in dialysis patients have been described. These include arsenic, barium, cadmium, chromium, lead, mercury, selenium, and silver. Water deionization removes most trace elements, except zinc and lead.[276] Standards for dialysate water have been devised, based upon lowest toxic levels reported in the dialysis literature and upon the Environmental Protection Agency regulations for toxic substances.[286] These standards are shown in Table 16–10. Water should be tested regularly to ensure adequate water purity.

Table 16–10. Recommended Product Water Standard for Hemodialysis

Substance	Maximum Concentration (mg/liter)
Aluminum	1.0×10^{-2}
Arsenic	5.0×10^{-3}
Barium	1.0×10^{-1}
Cadmium	1.0×10^{-3}
Chromium	1.4×10^{-2}
Copper	1.0×10^{-1}
Fluoride	2.0×10^{-1}
Lead	5.0×10^{-3}
Mercury	2.0×10^{-4}
Selenium	9.7×10^{-2}
Silver	5.0×10^{-3}
Sulfate	100
Zinc	1.0×10^{-1}

From Keshaviah P, Luehmann DA: Overview of the FDA Contract Report: Investigation of the risks and hazards associated with hemodialysis devices. In Issues in Hemodialysis. Copyright Association for the Advancement of Medical Instrumentation, Arlington, VA, 1981, used with permission.

CONTINUOUS AMBULATORY PERITONEAL DIALYSIS (CAPD)

For many years, peritoneal dialysis was the poor country cousin to the more flashy hemodialysis. Hemodialysis treatments required only 12 to 18 hours of therapy each week, while intermittent peritoneal dialysis required 36 to 40 hours each week. The efficiency of hemodialysis far outstripped intermittent peritoneal dialysis: weekly clearance rates for small (urea) and middle size (vitamin B_{12}) molecules were twice as high with hemodialysis compared to intermittent peritoneal dialysis. While many nephrologists thought about ways to increase the efficiency of intermittent peritoneal dialysis,[4,287] it was clear that, at best, peritoneal dialysance was only a fraction of hemodialysance. Creative thinking was required to change our focus away from efficiency of solute removal to a more comprehensive view of renal replacement therapy.

In 1976 Popovich, Moncrief, and colleagues[288,289] proposed an entirely new way to look at artificial kidneys. They expounded a theoretical analysis of steady-state balance between metabolite generation and removal through dialysis. They reasoned that if low efficiency peritoneal dialysis were performed, and if the rate of urea and other metabolite removal were sufficient to balance their generation, the steady state would be maintained and patients might remain healthy. In order to remove 5 to 8 g of urea each day, dialysis with 8.5 ml/min (12 liters/day) of dialysate which is allowed continuous equilibration with the peritoneal capillaries, would be necessary. This was accomplished by five daily exchanges of 2 liters each, using hypertonic dialysate to increase the drainage volume to 12 liters/day. Each exchange lasted for approximately 4 hours. Levels of urea, creatinine, uric acid, potassium, calcium, and phosphorus came to and remained at steady state as predicted by the hypothesis. The plasma concentration of these metabolites was approximately the same as the postdialysis concentrations of hemodialysis patients. This technique abandons concern about dialysis efficiency in favor of the mass effect of inefficient but continuous therapy, and with dramatic results.[5,205,290-293] Not only did patients feel well on this protocol, but the clearances of middle and large size molecules increased 2 to 6-fold compared to intermittent peritoneal dialysis or hemodialysis. Daily volume control was usually easy to maintain, potassium and phosphorus balance was often possible without severe dietary restriction or oral phosphate binders, serum calcium and bicarbonate levels rose to normal, and the hematocrit rose in many patients. Despite a high level of protein loss through the dialysate, the serum albumin concentration remained normal. The incidence of peritonitis, the major complication of continuous ambulatory peritoneal dialysis has been reduced substantially by patient education, use of plastic bags for dialysate, titanium connectors, and other promising devices to eliminate contamination when dialysate is exchanged.

Advantages of continuous ambulatory peritoneal dialysis include a continuous steady state, increased clearance of middle size molecules thought by some to play a role in uremic toxicity,[13] no need for blood access or machine treatment, and potential economic savings if fewer patients require in-center labor-intensive treatment. In addition, even should the effective peritoneal surface of exchange decrease with time, small molecules like urea, which equilibrate quickly, would still be at equilibrium during long dwell periods, and modestly decreased large molecular weight clearances would still be severalfold higher than with intermittent peritoneal dialysis or hemodialysis.[291] In fact, follow-up studies of continuous ambulatory peritoneal dialysis patients have shown that peritoneal transport is unchanged despite frequent bouts of peritonitis.[294,295] For all solutes with molecular weights >100 steady-state concentrations for continuous ambulatory peritoneal dialysis are lower than for hemodialysis when 4 or 5 daily two-liter exchanges are used.[5] Continuous lavage with hypertonic solutions may increase peritoneal permeability, since creatinine and vitamin B_{12} clearances are higher in continuous ambulatory peritoneal dialysis patients than in intermittent peritoneal dialysis.[295]

Patients and sometimes their families are instructed to drain the dialysate, connect the peritoneal catheter to a fresh bag of dialysate, instill the dialysate, and to repeat this antiseptic procedure four times daily. Peritonitis can be managed at home in many cases when the patient adds antibiotic to the infused dialysate. While the long-term effects of protein and large molecule loss, constant glucose infusion, high serum triglyceride levels, and frequent peritonitis are not known, continuous ambulatory peritoneal dialysis has attracted thousands of patients all over the world because of ease of administration and because it allows a more normal life style.

Fluid and Solute Removal and CAPD

During peritoneal dialysis, an ultrafiltrate of plasma moves across the membrane into the dialysate when the dialysate is hypertonic with respect to plasma. Dialysate is designed to be hypertonic by the addition of glucose in concentrations of 15 to 42.5g/liter. As dialysis proceeds, the dialysate osmolality falls for two reasons: fluid moves into the peritoneal space, and glucose is absorbed into the plasma.

When plasma and dialysate osmolalities are equal, ultrafiltration ceases. Thereafter, as glucose absorption continues, the dialysate becomes hypotonic with respect to the plasma, and fluid moves from dialysate to plasma. Fluid that remains in the peritoneal space for long periods of time is reabsorbed slowly. When 2 liters of 1.5 percent (15 g/liter) dextrose solution is used, an average ultrafiltrate of 331 ml collects 140 minutes after dialysis begins, and thereafter is reabsorbed at an average rate of 0.58 to 0.68 ml/min.[19,296] Thus the actual volume of ultrafiltrate removed after a 6-hour dwell of 1.5 percent solution is ~180 ml. When 2 liters of 4.25 percent dextrose solution is infused, an average of 1028 ml ultrafiltrate collects 4 hours following instillation and thereafter declines by 0.87 ml/min. Since the effective membrane surface area and rate of glucose absorption vary considerably from patient to patient,[6] ultrafiltration rates must be measured empirically in each patient, and a protocol to select appropriate solutions must be designed individually.

Solute flux is determined primarily by the mass transfer-area coefficient. The dialysate (D) concentration of urea approaches that of the plasma (P) concentration (D:P ratio = 0.9) after 5 hours of 1.5 percent dialysate dwell,[26] but larger solutes are not at equilibrium with either 1.25 or 4.25 percent solutions. For example, after 5 hours the dialysis : plasma ratio for creatinine is 0.78 and for inulin is 0.36.[26] Net solute removal for most metabolites continues well beyond 4 hours. Hypertonic dialysate may increase membrane permeability and thus the mass transfer-area coefficient.[12] The increased diffusion results in increased clearance measurements for urea, creatinine, and insulin when 4.25 percent solution is used.[205]

A small component of solute flux is convective and determined by the sieving coefficient. The dialysate : plasma sodium concentration ratio falls below 1, particularly when 4.25 percent solution is used[26,296]; this effect is still evident many hours after infusion.[26] However, a recent study of sieving in continuous ambulatory peritoneal dialysis patients shows this effect to be blunted and short-lived.[296] Most continuous ambulatory peritoneal dialysis patients do not develop hypernatremia and increased thirst.

The amount of sodium removed is proportional to the serum sodium concentration and the ultrafiltration rate.[206] An estimate of net sodium removal can be made based upon these variables. When the serum sodium concentration is 140 mEq/liter, four 1.5 percent exchanges will remove ~150 mEq/day, while four 4.25 percent exchanges results in more than 300 mEq/day sodium efflux.

Potassium

The mass transfer-area coefficient for potassium is high, and virtually all potassium movement can be ascribed to diffusion. Therefore, the dialysate : plasma potassium ratio is high (>0.7) after only 2 hours and is not different whether 1.5 or 2.6 percent solutions are used.[296] The highest the dialysate : plasma potassium concentration ratio reaches after 10 hours is 0.91, and at all times this ratio is less than that for sodium.[206,296] When more hypertonic 4.25 percent solution is used, the dialysate : plasma potassium ratio is lower early in the exchanges, a result of the sieving effect.[296] When the plasma potassium concentration is 4 to 5 mEq/liter, CAPD can remove 30 to 45 mEq/day of potassium. Therefore, patients may eat a fairly normal diet containing 30 to 45 mEq/d of potassium and remain in equilibrium.

Acid-Base Homeostasis

A major advantage of continuous dialysis when compared to intermittent therapy is the steady state it provides. While patients receiving intermittent peritoneal dialysis or hemodialysis often develop recurrent acidemia before each treatment, continuous ambulatory peritoneal dialysis prevents this complication.[159,297] When a group of patients was switched from intermittent peritoneal dialysis to CAPD, the mean plasma bicarbonate concentration rose from 22.3 mEq/liter (preintermittent peritoneal dialysis) to 26.5 mEq/liter (post-CAPD).[297] The selection of dialysate base is important in CAPD. When lactate is used, serum bicarbonate levels are normal (27.7 mEq/liter) and serum lactate levels are low. When acetate is used, the serum bicarbonate level (29.5 mEq/liter) and the serum acetate level are elevated.[159] Lactate is therefore the preferred buffer for CAPD.

Nutrition, Glucose Metabolism, and Trace Metals

Continuous ambulatory peritoneal dialysis provides 30 percent of the daily caloric intake by constant glucose absorption, and patients reduce dietary intake to 20 to 30 kcal/kg.[298] In addition to this lower caloric ingestion, CAPD patients also have a low protein intake of 0.7 to 0.9 g/kg/day, perhaps a result of glucose-induced appetite reduction. Since large quantities of protein are lost each day in the dialysate[296,299,300] (the amount is proportional to the serum protein concentration and body surface area), the long-term risk of protein malnutrition is of real concern. While short-term nitrogen balance studies show that most patients are in positive nitrogen balance[298] and serum albumin concentration remains stable,[301] studies of CAPD patients after one year show a 15 percent decline of total body nitrogen.[302,303] In addition, one study of five CAPD patients showed that after 1 to 7 months of treatment glucose tolerance was impaired.[299] Patients demonstrated elevated glucose levels and a reduced rate of insulin secretion in response to an oral glucose load. One possible solution to this problem is to find an osmotically active substance to substitute for glucose in the dialysate. Sorbitol,[304] fructose,[299,305] and xylitol[306] have been studied, but each has drawbacks and they have not been used widely. Early studies with the use of amino acids in the dialysate suggest that they are as effective osmotic agents as dextrose, do not alter diffusive metabolite transport, and may reduce hypoproteinemia.[307] If such solutions can be prepared cost effectively, wider study of their use would be of great interest.

The plasma concentrations of aluminum, fluoride, zinc, and copper did not rise significantly after 6 months of CAPD treatment,[299] although fluoride levels were significantly above the normal range. Longer-term studies of trace metal metabolism in CAPD patients are needed, but no clinically important syndromes have been reported to suggest disorders of these ions.

REFERENCES

1. Gotch FA: Hemodialysis. Technical and kinetic considerations. p. 1672. In Brenner BM and Rector FC (eds): The Kidney, 1st ed. WB Saunders, Philadelphia, 1976
2. Henderson LW. Hemodialysis: Rationale and physical principles. p. 1643. In Brenner BM and Rector FC (eds): The Kidney, 1st ed. WB Saunders, Philadelphia, 1976
3. Henderson LW, Colton CK, Ford CA: Kinetics of hemodiafiltration. II. Clinical characterization of a new blood cleansing modality. J Lab Clin Med 85:372, 1975
4. Nolph KD, Popovich RP, Ghods AJ, et al: Determinants of low clearances of small solutes during peritoneal dialysis. Kidney Int 13:117, 1978
5. Nolph KD, Miller F, Rubin J, et al: New directions in peritoneal dialysis concepts and applications. Kidney Int 18(Suppl 10):S-111, 1980
6. Boen ST: Kinetics of peritoneal dialysis. A comparison with the artificial kidney. Medicine (Baltimore) 40:243, 1961
7. Miller FN, Nolph KD, Harris PD, et al: Comparison of the effects of altered peritoneal dialysis solutions on the microcirculation of the rat and on peritoneal clearances in man. Kidney Int 15:630, 1979
8. Nolph KD, Ghods A, Brown P, et al: Effects of nitroprusside on peritoneal mass transfer

coefficients and microvascular physiology. Trans Am Soc Artif Intern Organs 23:210, 1977
9. Karnovsky MJ: The ultrastructural basis of transcapillary exchanges. p. 64. In Biological Interfaces: Flows and Exchanges. Little, Brown, Boston, 1968
10. Cetran RS: The fine structure of the microvasculature in relation to normal and altered permeability. pp. 249–275. In Reeve, Guyton (eds). Physical Bases of Circulatory Transport: Regulation and exchange. WB Saunders, Philadelphia, 1967
11. Finkelstein FO, Kliger AS: Enhanced efficiency of peritoneal dialysis using rapid, small volume exchanges. Am Soc Artif Intern Organc J 2:103, 1979
12. Henderson LW, Nolph KD: Altered permeability of the peritoneal membrane after using hypertonic peritoneal dialysis fluid. J Clin Invest 43:992, 1969
13. Babb AL, Popovich RP, Christopher TG, et al: The genesis of the square meter hour hypothesis. Trans Am Soc Artif Intern Organs 17:81, 1971
14. Tenckhoff H, Ward G, Boen ST: The influence of dialysate volume and flow rate on peritoneal clearance. Proc Eur Dial Transplant Assoc 2:113, 1965
15. Brown EA, Kliger AS, Goffinet J, et al: Effect of hypertonic dialysate and vasodilator on peritoneal dialysis clearances in the rat. Kidney Int 13:271, 1978
16. Nolph KD, Ghods AJ, VanStone J, et al: The effects of intraperitoneal vasodilators on peritoneal clearances. Trans Am Soc Artif Intern Organs 22:586, 1976
17. Finkelstein, Yap P, Kliger AS: Effect of nitroprusside on peritoneal dialysis. Yale J Biol Med 53:127, 1980
18. Henderson LW: Peritoneal ultrafiltration dialysis. Enhanced urea transfer using hypertonic peritoneal dialysis fluid. J Clin Invest 45:950, 1966
19. Pyle WK, Moncrief JW, Popovich RP: Peritoneal transport evaluation in CAPD. p 35. In Moncrief JW, Popovich RP (eds): CAPD update. Masson, New York, 1981
20. Nolph KD, Hano JE, Teschan PE: Peritoneal sodium transport during hypertonic peritoneal dialysis: Physiologic mechanisms and clinical implications. Ann Intern Med 70:931, 1969
21. Ribot S, Jacobs MG, Frankel HJ, et al: Complications of peritoneal dialysis. Am J Med Sci 252:505, 1966
22. Boyer J, Gill GN, Epstein FH: Hyperglycemia and hyperosmolality complicating peritoneal dialysis. Ann Intern Med 67:568, 1967
23. Gault MH, Ferguson EL, Sidhu JS, et al: Fluid and electrolyte complications of peritoneal dialysis. Ann Intern Med 75:253, 1971
24. Cairns, KB, Porter GA, Kloster FE, et al: Clinical and hemodynamic results of peritoneal dialysis for severe cardiac failure. Am Heart J 76:229, 1968
25. Miller RB, Tassistro CR: Peritoneal dialysis. N Engl J Med 281:745, 1969
26. Nolph KD, Twardowski ZJ, Popovich RP, et al: Equilibration of peritoneal dialysis solutions during longdwell exchanges. J Lab Clin Med 93:246, 1979
27. Ahearn DJ, Nolph KD: Controlled sodium removal with peritoneal dialysis. Trans Am Soc Artif Intern Organs 28:423, 1972
28. Henderson LW: Symptomatic hypotension during hemodialysis. Kidney Int 17:571, 1980
29. delGreco F, Shere J, Simon NM: Hemodynamic effects of hemodialysis in chronic renal failure. Trans Am Soc Artif Intern Organs 10:353, 1964
30. delGreco F, Simon NM, Roguska J, et al: Hemodynamic studies in chronic uremia. Circulation 40:87, 1969
31. Goss JE, Alfrey AC, Vogel JHK, et al: Hemodynamic changes during hemodialysis. Trans Am Soc Artif Intern Organs 13:68, 1967
32. Kim KE, Neff M, Cohen B, et al: Blood volume changes and hypotension during haemodialysis. Trans Am Soc Artif Intern Organs 16:508, 1970
33. Endou K, Kamijima J, Kakubari Y, et al: Hemodynamic changes during hemodialysis. Cardiology 63:175, 1978
34. Fitzsimons JT, Simons BJ: The effect of angiotensin on drinking in the rat. J Physiol (Lond) 196:39P, 1968
35. Brown JJ, Curtis JR, Lever AF, et al: Plasma renin concentration and the control of blood pressure in patients on maintenance haemodialysis. Nephron 6:329, 1969

36. Schalekamp MA, Beevers DG, Briggs JD, et al: Hypotension in chronic renal failure. Am J Med 55:379, 1973
37. Bergstrom J, Asaba H, Furst P, et al: Dialysis ultrafiltration and blood pressure. Proc Eur Dial Transplant Assoc 13:293, 1976
38. Rouby JJ, Rottembourg J, Durande JP, et al: Hemodynamic changes induced by regular hemodialysis and sequential ultrafiltration hemodialysis: A comparative study. Kidney Int 17:801, 1980
39. Wehle B, Asaba H, Castenfors J, et al: Hemodynamic changes during sequential ultrafiltration and dialysis. Kidney Int 15:411, 1979
40. Shaldon S, Beau MC, Deschoot P, et al: Vascular stability during hemofiltration. Trans Am Soc Artif Intern Organs 26:391, 1980
41. Graefe U, Follette WC, Vizzo JE, et al: Reduction in dialysis-induced morbidity and vascular instability with the use of bicarbonate in dialysate. Clin Dial Transplant Forum 6:203, 1976
42. Graefe U, Milutinovich J, Follette WC, et al: Less dialysis-induced morbidity and vascular instability with bicarbonate in dialysate. Ann Intern Med 88:332, 1978
43. Raja R, Kramer M, Rosenbaum JL, et al: Prevention of hypotension during iso-osmolar hemodialysis with bicarbonate dialysate. Trans Am Soc Artif Intern Organs 26:375, 1980
44. Raja RM, Kramer MS, Rosenbaum JL, et al: High sodium dialysate with addition of chloride, acetate and bicarbonate. Trans Am Soc Artif Intern Organs 27:36, 1981
45. Fournier G, Man NK: Prevention of hemodialysis-induced hypoxemia by use of bicarbonate-containing dialysate. Kidney Int 17:701, 1980
46. Keshaviah P, Himes M, Ilstrup K, et al: Hypotension during iso-osmotic dialysis. Kidney Int 21:170, 1982
47. Leenen FHH, Budd AJ, Smith DL, et al: Blood pressure and cardiac function during bicarbonate and acetate hemodialysis. Kidney Int 21:172, 1982
48. VanStone JC, Cook J: The effect of replacing acetate with bicarbonate in the dialysate of stable chronic hemodialysis patients. Proc Clin Dial Transplant Forum 8:103, 1978
49. Wehle B, Asaba H, Castenfors J, et al: Influence of dialysate composition on cardiovascular function in isovolaemic hemodialysis. Proc Eur Dial Transplant Assoc 18:153, 1981
50. Arieff AI, Park R, Leach WJ, et al: Pathophysiology of experimental lactic acidosis in dogs. Am J Physiol 239:F135, 1980
51. Bischel MD, Scoles BG, Mohler JG: Evidence for pulmonary microembolization during hemodialysis. Chest 67:335, 1975
51a. Park R, Arieff A: Lactic acidosis: Current concepts. Clin Endocrin Metab 12:339, 1983
52. Craddock PR, Fehr J, Brigham KL, et al: Complement and leukocyte-mediated pulmonary dysfunction in hemodialysis. N Engl J Med 296:769, 1977
53. Aurigemma NM, Feldman NT, Gottlieb M, et al: Arterial oxygenation during hemodialysis. N Engl J Med 297:871, 1977
54. Dolan MJ, Whipp BJ, Davidson WD, et al: Hypopnea associated with acetate hemodialysis: Carbon dioxide-flow-dependent ventilation. N Engl J Med 305:72, 1981
55. Sherlock JE, Yoon Y, Ledwith JW, et al: Respiratory gas exchange during hemodialysis. Proc Clin Dial Transplant Forum 2:171, 1972
56. Letteri JM, Sherlock JE, Ledwith JW: Blood gas analysis during hemodialysis. Chest 69:246, 1976
57. Sherlock JE, Ledwith J, Letteri J: Hypoventilation and hypoxemia during hemodialysis: Reflex response to removal of CO_2 across the dialyzer. Trans Am Soc Artif Intern Organs 23:406, 1977
58. Nissenson AR: Prevention of dialysis-induced hypoxemia by bicarbonate dialysis. Trans Am Soc Artif Intern Organs 26:339, 1980
59. Patterson RW, Nissenson AR, Miller J, et al: Hypoxemia and pulmonary gas exchange during hemodialysis. J Appl Physiol 50:259, 1981
60. Eiser AR, Jayamanne D, Koksong C, et al: Contrasting alterations in oxygen consumption and respiratory quotient during acetate and bicarbonate hemodialysis. Kidney Int 19:145, 1981
61. Tolchin N, Roberts JL, Lewis EJ: Respiratory gas exchange by high-efficiency hemodialyzers. Nephron 21:137, 1978
62. Nissenson AR, Patterson RW, Narins RG,

et al: Dialysis-induced hypoxemia is due to increased O_2 consumption and CO_2 dialysance with normal lungs. Am Soc Nephrol 11:47A, 1978
63. Gotch F: Discussion of dialysis induced hypoxemia. Trans Am Soc Artif Intern Organs 26:342, 1980
64. Sherlock JE: Discussion of dialysis induced hypoxemia. Trans Am Soc Artif Intern Organs 26:342, 1980
65. Ahmad S, Pagel M, Shen F, et al: The role of hypoxemia in the expression of acetate intolerance. Kidney Int 19:140, 1982
66. Abu-Hamdan DK, Mahajan SK, Desai S, et al: Hypoxemia during bicarbonate dialysis. Kidney Int 19:140, 1981
67. Maierhofer W, Maymon HL, Woods MP, et al: Hypoxemia during hemodialysis: Effects of hourly changes in bath composition. Kidney Int 21:173, 1982
68. Eiser AR, Jayamrune DS, Neff MS, et al: Cause of hypoxemia during hemodialysis (letter). N Engl J Med 305:1351, 1981
69. Rohmer D, Nassri M, Sherlock J, et al: A comparison of the respiratory dynamics during hemodialysis using acetate and bicarbonate dialysate in a sorbent regenerative system. Trans Am Soc Artif Intern Organs 27:176, 1981
70. Brautbar N, Shinaberger JH, Miller JH, et al: Hemodialysis hypoxemia: Evaluation of mechanisms utilizing sequential ultrafiltration-dialysis. Nephron 26:96, 1980
71. Jacob AL, Gavellas G, Zarco R, et al: Leukopenia, hypoxia, and complement function with different hemodialysis membranes. Kidney Int 18:505, 1980
72. Jones RH, Broadfield JB, Parsons V: Arterial hypoxemia during hemodialysis for acute renal failure in mechanically ventilated patients: Observations and mechanisms. Clin Nephrol 14:18, 1980.
73. Heneghan WF, Brunswick JW, Oh MS, et al: Dialysis hypoxemia causes hypotension. Kidney Int 21:169, 1982
74. Port FK, Johnson WJ, Klass DW: Prevention of dialysis disequilibrium syndrome by use of high sodium concentration in the dialysate. Kidney Int 3:327, 1973
75. Wehle B, Asaba H, Castenfors J, et al: The influence of the dialysis fluid composition on the blood pressure response during dialysis. Clin Nephrol 10:62, 1978
76. Boquin E, Parnell S, Grondin G, et al: Crossover study of the effects of different dialysate sodium concentrations in large surface area, short term dialysis. Proc Clin Dial Transplant Forum 7:48, 1977
77. Levine J, Falk B, Henriquez M, et al: Effects of varying dialysate sodium using large surface area dialyzers. Trans Am Soc Artif Intern Organs 24:139, 1978
78. Bergstrom J: Hemodialysis induced hypotension. Int J Artif Organs 1:204, 1979
79. VanStone JC, Bauer J, Carey J: The effect of dialysate sodium concentration on body fluid distribution during hemodialysis. Trans Am Soc Artif Intern Organs 26:383, 1980
80. Kjellstrand CM: Osmolar changes during dialysis. Int J Artif Organs 3:251, 1980
81. Kjellstrand CM, Rosa AA, Shideman JR: Hypotension during hemodialysis. Osmolality fall is an important pathogenetic factor. Am Soc Artif Intern Organs J 3:11, 1980
82. Rodrigo R, Shideman J, McHugh R, et al: Osmolality changes during hemodialysis. Ann Intern Med 86:554, 1977
83. Henrich WL, Woodard TD, Blachley JD, et al: Role of osmolality in blood pressure stability after dialysis and ultrafiltration. Kidney Int 18:480, 1980
84. Akbar S, Gronidin G, Schauerte J, et al: Fluid removal during hemodialysis—Which method? Trans Am Soc Artif Intern Organs 24:667, 1978
85. Schuenemann B, Borghardt J, Falda Z, et al: Reactions of blood pressure and body spaces to hemofiltration treatment. Trans Am Soc Artif Intern Organs 24:687, 1978
86. Raja R, Henriquez M, Kramer M, et al: Intradialytic hypotension—Role of osmolar changes and acetate influx. Trans Am Soc Artif Intern Organs 25:419, 1979
87. Aizawa Y, Hirasawa Y, Shibata A: A fall of plasma osmolality created at dialyses and its possible effect on circulating blood volume. Clin Nephrol 12:269, 1979
88. Shaldon S. Deschodt G, Beau MC, et al: The importance of serum osmotic changes in symptomatic hypotension during short hemodialysis. Proc Clin Dial Transplant Forum 8:184, 1978
89. Keshaviah P, Ilstrup E, Constantini R, et

al: The influence of ultrafiltration and diffusion on cardiovascular parameters. Trans Am Soc Artif Intern Organs 26:328, 1980
90. Goldberger S, Thompson A, Guha A, et al: Autonomic nervous dysfunction in chronic renal failure. Clin Res 19:531, 1973
91. Ewing DJ, Winney R: Autonomic function in patients with chronic renal failure on intermittent hemodialysis. Nephron 15:424, 1975
92. Kersh ES, Kronfield SJ, Unger A, et al: Autonomic insufficiency in uremia as a cause of hemodialysis induced hypotension. N Engl J Med 290:650, 1974
93. Lilley JJ, Golijen J, Stone RA: Adrenergic regulation of blood pressure in chronic renal failure. J Clin Invest 57:1190, 1975
94. Cannella G, Picotti GB, Mioni G: Blood pressure behaviour during dialysis and ultrafiltration—A pathogenic hypothesis on hemodialysis induced hypotension. Int J Artif Organs 1:69, 1978
95. Korchik WP, Demaster EG, Brown DC: Plasma norepinephrine and hemodialysis. Kidney Int 12:484, 1977
96. Korchik WP, Brown DC, DeMaster EG: Hemodialysis induced hypotension. Int J Artif Organs 1:151, 1978
97. Corder CN, Sharma J, McDonald RH Jr: Variable levels of plasma catecholamines and dopamine β-hydroxylase in hemodialysis patients. Nephron 25:267, 1979
98. Henrich WL, Katz FH, Molinoff PB, et al: Competitive effects of hypokalemia and volume depletion on plasma renin activity, aldosterone and catecholamine concentrations in hemodialysis patients. Kidney Int 12:279, 1977
99. Nies AS, Robertson D, Stone WJ: Hemodialysis hypotension is not the result of uremic peripheral autonomic neuropathy. J Lab Clin Med 94:395, 1979
100. Widmer B, Gerhardt RE, Harrington JT, et al: Serum electrolyte and acid-base composition: The influence of graded degrees of chronic renal failure. Arch Int Med 139: 1099, 1102, 1979
101. Freeman RM, Richards CJ: Studies on sulfate in endstage renal disease. Kidney Int 15:167, 1979
102. Michalk D, Klare B, Manz F, et al: Plasma inorganic sulfate in children with chronic renal failure. Clin Nephrol 16:8, 1981
103. Gonick HC, Kleeman CR, Rubini ME, et al: Functional impairment in chronic renal disease. II. Studies of acid excretion. Nephron 6:28, 1969
104. Schwartz WB, Hall PW III, Hays RM, et al: On the mechanism of acidosis in chronic renal disease. J Clin Invest 38:39, 1959
105. Goodman AD, Lemann J Jr, Lennon EJ, et al: Production, excretion and net balance of fixed acid in patients with renal acidosis. J Clin Invest 44:495, 1965
106. Lemann J Jr, Lennon EJ: Role of diet, gastrointestinal tract and bone in acid–base homeostasis. Kidney Int 1:275, 1972
107. Albright F, Feifenstein EC: The Parathyroid Glands and Metabolic Bone Disease. p 242. Williams & Wilkins, Baltimore, 1948
108. Albright F, Reitenstein EC: The Parathyroid Glands and Metabolic Bone Disease. p 242. Williams & Wilkins, Baltimore, 1948
109. Litzow JR, Lemann J Jr, Lennon EJ: The effect of treatment of acidosis on calcium balance in patients with chronic azotemic renal disease. J Clin Invest 46:280, 1967
110. Stanbury SW, Lumb GA: Metabolic studies of renal osteodystrophy. I. Calcium, phosphorus and nitrogen metabolism in rickets, osteomalacia and hyperparathyroidism complicating chronic uremia and in the osteomalacia of the adult Fanconi syndrome. Medicine (Baltimore) 41:1, 1962
111. Pellegrino Ed, Biltz RM: The composition of human bone in uremia. Observations on the reservoir functions of bone and demonstration of a labile fraction of bone carbonate. Medicine (Baltimore) 44:397, 1965
112. Lemann J Jr, Litzow JR, Lennon EJ: The effects of chronic acid loads in normal man. Further evidence for the participation of bone mineral in the defense against chronic metabolic acidosis. J Clin Invest 45:1608, 1966
113. Burnell JM: Changes in bone sodium and carbonate in metabolic acidosis and alkalosis in the dog. J Clin Invest 50:327, 1971
114. Kaye M, Frueh AJ, Silverman M: A study of vertebral bone powder from patients with chronic renal failure. J Clin Invest 49:442, 1970
115. Fraley DS, Adler S: An extrarenal role for

parathyroid hormone in the disposal of acute acid loads in rats and dogs. J Clin Invest 63:985, 1979
116. McSherry E, Morris RC Jr: Attainment of normal stature with alkali therapy in infants and children with classic renal tubular acidosis. J Clin Invest 61:509, 1978
117. Earnest DL, Sadler JH, Ingram RH, et al: Acid-base balance in chronic hemodialysis. Trans Am Soc Artif Intern Organs 14:434, 1968
118. Harrington JT, Cohen JJ: Metabolic acidosis. p 196. Cohen JJ, Kassirer JP (eds): Acid–Base. Little, Brown, Boston, 1982
119. Weller JM, Swan RC, Merrill JP: Changes in acid-base balance of uremic patients during hemodialysis. J Clin Invest 32:729, 1953
120. Cowie J, Lambie AT, Robson JS: The influence of extracorporeal dialysis on the acid-base composition of blood and cerebrospinal fluid. Clin Sci 23:397, 1962
121. Blumentals, AS, Eichenholz A, Mulhausen RO: Acid-base changes during hemodialysis. Metabolism 14:667, 1965
122. Henderson LW, Rodriquez B, Bluemle LW Jr: Factors influencing blood pH changes during extracorporeal dialysis in patients with chronic renal failure. Trans Am Soc Artif Intern Organs 12:193, 1966
123. Morrell MT, Parsons FM: Acid–base regulation by dialysis. Br J Surg 55:154, 1968
124. Rosenbaum BJ, Coburn JW, Shinaberger JH, et al: Acid-base status during the interdialytic period in patients maintained with chronic hemodialysis. Ann Intern Med 71: 1106, 1969
125. Graziani G, Ponticelli C, diFilippo G, et al: Acid-base changes in hemodialysis. Br Med J 3:163, 1970
126. Blumberg A, Marti HR: Mechanism of post-dialysis hyperventilation in patients with chronic renal insufficiency. Clin Nephrol 5:119, 1976
127. Hamilton RW, Epstein PE, Henderson LW, et al: Control of breathing in uremia: Ventilatory response to CO_2 after hemodialysis. J Appl Physiol 41:216, 1976
128. van Ypersele de Strihou C, Frans A: The pattern of respiratory compensation in chronic uremic acidosis. Nephron 7:37, 1970
129. Tolchin N, Roberts JL, Hayashi J, et al: Metabolic consequences of high mass-transfer hemodialysis. Kidney Int 11:366, 1977
130. Lewis EJ, Tolchin N, Roberts JL: Estimation of the metabolic conversion of acetate to bicarbonate during hemodialysis. Kidney Int 18(suppl 10):S-51, 1980
131. Keshaulah P, Cadwell K, Wathen R, et al: Acid base changes in sequential therapy. Proc Dial Transplant Forum 7:53, 1977
132. Peters JP Jr: The response of the respiratory mechanism to rapid changes in the reaction of the blood. Am J Physiol 44:84, 1917
133. Gibson GJ, Streeton JA: Ventilatory responses and acute acid-base changes in response to inhaled carbon dioxide in patients with chronic renal failure on long term haemodialysis. Respiration 30:389, 1973
134. Taccone-Gallucci M, Mazzarella V, Morosetti M, et al: Evaluation of acid-base balance and pO_2 with acetate dialysis in non-uremic patients. Int J Artif Organs 5:145, 1982
135. Mion CM, Hegstrom RM, Boen ST, et al: Substitution of sodium acetate for sodium bicarbonate in the bath fluid for hemodialysis. Trans Am Soc Artif Intern Organs 10:110, 1964
136. Mudge GH, Manning JA, Gilman A: Sodium acetate as a source of fixed base. Proc Soc Exp Biol Med 71:136, 1949
137. Bjoeldager PAL, Christiansen E, Jensen HA, et al: Improved effect of hemodialysis on acidemic patients from an acetate concentration of 38 mmol/L. Nephron 27:142, 1981
138. Vreman HJ, Assomull VM, Kaiser BA, et al: Acetate metabolism and acid-base homeostasis during hemodialysis: Influence of dialyzer efficiency and rate of acetate metabolism. Kidney Int 18(Suppl 10):S62, 1980
139. Eliahou HE, Feng PH, Weinberge U, et al: Acetate and bicarbonate in the correction of uremic acidosis. Br Med J 4:399, 1970
140. Lindquist F: Production and utilization of free acetate in man. Nature 193:579, 1962
141. Kveim M, Nesbakken R: Utilization of exogenous acetate during hemodialysis. Trans Am Soc Artif Intern Organs 21:138, 1975
142. Port FK, Easterling RE: Evaluation of acetate tolerance during highly efficient hemodialysis. Proc Dial Transplant Forum 5:128, 1975
143. Novello A, Kelsch RC, Easterling RE: Ace-

tate intolerance during hemodialysis. Clin Nephrol 5:29, 1976
144. Kaiser BA, Potter DE, Bryant RF, et al: Acid–base changes and acetate metabolism during routine and high efficiency hemodialysis in children. Kidney Int 19:70, 1981
145. Egan JD, Wells IC: Acetate intolerance and an inhibitor of acetate utilization in hemodialysis patients. Clin Chem 25:379, 1979
146. Harrington JT, Kassirer TP: Dialysis, hypothermia, blood transfusion. In Cohen JJ, Kassirer JP (eds): Acid–Base. Little, Brown Boston, 1982
147. Kirkendoe PK, Pearson JE, Bower JD, et al: Myocardial depressant effects of sodium acetate. Cardiovasc Res 12:127, 1978
148. Llang CS, Lowenstein JM: Metabolic control of the circulation. Effects of acetate and pyruvate. J Clin Invest 62:1029, 1978
149. Aizawa Y, Ohmori T, Imai K, et al: Depressant action of acetate upon the human cardiovascular system. Clin Nephrol 8:477, 1977.
150. Ei K, Hanai I, Horiuchi T, Hanai J, et al: Hemodialysis-associated asthma in a renal failure patient. Nephron 25:247, 1980
151. Uldall PR, Kennedy I, Craske H, et al: A double blind controlled trial of acetate versus bicarbonate dialysate in ESRD. Kidney Int 19:161, 1981
152. Borges H, Fryd D, Kjellstrand C: Bicarbonate is not better than acetate in acute dialysis. Kidney Int 19:144, 1980
153. Posen GA, Mikhael R: Dialysis-related hypotension: Etiology and prevention. Kidney Int 19:393, 1981
154. Kirkendol PK, Devia CJ, Bower JD, et al: A comparison of the cardiovascular effects of sodum acetate, sodium bicarbonate and other potential sources of fixed base in hemodialysate solutions. Trans Am Soc Artif Intern Organs 23:399, 1977
155. Cambi V, Arisi L, Biasini A, et al: Improvement of intradialytic tolerance with low-volume dialysis and bicarbonate buffering of dialysate. Kidney Int 18(suppl 10) S56, 1980
156. Gotch FA, Sargent JA: Measurement of H^+ balance (H^+b) during acetate and bicarbonate dialysis (AD,BD) therapy. Kidney Int 16:887, 1979
157. Dixon SR, McKean WI, Pryor JE, et al: Changes in acid–base balance during peritoneal dialysis with fluid containing lactate ions. Clin Sci 39:51, 1970
158. Burns RO, Henderson LW, Hager EB, et al: Peritoneal dialysis. Clinical experience. N Engl J Med 267:1060, 1962
159. LaGreca G, Biasioli S, Chiaramonte S, et al: Acid–base balance on peritoneal dialysis. Clin Nephrol 16:1, 1981
160. Miller FN, Nolph KD, Joshus IG, et al: Hyperosmolality, acetate and lactate: Dilatory factors during peritoneal dialysis. Kidney Int 20:397, 1981
161. Ramos D, Hammeke M, Bierman MH: The importance of dialysate titratable acidity for acid–base balance in intermittent peritoneal dialysis. Kidney Int 21:176, 1982
162. Sekar T, Moorthi DS, Gelman ML, et al: Pulmonary function testing during peritoneal dialysis. Kidney Int 19:140, 1982
163. Harrington JT, Kassirer JP. Metabolic alkalosis. p 291. In Cohen JJ, Cassirer JP (eds): Acid–Base. Little, Brown, Boston, 1982
164. Miller PD, Berns AS: Acute metabolic alkalosis perpetuating hypercarbia. A role for acetazolamide in chronic obstructive pulmonary disease. JAMA 238:2400, 1977
165. Swartz RD, Jacobs JF Jr: Modified dialysis for metabolic alkalosis. Ann Intern Med 88:432, 1978
166. Ayus JC, Olivero JJ, Adrogue HJ: Alkalemia associated with renal failure. Correction by hemodialysis with low-bicarbonate dialysate. Arch Intern Med 140:513, 1980
167. Swartz RD, Rubin JE, Brown RS, et al: Correction of postoperative metabolic alkalosis and renal failure by hemodialysis. Ann Intern Med 86:52, 1977
168. Oliva PB: Lactic acidosis. Am J Med 48:209, 1970
169. MacLeod J Jr, Hoover DH: Studies in experimental glycosuria. XII. Lactic acid production in the blood following the injection of alkaline solutions of dextrose or of alkaline solutions alone. Am J Physiol 42:461, 1917
170. Haldi J: Lactic acid in blood and tissue following intravenous injection of sodium bicarbonate. Am J Physiol 106:134, 1933
171. Arieff AL, Leach WJ, Lazarowitz VC: Systemic effects of $NaHCO_3$ in experimental lactic acidosis. Am J Physiol 242:F586, 1982
172. Fraley DS, Adler S, Bruns FJ, et al: Stimulation of lactate production by administration

of bicarbonate in a patient with a solid neoplasm and lactic acidosis. N Engl J Med 303:1100, 1980

172a. Park R, Arieff AI: Treatment of lactic acidosis with dichloroacetate in dogs. J Clin Invest 70:853, 1982

172b. Stacpoole PW, Harman EM, Curry SH, et al: Treatment of lactic acidosis with dichloroacetate. New Engl J Med 309:390, 1983

173. Sheppard JM, Lawrence JR, Oon RCS, et al: Lactic acidosis: Recovery associated with use of peritoneal dialysis. Aust NZ J Med 2:389, 1972

174. Hayat JC: The treatment of lactic acidosis in the diabetic patient by peritoneal dialysis using sodium acetate: A report of two cases. Diabetologia 10:485, 1974

175. Vaziri ND, Ness R, Wellikson L, et al: Bicarbonate-buffered peritoneal dialysis. An effective adjunct in the treatment of lactic acidosis. Am J Med 67:392, 1979

176. Vaziri ND, Warner AS: Peritoneal dialysis clearance of endogenous lactate. J Dial 3:107, 1979

177. Breborowicz A, Szule R: Removal of endogenous lactates via the peritoneum in experimental lactic acidosis. Intensive Care Med 7:297, 1981

178. Foulks CJ, Wright LF: Successful repletion of bicarbonate stores in ongoing lactic acidosis: A role for bicarbonate-buffered peritoneal dialysis. South Med J 74:1162, 1981

179. Gudis S, Mangi S, Feinroth M, et al: Rapid correction of severe lactic acidosis with massive isotonic bicarbonate infusion and simultaneous ultrafiltration. Kidney Int 21:168, 1982

180. Adrogue HJ, Madias NE: Changes in plasma potassium concentration during acute acid–base disturbances. Am J Med 71:456, 1981

181. Kliger AS, Hayslett JP: Disorders of potassium balance. p 170. In Brenner BM, Stein JH (eds): *Acid-Base and Potassium Homeostasis.* Churchill Livingstone, New York, 1978

182. Bourgoignie JJ, Kaplan M, Pincus J, et al: Renal handling of potassium in dogs with chronic renal insufficiency. Kidney Int 20:482, 1981

183. Hayes CP Jr, Robinson RR: Fecal potassium excretion in patients on chronic intermittent dialysis. Trans Am Soc Artif Intern Organs 11:242, 1965

184. Hayes CP, McLeod MI, Robinson RR: An extrarenal mechanism for the maintenance of potassium balance in severe chronic renal failure. Trans Assoc Am Physicians 80:207, 1967

185. Kliger AS, Binder HJ, Bastl C, et al: Demonstration of active potassium transport in the mammalian colon. J Clin Invest 67:1189, 1981

186. Brennen BL, Yasumura S, Letteri JM, et al: Total body electrolyte composition and distribution of body water in uremia. Kidney Int 17:364, 1980

187. Berlyne GM, vanLaetham L, Ben Ari J: Exchangeable potassium and renal potassium handling in advanced chronic renal failure in man. Nephron 8:264, 1971

188. Knochel JP, Seldin DW: The pathophysiology of uremia. p 2152. In Brenner BM, Rector FC Jr (eds): *The Kidney,* 2nd ed. WB Saunders, Philadelphia, 1981

189. Bilbrey GL, Carter NW, White MG, et al: Potassium deficiency in chronic renal failure. Kidney Int 4:423, 1973

190. Schultze RG, Taggart DD, Shapiro H, et al: On the adaptation in potassium excretion associated with nephron reduction in the dog. J Clin Invest 50:1061, 1971

191. Winkler AW, Haff HE, Smith PK: The toxicity of orally administered potassium salts in renal insufficiency. J Clin Invest 20:119, 1941

192. Weidmann P, Maxwell MH, Lupu AN: Plasma aldosterone in terminal renal failure. Ann Intern Med 78:13, 1973

193. Dluhy RG, Axelrod L, Underwood RH, et al: Studies of the control of plasma aldosterone concentration in normal man. J Clin Invest 51:1950, 1972

194. Bastl C, Hayslett JP, Binder HJ: Increased large intestinal secretion of potassium in renal insufficiency. Kidney Int 12:9, 1977

195. Bia MJ, Tyler KA, DeFronzo RA: Regulation of extrarenal potassium homeostasis by adrenal hormones in rats. Am J Physiol 242:F641, 1982

196. Sterns RH, Feig PU, Pring M, et al: The disposition of intravenous potassium in anuric man. A kinetic analysis. Kidney Int 15:651, 1979

197. McCaa RE, Bower JD, McCaa CS: Relative influence of acute sodium and volume depletion on aldosterone secretion in nephrectomized man. Circ Res 33:555, 1973
198. Ksiazek A: Dopamine-beta-hydroxylase activity and catecholamine levels in the plasma of patients with renal failure. Nephron 24:170, 1979
199. DeFronzo R: Pathogenesis of glucose intolerance in uremia. Metabolism 27:1866, 1978
200. Bia MJ, DeFronzo RA: Extrarenal potassium homeostasis. Am J Physiol 240:F257, 1981
201. Morgan AG, Burkinshaw L, Robinson PJA, et al: Potassium balance and acid-base changes in patients undergoing regular haemodialysis therapy. Br Med J 1:779, 1970
202. Feig PU, Shook A, Sterns RH: Effect of potassium removal during hemodialysis on the plasma potassium concentration. Nephron 27:25, 1981
203. Wiegand CF, Davin TD, Raij L, et al: Severe hypokalemia induced by hemodialysis. Arch Intern Med 141:167, 1981
204. Brown ST, Ahearn DJ, Nolph KD: Potassium removal with peritoneal dialysis. Kidney Int 4:67, 1973
205. Popovich RO, Moncrief JW, Nolph KD, et al: Continuous ambulatory peritoneal dialysis. Ann Intern Med 88:449, 1978
206. Nolph KD, Sorkin ML, Moore H: Autoregulation of sodium and potassium removal during continuous ambulatory peritoneal dialysis. Trans Am Soc Artif Intern Organs 26:334, 1980
207. Lyman N, Walcer R, Mulgaonkar S, et al: Glucose-K^+ relationships during continuous ambulatory peritoneal dialysis. Effects of intraperitoneal insulin. Kidney Int 21:172, 1982
208. Tyler K, DeFronzo R, Bia M: Adrenergic control of extrarenal potassium tolerance is mediated by a β-2 receptor. Kidney Int 21:159, 1982
209. Sandstead HH: Trace elements in uremia and hemodialysis. Am J Clin Nutr 1501, 1980
210. Berlyne GM, Ben-Ari J, Pest D, et al: Hyperaluminaemia from aluminum resins in renal failure. Lancet 2:494, 1970
211. Alfrey AC, LeGendre GR, Kaehny WD: Dialysis encephalopathy syndrome: Possible aluminum intoxication. N Engl J Med 294:184, 1976
212. Platts NM, Goode GC, Hislop JS: Composition of the domestic water supply and the incidence of fractures and encephalopathy in patients on home dialysis. Br Med J 2:657, 1977
213. Elliott HL, Dryburgh R, Fell GS, et al: Aluminum toxicity during regular hemodialysis. Br Med J 1:1101, 1978
214. Pierides AM, Edwards WA Jr, Cullum UX, et al: Haemodialysis encephalopathy with osteomalacic fractures and muscle weakness. Kidney Int 18:115, 1980
215. Parsons V, Davies C, Goode C, et al: Aluminum in bone from patients with renal failure. Br Med J 4:273, 1971
216. Dunea G, Mahurkar S, Mamdani B, et al: Role of aluminum in dialysis dementia. Ann Intern Med 88:502, 1978
217. Rosas VV, Port FK, Rutt WM: Progressive dialysis encephalopathy from dialysate aluminum. Arch Intern Med 138:1375, 1978
218. Platts MM, Moarhead JH, Greech P: Dialysis dementia. Lancet 2:157, 1973
219. Flendrig JA, Kruis H, Das A: Aluminum intoxication: The cause of dialysis dementia? Proc Eur Dial Transplant Assoc 13:355, 1976
220. Clarkson EM, Luck VA, Hynson WV, et al: The effect of aluminum hydroxide on calcium, phosphorus and aluminum balances, the serum parathyroid hormone concentration and the aluminum content of bone in patients with chronic renal failure. Clin Sci 43:519, 1972
221. Mayor GH, Keiser JA, Mukdani, et al: Aluminum absorption and distribution. Effect of parathyroid hormone. Science 197:1187, 1977
222. Gorsky JE, Dietz AA, Spencer H, et al: Metabolic balance of aluminum studied in six men. Clin Chem 25:1739, 1979
223. Wallace MR: Correction of high serum aluminum in a patient on maintenance hemodialysis. NZ Med J 93(684):335, 1981
224. McDermott JR, Smith AI, Ward MR, et al: Brain aluminum concentration in dialysis encephalopathy. Lancet 1:901, 1978
225. Kaehny WD, Alfrey AC, Holman RE, et al: Aluminum transfer during haemodialysis. Kidney Int 12:361, 1977

226. Gorsky JE, Dietz AA: Aluminum concentrations in serum of hemodialysis patients. Clin Chem 27:932, 1981
227. Alfrey AC, Mishell JM, Burks J, et al: Syndrome of dyspraxia and multifocal seizures associated with chronic hemodialysis. Trans Am Soc Art Intern Organs 18:257, 1972
228. DeBoni U, Otvos A, Scott JW, et al: Neurofibrillary degeneration induced by systemic aluminum. Acta Neuropathol 35:285, 1976
229. Klatzo I, Wisniewski HM, Streicher EJ: Experimental production of neurofibrillary degeneration. J Neuropathol Exp Neurol 24:187, 1965
230. Arieff AI, Cooper JD, Armstrong D, et al: Dementia, renal failure and brain aluminum. Ann Intern Med 90:741, 1979
231. Rosati G, DeBastiani P, Gilli P, et al: Oral aluminum and neuropsychological functioning. J Neurol 223(4):251, 1980
232. Drueke T: Dialysis osteomalacia and aluminum intoxication. Nephron 26:207, 1980
233. Ward MD, Feest TG, Ellis HA, et al: Osteomalacic dialysis osteodystrophy: Evidence for a water-bone etiological agent, probably aluminum. Lancet 1:841, 1978
234. Parkinson IS, Ward MK, Ferst TG, et al: Fracturing dialysis osteodystrophy and dialysis encephalopathy. Lancet 1:406, 1979
235. Ellis HA, McCarthy JH, Herrington J: Bone aluminum in haemodialyzed patients and in rats injected with aluminum chloride: Relationship to impaired bone mineralization. J Clin Pathol 321:832, 1979
236. Walker GS, Aaron JE, Peacock M, et al: Dialysate aluminum concentration and renal bone disease. Kidney Int 21:411, 1982
237. Alfrey AC, Hegg A, Miller N, et al: Interrelationship between calcium and aluminum metabolism in dialyzed uremic patients. Mineral Electrolyte Metab 2:81, 1979
238. Cournot-Witmer G, Zingraff J, Bourdon R, et al: Aluminum and dialysis bone disease. Lancet 2:795, 1979
239. Cournot-Witmer G, Zingraff J, Plachot JJ, et al: Aluminum localization in bone from hemodialyzed patients: Relationship to matrix mineralization. Kidney Int 20:375, 1981
240. Pierides AM, Skillen AW, Ellis HA: Serum alkaline phosphatase in azotemic and hemodialysis osteodystrophy: A study of iso-enzyme patterns, their correlation with bone histology, and their changes in response to treatment with $1\alpha(OH)D_3$ and $1,25(OH)_2D_3$. J Lab Clin Med 93:899, 1977
241. Maloney NA, Ott SM, Alfrey AC, et al: Histological quantitation of aluminum in iliac bone from patients with renal failure. J Lab Clin Med 99:206, 1982
242. Delmez JA, Schwartz JC, Harter HR, et al: Does strict phosphorus control potentiate osteomalacia in chronic hemodialysis patients? Kidney Int 21:166, 1982
243. Guillot AP, Hood VL, Ringe CF, et al: The use of magnesium-containing phosphate binders in patients with end-stage renal disease on maintenance hemodialysis. Nephron 30:114, 1982
244. Randall RE Jr: Magnesium metabolism in chronic renal disease. Ann NY Acad Sci 162:831, 1969
245. Mahler DJ, Walsh JR, Hayme GD: Magnesium, zinc and copper in dialysis patients. Am J Clin Pathol 56:17, 1971
246. Antoniou LD, Shalhoub RJ, Elliott S: Zinc tolerance tests in chronic uremia. Clin Nephrol 16:181, 1981
247. Schreiner GE, Maher JF, Freeman RB, et al: Problems of hemodialysis. Proc Int Congr Nephrol 3:316, 1967
248. Halsted JA, Smith JC Jr, Irwin MI: A conspectus of research on zinc requirements of man. J Nutr 104:345, 1974
249. Tsukamoto Y, Iwanami S, Marumo F: Disturbances of trace element concentrations in plasma of patients with chronic renal failure. Nephron 26:174, 1980
250. Mansouri K, Halsted JA, Gombos EA: Zinc, copper, magnesium and calcium in dialyzed and non-dialyzed uremic patients. Arch Intern Med 125:88, 1970
251. Casey CE, Moser MC, Hambidge KM, et al: Zinc, copper and vitamin A in pediatric dialysis. J Pediatr 98:434, 1981
252. Prasad AS, Miale A Jr, Farid Z, et al: Biochemical studies on dwarfism, hypogonadism and anemia. Arch Intern Med 111:407, 1963
253. Sandstead HH, Prasad AS, Schulert AR, et al: Human zinc deficiency, endocrine manifestations and response to treatment. Am J Clin Nutr 20:422, 1967
254. Antoniou LD, Shalhoub RJ, Sudhakar T,

et al: Reversal of uraemic impotence by zinc. Lancet 2:895, 1977
255. Mahajan SK, Prasad AS, Briggs WA, et al: Effect of zinc therapy on sexual dysfunction in hemodialysis patients. Trans Am Soc Artif Intern Organs 26:139, 1980
256. Brook AC, Johnston DG, Ward MK, et al: Absence of a therapeutic effect of zinc in the sexual dysfunction of haemodialyzed patients. Lancet 2:618, 1980
257. Zetin M, Stowe RA. Effects of zinc in chronic hemodialysis. Clin Nephrol 13:20, 1980
258. Henkin RI, Schlechter PJ, Hoye R, et al: Idiopathic hypogeusia with dysgeusia, hyposmia, and dysosmia. A new syndrome. JAMA 217:434, 1971
259. Henkin RI, Schechter PJ, Friedewald WT: A double blind study of the effects of zinc sulfate on taste and smell dysfunction. Am J Med Sci 272:285, 1976
260. Atkin-Thor E, Goodard BW, O'Nion J, et al: Hypogeusia and zinc depletion in chronic dialysis patients. Am J Clin Nutr 31:1948, 1978
261. Mahajan SK, Prasad AS, Lambujen J, et al: Improvement of uremic hypogeusia by zinc: A double blind study. Am J Clin Nutr 33:1517, 1980
262. O'Nion JV, Atkin-Thor E, Rothert SW, et al: Effect of zinc supplementation on red blood cell zinc, serum zinc, taste activity and dietary intake in zinc deficient dialysis patients. Dial Transplant 7:1208, 1978
263. Vreman JH, Venter C, Leegwater J, et al: Taste, smell and zinc metabolism in patients with chronic renal failure. Nephron 26:163, 1980
264. Ciechanover M, Peresecenschi G, Aviram A, et al: Malrecognition of taste in uremia. Nephron 26:20, 1980
265. Moynahan EJ: Acrodermatitis enteropathica. A lethal inherited human zinc deficiency disorder. Lancet 2:399, 1974
266. Gross RL, Osdin N, Fong L, et al: Depressed immunological function in zinc-deprived rats as measured by nitrogen response of spleen, thymus, and peripheral blood. Am J Clin Nutr 32:1260, 1979
267. Antoniou LD, Shalhoub RJ, Schechter GP: The effect of zinc on cellular immunity in chronic uremia. Am J Clin Nutr 34:1912, 1981
268. Briggs WA, Pederson MM, Mahajan SK, et al: Lymphocyte and granulocyte function in zinc-tested and zinc deficient hemodialysis patients. Kidney Int 21:827, 1982
269. Lyle WH: Chronic dialysis and copper poisoning. N Engl J Med 276:1209, 1967
270. Blomfield J, McPherson J, George CRP: Active uptake of copper and zinc during haemodialysis. Br Med J 2:141, 1969
271. Barbour BH, Bischel M, Abrams DE: Copper accumulation in patients undergoing chronic hemodialysis. The role of cuprophan. Nephron 8:455, 1971
272. Ivanovich P, Manzler A, Drake R: Acute hemolysis following hemodialysis. Trans. Am Soc Artif Intern Organs 15:316, 1969
273. Matter BJ, Pederson J, Psimenos G, et al: Lethal copper intoxication in hemodialysis. Trans Am Soc Artif Intern Organs 15:309, 1969
274. Manzler AD, Schreiner AW: Copper-induced acute hemolytic anemia. Ann Intern Med 73:409, 1970
275. Bustamante J, Martin-Mateo MC, DePaula-dePedro A, et al: Changes in copper and ceruloplasmin in chronic renal insufficiency treated by hemodialysis and peritoneal dialysis. Nephron 22:312, 1978
276. Salvadeo A, Minoia C, Segdgni S, et al: Trace metal changes in dialysis fluid and blood of patients on hemodialysis. Int J Artif Organs 2:17, 1979
277. Taves DR, Terry R, Smith FA, et al: Use of fluoridated water in long-term hemodialysis. Arch Intern Med 115:167, 1965
278. DeVeber GA, Oreopoulos DG, Rabinovich S, et al: Changing pattern of renal osteodystrophy with chronic hemodialysis. Trans Am Soc Artif Intern Organs 16:479, 1970
279. Rashid A, Posen GA, Gray D, et al: Bone disease in patients dialyzed with untreated water. Med Instrum 8:209, 1974
280. Jowsey JK, Johnson WJ, Taves DR, et al: Effects of dialysate calcium and fluoride on bone disease during regular hemodialysis. J Lab Clin Med 79:204, 1972
281. Johnson WJ, Taves DR: Exposure to excessive fluoride during hemodialysis. Kidney Int 5:451, 1974
282. Curdy PE, Gagnon R, Taves DR, et al: Bone disease in hemodialysis patients with particular reference to the effect of fluoride. Trans Am Soc Artif Intern Organs 20:197, 1974

283. Lough J, Noonan R, Gagnon R, et al: Effects of fluoride on bone in chronic renal failure. Arch Pathol Lab Med 99:484, 1975
284. Oreopoulos DG, Taves DR, Rabinovich S, et al: Fluoride and dialysis osteodystrophy: Results of a double blind study. Trans Am Soc Artif Intern Organs 20:203, 1974
285. Comty C, Luehmann D, Wathan R, et al: Prescription water for chronic hemodialysis. Trans Am Soc Artif Intern Organs 20:189, 1974
286. Keshaviah P, Luehmann DA: Overview of the FDA Contract Report: Investigation of the risks and hazards associated with hemodialysis devices. p 7. In Association for the Advancement of Medical Instrumentation, *Issues in Hemodialysis.* Arlington, VA, 1981
287. Kliger AS: Current concepts in peritoneal dialysis. Nephron 27:209, 1981
288. Popovich RP, Pyle WK, Moncrief JW, et al: Preliminary verification of the low dialysis clearance hypothesis via a novel equilibrium peritoneal dialysis technique. Proc Australas Conf Heat Mass Transfer 2:217, 1977
289. Popovich RP, Moncrief JW, Decherd JF, et al: Clinical development of the low dialysis clearance hypothesis via equilibrium peritoneal dialysis. Proc Annu Contractors Conf, Artif Kidney Programs NIAMDD 10:123, 1977
290. Moncrief JW, Nolph KD, Rubin J: Additional experience with continuous ambulatory peritoneal dialysis (CAPD). Trans Am Soc Artif Intern Organs 24:476, 1978
291. Nolph KD, Popovich RP, Moncrief JW: Theoretical and practical implications of continuous ambulatory peritoneal dialysis. Nephron 21:117, 1978
292. Oreopoulos DG, Robson M, Taller B, et al: Continuous ambulatory peritoneal dialysis: A new era in the treatment of chronic renal failure. Clin Nephrol 11:125, 1979
293. Faller B, Marichal JF: Treatment of chronic renal failure: Situation of CAPD. Int J Artif Organs 3:243, 1980
294. Rubin J, Nolph K, Arfania D, et al: Follow-up of peritoneal clearances in patients undergoing continuous ambulatory peritoneal dialysis. Kidney Int 16:619, 1979
295. Farrell PC, Randerson DH: Membrane permeability changes in long-term CAPD. Trans Am Soc Artif Intern Organs 26:197, 1980
296. Twardowski Z, Ksiazek A, Majdan M, et al: Kinetics of continuous ambulatory peritoneal dialysis (CAPD) with four exchanges per day. Clin Nephrol 15:119, 1981
297. Madden MA, Zimmerman SW, Simpson DP: Longitudinal comparison of intermittent versus continuous ambulatory peritoneal dialysis, in the same patients. Clin Nephrol 16:293, 1981
298. Gahl GM, v. Baeyer H, Riedinger R, et al: Caloric intake and nitrogen balance in patients undergoing CAPD. p 87. In Moncrief JW, Popovich RP (eds): CAPD update. Masson, New York, 1981
299. Arinsfrong VW, Buschmann V, Ebert R, et al: Biochemical investigations of CAPD plasma levels of trace elements and amino acids and impaired glucose tolerance during the course of treatment. Int J Artif Organs 3:237, 1980
300. Gahl GM, Schurig R, Becker H, et al: Clinical and metabolic aspects of continuous ambulatory peritoneal dialysis. Int J Artif Organs 3:245, 1980
301. Rubin J, Flynn MA, Nolph KD: Total body potassium—A guide to nutritional health in patients undergoing continuous ambulatory peritoneal dialysis. Am J Clin Nutr 34:94, 1981
302. Williams P, Harrison J, McNeill K, et al: Continuous ambulatory peritoneal dialysis. (Letter.) Am J Clin Nutr 34:2854, 1981
303. Williams P, Kay R, Harrisson J, et al: Total body nitrogen and potassium changes in patients undergoing continuous ambulatory peritoneal dialysis. Kidney Int 21:182, 1982
304. Yutuc W, Ward G, Shilipetar G, et al: Substitution of sorbitol for dextrose in peritoneal irrigation fluid. A preliminary report. Trans Am Soc Artif Intern Organs 13:168, 1967
305. Raja RM, Kramer MS, Manchanda R, et al: Peritoneal dialysis with fructose dialysate: Prevention of hyperglycemia and hyperosmolality. Ann Intern Med 79:511, 1973
306. Tsan-Shin Y, Jen-Tse C, Wan-Yu C: Studies on peritoneal dialysis. J Formosa Med Assoc 69:20, 1970
307. Oreopoulos DG, Balfe JW, Khanna R, et al: Further experience with the use of amino acid containing dialysate (amino-dianeal) in peritoneal dialysis. p. 109. In Moncrief JW, Popovich, RP (eds): CAPD Update. Masson, New York, 1981

17

Gastrointestinal Disorders

John Dobbins

The gastrointestinal tract plays an important role in fluid, electrolyte, and acid–base balance. The intestine has to absorb about 10 liters of fluid per day. While this is a paltry amount compared with what the kidneys absorb, failure to absorb this fluid can result in significant water, acid–base, and electrolyte imbalance and great discomfort, as anyone with severe diarrhea can testify.

Of the 10 liters of fluid that the intestine absorbs per day, only 2 to 3 liters is ingested fluid. The remainder represents endogenous secretions of salivary, gastric, pancreatic, biliary, and enteric origin. Since gastric secretions are acidic, failure to absorb this fluid will result in systemic alkalosis. In contrast, pancreatic secretions are alkaline; failure to absorb this fluid will lead to the development of systemic acidosis.

The burden of absorbing endogenous secretion plus ingested nutrients falls upon the small intestine and colon. For this reason, emphasis will be placed on the pathophysiology of water and electrolyte transport in small intestine and colon in subsequent sections. The jejunum absorbs about 60 percent of the fluid load, the ileum 20 percent, and the colon 20 percent. The normal stool contains only about 100 ml water; thus the overall efficiency of absorption is about 99 percent. Absorptive efficiency is greatest in the colon and least in the jejunum. The colon absorbs 95 percent of the 2 liters presented to it daily, whereas the jejunum and ileum have only a 50 to 60 percent absorptive efficiency. Efficiency of absorption may be related in part to the permeability or leakiness of the intercellular tight junctions.

The intestine and colon can secrete as well as absorb fluid and electrolytes. Passive secretion normally occurs in the jejunum in response to the osmotic content of food intake. Active secretion can also occur, resulting in diarrhea if sufficiently large. The biologic advantage to the host of this secretory process is unclear. However, the involvement of the second messengers, cyclic nucleotides and calcium, in active secretion suggests a regulatory role of the gut in fluid and electrolyte homeostasis, if not now, then perhaps in our amphibian past.

The rectal gland of the shark exemplifies this principle. This sea-residing amphibian is constantly ingesting large amounts of hypertonic salt solution. The development of the specialized chloride-secreting rectal gland permits the shark to maintain a normal internal electrolyte milieu despite the high concentration of NaCl in the fluid it ingests. Speculation aside, alterations in active anion secretion by the intestine and colon can have profound metabolic effects in humans. Patients with cholera can excrete up to 20 liters of diarrheal fluid per day, which may cause life-threatening dehydration and marked disturbances in acid–base and electrolyte homeostasis.

WATER AND ELECTROLYTE TRANSPORT: GENERAL

Water Transport

Water movement across the intestinal mucosa is determined by osmotic and hydrostatic pressure gradients, hence is entirely passive. Although hydrostatic pressure is a determinant of water movement and can be altered experimentally,[1,2] there is no evidence that significant alterations in hydrostatic pressure occur in health or diarrheal diseases. Thus, alterations in osmotic gradients are the major determinant of changes in water movement. Since osmotic gradients are determined by solute movement across the mucosa, solute transport will be discussed in some detail. Although any nonwater molecule qualifies as a solute, the major intestinal solutes are Na, K, H, Cl, HCO_3, carbohydrates, small organic acids, amino acids, and di- and tripeptides.

Electrolyte Transport

Electrolyte transport is determined by (1) the electrochemical gradients across the extracellular pathway and the brush border and basolateral membranes; (2) the ability of the electrolyte to traverse these membranes and the extracellular pathway; and (3) the presence of energy-requiring electrolyte pumps. Electrolyte transport can thus be broken down into two components: (1) energetics, or those factors that determine the electrochemical gradients; and (2) kinetics, or the mechanism(s) by which electrolytes traverse membranes and extracellular spaces.

ENERGETICS

Na–K Pump

An energy-requiring Na–K exchange pump is located on the basolateral membrane of all intestinal epithelial cells and is of crucial importance in establishing electrochemical gradients that regulate electrolyte transport.[3-5] This pump, intimately related to the enzyme Na–KATPase, is able to transport Na and K against their electrochemical gradients. It is responsible for the steep chemical gradients that exist for these electrolytes across the basolateral membrane. Na is pumped out of the cell and K into the cell. The usual exchange ratio is 3 Na:2 K.[6] Thus, there is net transfer of charge across the basolateral membrane, and the interior of the cell is negatively charged compared with either the lumen of the intestine or the blood (−35 mV).[1,7,8] As a result of this pump, intracellular Na is maintained at a relatively low concentration (15 mEq/liter) compared with extracellular Na (140 mEq/liter), and intracellular K is maintained at a high concentration compared with extracellular K.

The Na–K pump is not only important for Na and K: virtually all ion intestinal transport appears to be linked in some fashion to the activity of this pump. Indeed, transport (both absorption or secretion) nearly completely ceases when Na–K-ATPase is inactivated by metabolic (ATP deprivation) or transport (blockage of transport) inhibitors.[1,9] Thus, the enzyme Na–K-ATPase plays a crucial role in both normal intestinal electrolyte transport and in the abnormalities that result from gastrointestinal disorders.

Ca Pump

Ca-ATPase is present on the basolateral membrane of intestinal enterocytes.[10,11] Its role in electrolyte transport or even in maintaining intercellular Ca levels is unknown. It presumably pumps Ca out of the cell in order to maintain low intracellular Ca levels. Because so little is known about the physiologic role of this enzyme in intestinal electrolyte transport, it will not be discussed further here. However, an important role for this enzyme may become apparent in the future.

K–H Pump

K–H ATPase is an important transport enzyme that regulates acid secretion by the stomach.[12] Located on the apical membrane of parietal cells, it catalyzes the exchange of K for protons. K in the mucosal solution enters the cell and protons exit. Recently evidence suggests that K–H ATPase also may be present on the apical membrane in the colon.[13,14] The importance of this enzyme in K transport, however, remains to be determined.

KINETICS

Extracellular

Extracellular transport, which is by definition passive and noncarrier mediated, plays a crucial role in the small intestine, which is a relatively leaky epithelium.[1,7] Extracellular transport is thought to be determined primarily by the permeability of the tight junction to electrolytes and water.[7] The jejunum is most permeable, followed by the ileum; the distal colon is least permeable.[15-17] Thus, there is a progressive decrease in permeability as one progresses down the intestine to the rectum. This phenomenon may be important for the formation of solid fecal matter.

Transcellular

Channels. Channels or pores undoubtedly play an important role in the regulation of electrolyte transport. However, because of technical problems, little is known about their function in the intestine. To characterize channels carefully, one must gain access to the intracellular space. Intracellular microelectrode studies are difficult to perform in the intestine and few have been attempted. Studies with brush border and basolateral membrane vesicles are providing some information. For example, it has recently been demonstrated that there is a chloride conductive channel in the brush border membrane of the rat small intestine.[18]

A channel can be considered in its simplest form as a water-filled hole in the lipid bilayer of the cell membrane, through which electrolytes can move by simple diffusion. Channels can be more complex with such features as ion selectivity, saturation kinetics, and competitive inhibition. Movement through a channel may be so restrictive (single-file diffusion) that one might argue whether it is a channel or a carrier. Aside from the Cl channel, other examples are K-conductive channels in the brush border and basolateral membrane[19] and an amiloride-sensitive, mineralocorticoid-inducible Na channel in the brush border membrane[20] of the colon.

Carriers. Carrier-mediated transport is a major mechanism of intestinal nutrient and electrolyte transport. The three cation pumps—Na–K, Ca, and K–H—are examples of carrier-mediated transport processes that can result in active transport. Non-energy-requiring carriers that facilitate passive transport are numerous: Na-glucose, Na-amino acid, Na-PO_4 cotransport, Na–H exchange, and Cl-HCO_3 exchange, to name a few, Carrier-mediated transport can be simply defined as transmembrane transport that requires a specialized transport protein, with transport dependent on a number of factors (e.g., affinity, selectivity, inhibition) that can be defined in kinetic terms.

SALIVARY, GASTRIC, BILIARY, AND PANCREATIC SECRETION

Salivary Glands

Saliva accounts for about 1500 ml of the 10 liters the intestine absorbs per day. The parotid glands account for most of this quantity. Fluid and electrolyte secretion by the parotids is probably similar to secretory mechanisms in the pancreas and intestine (see below).

Stomach

The parietal cells in the stomach secrete HCl. They do so by means of a K:H pump on the luminal membrane.[12] In the resting state, the luminal membrane of the parietal cell has many infoldings, and there are intracellular vesicles in close proximity to the invaginated luminal membrane. KCl accumulates in these vesicles and invaginations, probably passively through conductive channels. The K:H pump actively pumps K out of these vesicles in exchange for H. Thus, HCl accumulates in these vesicles and invaginations. During stimulation, the vesicles fuse with the luminal membrane, the infoldings decrease dramatically, and HCl is extruded into the gastric lumen. HCl concentration can be as high as 150 mM; potassium concentration is usually ~10 mM. There is an inverse relationship between Na and H concentration in gastric juice.[21] The source of Na has not been established and may be of nonparietal cell origin. The stomach normally secretes about 2 to 3 liters/day. If none of the secreted hydrogen ion were reabsorbed, ~400 to 500 mEq of acid would be lost each day, and profound metabolic alkalosis would ensue.

Three receptors have been found on the parietal cell. All stimulate acid secretion and have been named after the hormone with which they bind: gastrin, acetylcholine (Ach), and histamine receptor.[22] There is synergism between the histamine receptor and the other two receptors such that stimulation of the histamine receptor and one of the other receptors results in acid secretion greater than the additive effect of stimulating either receptor singly.[22] There is no synergism between the gastrin and acetylcholine receptors. This synergism is thought to explain in part the ability of H_2 antagonists, such as cimetidine, to inhibit acid secretion stimulated by any mechanism.

Pancreas

The pancreas normally secretes about 1500 ml of HCO_3-rich fluid per day. At high flow rates, the HCO_3 concentration approaches 150 mEq/liter with a pH of 8.3. The mechanism of HCO_3 secretion is not known; a Na:H pump on the luminal membrane of pancreatic ductular cells has been proposed on the basis of studies performed in the rabbit.[23] There is a reciprocal relationship between Cl and HCO_3 concentration in pancreatic fluid that is dependent on flow rate.[24] At low flow rate, Cl is the major anion. Three theories have been proposed to explain this phenomenon. The most simple states that Cl:HCO_3 exchange occurs along the pancreatic duct and would be greatest at low flow rates.[25] A second hypothesis suggests that Cl is contributed by one cell type and HCO_3 by another, the final concentrations being determined by the relative contributions of each cell type.[26]

Bile

Biliary secretion amounts to ~500 ml/day. Bile acids are a major determinant of bile flow. The mechanism(s) of biliary secretion are poorly understood because of inaccessability of the canaliculus and canalicular membrane for study.[27] The electrolyte composition of bile is similar to plasma, except for the presence of bile acids.[28]

INTESTINAL TRANSPORT

Jejunum

ABSORPTION

The jejunum is a leaky epithelium the major function of which is nutrient absorption rather than fluid and electrolyte transport.[1,15] The tight junctions in the jejunum are quite leaky to the major electrolytes, so much so in fact that very little transmembrane potential is generated despite the presence of an active Na pump. The basal PD transmembrane potential in the jejunum is only 1 to 2 mV. Because of this leakiness, the jejunum cannot transport Na against steep electrochemical gradients. The tight junctions are less permeable to nutrients such as glucose, amino acids, and small peptides. Thus the jejunum efficiently absorbs these nutrients.

Jejunal absorptive mechanisms are depicted in Figure 17–1. The Na pump generates a low intracellular Na concentration (15 mEq/liter). In addition, the intracellular space is negatively charged (−35 mV) compared with the mucosal and serosal solutions. Thus, there is a favorable electrochemical gradient for Na entry into the enterocyte.[1] Glucose, amino acid, and small peptides are transported across the brush border membrane by a Na cotransport mechanism (Fig. 17–1). These nutrients can be transported uphill against their concentration gradients into the cell as a result of the downhill electrochemical gradient for Na that exists across the brush border membrane due to the action of the Na pump.[29] The nutrient cotransport step across the brush border is passive, dependent on the Na gradient across the brush border, which in turn is generated by the activity of the Na pump. The energy-requiring step, Na extrusion, occurs at the basolateral membrane. No glucose absorption would occur in the absence of a favorable Na gradient. Finally, it should be noted that carrier-mediated Na-glucose cotransport, being totally passive, can occur in either direction, as a function of the concentration gradients. Thus, Na and glucose secretion could occur via this carrier, provided that Na and/or glucose concentration are greater inside the cell than in the lumen. The exit of glucose and amino acids across the basolateral membrane is passive and carrier mediated but Na independent.[31,70]

The leaky epithelium found in the jejunum may be important in nutrient absorption. Na can be recycled during nutrient absorption. Once Na-glucose absorption occurs, Na is pumped into the lateral intercellular space, where it can leak back into the mucosal solution to be reutilized in nutrient absorption (Fig. 17–1). This is analogous to the enterohepatic circulation of bile acids.

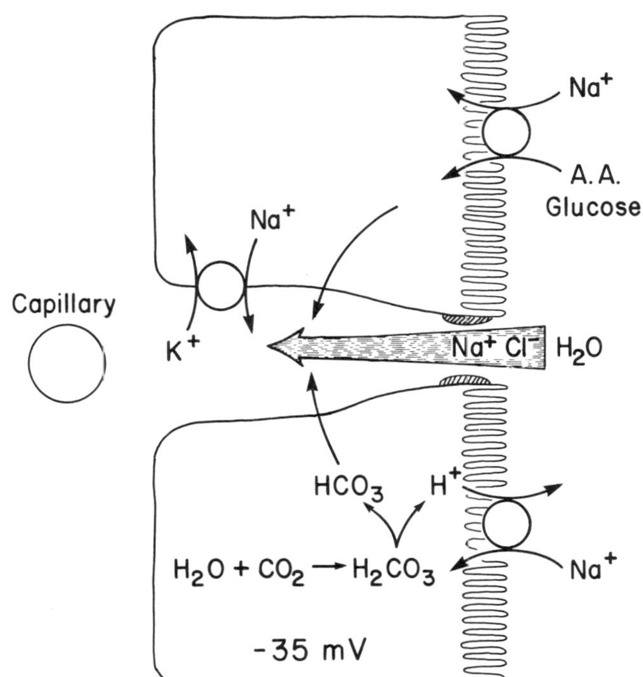

Fig. 17–1. Jejunal absorptive mechanisms. See text for a detailed explanation.

HCO_3 is also absorbed by a Na-coupled mechanism. It should be pointed out that Na–HCO_3 cotransport is indistinguishable from Na:H exchange, which is the probable mechanism by which HCO_3 is absorbed.[32] Like Na-glucose cotransport, this is a passive carrier system with transport being determined by the gradients of Na and HCO_3 (H^+) across the brush border membrane. HCO_3 exit across the basolateral membrane may occur by an anion-exchange process.[33]

No evidence for carrier-mediated transport of Cl across the brush border membrane exists; it is thought that Cl absorption occurs via the extracellular route in response to the potential generated by active Na transport. Cl:OH exchange (H:Cl cotransport) has been described in the rat small intestine,[7] but this is probably an ileal process.[34] K transport in the jejunum appears to be passive and extracellular.

In summary, nutrient and electrolyte absorption in the jejunum is largely dependent on Na and the Na pump (Fig. 17–1). Once nutrients and HCO_3 have entered the enterocyte against their electrochemical gradients (driven by the downhill gradient for Na), they can exit the enterocyte down their electrochemical gradient, and move into the lateral intercellular space. As a result, the osmotic pressure in the lateral intercellular space rises, thereby providing a driving force for water movement. Water can move into the lateral intercellular space via either the transcellular or extracellular route. Movement through extracellular route can result in further electrolyte absorption, by the process of convection or solvent drag (Fig. 17–1).

SECRETION

The jejunum secretes chloride[35] probably by the same mechanism as occurs in the ileum.[9] Since Cl secretion has been more extensively investigated in the ileum, this process will be described subsequently. HCO_3 secretion by the duodenum has been studied in some species. In bullfrog duodenum, HCO_3 secretion appears to occur by a mechanism similar to that involved in Cl secretion. In amphiuma, duodenal HCO_3 secretion appears to be the result from Cl:HCO_3 exchange on the basolateral membrane followed by diffusion of HCO_3 across the brush border membrane.[36]

Ileum

ABSORPTION

Absorption of nutrients in the ileum is essentially identical to that in the jejunum. The ileum is a slightly tighter epithelium than the jejunum and develops transepithelial potentials of 2 to 4 mV in the basal state. Thus, there is less backleak of electrolytes through the tight junction and less solvent drag during absorption.[15] Carrier-mediated Na-coupled transport of bile acids occurs across the brush

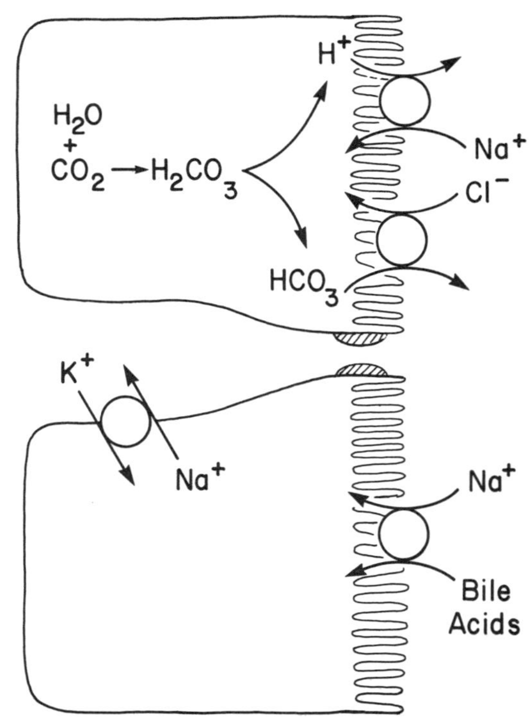

Fig. 17–2. Na and Cl transport mechanisms in the ileum. See text for discussion.

border in the ileum, but not in the jejunum.

Na:H exchange is present on the brush border in the ileum, as in the jejunum.[37] Cl:HCO_3 and Cl:OH exchange are also present in the ileum, unlike the jejunum (Fig. 17–2).[18,38] The net effect of Na:H and Cl:HCO_3 or Cl:OH exchange is Na and Cl transport across the brush border. This probably accounts for the apparent Na–Cl cotransport observed with intact tissue in vitro.[39] Using brush border membrane vesicles, Fan et al.[40] have found evidence for Na–Cl cotransport, but this has not been confirmed in investigations by Knickelbein et al.[37] or by Liedtke et al.[41] In vivo studies in human subjects suggest that Na and Cl transport occurs by dual exchangers, as illustrated in Figure 17–2.[42] Cl exit across the basolateral membrane has not been elucidated.

SECRETION

The ileum can secrete Cl and HCO_3, probably by similar mechanisms. Under stimulated conditions, such as observed after vasoactive intestinal polypeptide (VIP) or cholera enterotoxin administration, Cl secretion is observed in vitro, whereas HCO_3 secretion is observed in vivo. The reason for this discrepancy is not apparent.

Cl secretion probably occurs as illustrated in Figure 17–3.[9] Cl enters the enterocyte across the basolateral membrane coupled to Na. The driving force for this entry is the electrochemical gradient for Na that exists across the basolateral membrane because of the action of the Na pump. This Na–Cl cotransport is another example of secondary active transport. Cl accumulates inside the cell against its electrochemical gradient; that is, the intracellular concentration of Cl is greater than can be explained by the Nernst equation. Cl then exists passively from the cell across the brush border membrane. Na is pumped back into the lateral intercellular space; the net effect is electrogenic Cl secretion. HCO_3 secretion probably occurs by a similar mechanism.[43] Cl exit across the brush border membrane most likely occurs via a Cl-conductive channel.[44,45] The permeability of this Cl-

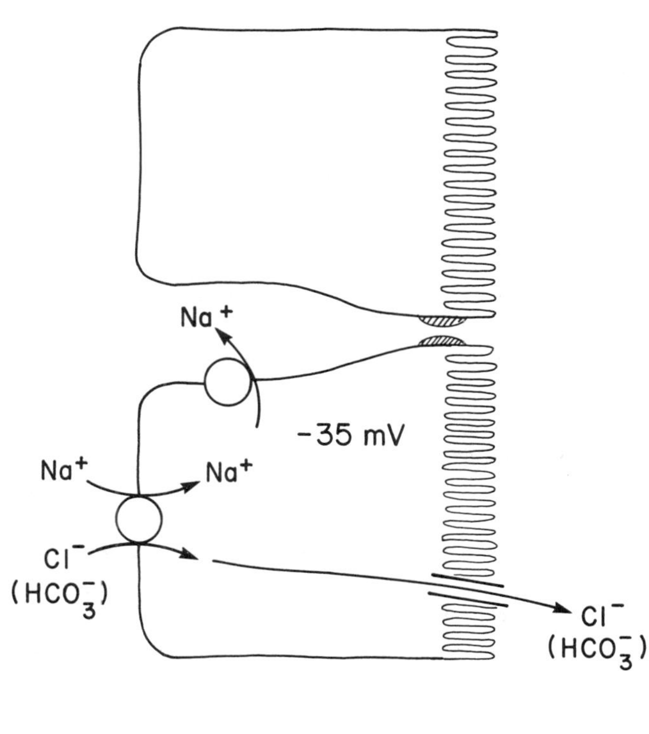

Fig. 17–3. Cl secretion by epithelial tissues. See text for discussion.

conductive channel appears to be regulated by intracellular mediators of electrolyte transport. Similar mechanisms exist in the duodenum, jejunum, and colon.

It has been pointed out that the ileum can absorb (Fig. 17–2) and secrete (Fig. 17–3) Cl. These processes are quite similar, differing only in the sites at which Cl entry and exit are located on the enterocyte. Current evidence suggests that Cl absorption (Fig. 17–2) occurs on villous or surface cells and that Cl secretion (Fig. 17–3) occurs in crypt cells.[46] Some studies, however, suggest that both Cl absorption and secretion can occur in villous cells.[47,48]

Colon

ABSORPTION

The colon, especially the distal colon, is a much tighter epithelium than the jejunum or ileum and can develop transepithelial potentials of ≥30 mV.[17,49] The colon is therefore, much more efficient than the small intestine in its ability to absorb water. This property is partly responsible for the solid stool produced by healthy persons. In contrast, patients with an ilestomy always have liquid stools.

Sugars and amino acids are not absorbed in the colon by carrier-mediated mechanisms as in the small intestine. The colon can, however, absorb some of the bacterial degradation products of carbohydrates and short-chain fatty acids, such as butyric and acetic acid. These fatty acids appear to be absorbed by passive nonionic diffusion or fatty acid:HCO_3 exchange, and possibly by sodium cotransport.[50,51]

Na transport across the brush border membrane also occurs via a conductive channel that is inducible by aldosterone and blocked by amiloride (Fig. 17–4).[20] There appears to be no direct or indirect coupling between Na and Cl or HCO_3 transport in the distal colon as in the jejunum and ileum. Cl–HCO_3 exchange is present in the distal colon, which

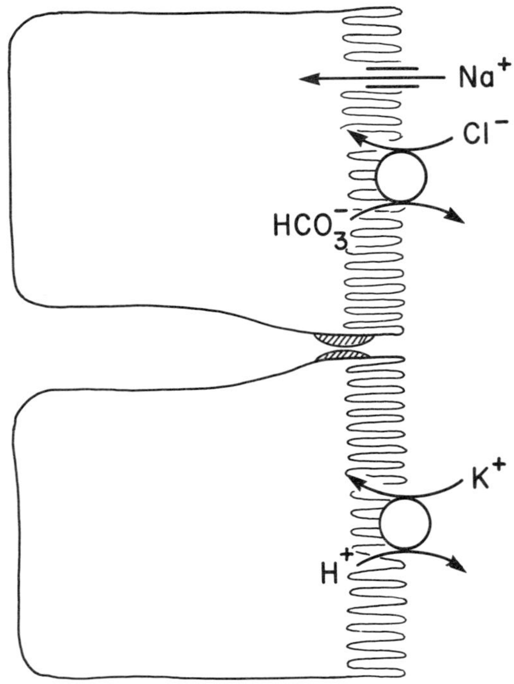

Fig. 17–4. Colonic electrolyte transport.

is responsible for active Cl absorption and HCO_3 secretion in the distal colon (Fig. 17–4). This Cl:HCO_3 exchange is insensitive to ouabain or Na removal.[52,53] The colon can actively absorb K and appears to do so by a brush border K:H pump, which is probably identical to the K:H pump in the stomach responsible for acid secretion.[13,14]

SECRETION

The colon can secrete Cl by a similar mechanism as the ileum (Fig. 17–3).[54] The colon can also secrete potassium, and this process is stimulated by both aldosterone and glucocorticoids.[55,56] Potassium secretion is closely linked to the activity of Na:K-ATPase located in the basolateral membrane.

The transport properties of the colon are not uniform throughout its lengths. The proximal colon is leakier than the distal colon and is therefore more similar to the ileum in its transport properties[57] (Fig. 17–3). Under basal conditions, K secretion occurs in the proximal colon, whereas K absorption takes place in the distal colon.[58]

INTRACELLULAR MEDIATORS OF INTESTINAL ELECTROLYTE TRANSPORT

cAMP

Cyclic adenosine monophosphate (cAMP) is the best characterized of the intracellular mediators of electrolyte transport. Many neurohumoral agents, enterotoxins, and laxatives appear to exert their effect on electrolyte transport by increasing the intracellular level of cAMP. This increase in intracellular cAMP concentration affects electrolyte transport in two ways: (1) by blocking coupled (direct or indirect) entry of Na and Cl across the brush border (presumably in villous cells) (Fig. 17–3); and (2) by increasing the permeability of the Cl conductive channel on the brush border membrane (presumably in crypt cells).[39,44,45] These two effects result in an inhibition of Na and Cl absorption and the stimulation of Cl (HCO_3) secretion. Increasing intracellular cAMP levels do not block Na-coupled glucose and amino acid entry across the brush border membrane. This observation provides the basis for the use of oral glucose–electrolyte solutions in the treatment of severe diarrheal diseases mediated by cAMP, such as cholera. The effect of decreasing intracellular levels of cAMP, if any, is unknown.

cGMP

Although it is not as convincing as for cAMP, evidence is accumulating that cyclic guanosine monophosphate (cGMP) may function as an intracellular mediator of electrolyte transport as well.[59-61] When intracellular levels of cGMP rise, coupled Na and Cl absorption is inhibited and Cl secretion is stimulated.. The effect of decreasing cGMP levels is unknown.

Calcium

Intracellular calcium is possibly the most important regulator of ion transport. Unlike the cyclic nucleotides, raising and lowering the calcium concentration both affect transport. Furthermore, there is some evidence that cAMP may mobilize intracellular calcium.[62] Thus, it is possible that calcium is the final mediator of cyclic nucleotide-induced changes in ion transport.[63] Increasing intracellular calcium levels has the same effect as cyclic nucleotides in blocking Na and Cl entry into the cell and in stimulating Cl (HCO_3) secretion. In contrast, decreasing intracellular calcium levels stimulates Na and Cl absorption.

Serotonin and cholinergic agonists have been found to increase intracellular calcium levels by increasing Ca entry from the extracellular space; in essence, they act as calcium ionophores.[64,65] Calcium channel blockers, such as verapamil and nifedipine, stimulate absorption, presumably by lowering intracellular calcium levels.[66] Dopamine and alpha-2-adrenergic agonists stimulate absorption, probably by acting as calcium channel blockers.[67] Of interest, the effect of A23187, a calcium ionophore, is blocked by indomethacin, a cyclooxygenase inhibitor.[68] Since calcium is required for prostaglandin formation, the role of prostaglandins in calcium-mediated changes in electrolyte transport will have to be determined. Many prostaglandins, including PGE_2, are known to increase cAMP levels.

NEUROHUMORAL CONTROL OF INTESTINAL ION TRANSPORT

A number of endogenous substances are known to affect electrolyte transport. These can broadly be defined as neurohumoral agents, although some do not fit into the classic definition of either neurotransmitters or hormones. We have divided these agents into two categories: those that stimulate secretion and those that enhance absorption[69] (Table 17–1).

Table 17–1. Neurohumoral Agents That Alter Fluid and Electrolyte Transport

Secretagogues	Absorptagogues
Arachidonic acid metabolites	Somatostatin
Prostaglandin E_1 and E_2,	Enkephalin
HETE, HPETE	Adrenergic agonists
Vasoactive intestinal peptide	Dopamine
Secretin	Glucocorticoids
Serotonin	Angiotensin
Cholinergic agonists	
Calcitonin	
Gastric inhibitory peptide	
Glucagon	
Cholecystokinin	
Substance P	
Bombesin	
Motilin	
Bradykinin	
Neurotensin	

Secretogogues[69]

Prostaglandin E_1 and E_2, 5-hydroxyeicosatetraenoic acid (HETE), and 5-hydroperoxyeicosatetraenoic acid (HPETE) are potent secretogogues.[70,71] PGE_1 and PGE_2 appear to act by increasing adenylate cyclase activity,[70] while the effect of HETE and HPETE on cyclic nucleotides has not been determined. Bradykinin stimulates PGE_2 production[72] and secondarily adenylate cyclase activity.

Vasoactive intestinal polypeptide,[73,74] adenosine, and ATP also stimulate adenylate cyclase.[75,76] Serotonin and cholinergic agonists act as calcium ionophores.[64,65] The mechanism of action of the other agents listed in Table 17–1 has not been determined.

Absorptagogues[69]

Somatostatin, enkephalins and other opiates, dopamine, and adrenergic agonists generally have the opposite effect on ion transport exhibited by the cyclic nucleotide- and calcium-mediated secretogogues. Thus, they enhance coupled Na and Cl absorption and probably inhibit electrogenic Cl (HCO_3) secretion.[77] These agents, however, have not been shown to affect cyclic nucleotide levels. Dopamine acts as a calcium channel blocker. Since dopamine acts primary as an alpha-adrenergic agonist, it is likely that alpha-adrenergic agonists will act as calcium channel blockers as well.[67]

Glucocorticoids have multiple effects: they stimulate Na–K-ATPase located on the basolateral membrane, increase brush border Na:H exchange, and inhibit prostaglandin formation.[78-80] Mineralocorticoids stimulate Na transport across the brush border membrane.[20] Prostacyclin has only been studied in vivo.[81]

PATHOPHYSIOLOGY OF DIARRHEA

Definition of Diarrhea

Diarrhea results from an excess of water in the stool and essentially represents malabsorption of water. Normal stool is about 75 percent water, and weighs 100 to 200 g/day. An excess of water in stool will cause an increase in stool weight. Thus, diarrhea can be defined as fecal weight >225 to 250 g/24 hr. Fecal weight is also a useful way to quantitate the severity of the diarrhea. Note that diarrhea is not determined by the number or frequency of bowel movements. Patients with the irritable bowel syndrome can have numerous movements in a 24-hour period, yet their 24-hour stool weight is normal or only slightly increased.[82] These persons, by definition, have little or no diarrhea.

Mechanism of Diarrhea

Since water is absorbed passively, excess water in stool must be due to excess solute in stool. Excess solute in the stool can result from (1) decreased absorption of ingested solute, or (2) electrolyte secretion by the intestine (Fig. 17–5). A classic example of decreased absorption of an ingested solute is lactose intolerance. Lactose (and its breakdown products due to bacterial degradation) are incompletely absorbed, leading to excess

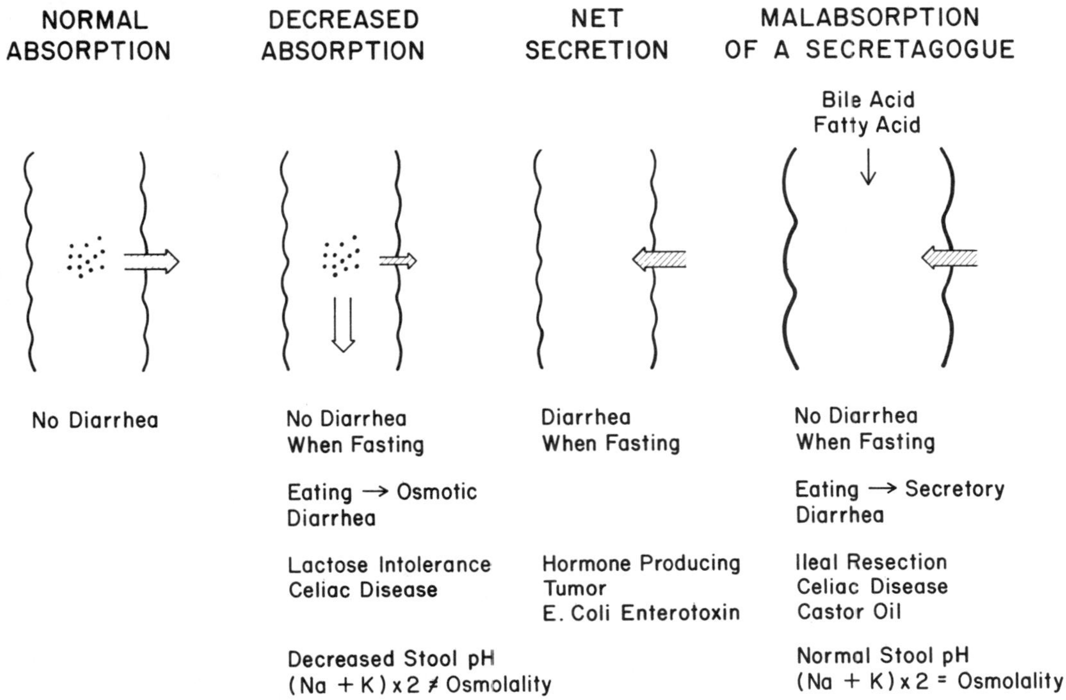

Fig. 17–5. Mechanisms of diarrhea.

solute and secondarily excess water in the stool. This type of diarrhea is frequently called an osmotic diarrhea, although technically all diarrhea is osmotic; obviously it does not occur under fasting conditions. Since bacteria convert lactose and other carbohydrates into organic acids, the pH of the stool in carbohydrate malabsorption will frequently be acidic (pH as low as 5).

Another characteristic of "osmotic diarrhea" is that the usual stool electrolytes (i.e., Na, K, and accompanying anions) do not account for all the stool osmolality (stool is usually isosmotic with serum). Since HCO_3 cannot be accurately determined in fecal fluid unless it is collected under oil, a convenient way to determine whether stool electrolytes account for the osmolarity is to measure Na and K in fecal fluid and to multiply by 2 to account for the anions. If this number is significantly less than the measured osmolarity, then an osmotic gap exists, which must be due to an unmeasured solute in the stool. In carbohydrate malabsorption, the sugar and its bacterial degradation products are the unmeasured solute. With magnesium-containing laxative use, magnesium is the unmeasured solute.

A classic example of diarrhea due to electrolyte secretion is *Escherichia coli* enterotoxin-induced diarrhea (see Fig. 17–5). This type of diarrhea is frequently called a secretory diarrhea. If severe enough, diarrhea will persist with fasting. Fecal osmolality can be accounted for by fecal electrolytes, $(Na + K) \times 2$. A variant of secretory diarrhea is malabsorption of a secretagogue (see Fig. 17–5). Classic examples are bile acid and fatty acid diarrhea. Fatty acids are normally absorbed throughout the small intestine, and bile acids are absorbed by the terminal ileum. When these substances are not absorbed in the small intestine, they act as secretagogues while passing through the colon. Like osmotic diarrhea, no diarrhea occurs with fasting because bile acids are stored in the gallbladder. Similarly if fatty foods have not been ingested, fatty acid malabsorption will not occur. Unlike osmotic diarrhea, however, stool electrolytes account for the osmolarity and stool pH is normal (see Fig. 17–5).

Etiology of Diarrhea

There are four major causes of diarrhea, each of which can cause fluid, electrolye or acid–base disorders.

Secretagogues

There are three major categories of secretagogues, that is, agents that stimulate secretion.

BACTERIAL ENTEROTOXINS. Many bacteria have been found to produce enterotoxins; these are listed in Table 17–2.[83-89] Table 17–2 also lists the intracellular mediators believed to be responsible for the diarrhea. It should be noted that some bacteria make more than one enterotoxin. For instance, *E. coli* can produce either a heat-labile or heat-stable enterotoxin. The heat-labile enterotoxin increases cAMP production and the heat-stable enterotoxin increases cGMP production. Some enterotoxins are cytotoxic, such as that produced by *Staphlococcus aureus.* Although the precise role of cytotoxicity in producing diarrhea is poorly understood for most bacteria, *Clostridium difficile* enterotoxin has been shown to produce a marked inflammatory response in the intestinal mucosa. *Clostridium difficile* also makes an enteroxtoxin that is not cytotoxic[88] and that may induce diarrhea by increasing intracellular calcium levels.[89]

NEUROHUMORAL AGENTS. A number of hormones and/or neurotransmitters can stimulate electrolyte secretion (Table 17–1). Vasoactive intestinal peptide is the leading candidate as the cause of most cases of pancreatic cholera. One-third of patients with medullary carcinoma of the thyroid complain of diarrhea, which is believed to result from high circulating calcitonin levels. Diarrhea is frequently present in the carcinoid syndrome and is associated with serotonin hypersecretion. Diabetic diarrhea may be due to autonomic neuropathy,[90] which leads to an imbalance between adrenergic innervation (i.e., stimulates absorption) and cholinergic innervation (i.e., stimulates secretion) in the intestine. The remaining secretagogues listed in Table 17–1 have not yet been associated with a clinical syndrome.

LAXATIVES (DETERGENTS). Many laxatives act as secretagogues[87,91] (Table 17–3). Bile acids can be thought of as endogenous laxatives. Dihydroxy bile acids stimulate electrolyte se-

Table 17–2. Bacterial Enterotoxins That Stimulate Secretion

Bacterial Agent	Mediator	Cytotoxic
Vibrio cholera	cAMP	
Escherichia coli		
Heat labile	cAMP	
Heat stabile	cGMP	
Bacillus cereus	cAMP	
Staphylococcus aureus		+
Clostridium perfringens		+
Shigella		+
Yersinia enterocolitica	cGMP	
Klebsiella pneumoniae		
Enterobacteria cloacae		
Clostridium difficile	Calcium	+
Pseudomonas aeruginosa		
Aeromonas hydrophilia		

Table 17–3. Laxatives (Detergents) That Stimulate Secretion

Laxative	Mediator
Dihydroxy bile acids	cAMP
Fatty acids	cAMP
Hydroxy fatty acids	cAMP
(ricinoleic acid)	cAMP
Dioctyl sodium sulfosuccinate	cAMP
Senokot	Calcium
Bisacodyl	
Oxyphenisatin	
Phenolphthalein	
Anthraquinones	

Adapted from Gorbach SL: Infectious Diarrhea. p. 925. In Sleisenger MH, Fordtran JS (eds): Gastrointestinal Disease. 3rd Ed. WB Saunders, Philadelphia, 1983.

cretion in the colon, and malabsorption of bile acids will result in bile acid diarrhea. Long-chain (dietary) fatty acids also stimulate colonic electrolyte secretion. Thus, any disease causing steatorrhea can result in fatty acid diarrhea. Hydroxy fatty acids are potent secretagogues. The major fatty acid in castor oil is ricinoleic acid, a hydroxy fatty acid. Medium-chain fatty acids do not stimulate intestinal secretion. Dioctyl sodium sulfosuccinate (Colase) increases cAMP content in colonic mucosa, as do bile acids and fatty acids.[91] Senokot (senna) may work by increasing intracellular calcium concentration.[92]

Loss of Absorptive Cells

Loss of intestinal absorptive cells results in diarrhea because of (1) loss of brush border enzymes that hydrolyze carbohydrate and peptides; (2) loss of Na-cotransport carriers that transport glucose, amino acids, HCO_3, and Cl across the brush border membrane; and (3) uncovering of secretory crypt cells. The classic example is celiac sprue, but a much more common cause is viral gastroenteritis. In many forms of viral enteritis, the virus invades the villous cells, resulting in their destruction. This leads to villous atrophy and crypt hypertrophy.[93,94] However, not all viruses produce this spruelike picture, and the mechanism of diarrhea with these agents remains to be clarified.

Inflammation of the Bowel

Inflammatory bowel disease can result from bacterial or parasitic invasion, cytotoxins, radiation, or ischemic damage, or it may be idiopathic. Prostaglandins and other arachidonic acid metabolites are generated as part of the inflammatory response. Inflammation stimulates production of two classes of arachidonic acid metabolites. Arachidonic acid can be metabolized by the enzyme cyclooxygenase to produce the classic prostaglandins and prostacyclin. In this class of compounds, PGE_1 and PGE_2 have been shown to stimulate adenylate cyclase and active anion secretion. Arachidonic acid can also be metabolized by the enzyme lipoxygenase to produce the class of compounds known as the leukotrienes. In this group two substances, HETE and HPETE, have been demonstrated to be intestinal secretagogues.[71] Glucocorticoids block the mobilization of arachidonic acid from phospholipid by inhibiting phospholipase A_2 and will therefore block the synthesis of both classes of arachidonic acid metabolites. Nonsteroidal antiinflammatory agents such as aspirin and indomethacin inhibit cyclooxygenase, thus blocking production of the classic prostaglandins.

In an animal model of *Salmonella* enteritis fluid secretion by the involved ileum has been shown to result from increased prostaglandin E_2 production and increased adenylate cyclase activity. Indomethocin treatment lowers prostaglandin E_2 levels, decreases adenylase cyclase activity, and inhibits fluid secretion by the ileum.[95,96] Pretreatment of the animals with nitrogen mustard to block the inflammatory response also blocks the increase in fluid secretion.[97] In colonic tissue obtained by biopsy of patients with active ulcerative colitis, increased production of the prostaglandin E series has been demonstrated, which can be inhibited by glucocorticoids and by 5-aminosalicylate.[98] Sulfasalazine has been used effectively in the treatment of idiopathic inflammatory bowel disease. This agent is split by colonic bacteria into sulfapyridine and 5-aminosalicylate, the later of which is a potent inhibitor of prostaglandin synthesis.

Ingestion of a Poorly Absorbed Solutes

Ingestion of such compounds as mannitol, sorbitol, lactulose, sulfate, and magnesium, which are poorly absorbed by the gastrointestinal tract, will lead to an osmotic diarrhea.

Table 17–4. Clinical Presentation of Acute Infectious Diarrhea

	Response	
Clinical Feature	Noninflammatory[a]	Inflammatory[b]
Location of infection	Jejunum	Ileum and colon
Clinical syndrome	Vomiting Diarrhea	Fever and diarrhea Fever and dysentery
Location of pain	Mid-abdominal	Lower abdominal
Volume of diarrhea	Large	Large or small
Blood in stools	Rare	Very common
White blood cells in stool	Rare	Very common
Proctoscopy	Normal	Hemorrhagic, friable

Adapted from Gorbach SL: Infectious Diarrhea. p. 925. In Sleisenger MH, and Fordtran JS (eds): Gastrointestinal Disease. 3rd Ed. WB Saunders, Philadelphia, 1983.

[a] *Noninflammatory origin:* virus; toxigenic bacteria, including *Staphylococcus* aureus, *Escherichia coli, Bacillus cereus; Giardia.*

[b] *Inflammatory origin:* invasive bacteria, including *Salmonella* and Campylobacter, as well as the toxin-producing *Shigella* and *Yersinia;* also amebiasis.

Evaluation of Acute Infectious Diarrhea

Acute infectious diarrhea can be divided into two categories: those that produce an inflammatory response and those that do not.[84] The characteristic clinical features of these two categories are listed in Table 17–4. Organisms that produce inflammation frequently require antibiotic treatment, whereas those that do not are usually milder and self-limiting and can frequently be treated symptomatically.

Evaluation of Chronic Diarrhea

Chronic diarrhea can result from a large number of disease processes (Table 17–5), the evaluation of which cannot be delineated by a simple set of procedures. A good history and physical examination should point to the performance of necessary selected diagnostic tests. If the diagnosis is not apparent after a careful history taking, physical examination, and initial screening laboratory procedures, it may be helpful to determine whether the diarrhea is osmotic or secretory. If diarrhea persists with fasting and if the fecal electrolytes (Na + K) × 2 equal the fecal osmolality, then the diarrhea is secretory in nature. Secretory diarrheas that defy the usual workup are usually due to either hormone-producing tumors or surreptitious laxative abuse.[82]

SYSTEMIC EFFECTS OF DIARRHEA

The effect of diarrhea on fluid, electrolyte, and acid–base equilibrium depends on the type, duration, and severity of the diarrhea, as well as the host response. For example, if shock occurs as a result of severe diarrhea, then renal failure and lactic acid production may result in systemic acidosis (see Chapter 7) and hyperkalemia. Contraction of the extracellular volume due to diarrhea may result in contraction alkalosis and hypokalemia (see Chapters 9 and 7). If diarrheal losses are replaced primarily with water, hyponatremia (see Chapter 5) may result from water retention secondary to the secretion of antidiuretic hormone and enhanced proximal tubular salt and water reabsorption, limiting sodium delivery to the more distal diluting sites (thick ascending limb of Henle and early distal tubule).

Osmotic Diarrhea

The most common cause of osmotic diarrhea is carbohydrate malabsorption. The unabsorbed carbohydrate is converted by colonic

Table 17-5. Causes of Chronic Diarrhea

Malabsorption syndromes	
	Lactose intolerance
	Biliary tract obstruction
	Bacterial overgrowth
	Pancreatic insufficiency
	Mucosal disease
	Celiac disease
	Lymphoma
	Lymphangiectasia
Inflammatory bowel disease	
	Ulcerative colitis
	Crohn's disease
	Radiation
	Ischemia
Infection	
	Giardia
	Amebiasis
Postsurgical	
	Gastrectomy–Vagotomy
	Cholecystectomy
	Ileal resection
Hormone-producing tumors	
	Zollinger-Ellison syndrome (gastrin)
	Pancreatic cholera (vasoactive intestinal polypeptide)
	Medullary carcinoma of the thyroid (calcitonin)
	Carcinoid syndrome (serotonin)
Surreptitious laxative or diuretic abuse	
Irritable bowel syndrome	
Miscellaneous	
	Villous adenoma
	Hyperthyroidism
	Addison's disease
	Drug related

bacteria to short-chain fatty acids, such as butyric acid and acetic acid. These organic solutes produce an osmotic gap, that is, stool osmolality is significantly greater than that which can be accounted for by stool electrolytes (Na + K and their anions). This results in hyponatric fluid loss, which may produce severe hypernatremia. It should be emphasized that osmotic diarrhea, like an osmotic diuresis (see Chapter 25), is characterized by two distinct disturbances. The first is water loss in excess of sodium. This causes an increase in the plasma osmolality, and the resultant hypertonicity will produce an osmotic shift of water out of cells, leading to intracellular dehydration. Brain function may become seriously impaired, and confusion, central nervous system depression, seizures, and coma may develop (see Chapter 21). The second problem complicating osmotic diarrhea is sodium loss and the resultant intravascular volume depletion. Resultant organ hypoperfusion may lead to acute tubular necrosis, stroke, myocardial infarction, ischemic bowel, or pancreatitis.

Treatment of the patient with hypertonic dehydration involves first the restoration of the intravascular volume with normal saline (and colloid, if indicated). It should be remembered that normal saline will be hypotonic compared with the patient's plasma tonicity. The isotonic saline should be administered as rapidly as possible to correct orthostatic changes and restore tissue perfusion. Once the sodium deficit has been corrected, free water (usually in the form of 5 percent dextrose in water) can be administered to correct the free water losses. Normally half the water deficit is restored within the first 12 to 16 hours and the remainder in the subsequent 24 to 36 hours (see Chapter 21 for a more detailed discussion of therapy). Care should be taken not to correct the water losses too quickly, since the buildup of idiogenic osmoles within the brain will obligate a significant intracerebral water shift, and cerebral edema may ensue.

Most patients with diarrhea, be it osmotic or secretory, will have lost significant amounts of potassium in the stool; therefore, adequate potassium replacement should be given to prevent hypokalemia. The plasma potassium concentration and urine output should be followed carefully. If acute tubular necrosis develops, potassium replacement may have to be curtailed abruptly. One must also keep in mind that hypokalemia protects against hypocalcemia, which also may be present in such patients. If potassium is administered before the hypocalcemia has been corrected, tetany and seizures may be precipitated.

Acid–base disturbances will be discussed in more detail in the subsequent section on secretory diarrhea. It should be noted that in certain of the osmotic diarrhea states, organic acids produced by bacterial fermentation may result in systemic acidosis by reacting with fecal HCO_3 to produce the sodium salt of the organic acid. Organic anion in stool would then be equivalent to HCO_3, and HCO_3 depletion could occur. The organic acids produced by bacterial fermentation can be absorbed by passive nonionic diffusion and/or organic anion:HCO_3 exchange. Either mechanism results in HCO_3 loss, which may result in systemic acidosis.

Acidic fecal content will also lead to an increase in stool NH_3 excretion. NH_3 is protonated to NH_4^+ in an acidic environment. Since NH_4^+ cannot be absorbed as easily as NH_3, fecal ammonium excretion will increase. This phenomenon is made use of in the treatment of hepatic encephalopathy with the nonabsorbable carbohydrate, lactulose.

Osmotic diarrhea due to carbohydrate malabsorption, resulting in fluid, electrolyte, or acid–base disorders, is primarily a problem seen in infants. Older children and adults rarely develop systemic effects from carbohydrate intolerance.

Secretory Diarrhea

Secretory diarrhea results from inhibition of coupled Na and Cl absorption and active anion (Cl, HCO_3) secretion by the intestine or colon. Fecal osmolality can be accounted for by fecal electrolytes (Na + K and their anions). Thus, no fecal osmotic gap is present. Isotonic contraction of the extracellular volume occurs and serum Na does not change unless water is used to replete losses, in which case hyponatremia may develop. The treatment of isotonic dehydration involves the infusion of normal saline to restore intravascular volume and adequate potassium replacement.

Acid–base disturbances will depend in part on the relative losses of Cl and HCO_3. If the HCO_3:Cl ratio in fecal fluid is greater than that in plasma, a hyperchloremic metabolic acidosis will develop. If the ratio is less than that in plasma, metabolic alkalosis will occur. Fordtran states, "If the sum of sodium plus potassium minus chloride [in fecal fluid] is greater than the plasma concentration of bicarbonate, the patient must be losing bicarbonate or its equivalent and the result is to acidify body fluids. On the other hand, if the sum of sodium plus potassium minus chloride is less than plasma bicarbonate acid in some form is being lost, and this tends to produce alkalosis."[99] Bicarbonate in fecal fluid is usually not measured, because to do so accurately, fecal material would have to be collected under oil to prevent the loss of CO_2. In general, most diarrheal states are associated with the development of a hyperchloremic metabolic acidosis (see Chapter 7).

Whether or not one decides to administer bicarbonate to patients with diarrhea and metabolic acidosis will depend upon the severity of the acidemia. If the plasma HCO_3^- is >10 mEq/liter and the blood pH >7.1, correct the underlying cause of the diarrhea and the acidosis will correct itself spontaneously. It must be remembered, however, that these patients may be profoundly volume contracted and may require large amounts (3 to 5 liters) of normal saline. This may result in a dilution acidosis (see Chapter 7). Therefore, all replacement fluid should contain a bicarbonate concentration that is at least equivalent to the patient's plasma bicarbonate. If the patient presents with severe metabolic acidosis (plasma HCO_3^- <8 to 10 mEq/liter and blood pH <7.15), enough bicarbonate should be given to increase the plasma HCO_3^- concentration to 13 to 15 mEq/liter and the blood pH to >7.20.

In unusual circumstances diarrhea may be associated with the development of metabolic alkalosis. If intestinal transport is particularly rapid, upper gastrointestinal fluid may be lost and a metabolic alkalosis may develop. Occasional patients with laxative abuse (milk of magnesia) also may present with a metabolic alkalosis. In the syndrome of congenital chloridorrhea, metabolic alkalosis also may develop. This is a rare disease in which the Cl:HCO_3 exchange in the ileum and colon is not present.[100] The Na:H exchange is intact; thus Na is absorbed in exchange for H and the net effect is HCl loss in the stool and the development of a metabolic alkalosis.

The potassium concentration in normal stool is high, and may be as much as 120 mEq/liter. The high fecal K concentration presumably results from active K secretion coupled to Na absorption.[55,56,58] With diarrhea, the K concentration falls; when the volume of diarrhea is greater than 2 liters/day, it tends to approach the plasma concentration. Thus, fecal losses of K tend to be considerably less than that of Na in secretory diarrhea. The decrease in fecal K concentration in diarrhea is presumably due to decreased Na absorption by the colon. The latter results from a variety of factors, including intrinsic colonic disease, rapid fluid movement through a normal colon, and dilution of the fecal sodium concentration, leading to a larger concentration gradient against which it must be pumped. Nonetheless, hypokalemia is frequently seen in severe diarrhea, even though the K concentration in fecal fluid is considerably less than that of Na. This hypokalemia is largely due, to volume contraction and resultant hyperaldosteronism, which stimulates renal potassium excretion. In rare instances, hyperkalemia may be seen in severe diarrhea. The explanation of this event is not clear, but one should always exclude metabolic acidemia, renal failure, and intravascular hemolyis that may result from concomitant phosphate depletion.

Magnesium and Calcium

Magnesium and calcium transport are not known to be affected by the intracellular mediators of electrolyte (cyclic nucleotides and calcium) transport. No abnormality in the transport of these ions occurs in uncomplicated cases of secretory diarrhea such as that induced by bacterial enterotoxins and other secretagogues. However, reduced absorption of calcium and magnesium can occur in gastrointestinal diseases in which there is (1) vitamin D deficiency or resistance, (2) mucosal disease such as celiac sprue or Crohn's disease, (3) intestinal resection or bypass, or (4) steatorrhea (fecal calcium and magnesium are lost as fatty acid soaps). Many of the intestinal diseases listed in Table 17–5 can cause one or more of the preceding four abnormalities. In most of the conditions associated with decreased calcium and magnesium absorption, steatorrhea also will be present. Decreased dietary intake may contribute to deficiency of these ions, as in postgastrectomy syndrome and alcoholism. The systemic consequences of hypocalcemia and hyponmagnesemia are discussed in Chapters 10 and 11, respectively.

Nephrolithiasis

An increased incidence of both uric acid and calcium oxalate nephrolithiasis occurs in patients with chronic diarrheal diseases, such as ulcerative colitis and Crohn's disease and in those with jejunoileal bypass for obesity.[101] This phenomenon is particularly apparent in patients who have undergone intestinal resection or bypass.[102]

Uric acid stones are particularly common in patients who have had a colectomy for ulcerative colitis.[103,104] These patients appear to have a chronic metabolic acidosis, secondary to bicarbonate loss in the ileostomy fluid. This results in an acidic urine, favoring uric acid precipitation. Such patients are also mildly volume contracted and will, therefore, excrete a concentrated urine.

Calcium oxalate stones are frequently seen in patients who have undergone intestinal resection or bypass. These patients have been found to have increased absorption of dietary oxalate.[101] This enhanced absorption results from two factors: (1) increased solubility of dietary oxalate, and (2) increased permeability of the colon to oxalate within the intestinal lumen.[101] Increased solubility of oxalate is a result of steatorrhea. Normally, dietary oxalate combines with dietary calcium to form an insoluble precipitate that cannot be absorbed. When steatorrhea is present, fatty acids combine with calcium to form soaps, leaving less calcium to combine with oxalate. Consequently, more oxalate remains in solution and is available for absorption. Increased intestinal permeability to oxalate is a result of the effect of bile acids and fatty acids on the colonic mucosa. When these substances are not absorbed in the small intestine because of disease, resection, or bypass, they spill into the colon and cause a nonspecific increase in the permeability of the colon to small solutes.[105] This increased permeability probably results from the binding to and removing of calcium by the bile acids and fatty acids from the tight junctions between colonocytes, thereby decreasing the integrity of these structures.

Present evidence indicates that the major site of increased oxalate absorption is the colon. This is probably because bile acids and fatty acids do not increase permeability and thus oxalate absorption in the small intestine. Whatever the mechanism, patients with a total colectomy do not have increased absorption of dietary oxalate.[106]

Patients with enteric hyperoxaluria also have other urinary abnormalities that may contribute to stone formation. They have low levels of urinary magnesium and very low levels of urinary citrate.[107] Citrate is a calcium chelator, hence will prevent formation of calcium oxalate crystals. Magnesium increases the solubility of calcium oxalate in urine.

SYSTEMIC EFFECTS OF OTHER GASTROINTESTINAL DISORDERS

Loss of Gastric Juice

Loss of gastric juice can result from any disorder resulting in vomiting, such as gastric outlet obstruction, or from removal of gastric juice with a nasogastric or gastrostomy tube. Since gastric juice contains significant amounts of sodium, potassium, and HCl, its loss may lead to Na and K deficiency and systemic alkalosis.

The generation of the metabolic alkalosis results from a variety of physiologic alterations: (1) direct loss of HCl per se; (2) fluid loss resulting in contraction of the extracellular fluid volume around a fixed amount of bicarbonate; (3) hyperaldosteronism, which augments distal hydrogen ion secretion. and (4) hypokalemia, which causes a shift of potassium out of cells in exchange for hydrogen. Once the metabolic alkalosis has been generated, it will be maintained by volume contraction and hypokalemia, both of which increase the $T_m HCO_3$ in the proximal tubule.

The origin of hypokalemia is multifactorial. Potassium loss in the gastric juice is usually modest. The primary route of the potassium loss is via increased renal excretion. Initially, the plasma HCO_3 concentration will rise faster than the rise in $T_m HCO_3$ in the kidney. During this disequilibrium state, excessive amounts of HCO_3 will be excreted in the urine, obligating the excretion of K and Na in order to maintain electrical neutrality. In addition, volume concentration will cause secondary hyperaldosteronism, which will stimulate distal tubular potassium secretion. Metabolic alkalosis per se also has been shown to augment K secretion directly by the kidney. In addition, metabolic alkalosis will cause a shift of potassium into cells. A more detailed discussion of the pathogenesis of hypokalemia and metabolic alkalosis after vomiting can be found in Chapters 7 and 9.

The treatment of metabolic alkalosis in patients with upper gastrointestinal losses is adequate replacement with isotonic NaCl plus KCl. Volume correction and normalization of the plasma K concentration will decrease the $T_m HCO_3$ and allow the kidney to excrete the retained bicarbonate. In occasional circumstances one may wish to correct the metabolic alkalosis by giving dilute HCl. If the metabolic alkalosis results from nasogastric suction and this can not be discontinued, an H_2 receptor antagonist such as cimetidine can be administered. Cimetidine will block HCl secretion and, to a lesser extent, volume secretion by the stomach. This therapy has proved useful in managing the systemic alkalosis that results from prolonged nasogastric suction.

Loss of Pancreatic Juice

Loss of pancreatic juice can occur when there is a fistula from the pancreas to the abdominal wall. This rare occurrence is usually a complication of surgery on the pancreas or may result from drainage of a pancreatic pseudocyst through the abdominal wall. Since pancreatic juice is rich in bicarbonate, systemic acidosis may occur. Treatment involves adequate replacement with sodium bicarbonate.

REFERENCES

1. Humphreys MH, Earley LE: The mechanism of decreased intestinal sodium and water absorption after acute volume expansion in the rat. J Clin Invest 50:2355, 1971
2 Yablonski ME, Lifson N: Mechanism of production of intestinal secretion by elevated venous pressure. J Clin Invest 57:904, 1976
3. Schultz SG, Frizzel RA, Nellans HN: Ion transport by mammalian small intestine. Annu Rev Physiol 36:51, 1974
4. Stirling CE: Radioautographic localization of sodium pump sites in rabbit intestine. J Cell Biol 53:704, 1972
5. Fujita M, Ohta H, Kawai K, et al: Differential isolation of microvillous and basolateral plasma membranes from intestinal mucosa: Mutually exclusive distribution of digestive enzymes and ouabain-sensitive ATPase. Biochim Biophys Acta 274:336, 1972
6. Kirk KL, Halm DR, Dawson DC: Active sodium transport by turtle colon via an electrogenic Na–K exchange pump. Nature 287:237, 1980
7. Frizzell, RA, Schultz SG: Ionic conductances of extracellular shunt pathway in rabbit ileum. Influence of shunt on transmural Na transport and electrical potential differences. J Gen Physiol 59:318, 1972
8. Rose RC, Schultz SG: Studies on the electrical potential profile cross rabbit ileum. Effects of sugars and amino acids on transmural and transmucosal electrical potential differences. J Gen Physiol 57:639, 1971
9. Frizzell, RA, Field, M, Schultz SG: Sodium-coupled chloride transport by epithelial tissues. Am J Physiol 236:F1, 1979
10. Nellans HN, Popovitch JE: Calmodulin-regulated, ATP-driven calcium transport by basolateral membranes of rat small intestine. J Biol Chem 256:9932, 1982
11. Hildman B, Schmidt A, Murer H: Ca^{++}-transport across baso-lateral plasma membranes from rat small intestinal cells. J Membr Biol 65:55, 1979
12. Forte JG, Machen TE, Obrink KJ: Mechanisms of gastric H^+ and Cl^- transport. Annu Rev Physiol 42:111, 1980
13. Wills NK, Biagi B: Active potassium transport by descending colon epithelium. J Membr Biol 64:195, 1982
14. Gustin MC, Goodman DBP: Characterization of the phosphorylated intermediate of the K^+-ouabain-insensitive ATPase of the rabbit colon brush-border membrane. J Biol Chem 257:9629, 1982
15. Fordtran JS, Rector FC, Ewton MF, et al: Permeability characteristics of the human small intestine. J Clin Invest 44:1935, 1965
16. Fordtran JS, Rector FC, Locklear TW, et al: Water and solute movement in the small intestine of patients with sprue. J Clin Invest 46:287, 1967
17. Billich CO, Levitan R: Effects of sodium concentration and osmolality on water and electrolyte absorption from the intact human colon. J Clin Invest 48:1336, 1969
18. Liedtke CM, Hopfer V: Mechanism of Cl^- translocation across small intestinal brush-border membrane. II. Demonstration of Cl^-–OH^- exchange and Cl^- conductance. Am. J Physiol, 242:G272, 1982
19. Kirk KL, Halm DR, Dawson DC: Active sodium transport by turtle colon via an electrogenic Na–K exchange pump. Nature 287:237, 1980
20. Will PC, Lebowitz JL, Hopfer U: Induction of amiloride-sensitive sodium transport in the rat colon by mineralocorticoids. Am J Physiol 238:F261, 1980
21. Hunt JN, Wan B: Electrolytes of mammalian gastric juice. p. 781. In Code CF (ed). Handbook of Physiology. Vol. II, Sect. 6. Washington, DC, American Physiological Society, 1967
22. Soll AH: Physiology of isolated canine parietal cells: Receptors and effectors regulating function. p. 673. In Johnson LR (ed): Physi-

ology of the Gastrointestinal Tract. Raven Press, New York, 1981

23. Swanson CH, Solomon AK: Micropuncture analysis of the cellular mechanisms of electrolyte secretion by the in vitro rabbit pancreas. J Gen Physiol 65:22, 1975
24. Bro-Rasmussen F, Killmann SA, Thaysen JH: The composition of pancreatic juice as compared to sweat, parotids, saliva and tears. Acta Physiol Scand 37:97, 1956
25. Meyer, JH: Pancreatic physiology. p. 1398. In Fortran JS, Sleisenger MH (eds): Gastrointestinal Disease. 2nd ed. WB Saunders, Philadelphia, 1978
26. Lightwood R, Reber HA: Micropuncture study of pancreatic secretion in the cat. Gastroenterology 76:61, 1977
27. Blitzer BL, Boyer JL: Cellular mechanisms of bile formation. Gastroenterology 82:346, 1982
28. Erlinger S: Secretion of bile. p. 93. In Schiff, L, Schiff ER (eds): Diseases of the Liver. 5th ed. JB Lippincott, Philadelphia, 1982
29. Schultz SG: Ion-coupled transport across biological membranes. p. 273. In Andreoli TE, Hoffman JF, Fanestil DD (eds): Membrane Physiology. Plenum Press, New York, 1980
30. Hopfer V, Sigrist-Nelson K, Ammann E, et al: Differences in neutral amino acid and glucose transport between brush border and basolateral plasma membrane of intestinal epithelial cells. J Cell Physiol 89:805, 1976
31. Murer H, Kinne R: The use of isolated membrane vesicles to study epithelial transport processes. J Membr Biol 55:81, 1980
32. Turnberg LA, Fordtran JS, Carter NW, et al: Mechanism of bicarbonate absorption and its relationship to sodium transport in the human jejunum. J Clin Invest 49:548, 1970
33. White JF, Imon MA: A role for basolateral anion exchange in active jejunal absorption of HCO_3. Am J Physiol 244:G397, 1983
34. Gunter RD, Wright EM: Na^+, Li^+, and Cl^- transport by brush border membranes from rabbit jejunum. J Membr Biol 74:85, 1983
35. Davis GR, Santa Ana CA, Morawski S, et al: Active chloride secretion in the normal human jejunum. J Clin Invest 66:1326, 1980
36. White JF, Imon MA: Intestinal HCO_3 secretion in amphiuma: Stimulation by mucosal Cl and serosal Na. J. Membr Biol 68:207, 1982
37. Knickelbein R, Aronson PS, Atherton W, et al: Na and Cl transport across rabbit ileal brush border. I. Evidence for Na:H exchange. Am J Physiol 245:G504, 1983
38. Knickelbein RG, Aronson PS, Dobbins JW: Na-H and Cl-HCO_3 exchange in rabbit ileal brush border membrane vesicles. Fed Proc 41:1494, 1982
39. Nellans HN, Frizzell RA, Schultz SG: Coupled sodium-chloride influx across the brush border of rabbit ileum. Am J Physiol 226:467, 1973
40. Fan C-C, Faust RG Powell DW: Coupled sodium-chloride transport by rabbit ileal brush-border membrane vesicles. Am J Physiol 244:G375, 1983
41. Liedtke CM, Hopfer V: Mechanism of Cl^- translocation across small intestinal brush-border membrane. I. Absence of Na^+-Cl^- cotransport. Am J Physiol 242:G263, 1972
42. Turnberg LA, Bieberdorf FA, Morawski SG, et al: Interrelationships of chloride, bicarbonate, sodium and hydrogen transport in the human ileum. J Clin Invest 49:557, 1970
43. Simson JNL, Merhair A, Silen W: Alkaline secretion by amphibian duodenum. III. Effects of DBcAMP, theophylline and prostaglandins. Am J Physiol 241:G528, 1981
44. Frizzell RA, Welsh MJ, Smith PL: Hormonal control of chloride secretion by canine tracheal epithelium: An electrophysiologic analysis. Ann NY Acad Sci 372:558, 1981
45. Welsh MJ: Intracellular chloride activities in canine tracheal epithelium. Direct evidence for sodium-coupled intracellular chloride accumulation in a chloride-secretion epithelium. J Clin Invest 71:1392, 1983
46. Field M: Secretion of electrolytes and water by mammalian small intestine. p. 963. In Johnson LR (ed): Physiology of the Gastrointestinal Tract. Raven Press, New York, 1981
47. Donowitz M, Madara JL: Effect of extracellular calcium depletion on epithelial structure and function in rabbit ileum: A model for selective crypt or villus epithelial cell damage and suggestion of secretion by villus epithelial cells. Gastroenterology 83:1231, 1982
48. Holman GD, Naftalin RJ, Simmons NL, et al: Electrophysiological and electron-microscopical correlations with fluid and electro-

lyte secretion in rabbit ileum. J Physiol (Lond) 290:367, 1979
49. Rask-Madsen J: Simultaneous measurement of electrical polarization and electrolyte transport by the entire normal and inflamed human colon during in vivo perfusion. Scand. J. Gastroenterol 8:327, 1973
50. Ruppin H, Bar-Meir S, Soergel KH, et al: Absorption of short-chain fatty acids by the colon. Gastroenterology 78:1500, 1980
51. Vmesak Y, Yajima T, Yokokura T, et al: Effect of organic acid absorption on bicarbonate transport in rat colon. Pfluegers Arch 379:43, 1979
52. Binder HJ, Rawlins CL: Electrolyte transport across isolated large intestinal mucosa. Am J Physiol 225:1223, 1973
53. Frizzell RA, Koch MJ, Schultz SG: Ion transport by rabbit colon. I. Active and passive components. J Membr Biol 27:297, 1976
54. Heintze K, Stewart CP, Frizzell RA: Sodium-dependent chloride secretion across rabbit descending colon. Am J Physiol 244:G357, 1983
55. Foster ES, Sandle GI, Hayslett JP, et al: Cyclic adenosine monophosphate stimulates active potassium secretion in rat colon. Gastroenterology 84:324, 1983
56. Foster ES, Zimmerman TW, Hayslett JP, et al: Corticosteroid alteration of active electrolyte transport in rat distal colon. Am J Physiol 245:G668, 1983
57. Sellin J, DeSoignie R: Rabbit proximal colon: A distinct transport epithelium. Gastroenterology 84:1304, 1983
58. Kliger AS, Binder HJ, Bastl C, et al: Demonstration of active potassium transport in the mammalian colon. J Clin Invest 67:1189, 1981
59. Field M, Graf LH, Laird WJ, et al: Heat stable enterotoxin of Escherichia coli: In vitro effects of guanylate cyclase activity, cyclic GMP concentration, and ion transport in small intestine. Proc Natl Acad Sci (USA) 75:2800, 1978
60. Marnane WG, Tai Y-H, Decker RA, et al: Methyl-prednisolone stimulation of guanylate cyclase activity in rat small intestinal mucosa: Possible role in electrolyte transport. Gastroenterology 81:90, 1981
61. Brasitas TA, Field M, Kimberg DV: Intestinal mucosal cyclic GMP; regulation and relation to ion transport. Am J Physiol 231:275, 1976
62. Frizzell RA: Active chloride secretion by rabbit colon: Calcium-dependent stimulation by ionophore A23187. J Membr Biol 35:175, 1977
63. Ilundain A, Naftalin RJ: Role of Ca^{2+}-dependent regulator protein in intestinal secretion. Nature 279:446, 1979
64. Donowitz M, Asarkof N, Pike G: Calcium dependence of serotonin induced changes in rabbit ileal electrolyte transport. J Clin Invest 6:341, 1980
65. Zimmerman TW, Dobbins JW, Binder HJ: Role of calcium in the regulation of colonic secretion in the rat. Am J Physiol 244:G552, 1983
66. Donowitz M, Asarkof N: Calcium dependence on basal electrolyte transport in rabbit ileum. Am J Physiol 243:G28, 1982
67. Donowitz M, Cusolito S, Battisti L, et al: Dopamine stimulation of active Na and Cl absorption in rabbit ileum. Interaction with α_2-adrenergic receptors and specific dopamine receptors. J Clin Invest 69:1008, 1982
68. Smith PL, Blumberg JB, Stoff JS, et al: Antisecretory effects of indomethacin on rabbit ileal mucosa in vitro. Gastroenterology 80:356, 1981
69. Tapper EJ: Local modulation of intestinal ion transport by enteric neurons. Am J Physiol 244:G457, 1983
70. Kimberg DV, Field M, Johnson J, et al: Stimulation of intestinal mucosal adenyl cyclase by cholera enterotoxin and prostaglandins. J Clin Invest 50:1218, 1971
71. Musch MW, Miller RJ, Field M, et al: Stimulation of colonic secretion by lipoxygenase metabolites of arachidonic acid. Science 217:1255, 1982
72. Musch MW, Kachur JF, Miller RJ, et al: Bradykinin-stimulated electrolyte secretion in rabbit and guinea pig intestine. J Clin Invest 71:1073, 1983
73. Schwartz CJ, Kimberg DV, Sheerin HE, et al: Vasoactive intestinal peptide stimulation of adenylate cyclase and active electrolyte secretion in intestinal mucosa. J Clin Invest 54:536, 1974
74. Binder HJ, Lemp GF, Gardner JD: Receptors for vasoactive intestinal peptide and se-

cretion on small intestinal epithelial cells. Am J Physiol 238:G190, 1980
75. Korman LY, Lemp GF, Jackson MJ, et al: Mechanism of action of ATP on intestinal epithelial cells. Cyclic AMP-mediated stimulation of active ion transport. Biochim Biophys Acta 721:47, 1982
76. Dobbins JW, Laurenson JP, Forrest JN: Effect of adenosine and adenosine analogs on ion transport in rabbit ileum. Gastroenterology 84:1138A, 1983
77. Dobbins JW, Dharmsathaphorn K, Racusen L, et al: The effect of somatosatin and enkephalin on ion transport in the intestine. Ann NY Acad Sci 372:594, 1981
78. Charney AN, Donowitz M: Prevention and reversal of cholera enterotoxin-induced intestinal secretion by methylprednisolone induction of Na^+–K^+-ATPase. J Clin Invest 57:1590, 1976
79. Freiberg MJ, Kinsella J, Sacktor B: Glucocorticoids increase the Na^+–H^+ exchange and decrease the Na^+ gradient-dependent phosphate-uptake systems in renal brush border membrane vesicles. Proc Natl Acad Sci (USA), 79:4932, 1982
80. Hong SL, Levine L: Inhibition of arachidonic acid release from cells as the biochemical action of anti-inflammatory corticosteroids. Proc Natl Acad Sci (USA) 73:1730, 1976
81. Robert A, Hanchar AJ, Lancaster C, et al: Prostacyclin inhibits enteropooling and diarrhea. p. 147. In Vane JR, Bergstrom S (eds): Prostacyclin. Raven Press, New York, 1979
82. Read NW, Kregs GJ, Read MG, et al: Chronic diarrhea of unknown origin. Gastroenterology 78:264, 1980
83. Rao MC, Guandalini S, Laird WJ, et al: Effects of heat-stable enterotoxin of yersinia enterocolitic on ion transport and cyclic guanosine 3′, 5′-monophosphate metabolism in rabbit ileum. Infect Immun 26:875, 1979
84. Gorbach SL: Infectious Diarrhea. p. 925. In Sleisenger MH, Fordtran JS (eds): Gastrointestinal Disease. 3rd Ed. WB Saunders, Philadelphia, 1983
85. Pai CH, Mors V: Production of enterotoxin by yersinia enterocolitica. Infect Immun 19:908, 1978
86. Plotkin GR, Kluge RM, Waldman RH: Gastroenteritis: Etiology, pathophysiology and clinical manifestations. Medicine (Baltimore) 58:95 1979
87. Binder HJ: Absorption and secretion of water and electrolytes by small and large intestine. p. 811. In Sleisenger MH, Fordtran JS (eds): Gastrointestinal Disease. 3rd Ed. WB Saunders, Philadelphia, 1983
88. Lyerly DM, Lockwood DE, Richardson SH, et al: Biological Activities of toxin A and B of Clostridium difficile. Infect Immun 35:1147, 1982
89. Hughes S, Warhurst G, Turnberg LA, et al: Clostridium difficile toxin-induced intestinal secretion in rabbit ileum in vitro. Gut 24:94, 1983
90. Chang EB, Bergenstal RM, Field M: Diabetic diarrhea. Loss of adrenergic regulation of intestinal fluid and electrolyte transport. Gastroenterology 84:1121A, 1983
91. Donowitz M: Current concepts of laxative action: Mechanisms by which laxatives increase stool water. J Clin Gastroenterol 1:77, 1979
92. Donowitz M, Wirks J, Battisti L: Senokot inhibits active Na and Cl transport in rat descending colon by a Ca^{++} dependent mechanism: A new mechanism of laxative action. Gastroenterology 84:1139A, 1983
93. Shepherd, RW, Gall DG, Butler DG, et al: Determinants of diarrhea in viral enteritis. Gastroenterology 76:21, 1979
94. Shepherd RW, Butler DG, Cutz E, et al: The mucosal lesion in viral enteritis. Gastroenterology 76:770, 1979
95. Giannella RA, Formal SB, Dammin GJ, et al: Pathogenesis of salmonella-mediated intestinal fluid secretion. Gastroenterology 69:1238, 1975
96. Giannella RA, Drake KW, Luttrell M: Possible role of prostaglandins in salmonella-mediated intestinal secretion. Gastroenterology 80:1155A, 1981
97. Giannella RA: Importance of the inflammatory reaction in salmonella-mediated intestinal secretion. Infect Immun 23:140, 1979
98. Rachmilewitz D: Prostaglandins and diarrhea. Dig Dis Sci 25:897, 1980
99. Krejs GJ, Fordtran JJ: Physiology and pathophysiology of ion and water movement in the human intestine. p. 297. In Sleisenger MH, Fordtran JJ (eds): Gastrointestinal Dis-

ease. 2nd Ed. WB Saunders, Philadelphia, 1978

100. Holmberg C, Perheentupa J, and Launiala K: Colonic electrolyte transport in health and in congenital chloride diarrhea. J Clin Invest 56:302, 1978
101. Dobbins JW: Oxalate and intestinal disease. J Clin Gastroenterol 1:165, 1979
102. Dobbins JW, Binder HJ: Derangements of oxalate metabolism in gastrointestinal disease and their mechanisms. p. 505. In Glass GBJ (ed): Progress in Gastroenterology. Vol. 3. Grune & Stratton, New York, 1977
103. Deren JJ, Porush JG, Levit MF, et al: Nephrolithiasis as a complication of ulcerative colitis and regional enteritis. Ann Intern Med 56:843, 1962
104. Badenoch AW: Uric acid stone formation. Br J Urol 32:374, 1960
105. Dobbins JW, Binder HJ: Effect of bile salts and fatty acids on the colonic absorption of oxalate. Gastroenterology 70:1069, 1976
106. Dobbins JW, Binder HJ: The importance of the colon in enteric hyperoxaluria. N Engl J Med 296:298, 1977
107. Rudman D, Dedonis JL, Fountain MT, et al: Hypocitraturia in patients with gastrointestinal malabsorption. N Engl J Med 303:657, 1980

18

Acid–Base and Electrolyte Disorders Associated with Endocrine Disease: Pituitary and Thyroid

Arnold M. Moses
Stanley A. Blumenthal
David H. P. Streeten

CENTRAL DIABETES INSIPIDUS AND PRIMARY POLYDIPSIA

Clinical Features and Pathophysiology

Central or neurogenic diabetes insipidus is due to impaired renal conservation of water that results from deficient vasopressin release and low levels of circulating arginine vasopressin in response to normal physiologic stimuli. Polyuria, excessive thirst, and polydipsia are the major clinical features. Eneuresis may be an important feature in children. These symptoms are usually sudden in onset both when the disorder first appears and whenever the effects of administered vasopressin disappear during therapy of patients with the disorder. In severe cases, the urine is pale in color and its volume may be immense ($\leq$ 16 to 20 liters/day), requiring the patient to void at intervals of 30 to 60 minutes throughout the day and night. More frequently, however, the urine volume is only mildly to moderately excessive (2.5 to 6 liters/day), and occasionally the polyuria may be so minor as to cause no complaints. Urinary concentration is well below that of serum in severe cases, but may be higher (290 to 600 mOsm/kg) in patients with mild diabetes insipidus. Patients who fail to empty their bladders adequately because of urethral obstruction or other reasons may develop enlarged atonic bladders, hydroureter, hydronephrosis, and renal failure. These features are more common in patients with nephrogenic diabetes insipidus.

Prevention of dehydration, particularly in patients with severe polyuria, is dependent on an intact thirst mechanism. The usual stimulus for thirst is an elevated plasma osmolality, but the level of plasma osmolality necessary for thirst to occur is appreciably higher than that which is necessary for stimulation of vasopressin release.[1] As a consequence, patients with uncontrolled diabetes insipidus imbibe large quantities of fluids, preferably cold, and often go to great trouble to secure refrigerated fluids. Normal function of the thirst center ensures that polydipsia closely matches polyuria, so that dehydration is seldom detectable except by a slight elevation of serum sodium concentration. However, when adequate replenishment of water loss is interfered with, dehydration may become severe, causing weakness, fever, psychic disturbances, prostration, and even death. These features are associated with an elevated serum osmolality and sodium concentration, the latter sometimes exceeding 180 mEq/liter. Adipsia or hypodipsia may result from impaired function of the hypothalamic thirst center because of extension of the same abnormality that caused the diabetes insipidus, or dehydration may occur during periods of unconsciousness.

Pregnancy may decrease the sensitivity to small circulating amounts of arginine vasopressin and aggravate the syndrome of central diabetes insipidus.[2] In contrast, the need for therapy may decrease markedly during lactation.[2] Since oxytocin is produced by hypothalamic neurons, there has been some concern about its adequacy in pregnant patients with diabetes insipidus. However, it is very unusual for them to have either impaired uterine contractions during labor or impaired milk ejection.

For conceptual purposes four types of diabetes insipidus can be defined (Fig. 18–1). Patients of the first type show very little rise in urine osmolality with increasing plasma osmolality during water deprivation and no evidence of arginine vasopressin release during hypertonic saline infusion. They are essentially devoid of releasable arginine vasopressin. The second type of patient has an abrupt increase in urine osmolality during dehydration, but there is no evidence of an osmotic threshold during saline infusion. These patients have a defective osmoreceptor mechanism, but are capable of releasing arginine va-

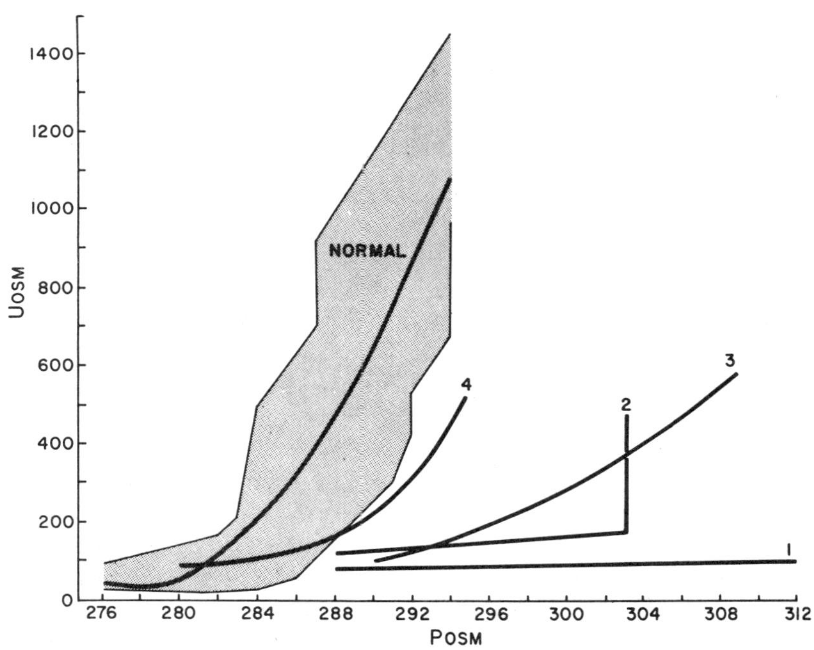

Fig. 18–1. Relationship between plasma and urine osmolality in normal adult subjects (shaded area) and four hypothetical types of patients with central diabetes insipidus. (From Streeten DHP, Moses AM, Miller M: Disorders of the neurohypophysis. p. 604. In Petersdorf RG, Adams RD, Braunwald E, et al (eds): Harrison's Principles of Internal Medicine. 10th Ed. McGraw-Hill, New York, 1983. © 1983, McGraw-Hill. Used with the permission of the McGraw-Hill Book Company.)

sopressin in response to the hypovolemic stimulus resulting from severe dehydration. Selective osmoreceptor failure has been recognized for years based on the observation that some patients with diabetes insipidus have an antidiuretic response to nicotine, but not to hypertonic saline.[3,4] The third type of patient has some rise in urine osmolality with increasing plasma osmolality and has an elevated osmotic threshold for arginine vasopressin release. These patients have a sluggish arginine vasopressin release mechanism and may be said to have a high set osmoreceptor. The fourth type of patient has urine and plasma osmolality coordinates just to the right of normal and a normal osmotic threshold. Arginine vasopressin release in these patients is initiated at a normal plasma osmolality but is subnormal in amount. Therefore, an increased osmotic stimulus is required to release sufficient arginine vasopressin for maximal antidiuresis. The second to fourth type of patients may develop a good antidiuresis in response to nausea, nicotine, chlorpropamide, or clofibrate, indicating that there is sufficient synthesis and storage of arginine vasopressin to allow for adequate urinary concentrating ability in the presence of an appropriate stimulus to arginine vasopressin release. In rare instances patients of the second to fourth types may have largely asymptomatic hypernatremia with little or no evidence of diabetes insipidus. For this to occur, the thirst mechanism has to be impaired. Otherwise, the patients will drink before an effective stimulus for vasopressin release is attained and polyuria results.

During the past 11 years, using modern techniques, we have investigated more than 100 patients with long-standing central diabetes insipidus, defined as being present for more than 6 months or until the patient died (Table 18–1). The median age of onset was 22.5 years, and 60 percent of the patients were male. The largest group was idiopathic (27 percent), followed closely by patients who developed diabetes insipidus before or after surgery for

Table 18–1. Long-Standing Central Diabetes Insipidus[a,b]

Cause	No. of Cases	Males	Females	Age of Onset (Years)	
				Median	Range
Histiocytosis	4	2	2	2	1–20
Primary brain tumor[c]					
Postop DI[d]	13	6	7	12	2–25
Preop DI[d]	14	12	2	17	3–58
Idiopathic	28	19	9	17	Infancy to 66
Head trauma	18	12	6	22	5–48
Anoxemic encephalopathy	5	2	3	37	15–73
Nonfunctioning pituitary tumor (pre- or postop)	5	4	1	38	15–41
Ruptured cerebral aneurysm	1	1	0	39	—
Sarcoidosis	1	0	1	42	—
Posthypophysectomy for treatment of Cushing's disease, acromegaly, diabetic retinopathy, cancer	7	1	6	46	24–68
Metastatic malignancy	8	5	3	57	32–71
Total:	104	64	40		

[a] Diagnosed during the period 1972–1983 at SUNY, Upstate Medical Center.
[b] Categories arranged in order of increasing median age of onset.
[c] Group consisted of 16 patients with craniopharyngeomas, six with pinealomas, and five with gliomas.
[d] DI, diabetes insipidus.

primary brain (extrapituitary) tumors (26 percent). Patients who developed diabetes insipidus after head trauma constituted the third largest group (18 percent). Eight percent of the patients had metastatic tumors to the hypothalamus, and 7 percent developed diabetes insipidus after hypophysectomy for treatment of pituitary hypersecretion, diabetic retinopathy or cancer. Five percent developed diabetes insipidus before or after surgery for nonfunctioning pituitary tumors, and the same number developed the disease from cerebral hypoperfusion. Four percent had histocytosis, and the remaining cases were due to sarcoidosis or to a ruptured cerebral aneurysm. Rare causes that have been reported but that we have not observed include thrombotic thrombocytopenic purpura,[5] pituitary apoplexy,[6] postpartum pituitary necrosis,[7,8] Wegener's granulomatosis,[9] and systemic blastomycosis.[10]

Our youngest group of patients developed diabetes insipidus from histiocytosis X. The patterns of abnormal water metabolism in these patients have been well described.[11] The next youngest group of our patients developed diabetes insipidus as a result of primary brain tumors. Of the patients in this group who developed diabetes insipidus before surgery, one-half also had evidence of anterior pituitary deficiency. Of those in whom permanent diabetes insipidus developed after surgery, 87 percent also developed evidence of anterior pituitary deficiency. In a study of 135 consecutive patients who underwent craniotomy, Balestrieri et al.[12] found that diabetes insipidus occurs almost exclusively in patients operated on for pituitary and/or hypothalamic disease. Removal or destruction of the posterior pituitary from surgical or other causes causes permanent diabetes insipidus only if there is degeneration of the neurons of the supraoptic and/or paraventricular nuclei. An intact stalk is able to release vasopressin adequately in response to physiologic stimuli.[13]

One-third of the patients classified in Table 18–1 as having idiopathic diabetes insipidus had one or more additional abnormalities (Table 18–2). The other endocrine abnormalities probably reflect hypothalamic disease beyond the supraoptic and/or paraventricular nuclei. A thickened infundibular stalk on computed tomography (CT) scan of the brain has previously been reported in patients with diabetes insipidus,[14] but there is no information available relating the relationship of this finding to the cause of the diabetes insipidus. It is our belief that in the future patients with diabetes insipidus with any of the findings listed in Table 18–2 should be classified as having diabetes insipidus, cause to be determined. These patients should be examined more frequently and carefully than patients who have no abnormalities other than diabetes insipidus.

Table 18–2. Additional Endocrinologic, Neurologic, or Radiologic Findings in Patients Classified as Having Idiopathic Diabetes Insipidus

N	Disorder
4	Thyroid-stimulating hormone deficiency
3	Galactorrhea or increased prolactin levels
2	Growth hormone deficiency
2	Adrenocorticotropin deficiency
2	Gonadotropin deficiency
2	Thickened infundibular stalk on computed tomography scan
1	Questionably enlarged sella turcica
1	Abnormal cerebrospinal fluid
1	Narcolepsy
1	Cerebral palsy

Idiopathic diabetes insipidus usually occurs sporadically but may be inherited either as an autosomal dominant or as an X-linked recessive disorder.[15,16] Pathologic studies in several patients with idiopathic diabetes insipidus including the inherited type have disclosed a striking depletion of the Nissl granules and in the number of neurons in the supraoptic and paraventricular nuclei.[16] Some patients with idiopathic diabetes insipidus have circulating antibodies to vasopressin producing cells of the hypothalamus,[17] thus suggesting an immunologic origin for the disease. In five members of a single family with hereditary diabetes insipidus, arginine vasopressin and its specific neurophysin have been shown to be absent from the urine and serum respectively, while oxytocin and its neurophysin were sometimes present.[18] Familial or genetically transmitted diabetes insipidus may coexist with diabetes mellitus.[19,20] Idiopathic diabetes insipidus is almost always permanent. However, we observed one patient with idiopathic diabetes insipidus who spontaneously reverted to normal after approximately 10 months of the disease.

Diabetes insipidus is a well-recognized complication of blunt head trauma. The clinical data on 18 of our patients who had this problem for more than 6 months or until they died are listed on Table 18–3. This type of diabetes insipidus is occurring with increasing frequency, probably due to improved medical care for head trauma victims which has resulted in survival of patients who previously would have died from severe neurologic damage. The problem is usually recognized as early as 12 or 24 hours after the accident.[21] Delays in diagnosis occur when head trauma does not appear to be severe, when the patient is admitted to a surgical service other than neurosurgery, or when the patient has unrecognized adrenal insufficiency. Since glucocorticoids are essential for the development of marked hypotonic polyuria,[22–26] the diabetes insipidus in these patients becomes evident only after the initiation of steroid therapy. A question may arise about trauma as a possible cause of diabetes insipidus when multiple head injuries occur in someone like a professional prizefighter, especially if symptoms are first noted weeks or months after the last episode of trauma. The diabetes insipidus caused by trauma may persist for anywhere from several hours to the duration of the patient's life. Traumatic diabetes insipidus is usually permanent if the patient does not recover by 4 to 6 months. However, we have had patients who improved to the point of not requiring therapy after intervals of 2, 3, and 10 years. The data on one of our cases who continued to improve for at least 2½ years are depicted in Figure 18–2. During that period, his urine concentrating ability improved in relationship to his plasma osmolality, his urine volume decreased from 11.1 to 1.76 liters/day, while his saline-induced osmotic threshold decreased from 314.8 to 291.3 mOsm/kg. Therapy was discontinued between the second and third dehydration tests. The patient's serum sodium concentration remained slightly elevated. When patients like this have partial antidiuretic hormone deficiency, as he did between the second and third dehydration tests, the sensitivity of the thirst mechanism determines the degree of polydipsia and polyuria. Since such patients can concentrate urine with a supranormal osmotic stimulus, they may have severe polydipsia and polyuria if the thirst mechanism is sensitive or a high-set osmoreceptor or essential hypernatremia if the thirst sensation is blunted.

Most of our patients who developed long-standing traumatic diabetes insipidus had substantial neurologic damage (Table 18–3). There was a high incidence of damage to the first and second cranial nerves. Three patients had loss of smell, while six had damage to

Table 18–3. Clinical Data on 18 Patients with Long-Standing Traumatic Diabetes Insipidus[a]

Age of onset (median 22 years, range 5–48 years)
Sex (12 M, 6 F)
Cause
Automobile accident (13)
Fall from bicycle, motorcycle accident, industrial explosion, falling house, falling tree (1 each)
Skull fracture (13)
Permanent[b] endocrine abnormality, other than diabetes insipidus (8)
Deficient thyroid-stimulating hormone (5), (gonadotropins (5); adrenocorticotropic hormone, (3); human growth hormone, (3)
Increased prolactin (4)
Permanent[b] neurologic damage (9)
Cranial nerves (8)
First cranial nerve (3)
Second cranial nerve or optic chiasm (6)
Other cranial nerves (3)
Hemiparesis (2)
Massive diffuse brain damage, carotid-cavernous fistula, adipsia, ataxia (1 each)
Loss of consciousness (None in 1 patient, minutes to months in remainder)

[a] Numbers in parentheses represent number of patients affected.

[b] Permanent is considered 6 months or longer.

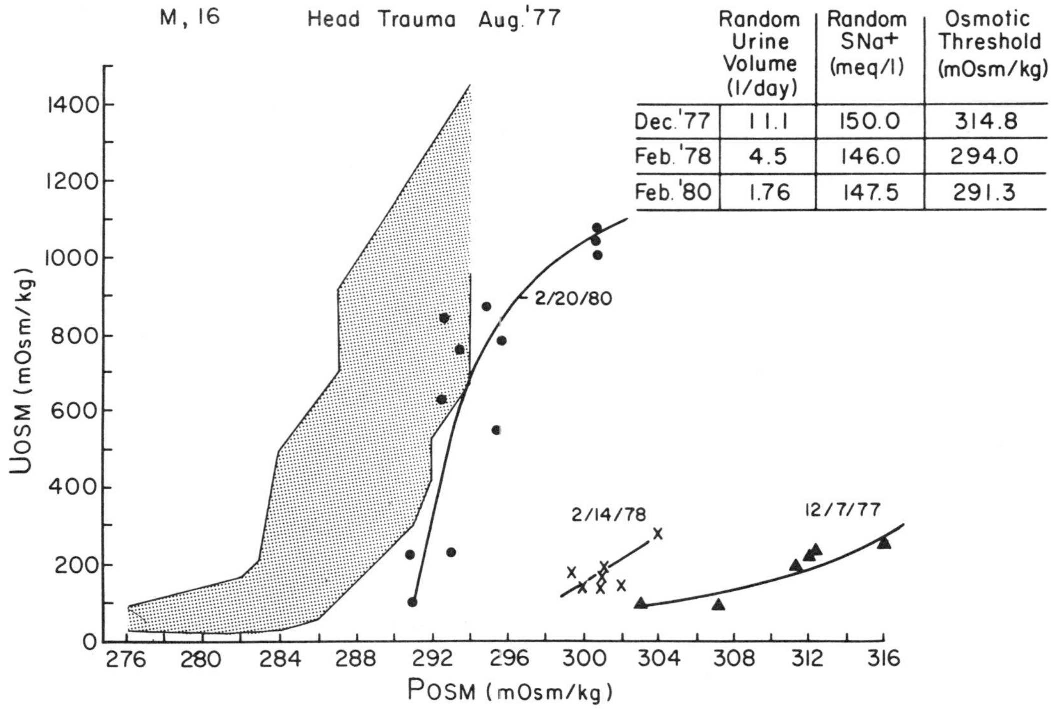

	Random Urine Volume (l/day)	Random SNa+ (meq/l)	Osmotic Threshold (mOsm/kg)
Dec.'77	11.1	150.0	314.8
Feb.'78	4.5	146.0	294.0
Feb.'80	1.76	147.5	291.3

Fig. 18–2. Plasma and urine osmolality relationships over a 26-month period in a patient with traumatic diabetes insipidus. Urine volumes and osmotic threshold values improved progressively during this period, while plasma sodium improved slightly but remained elevated. (Slightly modified and reproduced with permission from Moses AM, Norman DD: Diabetes Insipidus and Syndrome of Inappropriate Antidiuretic Hormone Secretion (SIADH), in Stollerman GH, et al (eds): Advances in Internal Medicine, Volume 27. Copyright © 1982 by Year Book Medical Publishers, Inc., Chicago.)

the optic nerves or chiasm. Savino et al.[27] reported that one-half their patients who were evaluated for traumatic chiasmal syndromes developed diabetes insipidus at least transiently. A total of nine of our patients had permanent neurologic damage, while 13 had one or more skull fractures. There are cases, however, in whom the diabetes insipidus developed shortly after very minimal trauma. The degree of trauma to our patients has ranged from a minor fall causing only transitory unconsciousness and no skull fracture to unconsciousness for longer than 5 months associated with low electroencephalogram (EEG) activity. Thus, although substantial head trauma may alert the physician to anticipate diabetes insipidus as a complication, it may occur with any head injury.

Detailed assessment of anterior pituitary function in patients with traumatic diabetes insipidus usually requires a delay until the patient is medically stable. Almost all these patients initially receive adrenal steroid therapy to prevent or treat cerebral edema, and the detailed evaluation of thyroid, gonadal, and growth hormone function is often impractical or difficult during the initial hospitalization period. The endocrinologic data that could be obtained in our patients with long-standing traumatic diabetes insipidus are listed in Table 18–3. We should remember that adrenal insufficiency masks the manifestations of antidiuretic hormone deficiency and the three patients with adrenocorticotropic hormone (ACTH) deficiency would not have expressed the hypotonic polyuria of antidiuretic hormone deficiency until they were treated with glucocorticoids. Barreca et al.[28] recently reviewed their experience with anterior pituitary abnormalities in 10 patients with traumatic diabetes insipidus and found that eight patients were deficient in one or more of the anterior lobe hormones.

Anoxemia or cerebral hypoperfusion is another cause of diabetes insipidus that is being described more frequently. At least nine cases have been reported,[29-33] and we have studied five additional patients (Table 18–4). The previously reported patients had severe encephalomalacia almost always associated with brain death resulting from asphyxia, drug-induced respiratory failure, diabetic ketoacidosis, cardiac arrest, and shock due to penetrating thoracic trauma. Our five patients (two males, three females) ranged in age from 15 to 73 years and developed encephalopathy and diabetes insipidus from shock secondary to a gunshot wound of the chest, an embolus to the middle cerebral artery, hypertensive encephalopathy, and cardiopulmonary arrest. One of our patients who survived for 68 days after the criteria for brain death were satisfied had findings at autopsy characteristic of an advanced stage in the sequence of changes that follow brain infarction with prolonged preservation of systemic circulatory function.[34]

Only one of our patients had sarcoidosis. However, diabetes insipidus has been reported by others in patients with sarcoidosis.[35,36] Sarcoidosis may also cause two other states of hypotonic polyuria: primary polydipsia and acquired nephrogenic diabetic insipidus.[37,38]

Diabetic insipidus resulted from metastatic malignancy in eight cases. There were two cases, each with carcinoma of the lung and breast, and one case each from carcinoma of kidney and rectum, one carcinoma with an unknown primary site, and one patient with leukemia. Diabetes insipidus as a complication of leukemia, although rare, has been previously reported.[39,40] Thirty-nine cases of metastatic breast carcinoma causing diabetic insipidus have been reported by Yap et al.[41]

Hypernatremia is an uncommon disorder associated with or aggravated by a deficient water intake. Increased fluid losses may aggravate the problem but do not cause hypernatremia if the thirst mechanism is intact and water is available. Even in the unusual situation of sodium overload, hypernatremia is transient if the thirst mechanism is intact.

Hypernatremia may therefore develop with either a concentrated or dilute urine. The neurohypophyseal system may be intact, or there may be vasopressin deficiency of varying degrees for several reasons. Some patients may have a defective osmoreceptor mechanism, while other receptor mechanisms remain

Table 18–4. Clinical Data on Five of Our Patients in Whom Diabetes Insipidus Developed from Anoxemic Encephalopathy[a]

Patient Data	Cause	Time of Development of Diabetes Insipidus
M, 15	Gunshot wound of chest causing shock	24–36 hours after injury, causing marked neurologic abnormalities, including bilateral fixed dilated pupils and absence of respiration
F, 32	Embolus to left middle cerebral artery and uncal herniation	2½ days after initial paresis ~ 12 hours after fixed dilated pupils and decerebrate posturing
F, 37	Hypertensive encephalopathy	2 days after hyperreflexia and muscle twitching, 1 day after occipital blindness and severe obtundation, and 2–3 hours after development of severe brain stem dysfunction
M, 49[b]	Cardiopulmonary arrest	~ 3 hours after the arrest and development of brain death
F, 73	Cardiopulmonary arrest	24 hours after the arrest, causing fixed dilated pupils, absent reflexes and respiration, and failure of oculovestibular responses

[a] All patients had to be maintained on total life-support systems and were brain dead at time diabetes insipidus developed.

[b] Developed panhypopituitarism. Remainder of patients could not be evaluated for anterior pituitary function.

intact.[42-45] Some of these patients release arginine vasopressin from induced hypovolemia, while others release arginine vasopressin when blood pressure is decreased by drugs like trimethaphan. The osmotic threshold for vasopressin release may be absent or elevated.[46] Other patients with severe hypernatremia may have adipsia with impaired arginine vasopressin secretion at all levels of plasma osmolality, so that urine concentration is possible only when plasma osmolality is greatly increased.[47] It is possible that vasopressin deficiency may cause or aggravate adipsia or hypodipsia, since vasopressin has been shown in dogs to have a central dipsogenic action.[48] Severe hypernatremia causes a characteristic clinical picture with most of the symptoms being referable to the central nervous system.[49] (see also Chapter 21). In addition, fluid loss may lead to vascular collapse. There are a variety of vascular, neoplastic, and granulomatous causes of adipsic hypernatremia.[1] A milder form of this abnormality is asymptomatic or essential hypernatremia. This is generally associated with dilution as well as concentration of the urine around an elevated serum sodium concentration and may be equated with a high-set osmoreceptor mechanism. Normonatremia may be restored by the provision of an adequate water supply.[50] Most patients with myotonic dystrophy may have asymptomatic hypernatremia due to an impaired release of arginine vasopressin and stimulation of thirst by hypertonicity in association with an intact volume control of arginine vasopressin release.[51] We have found a similar situation in two patients with Kallmann's syndrome.[52]

We have had five patients with central diabetes insipidus who were unable to concentrate their urine even with very high levels of serum sodium, who were hypodipsic or adipsic. The clinical problem presented by these patients is severe. It is very impressive and frightening to have one of these patients obtunded or in shock with a serum sodium of 180 mEq/liter and absolutely no sensation of thirst. The patients can be maintained in the hospital with some difficulty by careful adjustment of fluid intake on the basis of urine volume, estimated insensible and sensible fluid losses, with modifications made according to body weight and serum electrolyte and osmolality determinations. However, it is very difficult to do this at home, and the results may be very poor. Although Bode et al.[53] reported that chlorpropamide may restore drinking behavior, it has not been successful in our patients.

Primary polydipsia is a state of hypotonic polyuria with suppressed arginine vasopressin levels secondary to excessive fluid intake. Any tendency toward polydipsia can be aggravated by thorazine or similar drugs, such as thioridazine, which cause dryness of the mouth.[54] Primary polydipsia is often psychogenic in origin with the symptoms being less consistent than in patients with central or nephrogenic diabetes insipidus. In fact, some patients with psychogenic polydipsia may have normal water balance for days or weeks, followed by periods of excessive water turnover. Primary polydipsia, presumably on a psychogenic basis, may occur in patients with anorexia nervosa and disappear when they begin to eat properly. Increased thirst and polydipsia due to increased renin and/or angiotensin levels may occur in patients with renal artery stenosis.[55] We have investigated two patients who apparently developed primary polydipsia from hypothalamic disease. One patient developed the syndrome soon after a severe blow to the head, and the second had thyroid deficiency on a hypothalamic basis together with elevated prolactin levels and thickening of the infundibular stalk. Unlike patients with psychogenic polydipsia who become bloated and uncomfortable when treated with antidiuretic hormone,[56] these patients with apparent organic polydipsia had markedly improved symptoms when treated with Pitressin tannate in oil or a synthetic vasopressin analogue, 1-deamino-8-D-arginine vasopressin (dDAVP). This improvement may be related to the effect of antidiuretic hormone on increasing salivary flow rates and amelioration of thirst in patients with diabetes insipidus.[57] This is apparently a peripheral action of antidiuretic hormone, since centrally administered vasopressin has a dipsogenic action in the dog.[48]

Animal Models

Diabetes insipidus has been reported to occur in dogs from trauma and from a variety of other lesions.[58]

Experimental animal models of polydipsia and polyuria have been produced, usually in rats, by the induction of lesions in the central nervous system. The polydipsia and polyuria that result from these lesions are of varying causes, ranging from severe diabetes insipidus following the placement of lesions in the supraopticohypophyseal tracts[13,59] and in ventromedial hypothalamic areas,[60] to mildly defective arginine vasopressin release following medial preoptic lesions,[61] to primary polydipsia following the placement of lesions in the septal and lateral preoptic areas.[62–65] Some hypothalamic lesions result in both diabetes insipidus and primary polydipsia.[66] As may sometimes occur in patients with traumatic or surgically induced diabetes insipidus, these lesioned animals may manifest a triphasic disturbance of water metabolism, that is, a brief diuresis followed by a short period of oliguria, followed by polyuria and polydipsia.

A genetic laboratory model of diabetes insipidus is the hereditary hypothalamic diabetes insipidus rat of the Brattleboro strain, which has an intrinsic defect in vasopressin synthesis and release. Hypothalamic diabetes insipidus in this strain is inherited as an autosomal semirecessive trait at a single gene locus. Three genotypes can be distinguished: Brattleboro homozygotes, often referred to as diabetes insipidus (di/di) rats, Brattleboro heterozygotes (di/+), and normal rats of the Long-Evans hooded strain, from which Brattleboro rats were derived. The average output of urine in Brattleboro homozygotes is equivalent to about 70 percent of the body weight per day, and the water intake is correspondingly high. The urine osmolality averages ~130 mOsm/kg, in contrast to normal Long-Evans rats, which have a urine output of about 3 percent of the body weight per day and which concentrate their urine to ~2200 mOsm/kg when they are eating and drinking ad libitum. Brattleboro heterozygotes, having one normal and one abnormal allele, show characteristics of water turnover that are intermediate between those of normal rats and Brattleboro homozygotes.

The neural lobe of the Brattleboro homozygous rat (di/di) is completely devoid of arginine vasopressin and its associated neurophysin. The lack of arginine vasopressin has been demonstrated by radioimmunoassay and by high-performance liquid chromatography with fluorescence detection.[67] The heterozygous rat (di/+) has slightly more than one-half the normal amount of arginine vasopressin in the neural lobe and the same fraction of the normal amount of vasopressin-associated neurophysin. The untreated homozygous Brattleboro rat is deficient in neural lobe oxytocin and its associated neurophysins, but these values are normalized when fluid turnover is reduced by treatment with exogenous vasopressin. Since a vasopressin prohormone containing both vasopressin and its neurophysin has been defined,[68] these observations support the concept that homozygous and heterozygous Brattleboro rats have, respectively, a complete or incomplete deficiency in the synthesis of the prohormone for arginine vasopressin, propressophysin. The one neuron–one hormone thesis[69] allows us to believe that Brattleboro rats have a specific defect in the magnocellular neurons that synthesize propressophysin. During 4 days of water, deprivation pituitaries of the di/+ rats are depleted of arginine vasopressin at 57 percent of the normal rate, and after 4 days of dehydration there is no longer a significant difference in pituitary vasopressin content between the di/+ and normal rats. There is only one-half the decrease in pituitary vasopressin per mOsm/kg rise in plasma concentration in the heterozygous rat as in the normal.[70] The impaired hormone release results in the excretion of greater amounts of more dilute urine in the heterozygous rats than the normal and the consequent higher plasma osmolality during water deprivation. Following a period of dehydration, heterozygous rats reaccumulate pituitary vasopressin at 38 percent of the normal rate.

Plasma and urinary arginine vasopressin values in normal and heterozygous Brattleboro rats (di/+) are remarkably parallel when the animals drink ad lib and when they are dehydrated, and the values for di/+ rats are approximately one-half of normal. Homozygous Brattleboro rats (di/di) have essentially no arginine vasopressin in plasma or urine when hydrated or dehydrated. Di/di Brattleboro rats are capable of concentrating their urine to ~1200 mOsm/kg on the second day of water deprivation. There are many similarities between the heterozygous Brattleboro rats and those with medial preoptic lesions, each being an incomplete arginine vasopressin deficiency model.

Homozygous and heterozygous Brattleboro rats have been used for many biochemical, physiologic, psychological, and pharmacologic experiments, and much of this work has been reviewed in a publication of a recent symposium which was devoted to the Brattleboro rat.[71]

Laboratory Features

The diagnosis of diabetes insipidus is based on evaluation of the hypothalamoneurohypophyseal system including both the osmoreceptor mechanism and the ability of arginine vasopressin to be released in consequence of the activation of this receptor. Stimuli such as nicotine, nausea, and hypotension may release arginine vasopressin and are useful in attempting to understand the underlying pathophysiologic abnormality in individual patients. However, the results are clinically irrelevant. It matters little to the patient with symptomatic diabetes insipidus if we determine that one or all of these nonphysiologic or extreme stimuli cause the release of arginine vasopressin.

The diagnostic procedures discussed in this section were developed in an effort to use the known physiological factors that influence vasopressin release as applied to the clinical setting. The appropriate tests, therefore, have to be clinically practical, readily available, rapid in performance, noninjurious to the patient and preferably inexpensive.

The early tests used for the laboratory diagnosis of diabetes insipidus were based on the presence or absence of a decrease in urine flow rate in patients being infused with hypertonic saline.[72,73] In an effort to define the plasma osmolality at which the release of arginine vasopressin was initiated, we modified the saline infusion tests and developed the concept of an osmotic threshold for vasopressin release by using 5 percent saline to raise the plasma osmolality in water-loaded subjects.[23] When a hydrated normal subject was infused with hypertonic saline at a constant rate, there was a linear rise in plasma osmolality with time and that after an interval depending on the infusion rate, concentration of saline, and initial plasma osmolality, there was an abrupt progressive fall in free water clearance without a change in solute or creatinine excretion. We defined the plasma osmolality at the initiation of antidiuresis under these conditions as the osmotic threshold for vasopressin release and found that it occurred in normal subjects at a mean value of 287.3 mOsm/kg (Fig. 18–3).[23,74]

Osmotic threshold studies are conducted by giving the subject a water load, 20 ml/kg, by mouth over a 15- to 20-minute period, and the water load is maintained with further fluid administration in amounts equal to the volumes of urine passed every 15 minutes. The patient should remain recumbent between voidings and should have an indwelling needle placed in each forearm, kept patent with dilute (1:1000) heparin solution. When urine volume became stable for at least three (preferably five or six) 15-minute periods, the patient is given a rapid intravenous infusion of 5 percent NaCl solution through a forearm needle.

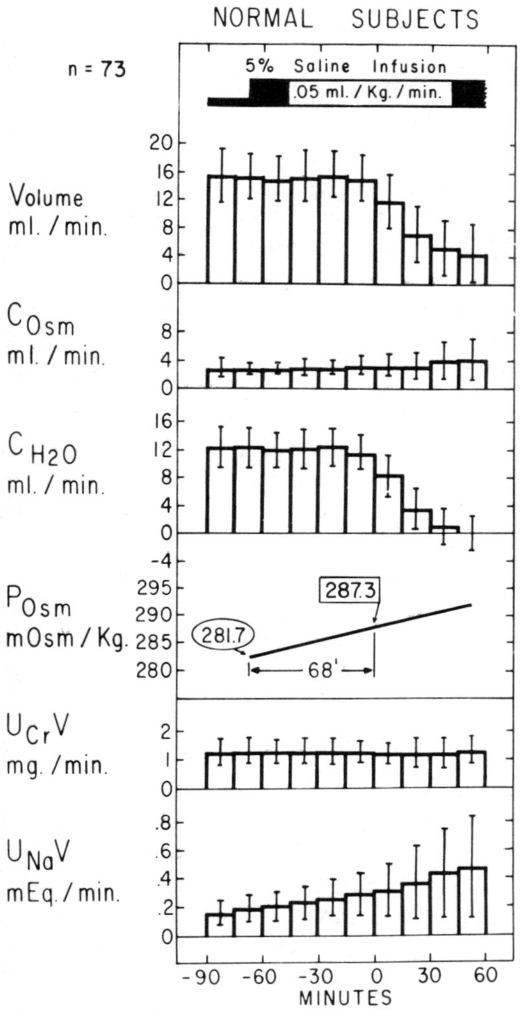

Fig. 18–3. Composite osmotic threshold studies in 73 normal subjects. Mean osmotic threshold is 287.3 mOsm/kg. (From Moses AM, Miller M: Diabetes insipidus. In Conn H, Conn R (eds): Current Diagnosis. Philadelphia, WB Saunders Co., 1971.

The 5 percent NaCl solution is administered by infusion pump at 0.05 ml/kg·min. During the saline infusion, serum samples are obtained every 15 minutes for osmolality measurements while the water load is maintained and urine collections are continued every 15 minutes. This procedure is continued until either 30 to 45 minutes after an abrupt reduction in urine flow indicating that the osmotic threshold has been reached, or until the infusion has continued for more than 2 hours, or until severe headache or discomfort supervenes, whichever comes first.

The free water clearance is calculated on each of the 15-minute urine samples before and during the hypertonic saline infusion. Free water clearance and not urine volume has to be used because an occasional patient substantially increases solute excretion (C_{osm}), and this masks the decrease in free water clearance (Fig. 18–4). When the osmotic threshold has been reached and arginine vasopressin has been released, there will be an obvious fall in free water clearance by >2 SD below the mean free water clearance in the control period. The serum osmolality at the beginning of that 15-minute collection period, measured by interpolation on the regression line relating serum osmolality with time, represents the osmotic threshold for arginine vasopressin release. In normal subjects this will be 284 to 291 (mean 287.3 ± SD 3.6) mOsm/kg. In patients with primary polydipsia the value is low or normal. In patients with diabetes insipidus an osmotic threshold may occur at an elevated plasma osmolality but is usually undetectable even if the serum osmolality is raised to very high levels (Fig. 18–5).

Other factors that may alter arginine vasopressin release include blood volume and blood pressure. These mechanisms are much less sensitive in altering hormone release and are considered backup mechanisms; they will not be discussed here in detail. Hypervolemia inhibits the release of arginine vasopressin and acts to raise the osmotic threshold for release of the hormone.[75] Cortisol and oxilorphan also raise the osmotic threshold for vasopressin release (Fig. 18–6).[23,76] In contrast, there is a lower osmotic threshold for vasopressin release when the osmotic stimulus is provided by dehydration than by infusion of 5 percent saline.[77] Pregnancy is another factor that may lower the osmotic threshold for vasopressin release.[60]

The first patients with diabetes insipidus whom we investigated had no attainable osmotic thresholds, but we soon recognized patients who had elevated osmotic thresholds

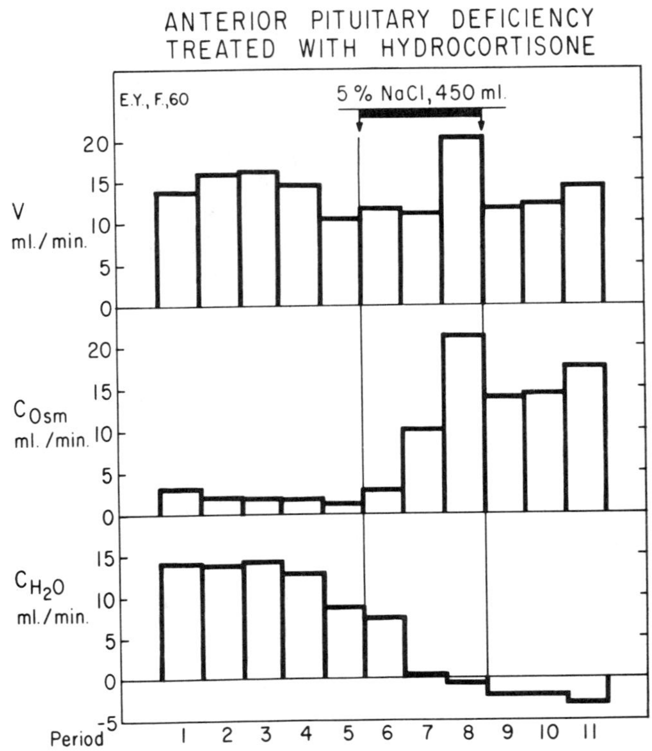

Fig. 18–4. Effect of hypertonic saline infusion in a patient with hypopituitarism treated with hydrocortisone. Note the apparent lack of antidiuretic response when the volume alone is considered. The decrease in free water clearance is masked by the marked increase in osmolal clearance. (From Moses AM, Streeten DHP: Differentiation of polyuric states by measurement of responses to changes in plasma osmolality induced by hypertonic saline infusions. Am J Med 42:368, 1967.)

(high-set osmoreceptor), and depending on the situation, mainly the sensitivity of the thirst mechanism, could be diagnosed as having either incomplete or partial diabetes insipidus or essential hypernatremia.[76] We rarely use the osmotic threshold test clinically, except where there is a problem in differentiating diabetes insipidus from primary polydipsia. In the latter condition the osmotic threshold is often low and slowly returns toward normal if fluids are restricted.

We next attempted to determine maximum urinary concentrating ability and to relate this to normality and to degrees of arginine vasopressin deficiency. The possibility of incomplete vasopressin deficiency had previously been claimed by Lipsett et al.[78,79] Since the maximal urinary concentrating capacity varies widely between patients, probably related to the osmolality of renal medullary interstitium, it is impossible to distinguish between deficiency and sufficiency of arginine vasopressin by the absolute level of urinary osmolality attained after specified periods of water deprivation. To overcome this problem, we modified existing dehydration tests[80] in an effort to develop a dehydration test not based on weight loss or time of water deprivation, but on the premise that normal subjects, regardless of maximal attainable urine osmolality, were limited in their maximum urine osmolality by their renal concentrating mechanism, while maximum urine osmolality in patients with impaired neurohypophyseal function was limited by the amount of arginine vasopressin releasable by water deprivation.[81] We found that in normal subjects, the injection of antidiuretic hormone after a plateau in urine osmolality had been attained produced no further rise in urine osmolality (Fig. 18–7, Table 18–5). In contrast, if vasopressin administration induced a further rise in urine osmolality after prolonged dehydration, there is a strong implication that vasopressin deficiency exists (Figs. 8 and 9; Table 18–5).

The test we described is performed by with-

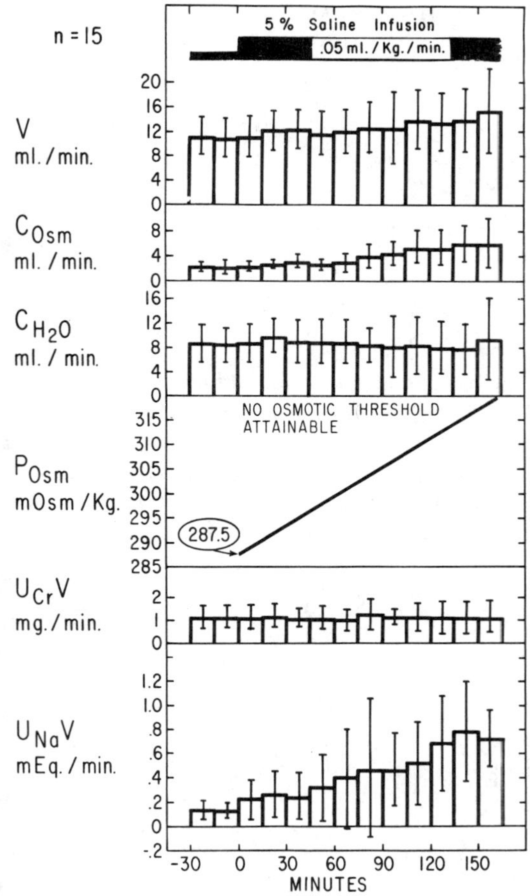

Fig. 18–5. Composite of 15 osmotic threshold studies in 10 subjects with diabetes insipidus, six of whom had combined pituitary deficiency. No osmotic threshold was attainable, even though the highest plasma osmolality in each instance ranged from 298 to 332 mOsm/kg. (From Moses AM, Streeten DHP: Differentiation of polyuric states by measurement of responses to changes in plasma osmolality induced by hypertonic saline infusions. Am J Med 42:368, 1967.)

holding fluids, usually from about 6 o'clock AM until the osmolality of successive hourly urine samples increases by <30 mOsm/kg, indicating that a plateau of urine concentration has been reached. Constancy of urine osmolality is usually reached by early afternoon. When the plateau is reached, a blood sample is obtained for osmolality and the patient is given aqueous Pitressin, 5 U by subcutaneous injection. Urine is collected at ½ hour and 1 hour after this injection for osmolality measurement. Body weights should be recorded at the beginning and end of the dehydration to determine the percentage of weight lost.

When neurohypophyseal reserve is normal, the maximal urinary osmolality after dehydration may be 800 to 1400 mOsm/kg in robust normal subjects, but may be only 450 to 800 mOsm/kg in chronically debilitated or malnourished persons. In all such subjects, urinary osmolality falls slightly or rises by less than 9 percent after administration of aqueous Pitressin (Fig. 18–9 and Table 18–5). Patients with primary polydipsia have values similar to those of the debilitated and malnourished subjects. In patients with severe diabetes insipidus, the maximum urinary osmolality which is reached before the Pitressin injection remains below serum osmolality. In those patients whose diabetes insipidus is partial or moderately severe, urinary osmolality generally rises above serum osmolality during dehydration. After the Pitressin injection in subjects whose endogenous vasopressin reserve is normal, urinary osmolality is never more than 9 percent higher than it was immediately before the injection. A Pitressin-induced rise in urinary osmolality of approximately 50 percent indicates the presence of vasopressin deficiency or central diabetes insipidus. Patients with nephrogenic diabetes insipidus show a subnormal rise in urinary osmolality after dehydration alone, rarely rising above serum osmolality, and a 0 to 45 percent rise in urinary osmolality after the Pitressin injection. Patients with primary polydipsia may be so overloaded with fluids that prolonged dehydration (more than 24 hours) may be needed before endogenous arginine vasopressin is released and urine is concentrated. In these patients, the finding that serum osmolality has not risen above the normal osmotic threshold indicates the need for more prolonged dehydration. This test is simple, generally available and safe even in patients with profound deficiency of arginine vasopressin, if severe dehydration is prevented by not allowing body weight to fall

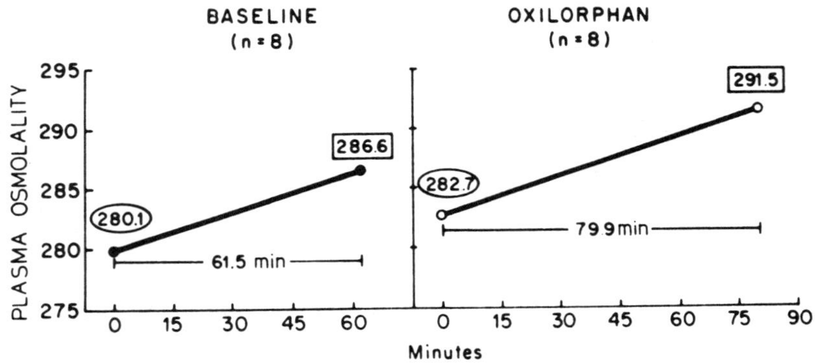

Fig. 18–6. Effect of 2 mg oxilorphan on the osmotic threshold for antidiuretic hormone (AVP) release in eight normal subjects. Drug treatment resulted in a significant prologation of the time necessary for hypertonic saline to cause an antidiuresis, and the osmotic threshold was significantly elevated. (From Miller M, Moses AM: Clinical states due to alteration of ADH release and action. p. 153. In Moses AM, Share L (eds): Neurohypophysis. S. Karger, Basel, 1977.)

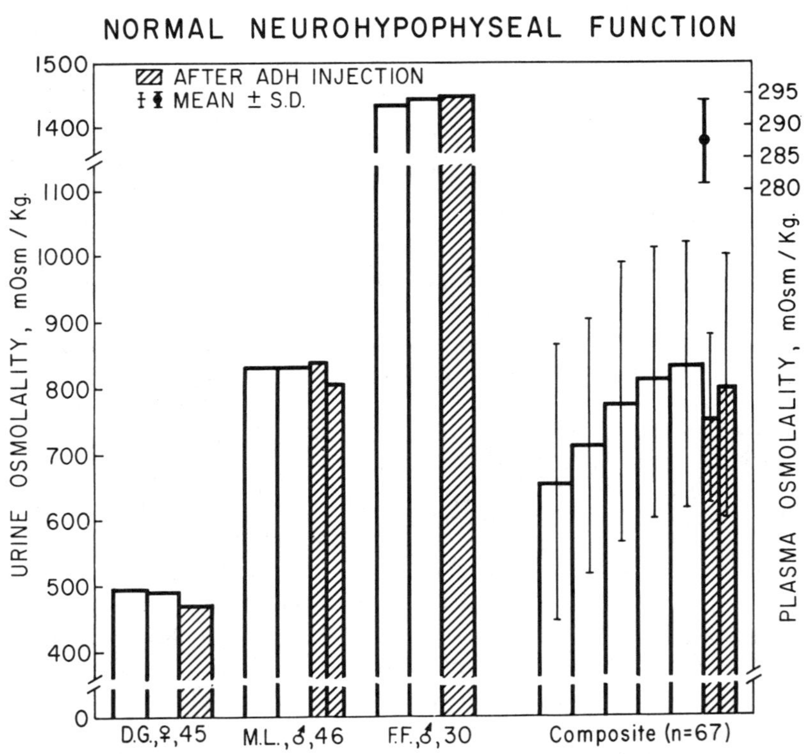

Fig. 18–7. Dehydration studies in three normal subjects and a composite of 67 studies in normal subjects demonstrating that the maximum urine osmolality varies from ~500 to 1400 mOsm/kg and that the injection of antidiuretic hormone (ADH) (5 U aqueous Pitressin) causes no further increase. (From Moses AM, Miller M: Diabetes insipidus. In Conn H, Conn R (eds): Current Diagnosis. Philadelphia, WB Saunders Co., 1971, pp. 705–710.)

Table 18–5. Interpretation of Dehydration Test

	Maximum $\frac{U_{osm}}{P_{osm}}$ Before Pitressin	Maximum $\frac{U_{osm}}{P_{osm}}$ After Pitressin	U_{osm} Increase After Pitressin (Percent)
Normal or primary polydipsia	>1	>1	<9
Partial ADH[a,b] deficiency	>1	>1	>9
Severe ADH[b] deficiency	<1	< or >1	>50
Nephrogenic diabetes insipidus	<1	<1	<45

[a] Note that these patients may have severe polyuria.
[b] ADH, antidiuretic hormone.

by more than 5 percent. It should be emphasized that the dehydration test could be abnormal with a normal osmotic threshold or vice versa, since one test measures factors related to initiation of arginine vasopressin release, while the other test determines factors related to maximum concentration of urine.

This test has provided much important information about the status of neurohypophyseal function in many patients, but it eventu-

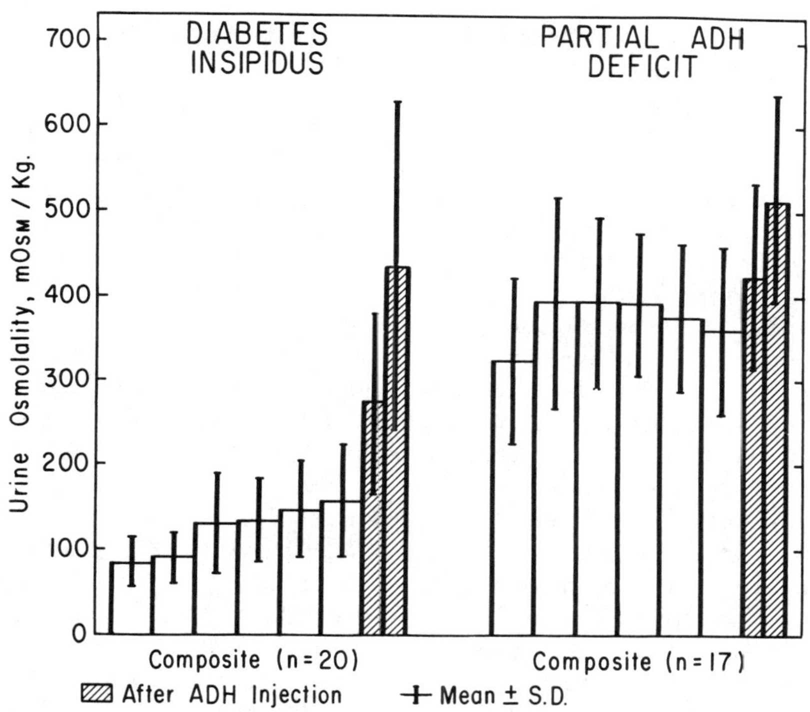

Fig. 18–8. Composite dehydration studies in patients with severe (left) and mild (right) antidiuretic hormone (ADH) deficiency. Both types of patients concentrate their urine more in response to exogenous ADH (5 U aqueous Pitressin) than to the amount of ADH released endogenously in response to dehydration. (From Moses AM, Miller M: Diabetes insipidus. In Conn H, Conn R (eds): Current Diagnosis. Philadelphia, WB Saunders Co., 1971, pp. 705–710.)

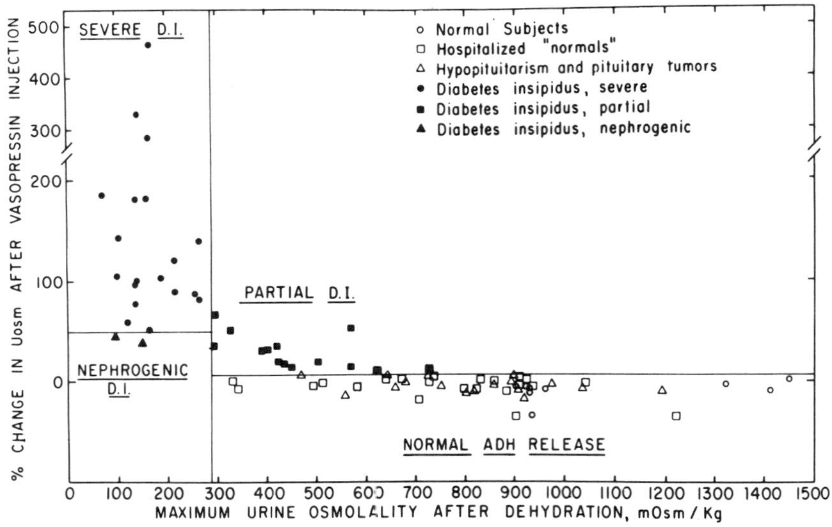

Fig. 18–9. Maximum urine osmolality after dehydration plotted against the percentage change in urine osmolality induced by injection of 5 U aqueous Pitressin. (From Miller M, Dalakos T, Moses AM, et al: Recognition of partial defects in antidiuretic hormone secretion. Ann Intern Med 73:721, 1970.)

ally became obvious that the urine osmolality attained during dehydration had to be related carefully to plasma osmolality.[21,76,82] For instance, patients were found who had apparently normal dehydration tests, but with high plasma osmolalities. Under random conditions, their thirst mechanisms might not allow them to get sufficiently dehydrated to concentrate the urine, so that under random conditions they would have hypotonic polyuria. If their thirst mechanism was insensitive, they would be classified as having a high-set osmoreceptor or essential hypernatremia. We collected plasma and urine osmolality data during water loading and dehydration and described a normal area indicated by the shaded areas in Figures 18–1 and 18–2. This permitted an assessment of the range of urine and plasma osmolality relationships under conditions similar to those encountered in day-to-day conditions of water balance. A similar relationship has been described for children.[83] In all relationships between plasma osmolality and arginine vasopressin release, the plasma osmolality is that which reflects the presence of biologically active particles, essentially sodium and its associated anions. Increased amounts of urea or glucose have to be corrected down to normal amounts, and appropriate corrections have to be made for substances such as ethanol which, like urea, have little or no effect on altering osmotic gradients across cell membranes.

The plasma, urine osmolality coordinates can be divided into four quadrants (Fig. 18–10). Points that fall in area II (hypertonic urine at an appropriate plasma osmolality) are normal, while points that fall in area IV (hypotonic urine with an elevated plasma osmolality) are abnormal and indicate the presence of central or nephrogenic diabetes insipidus. Except for patients with nephrogenic diabetes insipidus, the relationship between plasma and urine osmolality is similar to the relationship between plasma osmolality and urine arginine vasopressin. Points that fall in area I (dilute urine without an elevated plasma osmolality) are indeterminate. To clarify the clinical status of these patients, oral or intravenous fluids should be restricted and urine and plasma osmolality values determined hourly. If the withholding of fluids causes urine versus plasma osmolality coordinates to move into area IV, the patient has diabetes insipidus (central or nephrogenic). If initial urine and plasma osmolality coordinates are both dilute

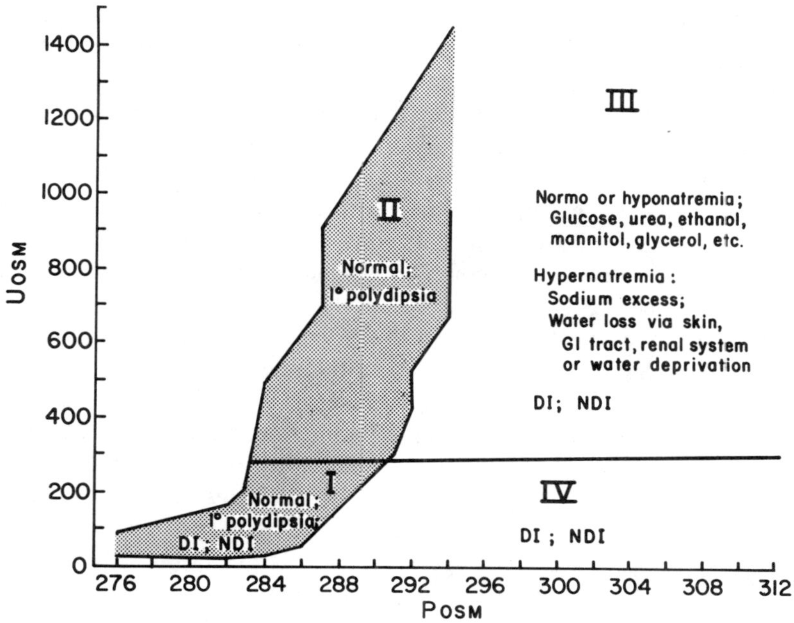

Fig. 18–10. Comparison of plasma and urine osmolalities with data from normal subjects in shaded area. Coordinates in area II indicate a normal concentrating mechanism, while coordinates in area IV indicate the presence of central or nephrogenic diabetes insipidus. Areas I and III are indeterminate and patients exhibiting such data should be dehydrated or hydrated as detailed in the text.

(area I), dehydration may cause the subsequent points to fall into a normal area, where urine is appropriately concentrated in relationship to plasma osmolality (area II). This would indicate that the hypotonic polyuria was due to overhydration in a patient with a normal neurohypophyseal mechanism. If dehydration causes the urine to become concentrated, but only at the expense of an elevated plasma osmolality (area III), the patient probably has an incomplete antidiuretic hormone deficiency. With water restriction, patients with primary polydipsia develop coordinates that fall within the normal area or within the low-set osmoreceptor area to the left of normal. When the pattern becomes clear, the test may be terminated before a plateau in urine osmolality is reached, or alternatively a formal dehydration test may be conducted as described. Patients with incomplete or partial diabetes insipidus may have severe polyuria under random conditions if the thirst mechanism is sensitive.

Another aspect of the formulation in Figure 18–10 is that when initial data fall within area III (hypertonicity or hypernatremia with concentrated urine), the gentle forcing of hypotonic fluids will cause subsequent points to fall within areas II or IV, generally permitting a definitive diagnosis to be established. If hydration causes osmolality coordinates to move into area II, the initial hypernatremia was due to water deprivation in a patient with normal neurohypophyseal function. If hydration causes the coordinates to move into area IV, the initial hypernatremia was due to a combination of inadequate water intake and a water-losing state. Some patients have chronic asymptomatic hypernatremia without definable cause and are said to have a high-set osmoreceptor mechanism for stimulation of thirst and vasopressin release, or essential hypernatremia.[1]

The use of plasma, urine osmolality coordinates does not permit differentiation between central and nephrogenic diabetes insipidus.

However, these two causes of hypotonic polyuria can usually be differentiated by the difference in the acute response of urine osmolality to the injection of aqueous Pitressin, or by the response to prolonged therapy with Pitressin tannate in oil or dDAVP nasal spray. When a definitive diagnosis is not possible by the use of these methods, measurement of plasma[44,84,85] or urinary arginine vasopressin[86] permits the diagnosis to be clearly established. In patients with renal disease, plasma rather than urinary arginine vasopressin measurements have to be used. Urinary arginine vasopressin is normal or supranormal relative to plasma osmolality in patients with nephrogenic diabetes insipidus (Fig. 18–11). In contrast, patients with central diabetic insipidus have very low levels of urinary arginine vasopressin in relationship to plasma osmolality. The use of the urinary arginine vasopressin versus urinary osmolality relationship, as depicted in Figure 18–12, also separates patients with central and nephrogenic diabetes insipidus.

These diagnostic points are usually quite straightforward. However, some patients have conflicting data. There should never be difficulty differentiating central and nephrogenic diabetes insipidus using the above criteria, including measurement of arginine vasopressin levels when necessary. Severe and incomplete central diabetes insipidus represent a contin-

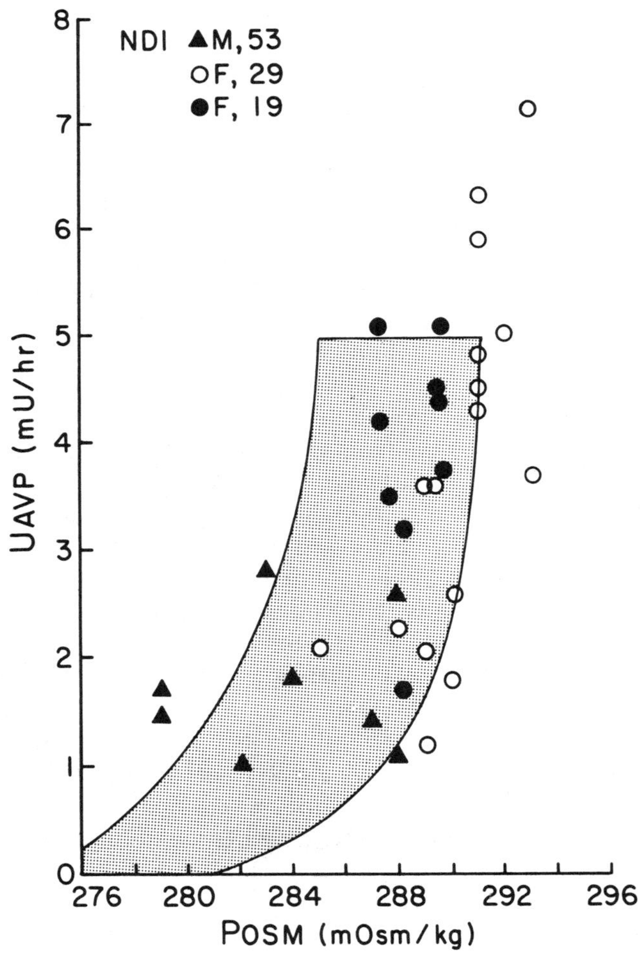

Fig. 18–11. Relationship between plasma osmolality and urine arginine vasopressin (AVP) in normal subjects (shaded area) and in patients with nephrogenic diabetes insipidus. Patients with central diabetes insipidus have points far to the right of normal.

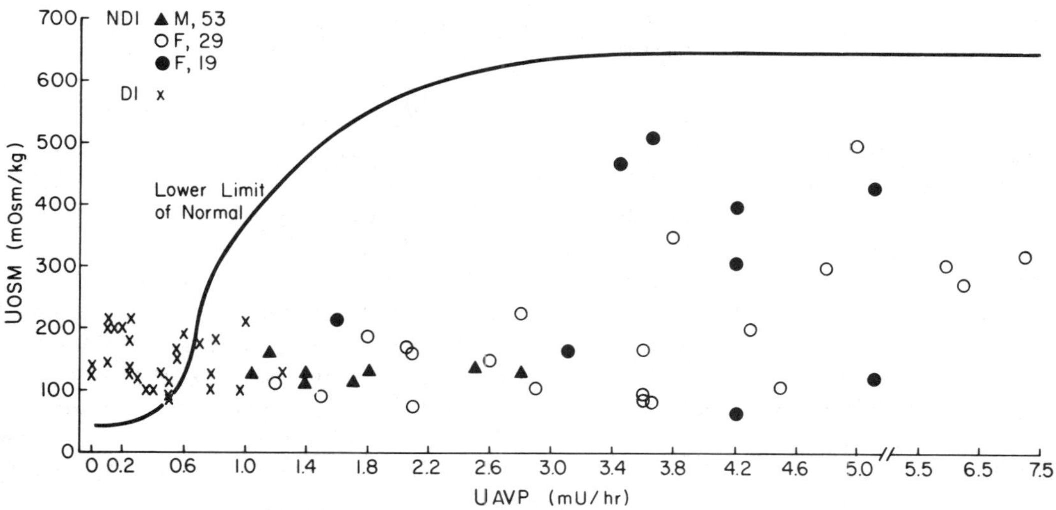

Fig. 18–12. Relationship between urine vasopressin excretion (U_{AVP}) and urine osmolality (U_{osm}) in normal subjects (lower limit depicted by line), in patients with central diabetes insipidus (crosses) whose U_{AVP} is almost always below 1 mU/hr and in patients with nephrogenic diabetes insipidus (circles) who excrete >1 mU AVP/hr. AVP, arginine vasopressin.

uum and are not clearly separable. The only clinical problem is whether or not to treat the patient. There may be difficulty at times differentiating between incomplete central diabetes insipidus and primary polydipsia. The response to therapy cannot be used as an ultimate criterion, because patients with primary polydipsia on an organic basis may markedly improve with antidiuretic hormone therapy, the improvement being related to an increased salivary flow rate and amelioration of thirst.[57] In essence, there is no single definitive diagnostic standard for the differential diagnosis of the hypotonic polyurias. The diagnosis has to be based on a combination of factors. Rarely, a definitive diagnosis cannot be established.

Treatment

Central diabetes insipidus may be treated by replacement therapy with various forms of vasopressin given parenterally (by nasal spray or by injection) or in mild to moderate deficiency, with oral agents that increase the action and/or the release of endogenous arginine vasopressin. Treatment with diuretics and sodium restriction is difficult to implement and only mildly effective and should be attempted only in patients with nephrogenic diabetes insipidus. The possibility of effectively treating the cause of the diabetes insipidus should always be borne in mind. Sarcoidosis may be treated with steroids,[87] Wegener's granulomatosis with cyclophosphamide,[9] and metastatic tumors to the hypothalamus by radiotherapy.

A synthetic analogue of arginine vasopressin, desmopressin, dDAVP, administered intranasally, is the most convenient and effective form of therapy for most patients. The appropriate dosage, usually 5 to 20 μg, is determined by observing the duration and extent of antidiuresis resulting from the intranasal instillation of 0.05, 0.1, or 0.2 ml of the dDAVP solution (100 μg/ml) using the plastic cannula that is provided. Optimal dosage should control polyuria and polydipsia for at least 12 hours, permitting the administration of the drug once or twice daily and permitting the patient to sleep without interruption by nocturia.[88,89] An injectable form of dDAVP may be used in patients who have nasal obstruction or damaged mucosa.[90] When injected subcutaneously, 0.5 μg dDAVP causes an antidiuresis for 10 hours, with each doubling of the dose to 4 μg, increasing the duration of action by 4 hours (Fig. 18–13). Both the intranasal and subcutaneous preparations of dDAVP are essentially devoid of side effects and are ideal agents for the treatment of central diabetes insipidus. The absence of vascular effects of dDAVP is due to substitution of D-arginine for the naturally occurring L-arginine, and the increased magnitude and duration of action of dDAVP is related to the removal of an amino group that causes resistance to enzymatic degradation. In addition, dDAVP is much less effective than arginine vasopressin in stimulating urinary excretion of prostaglandin E_2 (unpublished data). Since prostaglandin E_2 inhibits arginine vasopressin-induced activation of adenylate cyclase activity, the magnitude of antidiuresis caused by dDAVP may be enhanced by the limited stimulation of prostaglandin E_2. The antidiuretic response to dDAVP is further enhanced by treatment with indomethacin.[90]

Lypressin (lysine-vasopressin) nasal spray has a shorter duration of action (4 to 6 hours), requires administration at least three times daily, and usually does not prevent nocturia.[91] Intramuscular or subcutaneous injections of aqueous vasopressin (arginine vasopressin, aqueous Pitressin) are used in doses of 5 or 10 U, mainly for testing and for rapid and brief control of polyuria. The intramuscular injection of 2.5 or 5 U of vasopressin tannate in oil (Pitressin tannate) provides effective and reliable control of polyuria for 24 to 72 hours,[92] provided that the ampule is warmed and shaken so that the pituitary powder is suspended in the oil before being aspirated

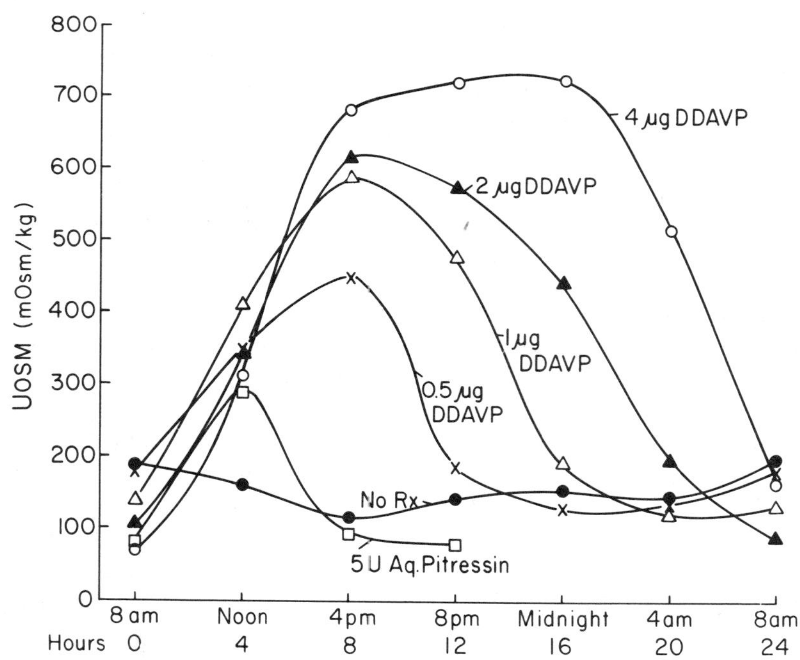

Fig. 18–13. Mean urine osmolality responses in six patients with central diabetes insipidus. Patients were untreated or given indicated amounts of aqueous Pitressin or 1-deamino-8-D-arginine vasopressin (dDAVP) subcutaneously. (From Moses AM, Moses LK, Notman DD, et al: Antidiuretic responses to injected desmopressin, alone and with indomethacin. J Clin Endocrinol Metab 52:910, 1981. © 1981 The Endocrine Society).

into the syringe. Some patients have allergic reactions to the animal proteins in Pitressin tannate. Because of the smooth muscle-constricting action of arginine vasopressin, Pitressin may cause abdominal cramps and headaches and may even cause serious cardiac accidents in patients with coronary artery insufficiency.[93] Posterior pituitary snuff causes severe nasal irritation and the development of miliary shadows in the lungs due to hypersensitivity,[94] hence is no longer recommended.

In our opinion, chlorpropamide is the most appropriate oral therapy for diabetes insipidus if it provides adequate control of polyuria. In doses of 200 to 500 mg/day it provides effective therapy in 30 to 50 percent of patients with central diabetes insipidus.[95,96] The antidiuretic effect ranges from none in patients who have no releasable arginine vasopressin to an extremely effective action that may even result in hyponatremia if fluid therapy is not carefully restricted (Fig. 18–14). Hyponatremia is particularly common in patients with anterior pituitary insufficiency[97] or if the drug is administered along with dDAVP.[98] On average, there is a 50 percent increase in urine osmolality and a 50 percent decrease in urine volume in patients treated with chlorpropamide.[99] Chlorpropamide may be administered in small doses (100 to 200 mg) together with small doses of other orally active agents.[100,101] The danger of hypoglycemia may limit the usefulness of chlorpropamide, especially in patients with pituitary insufficiency. Chlorpropamide may be very appropriate in those patients who have both diabetes mellitus and diabetes insipidus. The antidiuretic action of chlorpropamide is overcome by ethanol.[99,102]

Patients with central diabetes insipidus are often treated effectively with clofibrate.[103] However, it is not very popular because of the effectiveness of dDAVP nasal spray and for several other reasons as well. First, 2 g/day is usually less effective than 250 mg of chlorpropamide,[100] and it is rarely effective when chlorpropamide is ineffective. In addition, muscle damage may occur, and serum levels of muscle enzymes, such as creative

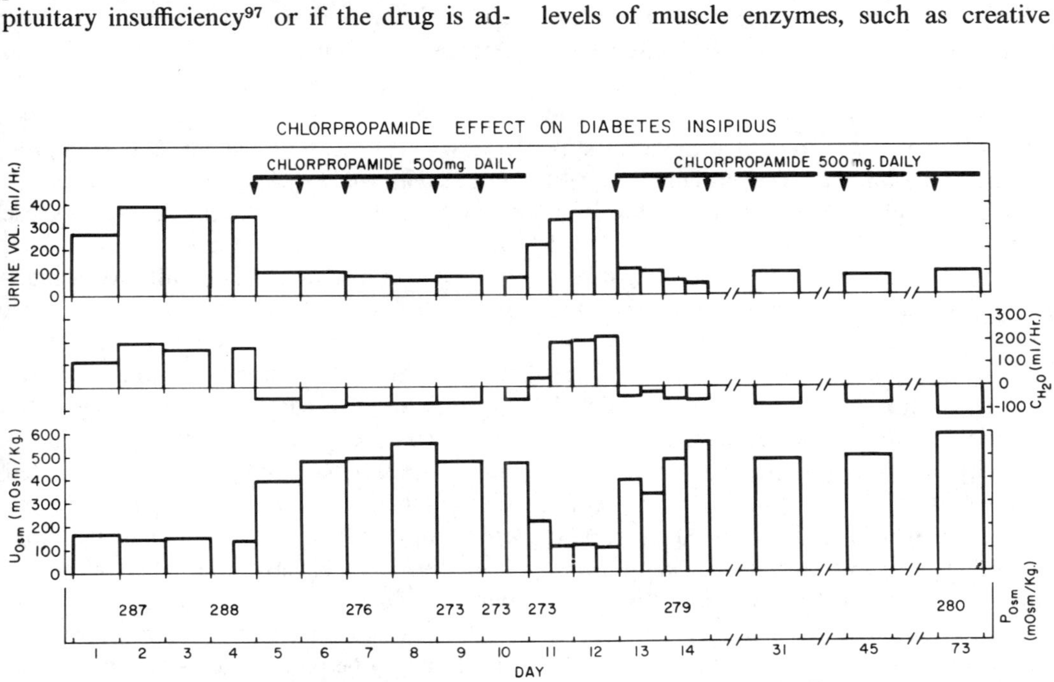

Fig. 18–14. Antidiuretic effect of chlorpropamide therapy in a patient with diabetes insipidus. Note that the antidiuresis was sufficient to cause plasma hypotonicity. (From Moses AM: Effects of sulfonylurea drugs on water metabolism. In Rifkin H (ed): Micronase (Glyburide), Pharmacological and Clinical Evaluation. Princeton, Excerpta Medica, 1975, p 105.)

phosphokinase, should be monitored, especially in patients who have hypothyroidism, a feature that favors development of myopathy.[104] Clofibrate may also increase the incidence of cholelithiasis[105] and has caused liver tumors in rodents.[106]

Carbamazepine is an effective treatment for many patients with diabetes insipidus.[107-110] The usual dose is 600 mg/day in divided doses, but less can be used if combined with other oral agents such as chlorpropamide.[111] In general, this drug has not been very popular for the oral treatment of diabetes insipidus because of the large variety and occasional severity of side effects. These reactions may involve many organ systems, including the neurologic, gastrointestinal, dermatologic, hematopoietic, cardiovascular, and genitourinary. The most severe side effect is aplastic anemia.

In general, diabetes insipidus that develops acutely after neurohypophyseal surgery or trauma should be monitored with urine volume and osmolality or specific gravity measurements hourly and treated with short-acting preparations such as aqueous vasopressin (Pitressin) as necessary (usually 5 U every 3 to 5 hours) to avoid both dehydration and overhydration. In chronic diabetes insipidus, intranasal desmopressin is usually the best drug. Frequency of doses is based on the duration of action of the drug in the patient being treated, as reflected by recurrence of polyuria and polydipsia when the action of the drug suddenly appears to be lost. There is generally no need to regulate fluid intake except to prevent overhydration when therapy is initiated. In patients whose diabetes insipidus is associated with a defective thirst, vasopressin should be given at the onset of polyuria; the intake of fluid should be recommended at regular intervals in known amounts defined by inhospital measurement of the volumes needed to maintain normal levels of plasma osmolality and body weight.

Patients with psychogenic polydipsia generally do not complain of polydipsia or polyuria, and treatment should be directed toward the underlying emotional condition. This problem is more important if the patient has a tendency toward dilutional hyponatremia because of heart failure or cirrhosis, or if the patient is being treated with water-retaining drugs (see Chapter 24). Patients with primary organic polydipsia may respond to various preparations of antidiuretic hormone. The effectiveness of antidiuretic hormone is probably due to the amelioration of thirst associated with increased salivary flow rate.[57]

SYNDROME OF INAPPROPRIATE ANTIDIURETIC HORMONE SECRETION

Clinical Features and Pathophysiology

Peters et al.[112] described a syndrome of cerebral salt wasting in patients with a variety of neurologic conditions. The original concept was that this syndrome resulted from ACTH deficiency or from central nervous system influences that impaired the kidney's ability to reabsorb salt. In fact, some cases may actually be due to renal salt wasting plus high plasma levels of ADH (see Chapter 21). However, subsequent studies classified the mechanism in most cases as being due to continual release of arginine vasopressin in spite of a subnormal plasma osmolality, that is, syndrome of inappropriate antidiuretic hormone secretion (SIADH). The classic features include hyponatremia and hypoosmolality of plasma, natriuresis, absence of edema or volume depletion, and normal renal, adrenal, and thyroid function. The urine is usually more concentrated than plasma, but when solute intake is markedly restricted, urine osmolality may be somewhat less than plasma osmolality, although never maximally dilute. Plasma or urinary arginine vasopressin levels may be clearly elevated or may be recognized as abnormal only in relation to the plasma osmolality.[113,114] The original concept of cerebral salt wasting may still apply to a selected group of hyponatremic patients who fulfill the laboratory criteria for

SIADH, but who also either have depleted intravascular volume[115] or a distal tubular abnormality that impairs the response to mineralocorticoid hormone (see Chapter 21).

In patients with SIADH, ingested fluids are retained, extracellular fluid volume is expanded, and dilutional hyponatremia develops. The dilutional hyponatremia is aggravated by several additional natriuretic mechanisms including suppression of renin and aldosterone secretion, as well as decrease in proximal tubular sodium reabsorption.[116,117] Because of the natriuresis, saline administration often fails to correct the hyponatremia unless the plasma volume is normalized by fluid restriction. This fact can be used diagnostically when the presence of SIADH is in doubt. In contrast with the prompt excretion of a sodium load in patients with SIADH, infused salt is retained when hyponatremia is due to volume depletion or edematous states. However, rare patients with SIADH who become markedly sodium depleted, as from persistent vomiting, may retain a sodium load until sodium depletion is corrected.[118] Marked sodium depletion can also decrease the characteristic natriuresis of SIADH.[118]

SIADH may result from or occur in association with many clinical disorders. The most common causes are malignant diseases, especially small cell or oat cell carcinomas of the lung. About two-thirds of patients with oat cell carcinoma have evidence of an impaired ability to excrete water, with the degree of impairment being related to the extent of malignant disease.[119] Malignant lung cells obtained from patients with SIADH are capable of synthesizing, storing, and releasing arginine vasopressin.[120] Chemical and biologic analyses of neoplasms have demonstrated arginine vasopressin identical to the hormone produced by the normal neurohypophyseal system.[120] In addition, vasopressin-associated neurophysin has been demonstrated in the blood and in the tumor tissue of patients with oat cell carcinoma.[121] Other malignancies associated with SIADH are carcinoma of the pancreas, duodenum,[116] and bladder,[122] lymphosarcoma, reticulum cell sarcoma,[123] Ewing's sarcoma,[124] Hodgkin's disease,[125] malignant histiocytosis,[126] and thymoma.[116] Some patients with SIADH due to tumor partially suppress arginine vasopressin release after water loading, possibly indicating a partial response of the neoplasms to this inhibitory stimulus.[114] It is possible that excess release of antidiuretic hormone from the neurohypophysis occurs in some of these patients.[114]

Nonmalignant pulmonary tissue possesses the capability to synthesize arginine vasopressin.[127] This may cause the hyponatremia that is a common feature of pulmonary tuberculosis. Arginine vasopressin is present in tuberculous lung tissue but not in uninvolved lung or in suspensions of tubercle bacilli.[127] Other pulmonary diseases that may be associated with SIADH are lung abscess, viral and bacterial pneumonia[128,129] and empyema.[130] SIADH may also occur in chronic obstructive disease, even when cardiac function is unimpaired. Hypercapnia and anoxemia may play a role in the excessive arginine vasopressin release.

Hyponatremia occurs in many patients with disorders of the central nervous system. Most of these patients have SIADH, but the possibility of the SIADH-like syndrome with decreased intravascular volume,[115] or of the low-set osmoreceptor mechanism,[1,131,132] must be borne in mind.

One of the most common causes of SIADH in patients with disorders of the central nervous system is craniofacial trauma. A recent review of 1808 patients admitted for this condition revealed a 4.6 percent incidence of SIADH, even though the patients were routinely fluid restricted.[133] The most common pathologic consequence of the trauma in these patients was chronic subdural hematoma. Other disorders of the central nervous system that cause SIADH include subarachnoid hemorrhage, cerebrovascular thrombosis, pituitary adenoma, hydrocephalus, and cerebral atrophy.[116,134] Acute encephalitis[135,136] and other infectious and inflammatory diseases of the central nervous system, such as tuberculous meningitis and purulent meningitis, may be accompanied by SIADH. Patients with Guillain-Barré syndrome,[116] lupus erythematosus,[137] and acute intermittent porphyria[138] may have hyponatremia due to SIADH. Acute psychosis,[139] physical and emotional stress,[140] and pain may also cause SIADH.

There is no clear mechanism to explain the SIADH in all patients with neurologic disease. However, there is evidence in monkeys that increased intracranial pressure can increase antidiuretic hormone release, and that under these circumstances antidiuretic hormone release is no longer inhibited by serum hypotonicity.[141]

Several drugs (other than antidiuretic hormone, its analogues, and oxytocin) may cause water retention and SIADH (Fig. 18–15). These drugs include sedatives, hypnotics, diuretics, nonsteroidal antiinflammatory agents, and a variety of other agents the actions of which are described in some detail in Chapter 24.

Symptoms of SIADH depend on both the severity of the hyponatremia and the rate at which it develops. Patients may have anorexia, followed frequently by nausea and sometimes by vomiting. Patients may become irritable, uncooperative, and confused. Lethargy, weakness, muscle cramps, extrapyramidal signs, convulsions, and coma may follow (see Chapter 23). Weight gain may be noted, but edema is rare. EEG changes may be present but are nonspecific. Symptoms of the hyponatremia usually improve shortly after its correction. However, symptoms may persist in some patients for as long as a week after correction of the electrolyte imbalance, and some patients may have permanent mental changes (see Chapter 21).

Diagnosis

The initial clue to the presence of SIADH is usually hyponatremia without evidence of edema, hypovolemia, or dehydration. In addi-

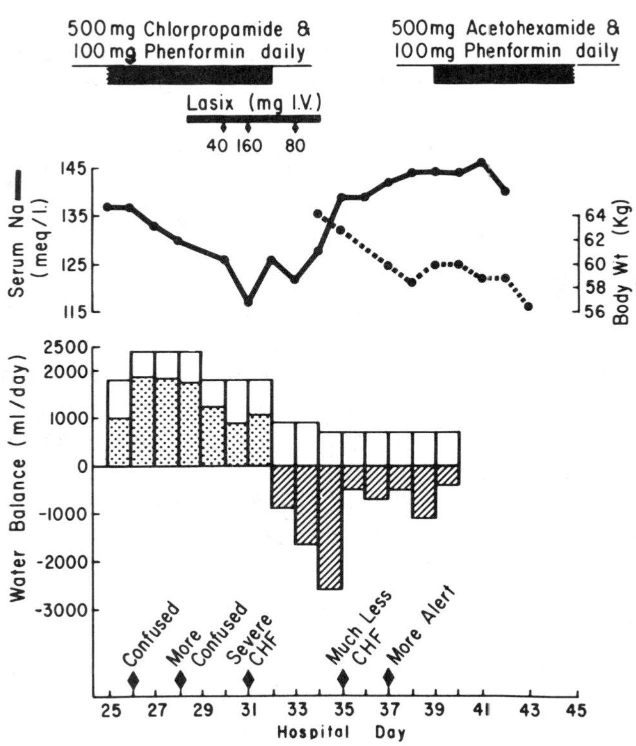

Fig. 18–15. Data on an elderly woman with congestive heart failure while being treated with chlorpropamide. During the course of treatment, progressive hyponatremia developed from water retention, causing a worsening clinical picture. After the drug was discontinued, prompt diuresis and weight loss occurred, as well as correction of hyponatremia in association with marked clinical improvement. (From Garcia M, Miller, M, Moses AM: Chlorpropamide-induced water retention in patients with diabetes mellitus. Ann Intern Med 75:549, 1971.)

tion to hyponatremia and hypoosmolality, patients often have low serum levels of urea nitrogen, uric acid, creatinine, and albumin. Urine osmolality usually excedes that of plasma. Urinary sodium concentrations >20 mEq/liter support the diagnosis of SIADH, although in the presence of extreme sodium depletion natriuresis may disappear.[116,118]

The definitive diagnosis of SIADH is, in a sense, based on eliminating the presence of other hyponatremic conditions. It is not the purpose of this chapter to review the differential diagnosis of hyponatremia (see Chapter 5). However, the various causes must be considered before SIADH is diagnosed; indeed, many of the hyponatremias, including the hypovolemic and edematous states, glucocorticoid deficiency, hypothyroidism, and some cases of low-set osmoreceptor syndrome, are caused in part by excessive circulating antidiuretic hormone.[25,142–144] However, these conditions should not be categorized as SIADH, as other factors contribute to the pathogenesis of their hyponatremia, and specific therapy should be directed toward the underlying diseases. The hyponatremia of Rocky Mountain spotted fever is a good example of a hypovolemic state that is easily confused with SIADH.[145]

Patients who have the laboratory features listed above who do not have other definable causes of hyponatremia and who do not have severe pain, hypotension, or other exogenous or nonosmotic stimuli that may cause release of arginine vasopressin can be considered to have SIADH particularly if they fail to excrete a water load properly. The failure to excrete a water load normally is of greatest value in differentiating patients with SIADH from those chronically ill patients with the sick cell syndrome or low-set osmoreceptor.[146] Water loading may be dangerous if the serum sodium concentration is <125 mEq/liter. The test is performed by administering a 20-ml/kg oral water load over 15 to 20 minutes with urine collected hourly for the next 4 hours while the patient is recumbent. A normal response is indicated by the excretion of more than 65 percent of the water by the end of 4 hours, with the urine osmolality falling to <100 mOsm/kg during the test. In some difficult cases, an evaluation of the relationship between plasma osmolality and plasma or urinary arginine vasopressin may help establish the diagnosis of SIADH.[114] However, many hyponatremic conditions other than classic SIADH have abnormal relationships between plasma osmolality and vasopressin. For instance, plasma arginine vasopressin is elevated in hyponatremic patients with extracellular volume depletion[147] and with cardiac failure and hepatic cirrhosis.[148,149] There is no way to avoid the conclusion that the diagnosis of SIADH must be based on an understanding and application of all the physiologic and pathologic factors involved in the release of arginine vasopressin.

Treatment

Definitive treatment must be directed toward eliminating the underlying problem. Water-retaining drugs should be replaced by agents that do not have this adverse side effect. Treatment of lung abscesses, pneumonia, or pulmonary tuberculosis with appropriate antimicrobial therapy results in gradual clearing of SIADH. In patients with SIADH due to malignancy, surgical resection, irradiation, or chemotherapy may be successful in alleviating water retention. Sometimes these measures should be carried out even when the malignancy cannot be cured, since treatment may correct life-threatening water intoxication and prevent the necessity for rigid fluid restriction. The disappearance of SIADH in these patients may be an indication of the success of the treatment.[119] Periodic water-loading tests may provide evidence of recurrent malignancy.

Patients with mild or moderate symptoms related to hyponatremia and water intoxication should have fluid intake restricted to ~600 to 800 ml/day. With this intake, urinary and insensible water losses usually result in a negative water balance. If water restriction is adequate, serum sodium and osmolality increase as body weight decreases. Patients with severe symptoms must be treated more vigorously. This is usually necessary only when the patient is symptomatic and serum sodium concentration is <120 mEq/liter, particularly if the development of the hyponatremia was acute. The intravenous administration of 515 mM (3 percent) NaCl solution at a rate calculated to raise the serum sodium by ~2 mEq/liter·hr to 130 mEq/liter constitutes appropriate therapy (see Chapter 21). Oral and parenteral fluids must continue to be restricted. Hypokalemia, when present, should be treated. Mild hypocalcemia is usually present but causes no symptoms and requires no specific therapy. The administration of furosemide along with saline has been advocated as a rapid means of treating patients with SIADH who are symptomatic with marked hyponatremia.[150] When furosemide is used, care must be taken to prevent the depletion of potassium and other electrolytes. There is evidence that the administration of urea to patients with SIADH may correct the sodium-losing tendency and, together with the osmotic diuresis, help resolve the hyponatremia.[151] The hyponatremia in some patients with SIADH may also be improved with desoxycorticosterone.[152] Once the hyponatremia has been improved, careful fluid restriction is necessary to prevent the recurrence of water intoxication.

No drugs are currently available to suppress arginine vasopressin release from malignant tumors. Diphenylhydantoin inhibits neurohypophyseal arginine vasopressin release acutely and was effective in the long-term treatment of one patient with SIADH due to skull fracture.[153] Several narcotic antagonists inhibit antidiuretic hormone release from the neurohypophysis of animals, and raise the osmotic threshold for vasopressin release in humans.[76] Their role in the treatment of SIADH remains to be determined in spite of success reported in two cases[76] (Fig. 18–16).

Lithium salts cause polyuria by interfering with the renal action of antidiuretic hormone and have thus been used for the treatment of SIADH.[154,155] Although such treatment may be effective in overcoming the effects of excessive antidiuretic hormone action, lithium may have serious toxicity, especially in patients with hyponatremia. The antibiotic demeclocycline also interferes with the renal action of antidiuretic hormone. This drug has

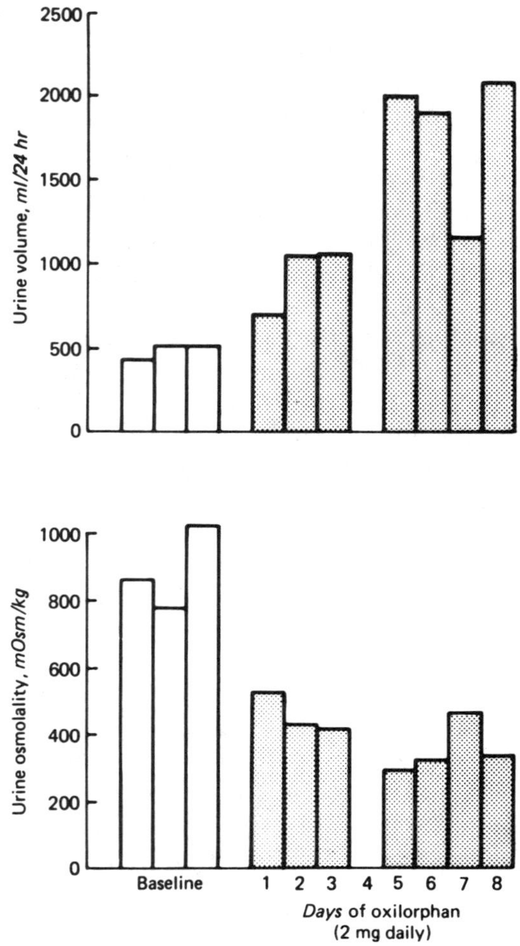

Fig. 18–16. Response to treatment with the narcotic antagonist oxilorphan in a 26-year-old man with chronic syndrome of inappropriate antidiuretic hormone secretion (SIADH) due to head trauma. During the 8 days of drug treatment there was a progressive increase in urine volume and decrease in urine osmolality. (Reprinted from Kidney International. Miller M, Moses AM: Drug-induced states of impaired water excretion. Kidney Int 10:96, 1976.)

been used successfully in the management of patients with SIADH[156] and may be more effective than lithium.[157] However, acute renal failure has been observed in patients with SIADH and cirrhosis who were treated with demeclocycline.[158,159] Fortunately, this complication usually disappears rapidly after discontinuation of the drug. Thus, demeclocycline in doses of 900 to 1,200 mg/day is often a useful adjunct in the management of patients with SIADH when fluid restriction is difficult and definitive therapy cannot be accomplished (Fig. 18–17). However, these patients must be carefully observed for evidence of renal failure, bacterial superinfection, and the development of dehydration and volume depletion. More specific means of inhibiting the action of arginine vasopressin will have to await the clinical application of aquaretics, which are vasopressin analogues that act to inhibit the antidiuretic action of arginine vasopressin.[160]

ELECTROLYTE AND WATER DISORDERS IN ADENOHYPOPHYSEAL DISEASE

Adenohypophyseal disease may affect body content and distribution of Na, K, and water through changes in the secretion of corticotropin and/or thyrotropin. Electrolyte effects of changes in the production of other pituitary hormones are seldom of clinical significance. The two important electrolyte manifestations of adenohypophyseal disease are hyponatremia and hypokalemia.

Hyponatremia in Adenohypophyseal Disease

Serum sodium concentration is usually normal in patients with mild pituitary disease, but hyponatremia may occur in the presence

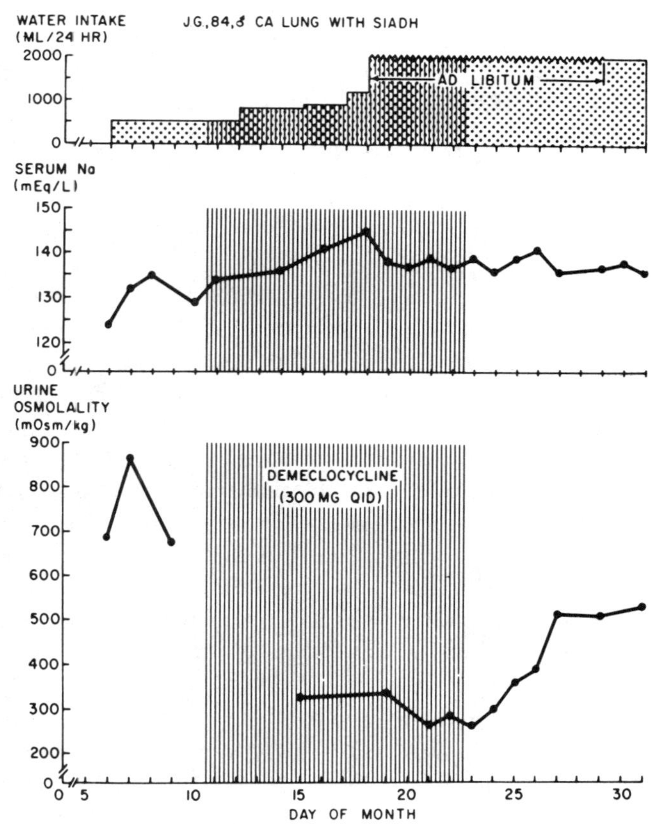

Fig. 18–17. Response to demeclocycline of a patient with syndrome of inappropriate antidiuretic hormone secretion (SIADH) due to lung carcinoma. Serum sodium became normal in 5 days and was maintained at a normal level without fluid restriction (From Moses AM, Miller M, Streeter DHP: Pathophysiologic and pharmacologic alteration in the release and action of ADH. Metabolism 25:697, 1976.)

of severe hypopituitarism,[161-164] mediated by glucocorticoid deficiency, hypothyroidism and/or concomitantly inappropriate antidiuretic hormone excess (SIADH). In patients with panhypopituitarism, hyponatremia is particularly likely to occur when sodium intake is reduced, or when sodium losses are increased by diuretic therapy or by diarrhea. Five of eight patients with hypopituitarism, studied on a 10-mEq sodium diet became hyponatremic.[161]

Hyponatremia (serum Na <125 mEq/liter) resulting from any cause may be manifested by a characteristic clinical syndrome:

1. Gastrointestinal symptoms (anorexia, nausea, and vomiting)
2. Cerebral features (malaise, lethargy, somnolence, confusion, stupor, coma, and convulsive seizures)
3. Muscular weakness and cramps

When the hyponatremia results predominantly from glucocorticoid deficiency rather than from hypothyroidism or SIADH, it is associated with hypovolemic manifestations, mediated by orthostatic hypotension: lightheadedness and palpitations in the upright posture, fainting spells, weakness, and fatigue.

GLUCOCORTICOID DEFICIENCY

The principal glucocorticoid in humans is hydrocortisone (cortisol), but small amounts of corticosterone are also secreted by the human adrenal. In rats, and most other rodents, corticosterone is the only glucocorticoid secreted in significant amounts. While most of the physiologic actions of cortisol and corticosterone are the result of their effects on glucocorticoid receptors, it should be recognized that these steroids do have some affinity for mineralocorticoid receptors through which they may have aldosteronelike actions.[165] This is particularly true of corticosterone, which has greater affinity than cortisol for mineralocorticoid receptors.

Effects of Cortisol Deficiency on Water Excretion

Adrenal insufficiency impairs the excretion of a water load[166-169] mainly because of cortisol deficiency, but probably also, to a minor extent, because of mineralocorticoid deficiency. The latter is present in some but not all patients with hypopituitarism and may result in extracellular fluid hypovolemia, stimulating antidiuretic hormone excess.[170-172] Although hypoadrenalism decreases the glomerular filtration rate, reduction in the glomerular filtration rate is far less important in impairing water excretion than are the associated abnormalities of renal tubular function.[168] Cortisol reduces proximal tubular reabsorption of sodium,[173] and cortisol deficiency increases Na reabsorption at this site, thereby decreasing the delivery of filtered Na to the diluting segment of the nephron. Thus, free water formation is diminished. However, the main effect of cortisol deficiency on water excretion occurs at the collecting tubule, where there is excessive permeability to water.[174,175] Since such an increase in distal tubular permeability to water is also seen in vasopressin excess, the possibility that this major mechanism of impaired water excretion might result from excessive vasopressin action has long been suspected.[167,176] Ahmed et al.[177] reported elevated blood levels of vasopressin, measured by bioassay, in adrenal insufficiency, and their observations have been widely confirmed by radioimmunoassay.[178-181] It seems likely that these elevated plasma vasopressin concentrations, which fail to fall after a water load, contribute significantly to the defect in water excretion in adrenal insufficiency. Thus, water excretion can almost be completely restored to normal by an antagonist of the hydroosmotic action of vasopressin in adrenalectomized rats[172] and is not even significantly impaired after 24 hours' glucocorticoid deficiency in homozygous Brattleboro rats with hereditary hypothalamic diabetes insipidus.[181] However, vasopressin excess is certainly not by any means the entire mechanism of the abnormal water excretion in chronic hypoadrenalism. Green et al.[182] have shown that the defects in water excretion after adrenalectomy are almost as severe in Brattleboro rats as in rats with normal vasopressin production. Restoration of normal excretion to adrenalectomized Brattleboro rats required not only glucocorticoid (prednisolone) administration, which alone increased urine flow rates to normal but failed to restore normal urinary diluting capacity, but mineralocorticoid (aldosterone) therapy as well, which improved flow rates insignificantly, but increased diluting capacity to normal.[182] Similar results were obtained in studies on adrenalectomized dogs.[183] Whether normal mineralocorticoid action is essential for the restoration of a normal excretory response to a water load in humans is unknown, but urinary flow rates are certainly normalized by cortisol alone in human subjects with adrenal insufficiency.[167,169] Glucocorticoids have pronounced natriuretic effects in adrenalectomized rats,[184] which are difficult to demonstrate in human subjects, but which probably account for the failure of free water clearance to increase normally during the excretion of a water load in glucocorticoid-treated adrenalectomized rats.

The mechanism whereby adrenal insufficiency increases vasopressin release has not been unequivocally determined. It may result from lack of the effect of glucocorticoids in raising the osmotic threshold for vasopressin release,[23] which in turn might be related to the extracellular dehydration and excessive intracellular hydration characteristic of adrenal insufficiency.[169,185–188]

Effects of Cortisol Deficiency on Sodium Excretion

Cortisol has important effects on renal excretion of sodium. Proximal tubular reabsorption of filtered sodium is reduced by cortisol, thus making more Na available for reabsorption and free water generation in the loop of Henle.[173] Large doses of cortisone and cortisol (~100 mg) cause retention of sodium in humans,[189,190] presumably because of effects on mineralocorticoid receptors in the loop of Henle or the distal tubule. Whether smaller amounts of cortisol might actually potentiate renal Na excretion in humans, as seen in the adrenalectomized rat,[184] is not clear. However, certain glucocorticoids, particularly triamcinolone, betamethasone, and 6-methylprednisolone, lack a consistent Na-retaining action[191] and may actually increase sodium excretion, leading to sodium depletion in human subjects.

Effects of Glucocorticoids on Distribution of Body Na and Water

In a series of experiments on adrenalectomized dogs, Swingle et al.[186,192] showed that steroids with glucocorticoid action (prednisolone) or with glucocorticoid and mineralocorticoid effects (2-methyl, 9α-fluorohydrocortisone) but not with mineralocorticoid action alone (deoxycorticosterone, aldosterone), would rapidly correct the severe hyponatremia, hyperkalemia, hypovolemia, hypotension, hemoconcentration, oliguria, and prerenal azotemia associated with profound adrenal insufficiency.

Dramatic correction of these abnormalities was accomplished by merely injecting the steroid, and without administering food, electrolytes, or fluids. These important observations provide seemingly incontrovertible evidence that glucocorticoid deficiency causes translocation of sodium and water out of the extracellular compartment, presumably into the cells, while glucocorticoid therapy reverses these shifts. Similar evidence of the maldistribution of Na and water and the excessive cellular hydration in adrenal insufficiency in rats has been adduced by Hegnauer and Robinson[188] and Frost and Talmage.[187] Only very limited information is available on the effects of glucocorticoids and mineralocorticoids on the distribution of Na and water in the human organism. Administration of a water load to patients with untreated adrenal insufficiency results in excessive erythrocyte swelling, resulting from entry of the administered water into these (and presumably other) cells.[169] This intracellular overhydration in patients with adrenal insufficiency can be prevented and corrected by the administration of cortisone.

THYROID HORMONE DEFICIENCY

Although hyponatremia is not a common feature of hypothyroidism, it is the major electrolyte abnormality which occurs in this disorder.[193-199] In rare instances, the reduction of serum sodium may be extreme. Thus, in a survey of 24 cases of hyponatremia and myxedema published between 1953 and 1979, serum sodium concentrations ranged from a high value of 129 mEq/liter to a low value of 103 mEq/liter.[200]

Hyponatremia in anterior pituitary disease is generally associated with ACTH deficiency.[161,201] It has not been reported in patients with isolated thyroid-stimulating hormone deficiency.[201-203] Nevertheless, pituitary hypothyroidism can seriously impair the excretion of a water load, thus increasing the risk of dilutional hyponatremia in commonly encountered clinical situations, for example, diuretic therapy, heart failure, and renal insufficiency.[144]

The hyponatremia of hypothyroidism is considered dilutional because total body sodium is increased.[204,205] Clinical observation supports this view. In response to the initiation of thyroid hormone replacement in patients with myxedema, renal plasma flow and glomerular filtration rate rapidly increase toward normal, a brisk diuresis of water and sodium occurs, and serum sodium concentration tends to rise.[204,206,207] Since blood volume is decreased in thyroid-deficient states, it must be assumed that the excess sodium is retained in an extravascular compartment.[208,209] One suggestion is that it is bound to extracellular mucopolysaccharide and is therefore unavailable for renal excretion.[210]

The pathogenesis of sodium retention in hypothyroidism not complicated by heart failure is still far from clear. One possibility is that renal plasma flow and glomerular filtration rate are sufficiently reduced to permit virtually complete reabsorption of the filtered sodium load.[211-213] Another possibility is that proximal tubular sodium reabsorption is enhanced under the stimulus of a contracted blood volume. Whatever the cause(s) of sodium retention, counterregulatory mechanisms eventually restore normal sodium balance. This explains why hypothyroid patients fail to gain weight on a high-salt diet and appear to have no difficulty excreting an intravenous salt load.[209,214]

Several animal studies have suggested that hypothyroidism interferes with sodium conservation because it deprives the renal tubules of the direct antinatriuretic action of thyroid hormone. Taylor and Fregly[215] reported that hypothyroid (propylthiouracil-treated) rats fed a salt-poor diet excreted excessive amounts of sodium after water or saline loading. The natriuresis was not abolished by administration of desoxycorticosterone acetate or aldosterone. Bradley et al.[216] demonstrated a significant degree of glomerulotubular imbalance (i.e., normal glomeruli, shortened proximal tubules) in microdissected nephrons from medically thyroidectomized (^{131}I-treated) rats and suggested that this was the morphologic basis for Taylor's observation. In a similar animal model, Holmes and DiScala[217] reported exaggerated natriuresis in response to 5 percent saline infusion, and Michael et al.,[218] employing both micropuncture techniques and standard clearance measurements, found impairment of proximal tubular sodium reabsorption. It is doubtful, however, that these disturbances in renal function, which would tend to cause sodium depletion, are relevant to the pathogenesis of the dilutional hyponatremia seen in hypothyroid patients.

A recent review discusses the possibility that the hyponatremia of hypothyroidism may be related to intracellular accumulation of sodium.[219] This is based on the findings of

Edelman and Ismail-Beigi that administration of triiodothyronine to hypothyroid or euthyroid rats significantly lowered intracellular Na^+/K^+ ratios in liver, diaphragm, and heart.[220] Presumably, triiodothyronine augmented the activity of Na–K-ATPase in these tissues. It is unlikely, however, that sequestration of sodium in cells could account for the hyponatremia associated with hypothyroidism. If sodium were to accumulate intracellularly as a consequence of thyroid deficiency, osmotic equilibrium would soon be restored by the transfer of water into cells. The ultimate result would be an increase in cell volume rather than hyponatremia.

Water retention is the principal cause of hyponatremia in thyroprival states. In this regard, studies of hypothyroid patients have documented: (1) reduction in renal plasma flow and glomerular filtration rate; and (2) functional defects indicative of impaired renal water excretion (e.g., diminished free water clearance, failure to achieve maximal urinary dilution, and delayed excretion of a water load).[221-224] The latter findings have been attributed to nonhormonal alterations in the handling of water by the kidneys and/or to the antidiuretic action of inappropriately elevated plasma vasopressin levels.

Role of Renal Mechanisms in Water Retention

Emmanouel et al.[225] investigated water metabolism in surgically or medically thyroidectomized rats with reduced clearances of inulin, free water, and sodium. When distal delivery of sodium was augmented by intravenous infusion of a carbonic anhydrase inhibitor or by removal of one kidney, free water clearance was greatly increased. These results were taken to mean that the major cause of diminished water excretion in hypothyroidism is a reduction in glomerular filtration rate that limits the delivery of glomerular filtrate to the distal diluting segment. This conclusion is consistent with the potent diuretic action of thyroid hormone in hypothyroid patients. Table 18–6 illustrates this action.[221]

Role of Vasopressin Excess in Water Retention

Schrier and Goldberg[226] have suggested that severe hypothyroidism stimulates vasopressin secretion through baroreceptor pathways (i.e., by reducing cardiac output). The evidence that elevated plasma vasopressin levels contribute

Table 18–6. Comparative Data in 11 Myxedematous Subjects Before and After Thyroid Hormone Therapy

	Subjects		
Data	Myxedematous	Treated Myxedematous	*p*
Creatinine clearance (ml/min)	66.1 ± 5.3	76.3 ± 4.5	<0.005
Sodium (mEq/liter)	136.3 ± 1.3	141.0 ± 1.2	<0.01
Weight (kg)	72.6 ± 5.7	67.1 ± 5.0	<0.01
Percent water excreted hours after ingestion			
Hour 2	44.1 ± 7.2	80.5 ± 9.8	<0.01
Hour 3	60.6 ± 9.3	100.1 ± 12.5	<0.025
Hour 4	77.5 ± 10.3	110.8 ± 11.9	<0.025

Source: Reproduced with permission from De Rubertis FR, Michelis MF, Bloom ME, et al: Impaired water excretion in myxedema. Am J Med 51:41, 1971.

to water retention in hypothyroidism can be summarized as follows:

1. Some hyponatremic myxedematous patients have fulfilled the diagnostic criteria for the syndrome of inappropriate vasopressin secretion (SIADH), that is, normal pituitary–adrenal axis, normal renal function, absence of heart failure or liver disease, low serum osmolality in conjunction with a high urine osmolality, and natriuresis in the face of hyponatremia.[196,227,228]

2. In the patient described by Goldberg and Reivich,[228] administration of ethanol, a known inhibitor of vasopressin secretion, caused transient dilution of the urine.

3. Skowsky et al.[144,229] found elevated plasma vasopressin levels in a group of hypothyroid patients and a 10-fold increase in vasopressin production rates in thyroidectomized sheep (see Table 18–7).

It should be emphasized that the evidence supporting an etiologic role for SIADH in the hyponatremia of hypothyroidism is not entirely persuasive. The inconclusive nature of this evidence can be illustrated by several citations from the literature.

1. Clinical data in the patient reported by Curtis (urinary sodium concentration 2.8 mEq/liter, serum sodium concentration 105 mEq/liter) and in the patient reported by Kiode et al. (serum sodium 115 mEq/liter, plasma vasopressin concentration immeasurably low) indicate that SIADH is not invariably present, even in severe myxedema.[193,199]

2. Goldberg's finding that ethanol permitted the elaboration of urine hypotonic to plasma in one hypothyroid patient with SIADH could not be duplicated in six hypothyroid patients studied by Lohavichan et al.[230]

3. Emmanouel et al.[225] found an increase in free water clearance in hypothyroid Brattleboro (vasopressin-deficient) rats when distal sodium delivery was increased by a carbonic anhydrase inhibitor.

4. In the study by Skowsky and Kikuchi,[144] individual patients showed a poor correlation between plasma vasopressin levels and the efficiency with which a water load was excreted. Patient 5 was one of the poorest water excretors among the 20 patients reported by Skowski (24.8 percent of the water load excreted in 4 hours), but nevertheless had a relatively normal plasma vasopressin concentration (2.7

Table 18–7. Blood Half-time, Volume of Distribution, Serum Concentration, and Production Rate of Arginine Vasopressin, and Serum Osmolality in Euthyroid and Thyroidectomized Sheep

Sheep	Weight (kg)	Serum Osmolality (mosml/kg)	Blood $t_{1/2}$ (min)	Volume of Distribution (liters)	Arginine Vasopressin Concn. (μU/ml)	AVP Production Rate	
						mU/hr	mU/kg·hr
Euthyroid							
E-1	60	298	19.1	6.33	0.9	12.4	0.21
E-2	68	301	19.8	5.65	1.2	14.2	0.21
E-3	64	303	18.9	5.72	1.4	17.6	0.28
Mean	64.0	301	19.3	5.90	1.2	14.7	0.23
SEM	2.3	1.5	0.3	0.22	0.1	1.5	0.02
Thyroidectomized							
T-1	60	263	12.4	7.11	6.0	140.6	2.34
T-2	67	282	7.9	8.92	5.1	241.9	3.61
T-3	64	271	10.0	7.75	6.1	192.9	3.01
T-4	58	268	8.2	8.84	3.2	139.4	2.40
T-5	65	274	8.8	8.21	4.9	185.6	2.86
Mean	62.8	272	9.5	8.15	5.1	180.1	2.84
SEM	1.7	3.2	0.8	0.33	0.5	19.0	0.3

Source: Reproduced with permission from Skowsky WR, Fisher DA: Arginine vasopressin secretion in thyroidectomized sheep. Endocrinology 100:1022, 1977.

μU/ml). On the other hand, patients 15 and 18 (respective plasma vasopressin levels, 11.6 μU/ml and 12.5 μU/ml) showed excellent responses to water loading (cummulative 4-hour water excretion 88.2 percent and 80.6 percent, respectively).

The degree to which vasopressin excess contributes to water retention in hypothyroidism could be readily determined if we possessed a selective inhibitor of the antidiuretic action of vasopressin. Such inhibitors have already been administered to experimental animals and may become available for clinical use in the future.[160]

THERAPY OF HYPONATREMIA IN HYPOPITUITARISM

Replacement therapy with hydrocortisone or other glucocorticoids will usually restore serum Na concentration to the normal range within several hours or 2 to 3 days.[161–163] If serum Na is very low (<115 mEq/liter) and associated with coma or convulsions, a slow infusion of 515 mM (3 percent) saline solution (see Chapter 21) will accelerate the return of the serum Na concentration toward normal.

When hypothyroidism is severe and might be contributing to the hyponatremia, it should be treated with gradually increasing doses of l-thyroxine. An excellent symptomatic response is the usual result of appropriate therapy.

Hypokalemia in Adenohypophyseal Disease

The main circumstances in which adenohypophyseal disease may result in hypokalemia is in association with Cushing's syndrome. Hypokalemia is a common feature of hypercortisolism and may be associated with a reduction in exchangeable body potassium. Its clinical manifestations are probably limited to the muscular weakness and fatigue, which are well-known features of Cushing's syndrome.

PATHOPHYSIOLOGY

There are no definitive data on the cellular mechanisms whereby excessive plasma cortisol concentrations lead to hypokalemia. Presumably either or both of two mechanisms might be operative:

1. Very high plasma and tissue concentrations of cortisol, probably acting through the mineralocorticoid receptors in the renal tubule,[165] result in excessive potassium excretion.[189–191] The consequent losses of potassium cause hypokalemia and reduction of cellular potassium. Skeletal muscle weakness is one obvious consequence, but potassium depletion probably has adverse effects as well on the function of the brain, the myocardium, and other cellular tissues.
2. The antianabolic action of high concentrations of cortisol results in reduction of cellular protein and potassium content of the muscle and probably of most other body tissues.[165,191] These compositional changes would be expected to reduce strength and impair function of the affected tissues.

Appropriate therapy of the underlying hypercortisolism will always reverse the potassium depletion and hypokalemia, as well as the deleterious effects of these abnormalities within a few weeks. Before the beneficial effects of therapy of the hypercortisolism become apparent, potassium supplementation is advisable.

ACKNOWLEDGMENT

This work was supported by grant RR-229 from the General Clinical Research Centers Program of the Division of Research Resources of the National Institutes of Health.

REFERENCES

1. Robertson GL, Aycinena P, Zerbe RL: Neurogenic disorders of osmoregulation. Am J Med 72:339, 1982
2. Scheer RL, Raisz LG, Lloyd CW: Changes in diabetes insipidus during pregnancy and lactation. J Clin Endocrinol Metab 19:805, 1959
3. Cates JE, Garrod O: The effect of nicotine on urinary flow in diabetes insipidus. Clin Sci 10:145, 1951
4. Dingman JF, Benirschke K, Thorn GW: Studies of neurohypophyseal function in man. Diabetes insipidus and psychogenic polydipsia. Am J Med 23:226, 1957
5. Van Slyck EJ, Jurgensen JC, Cargill JW: Diabetes insipidus complicating thrombotic thrombocytopenic purpura. JAMA 209:768, 1969
6. Veldhuis JD, Hammond JM: Endocrine function after spontaneous infarction of the human pituitary: Report, review, and reappraisal. Endocrinol Rev 1:100, 1980
7. Schwartz AR, Leddy AL: Recognition of diabetes insipidus in postpartum hypopituitarism. Obstet Gynecol 59:394, 1982
8. Baylis PH, Milles JJ, London DR, et al: Postpartum cranial diabetes insipidus. Br Med J 280:20, 1980
9. Haynes BF, Fauci AS: Diabetes insipidus associated with Wegener's granulomatosis successfully treated with cyclophosphamide. N Engl J Med 299:764, 1978
10. Kelly PM: Systemic blastomycosis with associated diabetes insipidus. Ann Intern Med 96:66, 1982
11. Helbock H, Krivit W, Nesbit ME Jr: Patterns of anti- diuretic function in diabetes insipidus caused by histiocytosis X. J Lab Clin Med 78:194, 1971
12. Balestrieri FJ, Chernow B, Rainey TG: Postcraniotomy diabetes insipidus. Who's at risk? Crit Care Med 10:108, 1982
13. László FA, de Weid D: Antidiuretic hormone content of the hypothalamo-neurohypophysial system and urinary excretion of antidiuretic hormone in rats during the development of diabetes insipidus after lesions in the pituitary stalk. J Endocrinol 36:125, 1966
14. Manelfe C, Louvet JP: Computed tomography in diabetes insipidus. J Comput Assist Tomogr 3:309, 1979
15. Blotner H: Primary or idiopathic diabetes insipidus: A system disease. Metabolism 7:191, 1958
16. Braverman LE, Mancini JP, McGoldrick DM: Hereditary idiopathic diabetes insipidus. A case report with autopsy findings. Ann Intern Med 63:503, 1965
17. Scherbaum WA, Bottazzo GF, Slater JDH: Autoantibodies to vasopressin-producing cells of human hypothalamus in idiopathic diabetes insipidus. (Abst.) Program of the 64th Annual Meeting of the Endocrine Society, San Francisco, June 1982
18. Legros JJ, Crabbe J: Serum neurophysins in familial central diabetes insipidus. J Clin Endocrinol Metab 47:1065, 1978
19. Bretz GW, Baghdassarian A, Graber JD, et al: Coexistence of diabetes mellitus and insipidus and optic atrophy in two male siblings. Am J Med 48:398, 1970
20. Gossain VV, Sugawara M, Hagen GA: Coexistent diabetes mellitus and diabetes insipidus, a familial disease. J Clin Endocrinol Metab 41:1020, 1975
21. Notman DD, Mortek MA, Moses AM: Permanent diabetes insipidus following head trauma: Observations on ten patients and an approach to diagnosis. J Trauma 20:599, 1980
22. Moses AM, Gabrilove JL, Soffer LJ: Simplified water loading test in hypoadrenocorticism and hypothyroidism. J Clin Endocrinol Metab 18:1413, 1958
23. Aubry RH, Nankin HR, Moses AM, et al: Measurement of the osmotic threshold for vasopressin release in human subjects, and its modification by cortisol. J Clin Endocrinol Metab 25:1481, 1965
24. Moses AM, Miller M: Osmotic influences on the release of vasopressin. P. 225. In Greep RO, Astwood EB, Knobil E, et al. (eds): Handbook of Physiology. Sect. 7: Endocrinology. Vol. IV: The Pituitary Gland and Its Neuroendocrine Control. Part 1. American Physiological Society, Washington, DC, 1974
25. Quintanilla AP, Delgado-Butron C, Zeballos J: Renal hemodynamics and water excretion in Addison's disease. Metabolism 25:419, 1976

26. Boykin J, de Torrenté A, Erickson A, et al: Role of plasma vasopressin in impaired water excretion of glucocorticoid deficiency. J Clin Invest 62:738, 1978
27. Savino PJ, Glaser JS, Schatz NJ: Traumatic chiasmal syndrome. Neurology (NY) 30:963, 1980
28. Barreca T, Perria C, Sannia A, et al: Evaluation of anterior pituitary function in patients with posttraumatic diabetes insipidus. J Clin Endocrinol Metab 51:1279, 1980
29. Taubin H, Matz R: Cerebral edema, diabetes insipidus, and sudden death during the treatment of diabetic ketoacidosis. Diabetes 17:108, 1968
30. Machiedo G, Bolanowski PJP, Bauer J, et al: Diabetes insipidus secondary to penetrating thoracic trauma. Ann Surg 181:31, 1975
31. Moyson F: Anoxie cérébrale et diabète insipide après inhalation d'un corps étranger chez l'enfant. Ann Chir Infant 16:241, 1975
32. Glauser FL: Diabetes insipidus in hypoxemic encephalopathy. JAMA 235:932, 1976
33. Rothschild M, Shenkman L: Diabetes insipidus following cardiorespiratory arrest. JAMA 238:620, 1977
34. Parisi JE, Kim RC, Collins GH, et al: Brain death with prolonged somatic survival. N Engl J Med 306:14, 1982
35. Winnacker JL, Becker KL, Katz S: Endocrine aspects of sarcoidosis. N Engl J Med 278:427, 1968
36. Bruning PF, Koster HG, Hekster REM, et al: Sarcoidosis presenting with diabetes insipidus followed by acute cranial nerve syndrome. Acta Med Scand 205:441, 1979
37. Panitz F, Shinaberger JH: Nephrogenic diabetes insipidus due to sarcoidosis without hypercalcemia. Ann Intern Med 62:113, 1965
38. Stuart CA, Neelon FA, Lebovitz HE: Disordered control of thirst in hypothalamic–pituitary sarcoidosis. N Engl J Med 303:1078, 1980
39. Betkerur U, Shende A, Lanzkowsky P: Acute myeloblastic leukemia presenting with diabetes insipidus. Am J Med Sci 273:325, 1977
40. Kornberg A, Zimmerman J, Matzner Y, et al: Acute lymphoblastic leukemia: Association with vasopressin-responsive diabetes insipidus. Arch Intern Med 140:1236, 1980
41. Yap HY, Tashima CK, Blumenschein GR, et al: Diabetes insipidus and breast cancer. Arch Intern Med 139:1009, 1979
42. DeRubertis FR, Michelis MF, Beck N, et al: "Essential" hypernatremia due to ineffective osmotic and intact volume regulation of vasopressin secretion. J Clin Invest 50:97, 1971
43. Halter JB, Goldberg AP, Robertson GL, et al: Selective osmoreceptor dysfunction in the syndrome of chronic hypernatremia. J Clin Endocrinol Metab 44:609, 1977
44. Kimura T, Matsui K, Sato T, et al: Relationship between plasma osmolality and plasma concentration of antidiuretic hormone in normal subjects, patients with chronic renal diseases, and patients with central diabetes insipidus. Tohoku J Exp Med 113:77, 1974
45. Brezis M, Weiler-Ravell D: Hypernatremia, hypodipsia and partial diabetes insipidus: A model for defective osmoregulation. Am J Med Sci 279:37, 1980
46. Mahoney JH, Goodman AD: Hypernatremia due to hypodipsia and elevated threshold for vasopressin release. Effects of treatment with hydrochlorothiazide, chlorpropamide and tolbutamide. N Engl J Med 279:1191, 1968
47. Sridhar CB, Calvert GD, Ibbertson HK: Syndrome of hypernatremia, hypodipsia and partial diabetes insipidus: A new interpretation. J Clin Endocrinol Metab 38:890, 1974
48. Szczepańska-Sadowska E, Sobocińska J, Sadowski B: Central dipsogenic effect of vasopressin. Am J Physiol 242:R372, 1982
49. Arieff AI, Guisado R: Effects on the central nervous system of hypernatremic and hyponatremic states. Kidney Int 10:104, 1976
50. Smitz S, Legros JJ: Hypodipsie et dysfonction sélective des osmorécepteurs dans le syndrome d'hypernatremié. CR Soc Biol (Paris) 175:874, 1981
51. Smals AGH, Kloppenborg PWC: Hypernatraemia in human myotonic dystrophy. Neth J Med 23:95, 1980
52. Hochberg Z, Moses AM, Miller M, et al: Altered osmotic threshold for vasopressin release and impaired thirst sensation: Additional abnormalities in Kallmann's syndrome. J Clin Endocrinol Metab 55:779, 1982
53. Bode HH, Harley BM, Crawford JD: Restoration of normal drinking behavior by chlor-

propamide in patients with hypodipsia and diabetes insipidus. Am J Med 51:304, 1971
54. Rao KJ, Miller M, Moses, AM: Water intoxication and thioridazine (Mellaril). Ann Intern Med 82:61, 1975
55. Rogers PW, Kurtzman NA: Renal failure, uncontrollable thirst, and hyperreninemia. JAMA 225:1236, 1973
56. Barlow ED, De Wardener HE: Compulsive water drinking. Q J Med 28:235, 1959
57. Pasqualini RQ, Codevilla A: Thirst-suppressing (antidipsetic) effect of Pitressin in diabetes insipidus. Acta Endocrinol (Copenh) 30:37, 1959
58. Sasaki S, Suzuki N: Ultrastructure of the neurohypophysis in dogs with diabetes insipidus and normal dogs. Jpn J Vet Sci 42:465, 1980
59. Smith RW, McCann SM: Alterations in food and water intake after hypothalamic lesions in the rat. Am J Physiol 203:366, 1962
60. Durr JA, Stamoutsos B, Lindheimer MD: Osmoregulation during pregnancy in the rat. Evidence for resetting of the threshold for vasopressin secretion during gestation. J Clin Invest 68:337, 1981
61. van Gemert M, Miller M, Carey RJ, et al. Polyuria and impaired ADH release following medial preoptic lesioning in the rat. Am J Physiol 228:1293, 1975
62. Harvey JA, Hunt HF: Effects of septal lesions on thirst in the rats as indicated by water consumption and operant responding for water reward. J Comp Physiol Psychol 59:49, 1965
63. Lubar JF, Boyce BA, Schaefer CF: Etiology of polydipsia and polyurea in rats with septal lesions. Physiol Behav 3:289, 1968
64. Fitzsimons JT: Thirst. Physiol Rev 52:468, 1972
65. Carey RJ, Procopio G: Differential effects of septal, preoptic and habenula ablations on thirst-motivated behavior in rats. J Comp Physiol Psychol 86:1163, 1974
66. Rolls BJ: Drinking by rats after irritative lesions in the hypothalamus. Physiol Behav 5:1385, 1970
67. Möhring J, Böhlen P, Schoun J, et al: Comparison of radioimmunoassay, chemical assay (HPLC) and bioassay for arginine vasopressin in synthetic standards and posterior pituitary tissue. Acta Endocrinol (Copenh) 99:371, 1982
68. Pickering BT: Prohormones for vasopressin. Nature 295:280, 1982
69. Morris JF, Sokol HW, Valtin H: One neuron—one hormone? Recent evidence from Brattleboro rats. P. 58. In Moses AM, Share L (eds): Neurohypophysis. S. Karger, Basel, 1977
70. Moses AM, Miller M: Accumulation and release of pituitary vasopressin in rats heterozygous for hypothalamic diabetes insipidus. Endocrinology 86:34, 1970
71. Sokol HW, Valtin H (Eds): The Brattleboro rat. NY Acad Sci 394:1, 1982
72. Hickey RC, Hare K: The renal excretion of chloride and water in diabetes insipidus. J Clin Invest 23:768, 1944
73. Carter AC, Robbins J: The use of hypertonic saline infusions in the differential diagnosis of diabetes insipidus and psychogenic polydipsia. J Clin Endocrinol 7:753, 1947
74. Moses AM, Streeten DHP: Differentiation of polyuric states by measurement of responses to changes in plasma osmolality induced by hypertonic saline infusions. Am J Med 42:368, 1967
75. Moses AM, Miller M, Streeten DHP: Quantitative influence of blood volume expansion on the osmotic threshold for vasopressin release. J Clin Endocrinol Metab 27:655, 1967
76. Miller M, Moses AM: Clinical states due to alteration of ADH release and action. P. 153. In Moses AM, Share L (eds): Neurohypophysis. S. Karger, Basel, 1977
77. Moses AM, Miller M: Osmotic threshold for vasopressin release as determined by saline infusion and by dehydration. Neuroendocrinology 7:219, 1971
78. Lipsett MB, MacLean JP, West CD, et al: An analysis of the polyuria induced by hypophysectomy in man. J Clin Endocrinol 16:183, 1956
79. Lipsett MB, Pearson OH: Further studies of diabetes insipidus following hypophysectomy in man. J Lab Clin Med 49:190, 1957
80. Dashe AM, Cramm RE, Crist CA, et al: A water deprivation test for the differential diagnosis of polyuria. JAMA 185:699, 1963
81. Miller M, Dalakos T, Moses AM, et al: Recognition of partial defects in antidiuretic hor-

mone secretion. Ann Intern Med 73:721, 1970
82. Moses AM, Notman DD: Diabetes insipidus and syndrome of inappropriate antidiuretic hormone secretion (SIADH). Adv Intern Med 27:73, 1982
83. Richman RA, Post EM, Notman DD, et al: Simplifying the diagnosis of diabetes insipidus in children. Am J Dis Child 135:839, 1981
84. Skowsky WR, Rosenbloom AA, Fisher DA: Radioimmunoassay measurement of arginine vasopressin in serum: Development and application. J Clin Endocrinol Metab 38:278, 1974
85. Zerbe RL, Robertson GL: A comparison of plasma vasopressin measurements with a standard indirect test in the differential diagnosis of polyuria. N Engl J Med 305:1539, 1981
86. Miller M, Moses AM: Urinary antidiuretic hormone in polyuric disorders and in inappropriate ADH syndrome. Ann Intern Med 77:715, 1972
87. Shealy CN, Kahana L, Engel FL, et al: Hypothalamic–pituitary sarcoidosis. A report on four patients, one with prolonged remission of diabetes insipidus following steroid therapy. Am J Med 30:46, 1961
88. Robinson AG: DDAVP in the treatment of central diabetes insipidus. N Engl J Med 294:507, 1976
89. Cobb WE, Spare S, Reichlin S: Neurogenic diabetes insipidus: Management with dDAVP (1-desamino-8-D-arginine vasopressin). Ann Intern Med 88:183, 1978
90. Moses AM, Moses LK, Notman DD, et al: Antidiuretic responses to injected desmopressin, alone and with indomethacin. J Clin Endocrinol Metab 52:910, 1981
91. Moses AM: Synthetic lysine vasopressin nasal spray in the treatment of diabetes insipidus. Clin Pharmacol Ther 5:422, 1964
92. Greene JA, January LE. Diabetes insipidus treated by the subcutaneous administration of a suspension of pitressin tannate in oil. JAMA 115:1183, 1940
93. Slotnik IL, Teigland JD: Cardiac accidents following vasopressin injection (Pitressin). JAMA 146:1126, 1951
94. Mahon WE, Scott DJ, Ansell G, et al: Hypersensitivity to pituitary snuff with miliary shadowing in the lungs. Thorax 22:13, 1967
95. Arduino F, Ferraz FPJ, Rodrigues J: Antidiuretic action of chlorpropamide in idiopathic diabetes insipidus. J Clin Endocrinol Metab 26:1325, 1966
96. Moses AM, Numann P, Miller M: Mechanism of chlorpropamide-induced antidiuresis in man: Evidence for release of ADH and enhancement of peripheral action. Metabolism 22:59, 1973
97. Aasen G, Frey HMM: Excessive sensitivity to the hyponatremic effect of chlorpropamide in a patient with diabetes mellitus and anterior pituitary insufficiency. Acta Med Scand 208:233, 1980
98. Valkusz Z, Laczi F, László FA: Development of the Schwartz–Bartter syndrome after the administration of chlorpropamide and 1-deamino-8-D-arginine vasopressin. Endokrinologie 79:345, 1982
99. Miller M, Moses AM: Mechanism of chlorpropamide action in diabetes insipidus. J Clin Endocrinol Metab 30:488, 1970
100. Thompson P Jr, Earll JM, Schaaf M: Comparison of clofibrate and chlorpropamide in vasopressin-responsive diabetes insipidus. Metabolism 26:749, 1977
101. Manns M, Schneider J, Meyer zum Büschenfelde K-H: Treatment of diabetes insipidus complicated by diabetes mellitus with chlorpropamide and clofibrate. Klin Wochenschr 58:847, 1980
102. Yamamoto T: Diabetes insipidus and drinking alcohol. N Engl J Med 294:55, 1976
103. Moses AM, Howanitz J, vanGemert M, et al: Clofibrate-induced antidiuresis. J Clin Invest 52:535, 1973
104. Matsukura S, Matsumoto J, Chihara K, et al: Clofibrate-induced myopathy in patients with diabetes insipidus. Endocrinol Jpn 27:401, 1980
105. Oliver MF: Cholesterol, coronaries, clofibrate and death. N Engl J Med 299:1360, 1978
106. Gardner S, Novitch M, Pines WL, et al: New label restriction and boxed warning on clofibrate. FDA Drug Bull 9:14, 1979
107. Bonnici F: Antidiuretic effect of clofibrate and carbamazepine in diabetes insipidus: Studies on free water clearance and response

to a water load. Clin Endocrinol 2:265, 1973
108. Czakó L, László FA: Antidiuretic effect of carbamazepine in diabetes insipidus. Int J Clin Pharmacol 11:58, 1975
109. Kimura T, Matsui K, Sato T, et al: Mechanism of carbamazepine (Tegretol)-induced antidiuresis: Evidence for release of antidiuretic hormone and impaired excretion of a water load. J Clin Endocrinol Metab 38:356, 1974
110. Leiba S, Rusecki Y, Ber A, et al: The antidiuretic effect of Tegretal in diabetes insipidus. J Israel Med Assoc 89:460, 1975
111. Radó JP: Combination of carbamazepine and chlorpropamide in the treatment of "hyporesponder" pituitary diabetes insipidus. J Clin Endocrinol Metab 38:1, 1974
112. Peters JP, Welt LG, Sims EAH, et al: A salt-wasting syndrome associated with cerebral disease. Trans Assoc Am Physicians 63:57, 1950
113. Robertson GL, Athar S: The interaction of blood osmolality and blood volume in regulating plasma vasopressin in man. J Clin Endocrinol Metab 42:613, 1976
114. Zerbe R, Stropes L, Robertson G: Vasopressin function in the syndrome of inappropriate antidiuresis. Annu Rev Med 31:315, 1980
115. Nelson PB, Seif SM, Maroon JC, et al: Hyponatremia in intracranial disease: Perhaps not the syndrome of inappropriate secretion of antidiuretic hormone (SIADH). J Neurosurg 55:938, 1981
116. Bartter FC, Schwartz WB: The syndrome of inappropriate secretion of antidiuretic hormone. Am J Med 42:790, 1967
117. Clift GV, Schletter FE, Moses AM, et al: Syndrome of inappropriate vasopressin secretion. Studies on the mechanism of the hyponatremia in a patient. Arch Intern Med 118:453, 1966
118. DeTroyer A, Bonnyns M, Demanet JC: Extreme salt depletion in a patient with the syndrome of inappropriate antidiuresis. Acta Clin Belg 34:140, 1979
119. Comis RL, Miller M, Ginsberg SJ: Abnormalities in water homeostasis in small cell anaplastic lung cancer. Cancer 45:2444, 1980
120. George JM, Capen CC, Phillips AS: Biosynthesis of vasopressin in vitro and ultrastructure of a bronchogenic carcinoma. Patient with the syndrome of inappropriate secretion of antidiuretic hormone. J Clin Invest 51:141, 1972
121. Cheng KW, Friesen HG: Studies of human neurophysin by radioimmunoassay. J Clin Endocrinol Metab 36:553, 1973
122. Kaye SB, Ross EJ: Inappropriate anti-diuretic hormone (ADH) secretion in association with carcinoma of bladder. Postgrad Med J 53:274, 1977
123. Miller R, Ashkar FS, Rudzinski DJ: Inappropriate secretion of antidiuretic hormone in reticulum cell sarcoma. South Med J 64:763, 1971
124. Zimbler H, Robertson GL, Bartter FC, et al: Ewing's sarcoma as a cause of the syndrome of inappropriate secretion of antidiuretic hormone. J Clin Endocrinol Metab 41:390, 1975
125. Cassileth PA, Trotman BW: Inappropriate antidiuretic hormone in Hodgkin's disease. Am J Med Sci 265:233, 1973
126. Simpson CD, Aitken SE: Malignant histiocytosis associated with SIADH and retinal hemorrhages. Canad Med Assoc J 127:302, 1982
127. Vorherr H, Massry SG, Fallet R, et al: Antidiuretic principle in tuberculous lung tissue of a patient with pulmonary tuberculosis and hyponatremia. Ann Intern Med 72:383, 1970
128. Rosenow EC III, Segar WE, Zehr JE: Inappropriate antidiuretic hormone secretion in pneumonia. Mayo Clin Proc 47:169, 1972
129. Spanos A, Spry CJ: Inappropriate secretion of antidiuretic hormone with chronic chest infections. Br Med J 3:785, 1974
130. Petty BG, Smith CR: The syndrome of inappropriate secretion of antidiuretic hormone associated with anaerobic thoracic empyema. Am Rev Respir Dis 115:685, 1977
131. Penney MD, Murphy D, Walters G: Resetting of osmoreceptor response as cause of hyponatraemia in acute idiopathic polyneuritis. Br Med J 2:1474, 1979
132. Hammer M: Defects in osmoregulation of vasopressin secretion. Acta Med Scand 211:133, 1982
133. Dóczi T, Tarjányi J, Huszka E, et al: Syndrome of inappropriate secretion of antidiuretic hormone (SIADH) after head injury. Neurosurgery 10:685, 1982
134. Greiss KC, Moses AM, Krieger DT: Pituitary adenoma associated with inappropriate

antidiuretic hormone secretion. Acta Endocrinol (Copenh) 76:59, 1974
135. Siersbaek-Nielsen K, Hansen JM, Reisby N, et al: Increased urinary excretion of antidiuretic material in encephalitis. Acta Neurol Scand 46:648, 1970
136. Rovit RL, Sigler MH: Cerebral hyponatremia secondary to excess secretion of antidiuretic hormone in a patient with herpes simplex encephalitis. Trans Am Neurol Assoc 88: 264, 1963
137. Kaplan AP, Curl FD, Decker JL: Central hyperventilation and inappropriate antidiuretic hormone secretion in systemic lupus erythematosus. Am J Med 48:661, 1970
138. Lipschutz DE, Reiter JM: Acute intermittent porphyria with inappropriately elevated ADH secretion. JAMA 230:716, 1974
139. Raskind MA, Orenstein H, Christopher TG: Acute psychosis, increased water ingestion and inappropriate antidiuretic hormone secretion. Am J Psychiatry 132:907, 1975
140. Moran WH Jr, Miltenberger FW, Shuayb WA, et al: The relationship of antidiuretic hormone secretion to surgical stress. Surgery 56:99, 1964
141. Gaufin L, Skowsky WR, Goodman SJ: Release of antidiuretic hormone during mass-induced elevation of intracranial pressure. J Neurosurg 46:627, 1977
142. Humes HD, Gottlieb MN, Brenner BM: The kidney in congestive heart failure. In Brenner BM, Stein JH (eds): Contemporary Issues in Nephrology. Vol 1. Churchill Livingstone, New York, 1978
143. Levy M: The kidney in liver disease. In Brenner BM, Stein JH (eds): Contemporary Issues in Nephrology. Vol 1. Churchill Livingstone, New York, 1978
144. Skowsky WR, Kikuchi TA: The role of vasopressin in the impaired water excretion of myxedema. Am J Med 64:613, 1978
145. Kaplowitz LG, Robertson GL: Hyponatremia in Rocky Mountain Spotted Fever: Role of antidiuretic hormone. Ann Intern Med 98:334, 1983
146. DeFronzo RA, Goldberg M, Agus ZS: Normal diluting capacity in hyponatremic patients. Reset osmostat or a variant of the syndrome of inappropriate antidiuretic hormone. Ann Intern Med 84:538, 1976
147. Shimizu K, Hoshino M: Application of vasopressin radioimmunoassay to clinical study: Role of vasopressin in hypo- and hypernatremia and some other disorders of water metabolism. Contrib Nephrol 9:42, 1978
148. Bichet D, Szatalowicz V, Chaimovitz C, et al: Role of vasopressin in abnormal water excretion in cirrhotic humans. Ann Intern Med 96:413, 1982
149. Riegger GAJ, Liebau G, Kochsiek K: Antidiuretic hormone in congestive heart failure. Am J Med 72:49, 1982
150. Hantman D, Rossier B, Zohlman R, et al: Rapid correction of hyponatremia in the syndrome of inappropriate secretion of antidiuretic hormone. An alternative treatment to hypertonic saline. Ann Intern Med 78:870, 1973
151. Decaux G, Brimioulle S, Genette F, et al: Treatment of the syndrome of inappropriate secretion of antidiuretic hormone by urea. Am J Med 69:99, 1980
152. Weizman Z, Goitein K, Amit Y, et al: Combined treatment of severe hyponatremia due to inappropriate antidiuretic hormone secretion. Pediatrics 69:610, 1982
153. Tanay A, Yust I, Peresecenschi G, et al: Long-term treatment of the syndrome of inappropriate antidiuretic hormone secretion with phenytoin. Ann Intern Med 90:50, 1979
154. White MG, Fetner CD: Treatment of the syndrome of inappropriate secretion of antidiuretic hormone with lithium carbonate. N Engl J Med 292:390, 1975
155. Finsterer U, Beyer A, Jensen U, et al: The syndrome of inappropriate secretion of antidiuretic hormone (SIADH)—Treatment with lithium. Intensive Care Med 8:223, 1982
156. DeTroyer A: Demeclocycline. Treatment for syndrome of inappropriate antidiuretic hormone secretion. JAMA 237:2723, 1977
157. Forrest JN, Cox M, Hong C, et al: Superiority of demeclocycline over lithium in the treatment of chronic syndrome of inappropriate secretion of antidiuretic hormone. N Engl J Med 298:173, 1978
158. Padfield PL, Morton JJ, Hodsman GP: Demeclocycline in the treatment of the syndrome of inappropriate antidiuretic hormone release: with measurement of plasma ADH. Postgrad Med J 54:623, 1978
159. Carrilho F, Bosch J, Arroyo V, et al: Renal

failure associated with demeclocycline in cirrhosis. Ann Intern Med 87:195, 1977

160. Kinter LB, Stassen F, Horner E, et al: Vasopressin antagonist—associated aquaresis in primates. Kidney Int 23:259, 1983
161. Bethune JE, Nelson DH: Hyponatremia in hypopituitarism. N Engl J Med 272:771, 1965
162. Davis BB, Bloom ME, Field JB, et al: Hyponatremia in pituitary insufficiency. Metabolism 18:821, 1969
163. Liberman B, Wajchenberg BL, Pieroni RR: Water and electrolyte metabolism in adrenal and pituitary insufficiency. II. Effect of gluco- and mineralocorticoid adrenal steroids on sodium metabolism, with special reference to exchangeable sodium. Metabolism 15:992, 1966
164. Spital A: Hyponatremia in adrenal insufficiency: Review. Pathogenetic mechanisms. South Med J 75:581, 1982
165. Baxter JD, Tyrrell JB: The adrenal cortex. P. 385. In Felig P, Baxter JD, Broadus AE, et al: (eds): Endocrinology and Metabolism. McGraw-Hill, New York, 1981
166. Robinson FJ, Power MH, Kepler EJ: Two new procedures to assist in the recognition and exclusion of Addison's disease: a preliminary report. Mayo Clin Proc 16:577, 1941
167. Slessor A: Studies concerning the mechanism of water retention in Addison's disease and in hypopituitarism. J Clin Endocrinol 11: 700, 1951
168. Kleeman CR, Maxwell MH, Rockney RE: Mechanisms of impaired water excretion in adrenal and pituitary insufficiency. I. The role of altered glomerular filtration rate and solute excretion. J Clin Invest 37:1799, 1958
169. Dingman JF, Streeten DHP, Thorn GW: Effect of cortisone on the abnormal distribution of intravascular water in adrenal cortical insufficiency in man. J Lab Clin Med 49:7, 1957
170. Gill JR Jr, Gann DS, Bartter FC: Restoration of water diuresis in Addisonian patients by expansion of the volume of extracellular fluid. J Clin Invest 41:1078, 1962
171. Cutler RE, Kleeman CR, Koplowitz J, et al: Mechanisms of impaired water excretion in adrenal and pituitary insufficiency. III. The effect of extracellular or plasma volume expansion, or both, on the impaired diuresis. J Clin Invest 41:1524, 1962
172. Ishikawa SE, Schrier RW: Effect of arginine vasopressin antagonist on renal water excretion in glucocorticoid and mineralocorticoid deficient rats. Kidney Int 22:587, 1982
173. Yunis SL, Berkowitz, DD, Stein RM, et al: Renal tubular effects of hydrocortisone and aldosterone in normal hydropenic man; comments on sites of action. J Clin Invest 43: 1668, 1964
174. Raisz LG, McNeely WF, Saxon L, et al: The effects of cortisone and hydrocortisone on water diuresis and renal function in man. J Clin Invest 36:767, 1957
175. Ackerman GL, Miller CL: Role of hypovolemia in the impaired water diuresis of adrenal insufficiency. J Clin Endocrinol Metab 30: 252, 1970
176. Dingman JF, Despointes R: Adrenal steroid inhibition of vasopressin release from the neurohypophysis of normal subjects and patients with Addison's disease. J Clin Invest 39:1851, 1960
177. Ahmed ABJ, George BC, Gonzalez-Auvert C, et al: Increased plasma arginine vasopressin in clinical adrenocortical insufficiency and its inhibition by glucosteroids. J Clin Invest 46:111, 1967
178. Share L, Travis RH: Plasma vasopressin concentration in the adrenally-insufficient dog. Endocrinology 86:196, 1970
179. Boykin J, De Torrenté A, Erickson A, et al: Role of plasma vasopressin in impaired water excretion of glucocorticoid deficiency. J Clin Invest 62:738, 1978
180. Mandell, IN, DeFronzo RA, Robertson GL, et al: Role of plasma arginine vasopressin in the impaired water diuresis of isolated glucocorticoid deficiency in the rat. Kidney Int 17:186, 1980
181. Linas SL, Berl T, Robertson GL, et al: Role of vasopressin in the impaired water excretion of glucocorticoid deficiency. Kidney Int 18:58, 1980
182. Green HH, Harrington AR, Valtin H: On the role of antidiuretic hormone in the inhibition of acute water diuresis in adrenal insufficiency and the effects of gluco- and mineralocorticoids in reversing the inhibition. J Clin Invest 49:1724, 1970
183. Kleeman CR, Czaczkes JW, Cutler R: Mechanisms of impaired water excretion in adrenal and pituitary insufficiency. IV. Antidiuretic hormone in primary and secondary

adrenal insufficiency. J Clin Invest 43:1641, 1964

184. Streeten DHP, Pont ME, Conn JW: Effects of hydrocortisone on urinary excretion of sodium in adrenalectomized rats. J Lab Clin Med 46:729, 1955
185. Swingle WW, Pfiffner JJ, Vars HM, et al: The effect of fluid deprivation and fluid intake upon the revival of dogs from adrenal insufficiency. Am J Physiol 108:144, 1934
186. Swingle WW, Brannick LS, Osborn M, et al: Effect of gluco- and mineralocorticoid adrenal steroids on fluid and electrolytes of fasted adrenalectomized dogs. Proc Soc Exp Biol Med 96:446, 1957
187. Frost RC, Talmage RV: Fluid and electrolyte shifts in the hydrated adrenalectomized rat. Endocrinology 49:606, 1951
188. Hegnauer AH, Robinson EJ: The water and electrolyte distribution among plasma, red blood cells, and muscle after adrenalectomy. J Biol Chem 116:769, 1936
189. Thorn GW, Renold AE, Morse WI, et al: Highly potent adrenal cortical steroids: Structure and biologic activity. Ann Intern Med 43:979, 1955
190. Mills JN, Thomas S, Williamson KS: The acute effect of hydrocortisone, deoxycorticosterone and aldosterone upon the excretion of Na, K and acid by the human kidney. J Physiol (Lond) 151:312, 1960
191. Liddle GW: Effects of anti-inflammatory steroids on electrolyte metabolism. Ann NY Acad Sci 82:854, 1959
192. Swingle WW, DaVanzo JP, Crossfield HC, et al: Glucocorticoids and maintenance of blood pressure and plasma volume of adrenalectomized dogs subjected to stress. Proc Soc Exp Biol Med 100:617, 1959
193. Curtis RH: Hyponatremia in primary myxedema. Ann Intern Med 44:376, 1956
194. Forester CF: Coma in myxedema. Arch Intern Med 111:734, 1963
195. Holvey DN, Goodner CJ, Nicoloff JT, et al: Treatment of myxedema coma with intravenous thyroxine. Arch Intern Med 113:89, 1964
196. Chinitz A, Turner FL: The association of primary hypothyroidism and inappropriate secretion of the antidiuretic hormone. Arch Intern Med 116:871, 1965
197. Mataverde AQ, Abbasi AA, Hossain Z, et al: Hydrochlorothiazide-induced water intoxication in myxedema. JAMA 230:1014, 1974
198. Robles-Valdes C, Mayans JAR, Lomeli JIA: Severe hyponatremia in congenital hypothyroidism. J Pediatr 94:631, 1979
199. Koide Y, Oda K, Shimizu K, et al: Hyponatremia without inappropriate secretion of vasopressin in a case of myxedema coma. Endocrinol Jpn 29:363, 1982
200. Shalev O, Naparstek Y, Brezis M, et al: Hyponatremia in myxedema: A suggested therapeutic approach. Israel J Med Sci 15:913, 1979
201. Odell WD: Isolated deficiencies of anterior pituitary hormones. JAMA 197:1006, 1966
202. Miyai K, Azukizawa M, Kumahara Y: Familial isolated thyrotropin deficiency with cretinism. N Engl J Med 285:1043, 1971
203. Sachson R, Rosen SW, Cuatrecasas P, et al: Prolactin stimulation by thyrotropin-releasing hormone in a patient with isolated thyrotropin deficiency. N Engl J Med 287:972, 1972
204. Munro DS, Renschler H, Wilson GM: Exchangeable potassium and sodium in hyperthyroidism and hypothyroidism. Metabolism 7:124, 1958
205. Aikawa JK: The nature of myxedema. Alterations in the serum electrolyte concentrations and radiosodium space and in the exchangeable sodium and potassium contents. Ann Intern Med 44:30, 1956
206. Hlad CJ, Bricker NS: Renal function and I^{131} clearance in hyperthyroidism and myxedema. J Clin Endocrinol Metab 14:1539, 1954
207. Means JH, DeGroot LJ, Stanbury JB: The Thyroid and Its Diseases. 3rd Ed. McGraw-Hill, New York, 1963 p 329
208. Gibson JG, Harris AW: Clinical studies of the blood volume. V. Hyperthyroidism and myxedema. J Clin Invest 18:59, 1939
209. Vaamonde CA, Sebastianelli MJ, Vaamonde LS, et al: Impaired renal tubular reabsorption of sodium in hypothyroid man. J Lab Clin Med 85:451, 1975
210. Katz AI, Emmanouel DS, Lindheimer MD: Thyroid hormone and the kidney. Nephron 15:223, 1975
211. Yount EY, Little JM: Renal clearance in patients with myxedema. J Clin Endocrinol Metab 15:343, 1955
212. Corcoran AC, Page IH: Specific renal func-

tions in hyperthyroidism and myxedema. Effects of treatment. J Clin Endocrinol 7:801, 1947

213. Ford RV, Owens JC, Curd GW, et al: Kidney functions in various thyroid states. J Clin Endocrinol Metab 21:548, 1961
214. Davies CE, Mackinnon J, Platts MM: Renal circulation and cardiac output in "low-output" heart failure and in myxedema. Br Med J 2:595, 1952
215. Taylor RE, Fregly MJ: Renal response of propylthiouracil-treated rats to injected mineralocorticoids. Endocrinology 75:33, 1964
216. Bradley SE, Bradley GE, Stephen F: Role of structural imbalance in the pathogenesis of renal dysfunction in the hypothyroid rat. Trans Assoc Am Physicians 85:344, 1972
217. Holmes EW, DiScala VA: Studies on the exaggerated natriuretic response to a saline infusion in the hypothyroid rat. J Clin Invest 49:1224, 1970
218. Michael UF, Barenberg RL, Chavez R, et al: Renal handling of sodium and water in the hypothyroid rat. J Clin Invest 51:1405, 1972
219. Schrier RW, Berl T: Nonosmolar factors affecting renal water excretion. N Engl J Med 292:86, 1975
220. Edelman IS, Ismail-Beigi F: Thyroid thermogenesis and active sodium transport. Recent Prog Horm Res 30:235, 1974
221. DeRubertis FR, Michelis MF, Bloom ME, et al: Impaired water excretion in myxedema. Am J Med 51:41, 1971
222. Bleifer KH, Belsky JL, Saxon L, et al: The diuretic response to administered water in patients with primary myxedema. J Clin Endocrinol Metab 20:409, 1960
223. DiScala VA, Kinney MJ: Effects of myxedema on the renal diluting and concentrating mechanism. Am J Med 50:325, 1971
224. Crispell KR, Parson W, Sprinkle P: A cortisone-resistant abnormality in the diuretic response to ingested water in primary myxedema. J Clin Endocrinol Metab 14:640, 1954
225. Emmanouel DS, Lindheimer MD, Katz AI: Mechanism of impaired water excretion in the hypothyroid rat. J Clin Invest 54:926, 1974
226. Schrier RW, Goldberg JP: The physiology of vasopressin release and the pathogenesis of impaired water excretion in adrenal, thyroid, and edematous disorders. Yale J Biol Med 53:525, 1980
227. Pettinger WA, Talner L, Ferris TF: Inappropriate secretion of antidiuretic hormone due to myxedema. N Engl J Med 272:362, 1965
228. Goldberg M, Reivich M: Studies on the mechanism of hyponatremia and impaired water excretion in myxedema. Ann Intern Med 56:120, 1962
229. Skowsky WR, Fisher DA: Arginine vasopressin secretion in thyroidectomized sheep. Endocrinology 100:1022, 1977
230. Lohavichan C, Carroll KE, Sebastianelli MJ, et al: The failure of alcohol to improve impaired water diuresis in myxedema. Clin Res 18:508 1970

19

Acid–Base and Electrolyte Disorders Associated with Adrenal Disease

Anthony Sebastian Ira Kurtz
Morris Schambelan Rosemary E. Hernandez
Henry N. Hulter Edward G. Biglieri
Curtis Morris

Sodium, chloride, potassium, and acid–base homeostasis in humans is dependent in part on the mineralocorticoid activity of steroid hormones secreted by the adrenal cortex. The mineralocorticoid activity of adrenal steroids is reflected in the electrolyte and acid–base composition of the cellular and extracellular fluid compartments and in the volume of the arterial blood compartment. Aldosterone is the only adrenal steroid known to participate in the physiologic feedback regulation of electrolyte and volume homeostasis. Disorders of the adrenal gland that result in subnormal or supernormal rates of mineralocorticoid secretion lead to abnormalities in extracellular fluid volume and blood pressure and to abnormalities of plasma electrolyte and acid–base composition. Conversely, extraadrenal disorders that result in abnormalities of effective arterial blood volume or plasma electrolyte and acid–base composition alter the rate of aldosterone secretion; the altered rate of aldosterone secretion in turn modifies the clinical expression of the primary disorder. This chapter considers the clinical and pathophysiologic features of syndromes of mineralocorticoid excess and deficiency in the context of our current understanding of the physiologic effects of mineralocorticoid hormones on acid–base and electrolyte metabolism.

PHYSIOLOGIC EFFECTS OF MINERALOCORTICOID HORMONES

By direct or indirect mechanisms, mineralocorticoid hormones (MCH) modulate transepithelial transport of Na^+, K^+, H^+ (HCO_3^-), Cl^-, Ca^{2+}, Mg^{2+}, and H_2O. Target epithelia are present in kidney, large bowel, sweat glands, and salivary ducts. The renal effects of mineralocorticoid hormones provide the critical regulatory influence on mineral homeostasis in humans who are not excreting copious amounts of sweat or liquid stool. The renal response to mineralocorticoid hormones reflects specific effects on the tubules that can occur independently of measured changes in glomerular filtration rate or renal hemodynamics.[1,2] Renal functional responses attributed to mineralocorticoid hormone have been reported to occur in the distal nephron of dogs,[3] in the proximal and distal convoluted tubules of rats,[4,5] in the connecting tubules of rabbits,[6] in the cortical collecting tubules of rabbits,[6-8] and in the medullary collecting ducts of rabbits[9,10] and rats.[11,12] It is questionable whether the observed proximal tubular effects of aldosterone have homeostatic significance. Studies of isolated nephron segments in the rabbit indicate that the cortical collecting tubules are responsive to mineralocorticoid hormone but that the early segments of the distal convoluted tubules are not.[7] Earlier studies that revealed an effect of mineralocorticoid hormones in the distal convoluted tubule[4,5] may have reflected changes occurring in the initial collecting tubules. At least two cell types—light and dark cells—have been identified in the collecting tubules.[13] It is not known whether both cell types respond to mineralocorticoid hormone.

The urinary bladder of the toad[14,15] and of the freshwater turtle[16] also has been found to respond to mineralocorticoid hormone. These epithelia have morphologic and functional characteristics similar to those of mammalian collecting duct epithelia and have been used extensively as a model for studies of mineralocorticoid hormone action.

Cellular Action of Mineralocorticoid Hormone

SODIUM TRANSPORT

The effects of MCH on ion and water transport at the cellular level have been studied in toad and turtle bladders and in isolated segments of mammalian renal tubules. Mineralocorticoid hormone increases sodium reabsorption despite opposing transepithelial electrical gradient (lumen-negative) and chemical gradient (Na^+ concentration lower in lumen than in peritubular fluid), that is, MCH stimulates active transport of Na^+.[17] The stimulation of active Na^+ transport increases the lumen-negative transtubular electrical potential difference, hence the transport process is electrogenic.[7] In studies of isolated perfused tubule segments (from rabbits), the transtubular potential difference is normally lumen negative and its magnitude is increased by MCH, as is the rate of Na^+ absorption, in the cortical collecting tubule,[7,8] but not in the outer medullary collecting tubules. The latter is normally either at near zero potential or is lumen positive, shows evidence of no net Na^+ transport, and is unresponsive to MCH in respect to alteration in Na^+ transport rate or transtubular potential difference.[8] The increased lumen-negative potential may account in part for the stimulation of H^+ and K^+ secretion observed in response to MCH, but aldosterone can stimulate secretion of these ions even when the effect of the hormone on Na^+ transport is prevented.[16,18,19] Furthermore, aldosterone stimulates H^+ secretion in a segment of the rabbit medullary collecting duct in which sodium transport is not stimulated by aldosterone.[9,10] Mineralocorticoid hormone stimulates net Cl^- reabsorption in isolated perfused collecting tubules of rabbits.[20] Aldosterone enhances the effect of vasopressin to increase transepithelial water movement in the toad bladder.[21]

According to current concepts, the alterations in transport induced by MCH are mediated by molecular-ionic events at the luminal and peritubular cell membranes. Transepithelial transport of Na^+ from lumen to cell along a favorable electrical and chemical (concentration) gradient is followed by active extrusion of Na^+ into peritubular fluid by an Na^+–K^+ exchange pump on the peritubular membrane. Mineralocorticoid hormone increases both the permeability of the luminal cell membrane to Na^+ and K^+ and the rate of peritubular Na^+–K^+ exchange.[22-24] The rate of transport of Na^+ across the peritubular membrane is increased at least in part by promoting increased cellular entry of Na^+ from the lumen. The peritubular transport process entails hydrolysis of adenosine triphosphate (ATP) by an enzyme activated by increasing concentrations of Na^+ (cell) or K^+ (peritubular fluids): Na^+–K^+-ATPase.[25] This enzyme is present in highest concentration in the peritubular cell membrane and has been identified as the Na^+–K^+-exchange pump. In studies on discrete nephron segments in rabbits, MCH increases Na^+–K^+-ATPase activity only in the cortical collecting tubule and in the so-called connecting segment, located between the end of the distal convoluted tubule and the beginning of the cortical collecting tubule.[6] The possibility has been considered that MCH-induced renal Na^+–K^+-ATPase activity reflects a direct effect of MCH that is prerequisite to MCH-induced Na^+ transport; despite numerous investigations, however, the available evidence neither supports nor excludes this possibility conclusively. Recent studies conflictingly report that preclusion of cellular uptake of Na^+ does[26] and does not[27] inhibit MCH stimulation of Na^+–K^+-ATPase activity. Evidence has been adduced that MCH increases the supply of ATP and alters the coupling between ATP utilization and the transport process in such a way as to increase the efficiency of energy used for transport.[28]

The results of recent studies indicate a close relationship between the distal nephron Na^+ reabsorption mechanism and the activity of the renal kallikrein–kinin system.[29] Renal kallikrein is a proteolytic enzyme that catalyzes the formation in the kidney of a vasoactive peptide, kallidin (lysl-bradykinin), from a precursor (kininogen) of renal origin. Kallikrein is localized histochemically in the apical border of cortical distal nephron cells and is excreted in the urine in increased amounts in response to administration of mineralocorticoid hormones. In vitro studies indicate that kallikrein activity is inhibitable by amiloride and that like amiloride other inhibitors of kallikrein activity inhibit transepithelial transport of Na^+ in aldosterone responsive urinary epithelia (e.g., the toad bladder).[29,30] It is tempting to speculate that luminal membrane-bound kallikrein in the aldosterone-sensitive segments of the distal nephron comprises or controls the Na^+ entry channels, which are increased in number in response to aldosterone and are inhibited by amiloride.

HYDROGEN ION TRANSPORT

The cellular mechanism of acidification in the mammalian distal nephron has not been defined. A widely adopted working model has been derived from in vitro studies of the urinary bladder of the Colombian toad and the freshwater turtle, H^+-secreting epithelia that resemble the mammalian collecting tubules and ducts (in contradistinction to more proximal nephron segments) with respect to embryologic origin and certain characteristics of structure and function.[15,31,32,32a] In these epithelia, the H^+ secretory mechanism is electrogenic, that is, it is capable of transporting a net positive charge into the lumen; it is not dependent on Na^+ resorption, although the rate of H^+ secretion may be influenced by the rate of active Na^+ resorption, which determines the magnitude of the transepithelia electrical potential difference promoting or opposing H^+ secretion. Secretion of H^+ occurs even under conditions in which Na^+ transport is prevented and no favorable transepithelial electrical potential difference is permitted to develop. Under these conditions, the rate of H^+ secretion decreases in response to an increase in the transepithelial H^+ concentration gradient against which H^+ is secreted; when the H^+ concentration in the mucosal fluid is approximately 1000 times greater (i.e., 3.0 pH units less) than that in the serosal fluid, the net rate of H^+ secretion is reduced to zero (Fig. 19–1). This reflects cessation of unidirectional H^+ secretion from cell to lumen; backleak of H^+ from the mucosal fluid into the cell or serosal fluid is negligible. The magnitude of the transepithelial H^+ concentration gradient required to nullify net H^+ secretion is an index of the "driving force" (proton-motive force) of the H^+ secretory pump. The rate of H^+ secretion when the transepithelial H^+

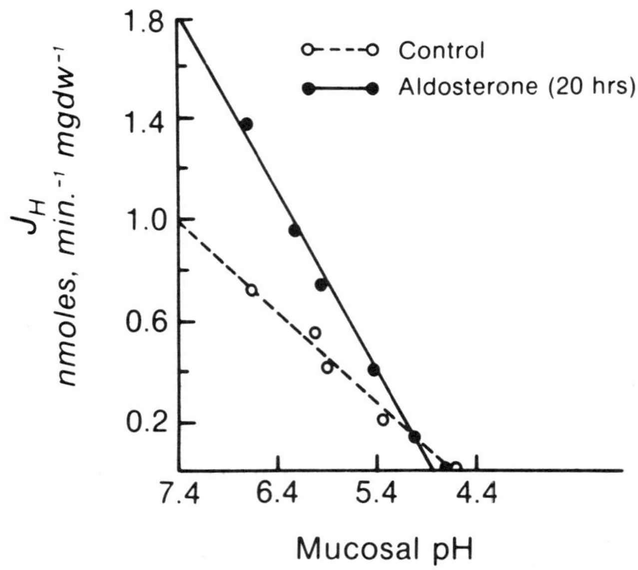

Fig. 19–1. The relationship of H^+ secretion (J_H) to the applied pH gradient (against which H^+ is secreted) in ouabain-treated freshwater turtle (*Pseudemys scripta*) bladders studied under short-circuit conditions in both control (○, freshly pithed) and aldosterone-treated (●, 20 hours) hemibladders. Aldosterone increased the rate of H^+ secretion at nonlimiting H^+ concentration gradients (increased slope), but did not alter the applied H^+ gradient at which net H^+ secretion ceases (the proton-motive force of the pump). (From Al-Awqati Q: Effect of aldosterone on the coupling between H^+ transport and glucose oxidation. J Clin Invest 60:1240, 1977. By permission of the American Society for Clinical Investigation.)

concentration gradient is nonlimiting represents an index of the conductance of H^+ through the active transport pathway. Aldosterone increases the rate of H^+ secretion at nonlimiting transepithelial H^+ concentration gradients, that is, it increases the conductance of H^+ in the active transport pathway. It does not influence the proton-motive force of H^+ secretory pump (Fig. 19–1).[16] In the mucosal border of the turtle bladder, a reversible proton-translocating ATPase can function as an H^+ pump that can account for urinary acidification.[33]

A characteristic of electrogenic H^+ secretion is dependence of the secretory rate on the transepithelial electrical potential difference.[34] The net rate of H^+ secretion is modulated by the transepithelial electrical potential difference, which is ordinarily determined in part by the net rate of sodium resorption. In the absence of a transepithelial H^+ concentration gradient, H^+ secretion can be nullified by an unfavorable transepithelial electrical gradient (lumen-positive) that is energetically equivalent to the H^+ concentration gradient that nullifies H^+ secretion in the absence of an electrical gradient.[35] Aldosterone stimulation of H^+ secretion is at least in part due to the increased lumen-negative electrical potential that results from aldosterone stimulation of active sodium reabsorption.

Recent studies of acidification of luminal fluid by the rabbit cortical collecting tubule perfused in vitro indicate that the physiologic characteristics of the H^+ secretory mechanism in the mammalian distal nephron are similar to those defined in the urinary bladder of the toad and turtle.[18] The data support the existence of a distinct acidification mechanism that is both active and electrogenic. Electrogenic H^+ secretion is stimulated by pretreatment of the animals with MCH.[18] Mineralocorticoid hormone stimulation of H^+ secretion in the rabbit cortical collecting tubule is due to (1) MCH stimulation of active sodium reabsorption since, in the presence of luminal sodium, MCH administration is associated with a large and significant increase in lumen-negative electrical potential and (2) a more direct effect on the proton secretory mechanism since, in the absence of luminal sodium, MCH administration results in a large and significant increase in lumen-positive electrical potential attributable to H^+ secretion.[18]

In outer medullary collecting tubules, unlike the circumstance in cortical collecting tubules, MCH does not stimulate Na^+ reabsorption, nor does it alter the transtubular electrical potential difference, which is oriented lumen-positive in the collecting tubules located in the inner stripe of the outer medulla.[8] The lumen-positive potential results from electrogenic H^+ secretion, which occurs despite the absence of Na^+ reabsorption, but is accompanied by Cl^- secretion at nearly identical rates.[10,36,37] Aldosterone stimulates H^+ secretion in this nephron segment.[9] Adrenalectomy reduces the rate of H^+ secretion, and aldosterone replacement restores the rate, suggesting that normal levels of aldosterone secretion maintain the normal rate of H^+ secretion in this nephron segment.[9] The intrinsic H^+ secretory capacity of this nephron segment exceeds that of the cortical collecting tubule and approaches 25 percent of that of the proximal convoluted tubule.[36] Thus, MCH-stimulated H^+ secretion in the outer medullary collecting tubule may be the major determinant of distal nephron H^+ secretion rates in the mammalian kidney under ordinary physiologic conditions and in physiologic and pathologic states of altered mineralocorticoid levels.

POTASSIUM TRANSPORT

The specific effects of mineralocorticoid hormone on transepithelial transport of K^- have not been studied as extensively as those of Na^+. In the lumen-negative post-macula densa segments of the distal nephron, principally the collecting tubules and ducts and late distal convoluted tubules, the K^+ secretory process can be subdivided into several components: (1) active cellular uptake of K^+ at the peritubular membrane mediated by Na^+–K^+-ATPase; (2) passive diffusion of K^+ from cell to lumen along a favorable electrochemical gradient; and (3) active cellular uptake of K^+ from the lumen by a pump presumed to be located in the luminal membrane. Indirect evidence suggests that in the collecting duct segments, K^+ secretion is mediated by the principal cells, whereas K^+ reabsorption is mediated by the intercalated cells.[38,39] By increasing Na^+ reabsorption, MCH increases the lumen-negative transtubular electrical potential difference in the cortical collecting tubule, where it is known that K^+ secretion correlates positively with the magnitude of the transtubular potential difference and rate of Na^+ reabsorption.[40] Mineralocorticoid hormone also appears to increase the permeability of the luminal membrane to K^+[23,24] and the rate of cellular uptake of K^+ at the peritubular membrane, secondary to increased Na^+–K^+-ATPase activity,[23] the effects of which would facilitate the K^+ secretory response to increased transtubular potential difference.

Mineralocorticoid–Antidiuretic Hormone Interactions

Potentiation by aldosterone of the hypo-osmotic effect of vasopressin appears to be mediated by more than one mechanism: (1) inhibition of cyclic nucleotide phosphodiesterase activity with resultant diminution of cyclic adenosine monophosphate cAMP degradation[41] and (2) inhibition of prostaglandin E synthesis, which ordinarily inhibits vasopressin-induced cAMP.[42] Greater potentiation occurs with adrenal steroids that have greater glucocorticoid potency than aldosterone, raising the possibility that this effect of aldosterone is mediated by its glucocorticoid activity.

Subcellular Mechanisms of Steroid Action

A biochemical basis for the distinction between glucocorticoid and mineralocorticoid activity is provided by studies of the mechanism of steroid action at the subcellular level. The steroid crosses the cell membrane, presumably by simple diffusion, where it binds to high-affinity receptor proteins in the cytoplasm of the appropriate target tissue.[43] Studies in rat kidney tissue have suggested that there are multiple steroid hormone-binding sites.[44] Hormones classified as mineralocorticoid or glucocorticoid on the basis of their physiologic effects bind with different affinities to the various receptor sites. The mineralocorticoid and glucocorticoid potency of a particular steroid hormone correlates with its relative affinity for the so-called mineralocorticoid and glucocorticoid receptors.[45] Steroid action is dependent on the formation of an active steroid–receptor complex for subsequent initiation of genetic action.[46] Steroids with stimulatory (agonist) properties in a given tissue generate a steroid–receptor complex that is transferred to the cell nucleus. Studies with inhibitors of DNA-dependent RNA synthesis and inhibitors of synthesis of ribosomal protein suggest that the formation of an aldosterone-induced protein plays a primary role in mediating the Na^+ transport effects of the hormone.[47-49]

Steroids that act as competitive antagonists (e.g., progesterone, 17α-hydroxyprogesterone, and spironolactone) bind with high affinity to the MCH receptor, but fail to initiate the subsequent steps required for MCH action.[50] On the basis of autoradiographic studies in isolated nephron segments from rabbits, it has been concluded that in the cortical collecting tubule aldosterone binds predominantly to mineralocorticoid sites, whereas in the loop of Henle, distal convoluted tubule, and medullary collecting duct, aldosterone binds to both mineralocorticoid and glucocorticoid sites.[51-53]

SYNDROMES OF MINERALOCORTICOID HORMONE EXCESS (TABLE 19–1)

Experimental States of Mineralocorticoid Hormone Excess

Acute parenteral administration of large amounts of MCH in humans results in a reduction in the urinary excretion rates of Na^+ and Cl^- and an increase in the excretion rate of K^+ and net acid.[54-56] With continued administration (days or weeks), extracellular fluid volume and Na^+ concentration increase and K^+ depletion and hypokalemia occur.[57,58] In subjects ingesting normal amounts of Na^+ and K^+ the plasma bicarbonate concentration is not significantly changed, however, despite prolonged (3 months) administration of even 10 times the normal amount of aldosterone.[57] In dogs the alkalosis-producing effect of MCH is potentiated by deprivation of dietary K^+.[59,60] Similar potentiation may occur in man because in patients with primary aldo-

Table 19–1. Clinical Spectrum of Syndromes of Mineralocorticoid Hormone Excess

- Primary MCH excess
  - Primary aldosteronism
    - Aldosterone-producing adenoma
    - Idiopathic hyperplasia
    - Aldosterone-producing carcinoma
    - Glucocorticoid-suppressible hyperaldosteronism
  - Adrenal enzyme defects
    - 11β-hydroxylase deficiency
    - 17α-hydroxylase deficiency
  - Cushing's syndrome
    - Ectopic ACTH syndrome
    - Adrenal carcinoma
    - Adrenal adenoma
    - Hypothalamic–pituitary (Cushing's disease)
  - Other MCH hormones
    - Licorice
    - Carbenoxolone
    - (?) Low-renin essential hypertension
- Secondary MCH excess
  - Physiologic
    - Sodium depletion (vomiting, diarrhea)
    - Hemorrhage
    - Pregnancy
  - Pathophysiologic
    - Nonhypertensive
      - edematous states (cirrhosis, congestive heart failure, nephrotic syndrome)
      - Bartter's syndrome
      - Renal tubular acidosis
      - Diuretic therapy
    - Hypertensive
      - Accelerated hypertension
      - Renovascular hypertension
      - Renin-secreting tumor
      - End-stage renal failure
      - Post-transplant hypertension
      - Estrogen therapy
- Pseudohypermineralocorticoidism
  - Liddle's syndrome

Abbreviations: ACTH, adrenocorticotropism; MCH, mineralocorticoid hormone.

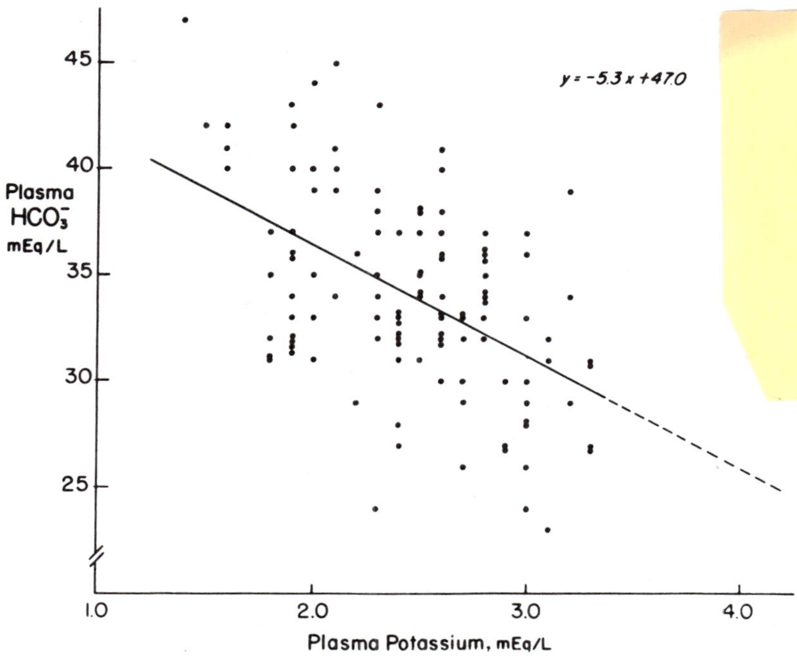

Fig. 19–2. The relationship of plasma bicarbonate concentration with plasma potassium concentration in 111 published patients with primary aldosteronism without evidence of a complicating acid–base or electrolyte disturbance. (From Kassirer JP, London AM, Goldman DM, et al: On the pathogenesis of metabolic alkalosis in hyperaldosteronism. Am J Med 49:306, 1970.)

steronism the severity of metabolic alkalosis is proportional to the degree of potassium depletion as indicated by the serum K^+ concentration (Fig. 19–2).[57]

The reduction in urinary excretion of Na^+ and Cl^- that occurs after initiation of MCH administration does not persist with continued hormone administration. The expansion of extracellular fluid volume that occurs as NaCl is retained initiates physiologic events that increase the filtered load of Na^+ and decrease the fraction of the filtered load of Na^+ reabsorbed by the renal tubules. As a consequence, after an initial decrement, the urinary excretion rates of Na^+ and Cl^- return to baseline values. Prior restriction of the amount of NaCl in the diet diminishes the initial decrement and prolongs the period of Na^+ and Cl^- retention, perhaps because a critical level of volume expansion is required to reestablish the steady state.[58] Alterations in renal hemodynamics, interstitial hydrostatic pressure, plasma oncotic pressure, and plasma concentration of natriuretic substances have been implicated in mediating the reduction in fractional Na^+ reabsorption that permits establishment of the steady state.[61] The mediating mechanism is not dependent on a decline of aldosterone-stimulated Na^+ reabsorption in the cortical collecting duct.[62] The precise intrarenal physiologic mechanisms that mediate the reestablishment of Na^+ and Cl^- balance have not been elucidated, and conflicting observations remain to be resolved.

The magnitude of the kaliuretic response to MCH administration in normal subjects is influenced by the amount of NaCl in the diet.[58] Prior restriction of Na^+ intake limits the kaliuretic (and acid excretory) response, and prior supplementation with Na^+ and Cl^- exaggerates the response. With continued MCH administration, kaliuresis may persist beyond the transition period wherein Na^+ balance is reestablished. Chronic K^+ depletion stimulates thirst,[63] decreases renal concentrating ability,[63,64] and leads to polyuria. It reversibly decreases renal blood flow and glomerular filtration rate,[65] increases renal ammonia production,[66] and impairs renal conservation of Cl^-.[67]

Primary Aldosteronism

The syndrome of primary aldosteronism is recognized by the classic findings of hypertension, hypokalemia, metabolic alkalosis, hyperaldosteronism, and suppressed plasma-renin activity.[68,69] Hypertension occurs in part as a consequence of expanded extracellular fluid volume.[70] Administration of mineralocorticoid antagonists (e.g., spironolactone) and other natriuretic agents usually ameliorates the hypertension.[71] When spironolactone treatment is discontinued abruptly in patients with primary aldosteronism, hypertension recurs promptly because total body Na^+ stores and plasma volume again become supernormal.[72] With continued observation, plasma volume tends to return toward normal levels, but hypertension persists. Whether factors other than plasma volume expansion contribute to hypertension in states of chronic MCH excess remains to be established.

Hypokalemia resulting from renal K^+ wasting is characteristic of primary aldosteronism and is often the disturbance by which such patients are recognized clinically. Administration of large amounts of dietary NaCl tends to exacerbate renal K^+ wasting and hypokalemia because the kaliuretic response to MCH is amplified by increased delivery of tubular fluid to the K^+ secretory sites in the distal nephron[73] and because expansion of extracellular fluid volume fails to suppress aldosterone production normally in patients with primary aldosteronism.[74,75] Conversely, restriction of dietary NaCl reduces renal K^+ wasting and ameliorates hypokalemia. Some patients with primary aldosteronism may not have frank hypokalemia despite normal amounts of dietary NaCl, but in contrast to normal subjects, such patients become hypokalemic when dietary Na^+ intake is further increased.

Adrenal Enzyme Defects

Genetically transmitted deficiencies of the enzymes required for adrenal steroid biosynthesis lead to distinct clinical syndromes of disturbed MCH production. In two such enzyme-deficiency states, 11β- and 17α-hydroxylase deficiency,[76–79] impaired cortisol production results in increased ACTH secretion and secondary increased production of deoxycorticosterone (DOC), which produces a typical syndrome of mineralocorticoid excess. In 11β-hydroxylase deficiency, conversion of DOC to corticosterone and its derivatives is impaired, hence corticosterone, 18-hydroxycorticosterone, and/or aldosterone may be deficient. In 17α-hydroxylase deficiency, conversion of DOC to its derivatives is not enzymatically blocked, hence corticosterone levels are markedly elevated and may contribute to the hypermineralocorticoid state. Despite the intact enzymatic pathway to aldosterone, aldosterone production is generally subnormal, presumably as a consequence of the reduced plasma renin activity and the hypokalemia that occur due to the hypermineralocorticoid state.[80]

Although the mineralocorticoid potency of DOC is less than that of aldosterone, the levels of DOC present in patients with these two disorders appear sufficiently great to account for the hypermineralocorticoid state. In studies using renal mineralocorticoid receptors incubated in the presence of normal plasma-binding proteins, the estimated mineralocorticoid potency of DOC is approximately one-sixth that of aldosterone and accounts for little or no receptor occupancy at normal plasma concentrations (5 to 10 ng/dl).[45] At plasma levels of DOC comparable to those observed in patients with these two enzyme deficiency states (200 to 500 ng/dl),[81] major receptor occupancy has been demonstrated. It has been hypothesized that the increased levels of corticosterone and 11-deoxycortisol may compete with DOC for available binding sites on the circulating corticosteroid-binding globulin and may therefore make more free DOC available for interaction with the mineralocorticoid receptor.[81]

These two syndromes may be readily distinguished in the clinical setting by their different effects on sexual development. In the 17α-hydroxylase deficiency syndrome, biosynthesis of adrenal and gonadal androgen and estrogen is impaired, inhibiting normal sexual maturation. Genotypic female patients fail to undergo menarche or to develop secondary sexual characteristics.[76] Genotypic male patients become pseudohermaphrodites as a consequence of androgen deficiency in utero.[79,82] In the 11β-hydroxylase deficiency syndrome, the enzymatic steps required for the synthesis of adrenal sex steroids are unimpaired. The increased adrenocorticotropic hormone (ACTH) level stimulates increased production of adrenal androgen, frequently causing virilism.[77] In both syndromes, glucocorticoid hormone replacement therapy inhibits ACTH secretion and resultant excess MCH production and ameliorates the hypermineralocorticoid state. In patients with the 11β-hydroxylase deficiency syndrome, androgen production diminishes and signs of virilization tend to disappear.

Cushing's Syndrome

Glucocorticoid hormone excess characteristically results in obesity, carbohydrate intolerance, muscle wasting, osteoporosis, and mild hirsutism. Hypertension and the electrolyte abnormalities of typical hypermineralocorticoidism may occur but are rarely severe. Because the severity of the hypokalemia and metabolic alkalosis in patients with Cushing's syndrome can be directly related to the degree of elevation of plasma cortisol,[83] it has been suggested that the electrolyte abnormalities reflect the mineralocorticoid activity of cortisol. Although cortisol has only 0.4 percent of the mineralocorticoid activity of aldosterone when measured in the presence of normal amounts of plasma-binding proteins,[45] the plasma concentrations may become sufficiently great to have a considerable mineralocorticoid effect.

In a patient with marked hypertension and hypokalemia, the presence of a more potent mineralocorticoid hormone than cortisol should be suspected. Elevated DOC levels, as high as those observed in patients with the 17α-hydroxylase deficiency syndrome, have been reported in patients with Cushing's syndrome caused by malignancy of adrenal[84] or extraadrenal (ectopic ACTH syndrome) origin.[85] Less commonly, aldosterone is also elevated and probably contributes to the severity of the hypermineralocorticoid state.[85] One of the consequences of excess amounts of DOC and/or aldosterone is suppressed plasma renin activity, which is ordinarily normal or increased in patients with Cushing's syndrome caused by benign adrenal hyperplasia. Thus, the finding of suppressed plasma renin activity in a patient with Cushing's syndrome should also suggest the presence of a potent mineralocorticoid hormone.[86]

Pseudohyperaldosteronism

In 1963 Liddle et al.[87] described a familial disorder in which the clinical manifestations closely resembled those resulting from an aldosterone-producing adenoma of the adrenal glands (primary aldosteronism), but in which the measured rate of aldosterone secretion and excretion was greatly subnormal. The presenting findings were hypertension, hypokalemia due to renal potassium wasting, and metabolic alkalosis. Consideration was given to the possibility that these findings reflected the renal action of an unidentified mineralocorticoid present in abnormally increased concentrations, but this possibility was excluded by the observation that urinary electrolyte excretion was unchanged after administration of large amounts of a mineralocorticoid antagonist (spironolactone).

It was proposed that the primary abnormality was a renal tubular transport defect characterized by hyperabsorption of sodium (resulting in extracellular fluid volume expansion, hypertension, and suppression of renin and aldosterone secretion) and hypersecretion of potassium and hydrogen ion (resulting in hypokalemia and metabolic alkalosis). Consistent with this proposal is the finding that hypokalemia, alkalosis, and hypertension are corrected during chronic administration of triamterene or amiloride,[87-89] diuretic agents that cause natriuresis and renal potassium retention by a direct tubular effect that is not dependent on the presence of mineralocorticoids. The nature of the proposed defect of the renal tubule has not been elucidated, but its localization to post-macula densa segments of the distal nephron would be in accord with the known segmental localization of the renal action of amiloride and triamterene.

Recently, Rodriguez et al.[88] reported the results of extensive studies carried out in a patient with a syndrome similar to that of the patient reported by Liddle et al.[87] Plasma renin concentration and plasma aldosterone concentration were markedly subnormal, confirming that the renin–angiotensin–aldosterone system was suppressed. The presence of an unidentified adrenal mineralocorticoid was excluded by the observation that renal potassium wasting was not ameliorated during chronic administration of a potent inhibitor of adrenal steroid biosynthesis, aminoglutethimide. Furthermore, no abnormal steroid metabolites were detected in the urine by mass spectroscopy. Renal potassium wasting and hypertension were ameliorated in response to dietary restriction of sodium, a finding consistent with the primary defect proposed by Liddle et al.[87] as the cause in this syndrome: It would be predicted that during dietary sodium restriction hyperabsorption of sodium in the distal nephron would be limited consequent to a reduction in distal delivery of sodium, hence body sodium stores and the rate of distal nephron sodium-dependent potassium secretion would be reduced.

Abnormally increased rates of reabsorption of sodium and secretion of potassium and hydrogen ion might reflect a defect in the operation of a normal mechanism that ordinarily imposes a partial tonic inhibition of sodium reabsorption and potassium and hydrogen ion secretion. In distal nephron segments normally responsive to aldosterone, such a normal inhibitory mechanism might in turn be normally suppressed by aldosterone, or specifically, by aldosterone-induced protein. The suppression might account for the normal action of aldosterone to stimulate sodium reabsorption and potassium and hydrogen ion secretion. The possible existence of such an aldosterone-suppressible tonic inhibitory control mechanism has been provided by the results of in vitro studies of the effect of protein inhibitors on aldosterone-modulated transepithelial hydrogen ion transport in toad bladders.[90] Conceivably, Liddle's syndrome might result from the loss of this postulated control mechanism.

Secondary Hyperaldosteronism

Hyperaldosteronism characteristically occurs in states of reduced effective arterial blood volume, where there is activation of the renin–angiotensin system.[91] The resultant increases in plasma aldosterone concentration stimulate renal tubular reabsorption of Na^+ and Cl^- and thereby tend to restore normal effective blood volume. When hypovolemia is of extrarenal origin (vomiting, diarrhea, or hemorrhage) and renal tubular reabsorption of Na^+ and Cl^- is not specifically impaired, the Na^+-retaining effect of hypermineralocorticoidism is manifested by reduced urinary excretion rates of Na^+ that persist until effective arterial blood volume is restored. Provision of adequate amounts of dietary NaCl may effect normalization of effective arterial blood volume. The Na^+-retaining effect of hypermineralocorticoidism does not reduce excretion rates of Na^+ when hypovolemia is caused predominantly by impaired renal tubular reabsorption of Na^+ and Cl^-, as in diuretic administration, Bartter's syndrome, and some types of renal tubular acidosis. When the reduction in effective arterial blood volume is due to congestive heart failure, cirrhosis, nephrotic syndrome, or other similar disorders, provision of dietary NaCl leads to progressive expansion of extracellular fluid volume and edema without restoration of effective blood volume.

Hyperaldosteronism secondary to activation of the renin–angiotensin system also occurs in patients with accelerated hypertension, renovascular or segmental renal lesions, and rarely, renin-secreting neoplasms.[91] Activation of the renin–angiotensin–aldosterone system in the absence of hypovolemia results in hypertension.

The exact contribution of excess MCH production to the pathophysiology observed in states of secondary hyperaldosteronism is not always clear. Hypertension persisted despite adrenalectomy in a patient with a renin-secreting tumor[92] and in animals with experimental renovascular hypertension.[93] Reduction of Na^+ excretion and edema formation can occur in patients who have cardiac, renal, or hepatic disease without evidence of increased aldosterone secretion.[94] Potassium wasting persists despite sustained correction of secondary hyperaldosteronism in some patients with type 1 renal tubular acidosis[95] and in some patients with Bartter's syndrome.[96] In these disorders, however, it seems likely that the secondary aldosteronism serves to amplify the consequences of the primary defect responsible for renal potassium wasting.

Bartter's Syndrome and Other Syndromes of Renal Potassium Wasting (Table 19–2)

In 1962 Bartter et al.[97] described a unique syndrome characterized by hypokalemia due to renal potassium wasting; chloride-resistant metabolic alkalosis; increased circulating angiotensin II and urine aldosterone in the absence of edema, hypertension, or clinically overt hypovolemia; subnormal pressor responsiveness to intravenously infused angiotensin II; ADH-resistant renal concentrating defect; hypertrophy and hyperplasia of the juxtaglomerular apparatus of the kidney; and growth retardation. Subsequently, hyperreninemia was determined to be a characteristic feature of the syndrome. Since the original description of the syndrome in two children, approximately 100 additional cases have been reported in both children and adults.

The following additional abnormalities occur frequently but not invariably: hypomagnesemia; hyperuricemia; increased urinary excretion of prostaglandin E_2 (PGE_2), and other prostaglandins of renal origin.[98] Both the renal histopathologic findings and the finding of subnormal pressor responsiveness to angiotensin II have been observed in disorders of extrarenal origin that cause hypokalemia (e.g., familial chloride diarrhea, chronic surreptitious vomiting, chronic laxative abuse) and are not considered of primary pathogenetic significance.

The primary pathogenetic mechanism of Bartter's syndrome remains unresolved. Bartter and associates interpret the available data as indicating that the proximate cause of the syndrome is abnormally reduced sodium chloride reabsorption in the thick ascending limb of the loop of Henle.[99] Other investigators have provided evidence that the primary abnormality is an impairment of sodium chloride reabsorption in the proximal convoluted tubule, and still others have proposed that impaired reabsorption of potassium in post-macula densa segments of the distal nephron could lead to the characteristic features of Bartter's syndrome.[100] Furthermore, it remains unresolved whether the same primary pathogenetic mechanism underlies all reported cases diagnosed as Bartter's syndrome.

Considerations of the pathophysiology of Bartter's syndrome have focused on the pathogenesis of renal potassium wasting, the dysfunction that gives rise to the predominant clinical manifestations. There is no compelling evidence that hyperaldosteronism is critical

Table 19–2. Renal Potassium Wasting Caused by Distal Nephron Dysfunction: Mechanisms and Classification

- Abnormally reduced passive reabsorption of potassium in the thick ascending limb of the loop of Henle secondary to inhibition of active chloride reabsorption
  - Loop diuretics (furosemide, ethacrynic acid)
  - ? Bartter's syndrome
  - ? Magnesium depletion
- Hypersecretion of potassium in postmacula densa distal nephron
  - Hypermineralocorticoidism in the setting of normal or supernormal rates of delivery of water and sodium chloride to the distal nephron
    - Hypertensive states
      - Primary aldosteronism
      - Cushing's syndrome
      - Hypertensive forms of congenital adrenal hyperplasia (17α-hydroxylase deficiency, 11β-hydroxylase deficiency)
      - Malignant hypertension
      - Renovascular hypertension
      - Renin-secreting tumor
    - Renal transport defects
      - Bartter's syndrome
      - Thiazides and loop diuretics
      - Type 1 renal tubular acidosis
      - Magnesium depletion
    - Metabolic acidosis of extrarenal origin (ammonium chloride, HCl)
  - Markedly supernormal rates of delivery of water and sodium salts of poorly reabsorbable anions in the setting of normal or increased circulating aldosterone
    - Carbenicillin, penicillin, nafcillin
    - Type 2 renal tubular acidosis
    - Metabolic alkalosis of extrarenal origin
    - Metabolic acidosis of extrarenal origin (organic acidoses, H_2SO_4)
    - Carbonic anhydrase inhibition
  - Pseudohyperaldosteronism (hyperaldosteronism-like states unassociated with endogenous mineralocorticoid excess and characterized by aldosterone deficiency)
    - Liddle's syndrome
    - Licorice gluttony
    - Exogenous mineralocorticoids
    - Carbenoxolone
  - Defect of luminal membrane resulting in leakage of cellular potassium into lumen
    - Amphotericin nephrotoxicity
    - Toluene nephrotoxicity
    - ? Bartter's syndrome
- Impaired active reabsorption of potassium secondary to defect of luminal membrane in postmacula densa distal nephron
  - ? Bartter's syndrome

to the causation of renal potassium wasting in Bartter's syndrome, although the degree of hyperaldosteronism may determine the severity of renal potassium wasting. Renal potassium wasting has been observed to persist when the secretion rate of aldosterone was reduced by administration of an inhibitor of aldosterone biosynthesis as well as by maneuvers that suppress renin secretion.[96] However, it remains uncertain in these instances whether the degree of suppression of aldosterone secretion was of sufficient magnitude to exclude aldosterone stimulation of renal potassium secretion as a factor contributing to the severity of the renal potassium wasting. It is conceivable that even small amounts of circulating aldosterone are sufficient to promote renal potassium wasting in patients with Bartter's syndrome despite renal potassium wasting in one patient after adrenalectomy.[100]

In those patients with Bartter's syndrome in whom the secretion rate of aldosterone is not greatly increased, the occurrence of renal potassium wasting might be accounted for as a consequence of delivery of an abnormally large amount of sodium and water to the potassium-secreting segments of the distal nephron. Increased distal delivery of sodium and water could result from an impairment in the reabsorption of filtered sodium and water in the proximal tubule, loop of Henle, or distal convoluted tubule. The finding that renal potassium wasting persists in patients with Bartter's syndrome under conditions of restriction of dietary intake of sodium has been interpreted as evidence in support of this possibility.[97] This interpretation is based on the consideration that restriction of dietary sodium corrects renal potassium wasting in patients with primary aldosteronism, who are presumed not to have abnormally increased delivery of sodium to the aldosterone-responsive segments of the nephron during dietary sodium restriction. The interpretation can be questioned, however, since it is based on the assumption that dietary sodium restriction does not reduce distal sodium delivery appropriately in patients with Bartter's syndrome. Conceivably, in patients with Bartter's syndrome, restriction of dietary sodium appropriately reduces the delivery of sodium and water to the aldosterone-responsive segments of the nephron, yet renal potassium wasting persists owing to a defect in potassium transport not dependent on a supernormal distal delivery of sodium.

The hypothesis that the proximate cause of Bartter's syndrome is a defect in sodium chloride reabsorption in the thick ascending limb of Henle has been supported by the finding of impaired renal diluting ability in patients with the syndrome.[99] Normally, the thick ascending limb is quantitatively the most important segment of the nephron that results in the excretion of solute free water in response to water loading. During water loading, when release of antidiuretic hormone is normally suppressed, the renal clearance of solute free water (CH_2O) provides a reliable estimate of the rate at which solute (NaCl) is reabsorbed in the thick ascending limb. In several patients with Bartter's syndrome undergoing water loading, CH_2O has been subnormal in relationship to the amount of solute delivered to the diluting segment.[99] This finding has been interpreted as evidence that the rate at which NaCl is reabsorbed in the thick ascending limb is subnormal. An intrinsic impairment in the capacity of the thick ascending limb to reabsorb NaCl would imply an impairment in the active transport of chloride, the transport process postulated to provide the major, if not exclusive, driving force for sodium reabsorption in the thick ascending limb. Such an impairment might also reduce the rate of reabsorption of potassium in the thick ascending limb where normally as much as 30 to 40 percent of the filtered load of potassium may be reabsorbed secondary to active chloride reabsorption.[73] Diuretic agents that inhibit active chloride reabsorption in the thick ascending limb greatly increase the amount of potassium and sodium entering the distal convoluted tubule.[101] Indeed, chronic abuse of diuretic agents can lead to a syndrome resembling Bartter's syndrome.

However, the finding of impaired renal diluting ability in patients with Bartter's syndrome does not necessarily indicate an impairment of sodium chloride reabsorption in the distal nephron. During oral water loading, it is assumed that systemic levels of antidiuretic hormone are suppressed, and antidiuretic hormone-mediated water reabsorption throughout the distal nephron is minimized. In patients with Bartter's syndrome it is conceivable that antidiuretic hormone-mediated water reabsorption is not appropriately minimized during oral water loading, thereby resulting in impaired diluting ability. One reason for this may be that antidiuretic hormone secretion is not normally suppressed in response to water loading owing to nonosmotic factors stimulating antidiuretic hormone secretion. In the only patient reported in whom measurement of plasma antidiuretic hormone concentration was obtained during water loading,[102] antidiuretic hormone was undetectable. This finding may not be compelling, since plasma antidiuretic hormone concentration may have been significantly greater in the patient than in similarly studied normal subjects, and this difference may have been sufficient to account for the moderate impairment in renal diluting ability observed in the patient. It is also possible that appropriate suppression of antidiuretic hormone secretion occurs during water loading in patients with Bartter's syndrome, yet water reabsorption is not appropriately suppressed owing to (1) abnormal water reabsorption not dependent on antidiuretic hormone or (2) exaggerated renal responsiveness to antidiuretic hormone conditioned by unidentified intrarenal factors. Exclusion of inappropriate water reabsorption in the collecting duct is prerequisite to the interpretation that impaired renal diluting ability indicates a defect in NaCl reabsorption in the thick ascending limb of the loop of Henle.

Alternative mechanisms can be postulated to account for the pathogenesis of renal potassium wasting in Bartter's syndrome based on current concepts of distal nephron potassium transport. A defect of the luminal membrane in the collecting duct that results in leakage of cellular potassium into the lumen or that impairs active reabsorption of potassium from the lumen might result in renal potassium wasting that is not dependent on aldosterone but that is amplified by hyperaldosteronism. How such a defect could give rise to hyperreninemia and hyperaldosteronism without overt alterations in extracellular fluid volume and blood pressure must remain conjectural. It is possible that a primary potassium transport defect is shared by the epithelial cells of the macula densa segment of the distal nephron and that such a defect leads directly to increased renin secretion.

Magnesium depletion secondary to renal magnesium wasting might play a critical role in the causation of renal potassium wasting in some patients with Bartter's syndrome. Experimentally induced magnesium depletion in normal subjects results in reversible renal potassium wasting,[103] while chronic intravenous administration of magnesium can induce renal conservation of potassium in some patients with Bartter's syndrome.[102] Table 19–2 summarizes the potential mechanisms of renal potassium wasting that may be caused by distal nephron dysfunction and outlines a classification for the clinical spectrum of renal potassium-wasting syndromes.

SYNDROMES OF MINERALOCORTICOID HORMONE DEFICIENCY (Table 19–3)

Experimental States of Mineralocorticoid Hormone Deficiency

In dogs with isolated MCH deficiency the most prominent pathophysiologic features are hyponatremia and hypovolemia due to Na^+ wasting, hyperkalemia due to K^+ retention, and metabolic acidosis due to reduced net acid excretion.[104,105] The effect of aldosterone deficiency on the acidification process of the mammalian nephron has been studied in adrenalectomized dogs maintained postoperatively on physiologic replacement doses of glucocorticoid and mineralocorticoid hormones.[104] When the administration of mineralocorticoid hormones is discontinued, net acid excretion decreases, and hyperkalemia and hyperchloremic acidosis occur (Fig. 19–3). The reduction in net acid excretion is accounted for largely by reduction in urine ammonium excretion, which in turn appears to be due to diminished renal production of ammonia, since it occurs in the absence of an increase in urine pH or a decrease in urine flow. The reduction in ammonia production appears to be in part a response to hyperkalemia, since the excretion rate of ammonium correlates inversely with the plasma potassium concentration and does not decrease on discontinuation of mineralocorticoid if the occurrence of hyperkalemia is prevented by concomitantly restricting potassium intake.

The results of additional studies in the adrenalectomized dog indicate that aldosterone deficiency impairs the rate capacity of the distal nephron to secrete H^+ but does not impair its ability to generate normally steep lumen-to-blood H^+ concentration gradients. The H^+ concentration gradient-generating ability of

Table 19–3. Clinical Spectrum of Syndromes of Mineralocorticoid Hormone Deficiency and Resistance

- Aldosterone deficiency
  - Combined deficiency of aldosterone and adrenal glucocorticoid hormones
    - Addison's disease
    - Bilateral adrenalectomy
    - Inherited impairment of steroidogenesis: 21-hydroxylase deficiency (congenital adrenal hyperplasia)
  - Selective deficiency of aldosterone
    - Inherited impairment of aldosterone biosynthesis (corticosterone methyl oxidase deficiency)
    - Secondary to deficient renin secretion
      - Diabetic nephropathy
      - Chronic tubulointerstitial disease with glomerular insufficiency
      - Indomethacin administration
    - Chronic idiopathic hypoaldosteronism in adults and children
- Pseudohypoaldosteronism (attenuated renal response to aldosterone with secondary hyperreninemia and hyperaldosteronism)
  - Classic pseudohypoaldosteronism of infancy
  - Chronic tubulointerstitial disease with glomerular insufficiency salt-wasting nephritis
  - Drugs (spironolactone, amiloride, triamterene)
- Attenuated renal response to aldosterone + aldosterone deficiency
  - Selective tubule dysfunction with impaired renin secretion
  - Chronic tubulointerstitial disease with glomerular insufficiency
    - Associated deficient renin secretion
    - Renin status uncertain
  - Renal transplantation with deficient renin secretion
  - Lupus nephritis with deficient renin secretion

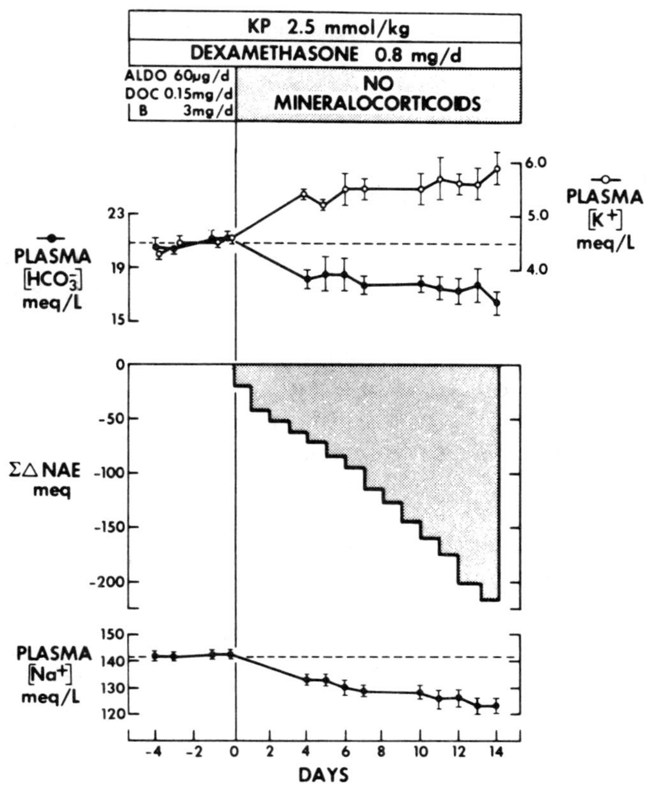

Fig. 19–3. Effect of mineralocorticoid discontinuation on plasma and urinary acid–base and electrolyte composition in adrenalectomized dogs maintained on dexamethasone without direct effort to maintain normal sodium balance or to prevent development of hyperkalemia. (From Hulter HN, Licht JH, Glynn RD, et al: Renal acidosis in mineralocorticoid deficiency is not dependent on NaCl depletion or hyperkalemia. Am J Physiol 236:F283, 1979.)

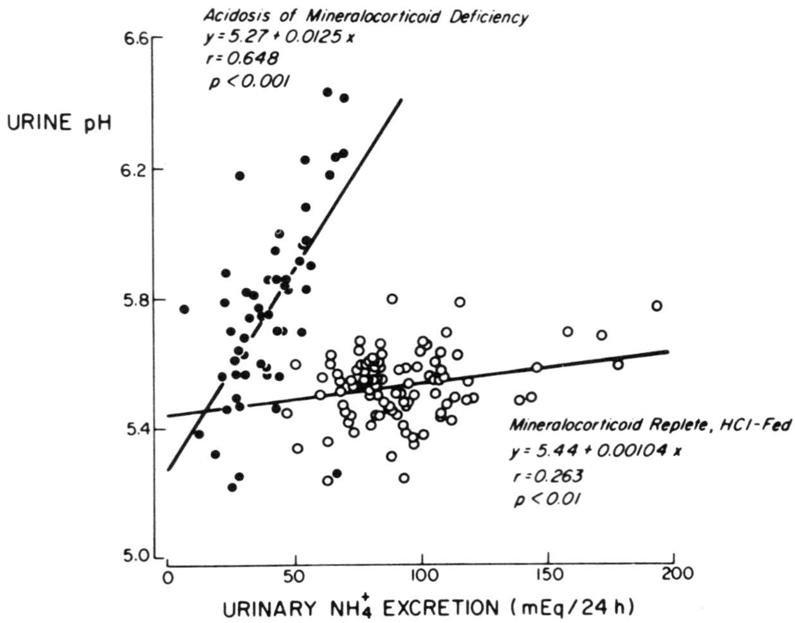

Fig. 19–4. Daily urine pH as a function of daily urinary ammonium excretion in mineralocorticoid-deficient glucocorticoid-replete adrenalectomized dogs ($N = 5$) and in mineralocorticoid-replete hydrochloric acid-fed dogs ($N = 8$) during steady-state metabolic acidosis. (From Hulter HN, Ilnicki LP, Harbottle JA, et al: Impaired renal H^+ secretion and NH_3 production in mineralocorticoid-deficient glucocorticoid-replete dogs. Am J Physiol 232:F136, 1977.)

the distal nephron is best assessed when luminal buffer concentration is low, as when renal production and urine excretion of ammonia are greatly reduced by hyperkalemia. Under these conditions, urine pH in mineralocorticoid-deficient dogs is not different from that in mineralocorticoid-replete dogs in which similar degrees of metabolic acidosis have been induced by exogenous acid feeding (Fig. 19–4). However, when the amount of luminal buffer is increased, the urine pH increases to a substantially greater degree in mineralocorticoid-deficient dogs than in mineralocorticoid-replete dogs, indicating that in the former group the secretion of H^+ increases at a blunted rate (Fig. 19–4). These findings in the dog are consistent with the results of in vitro studies in turtle bladders.[16]

In humans, similar studies have been performed in adrenalectomized patients in an attempt to investigate the renal and systemic acid–base consequences of mineralocorticoid deficiency in the absence of either glucocorticoid deficiency or parenchymal renal disease (Fig. 19–5).[106] Glucocorticoid replacement was provided with dexamethasone and mineralocorticoid replacement with fludrocortisone. After a control period, mineralocorticoid replacement was either discontinued or initiated. Net acid excretion and plasma total CO_2 decreased in each patient in whom mineralocorticoid was discontinued and increased in each patient in whom mineralocorticoid was initiated. The magnitude of the cumulative change in net acid excretion correlated with the basal rate of net acid excretion, hence presumably with the basal rate of endogenous acid production. The change in plasma total CO_2 correlated with the change in net acid excretion and the changes in net acid excretion cor-

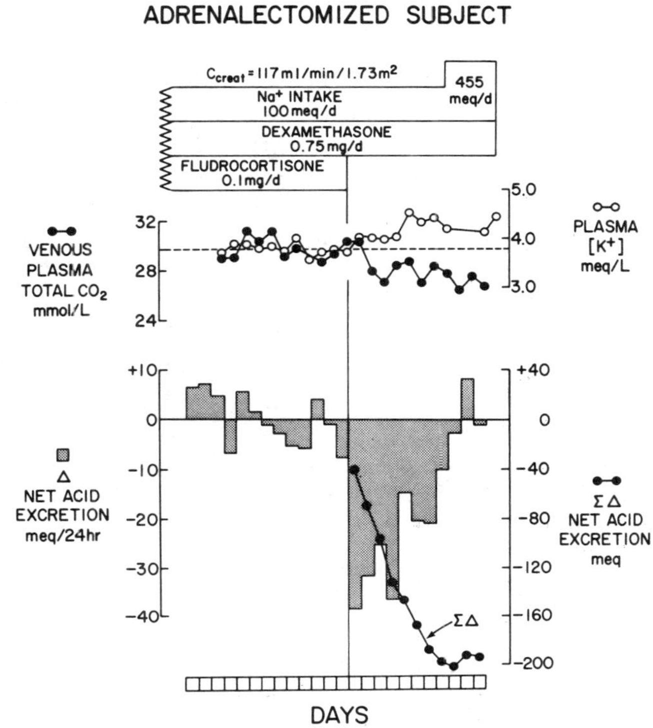

Fig. 19–5. Representative study of the effect of discontinuation of mineralocorticoid replacement therapy in an adrenalectomized patient without apparent intrinsic renal disease. (Top) The dashed curve represents the mean control value of both plasma total carbon dioxide and potassium concentration (P_K). Values of Δ net acid excretion (ΔNAE) represent the difference between the daily net acid and the mean control values. Values of ΣΔNAE represent the accumulated sum of the daily values of ΔNAE during the period of mineralocorticoid discontinuation. (Reprinted from Kidney International. Sebastian A, Sutton JM, Hulter HN, et al: Effect of mineralocorticoid replacement therapy on renal acid–base homeostasis in adrenalectomized patients. Kidney Int 18:762, 1980.)

related positively with the corresponding changes in sodium balance and negatively with the corresponding changes in potassium balance.

These findings provide the first evidence that renal acidification is under tonic stimulation by mineralocorticoid at levels of mineralocorticoid not exceeding those of normal subjects ingesting typical acid-producing diets with normal sodium and potassium content. The extent to which the tonic stimulation of renal acidification is mediated by a direct effect of mineralocorticoid on renal H^+ transport or by an indirect effect dependent on altered renal sodium and/or potassium transport was not determined. Nevertheless, the findings implicate mineralocorticoid deficiency as a significant renal acidosis-producing condition not dependent on the presence of renal disease or glucocorticoid deficiency, and potentially amplified when endogenous acid production is increased by diet or disease.

Generalized Adrenocortical Insufficiency

Generalized adrenocortical insufficiency (Addison's disease) occurs when, as a consequence of destruction of adrenocortical tissue, secretory rates of both MCH and glucocorticoid hormone are inadequate to meet the physiologic needs of the organism. The combined deficiency of cortisol and aldosterone results in a progressive syndrome that is usually fatal if untreated.

Cortisol deficiency results in anorexia, weight loss, weakness, apathy, and a general inability to withstand stress. Cortisol normally inhibits ACTH secretion, hence markedly elevated levels of ACTH are characteristic of Addison's disease. Mineralocorticoid deficiency results in impaired renal Na^+ conservation. If the Na^+ intake is sufficiently large, extracellular fluid volume can be maintained at normal or near normal levels. However, if the Na^+ intake is low or if extrarenal losses of Na^+ occur, the inability to conserve Na^+ maximally results in marked Na^+ deficits, hyponatremia, hypovolemia, and increased plasma renin levels.[107] Glucocorticoid deficiency may contribute further to the severity of the hypovolemia by redistribution of fluid between vascular and extravascular compartments.[108,109]

The failure of the kidney to correct hyponatremia in patients with Addison's disease by the excretion of urine that is appropriately dilute with respect to the prevailing level of plasma hypoosmolality appears to be a consequence of the deficiency of both MCH and glucocorticoid hormone. In MCH-deficient glucocorticoid-replete animals impaired renal-diluting ability is prevented by administration of sufficient amounts of NaCl to minimize extracellular fluid volume depletion.[110] Extracellular fluid volume depletion is associated with enhanced proximal reabsorption of filtrate and thereby with a decreased delivery of tubular fluid to the diluting segments of the distal nephron, which limits the rate of excretion of solute free water. Hypovolemia is also known to stimulate release of antidiuretic hormone,[111] which could further limit water excretion. Impaired diluting ability also occurs in patients who have glucocorticoid deficiency without MCH deficiency, such as those with panhypopituitarism or isolated ACTH deficiency; this abnormality is reversible by administration of small doses of glucocorticoid hormones.[112] Elevated levels of antidiuretic hormone have been observed in adrenalectomized dogs maintained only on MCH,[113] and the associated defect in water excretion has been attributed to impaired suppression of secretion of antidiuretic hormone secondary to hemodynamic factors (e.g., decreased left ventricular stroke volume).

Hyperkalemia and metabolic acidosis might be expected to occur in patients with Addison's disease as a consequence of a diminished mineralocorticoid effect on K^+ and H^+ secretion in the distal nephron. In adrenalectomized subjects with normal kidneys, ingesting liberal amounts of dietary Na^+ and Cl^- and receiving glucocorticoid hormone therapy, isolated MCH deficiency results in mild hyperkalemia or metabolic acidosis.[106]

A variety of pathologic processes involving the adrenal gland can result in generalized adrenocortical insufficiency: tuberculosis, histoplasmosis and other fungal diseases, metastatic carcinoma, amyloidosis, and bilateral adrenal hemorrhage. Addison's disease appears to occur most frequently as a component of an autoimmune process that results in selective atrophy of the adrenal cortex (idiopathic adrenal insufficiency), usually sparing the adrenal medulla.[114] Patients so affected often manifest evidence of other autoimmune processes affecting the thyroid, islet cells, gonads, and other tissues.

The diagnosis of adrenal insufficiency is confirmed by the finding of subnormal plasma cortisol and urinary 17-hydroxycorticoid levels after administration of ACTH and by increased baseline plasma ACTH concentration. Treatment with hydrocortisone or an equivalent glucocorticoid is required on a lifelong basis. Because aldosterone production is also decreased, MCH replacement is frequently added, but many patients may be maintained on a high Na^+ intake without MCH.

Adrenal Enzyme Defects Causing Mineralocorticoid Deficiency

Mineralocorticoid deficiency occurs in several of the congenital disorders of the adrenal gland characterized pathologically by diffuse bilateral enlargement of the adrenal cortex and collectively referred to as congenital adrenal hyperplasia. These disorders usually result from inherited defects in adrenal steroid biosynthesis inferred to result from adrenal enzyme defects. At least five different disorders have been recognized. The abnormal pattern and amounts of steroids secreted differ for each genotype and mediate a different clinical

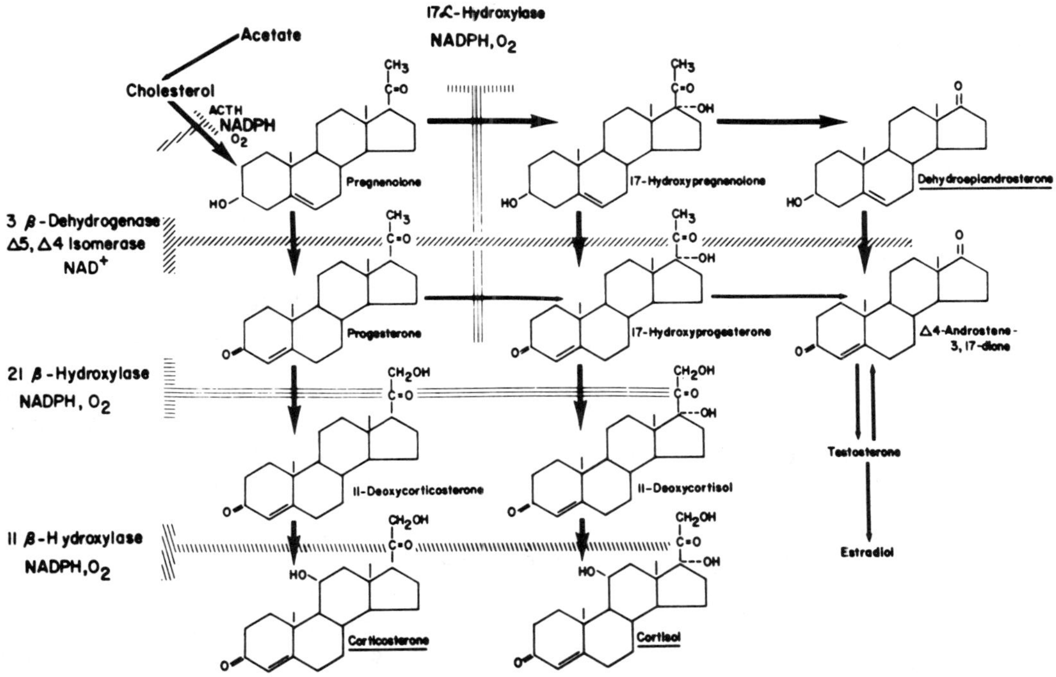

Fig. 19–6. Outline of hormone biosynthesis in the zona fasciculata and zona reticularis of the adrenal cortex. Major secretory products are underlined. Enzymes and cofactors for the reactions progressing down each column are shown on the left and from the first to the second column at the top of the chart. When a particular enzyme is deficient, hormone production is blocked at the points indicated by the shaded bars. (Reproduced, with permission, from Ganong WF: Review of Medical Physiology, 11th ed. Copyright 1983 by Lange Medical Publications, Los Altos, California.)

syndrome. The disordered secretion of steroids by the adrenal gland in these disorders leads to supernormal circulating levels of adrenocorticotropic hormones (ACTH and/or angiotensin), which influence the rate of secretion of the steroids by the defective gland and induce adrenal hyperplasia.

When the normal flow of steroid intermediates through the biosynthetic pathways is restricted because of deficient enzyme activity, steroids proximal to the point of restriction accumulate and appear in the peripheral circulation and in the urine along with their metabolites generated in the liver and kidney. The steroid biochemical consequences of restricting the normal biosynthetic pathway in the common forms of congenital adrenal hyperplasia are summarized in Figures 19–6 and 19–7.

21-HYDROXYLASE DEFICIENCY

The commonest form of congenital adrenal hyperplasia that results in MCH deficiency results from defective 21-hydroxylation in the zona fasciculata, and in some but possibly not all patients, also in the zona glomerulosa as well. Secretion by the zona fasciculata of all glucocorticoid and mineralocorticoid hormones (21-hydroxylated steroids) is subnormal, whereas secretion of progesterone and 17-hydroxyprogesterone (the normal substrates for 21-hydroxylation) is supernormal. Signs and symptoms of combined glucocorticoid and mineralocorticoid deficiency are commonly but not invariably present. The increased levels of 17-hydroxyprogesterone in the fasciculata cells result in overproduction of adrenal androgens (Fig. 19–6), causing clin-

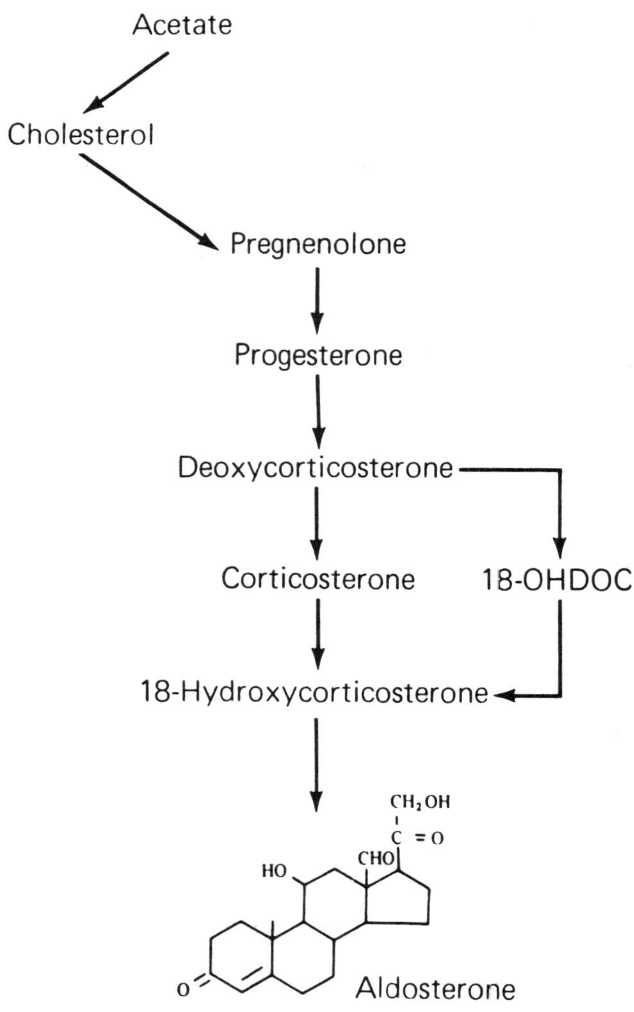

Fig. 19–7. Hormone synthesis in the zona glomerulosa. The steps from acetate to corticosterone are the same as in the zona fasciculata and reticularis. However, the zona glomerulosa contains the enzymes for converting corticosterone to aldosterone, whereas it lacks 17α-hydroxylase activity. 18-OHDOC, 18-hydroxydeoxycorticosterone. (Reproduced, with permission, from Ganong WF: Review of Medical Physiology, 11th ed. Copyright 1983 by Lange Medical Publications, Los Altos, California.)

ical virilization manifested as female pseudohermaphroditism or male precocious puberty, but differing greatly in severity among patients. The increased levels of 17-hydroxyprogesterone and progesterone in the peripheral circulation contribute to the clinical manifestations of mineralocorticoid insufficiency inasmuch as these steroids are mineralocorticoid receptor antagonists that inhibit the renal action of aldosterone.

Plasma and urine aldosterone concentrations and aldosterone secretion rates, reflecting aldosterone production uniquely by the zona glomerulosa, differ widely among patients. Normal,[115] subnormal,[115,116] and supernormal[115,117,118] levels have been reported. Likewise, the severity of clinical mineralocorticoid deficiency differs widely among patients. Two major clinical variants, so-called salt-losing and non-salt-losing forms of 21-hydroxylation deficiency, have been described, distinguished chiefly by the presence or absence of clinical evidence of sodium chloride depletion. The two variants are not associated with predictable differences in aldosterone levels, however. Aldosterone levels have been variously reported either as subnormal[115,116,119] or supernormal[115,118] in patients diagnosed as having the salt-losing variant. These levels have been reported as normal[118] or supernormal[117,119] in patients with the non-salt-losing variant. The cause of these differences in aldosterone levels has not been completely defined.

Supernormal levels of aldosterone are associated with supernormal levels of plasma renin in patients with 21-hydroxylation defect.[115,118] This combination has been interpreted as indicative of a functional state of mineralocorticoid insufficiency, especially hypovolemia, in these patients.[118] The functional state of mineralocorticoid insufficiency develops as a consequence of end-organ resistance to the action of mineralocorticoid, which occurs because the renal action of aldosterone is inhibited by high levels of 17-hydroxyprogesterone and progesterone. The stimulatory effect of renin–angiotensin hyperactivity on the zona glomerulosa promotes aldosterone production, with the result that peripheral aldosterone levels are maintained at supernormal levels. The end-organ antagonism to aldosterone is thereby mitigated, and concomitantly the physiologic state of mineralocorticoid insufficiency is mitigated. Many patients diagnosed as having the non-salt-losing variant of 21-hydroxylation deficiency evidence hyperreninemia and supernormal aldosterone levels. These patients do not evidence symptomatic sodium depletion, in particular, as long as dietary salt is not restricted.

The finding of supernormal levels of aldosterone in such patients does not necessarily imply that aldosterone biosynthesis in the zona glomerulosa is spared the genetic defect. Such a sparing of the zona glomerulosa would be suggested if the rate of aldosterone secretion were completely appropriate for the prevailing levels of stimulation of the zona glomerulosa by the renin–angiotensin system (and other trophic factors), but this has never been documented. Rather, it has been documented in many cases that aldosterone levels are not appropriately high, at least not appropriate in relationship to plasma renin activity.[115] Yet, this finding does not necessarily indicate a primary defect of the zona glomerulosa, since it is known that normally there are inhibitors of aldosterone secretion (e.g., dopamine) in the circulation, whereas it is not known what role such inhibitors play in determining the rates of aldosterone secretion in this disorder. Thus it remains unresolved whether there is genetic impairment of aldosterone biosynthesis in the zona glomerulosa in any variant of the syndrome of deficient 21-hydroxylation.

It is not certain that the primary genetic defect is the same in all patients with the syndrome of deficient 21-hydroxylation. Some investigators have inferred that the disturbance of adrenal steroid biosynthesis in at least some of these patients results from aberrant 11β-hydroxylation and is not due to a defective 21-hydroxylase.[120] The 11β-hydroxylase is aberrant in that it has preferential affinity toward the normal substrates of 21-hydroxylase, thereby forming 11-hydroxysteroids that are poor substrates for the 21-hydroxylase and thus eventuating in a deficiency of the normal products of 21-hydroxylation.[120]

CORTICOSTERONE METHYL OXIDASE DEFICIENCY

A deficiency in the mixed-function oxidase required for the final steps of aldosterone biosynthesis results in a syndrome of isolated mineralocorticoid deficiency characterized by salt wasting, hyperkalemia, and metabolic acidosis.[121–127] Examples of impaired hydroxylation of corticosterone to 18-hydroxycorticosterone and of subsequent dehydrogenation of 18-hydroxycorticosterone to aldosterone have been reported. The terms corticosterone methyl oxidase types 1 and 2 have been proposed to describe these enzyme deficiency states.[125] In patients with the type 2 defect, plasma levels of aldosterone may occasionally be in the normal range,[123] but these values should be considered inappropriately low for the marked degree of hyperreninemia and hyperkalemia. The presence of the type 2 defect can be established by the demonstration of an increase in the excretory rate of the major urinary metabolites of 18-hydroxycorticosterone and aldosterone.[125] Because these enzymes are not required for the biosynthesis of cortisol, there are no associated abnormalities in the levels of cortisol, ACTH, or adrenal androgen. The severity of the consequences of MCH deficiency in affected children can be minimized by the maintenance of a high salt intake or by MCH replacement therapy. Whereas the requirements for MCH and/or a high salt intake may decrease with age, the impaired ability to conserve Na^+ in response to a low salt intake persists.

Hyporeninemic Hypoaldosteronism

In adults, mineralocorticoid deficiency occurs in numerous renal and extrarenal disorders that cause diminished renal secretion of renin. This enzyme initiates a sequence of intravascular chemical reactions that result in the production of angiotensin II, the potent trophic hormone that stimulates production and secretion of aldosterone by the adrenal zona glomerulosa.[128-131] Under ordinary physiologic conditions in healthy subjects, angiotensin II provides a major tonic stimulatory effect on aldosterone secretion; hypoangiotensinemia attendant on diminished renin secretion leads to a clinically significant state of mineralocorticoid deficiency, so-called hyporeninemic hypoaldosteronism. In affected patients, mineralocorticoid deficiency is manifested as hyperkalemia characteristically and hyperchloremic metabolic acidosis commonly. Sodium depletion and renal sodium wasting are not invariably present,[130,132] however, and in some patients, total body sodium and extracellular fluid volume are supernormal.[132]

In 1980, DeFronzo[128] reviewed the findings in 81 reported cases of hyporeninemic hypoaldosteronism. On the basis of this review, the clinical features of hyporeninemic hypoaldosteronism can be summarized as follows:

1. Mean age: 65 ± 7 years.
2. Only 25 percent of such patients come to medical attention because of symptoms referable to hyperkalemia.
3. Fifty percent of such patients have unequivocal hyperchloremic metabolic acidosis.
4. Salt wasting is uncommon.
5. The insufficiency of aldosterone is usually only partial.
6. Cortisol levels and cortisol response to ACTH administration are normal.
7. Chronic renal insufficiency and diabetes mellitus are the two most common identifiable underlying disorders, with renal insufficiency most commonly caused by diabetic nephropathy or one of a variety of tubulointerstitial nephritides.

In an investigation of the prevalence of aldosterone deficiency in hyperkalemic patients with diffuse renal parenchymal disease and chronic renal insufficiency, Schambelan et al.[130] measured plasma and urine aldosterone levels in 31 such patients who had creatinine clearances ranging from 10 to 56 ml/min/1.73 m^2 and serum potassium concentrations ranging from 6.0 to 8.7 mEq/liter when dietary potassium was unrestricted at the time of initial diagnosis. None of the patients had cortisol deficiency. Urine aldosterone excretion ranged from 0.8 to 10.9 μg/24 hr when the subjects were in a steady state while ingesting a constant diet containing 108 to 128 mEq sodium and 30 to 64 mEq potassium. Under similar conditions in 29 normal subjects, urine aldosterone ranged from 4.2 to 15.6 μg/24 hr. By comparison with these values in normal subjects, 14 of the 31 patients had frank hypoaldosteronism. However, aldosterone excretion rates in patients with chronic hyperkalemia should be compared with values observed in normal subjects who also have chronic hyperkalemia, inasmuch as hyperkalemia per se ordinarily stimulates aldosterone secretion.[133-136] No such data are available in normal subjects with chronic experimental hyperkalemia. Therefore, in the patients with chronic renal insufficiency, aldosterone levels were evaluated by comparing the ratio of urine aldosterone excretion to the serum potassium concentration ($U_{aldo}V/S_K$) with the ratio ob-

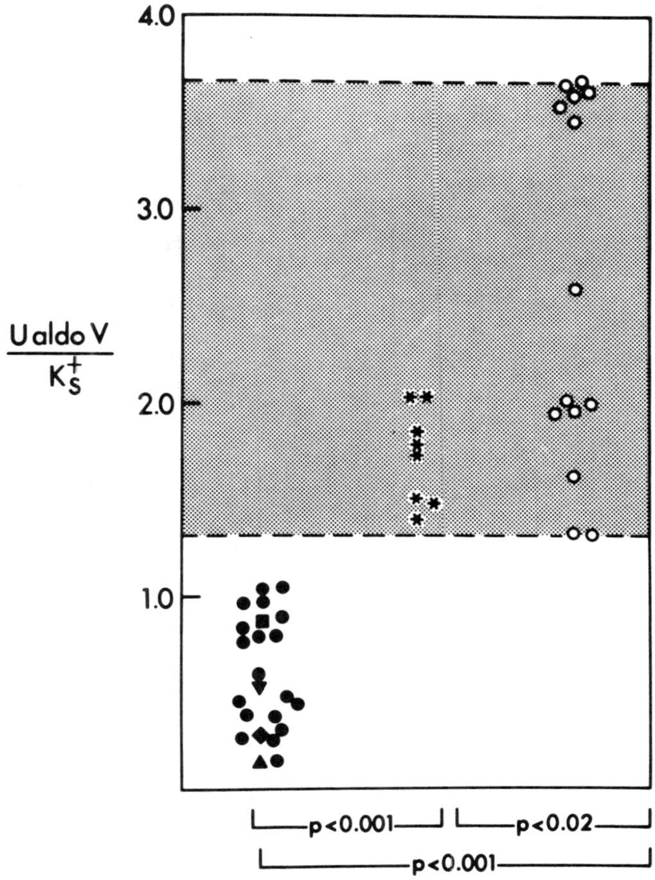

Fig. 19–8. Values for the ratio of urinary excretion of aldosterone-18-glucuronide to serum potassium concentration (U_{aldo}/S_K) in patients with hyperkalemia and chronic renal insufficiency (filled symbols and unfilled circles) and in normal subjects (unfilled triangles). Two subgroups of patients are identified: 23 patients (subgroup A) (filled symbols) in whom values of this ratio are below the range in normal subjects (shaded area) and eight patients (subgroup B) (unfilled circles) in whom the value of this ratio fell within the normal range. (Reprinted from Kidney International. Schambelan M, Sebastian A, Biglieri EG: Prevalence, pathogenesis, and functional significance of aldosterone deficiency in hyperkalemic patients with chronic renal insufficiency. Kidney Int 17:89, 1980.)

served in the normal subjects studied (Fig. 19–8). In 23 of the 31 patients, $U_{aldo}V/S_K$ was distinctly subnormal, and these patients were diagnosed as having hypoaldosteronism and designated subgroup A (Fig. 19–8). In the remaining eight patients, $U_{aldo}V/S_K$ was within the range observed in normal subjects, and these patients were designated subgroup B (Fig. 19–8).

Since the values of $U_{aldo}V/S_K$ in normal subjects who have chronic hyperkalemia are not known, the possibility could not be excluded that the patients in subgroup B also had hypoaldosteronism, but relatively less severe compared with that in subgroup A. Further evidence of hypoaldosteronism in subgroup B is the finding that normokalemic patients with chronic renal insufficiency characteristically have substantially higher concentrations of plasma aldosterone than were observed in the patients in subgroup B.[137–139] The results of the study by Schambelan et al.[130] indicate that hypoaldosteronism occurs commonly in patients with chronic renal insufficiency who have hyperkalemia.[130]

The results of the study by Schambelan et al.[130] also indicated clearly that aldosterone deficiency contributed to the pathogenesis of hyperkalemia in patients with chronic renal insufficiency. In subgroups A and B, a significant positive correlation was observed between the serum potassium concentration and the steady-state urinary excretion rate of potassium (Fig. 19–9). Urinary potassium excretion in the steady state is presumed to reflect net dietary load of potassium (diet minus stool potassium). A significantly greater degree of hyperkalemia was observed in the patients with hypoaldosteronism (subgroup A) than in those without overt hypoaldosteronism (sub-

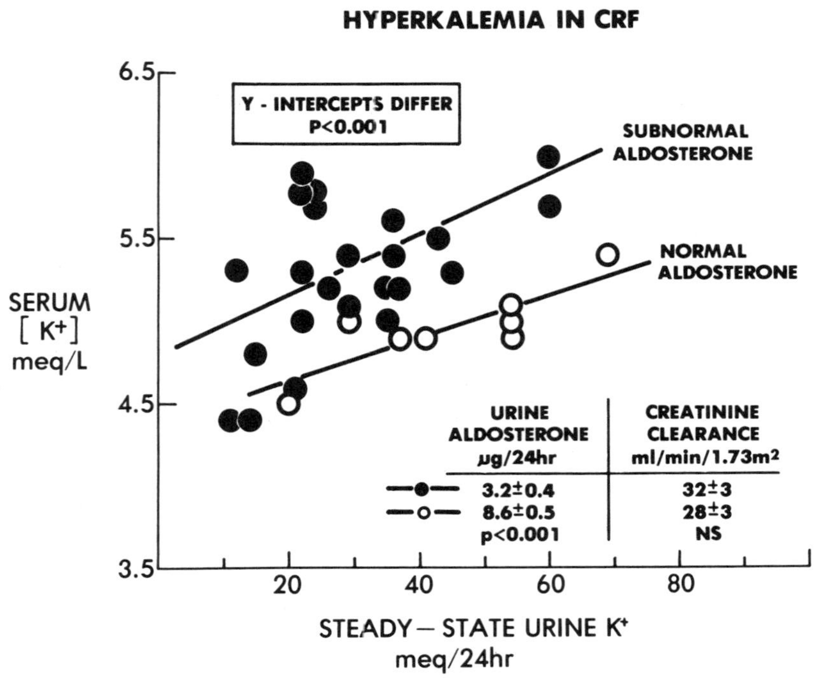

Fig. 19–9. Relationship between serum potassium concentration and urinary potassium excretion in patients with isolated hypoaldosteronism (subgroup A) (filled circles) and in patients with chronic renal insufficiency without hypoaldosteronism (subgroup B, unfilled circles). Regression lines show the significant positive correlation between these variables observed both in the patients in subgroup A ($y = 0.020x + 4.72$; $r = 0.56$; $p < 0.01$) and in those in subgroup B ($y = 0.013x + 4.38$; $r = 0.83$; $p < 0.01$). The y intercept was significantly greater ($p < 0.001$) in the patients in subgroup A than it was in those in subgroup B, but the slopes did not differ significantly in the two groups (analysis of covariance).

group B) in relationship to the net dietary load of potassium (Fig. 19–9). It is conceivable that the presence of hyperkalemia in subgroup B, albeit of lesser severity than in subgroup A, is related to the relative degree of hypoaldosteronism in these patients. Viewed in another way, these data indicate that renal clearance of potassium is impaired in hyperkalemic patients with chronic renal insufficiency and that the magnitude of this impairment is related to the extent to which aldosterone secretion is subnormal.

The role of aldosterone deficiency in the pathogenesis of metabolic acidosis in patients with diffuse renal parenchymal disease and reduced glomerular filtration rate has been investigated in studies in which the potent mineralocorticoid fludrocortisone was administered to patients with hyperkalemic renal tubular acidosis and hypoaldosteronism in the setting of chronic tubulointerstitial nephritis.[140] Administration of physiologic amounts of fludrocortisone in some cases resulted in large increases in net acid excretion of sufficient magnitude to ameliorate substantially the degree of systemic acidosis. In the patients in whom glomerular filtration rate was not markedly subnormal, that is, those having a glomerular filtration rate of >30 ml/min), the increase in net acid excretion was due almost entirely to an increase in urinary ammonium excretion (Fig. 19–10). In the patients in

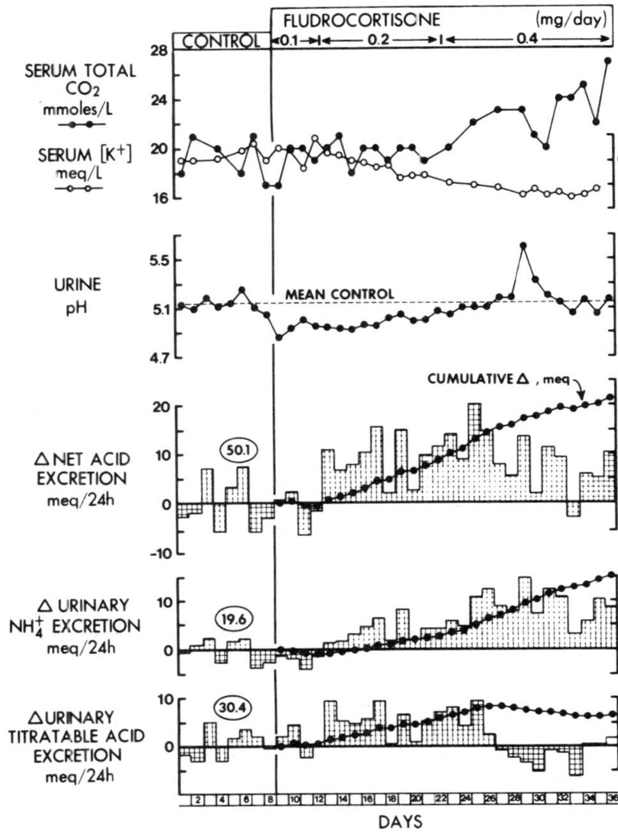

Fig. 19–10. Effect of fludrocortisone on serum carbon dioxide content and potassium concentration, urine pH and urinary titratable acid, and ammonium and net acid excretion in a patient with hyporeninemic hypoaldosteronism and chronic renal insufficiency (creatinine clearance, 36 ml/min per 1.73 m²). Systemic acidosis had not previously been treated. In the three bottom panels, the hatched bars represent the difference between the measured value of acid excretion and the mean value before therapy. The magnitude of these differences is indicated by the scale on the left-hand side of the panel. The mean control value is designated by the numerals within the ellipse. The accumulated values of the daily difference are shown by the solid circles and are indicated by the scale on the right-hand side of the panel. (Reprinted, by permission of the New England Journal of Medicine, from Sebastian A, Schambelan M, Lindenfeld S, et al: Amelioration of metabolic acidosis with fludrocortisone therapy in hyporeninemic hypoaldosteronism. N Engl J Med 297:576, 1977.)

whom glomerular filtration rate (and presumably also renal mass) was more markedly reduced, the contribution of urine ammonium excretion to the increase in net acid excretion was less; increased titratable acid excretion contributed substantially (Fig. 19–11). Analysis of the changes in urine pH and ammonium excretion indicated that administration of exogenous mineralocorticoid both augmented renal ammonia production and stimulated renal hydrogen ion secretion. The augmentation of ammonia production appeared to be due to the correction of hyperkalemia, but a more direct effect of mineralocorticoid on renal ammoniagenesis cannot be excluded. The findings in this investigation and the interpretation of the findings are described more fully in the following sections.

The results obtained in the study of one patient are summarized in Figure 19–11. The renal and systemic acid–base effects of chronic administration of a physiologic replacement dose of fludrocortisone (0.10 to 0.15 mg/day) are shown in a patient with chronic tubulointerstitial renal disease (creatinine clearance 13 ml/min per 1.73 m²) and hyporeninemic hypoaldosteronism. Fludrocortisone administration was associated with a reduction in urine pH, an increase in net acid excretion, and a substantial amelioration of systemic acidosis and hyperkalemia. The observed reduction in urine pH during fludrocortisone administration suggests that (1) despite the highly acidic urine during the pretreatment period, acidification was impaired owing to aldosterone deficiency and (2) mineralocorticoid replacement ameliorates the impairment by stimulation of H^+ secretion. Presumably the pretreatment

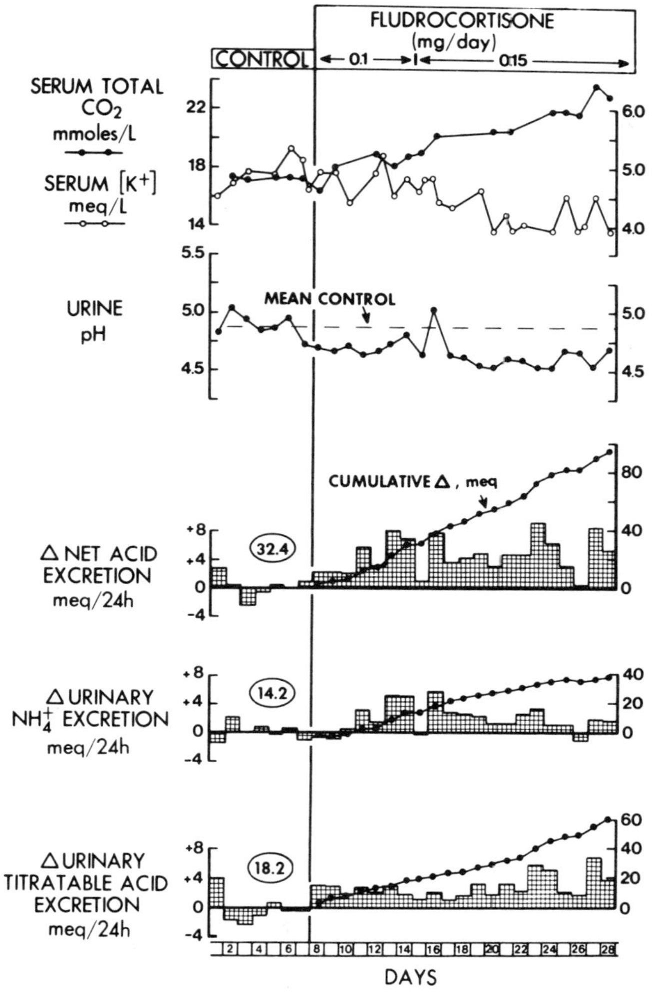

Fig. 19–11. Effect of orally administered fludrocortisone on serum carbon dioxide content and potassium concentration, urine pH and urinary titratable acid, and ammonium and net acid excretion in a patient with hyporeninemic hypoaldosteronism and chronic renal insufficiency (creatinine clearance 13 ml/min per 1.73 m^2). Systemic acidosis had not previously been treated. The severity of hyperkalemia had been mitigated before the study was initiated by the provision of a low-normal dietary intake of potassium. In the three bottom panels, the hatched bars represent the difference between the measured value of acid excretion and the mean value before therapy. The magnitude of these differences is indicated by the scale on the left-hand side of the panel. The mean control value is designated by the numerals within the ellipse. The accumulated values of the daily differences are shown by the solid circles and are indicated by the scale on the right-hand side of the panel. The observed reduction in urine pH during fludrocortisone administration suggests that, even though the urine was highly acidic in the pretreatment period, acidification was impaired owing to aldosterone deficiency and that mineralocorticoid replacement ameliorates the impairment by stimulation of H^+ secretion. Presumably the treatment values of urine pH would have been considerably higher had the pretreatment rate of renal ammonia production not been limited in this patient owing to a marked reduction in renal mass. (Reprinted, by permission of the New England Journal of Medicine, from Sebastian A, Schambelan M, Lindenfeld S, et al: Amelioration of metabolic acidosis with fludrocortisone therapy in hyporeninemic hypoaldosteronism. N Engl J Med 297:576, 1977.)

values of urine pH would have been considerably higher than those observed had the pretreatment rate of renal ammonia production not been limited in this patient owing to a marked reduction in renal mass.

In other patients with hyperkalemic metabolic acidosis and chronic renal insufficiency and hypoaldosteronism, administration of physiologic amounts of fludrocortisone has had little or no effect on acid–base balance, but administration of superphysiologic amounts has resulted in a substantial increase in net acid excretion and amelioration of systemic acidosis (Fig. 19–10).[140] The requirement for superphysiologic amounts of exogenous mineralocorticoid raises the possibility that in addition to deficiency of aldosterone, the kidney in some patients may be hyporesponsive to the action of aldosterone. This circumstance might not be specific for patients with chronic renal insufficiency who have hyperkalemic metabolic acidosis. Chronic renal disease may in some way limit the renal response to aldosterone, since the secretion rate and plasma concentration of aldosterone is commonly supernormal in patients with chronic renal insufficiency.[137-139] Thus failure to correct metabolic acidosis might reflect failure to administer hormone in an amount appropriate for the degree of renal insufficiency. This possibility is suggested by the finding of Daughaday and Rendleman[141] in an adrenalectomized patient with pyelonephritis that the amount of exogenous MCH required to maintain correction of acidosis and hyperkalemia increased greatly as the renal disease progressed. Failure to correct acidosis in some cases might also reflect an inadequate duration of hormone administration to achieve the requisite cumulative acid-excretory effect given that the number of functioning nephrons is greatly reduced.[140] Superphysiologic amounts of exogenous mineralocorticoid may be appropriate replacement therapy for patients with aldosterone deficiency and reduced numbers of functioning nephrons.

In patients with hyperkalemic metabolic acidosis and hypoaldosteronism in whom glomerular filtration rate is not markedly reduced (i.e., creatinine clearance >30 ml/min), the increase in net acid excretion observed during mineralocorticoid therapy is accounted for predominantly by increased urine ammonium excretion (Fig. 19–10). Urine pH decreased when mineralocorticoid therapy was initiated, but with continued therapy it increased in parallel with the observed increase in urine ammonium excretion (Figs. 19–10 and 19–12). These findings suggest that the rate of renal production of ammonia increased during mineralocorticoid therapy. A primary increase in ammonia production would result in an increase in the amount of ammonia diffusing into the tubular lumen, which would both augment the excretion of ammonium and, by increasing the amount of luminal buffer, raise urine pH. Urine ammonium excretion correlated inversely with serum potassium concentration (Fig. 19–12) and did not decrease on discontinuation of mineralocorticoid therapy if hyperkalemia was prevented from recurring by reduction of dietary potassium intake. Titratable acid and net acid excretion did decrease, however (Fig. 19–13). Thus, in patients with hypoaldosteronism and chronic renal insufficiency, administration of mineralocorticoid can augment both renal H^+ secretion and, by correction of hyperkalemia, renal ammonia production, and thereby ameliorate metabolic acidosis.

The results depicted in Figure 19–14 provide additional evidence that in patients with hyperkalemic metabolic acidosis and hypoaldosteronism, mineralocorticoid replacement therapy stimulates renal hydrogen ion secretion independently of its effect (direct or indirect) of stimulating renal ammonia production. Figure 19–14 shows the relationship between urine pH and urine ammonium excretion before initiation of fludrocortisone therapy and during the period of fludrocortisone therapy. During the pretreatment period, the relationship between these two variables was dictated by a decreasing rate of ammonium excretion associated with an increase in plasma potassium concentration, a non-

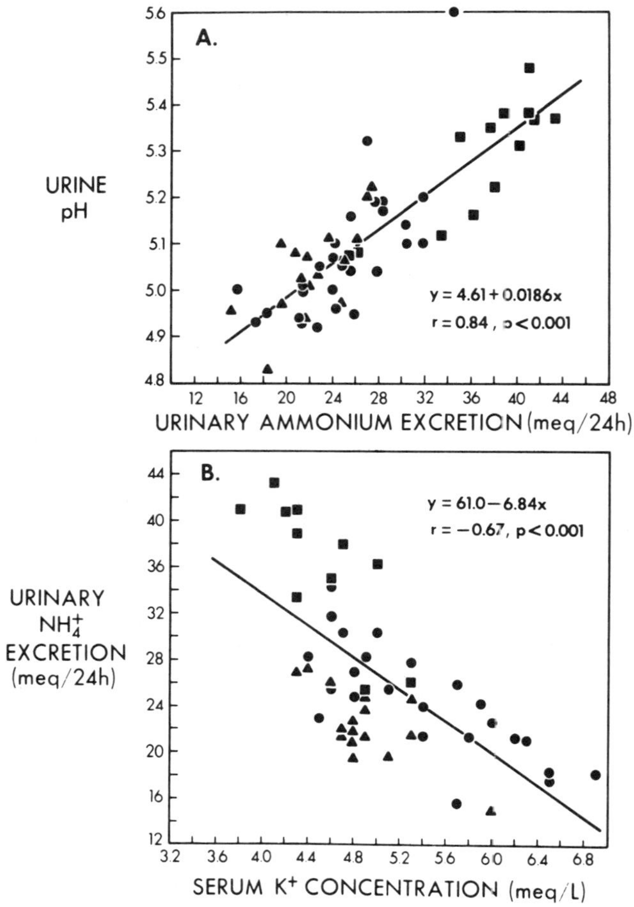

Fig. 19–12. Relationship between the rate of urinary ammonium excretion and serum potassium concentration (lower figure) and between urine pH and urinary ammonium excretion (upper figure) during oral administration of fludrocortisone therapy. These patients had hyporeninemic hypoaldosteronism without far advanced chronic renal insufficiency (creatinine clearance 35 to 44 ml/min per 1.73 m²). (Reprinted, by permission of the New England Journal of Medicine, from Sebastian A, Schambelan M, Lindenfeld S, et al: Amelioration of metabolic acidosis with fludrocortisone therapy in hyporeninemic hypoaldosteronism. N Engl J Med 297:576, 1977.)

steady-state condition caused by renal potassium retention. During the treatment period, the relationship between these two variables was dictated by an increasing rate of ammonium excretion associated with a decreasing plasma potassium concentration, a consequence of fludrocortisone-stimulated renal potassium excretion. During both periods, urine pH correlated positively with urine ammonium excretion, implying that the changes in urine pH reflected to a considerable extent the effect of corresponding changes in the rate of renal production of ammonia and the consequent changes in the availability of ammonia for diffusion into the urine. As shown in Figure 19–14, considerably smaller changes in urine pH occurred during the fludrocortisone treatment period than during the pretreatment period despite changes in the rate of renal production of ammonia that resulted in a similar range of urine ammonium excretion rates in the two periods. That is, the slope of the relationship between urine pH and urine ammonium excretion is considerably lower during fludrocortisone therapy than during the pretreatment period. Since urine pH is lower in relationship to urine buffer (ammonia) content during fludrocortisone therapy, it may be inferred that fludrocortisone in some way increases the capacity of the distal nephron to titrate luminal buffers. As previously discussed in relationship to the studies depicted in Figure 19–4, the slope of the positive correlation between urine pH and urine ammonium excretion can be taken as an index of the hydrogen ion secretory capacity of the distal

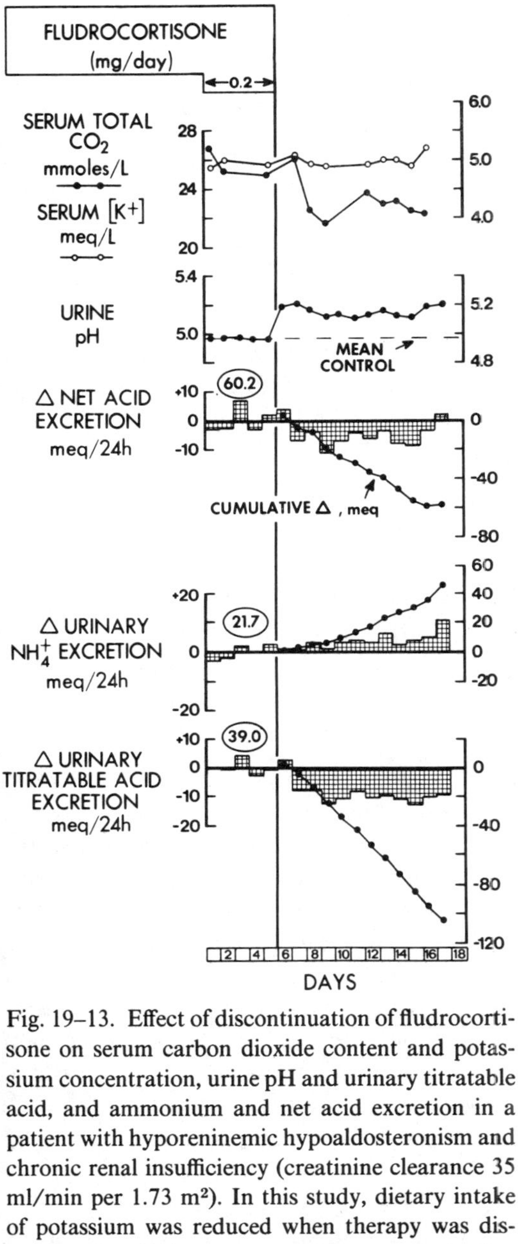

Fig. 19–13. Effect of discontinuation of fludrocortisone on serum carbon dioxide content and potassium concentration, urine pH and urinary titratable acid, and ammonium and net acid excretion in a patient with hyporeninemic hypoaldosteronism and chronic renal insufficiency (creatinine clearance 35 ml/min per 1.73 m²). In this study, dietary intake of potassium was reduced when therapy was discontinued, and the serum potassium concentration remained constant. The rate of urinary ammonium excretion did not decrease when therapy was discontinued, despite a sustained increase in urine pH. (Reprinted, by permission of the New England Journal of Medicine, from Sebastian A, Schambelan M, Lindenfeld S, et al: Amelioration of metabolic acidosis with fludrocortisone therapy in hyporeninemic hypoaldosteronism. N Engl J Med 297:576, 1977.)

nephron. In addition, the value of urine pH at very low or near-zero urine ammonium excretion rates can be taken as an index of the hydrogen ion concentration gradient-generating ability of the distal nephron. Thus, as in dogs and turtles, mineralocorticoid appears to increase the rate capacity of the distal nephron for hydrogen ion secretion when luminal buffer availability is not limiting, but does not affect the hydrogen ion concentration gradient-generating ability when luminal buffer availability is near zero.

Whereas treatment of patients with hyporeninemic hypoaldosteronism with MCH will correct hyperkalemia and hyperchloremic metabolic acidosis, such therapy may not always be indicated. For example, some patients are hypertensive and show increases in extracellular fluid volume and total exchangeable Na^+ content.[132] By increasing renal tubular reabsorption of NaCl, MCH treatment might exacerbate the degree of hypertension and might produce congestive heart failure in patients with limited cardiac reserve.

Administration of furosemide has recently been demonstrated to increase K^+ and net acid excretion and to substantially ameliorate hyperchloremia and metabolic acidosis in such patients.[142] The studies indicate that furosemide increases net acid excretion both by stimulating H^+ secretion and by increasing the availability of ammonia for titration of secreted H^+. In the patients studied, the magnitude of the acid excretory and kaliuretic effect of furosemide was directly correlated with the level of endogenous aldosterone. In those patients with the most severe degree of hypoaldosteronism, the ameliorative effect of furosemide was greatly enhanced by pretreatment with small doses of MCH.

Pseudohypoaldosteronism

The term pseudohypoaldosteronism has been employed to designate clinical conditions in which the signs and symptoms are suggestive of aldosterone deficiency but in which al-

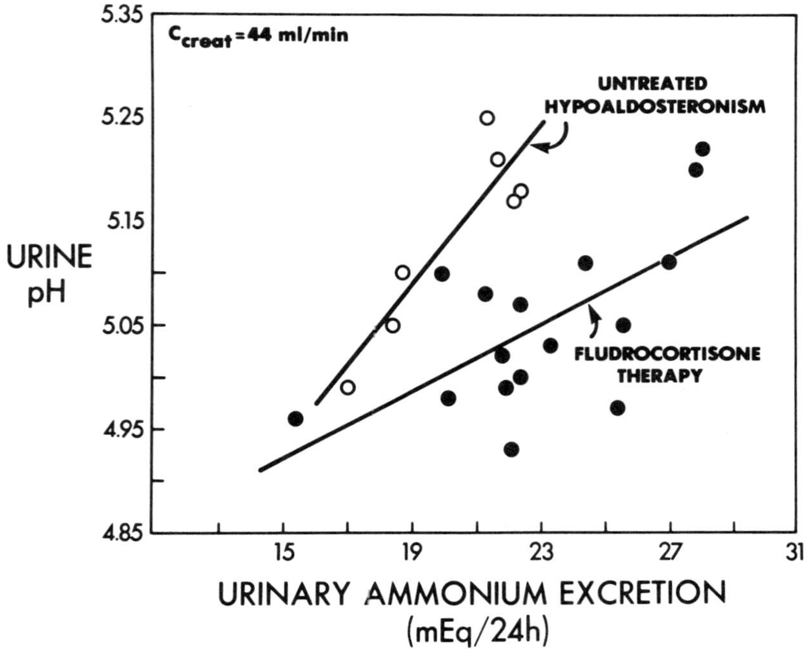

Fig. 19–14. Effect of mineralocorticoid replacement therapy in hyperkalemic metabolic acidosis and hypoaldosteronism. Urine pH and urine ammonium excretion (○) before and (●) during fludrocortisone therapy. See text for further explanation.

dosterone levels are supernormal and in which administration of exogenous mineralocorticoid is not ameliorative. A clinically distinctive form of pseudohypoaldosteronism occurs in infants as an apparently congenital (and in some cases, a familial) disorder characterized by failure to thrive, dehydration and hyponatremia due to renal salt wasting, hyperkalemia due to renal potassium retention, and renal tubular acidosis.[143-146] Plasma renin activity and plasma and urinary aldosterone concentrations are markedly elevated, plasma deoxycorticosterone and corticosterone concentrations are normal, and neither glucocorticoid deficiency nor excess is present. Mineralocorticoid refractoriness of renal sodium wasting and potassium retention is evident even during prolonged periods of parenteral administration of large amounts of deoxycorticosterone and aldosterone and oral administration of fludrocortisone. Supplementation of the diet with large amounts of sodium chloride can reverse hyponatremia and hyperkalemia, relieve symptomatology, and permit normal or improved growth. Characteristically, the severity of renal sodium wasting and potassium retention diminishes after the period of infancy, permitting discontinuation of sodium chloride supplements without recurrence of overt hyponatremia or hyperkalemia. Disordered renal handling of sodium and potassium persists, however, evidenced by recurrence of hyponatremia and hyperkalemia in response to restriction of dietary sodium chloride.[142]

The pathogenesis of classic pseudohypoaldosteronism of infancy has not been elucidated. In the single case reported by Cheek and Perry in 1958, it was postulated "that the defect may be due to a refractory state on the part of the [renal] tubules to endogenous salt-active steroids or mineralocorticoids."[143] Generalized adrenocortical insufficiency (Addison's disease) was excluded. Extensive investigations in a second case reported 1 year later by Donnell et al.[144] confirmed the absence of Addison's disease and demonstrated the presence of extraordinarily high concentrations of aldosterone in urine. Glomerular filtration rate was normal, there was no hyperaminoaciduria or glucosuria or increased renal clearance of phosphorus, renal concentrating and diluting ability grossly were unimpaired, and no structural abnormality was evident on intravenous pyelograms. These findings exonerating generalized glomerular and tubular dysfunction have been confirmed in subsequent reports, and examination of biopsied renal tissue has usually revealed only the presence of mild hyperplasia of the juxtaglomerular apparatus. Patients with classic pseudohypoaldosteronism of infancy are thus distinguishable from those with pseudohypoaldosteronism associated with generalized renal parenchymal structural damage such as salt-losing nephritis caused by methicillin nephritis or medullary cystic disease.

There has been relatively little study of the pathogenesis of the disease at the cellular level. The pathophysiologic manifestations of the disorder are consistent with a cellular defect that interferes with the action of aldosterone in those segments of the renal tubule normally responsive to aldosterone, specifically the collecting tubules and ducts. According to current concepts of the mechanism of action of aldosterone, induced alterations in transepithelial ion transport occur consequent to the binding of aldosterone to high-affinity stereospecific receptors in the cytoplasm. This event leads to modulation of DNA-dependent messenger RNA synthesis and consequent alterations in the cellular content of specific proteins, the so-called aldosterone-induced proteins, which modulate the ion transport mechanism.[147,148] In the only study of a patient with pseudohypoaldosteronism in which an attempt to examine binding of aldosterone in a target tissue was performed, the amount of tritiated aldosterone binding to mucosal cells obtained from the sigmoid colon was found to be similar to that observed in control subjects.[146]

In another report, a mineralocorticoid-responsive defect in transepithelial transport of sodium and potassium was demonstrated in multiple target organs of aldosterone, including salivary glands, sweat glands, and colon, as well as the kidney.[145] Available data on the electrolyte composition of sweat in other reported cases of pseudohypoaldosteronism suggest that sweat glands are either unresponsive to mineralocorticoid or subnormally responsive given the prevailing supernormal levels of circulating aldosterone.[143–145] In none of these cases, however, has the cellular mechanism of the defect in electrolyte transport been defined. Therefore, it remains to be determined whether a defect exists in the sequence of biochemical reactions initiated by binding of aldosterone to its receptor and culminating in the generation of aldosterone-induced proteins.

It has been suggested that the renal tubule dysfunction of classic pseudohypoaldosteronism results from a deficiency of sodium- and potassium-activated adenosine triphosphatase (Na^+–K^+-ATPase), the ubiquitous membrane-bound enzyme that provides the fundamental cellular mechanism for maintaining the normally low concentrations of sodium and high concentrations of potassium in the cytoplasm relative to those in the extracellular fluid compartment.[149] In the kidney, Na^+–K^+-ATPase is localized to the basolateral membranes of renal tubular cells in virtually every segment of the nephron and plays a critical role in net reabsorption of filtered sodium and net secretion of potassium by the renal tubule.[25,150]

Recent evidence suggests that it also plays a role in the acidification process of the distal nephron.[151] Virtually no renal Na^+–K^+-ATPase activity was detectable in either proximal or distal nephron segments obtained by microdissection of biopsied renal tissue from one patient with classic pseudohypoaldosteronism.[149] However, interpretation of this finding as indicative of a primary defect in renal Na^+–K^+-ATPase is questionable, since the specific activity of renal Na^+–K^+-ATPase is known to decrease under a variety of physiologic circumstances that reduce net renal sodium reabsorption. In adrenalectomized animals net renal sodium reabsorption as varied by alterations in sodium chloride intake appears to be a major determinant of the specific activity of Na^+–K^+-ATPase, and mineralocorticoid-induced increases in Na^+–K^+-ATPase activity appear to be secondary to stimulation of tubular sodium transport.[152]

In classic pseudohypoaldosteronism the spontaneously occurring apparent amelioration of renal sodium wasting and potassium retention during the postinfancy period is associated with persisting supernormal levels of plasma renin and aldosterone. In one patient with classic pseudohypoaldosteronism and persistent hyperaldosteronism who was studied at age 9 years, normonatremia and normokalemia were maintained without dietary supplements of sodium chloride, but hyponatremia and hyperkalemia recurred in response to administration of the mineralocorticoid antagonist, in this case spironolactone.[146] By contrast, chronic administration of spironolactone to normal subjects does not result in overt hyponatremia or hyperkalemia.[153] Presumably, renal resistance to the action of aldosterone was incomplete in the patient with pseudohypoaldosteronism, and the supernormal levels of circulating aldosterone observed before spironolactone administration contributed to the maintenance of normokalemia and normonatremia. It would be of interest to study adult patients who had classic pseudohypoaldosteronism as infants, since it is known that adults with total mineralocorticoid deficiency (secondary to bilateral adrenalectomy) do not become frankly hyponatremic or hyperkalemic as long as dietary sodium and potassium intake is normal.[106]

It is not certain that the same fundamental pathogenetic disturbance underlies classic pseudohypoaldosteronism of infancy in all reported cases, nor is it certain that a genetic abnormality is present in all cases. The familial occurrence of the disorder has been documented in only a small fraction of the reported cases. A higher incidence of familial occurrence might be detected if asymptomatic parents and grandparents were to be tested under conditions of dietary sodium chloride restriction. Several families have been described in which asymptomatic older siblings, parents, and grandparents were found to have abnormally increased plasma renin activity and/or plasma aldosterone concentration, suggesting the persistence of a disturbance in renal handling of sodium chloride that might be unmasked by restriction of dietary sodium chloride or by administration of an aldosterone antagonist.

Hyperkalemic Renal Acidosis Caused by Distal Nephron Chloride Hyperabsorption

In a wide spectrum of clinical disorders, chronic renal hyperkalemia and renal acidosis occur in the absence of diffuse renal parenchymal disease and reduced glomerular filtration rate (Table 19–3). In some of these conditions renal hyperkalemia and renal acidosis can be attributed to a deficiency of aldosterone and can be corrected by administration of exogenous MCH in physiologic replacement doses. In other conditions, aldosterone deficiency is not present, and hyperkalemia and acidosis persist despite administration of even superphysiologic doses of mineralocorticoids.

Such mineralocorticoid-resistant renal hyperkalemia and acidosis occurs in two distinctly different clinical syndromes: (1) classic pseudohypoaldosteronism of infancy, characterized by renal salt wasting and hypotension, and described in an earlier section of this review, and (2) a syndrome of chronic mineralocorticoid-resistant hyperkalemia and acidosis unaccompanied by renal salt wasting or hypotension, and frequently associated with hypertension. These two syndromes have been designated as types 1 and 2 pseudohypoaldosteronism, respectively. The primary abnormality of type 1 pseudohypoaldosteronism has been postulated to be a specific defect in the renal response to MCH, which accounts for

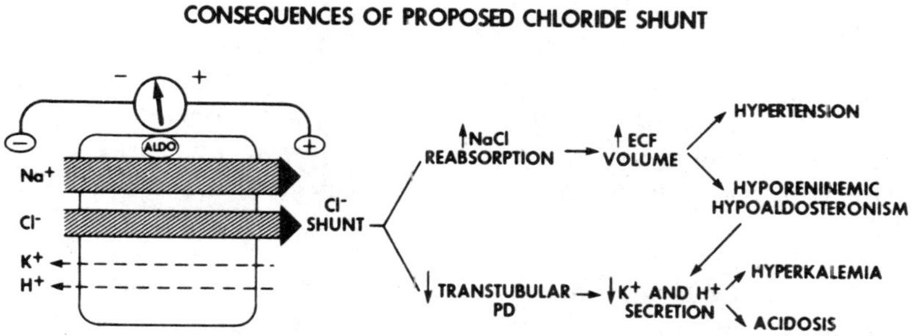

Fig. 19–15. Pathophysiologic consequences of abnormally increased distal nephron chloride reabsorption. (Reprinted from Kidney International. Schambelan M, Sebastian A, Rector FC Jr: Mineralocorticoid–resistant renal hyperkalemia without salt wasting (Type II pseudohypoaldosteronism): Role of increased renal chloride reabsorption. Kidney Int 19:716, 1981.)

the coexistence of salt wasting, potassium retention and acidosis. The primary abnormality in type 2 pseudohypoaldosteronism has been postulated by some investigators to be a specific defect of the renal secretory mechanism for potassium, which limits the kaliuretic response to MCH but not the sodium and chloride reabsorptive effect of the hormone, and which results in acidosis secondary to hyperkalemia.

Recent evidence indicates that mineralocorticoid-resistant renal hyperkalemia and acidosis in type 2 pseudohypoaldosteronism cannot be attributed to the absence of a renal potassium secretory mechanism, but instead may be dependent on the amount of chloride available for reabsorption in the distal nephron.[154] The findings suggest that the primary abnormality in this syndrome is a defect of the distal nephron that increases the reabsorptive avidity of the distal nephron for chloride, which (1) limits the sodium and mineralocorticoid-dependent voltage driving force for potassium and hydrogen secretion, resulting in hyperkalemia and acidosis, and (2) augments distal NaCl reabsorption, resulting in hyperchloremia, volume expansion, and hypertension (Fig. 19–15). Such a chloride shunt might arise as a result of an abnormal increase in the permeability of the distal nephron to chloride. Consistent with the presence of such a chloride shunt, restriction of dietary sodium chloride or administration of a chloruretic diuretic (furosemide, thiazide) was found to correct hyperkalemia and acidosis. Conceivably, a similar kind of chloride shunt might arise as a consequence of diffuse structural damage to the renal parenchyma as in patients with chronic tubulointerstitial disease or diabetic nephropathy who have renal hyperkalemic acidosis. This possibility provides an explanation for the frequent concomitance in these patients of hyporeninemic hypoaldosteronism (caused by hyperabsorption of NaCl and consequent extracellular fluid volume expansion) and a diminished acid-excretory and kaliuretic response to mineralocorticoid (caused by chloride shunting of the voltage driving force) and for the favorable therapeutic response to chronic administration of chloruretic diuretics.

ACKNOWLEDGMENTS

The studies in humans were carried out on the General Clinical Research Centers at Moffitt and San Francisco General Hospitals, University of California, San Francisco, and were supported by NIH grants RR 79, RR 83, AM 21605, AM 06415, AM 28643, AM 31626, HL 06285, HL, 11046, PHS-CCIC grant SF96-83, and a MRC (Canada) Fellowship (Dr. Kurtz). Special acknowledgment of the enabling contribution of Patricia Douglass.

REFERENCES

1. Garrod O, Davies SA, Cahill G Jr: The action of cortisone and desoxycorticosterone acetate on glomerular filtration rate and sodium and water exchange in the adrenalectomized dog. J Clin Invest 34:761, 1955
2. Yunis SL, Bercovitch DD, Stein RM, et al: Renal tubular effects of hydrocortisone and aldosterone in normal hydropenic man: Comment on sites of action. J Clin Invest 43:1668, 1974
3. Vander AJ, Malvin RL, Wilde WS, et al: Effects of adrenalectomy and aldosterone on proximal and distal tubular sodium reabsorption. Proc Soc Exp Biol Med 99:323, 1958
4. Hierholzer K, Wiederholt M, Stolte H: Hemmung der Natriumresorption im proximalen und distalen konvolut adrenalektomierter Ratten. Pfluegers Arch 291:43, 1966
5. Wiederholt M, Behn C, Schoormans W, et al: Effect of aldosterone on sodium and potassium transport in the kidney. J Steroid Biochem 3:151, 1972
6. Garg LC, Knepper MA, Burg, MB: Mineralocorticoid effects on Na-K-ATPase in individual nephron segments. Am J Physiol 240:F536, 1981
7. Gross JB, Imai M, Kokko JP: A functional comparison of the cortical collecting tubule and the distal convoluted tubule. J Clin Invest 55:1284, 1975
8. Stokes JB, Ingram MJ, Williams AD, et al: Heterogeneity of the rabbit collecting tubule: Localization of mineralocorticoid hormone action to the cortical portion. Kidney Int 20:341, 1981
9. Stone DK, Kokko JP, Jacobson HR: In-vitro stimulation of proton secretion by aldosterone. Kidney Int 21:240, 1982
10. Stone DK, Kokko JP, Jacobson HR: Sodium independence of proton secretion in medullary collecting duct. Clin Res 30:464A, 1982
11. Uhlich E, Baldamus CA, Ullrich KJ: Einfluss von Aldosteron auf den Natriumtransport in den Sammelrohren der Säugetierniere. Pfluegers Arch 308:111, 1969
12. Uhlich E, Halbach R, Ullrich KJ: Einfluss von Aldosteron auf den Ausstrom markierten Natriums aus den Sammelrohren der Ratte. Pfluegers Arch 320:261, 1970
13. Tisher CC: Anatomy of the kidney. p. 3. In Brenner BM, Rector FC Jr (eds): The Kidney. WB Saunders, Philadelphia, 1981
14. Lipton P, Edelman IS: Effects of aldosterone and vasopressin on electrolytes of toad bladder epithelial cells. Am J Physiol 221:733, 1971
15. Ludens JH, Fanestil DD: Aldosterone stimulation of acidification of urine by isolated urinary bladder of the Colombian toad. Am J Physiol 226:1321, 1974
16. Al-Awqati Q, Norby LH, Mueller A, et al: Characteristics of stimulation of H^+ transport by aldosterone in turtle urinary bladder. J Clin Invest 58:351, 1976
17. Crabbé J: Stimulation of active sodium transport by the isolated toad bladder with aldosterone in vitro. J Clin Invest 40:2103, 1961
18. Koeppen BM, Helman SI: Acidification of luminal fluid by the rabbit cortical collecting tubule perfused in vitro. Am J Physiol 242:F521, 1982
19. Lifschitz MD, Schrier RW, Edelman IS: Effect of actinomycin D on aldosterone-mediated changes in electrolyte excretion. Am J Physiol 224:376, 1973
20. Hanley MJ, Kokko JP: Study of chloride transport across the rabbit cortical collecting tubule. J Clin Invest 62:39, 1978
21. Handler JS, Preston AS, Orloff J: Effect of adrenal steroid hormones on the response of the toad's urinary bladder to vasopressin. J Clin Invest 48:823, 1969
22. Hierholzer K, Wiederholt M: Some aspects of distal tubular solute and water transport. Kidney Int 9:198, 1976
23. Koeppen B, Giebisch G: Microelectrode study of rabbit cortical collecting tubules (CCT): Effect of mineralocorticoid. Am Soc Nephro 15:167A, 1982
24. Stokes JB: Mineralocorticoid stimulation of K^+ transport by the cortical collecting tubule (CCT): Evidence for increased cell K^+ permeability. Am Soc Nephro 15:174A, 1982
25. Katz AI, Epstein FH: The role of sodium-potassium activated adenosine triphosphatase in the reabsorption of sodium by the kidney. J Clin Invest 46:1999, 1967
26. Petty KJ, Kokko JP, Marver D: Secondary effect of aldosterone on Na–K ATPase activity in the rabbit cortical collecting tubule. J Clin Invest 68:1514, 1981

27. Geering K, Girardet M, Bron C, et al: Hormonal regulation of (Na^+,K^+)-ATPase biosynthesis on the toad bladder. Effect of aldosterone and 3,5,3′-triiodo-L-thyronine. J Biol Chem 257:10338, 1982
28. Edelman IS, Fanestil DD: Mineralocorticoids. In Litwack G (ed): Biochemical Actions of Hormones. Academic Press, New York, 1970
29. Margolius HS, Chao J: Amiloride inhibits mammalian renal kallikrein and a kallikrein-like enzyme from toad bladder and skin. J Clin Invest 65:1343, 1980
30. Orce GC, Castillo GA, Margolius HS: Inhibition of short-circuit current in toad urinary bladder by inhibitors of glandular kallikrein. Am J Physiol 239:F459, 1980
31. Al-Awqati Q: H^+ transport in urinary epithelia. Am J Physiol 235:F77, 1978
32. Steinmetz PR: Cellular defects in urinary acidification and renal tubular acidosis. p. 987. In Andreoli TE, Hoffman JF, Fanestil DD (eds): Physiology of Membrane Disorders. Plenum, New York, 1978

32a. Ludens JH, Fanestil DD: Acidification of urine by the isolated urinary bladder of the toad. Am J Physiol 223:1338, 1972

33. Dixon TE, Al-Awqati Q: Urinary acidification in turtle bladder is due to a reversible proton-translocating ATPase. Proc Natl Acad Sci (USA) 76:3135, 1979
34. Berry CA, Warnock DG: Acidification in the in vitro perfused tubule. Kidney Int 22:507, 1982
35. Al-Awqati Q, Mueller A, Steinmetz PR: Transport of H^+ against electrochemical gradients in turtle urinary bladder. Am J Physiol 233:F502, 1977
36. Lombard WE, Jacobson HR, Kokko JP: Collecting duct bicarbonate transport: Comparison of cortical and medullary segments. Kidney Int 16:827, 1979
37. Stone DK, Seldin DW, Kokko JP, et al: Chloride dependence of medullary collecting duct acidification. Kidney Int 23:239, 1983
38. Stanton BA, Biemesderfer D, Wade JB, et al: Structural and functional study of the rat distal nephron: Effects of potassium adaptation and depletion. Kidney Int 19:36, 1981
39. Stetson DL, Wade JB, Giebisch G: Morphologic alterations in the rat medullary collecting duct following potassium depletion. Kidney Int 17:45, 1980
40. Stokes JB: Potassium secretion by cortical collecting tubule: Relation to sodium absorption, luminal sodium concentration, and transepithelial voltage. Am J Physiol 241: F395, 1981
41. Stoff JS, Handler JS, Preston AS, et al: The effect of aldosterone on cyclic nucleotide phosphodiesterase activity in toad urinary bladder. Life Sci 13:545, 1973
42. Zusman RM, Keiser HR, Handler JS: Adrenal steroids enhance vasopressin-stimulated water flow in the toad bladder by inhibiting prostaglandin E biosynthesis. Proc Am Soc Nephrol 10:127A, 1977
43. Feldman D, Funder JW, Edelman IS: Subcellular mechanisms in the action of adrenal steroids. Am J Med 53:545, 1972
44. Funder JW, Feldman D, Edelman IS: The roles of plasma binding and receptor specificity in the mineralocorticoid action of aldosterone. Endocrinology 92:994, 1973
45. Baxter JD, Schambelan M, Matulich DT, et al: Aldosterone receptors and the evaluation of plasma mineralocorticoid activity in normal and hypertensive states. J Clin Invest 58:579, 1976
46. Samuels HH, Tomkins GM: Relation of steroid structure to enzyme induction in hepatoma tissue culture cells. J Mol Biol 52:57, 1970
47. Crabbé J, De Weer P: Action of aldosterone on the bladder and skin of the toad. Nature 202:298, 1964
48. Edelman IS, Bogoroch R, Porter GA: On the mechanism of action of aldosterone on sodium transport: The role of protein synthesis. Proc Natl Acad Sci (USA) 50:1169, 1963
49. Fanestil DD, Edelman IS: On the mechanism of action of aldosterone on sodium transport: Effects of inhibitors of RNA and of protein synthesis. Fed Proc 25:912, 1966
50. Fanestil DD: Mode of spironolactone action: Competitive inhibition of aldosterone binding to mineralocorticoid receptors. Biochem Pharmacol 17:2240, 1968
51. Farman N, Vandewalle A, Bonvalet JP: Aldosterone binding in isolated tubules. I. Biochemical determination in proximal and distal parts of the rabbit nephron. Am J Physiol 242:F63, 1982

52. Farman N, Vandewalle A, Bonvalet JP: Aldosterone binding in isolated tubules. II. An autoradiographic study of concentration dependency in the rabbit nephron. Am J Physiol 242:F69, 1982
53. Vandewalle A, Farman N, Bencsath P and Bonvalet JP: Aldosterone binding along the rabbit nephron: An autoradiographic study on isolated tubules. Am J Physiol 240:F172, 1981
54. Lemann J Jr, Piering WF, Lennon EJ: Studies of the acute effects of aldosterone and cortisol on the interrelationship between renal sodium, calcium and magnesium excretion in normal man. Nephron 7:117, 1970
55. Mills JN, Thomas S, Williamson KS: The acute effect of hydrocortisone, deoxycorticosterone and aldosterone upon the excretion of sodium, potassium and acid by the human kidney. J Physiol (Lond) 151:312, 1960
56. Ross, EJ, Reddy WJ, Rivera A, et al: Effects of intravenous infusions of *dl*-aldosterone acetate on sodium and potassium excretion in man. J Clin Endocrinol Metab 19:389, 1959
57. Kassirer JP, London AM, Goldman DM, et al: On the pathogenesis of metabolic alkalosis in hyperaldosteronism. Am J Med 49: 306, 1970
58. Relman AS, Schwartz WB: The effect of DOCA on electrolyte balance in normal man and its relation to sodium chloride intake. Yale J Biol Med 24:540, 1952
59. Hulter HN, Sigala JF, Sebastian A: K^+ deprivation potentiates the renal alkalosis-producing effect of mineralocorticoid. Am J Physiol 235:F298, 1978
60. Kurtzman NA, White MG, Rogers PW: Pathophysiology of metabolic alkalosis. Arch Intern Med 131:702, 1973
61. Earley LE, Daugharty TM: Sodium metabolism. N Engl J Med 281:72, 1969
62. Schwartz GJ, Burg MB: Mineralocorticoid effects on cation transport by cortical collecting tubules in vitro. Am J Physiol 235:F576, 1978
63. Berl T, Linas SL, Aisenbrey GA, et al: On the mechanism of polyuria in potassium depletion: The role of polydipsia. J Clin Invest 60:620, 1977
64. Rubini JE: Water excretion in potassium-deficient man. J Clin Invest 40:2215, 1961
65. Abbrecht PH: Effects of potassium deficiency on renal function in the dog. J Clin Invest 48:432, 1969
66. Tannen RL: Relationship of renal ammonia production and potassium homeostasis. Kidney Int 11:453, 1977
67. Luke RG, Levitan H: Impaired renal conservation of chloride and the acid–base changes associated with potassium depletion in the rat. Clin Sci 32:511, 1967
68. Conn JW: Presidential address. II. Primary aldosteronism, a new clinical syndrome. J Lab Clin Med 45:3, 1955
69. Conn JW, Cohen EL, Rovner DR: Suppression of plasma renin activity in primary aldosteronism. JAMA 190:213, 1964
70. Biglieri EG, Forsham PH: Studies on the expanded extracellular fluid and responses to various stimuli in primary aldosteronism. Am J Med 30:564, 1961
71. Spark RF, Melby JC: Aldosteronism in hypertension. The spironolactone response test. Ann Intern Med 69:685, 1968
72. Wenting GJ, Man in't Veld AJ, Verhoeven RP, et al: Volume–pressure relationships during development of mineralocorticoid hypertension in man. Circ Res 40 (suppl):I–163, 1977
73. Wright FS: Sites and mechanisms of potassium transport along the renal tubule. Kidney Int 11:415, 1977
74. Biglieri EG, Slaton PE Jr, Kronfeld SJ, et al: Diagnosis of an aldosterone-producing adenoma in primary aldosteronism: An evaluative maneuver. JAMA 201:510, 1967
75. Kem DC, Weinberger MH, Mayes DM, et al: Saline suppression of plasma aldosterone in hypertension. Arch Intern Med 128:380, 1971
76. Biglieri EG, Herron MA, Brust N: 17-hydroxylation deficiency in man. J Clin Invest 45:1946, 1966
77. Bongiovanni AM, Root AW: The adrenogenital syndrome. N Engl J Med 268:1283, 1963
78. Gandy HM, Keutmann EH, Izzo AJ: Characterization of urinary steroids in adrenal hyperplasia: Isolation of metabolites of cortisol, compound S, and desoxycorticosterone from normotensive patient with adrenogenital syndrome. J Clin Invest 39:364, 1960
79. New MI, Seaman MP: Secretion rates of cor-

tisol and aldosterone precursors in various forms of congenital adrenal hyperplasia. J Clin Endocrinol Metab 30:361, 1970
80. Goldsmith O, Solomon DH, Horton R: Hypogonadism and mineralocorticoid excess. The 17-hydroxylase deficiency syndrome. N Engl J Med 277:673, 1967
81. Biglieri EG: Plasma deoxycorticosterone concentrations in the adrenal enzymatic deficiencies causing hypertension. P. 171. In New ME, Levine LS (eds): Juvenile Hypertension. Raven Press, New York, 1977
82. Mantero F, Busnardo B, Riondel A, et al: Hypertension artérielle, alcalose hypokaliémique et pseudohermaphrodisme mâle par déficit en 17-alpha-hydroxylase. Schweiz Med Wochenschr 101:38, 1971
83. Christy NP, Laragh JH: Pathogenesis of hypokalemic alkalosis in Cushing's syndrome. N Engl J Med 265:1083, 1961
84. Solomon SS, Swersie SP, Paulsen CA, et al: Feminizing adrenocortical carcinoma with hypertension. J Clin Endocrinol Metab 28:608, 1968
85. Schambelan M, Slaton PE Jr, Biglieri EG: Mineralocorticoid production in hyperadrenocorticism. Role in pathogenesis of hypokalemic alkalosis. Am J Med 51:299, 1971
86. Hogan MJ, Schambelan M, Biglieri EG: Concurrent hypercortisolism and hypermineralocorticoidism. Am J Med 62:777, 1977
87. Liddle GW, Bledsoe T, Coppage WS Jr: A familial renal disorder simulating primary aldosteronism but with negligible aldosterone secretion. Trans Assoc Am Physicians 76:199, 1963
88. Rodriguez JA, Biglieri EG, Schambelan M: Pseudohyperaldosteronism (PHA) with tubular resistance to mineralocorticoid hormone (MCH). Clin Res 29:567A, 1981
89. Wang C, Chan TK, Yeung, RTT, et al: The effect of trimaterene and sodium intake on renin, aldosterone, and erythrocyte sodium transport in Liddle's syndrome. J Clin Endocrinol Metab 52:1027, 1981
90. Ludens JH, Vaughn DA, Fanestil DD: Stimulation of urinary acidification by aldosterone and inhibitors of RNA and protein synthesis. J Membr Biol 40 (suppl):199, 1978
91. Biglieri EG, Stockigt JR, Schambelan M, et al: Secondary hyperaldosteronism. P. 283. In Page ID, Bumpus FM (eds): Angiotensin. Springer-Verlag, Berlin, 1974
92. Schambelan M, Howes EL Jr, Stockigt JR, et al: Role of renin and aldosterone in hypertension due to a renin-secreting tumor. Am J Med 55:86, 1973
93. Blair-West JR, Coghlan JP, Denton DA, et al: Effects of adrenal steroid withdrawal on chronic renovascular hypertension in adrenalectomized sheep. Circ Res 23:803, 1968
94. Chonko AM, Bay WH, Stein JH, et al: The role of renin and aldosterone in the salt retention of edema. Am J Med 63:881, 1977
95. Sebastian A, McSherry E, Morris RC Jr: Renal potassium wasting in renal tubular acidosis (RTA). Its occurrence in types 1 and 2 RTA despite sustained correction of systemic acidosis. J Clin Invest 50:667, 1971
96. Gill JR Jr, Frölich JC, Bowden RE, et al: Bartter's syndrome: A disorder characterized by high urinary prostaglandins and a dependence of hyperreninemia on prostaglandin synthesis. Am J. Med 61:43, 1976
97. Bartter FC, Pronove P, Gill JR Jr, et al: Hyperplasia of the juxtaglomerular complex with hyperaldosteronism and hypokalemic alkalosis. A new syndrome. Am J Med 33:811, 1962
98. Dunn MJ: Prostaglandins and Bartter's syndrome. Kidney Int 19:86, 1981
99. Gill JR Jr, Bartter FC: Evidence for a prostaglandin-independent defect in chloride reabsorption in the loop of Henle as a proximal cause of Bartter's syndrome. Am J Med 65:766, 1978
100. Trygstad CW, Mangos JA, Bloodworth JMB Jr, et al: A sibship with Bartter's syndrome: Failure of total adrenalectomy to correct the potassium wasting. Pediatrics 44:234, 1969
101. Giebisch G, Malnic G, Berliner RW: Renal transport and control of potassium excretion. p. 408. In Brenner BM, Rector FC Jr (eds): The Kidney. WB Saunders, Philadelphia, 1981
102. Baehler RW, Work J, Kotchen TA, et al: Studies on the pathogenesis of Bartter's syndrome. Am J Med 69:933, 1980
103. Shils ME: Experimental human magnesium depletion. Medicine (Baltimore) 48:61, 1969
104. Hulter HN, Ilnicki LP, Harbottle JA, et al: Impaired renal H^+ secretion and NH_3 production in mineralocorticoid-deficient gluco-

corticoid-replete dogs. Am J Physiol 232:F136, 1977
105. Kurtzman NA, White MG, Rogers PW: Aldosterone deficiency and renal bicarbonate reabsorption. J Lab Clin Med 77:931, 1971
106. Sebastian A, Sutton JM, Hulter HN, et al: Effect of mineralocorticoid replacement therapy on renal acid–base hemostasis in adrenalectomized patients. Kidney Int 18:762, 1980
107. Brown JJ, Fraser R, Lever AF, et al: Renin, angiotensin, corticosteroids, and electrolyte balance in Addison's disease. Q J Med 37:97, 1968
108. Haack D, Möhring J, Möhring B, et al: Comparative study on development of corticosterone and DOCA hypertension in rats. Am J Physiol 233:F403, 1977
109. Swingle WW, Parkins WM, Taylor AR, et al: Relation of serum sodium and chloride levels to alterations of body water in the intact and adrenalectomized dog, and the influence of adrenal cortical hormone upon fluid distribution. Am J Physiol 116:438, 1936
110. Ufferman RC, Schrier RW: Importance of sodium intake and mineralocorticoid hormone in the impaired water excretion in adrenal insufficiency. J Clin Invest 51:1639, 1972
111. Robertson GL, Mahr EA, Athar S, et al: Development and clinical application of a new method for the radioimmumoassay of arginine vasopressin in human plasma. J Clin Invest 52:2340, 1973
112. Agus ZS, Goldberg M: Role of antidiuretic hormone in the abnormal water diuresis of anterior hypopituitarism in man. J Clin Invest 50:1478, 1971
113. Berns AS, Pluss RG, Erickson AL, et al: Renin-angiotensin system and cardiovascular homeostasis in adrenal insufficiency. Am J Physiol 233:F509, 1977
114. Blizzard RM, Kyle M: Studies of the adrenal antigens and antibodies in Addison's sheep. J Clin Invest 42:1653, 1963
115. Keenan BS, Holcombe JH, Kirkland RT, et al: Sodium homeostasis and aldosterone secretion in salt-losing congenital adrenal hyperplasia. J Clin Endocrinol Metab 48:430, 1979
116. Bryan GT, Kliman B, Bartter FC: Impaired aldosterone production in "salt-losing" congenital adrenal hyperplasia. J Clin Invest 44:957, 1965
117. Beitins IZ, Bayard F, Kowarski A, et al: The effect of ACTH administration on aldosterone production in non salt-losing congenital adrenal hyperplasia. J Clin Endocrinol Metab 35:595, 1972
118. Horner JM, Hintz RL, Luetscher JA: The role of renin and angiotensin in salt-losing, 21-hydroxylase-deficient congenital adrenal hyperplasia. J Clin Endocrinol Metab 48: 776, 1979
119. Kowarski A, Finkelstein JW, Spaulding JS, et al: Aldosterone secretion rate in congenital adrenal hyperplasia. A discussion of the theories on the pathogenesis of the salt-losing form of the syndrome. J Clin Invest 44:1505, 1965
120. Finkelstein M, Shaefer JM: Inborn errors of steroid biosynthesis. Physiol Rev 59:353, 1979
121. Degenhart HJ, Frankena L, Visser HKA, et al: Further investigation of a new hereditary defect in the biosynthesis of aldosterone: Evidence for a defect in 18-hydroxylation of corticosterone. Acta Physiol Pharm 14:88, 1966
122. Katznelson D, Sack J, Kraiem Z, et al: Congenital hypoaldosteronism. Thirteen year follow-up in identical twins. Horm Res 11:22, 1979
123. Rösler A, Rabinowitz D, Theodor R, et al: The nature of the defect in a salt-wasting disorder in Jews of Iran. J Clin Endocrinol Metab 44:279, 1977
124. Rösler A, Theodor R, Boichis H, et al: Metabolic responses to the administration of angiotensin II, K and ACTH in two salt-wasting syndromes. J Clin Endocrinol Metab 44:292, 1977
125. Ulick S: Diagnosis and nomenclature of the disorders of the terminal portion of the aldosterone biosynthetic pathway. J Clin Endocrinol Metab 43:92, 1976
126. Ulick S, Gautier E, Vetter KK, et al: An aldosterone biosynthetic defect in a salt-losing disorder. J Clin Endocrinol Metab 24:669, 1964
127. Veldhuis JD, Kulin HE, Santen RJ, et al: Inborn error in the terminal step of aldosterone biosynthesis. Corticosterone methyl oxidase type II deficiency in a North American

pedigree. N Engl J Med 303:117, 1980
128. DeFronzo RA: Hyperkalemia and hyporeninemic hypoaldosteronism. Kidney Int 17: 118, 1980
129. Phelps KR, Lieberman RL, Oh MS, et al: Pathophysiology of the syndrome of hyporeninemic hypoaldosteronism. Metabolism 29:186, 1980
130. Schambelan M, Sebastian A, Biglieri EG: Prevalence, pathogenesis, and functional significance of aldosterone deficiency in hyperkalemic patients with chronic renal insufficiency. Kidney Int 17:89, 1980
131. Sebastian A, Hulter HN, Kurtz I, et al: Disorders of distal nephron function. Am J Med 72:289, 1982
132. Oh MS, Carroll HJ, Clemmons JE, et al: A mechanism for hyporeninemic hypoaldosteronism in chronic renal disease. Metabolism 23:1157, 1974
133. Cannon PJ, Ames RP, Laragh JH: Relation between potassium balance and aldosterone secretion in normal subjects and in patients with hypertensive or renal tubular disease. J Clin Invest 45:865, 1966
134. Dluhy RG, Axelrod L, Underwood RH, et al: Studies of the control of plasma aldosterone concentration in normal man. II. Effect of dietary potassium and acute potassium infusion. J Clin Invest 51:1950, 1972
135. Himathongkam T, Dluhy RG, Williams GH: Potassium-aldosterone–renin interrelationships. J Clin Endocrinol Metab 41:153, 1975
136. Laragh JH: Potassium, angiotensin and the dual control of aldosterone secretion. N Engl J Med 289:745, 1973
137. Berl T, Katz FH, Henrich WL, et al: Role of aldosterone in the control of sodium excretion in patients with advanced chronic renal failure. Kidney Int 14:228, 1978
138. Hené RJ, Boer P, Koomans HA, et al: Plasma aldosterone concentrations in chronic renal disease. Kidney Int 21:98, 1982
139. Weidmann P, Maxwell MH, Rowe P, et al: Role of the renin–angiotensin–aldosterone system in the regulation of plasma potassium in chronic renal disease. Nephron 15:35, 1975
140. Sebastian A, Schambelan M, Lindenfeld S, et al: Amelioration of metabolic acidosis with fludrocortisone therapy in hyporeninemic hypoaldosteronism. N Engl J Med 297:576, 1977
141. Daughaday WH, Rendleman D: Severe symptomatic hyperkalemia in an adrenalectomized woman due to enhanced mineralocorticoid requirement. Ann Intern Med 66:1197, 1967
142. Sebastian A, Schambelan M: Amelioration of type 4 renal tubular acidosis (RTA) in chronic renal failure (CRF) with furosemide (F). Kidney Int 12:534, 1977
143. Cheek DB, Perry JW: A salt wasting syndrome in infancy. Arch Dis Child 33:252, 1958
144. Donnell GN, Litman N, Roldan M: Pseudohypo-adrenalocorticism. Renal sodium loss, hyponatremia, and hyperkalemia due to a renal tubular insensitivity to mineralocorticoids. Am J Dis Child 97:813, 1959
145. Oberfield SE, Levine LS, Carey RM, et al: Pseudohypoaldosteronism: Multiple target organ unresponsiveness to mineralocorticoid hormones. J Clin Endocrinol Metab 48:228, 1979
146. Postel-Vinay M-C, Alberti GM, Ricour C, et al: Pseudohypoaldosteronism: Persistence of hyperaldosteronism and evidence for renal tubular and intestinal reponsiveness to endogenous aldosterone. J Clin Endocrinol Metab 39:1038, 1974
147. Baxter JD, Funder JW: Hormone receptors. N Engl J Med 301:1149, 1979
148. Ludens JH, Fanestil DD: The mechanism of aldosterone function. Pharmacol Ther 2:371, 1976
149. Bierich JR, Schmidt U: Tubular Na, K-ATPase deficiency, the cause of the congenital renal salt-losing syndrome. Eur J Pediatr 121:81, 1976
150. Silva P, Hayslett JP, Epstein FH: The role of Na-K-activated adenosine triphosphatase in potassium adaptation. Stimulation of enzymatic activity by potassium loading. J Clin Invest 52:2665, 1973
151. Westenfelder C, Birch FM, Baranowski RL, et al.: Effect of Na–K-ATPase on hydrogen ion and potassium secretion. Pfluegers Arch 386:161, 1980
152. Westenfelder C, Arevalo GJ, Baranowski RL, et al: Relationship between mineralocorticoids and renal Na^+–K^+ ATPase: Sodium reabsorption. Am J Physiol 233:F593, 1977

153. Manuel MA, Beirne GH, Wagnild JP, et al: An effect of spironolactone on urinary acidification in normal man. Arch Intern Med 134:472, 1974

154. Schambelan M, Sebastian A, Rector FC Jr: Mineralocorticoid-resistant renal hyperkalemia without salt wasting (type II pseudohypoaldosteronism): Role of increased renal chloride reabsorption. Kidney Int 19:716, 1981

155. Vandewalle A, Farman N, Bencsath P, et al: Aldosterone binding along the rabbit nephron: An autoradiographic study on isolated tubules. Am J Physiol 240:F172, 1981

20

Diabetic Comas

Mitchell L. Halperin
Marc B. Goldstein
Robert A. Bear
Robert G. Josse

The purpose of this chapter is to provide a general review of the pathophysiology of fluid, electrolyte, and acid–base metabolism that have a particular bearing on the syndromes of hyperosmolar hyperglycemic nonketotic coma, or simply nonketotic coma, and diabetic ketoacidosis. Approach to the fluid, electrolyte, and acid–base disturbances will be to discuss the pathophysiology of each individually and then to direct our attention to the diabetic coma syndromes to see how the metabolic disturbances collectively result in the individual clinical pictures. We have chosen to address the problem of hyperglycemia first because it is from this disturbance that many of the fluid and electrolyte aberrations arise, principally owing to the osmotic diuresis and intracellular fluid and extracellular fluid shifts.

OUTLINE OF THE PATHOPHYSIOLOGY OF FLUID AND ELECTROLYTE DISTURBANCES

Hyperglycemia in Comas Associated with Diabetes Mellitus

Since hyperglycemia is responsible for the major fluid and electrolyte disturbances in comas associated with diabetes mellitus, we shall discuss its pathophysiology in some detail. A rise in the extracellular fluid glucose concentration will occur if glucose input has exceeded its output from the extracellular fluid.

In order to evaluate glucose input, three sources must be analyzed: diet, hepatic glycogenolysis, and gluconeogenesis. Dietary input is variable, but it is usually easy to obtain semiquantitative information in this area. Most patients with nonketotic coma or diabetic ketoacidosis have only a limited dietary intake at presentation. Hepatic glycogenolysis and gluconeogenesis are controlled primarily by the hormonal balance—a fall in insulin and a rise in hormones with opposing actions (e.g., glucagon, catecholamines, glucocorticoids, and growth hormone) favor glucose synthesis. However, sustained hyperglycemia will not occur unless there is also a compromised glucose removal system. Glucose removal from the circulation is controlled primarily by its blood concentration. An elevated blood glucose concentration stimulates insulin release in normal subjects, and this leads to increased glucose removal, that is, conversion to glycogen and triglycerides or oxidation to produce adenosine triphosphatase (ATP). This sequence can be prevented if insulin fails to rise or if its actions are opposed. Loss of glucose can also occur in the urine. This loss is usually a function of the degree of hyperglycemia. In summary, hyperglycemia will occur in states in which the insulin response to an elevated glucose concentration is insufficient.

GLUCOSE INPUT

Diet

Two major dietary precursors can be converted to circulating glucose: carbohydrates and proteins. The former can be quantitatively converted to glucose, whereas only about 60 percent by weight of a mixed blend of dietary proteins can be metabolized to glucose.[1]

Production of Glucose from Endogenous Sources

Glucose production occurs primarily in the liver; hepatic glycogen can supply an emergency load of ~75 g glucose, and glucose can be synthesized via gluconeogenesis from three major endogenous precursors: muscle glycogen, glyceride glycerol, and body proteins. Muscle contains a total of 150 g of glycogen, but this must be recycled as lactate or alanine before conversion to glucose. As much as 25 g of glyceride glycerol can be metabolized to glucose per day; however, this supply is dependent on the degree of adipose tissue triglyceride mobilization (triglyceride is roughly 10 percent glycerol by weight). Body proteins supply amino acids, which may be converted into glucose; however, in quantitative terms, only about 75 g glucose can be formed from this precursor per day as the total daily nitrogen excretion in diabetic ketoacidosis under fasting conditions is usually <20 g and only 60 percent of these amino acids can yield glucose[1] (20 g N $\times$ 6.25 to convert N to protein $\times$ 0.60). In this discussion, we have ignored the Cori cycle, in which glucose is metabolized to lactate in peripheral tissues and the lactate is converted back to glucose via gluconeogenesis in the liver because there is not a large enough pool of lactate in the body to result in *net* accumulation of glucose (Fig. 20–1).

In summary, the maximum rate of net glucose production is 100 g (75 g from protein and 25 g from glyceride glycerol) plus the one-time contribution of glycogen; in addition, one must add the contribution of glucose precursors from the diet.

Gluconeogenesis also occurs in the kidney and is related to ammoniagenesis (for review, see ref. 2). Therefore, during metabolic acidosis or hypokalemia, not only the liver, but the kidney as well, may be a relatively important site for glucose production. Nevertheless, total net glucose production is as described above.

GLUCOSE REMOVAL SYSTEMS

Obligatory Glucose Oxidation

There is a mandatory need for water-soluble fuel oxidation to produce ATP in certain organs. The brain requires as much as 600 kcal water-soluble fuels (or 150 g glucose) per day. Ketone body anions can become the principal substrates for ATP synthesis in the brain during prolonged starvation (up to 75 percent of the total requirement), thereby decreasing the rate of glucose oxidation to carbon dioxide. When both hyperglycemia and ketosis are present, the brain may use more glucose than during the fasted state.

In diabetic ketoacidosis, glucose oxidation to carbon dioxide (i.e., flux through pyruvate dehydrogenase) is minimized in organs other than the brain, as this enzyme is inhibited when fatty acids and/or ketone bodies are oxidized (for review, see ref. 3). Glycolysis producing three-carbon intermediates re-formed into glucose does not result in net glucose appearance or disappearance. (Fig. 20–1).

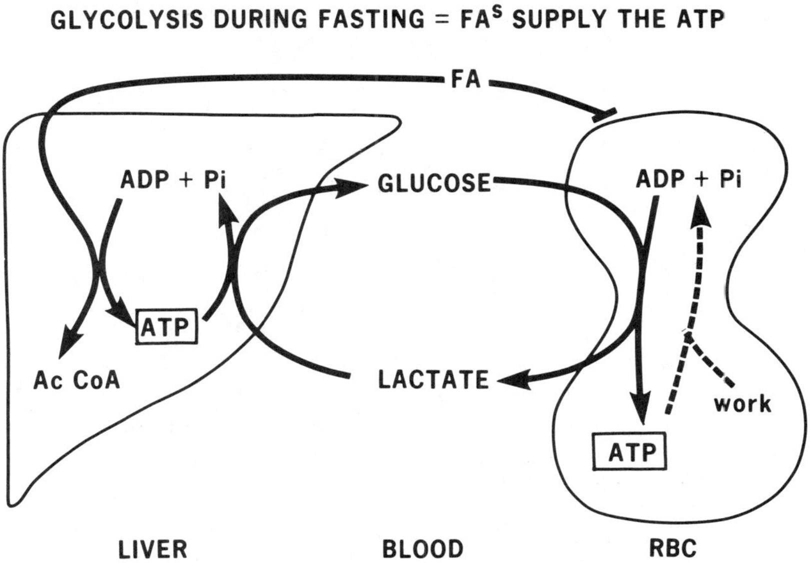

Fig. 20–1. In the red blood cell (RBC), adenosine triphosphate (ATP) is synthesized when glucose is converted to lactate. This lactate is delivered to the liver, where it is reconverted to glucose, which returns to the RBC completing the carbon (Cori) cycle without a net loss of glucose or lactate carbon. Since ATP, from fatty acid (FA) oxidation, is consumed during gluconeogenesis in the liver and ATP is produced from glycolysis in the RBC, there is in effect a net transfer of fat-derived energy from the liver to the RBC in this cycle.

Glycose Excretion in the Urine

Other than glucose oxidation in the brain, glycosuria represents the major process whereby glucose is "lost" from the body in diabetic ketoacidosis and nonketotic coma. Glucose is freely filtered at the glomerulus and the maximum rate of glucose reabsorption in the normal kidney is ~325 g/day this, might increase somewhat when there is a decrease in the extracellular fluid volume. Should the quantity of glucose filtered exceed 325 g/day, glucosuria develops. With a normal glomerular filtration rate of 180 liters/day, glucosuria will usually occur when the blood glucose concentration exceeds 180 mg/dl, the renal threshold. Glucose loss in the urine will result in the loss of calories and more specifically a potential energy fuel for the brain. However, on an acute basis these considerations are only of minor significance. Far more important are the renal sequelae of glycosuria, that is, large losses of sodium and potassium and disproportionately larger losses of water due to the osmotic diuresis (vide infra).

The quantity of glucose that should be excreted at a given blood glucose concentration and glomerular filtration rate is shown in Table 20–1. The data in Table 20–1 were derived using the following assumptions: (1) a constant rate of renal glucose reabsorption (325 g/day), (2) predicted spaces of glucose distribution,[4] (3) 150 g of glucose are oxidized in the brain, (4) a dietary intake of 225 g "glucose," and (5) a maximum rate of net endogenous glucose production of 100 g/day. Therefore, the total rate of glucose addition would be 325 g/day (225 g from the diet and 100 g from endogenous sources). Since only 150 g glucose can be oxidized, 175 g (325 − 150 g) must be excreted in the urine in order to remain in glucose balance.

Table 20–1. Effect of Hyperglycemia and Glomerular Filtration Rate on Glucose Excretion (g/day)

Plasma Glucose	GFR[a] (liters/day)					
(mg/dl)	180	150	100	75	50	25
200	35	0	0	0	0	0
300	215	125	25	0	0	0
400	395	275	75	0	0	0
500	575	425	175	50	0	0
600	755	575	275	125	0	0
750	1025	800	425	238	50	0
1000	1475	1175	675	425	175	0
1250	1925	1550	925	613	300	0
1500	2375	1925	1175	800	425	50

[a] GFR, glomerular filtration rate. All calculations, assume a maximum rate of glucose reabsorption of 325 g/day. In the presence of tubular damage, glucose reabsorption would decrease and renal glucose losses rise. Alternatively, if glucose reabsorption were significantly greater, glycosuria would fall.

Although Table 20–1 presents a theoretical formulation from which any given patient might deviate, several important general principles can be derived from it. First, in the presence of a normal glomerular filtration rate, an enormous glucose intake would be required to maintain very elevated plasma glucose concentrations. Such levels of glucose intake can occur with very unusual diets (with unusually large consumption of sugars), during peritoneal dialysis or during hypertonic glucose administration in parenteral nutrition. Therefore, in the absence of such a glucose intake, the patient with a blood sugar above 500 mg/dl must have a considerable reduction in glomerular filtration rate—a situation that almost universally occurs during the development of nonketotic coma and diabetic ketoacidosis. To give a quantitative aspect to the large amount of glucose input required in the presence of a normal glomerular filtration rate (180 liters/day), consider the requirements to maintain a plasma glucose at 500 mg/dl. At a glomerular filtration rate of 180 liters/day, the filtered load of glucose would be 900 g/day (5 g/liter and 180 liters/day) and, since only 325 g glucose can be reabsorbed, 575 g (900 − 325 g) will be lost in the urine. In addition, 150 g of glucose can be metabolized per day. Therefore, in this example, to remain in glucose balance 575 + 150, or 725 g glucose, would have to be added daily. If 100 g glucose can be produced from endogenous precursors, then 625 g must be ingested if renal function were to remain unchanged. Such conditions rarely if ever exist.

Second, reducing the glomerular filtration rate would have a considerable quantitative impact on the degree of hyperglycemia. Let us assume that a subject had a blood glucose of 500 mg/dl and a glomerular filtration rate of 150 liters/day and remained in glucose balance by ingesting 425 g of glucose/day (Table 20–1). If input and excretion were constant but glomerular filtration rate fell to 100 liters/day, glycemia would rise to 750 mg/dl. Further falls of glomerular filtration rate to 75 liters/day, then 50 liters/day, would result in steady-state glycemias of 1000 mg/dl and 1500 mg/dl, respectively. Thus, any situation that will reduce the glomerular filtration rate should result in a considerable rise in the blood glucose concentration.

Third, what are the combined effects of reducing the glomerular filtration rate and changing glucose input? Again, consider the patient with a plasma glucose of 500 mg/dl and glomerular filtration rate of 150 liters/day. Should the patient lose sufficient sodium to decrease the glomerular filtration rate by

50 to 100 liters/day, the glycemia would be maintained constant with considerably reduced glucose excretion, viz. 175 g vs 425 g; thus, decreased glucose input of this degree would serve only to maintain this elevated glycemia. It is readily appreciated that in the next step, hyperglycemia can worsen even dramatically, despite decreased glucose intake. A further decrease of glomerular filtration rate to 50 liters/day, with glucose excretion falling further to 50 g/day, would result in a glycemia of 750 mg/dl. This sequence is the typical evolution of a case of nonketotic coma. That is, despite progressively decreasing carbohydrate intake, the decreasing glomerular filtration rate will result in rising glycemia, often to extremely high levels.

Fourth, what are the therapeutic implications of increasing the glomerular filtration rate toward normal? In a patient with significant extracellular fluid volume contraction—the usual clinical setting—one would expect a significant fall in blood glucose concentration to accompany the intravenous saline-induced rise in the extracellular fluid volume and glomerular filtration rate even without any metabolic action of insulin to decrease glucose production or increase its metabolism. A patient with a blood glucose of 1500 mg/dl would have a glomerular filtration rate less than 20 percent of normal (Table 20–1). Total body glucose in such a patient is ~180 g (15 g/liter and ~12 liters glucose space because of the contracted extracellular fluid volume). Should this patient be treated vigorously with intravenous saline such that the glomerular filtration rate increased rapidly by 25 liters/day, the total body glucose would decline by ~15 g in the first hour and the extracellular fluid volume would be expanded by ~1 liter. The net result would be a fall in blood glucose of ~300 mg/dl.

In conclusion, it is important to consider quantitative influences on glucose metabolism and excretion in order to understand the implications of hyperglycemia. In the absence of an unusual diet, severe hyperglycemia indicates that the glomerular filtration rate is very low. A fall in glycemia could result from changes in glycosuria or extracellular fluid volume in addition to changes in glucose metabolism.

Water Metabolism in Comas Associated with Diabetes Mellitus

WATER DEFICIENCY IN DIABETES MELLITUS

Intracellular water deficiency can occur in diabetes mellitus because of decreased water intake or increased water loss and/or due to a shift of water from the intracellular fluid into the extracellular fluid secondary to hyperglycemia.

Water Intake

Normal subjects rarely suffer from water deficiency because of the action of the thirst center. However, decreased water intake is usually the result of a physical impairment (cannot get to water) and/or mental functional impairment (fails to appreciate water deficit). In the diabetic patient such factors as disturbed cerebrovascular function due to disease, hyperglycemia, severe acidosis, or hypoglycemia may play such a role. Although water losses in diabetic patients may be excessive, a normal person can keep up with these large water losses by increasing water intake. Therefore, if a diabetic has a total body water deficit, one should suspect a decreased water intake resulting from cerebral dysfunction or an inability to obtain water.

Distribution

Upon the induction of hyperglycemia (and relative insulin deficiency), the extracellular fluid osmolality rises. Therefore, in tissues requiring insulin for glucose entry (e.g., muscle), water must leave the intracellular fluid down an osmotic gradient until osmotic equilibration occurs, and these cells will shrink in size. However, glucose will enter certain cells (other than brain) and have a concentration that equals that in the extracellular fluid even in the absence of insulin.[5] Therefore, in these tissues (e.g., liver), there should be no net water movement out of the intracellular fluid. In fact, if the contribution to the tonicity of the extracellular fluid by solutes other than glucose (i.e., sodium) were to decrease as a result of water movement from the insulin-sensitive cells (muscle), water would actually move into the liver, down the effective osmotic gradient, and these cells would swell. Due to the metabolic disturbance of diabetes mellitus, other osmotically active substances may accumulate in various tissues.[6] Wherever these substances accumulate, osmolality will rise and may maintain osmotic equilibrium without loss of water from these cells.

The brain is particularly threatened by water deficits, as shrinkage of the brain can result in tearing of its vascular connections with the calvarium. In states of increased osmolality, brain tissue may have the capacity to increase intracellular osmoles, which will cause water to reenter brain cells and minimize potential shrinkage.[6] It is not clear whether this is a protective process that has evolved or whether these "idiogenic" osmoles are products of altered cell function. Approximately one-half the osmoles appear to be due to the entry of sodium, potassium, and chloride into the cell from the extracellular fluid; the remainder are osmoles that have been generated within the cell.

Water Loss

Increased water loss resulting in water deficiency is a common phenomenon in comas associated with diabetes mellitus. Water loss from nonrenal sources such as the gastrointestinal (GI) tract and skin may be substantial. However, the major source of water loss in the diabetic is the kidney because of the hyperglycemia-induced osmotic diuresis. Although the urine is usually slightly hypertonic (specific gravity ranges from 1.012 to 1.015), with the major osmole being glucose, there are also significant losses of sodium (40 to 60 mEq/liter, hyponatremic relative to the extracellular fluid) and potassium (30 to 50 mEq/liter) in this urine.

Diabetic patients may receive diuretic agents that inhibit electrolyte transport in the loop of Henle, such as furosemide and ethacrynic acid. These agents decrease the generation of a hypertonic renal medulla and thereby decrease the ability of the kidney to conserve water. In addition, certain renal medullary disorders occur more commonly in diabetic patients, including chronic interstitial nephritis, papillary necrosis, obstructive uropathy, and urinary tract infection. Hypokalemia may occur in diabetic patients and this may lead to changes limiting urinary concentrating ability. All these problems can contribute to a negative water balance.

WATER EXCESS IN DIABETES MELLITUS

Water excess in diabetes mellitus may come about as a result of increased water intake or decreased water excretion. In addition, there may be an apparent water excess due to shifting of water from the intracellular fluid to the extracellular fluid.

Increased Water Intake

Water intake may be increased in the diabetic with hyperglycemia (secondary to increased thirst with extracellular fluid volume contraction). This factor alone, however, is unlikely to lead to water excess. Hypotonic solutions are often used in therapy for the diabetic, but again, this is unlikely to lead to water excess.

Water Distribution

Hyperglycemia will lead to a net water shift from the intracellular fluid to the extracellular fluid because glucose does not freely enter all the intracellular fluid compartments. However, the water that shifts into the extracellular fluid is derived primarily from muscle, as there is no appreciable glucose concentration gradient across organs such as the liver. In fact, the liver will probably swell due to the hyponatremia produced by the water shift from muscle. One can predict the extent to which a given degree of hyperglycemia will lead to muscle dehydration and hyponatremia.[5] This calculation should include a consideration of this glucose distribution. In quantitative terms, a rise in blood glucose of 100 mg/dl should cause a 1.35-mEq/liter fall in plasma sodium concentration.

Water Loss

Many factors have the potential of limiting renal water excretion and some of these occur more commonly in diabetic patients (see Chapter 4). Decreased water loss can occur in diabetics who have a contracted extracellular fluid volume, which results in antidiuretic hormone release and a decreased delivery of sodium, chloride, and water to the diluting segment of the nephron, both of which reduce the amount of free water that can be excreted. In addition, if extracellular fluid volume contraction is severe, flow rate through the collecting duct will be reduced, and even in the absence of antidiuretic hormone, water will be reabsorbed. In considering extracellular fluid volume contraction, the important factor is the "effective" circulating volume. Diabetics who suffer from either congestive heart failure or the nephrotic syndrome have an increased total extracellular fluid volume with edema, but still have a reduced "effective" circulating volume, and will have all the limitations to water excretion.

There are many drugs, including certain oral hypoglycemic agents, which impair water excretion by causing the release of antidiuretic hormone or by potentiating or prolonging its action. Any of these drugs may be associated with water excess in the diabetic. In addition, diabetic patients often receive diuretic agents, and many diuretics (furosemide, ethacrynic acid, and thiazides) block the function of the diluting segments and thereby reduce the ability to excrete water. Excessive water intake (or administration) in conjunction with these diuretics will lead to water retention.

Finally, renal insufficiency commonly develops as a complication of diabetes mellitus; a decrease in renal function will lead to a decrease in the ability of the kidney to excrete a water load.

Sodium Metabolism in Diabetes Mellitus

SODIUM DEFICIENCY

Sodium deficiency may arise through decreased intake or increased losses. Decreased sodium intake may occur when low-sodium diets are prescribed for hypertension, congestive heart failure, or edema of the nephrotic syndrome. Also, sodium intake may be decreased if the patient is confused or does not have access to sufficient food containing sodium. In the presence of normal renal and adrenal function, the kidney responds to sodium deprivation with avid sodium reabsorption (urine Na <15 mEq/liter), thereby conserving the extracellular fluid volume. Increased losses are the cause of the more serious sodium deficiency states, and these losses may be from several sites. Gastrointestinal losses may be due to vomiting, diarrhea, or third-space effects (e.g., ileus, ascites). If diarrhea is the cause, there may be an accompanying metabolic acidosis due to sodium bicarbonate loss, whereas if vomiting is the source of sodium loss, there may be an associated metabolic alkalosis due to the hydrochloric acid loss and the extracellular fluid volume contraction. Loss via the skin can be significant; for example, vigorous exercise in a hot environment can result in sweat loss of up to 3 liters/hr.

Abnormal renal sodium losses are a frequent cause of extracellular fluid volume depletion. Renal sodium wasting may occur for a number of reasons. The most common is a glucose-induced osmotic diuresis, which also causes losses of water and potassium. Diuretic agents used as therapy for hypertension, congestive heart failure, and the nephrotic syndrome may also lead to sodium deficiency. The diabetic patient may have renal sodium wasting due to a wide variety of intrinsic renal diseases. Diabetics have a higher prevalence of pyelonephritis, which may progress to papillary necrosis, the resultant damage then leading to sodium loss in the urine. One must always bear in mind that decreased aldosterone action can occur in diabetes mellitus and is a cause of renal sodium wasting; hyperkalemia also occurs in this circumstance (for further discussion, see refs. 7 and 8 and Chapter 9). Also, renal sodium loss can be the direct result of insulin deficiency or secondary to ketonuria (for review, see ref. 9).

The serum sodium concentration directly reflects only the sodium:water ratio in the extracellular fluid. Therefore, sodium loss can be present with hypernatremia, a normal sodium concentration, or hyponatremia, depending on changes in water balance. For example, the patient with sodium depletion who has a large hypotonic fluid intake may well have hyponatremia due to diminished ability to excrete water. However, if the sodium losses are accompanied by water losses (e.g., osmotic diuresis) that exceed water intake, the patient may have hypernatremia. The urine sodium should be low (<15 mEq/liter) if sodium depletion is on a nonrenal basis, whereas a urine sodium >25 mEq/liter in a sodium-depleted state indicates renal sodium wasting. In the sodium-depleted state, the urine specific gravity should be high unless the patient has acute tubular necrosis (spec. grav., 1.010), has just received a diuretic (spec. grav., ≤ 1.010), or is undergoing an osmotic diuresis (spec. grav., 1.015). In a patient without underlying renal disease, sodium (and therefore extracellular fluid volume) depletion will lead to a larger elevation in the BUN than in the serum creatinine value (filtered urea will be reabsorbed under conditions of low urine flow). Underlying renal failure will be aggravated by coexistent sodium and extracellular fluid volume depletion, and this will also lead to a rise in BUN and creatinine. The hemoglobin and hematocrit will rise in the sodium-depleted patient (i.e., the patient with extracellular fluid volume contraction).

SODIUM EXCESS IN DIABETES MELLITUS

Sodium excess is not encountered unless the patient has cardiovascular hepatic or renal disease, as the kidney will excrete large sodium loads. The clinical manifestations of simple sodium excess are increased extracellular fluid volume as manifested by increased jugular or central venous pressure, edema, ascites, and possibly left ventricular failure, including a third heart sound and crackles in the chest. In contrast, hypoalbuminemia and sodium retention will have only the signs of interstitial fluid volume expansion (edema, ascites), whereas the vascular volume should be contracted. There are no specific laboratory manifestations of sodium excess, that is, the sodium concentration will reflect water balance, but the hemoglobin and hematocrit may fall with extracellular fluid volume expansion. Sodium intake should be stopped, and other conventional means to treat congestive heart failure should be instituted.

Potassium Metabolism in Coma Associated with Diabetes Mellitus

POTASSIUM DEFICIENCY

A fall in the extracellular fluid potassium concentration implies that either potassium input has decreased or its loss from the extracellular fluid has increased. Clinically significant potassium deficiency does not result from decreased potassium intake unless it is very prolonged as there are renal mechanisms for potassium conservation. Potassium loss from the extracellular fluid can reflect a shift of potassium into the intracellular fluid or it can be due to potassium excretion.

Potassium may enter the intracellular fluid after insulin action; in addition, a rise in blood pH leads to potassium entry and hydrogen ion exit from cells. Furthermore, bicarbonate may also cause potassium to shift into cells, apparently independent of a change in blood pH.[10]

Potassium losses can be conveniently divided into those that occur by renal or nonrenal mechanisms. Nonrenal mechanisms are via the gastrointestinal tract and are readily recognized by clinical assessment; this is aided by determining the urine potassium concentration. The urine potassium concentration should be <20 mEq/liter if the source of potassium loss is nonrenal, whereas if the source of the potassium loss is renal, the urine potassium concentration may be >40 mEq/liter. Renal potassium loss requires both sodium delivery to the distal nephron and aldosterone activity. The most common causes of renal potassium loss in patients with diabetes mellitus are either glucose-induced osmotic diuresis or the use of diuretics. The diuresis ensures sodium delivery to the distal nephron and the negative sodium balance causes extracellular fluid volume concentration, hence increased aldosterone release and action.

POTASSIUM EXCESS

A rise in the serum potassium concentration implies that potassium input has exceeded its loss. Hyperkalemia of a sustained nature does not usually occur from excessive oral or intravenous intake of potassium unless there is compromised renal excretion of this ion. In managing a patient with hyperkalemia, therefore, one should look for a cause of potassium transfer from the intracellular fluid or a cause for decreased renal excretion of potassium.

Although many factors can result in a potassium shift from the intracellular fluid to the extracellular fluid (see Chapter 9 for detailed discussion), in poorly controlled diabetics, cell necrosis and low basal insulin levels are probably the most important influences. Less important causes of a potassium shift could include a loss of intracellular anions (organic phosphates and protein anions) or a water shift due to hyperglycemia. Finally, much attention has been given to the intracellular buffering of hydrogen ions as a cause for a potassium shift. However, with weak organic acids such as ketoacids or lactic acid, which have anions that distribute in the intracellular fluid, a potassium shift is not a prominent feature of this buffering process.[11-13] Hyperkalemia is not generally observed in patients with lactic acidosis.

Factors reducing renal potassium excretion have been detailed in Chapter 9. Hyperkalemia generally accompanies renal insufficiency, which is a common complication of long-standing diabetes mellitus. Since distal sodium delivery and aldosterone are required for renal potassium secretion, decreased potassium secretion will occur with markedly enhanced proximal sodium reabsorption or reduced aldosterone activity. Reduced aldosterone activity may occur in diabetic patients for two major reasons. First, diabetes is often associated with renal medullary damage, and this may produce end-organ (cortical collecting duct) hyporesponsiveness to mineralcorticoid action. Second, a syndrome of hyporeninemic hypoaldosteronism has been described with increasing frequency in diabetic patients and is accompanied by hyperkalemia, metabolic acidosis, and subtle renal sodium wasting (for review, see refs. 7 and 8).

Acid–Base Disorders Associated with Coma in the Diabetic

Metabolic acidosis is the most common serious acid–base disorder complicating diabetes mellitus; ketoacidosis is the most common of these to be associated with coma. As discussed in Chapter 7, diabetic ketoacidosis is readily diagnosed by finding a wide unmeasured anion-gap type of metabolic acidosis in a hyper-

Table 20–2. Mean Blood Acid–Base Values in 83 Patients Presenting with Diabetic Ketoacidosis[a]

Parameter	Value (mEq/liter)[b]
pH	7.10
$[HCO_3^-]$[c]	16
β-Hydroxybutyrate	11
Acetoacetate	3
Lactate	4
Total organic anions[d]	18

[a] From Halperin ML, Bear RA, Hannaford M, et al: Selected aspects of the pathophysiology of metabolic acidosis in diabetes mellitus. Diabetes 30:781, 1981. Reproduced with permission from The American Diabetes Association, Inc.

[b] All units are expressed in milliequivalents per liter, except for pH.

[c] $[HCO_3^-]$, fall in plasma bicarbonate from the mean normal value of 24 mEq/liter. Hence, the mean bicarbonate concentration in these patients with diabetic ketoacidosis was 8 mEq/liter. This form of presentation permits the reader to compare directly the fall in bicarbonate concentration with the rise in organic anion concentration.

[d] Ketone body anions and lactate, hence total organic anions, were determined in 63 patients.

glycemic patient. Typical values are shown in Table 20–2. We shall discuss the pathophysiology of ketoacidosis by focusing the discussion on the hydrogen ion and the ketone body anion.

KETOACIDOSIS

Hydrogen Ion Concentration

PRODUCTION. The production of hydrogen ions (and ketone body anions) can be viewed as a two-component reaction. First, there is the provision of the substrate, free fatty acids from adipose tissue triglycerides. The second component of ketogenesis concerns the intrahepatic modifications that result in preferential oxidation of the circulating free fatty acids. This regulation is apparently induced via hormonal changes that influence the carnitine system in liver (for review, see ref. 14).

The maximum daily rate of ketoacid production is ~240 g, which is equivalent to 2400 mmol of hydrogen ion and ketone body anion production per day, a value that can greatly exceed the renal and nonrenal removal pathways. Therefore, in order to correct acidemia in diabetic ketoacidosis, the ketogenesis must be arrested promptly, by the administration of insulin.

Since patients with nonketotic coma have insulin deficiency and elevated levels of hormones that oppose the actions of insulin, they have the two prerequisites for enhanced ketogenesis, yet ketoacidosis is not a primary feature of nonketotic coma. Among the hypotheses considered to explain this phenomenon are that hormone-sensitive lipase is less active either because of a slightly, but not statistically significantly, higher insulin concentration, a higher number of insulin receptors than in diabetic ketoacidosis or that hyperglycemia is either antilipolytic or favors reesterification of free fatty acids in the adipocyte. However, the blood glucose concentration may be just as high in diabetic ketoacidosis. Partial support for an adipocyte locus for this phenomenon is that the blood free fatty acid level is lower in most but not all patients with nonketotic coma as compared to those with diabetic ketoacidosis.[15] Several findings favor a hepatic locus for the failure to observe ketoacidosis in nonketotic coma. Some patients have an adequate free fatty acid supply to the liver, and this is supported by the observation that some patients with nonketotic coma have both fatty livers and/or hypertriglyceridemia.[16] The hypothesis proposed to explain the low rates of hepatic ketogenesis are a relatively higher portal vein insulin concentration, a higher number of hepatic insulin receptors, and/or a preferential conversion of free fatty acid to hepatic triglyceride. The specific mechanisms have not been elucidated.

There is another consideration with respect to the apparent absence of ketoacidosis. Patients with this disorder often have a widened unmeasured anion gap of similar magnitude to that seen in diabetic ketoacidosis, but the clinical test for serum ketones is usually only weakly positive.[16] This means that there is not a marked acetoacetic acid acidosis. If lactic acidosis were also present, reflecting the poor oxygen delivery to tissues because of the marked extracellular fluid volume contraction, this would lead to the combination of lactic acidosis and β-hydroxybutyric acidosis and a false-negative test for serum ketones.[17] Although of possible importance, most cases in which lactate concentrations have been measured did not have large increases in this metabolite; however, the lactate:pyruvate ratios were increased. Therefore, to be certain, one should measure the β-hydroxybutyrate concentration directly to rule out this form of ketoacidosis.

In summary, because of the unpredictability of both the free fatty acid and insulin data, the absence of receptor data, and the heterogeneity of the patient population, the pathophysiology responsible for the low ketone body levels is still unclear.

DISTRIBUTION. In metabolic acidosis, about 60 percent of the hydrogen ion load is buffered in the intracellular fluid, whereas 40 percent is buffered in the extracellular fluid.[18] The decrease in the extracellular fluid bicarbonate content provides a quantitative estimate of the buffering in this compartment.

REMOVAL. Normal persons remain in acid–base balance because they excrete their daily acid load in the urine, largely as ammonium. In diabetic ketoacidosis, hydrogen ion production greatly exceeds its removal, and metabolic acidosis ensues. Significant removal of hydrogen ions also occurs as a consequence of the nonenzymatic conversion of acetoacetic acid to acetone and carbon dioxide. This pathway may be almost as important in quantitative terms as the renal pathway. Should the NADH/NAD increase (e.g., with hypoxia), the concentration of acetoacetic acid will fall and result in a lower rate of flux through the acetone pathway because the decarboxylation of acetoacetic acid is proportional to the acetoacetic acid concentration.

Ketoacid Anion Concentration

PRODUCTION. Ketone body anions and hydrogen ions are produced by the same biochemical process.

DISTRIBUTION. The free or undissociated β-hydroxybutyric acid achieves an equal concentration in the intracellular fluid and extracellular fluid. After dissociation, however, an extremely rapid process, the β-hydroxybutyrate anion and the hydrogen ion cannot cross this membrane as rapidly as the free acid and thus they have different concentrations in the intracellular fluid and extracellular fluid. If the dissociation constant is similar in both the intracellular fluid and extracellular fluid, it follows from both the law of mass action and the principle of nonionic diffusion that the products of $[H^+] \times [BHB^-$ (the β-hydroxybutyrate anion)] are equal in the intracellular fluid and extracellular fluid. (For a more detailed description, see refs. 19 and 20.)

In summary, although, ketoacids enter the intracellular fluid in the undissociated form, the eventual distribution of BHB^- and the H^+ depends on separate factors. For BHB^-, its concentration in the intracellular fluid will depend on the concentration of free acid (HBHB) and the intracellular fluid H^+ concentration. In contrast, the quantity of H^+ distributed in the intracellular fluid is a function of the quantity of intracellular fluid buffers, their pK values, and the intracellular fluid H^+ concentration.

REMOVAL. Ketone body anions are removed by metabolism, spontaneous decarboxylation, and renal excretion. Metabolism is the largest pathway and may account for 900 mmol/day. Both the metabolic and spontaneous decarboxylation pathways result in the production of a quantity of bicarbonate equal to the amount of ketone body anions consumed.

The renal handling of ketone bodies has been studied during fasting or after infusions, but it has not been studied in detail in diabetic ketoacidosis. Where studied, this excretion mechanism is independent of that of hydrogen ion. Ketone bodies are freely filtered and approximately 80 percent of this filtered load is reabsorbed without a tubular maximum. In diabetic ketoacidosis and nonketotic coma the glomerular filtration rate is markedly reduced due primarily to the extracellular fluid volume contraction. However excessive ketonuria may occur if the filtered load of lactate or acetylsalicylate is elevated or if there is a defect in proximal tubular function (for review, see ref. 19).

In severe diabetic ketoacidosis, it appears that more hydrogen ions than ketone body anions enter the intracellular fluid. Three implications may be drawn from these observations. First, the rise in the anion gap should be greater than the fall in the plasma bicarbonate concentration when patients with diabetic ketoacidosis are admitted. Failure to observe this change (Table 20–3) is probably the result of the renal excretion of ketone body anions exceeding that of ammonium. Second, on reversal of the diabetic ketoacidosis, more hydrogen ions than ketone body anions (or bicarbonate) would return to the extracellular fluid and would lead to a lesser rise in the plasma bicarbonate concentration than the fall in the anion gap. Oh et al.[21] recently described such a fall in the extracellular fluid bicarbonate plus ketone body anion contents after recovery from diabetic ketoacidosis. Third, for electroneutrality, some hydrogen ions must exchange across the cell membrane with cations such as potassium or sodium; however, in quantitative terms, there is only a small degree of po-

Table 20–3. Extracellular Fluid Bicarbonate and Organic Anion Data in Diabetic Ketoacidosis

Parameter	Normal Values	Value (mEq/liter)[a] Time (hr) 0	12–24	48+
ECF volume	15	12	15	15
[HCO_3^-]	24	8.5	18	24
Organic anion	1	17.5	1	1
ECF HCO_3^- content[b]	360	102	270	360
ECF OA content[c]	15	210	15	15
ECF HCO_3^- + OA contents[d]	375	312	285	375

[a] All units are expressed in milliequivalents per liter, except for ECF, which is in liters.

[b] ECF bicarbonate content is the product of the bicarbonate concentration and the ECF volume.

[c] ECF organic anion content is the product of the sum of β-hydroxybutyrate, acetoacetate, and lactate concentrations times the ECF volume. These values were derived from Table 20–2. Despite the fact that the fall in bicarbonate concentration was equal to the rise in organic anion concentration (Table 20–2), their contents were very different due to the change in ECF volume.

[d] The sum of ECF bicarbonate plus organic anion contents represents the total bicarbonate in the ECF after therapy. The fact that this content decreases after 12 to 24 hours probably reflects hydrogen ion movement into the ECF from the ICF as the ECF pH rises.

Abbreviations: ECF, extracellular fluid; ICF, intracellular fluid; OA, organic ion.

Source: Halperin ML, Bear RA, Hannaford M, et al: Selected aspects of the pathophysiology of metabolic acidosis in diabetes mellitus. Diabetes 30:781, 1981. Reproduced with permission from The American Diabetes Association, Inc.

tassium movement due to this effect in diabetic ketoacidosis.

METABOLIC ACIDOSIS WITH A NORMAL UNMEASURED ANION GAP IN DIABETES MELLITUS

Hyperchloremic metabolic acidosis in patients with diabetic ketoacidosis is present in virtually every case of diabetic ketoacidosis on admission and is due to an "indirect" loss of sodium bicarbonate (Tables 20–3 and 20–4). In addition, on recovery from diabetic ketoacidosis, hydrogen ions reenter the extracellular fluid from the intracellular fluid and thereby result in a further loss of extracellular fluid bicarbonate. For these reasons, a hyperchloremic metabolic acidosis should be expected with the usual successful initial therapy for diabetic ketoacidosis.

It is important to recall that the bicarbonate content in the extracellular fluid is the product of the bicarbonate concentration (amount/volume) and the total extracellular fluid volume. Therefore, 360 mEq of bicarbonate is present in the extracellular fluid in a typical patient, that is, 24 mEq/liter × 15 liter (see Table 20–3). For every milliequivalent of ketoacid added to the extracellular fluid, 1 mEq of bicarbonate is lost, 1 mEq of ketone body anion is gained, and the sum of bicarbonate plus ketone body anions remains constant. If we assume, for the moment, that the quantity of hydrogen ions and ketone body anions added to the extracellular fluid is equal at steady state, then the number of milliequivalents of bicarbonate lost must be equal to the number of milliequivalents of ketone body anions gained. It follows that 360 mEq of bicarbonate plus ketone body anions should be contained in the extracellular fluid at steady state during diabetic ketoacidosis. However, due principally to an osmotic diuresis, patients with diabetic ketoacidosis lose between 5 and 10 mEq sodium per kg body weight. As a round figure, we shall assume a 20 percent decline in the extracellular fluid volume, or

Table 20–4. Indirect Loss of Sodium Bicarbonate in Diabetic Ketoacidosis[a]

	Result	
Process	Gain to ECF	Loss from ECF
1. Gain of acid	$H^+ + KB^-$	
2. Buffering (loss of HCO_3^-) in ECF		$H^+ + HCO_3^- \rightarrow CO_2$
3. Anion excretion (loss of Na^+)[b]		$KB^- + Na^+ \rightarrow$ Urine
Sum of 1 + 2 + 3		$Na^+ + HCO_3^-$ loss

[a] In diabetic ketoacidosis, organic acids are added to the extracellular fluid. The hydrogen ions are buffered and the ketone body anions may be retained, metabolized, or excreted. The cycle describes hydrogen ions and ketone body anions produced and lost in equal quantities. Indirect loss of sodium bicarbonate occurs when there is a net loss of bicarbonate via the lungs and sodium in the urine to balance the electrical charge of the ketone body anions. Sodium loss in the urine is normally minimized because of ammonium excretion. The excretion of ammonium may be reduced in the diabetic because of either a primary renal disease, hyperkalemia, insufficient time for the adaptive changes in ammoniagenesis, or defects in hydrogen ion secretion.

[b] Should process 3 not occur, then an indirect loss of sodium bicarbonate would not occur. Two major alternatives can replace process 3. First, the ketone body anions may be completely reabsorbed by the kidney resulting in a simple anion-gap type of metabolic acidosis; second, the excretion of the ammonium salt of β-hydroxybutyric acid would cause the blood bicarbonate concentration to rise because the excretion of ammonium results in bicarbonate generation.

Abbreviations: ECF, extracellular fluid; KB, ketone body.

Source: Halperin ML, Bear RA, Hannaford M, et al: Selected aspects of the pathophysiology of metabolic acidosis in diabetes mellitus. Diabetes 30:781, 1981. Reproduced with permission from The American Diabetes Association, Inc.

a 3-liter deficit. This contraction of extracellular fluid volume should lead to an increase in the sum of the bicarbonate plus ketone body anion concentrations in diabetic ketoacidosis (i.e., 360 mEq/12 liters, or 30 mEq/liter).

However, as shown in Table 20–2, the mean sum of the bicarbonate and ketone body anion concentration in patients with diabetic ketoacidosis is only 26 mEq/liter, a value significantly less than would be predicted by the degree of extracellular fluid volume depletion. In other words, the fall in bicarbonate is greater than can be explained by the rise in unmeasured anions (i.e., ketone body anions). These observations suggest that a loss of extracellular fluid bicarbonate and/or ketone body anions has occurred during the development of diabetic ketoacidosis. Therefore, at presentation, patients with diabetic ketoacidosis have two factors contributing to the metabolic acidosis: (1) increased production of ketoacids; and (2) the loss of bicarbonate or potential bicarbonate, which will become more obvious after insulin therapy.

A number of mechanisms could explain this bicarbonate and/or ketone body anion deficit. Direct bicarbonate loss may occur via the gastrointestinal tract or the urine; the former is usually obvious to the clinician, although bicarbonate sequestration in the small intestine when there is an ileus may be more difficult to recognize. This complication can occur in diabetics who have marked potassium deficits or abdominal pathology. Direct loss of bicarbonate in the urine occurs when there is a defect in proximal tubular reabsorption of bicarbonate (proximal renal tubular acidosis); when uncomplicated, this disorder is characterized by the excretion of large quantities of bicarbonate in the urine (urine pH > 6.3). Proximal renal tubular acidosis is rare in diabetic patients, although it may be seen in association with severe hypophosphatemia. Bicarbonaturia may occur when carbonic anhydrase inhibitors are administered.

Ketonuria could lead to a decrease in the bicarbonate plus ketone body anion content, provided that the excretion of ketone body anions exceeds that of ammonium plus hydrogen ions. This might occur due to the presence, either singly or in combination, of four different circumstances (because ammonium excretion requires both NH_3 production and hydrogen ion secretion in the distal nephron): (1) reduced ammoniagenesis in the renal cortex due to kidney disease or hyperkalemia (for review, see ref. 21); (2) reduced medullary transfer of NH_3 from the loop of Henle to the collecting duct[22] (e.g., due to interstitial nephritis); (3) reduced hydrogen ion secretion in the distal nephron; and (4) presentation of a filtered load of ketones that is so large that even with the normal reabsorptive rate, ketonuria would exceed the augmented renal capacity for ammonium excretion.

When ketone body excretion exceeds that of net acid (NH_4 + titratable acid), the excess ketone body anions are excreted with sodium and potassium ions and the net result is an indirect loss of sodium bicarbonate. To understand the sequence of events resulting in the indirect loss of sodium bicarbonate, consider the following three steps (summarized in Table 20–4): (1) the addition of β-hydroxybutyric and acetoacetic acids to the extracellular fluid; (2) buffering of the hydrogen ions by bicarbonate with the resultant removal of carbon dioxide via the lungs; and (3) a loss of the ketone body anion in the urine along with sodium or potassium. Taken together, these events result in a net "indirect" loss of sodium bicarbonate from the extracellular fluid.

After successful therapy for diabetic ketoacidosis, the plasma bicarbonate concentration is ~20 mEq/liter. The mean bicarbonate plus potential bicarbonate content of the extracellular fluid is lower than anticipated in typical patients with diabetic ketoacidosis before therapy, despite the fact that the sum of their concentrations is 26 mEq/liter (Table 20–1). If the extracellular fluid volume is then reexpanded to normal with a bicarbonate-free solution (sodium plus potassium chloride) and all the excess ketone body anions oxidized to produce bicarbonate, the plasma bicarbonate concentration will be 20 percent below normal. In addition, hydrogen ion reentry into the extracellular fluid in excess of ketone body anions will lower this value even further (these hydrogen ions probably entered the extracellular fluid in exchange for sodium or potassium, Table 20–3). This bicarbonate deficit will be repaired by the renal excretion of ammonium chloride over the next 24 to 48 hours, provided that there is no primary renal defect.

TREATMENT OF METABOLIC ACIDOSIS: ALKALI THERAPY

Severe metabolic acidosis is a life-threatening situation. Specific therapy should be directed toward arresting hydrogen ion production; under some circumstances, sodium bicarbonate should be administered to remove hydrogen ions. General principles surrounding the use of bicarbonate therapy are as follows. See also Chapter 7.

Severity of the Acidosis

By comparing the data in lines 1–3 in Table 20–5, it can be seen that there is a more than simple additive rise in blood hydrogen ion concentration as the blood bicarbonate falls by 2-mEq/liter decrements. Hence, a patient is less able to tolerate an additional acid load if he or she already has a low serum bicarbonate concentration. Therefore, bicarbonate should probably be administered in metabolic acidosis if the rate of hydrogen ion production cannot be decreased markedly. In addition, bicarbonate therapy should be considered whenever the serum bicarbonate concentration is markedly reduced (i.e., <5 to 10 mEq/liter).

Degree of Hyperventilation

A patient who has severe metabolic acidosis (line 3, Table 20–5) is dependent on hyperventilation to maintain extracellular fluid hydrogen ion concentration in an acceptable range. Should the patient's ability to hyperventilate suddenly be compromised by a coughing spell, aspiration, or other event, the patient becomes markedly acidemic (line 4, Table 20–5). Therefore if such patients are at risk, they should receive bicarbonate to protect them from this lethal complication.

Regeneration of Bicarbonate

An important consideration in management of the patient with metabolic acidosis is whether the patient will be able to generate bicarbonate and how long it will take to raise the bicarbonate concentration. Once the metabolic disorder has been corrected, patients

Table 20–5. Rationale for Bicarbonate Therapy in Metabolic Acidosis: Role of the Severity of Acidosis and the Degree of Hyperventilation[a]

Condition	HCO_3^- (mEq/liter)	Blood Pa_{CO_2} (mm Hg)	$[H^+]$ (nEq/liter)	pH	Rise in $[H^+]$ (nEq/liter)
Metabolic acidosis	10	25	60	7.22	20
	8	23	69	7.16	29
	6	21	84	7.08	44
Metabolic acidosis and relative hypoventilation	6	35	140	6.85	100

[a] The patient is shown to have a progressive severe metabolic acidosis with the expected degree of hyperventilation indicated on lines 1–3. Since the normal blood hydrogen ion concentration is 40 nEq/liter, the blood hydrogen ion concentration is 20 nEq/liter above this value in line 1. Continued net hydrogen ion production causes the blood bicarbonate to fall by 2-mEq/liter decrements over the period of observation, and the patient hyperventilates to the expected degree. Note that the rise in blood hydrogen ion concentration has increased about two-fold during this period. A further two-fold rise in hydrogen ion concentration occurs when the patient hypoventilates (however, the blood Pa_{CO_2} is still <40 mm Hg). It follows that a patient with severe metabolic acidosis is very vulnerable, with respect to acidemia, to both continued hydrogen ion production and the lack of the appropriate degree of hypoventilation.

with lactic acidosis or ketoacidosis will be able to metabolize the lactate or ketoacid anions to neutral end products (CO_2, triglyceride, or glucose in the case of lactate) and thereby generate bicarbonate (1 mol of H^+ used for each mole of anion removed). This process will occur quickly after reversal of the metabolic disorder, and thus bicarbonate therapy will not be necessary if the metabolic acidosis is not severe (bicarbonate >10 mEq/liter) or complicated by respiratory acidosis. Similarly, patients who have sequestered bicarbonate-rich fluids in an ileus will be able to recover that bicarbonate once the ileus has been cured. By contrast, patients who have lost bicarbonate in the stool or urine (diarrhea or renal acidification defect) will not be able to regenerate bicarbonate quickly. If the renal acidification defect is transient or if the bicarbonate loss is via the gastrointestinal tract, the kidney will be able to generate bicarbonate by increasing net acid excretion. However, it may take several days for this to occur. Therefore, exogenous bicarbonate therapy will often be necessary for patients with a moderate or severe metabolic acidosis in association with a normal unmeasured anion gap or in patients with renal acidification defects.

Dangers of Bicarbonate Therapy

Bicarbonate administration is associated with potassium movement into cells; therefore, potassium deficits must be corrected coincident with bicarbonate therapy. If potassium deficits are very large, it is appropriate to begin aggressive potassium repletion (40 mEq/liter intravenous fluid) before starting bicarbonate therapy, especially if insulin is also being administered and the urine flow rate is brisk. In such cases, cardiac monitoring should be employed to detect arrhythmias due to hypokalemia. See Chapter 23.

Another major risk of bicarbonate therapy is that caused by the resultant extracellular fluid volume expansion owing to the sodium concentration in standard sodium bicarbonate preparations. In elderly patients, or in those with underlying cardiac disease, it is sometimes appropriate to use diuretics at the time of bicarbonate administration in order to minimize extracellular fluid volume expansion. However, in diabetic ketoacidosis this is not really a problem because of the marked extracellular fluid volume contraction.

In patients who have had a severe increased unmeasured anion-gap type of metabolic acidosis in whom large amounts of bicarbonate have been used, a significant metabolic alkalosis may develop once the disorder has been corrected and the ketoacid anions metabolized. In these cases, one should ensure that chloride and potassium deficits have been replaced so that the excess bicarbonate can be excreted rapidly by the kidneys.

Other factors often mentioned as dangers of sodium bicarbonate therapy include a shift in the oxygen–hemoglobin dissociation curve to the left and generation of a paradoxical cerebrospinal fluid acidosis. The former may lead to decreased oxygen delivery to tissues and the latter could lead to impaired cerebral function. These potential hazards are in our opinion overemphasized but can be minimized by partial correction of the metabolic acidosis. Finally, bicarbonate therapy through a central venous line or very rapid bicarbonate administration is not totally without risk, as bicarbonate concentrations and more importantly the PCO_2 in the fluid entering the heart may transiently be very high. Recent studies in an animal model of lactic acidosis have led to the caution that, in certain circumstances, bicarbonate therapy might have adverse effects.[23] In addition, in anorexic patients with lactic acidosis, alkali therapy may be associated with excessive tissue catabolism.[24]

SPECIFIC DISEASE STATES

Nonketotic Coma: Clinical Aspects

GENERAL FEATURES

Nonketotic coma is a clinical-biochemical entity characterized by marked hyperglycemia (most often > 600 mg/dl), hyperosmolality (usually > 350 mOsm/kg), the absence of marked ketonemia ("ketones" negative or positive only in undiluted plasma), and variable degrees of depression of the sensorium.[16] However coma in the usual sense is not a sine qua non of the physiologic derangement, although most patients will have some depression of sensorium. The diagnosis should be made long before a frankly comatose state has been reached. Even in the absence of coma, this state is to be regarded as an acute emergency. Early recognition and adequate management are necessary if the exceedingly high mortality rate is to be reduced. Indeed, the syndrome with coma should be largely preventable by anticipating the circumstances in which it is likely to develop.

The typical clinical presentation is in a patient over 50 years of age with non-insulin-dependent diabetes, who has other systemic disease (usually cardiovascular or renal) and is often under treatment with a variety of medications. The onset is insidious, and may be precipitated by an intercurrent illness, not necessarily related to the presence of glucose intolerance. The evolution initially involves significant hyperglycemia, glycosuria, natriuresis, and polyuria. The incomplete replacement of water and sodium losses and possibly excess carbohydrate intake then aggravate the hyperglycemia. The metabolic basis involves (1) inadequate insulin action to return the blood glucose concentration to normal; (2) a metabolic setting in which ketosis is not prominent; and (3) lowered glomerular filtration rate, such that glucosuria and glucose metabolism cannot eliminate sufficient glucose to maintain glycemia below 300 to 500 mg/dl.

It has been estimated that nonketotic coma occurs at one-sixth the frequency of diabetic ketoacidosis (for review, see ref. 25). Several hundred case reports have appeared in the literature, most of which have described aspects of severe cases in association with coma. The syndrome with coma undoubtedly occurs far more frequently than it is reported, since now only unusual concomitants merit publication. Many substantial series of reported cases were accumulated in single hospitals over 2- to 4-year periods, and further, since the syndrome without frank coma has been underemphasized, it must now be considered a relatively common problem.

Notwithstanding the increase in recognition of the syndrome, as well as improvements in management, the mortality rate remains distressingly high. In several large early series, it was about 50 percent (for review, see ref. 16). The lowest reported mortality rate thus far has been 20 percent in a series of 20 cases, seven of whom were comatose, 10 lethargic, and three alert on admission.[26] The syndrome is therefore one of considerable importance in terms of frequency of occurrence and of its high mortality and morbidity. However, many aspects of its pathophysiology and treatment remain controversial.

ETIOLOGIC FACTORS

Many of the patients affected are diabetic. However, an appreciable proportion of cases, usually with severe intercurrent disease and/or very unusual glucose loads, may show only a minimal abnormality of glucoregulation after convalescence. Although most commonly affected are non-insulin-dependent diabetics over 50 years of age, the syndrome has also been reported in young, insulin-dependent diabetics, and indeed may be the initial manifestation of the disease. Most often the syndrome is observed during the course of an acute intercurrent illness. Certainly any acute illness, particularly infective or gastrointestinal, would be capable of triggering the pathogenetic sequence in a susceptible individual. Too often, the acute illness receives full medical attention, and the insidious progression of the diuresis and water and electrolyte abnormalities go unnoticed.

The classic scenario would be that extracellular fluid volume contraction develops as the consequence of diuretic administration, of an acute febrile illness of the respiratory or urinary tracts, or of prolonged diarrhea, or it may occur with vomiting, preventing adequate fluid intake. The weakness resulting from any of these conditions would then exacerbate the patient's inability to maintain adequate fluid intake. In already hospitalized patients, the syndrome is seen most often in intensive care units. For example, with extensive burns covering 20 to 45 percent of body surface area, severe stress, fluid loss from a burn site, inability to maintain fluid intake, a tendency to treat with hyperosmolar glucose, and elevated catecholamine levels inhibiting insulin release all interact in its pathogenesis. In acute hemorrhagic pancreatitis, added to such factors is the direct inhibition of insulin secretion related to the extent of the disease process itself. If glucose influsion is added to impaired glucose utilization and augmented endogenous glucose production, the syndrome may occur.

Indeed, even without acute trauma, glucose administration in the very large amounts currently employed can precipitate the syndrome. This is especially true in the case of parenteral hyperalimentation as nutritional therapy. The same applies to certain defined formula "diets" or tube-feeding solutions which are hypercaloric and also contain high concentrations of carbohydrate. In these cases, an osmotic load inducing diarrhea may also contribute to the water loss. In peritoneal dialysis, the high glucose concentration in the dialysate, introduced to remove water from the patient by virtue of its hyperosmolality, results in the transfer of large amounts of glucose across the peritoneum. Where coexisting acute stress or diabetes are present, a hyperosmolar syndrome may develop. Even with insulin injection and insulin added to the dialysate, the cyclic challenges and prolonged duration of dialysis can present serious difficulties in maintaining glycemic control.

Many medications are capable of precipitating the hyperosmolar state via exacerbation of the pathogenetic sequence described. In some instances, there is suppression of insulin secretion (phenytoin, large doses of diazoxide, chlorpromazine), or extracellular fluid volume contraction induced by diuretics, which may alter carbohydrate tolerance by other mechanisms as well (e.g., catecholamines). High-dose corticosteroid therapy probably acts by increasing glucose production and impeding its clearance. In other cases, the precise mechanisms are not known.

Finally, in rare patients with thyrotoxicosis and Cushing's disease, nonketotic coma has been reported. The pathophysiology in thyrotoxicosis presumably relates to a decrease in glucose tolerance, mediated in part by the autonomic nervous system and to the tendency to lose sodium by excessive perspiration and frequent bowel movements. In endogenous hyperadrenocorticism, the pathophysiology is likely to be the same as during exogenous corticosteroid treatment.

DIAGNOSIS

During the evolution of nonketotic coma, the symptoms are those of the precipitating disorder plus those related to the osmotic diuresis and its consequences. The most important feature that merits reemphasis is the insidious development, which takes place over days to weeks. Thus, the polyuria, increase in thirst, weight loss, and mental changes may develop so slowly that the patient may not recognize them. This is in sharp contrast to the evolution of diabetic ketoacidosis. In this stage of evolution, clinical signs may be subtle and the diagnosis requires a high index of suspicion, supported by the essential laboratory tests. In the well-developed case, the essential clinical signs relate to extracellular fluid volume contraction, neurological disturbances, and the absence of signs of ketoacidodis. The intense extracellular fluid volume loss is often reflected in weight loss, dryness of mucous membranes, absence of sweating, decreased skin turgor, decreased jugular venous pressure, arterial hypotension, marked postural drop in blood pressure, and increase in pulse rate. Hyperthermia is often present, as distinct from hypothermia, which is often present in diabetic ketoacidosis. Frank circulatory insufficiency is present in the most severe cases. In this instance lactic acidosis may be superimposed. The level of consciousness varies from alertness through somnolence and from obtundation to coma. Periods of agitation may occur. Particularly noteworthy is the frequency of focal neurologic signs; those reported have included myoclonus of the extremities, focal motor seizures, Jacksonian seizures, and hemiparesis. Generalized convulsions can also be seen, and all add to the complexity of the presenting clinical picture. In addition, other neurologic changes such as aphasia, hyperreflexia, sensory defects, autonomic changes, and brain stem dysfunction can occur.[31] The foregoing are listed because (1) they are considerably less frequent in classic diabetic ketoacidosis, and (2) the diagnosis of the nonketotic coma can be delayed or missed by the urgency of treating these dramatic manifestations. Furthermore, postconvulsive acidosis may be superadded to the basic clinical picture, whether it be from the lactic acidosis component or from an aspiration pneumonitis.

Although a component of acidosis may be present, the absence of classic signs of acetone odor on the breath and Kussmaul respiration are useful in pointing clinically to nonketotic coma. However, rapid, shallow breathing has been commonly observed. The bedside diagnosis can be all but confirmed within minutes by the observation of a profoundly contracted extracellular fluid in a comatose patient who nonetheless passes large or appreciable volumes of urine, with marked glycosuria, absent or small amounts of ketonuria, a blood Dextrostix value above the interpretable range, and absent or small amounts of plasma ketones. It is important to note that the comatose diabetic patient should not have received intravenous glucose treatment before the observation of the Dextrostix result, and certainly not following it.

LABORATORY EVALUATION

Severe hyperglycemia(>600 mg/dl) is always present and may reach levels as high as 3000 mg/dl. Where the diagnosis is suspected, specific instruction to the biochemistry laboratory to perform multiple dilutions will aid in more rapid quantitation. The serum ketones are negative or weakly positive. The hyperosmolar syndrome may accompany ketoacidosis; in these cases, the serum ketones may or may not be strongly positive (note the false-negative test for ketones in β-hydroxybutyric acidosis.[17] The serum sodium concentration may be high, low, or within the normal range, depending on the magnitude of water losses relative to the intake. In one large series of 31 patients,[16] there were approximately equal numbers of patients in each category. Elevations have been reported as high as 190 mEq/liter, although values of 150 to 165 mEq/liter are more frequently observed. It is noteworthy that hyponatremia should accompany hyperglycemia, and that a correction factor may be employed to relate these changes; the expected decrease in serum sodium is 1.35 mEq/liter for every 100-mg/dl increase in glycemia above normal.[5]

While potassium depletion is universal in patients with this syndrome due to urinary losses secondary to the osmotic diuresis, the mean serum potassium was found to be 5.0, and only three of 33 patients had frank hypokalemia despite the fact that potassium deficits were greater than 100 mEq.[16] It is unlikely that acidemia was responsible for increasing the serum potassium; in fact, acidemia, correlated poorly with hyperkalemia in this series. Although the glomerular filtration rate was low at presentation, one cannot attribute the failure to find hypokalemia on renal failure per se because of the markedly negative potassium balance. The most likely cause for this failure to find hypokalemia is an altered potassium distribution, relatively higher in the extracellular fluid secondary to insulin deficiency. In any case, a net potassium deficit exists and requires careful surveillance during treatment.

The plasma osmolality—the single variable most closely correlated with the level of obtundation—should be measured or calculated. If measured, most often done by the technique of freezing point depression, remember that the sodium and glucose, are not the only solutes contributing (e.g., if alcohol has been ingested or if the BUN is elevated). The calculation is performed as described by Feig and McCurdy:[27]

$$P_{osm} = 2\ [\text{serum Na (mEq/liter)}] + \text{glucose (mg/dl)}/18 + \text{BUN mg/dl}/2.8$$

or

$$= 2\ [\text{serum Na (mEq/liter)}] + \text{glucose (mmol/liter)} + \text{urea (mmol/liter)}$$

Normal values according to this approach are 280 to 300 mOsm/kg H_2O. Typical values in nonketotic coma are in the range of 340 mOsm/kg H_2O, but values in excess of 400 mOsm/kg have been reported.

Metabolic acidosis is a prominent feature, as evidenced by the rise in the unmeasured anion gap ($Na - (Cl + HCO_3) = 34$ mEq/liter, normal value 12 ± 1 mEq/liter).[16] However, the serum bicarbonate concentration is usually only moderately reduced, reflecting the coexistent metabolic alkalosis secondary to the osmotic diuresis-induced loss of sodium and chloride and/or vomiting.

On occasion, the acidemia is severe; for example, four of the 33 patients reported[16] had a bicarbonate concentrations of ≤ 10 mEq/liter. The anion responsible for the elevated unmeasured anion gap is to some extent lactate, probably reflecting the extracellular fluid volume contraction. However, often a large proportion of the anions are unidentified. β-Hydroxybutyrate levels were not measured in this series of patients and may contribute in some cases to the unmeasured anions. There may also be short-chain fatty acids.[33]

The measurement of arterial blood pH, P_{CO_2}, and electrolytes is mandatory on first examination of the patient in order to elucidate the presence of acidosis, its severity, and associated causal and compensatory factors.

All patients are azotemic, with typical BUN levels of 87 ± 10 mg/dl.[16] Serum creatinine levels are also elevated ($5.5 + 1.1$ mg/dl). These values reflect not only the extracellular fluid volume contraction, but may also indicate the presence of intrinsic renal disease in many of the patients reported. The degree of blood volume contraction is also apparent in elevations of hemoglobin, hematocrit, and serum protein concentrations.

Estimation of the degree, nature, and (if possible) chronicity of the renal function impairment is also critical. Urine analysis, for the presence of protein, pH, and microscopic examination of the sediment, can provide an index of this estimation. Urine sodium and potassium concentrations are generally close to 50 mEq/liter. This measurement is not usually required urgently, but indicates the magnitude of ongoing sodium and potassium losses.

Serum enzymes of muscle origin are often elevated (SGOT, LDH, BHBDH, and CPK) and may rise even higher during rapid rehydration with hypotonic solutions.

The white blood cell count is frequently elevated, and the differential count may be useful in assessing the precipitating disorder. Where indicated, further studies may be carried out to elucidate the nature of concurrent disease states.

TREATMENT

The general strategy for management of all diabetic emergencies should include the immediate transfer of the patient to an intensive care unit. A single physician should be directly responsible for the patient, aided by qualified nursing and technical personnel and the facilities required for continuous surveillance of vital signs, neurologic status, electrocardiogram (ECG), and central venous pressure and for possible cardiopulmonary resuscitation.

The first priority of therapy is to correct the profound extracellular fluid volume depletion, which often will have resulted in circulatory collapse. This measure takes precedence over immediate insulin therapy. If there is significant hypokalemia, one should also begin potassium replacement. Once the blood pressure has been restored, one should begin to correct the water deficits. However, this should be done more slowly to prevent disproportionate expansion of brain cells.

Sodium

The most serious immediate threat to the patient is the circulatory collapse due to extracellular fluid volume contraction. One should aim to partially reexpand the extracellular fluid volume rapidly without worrying about inducing a rapid water shift into the intracellular fluid. Toward that end, isotonic saline (154 mM NaCl) should be administered initially to patients with manifestations of circulatory instability at rates that vary according to the clinical state. Since sodium losses in the patient with nonketotic coma are in the order of 10 mEq/kg in a 70-kg person, this loss is ~700 mEq, equivalent to ~5 liter of isotonic saline. Continuing losses due to the osmotic diuresis will increase the requirement for intravenous saline. One can calculate the total number of liters of osmotic diuresis that a patient with nonketotic coma can have, provided that no exogenous glucose is administered and that endogenous glucose production is 100 g/24 hr, or ~4 g/hr. The total glucose content in a patient with nonketotic coma and a glycemia of 1000 mg/dl (10 g/liter) is ~120 g (extracellular fluid volume 12 liter). Since each liter of urine in an osmotic diuresis contains ~30 g glucose and 50 mEq sodium, only 3 liter of urine could be produced—less if some glucose were metabolized—containing in addition 150 mEq sodium (i.e., requiring 1 liter of isotonic saline in addition to the above noted sodium deficit). Accordingly, administration of 2 liters of saline during the first hour or so would be an appropriate initial rate in the absence of elevated central venous pressure. As the extracellular fluid volume is restored with intravenous fluid administration, blood pressure will rise, and the glomerular filtration rate will increase, leading to a larger degree of glycosuria and a significant fall in blood glucose concentration as long as renal function has not been significantly compromised (e.g., acute tubular necrosis secondary to hypotension). The serum sodium concentration may rise initially, reflecting water movement into the intracellular fluid as a result of the fall in blood glucose concentration and the low sodium concentration in the urine during osmotic diuresis.

For every 100-mg/dl fall in blood glucose concentration, the extracellular fluid volume decreases ~100 ml. However, this reduction in extracellular fluid volume does not pose a problem when considered relative to the volume of saline administered.

Water

Once the extracellular fluid volume and circulatory status have sufficiently improved, the patient will still be hypertonic; the water deficit should now be corrected with the goal of replenishing the water deficits more slowly. This will allow time for the idiogenic osmoles gained by the brain to be dispersed.[31] There was previously some controversy as to the precise fluid to use and its route of administration. Balance studies have suggested that the fluid "lost" contains ~60 mEq/liter of monovalent cation. The most readily available intravenous fluid that approximates this level is 77 mmol/liter sodium chloride (half-normal). The average water deficit is about 24 percent of total body water, which would correspond to >8 liters in a 70-kg patient. With appropriate monitoring, one-half the estimated deficit, taking urinary losses into account, should be given during the first 12 hours, and the rest over a period of up to 24 to 48 hours. It would appear inappropriate to provide water as a glucose solution, even hypotonic, since the pathogenesis of the disorder relates to the inability to metabolize or excrete glucose adequately. The use of hypotonic fructose solution has been proposed as well, presumably because it does not require insulin for intracellular transport. However, significant loads of fructose will be rapidly converted to glucose, and fructose can radically decrease hepatic ATP and increase lactic acid production. In the presence of coma or obtundation, intragastric fluid delivery is contraindicated because of the danger of aspiration. Furthermore, while slow administration of distilled water intravenously has apparently been used, the dangers inherent in this practice and the limitations in rate and site of delivery are sufficient to discourage this as a general approach. Any hypertonic solution is contraindicated.

Potassium

Potassium depletion will be present even though the serum potassium may be normal or elevated at the time of presentation. Once therapy is under way, and especially once insulin has been started, potassium administration will be necessary. Most patients are oliguric initially; because some patients are hypotensive and may have suffered acute tubular necrosis, it is advisable in these cases to wait until a good urine output has been established before giving potassium, unless hypokalemia is present. Monitoring of the serum potassium and the ECG at regular intervals are the keys to timing and dosage. It is noteworthy that many of the electrocardiographic changes seen on admission, including ventricular extrasystoles, tachyarrhythmias, and ST segment and T wave abnormalities, often regress and disappear during reexpansion of the extracellular fluid volume. This is likely due to improved cardiac microcirculation, although other factors cannot be excluded.

Insulin

The major actions of insulin in patients with diabetic ketoacidosis are the inhibition of ketoacid production and reduction of the blood glucose concentration. The former action may not be important in nonketotic states. The latter can be accomplished to a major degree by saline infusion. Therefore, we do not think it necessary to give insulin immediately. In fact, there may be several adverse effects of insulin in this clinical situation: (1) Insulin will cause blood glucose (osmolality) to fall even more quickly and thus allow more water to enter brain cells, leading potentially to increased intracranial pressure; (2) insulin will promote potassium entry into cells and in these potassium-depleted patients may provoke dangerous hypokalemia; and (3) hypophosphatemia will be produced which may lead to impaired oxygen delivery to tissues (low 2,3-diphosphoglycerate (2,3-DPG) and renal tubular disorders. Therefore, in the absence of severe acidemia, it seems prudent to withhold initial insulin therapy until there is significant restoration of the extracellular fluid volume as well as of the potassium and phosphate deficits. As these patients with severe extracellular fluid volume contraction should have high levels of catecholamines (an antiinsulin hormone), even ketoacid formation may decrease with reexpansion of the extracellular fluid volume. Once extracellular fluid volume is significantly restored, usually within 4 hours, small doses of insulin should be used if hyperglycemia and severe glucose-induced osmotic diuresis persist. However, on the basis of our earlier discussion, it is likely that appropriate fluid repletion with a restored GFR may treat the hyperglycemia even in the absence of insulin therapy. If the clinician elects to administer insulin, an appropriate dose would be a bolus intravenous injection of 5 to 10 units followed by either continuous intravenous infusion of 5 units/hr or hourly 5-unit boluses. Doses should be adjusted according to response; in most cases, if such doses are needed at all, they are quite small. There are many different regimens for administering low dose insulin in diabetic coma. These are described in several review articles.[34,35]

It should be recognized that a controlled study to assess the optimum point at which to start insulin therapy has not been reported. The common recommendation is to use modest doses of insulin given early. In contrast, it is usually considered that patients with nonketotic coma are more sensitive to insulin than are patients with ketoacidosis. The current recommendations are thus based on the arguments related to insulin action as well as the following points: (1) the principal early mechanism by which glycemia falls is extracellular fluid reexpansion and increased renal excretion of glucose; (2) insulin is important to diminish ketoacidosis, and (3) excessively rapid fall in glycemia potassium and phosphate are very undesirable.

Glucose

As the glycemia approaches 250 mg/dl, 280 mM (5 percent) dextrose in water can be infused in order to replace the water deficit. Care should be taken to avoid inducing severe hyperglycemia.

It has been suggested that cerebral edema is more likely to occur as the plasma glucose levels approach normal and that insulin should be discontinued once glycemia reaches ~300 mg/dl. Since this recommendation is based on experimental and theoretical considerations[30,32] it would appear most prudent to individualize therapy and to modify insulin delivery rates to allow for slow reduction of glycemia between 300 mg/dl and normal, rather than to stop insulin therapy in all patients. If renal function is restored, and fluid input is adequate, the excretion of glucose will cause the glycemia to fall, without necessarily requiring exogenous insulin administration.

Underlying Disorders

Clearly, the nature of the precipitating or underlying disorders must be established and appropriate treatment begun concurrent with the above emergency measures. However, in light of the frequency of complications, it is proposed that the following be incorporated into management procedures.

PREVENTION OF BRONCHIAL OBSTRUCTIONS. The severe extracellular fluid volume contraction and respiratory muscle weakness contribute to the high incidence of bronchial obstruction with atelectasis and bronchopneumonia. Since any decrease in oxygenation or a further infective process could be fatal, it is strongly recommended that the humidity of inhaled air (or oxygen when indicated) be increased by standard methods. In addition, mouth, pharyngeal, and bronchial toilet should be performed, as well as appropriate physiotherapy.

PREVENTIVE NURSING CARE. Standard nursing practice for the comatose patient should include eye care, alternating pressure mattresses, and extreme care in management of urinary and intravenous catheters, since the immobility, extracellular fluid volume contraction, and hyperglycemia predispose to superinfection (do not insert a urinary catheter unless absolutely necessary). Such infection is commonly due to saprophytic organisms the virulence of which is enhanced by extreme hyperglycemia and the general debility of the patient.

The high incidence of complications, as well as the nature of the underlying disorders, contribute to the high mortality rate. Some of the complications are related to treatment itself and occur in the acute stage, whereas others become apparent only during convalescence. Management of each complication is beyond the scope of the present discussion.

Nonketotic coma should be largely preventable by an awareness of the circumstances in which it can arise and of the earlier stages of the syndrome. In particular, special attention must be paid in a diabetic patient over age 50 to the occurrence of any disease that will precipitate hyperglycemia and intense glycosuria, and especially when renal disease and treatment with drugs coexist. The early introduction of insulin treatment when hyperglycemia and glycosuria are not controllable by diet and oral agents in non-insulin-dependent adults might also reduce the incidence. Surveillance of glycemia, urine output, and glucosuria in all patients subjected to unusual stresses and/or receiving large carbohydrate loads will similarly lead to early recognition, and introduction of appropriate insulin therapy will further decrease the occurrence of the syndrome.

Diabetic Ketoacidosis

CLINICAL PRESENTATION

Diabetic ketacidosis is the mode of presentation of some previously undiagnosed diabetics, but more often it occurs in diabetics already receiving insulin. The precipitating causes include reduction or cessation of insulin therapy, intercurrent illnesses such as gastrointestinal disorders, pancreatitis, infections, and myocardial infarction, in situations wherein counterregulatory hormones may be present in excess (e.g., thyrotoxicosis, acromegaly, pregnancy, surgical stress, and hyperadrenocorticism), and finally following the intake of certain medications. In addition, emotional and psychological upheaval may precipitate episodes of diabetic ketoacidosis, especially in children.

The vast majority of the clinical manifestations of diabetic ketoacidosis are readily explained as the expected sequelae of the major biochemical changes: hyperglycemia, glycosuria, ketonemia, and metabolic acidosis. Most of the early signs and symptoms represent exacerbations of the classic clinical characteristics of poorly controlled diabetes. Thus the patient presents with a variable duration of thirst, polydipsia, polyuria, weakness, lethargy, and malaise. The persistent hyperglycemia causes an osmotic diuresis with water and electrolyte loss, resulting in extracellular fluid volume contraction which can lead to low blood pressure, postural hypotension, tachycardia, and reduced jugular and central venous pressure. In addition, the patient has reduced tissue turgor and dry mucous membranes, and the eyeballs may appear sunken and softer than normal. Anorexia, nausea, vomiting, and abdominal pain are frequent nonspecific gastrointestinal disturbances, especially common in children. These symptoms together with abdominal tenderness, decreased bowel sounds, sometimes guarding, and leukocytosis may be so severe as to mimic an acute abdominal emergency. Rebound tenderness is usually (but not universally) absent, and the presence of glycosuria and ketonemia should alert one to the correct diagnosis. With appropriate therapy, symptoms usually resolve in a matter of hours, the cause for the abdominal pain is not entirely clear, but in some cases it may be related to hypertriglyceridemia.

The metabolic acidosis caused by diabetic ketoacidosis results in an increased rate and depth of breathing (air hunger, Kussmaul respiration). In very severe acidemia, the hyperventilation may not be adequate, resulting in an acute worsening of the acidemia. The conversion of acetoacetic acid to acetone imparts the characteristic fruity odor to the breath. The severe acidemia may also have a negative inotropic effect on the heart and has been implicated as a cause of peripheral vasodilation, both of which can aggravate the hypotension from extracellular fluid volume contraction.

Not all the clinical findings, however, are completely explained in terms of the biochemical aberrations. Coma is only seen in fewer than 10 percent of patients with diabetic ketoacidosis, whereas as many as 20 percent may have no alteration in consciousness. Some degree of drowsiness is common, however. The state of consciousness does not correlate well with the concentrations of ketone bodies, electrolytes, hydrogen ions, or glucose. A much better correlation has been found between the level of stupor and coma and the serum osmolality.[16] See Chapter 23 for a discussion of the causes of coma in diabetic patients. Focal neurologic signs or seizures should not be attributed to ketoacidosis. Another feature of diabetic ketoacidosis that remains unexplained is hypothermia, even in the presence of infection. This fact together with the commonly seen leukocytosis make these two parameters invalid (at least initially) as definitive indicators of infection. Finally, the signs and symptoms of any precipitating disorder should be appreciated; in fact, these may dominate the clinical picture.

LABORATORY EVALUATION IN DIABETIC KETOACIDOSIS

Glucose and Ketone Bodies

Hyperglycemia, ketonemia, glycosuria, and ketonuria are four of the hallmarks in the laboratory diagnosis of diabetic ketoacidosis. The degree of hyperglycemia varies markedly and usually exceeds 250 mg/dl. Higher values can be seen if there is a marked reduction in the glomerular filtration rate or if the patient consumed a large carbohydrate intake just prior to admission. If the extracellular fluid volume, hence the blood volume, is markedly contracted, not only will there be an exaggerated degree of hyperglycemia, but glycosuria may be considerably reduced because the filtered load of glucose may not exceed the tubular capacity to reabsorb it. In rare cases, hyperglycemia may be less marked for other reasons, such as a reduced rate of gluconeogenesis secondary to the intake of ethanol or biguanides, exaggerated renal glycosuria, or self-imposed fasting by the patient.

In diabetic ketoacidosis, serum ketones are classically strongly positive up to a dilution of 1 in 8. However, only acetoacetate and acetone react with the clinical test reagents for ketone body detection (e.g., nitroprusside). If there is an increase in the redox (NADH: NAD) ratio (e.g., tissue hypoxia), the ketone bodies will be almost exclusively in the form of β-hydroxybutyrate. This latter compound is not detected by these clinical tests, and a specific enzymatic analysis will be necessary to establish the diagnosis of diabetic ketoacidosis.[17] Ketonuria may also be low or undetectable in patients with diabetic ketoacidosis and a markedly contracted extracellular fluid volume for two primary reasons: (1) the filtered load of ketones will be reduced when the glomerular filtration rate falls, and (2) the poor oxygen delivery will result in the conversion of acetoacetate to β-hydroxybutyrate. For these reasons, it is essential to analyze the anion gap and, if possible, to perform a direct β-hydroxybutyrate assay.

Plasma Sodium Concentration

In diabetic ketoacidosis, sodium deficiency is almost always present and usually amounts to 5 to 10 mEq/kg body weight. The true plasma sodium concentration (rule out factitious hyponatremia due to hypertriglyceridemia) is often reduced. Two major causes in addition to sodium depletion may play a role: (1) there is reduced ability to excrete ingested water as antidiuretic hormone is released in response to a contracted extracellular fluid volume, and (2) water is drawn osmotically, primarily from muscle cells, into the extracellular fluid due to hyperglycemia. Calculations indicate that the serum sodium concentration should fall 1.35 mEq/liter for every 100-mg/dl rise in blood glucose above normal.[5] However, some patients may not present with hyponatremia despite significant hyperglycemia and sodium depletion. In this group of patients, body fluids are hypertonic and indicate that water intake was significantly less than water loss. Special attention must be given to these patients during therapy.

Plasma Potassium Concentration

In diabetic ketoacidosis there is always a decrease in the total body potassium content, usually in the range of 5 to 10 mEq/kg body weight, even though hyperkalemia might be present. The principal reason for this loss is the glucose-induced osmotic diuresis that produces the combination of augmented distal sodium delivery and high aldosterone levels (secondary to extracellular fluid volume contraction). Typically, the urine potassium concentration is ~ 50 mEq/liter under these conditions. Loss of potassium can also occur via the gastrointestinal tract if vomiting, diarrhea, or an ileus is present. Despite the potassium deficiency, the plasma potassium concentration is usually not decreased, indicating that potassium has shifted from the intracellular fluid to the extracellular fluid compartment.

Several factors are important in altering the potassium distribution across the cell membrane in diabetic ketoacidosis. The most important factor causing potassium to leave the intracellular fluid compartment in diabetic ketoacidosis is a fall in the basal insulin concentration. Second, diabetic ketoacidosis may be precipitated by an underlying illness which could lead to cell necrosis, releasing potassium into the extracellular fluid. Since a larger quantity of hydrogen ions than ketone body anions appears to have entered the intracellular fluid during diabetic ketoacidosis, there will be some shift of potassium, but the quantity is very much smaller than most investigators have suggested.

Serum Bicarbonate Concentration and the Anion Gap

In diabetic ketoacidosis, the plasma bicarbonate concentration is reduced because β-hydroxybutyric and acetoacetic acids are added to the extracellular fluid. The degree to which the plasma bicarbonate concentration falls reflects primarily the extracellular fluid buffering of this acid load. The coexistence of additional acid–base disorders is diagnosed by evaluating the unmeasured anion gap relative to the fall in bicarbonate concentration and the P_{CO_2}. The data shown in Table 20–2 representing a fall in bicarbonate concentration equal to the rise in anion gap on the surface suggest that the anion gap type of metabolic acidosis is the sole or primary type of acid–base disturbance. However, as shown in Tables 20–3 and 20–4, these patients have a component of "indirect" sodium bicarbonate loss.

Blood pH, P_{CO_2}, and P_{O_2}

The patient with diabetic ketoacidosis is usually acidemic (pH < 7.35, $[H^+] > 45$ nM). There is a predictable hypocapnia depending on the degree of metabolic acidosis. (For a more detailed discussion, see Chapter 7.) The P_{O_2} should be somewhat elevated when corrected for temperature and P_{CO_2}, any reduction signifying intrinsic lung disease. Since hypothermia may occur in patients with diabetic ketoacidosis, one must take this into consideration when interpreting the values reported by the laboratory, because the measurements are made at 37°C.

BUN and Serum Creatinine

Since patients with diabetic ketoacidosis have a marked contraction of the extracellular fluid volume, there will be a reduction of the glomerular filtration rate. This is associated with elevated BUN and serum creatinine concentrations. The BUN is also influenced by other factors, such as protein intake, tissue catabolism, rate of gluconeogenesis, drugs, and urine flow rate, so it is less reliable as an index of changes in the glomerular filtration rate than is the serum creatinine.

Serum Phosphorus and Erythrocyte 2,3-DPG Levels

The presence of phosphorus deficiency in diabetic ketoacidosis has been known for several decades. The causes are multifactorial and include increased tissue catabolism, impaired glucose utilization and cellular phosphorus uptake leading to increased renal excretion, which is exacerbated by the metabolic acidosis. However, the phosphate concentration in the serum is usually in the normal range in patients presenting with diabetic ketoacidosis despite the marked total body phosphate deficiency, estimated to be between 0.5 and 1.3 mmol/kg body weight, which becomes evident early during therapy when very severe hypophosphatemia is commonly seen.

The erythrocyte 2,3-DPG levels are markedly reduced during diabetic ketoacidosis. The major implications of this finding relate to oxygen delivery to tissues—a low 2,3-DPG content increases the affinity of hemoglobin for oxygen. During acidemia this effect is partially counteracted by a lower affinity of hemoglobin for oxygen. It is therefore important, from a theoretical point of view at least, to be certain that phosphate is given early during treatment to restore the erythrocyte 2,3-DPG content and thereby the affinity of hemoglobin for oxygen to normal. Care should be taken, however, not to give too large or rapid infusions of phosphate, as these can lead to hypocalcemia and metastatic calcification. The possibility of side effects is significantly reduced if the dose is limited to 50 mmol of phosphate per 8 hours.

TREATMENT OF DIABETIC KETOACIDOSIS

Diabetic ketoacidosis is a medical emergency that demands urgent assessment and treatment. Mortality is influenced by the precipitating cause of diabetic ketoacidosis, the age of the patient, the level of consciousness, and the degree of acidosis, azotemia, and hyperglycemia. In most cases, the causes of death are infection, vascular thrombosis, and shock. Early diagnosis plus specific therapy for the underlying causes of diabetic ketoacidosis may further reduce the mortality. Successful treatment requires close, careful, continued supervision of the patient by a coordinated medical team, preferably in an acute care setting in which rapid and repeated clinical and biochemical evaluation can be undertaken. The aim of treatment should be the smooth restoration of the disturbed biochemical state; overly rapid correction is not necessarily beneficial and may result in its own complications.

A general approach to treatment could be made on the basis of the immediate threats to the patient's life as they appear during the course of diabetic ketoacidosis:

1. At the onset
   a. Severity of the acidemia
   b. Extracellular fluid volume contraction
   c. Profound hyper- or hypokalemia
   d. Underlying condition or precipitating event
2. During treatment
   a. Early
      i. Hypokalemia
      ii. Failure to respond to insulin
   b. Later
      i. Hypoglycemia
      ii. Cerebral edema
      iii. Recurrence of hyperglycemia and ketoacidosis

The underlying condition remains a continuing threat.

The patient should be given nothing by mouth; if comatose or stuporous, a nasogastric tube should be passed to aspirate the stomach contents, after endotreacheal intubation. Even if the patient is unable to pass urine readily, a bladder catheter should not be used, at least initially. All input and output data, critical clinical and laboratory parameters, and drugs administered should be recorded on a chronologic flow sheet. A large peripheral vein(s) should be chosen for the intravenous site and, if there is known cardiac disease or a cardiovascular complication, a central venous pressure (CVP) line should be inserted if accurate clinical information cannot otherwise be obtained.

Initially, one should repeat the biochemical evaluation hourly, following the blood sugar, serum ketones, electrolytes, unmeasured anions, and the blood pH and P_{CO_2}. If the initial arterial blood gas determinations demonstrate a normal Po_2 and an appropriate reduction of Pco_2, it is sufficient to do the subsequent pH and Pco_2 measurements on venous blood as long as there is no deterioration in the respiratory status.

Treatment can be divided into a number of aspects: fluid and electrolytes, insulin, bicarbonate, treatment of predisposing factors, and miscellaneous clinical problems. It is helpful to have a knowledge of the magnitude of the deficits to be expected in diabetic ketoacidosis. On average, there will be a deficit of 5 to 6 liters water, 500 mmol sodium, 350 mmol chloride, 300 to 1000 mmol potassium, 50 to 100 mmol each of phosphate and calcium, and 25 to 50 mmol magnesium. The calculated deficit of bicarbonate is 300 to 500 mmol initially, although a large part of this deficiency will be regenerated metabolically by the metabolism of the ketone bodies as the diabetic ketoacidosis is corrected. One should bear in mind that complete replacement of intracellular fluid deficits must await the resynthesis of the major intracellular fluid macromolecules.

Fluid and Electrolytes

Extracellular fluid volume contraction may be life threatening and therefore requires immediate attention. Rapid partial reexpansion of the extracellular fluid is an important feature in successful therapy of diabetic ketoacidosis. An average of ~3 to 4 liters of isotonic saline (154 mM NaCl) will be required to replace this deficit but one should also remember that an osmotic diuresis (~2 to 3 liters) will continue, especially early in therapy.

There is still some dispute about which is the most appropriate replacement fluid to use. The consensus of opinion now favors the early administration of 0.9 percent saline (154 mM NaCl) if the extracellular fluid volume is markedly contracted, even though the body is depleted of a hyponatremic fluid (i.e., more water than sodium has been lost). Despite the eventual occurrence of mild hypernatremia, one should quickly restore the extracellular fluid volume toward normal to correct the poor tissue perfusion with its tendency toward lactic acidosis and worsening acidemia. In addition, isotonic saline will prevent too rapid a fall in extracellular osmolality. If the patient is in shock, then plasma is an appropriate intravenous fluid. However, if hypernatremia is present on admission and the patient is not in shock, the initial therapy should be with hypotonic (0.45 percent) saline until hypernatremia is no longer a prominent feature.

An initial rate of 1 liter of isotonic saline/hour for the first 2 to 3 hours is usually sufficient in most cases of diabetic ketoacidosis. This rate of fluid replacement should continue with hourly clinical reassessments until the blood pressure is returned to near normal or until the jugular or central venous pressure is in the normal range (5 to 10 cm H_2O) and a brisk urine output is established. Oliguria may reflect a persistent inadequate intravascular volume or may be the initial manifestation of acute tubular necrosis.

After this acute replacement, the rate of fluid administration is decreased to 0.5 liters/hr. Older patients must be frequently reassessed for early signs of extracellular fluid volume overload and the development of congestive heart failure. It may be prudent in these cases to insert a CVP line for ease and accuracy of assessment and as a guide to further fluid therapy. One must bear in mind that the CVP provides right-sided measurements and that this is no substitute for auscultation of the heart and lungs in an effort to detect early signs of left-sided failure. When the plasma glucose falls below 250 mg/dl, glucose should be added to the infusate either as 5 percent dextrose in water or in 0.45 percent saline (depending on the extracellular fluid volume status and concurrent losses); the rate of infusion should be ~0.25 liters/hr. Further fluid therapy is determined by the clinical assessment, biochemical measurements, and calculated fluid losses.

Potassium depletion is a very important

electrolyte disturbance in diabetic ketoacidosis. Potassium deficits are conservatively reported to be ~5 mmol/kg, or 350 mmol in a 70-kg person. Despite the size of these losses the plasma potassium concentration is generally normal or elevated at the initial assessment. If it is decreased, a very severe state of potassium deficiency exists and patients are at high risk for life-threatening cardiac arrhythmias, as well as paralytic ileus, respiratory paralysis, and muscle weakness. The aims of potassium replacement are twofold: (1) to ensure a normal extracellular fluid potassium concentration during the acute stages of therapy, and (2) to replenish the total body (intracellular) potassium deficit. This latter component requires the reaccumulation of intracellular proteins and organic phosphates.

Once therapy is instituted, the plasma potassium concentration falls rapidly, often within the first hour. This is due to increased cellular potassium uptake consequent upon insulin action, continued urinary potassium loss, potassium entry into cells along with the gain of intracellular anions such as organic phosphates and proteins, correction of the acidosis and reentry of the potassium into the intracellular fluid, and dilution from reexpansion of extracellular fluid volume.

Early potassium replacement is appropriate. If the patient is hypokalemic or not markedly hyperkalemic and has a reasonable rate of urine output, then potassium supplementation is begun during the first hour or as soon as a serum determination is reported; 20 to 40 mmol potassium/hr may be given depending on the initial plasma potassium concentration. Care is needed when giving potassium, especially if there is oliguria. The ECG may serve as a useful, although not infallible, guide to changes in the plasma potassium concentration. While it is prudent to wait until an adequate urine output is established, patients with oliguria may still need cautious potassium supplementation, as the factors that produce hypokalemia during therapy are still operative. Potassium may be given as the chloride or as the phosphate salt or as is now recommended, a mixture of both. When diabetic ketoacidosis has been corrected, oral potassium supplementation should be continued to replenish the intracellular compartment.

Phosphate

The mean phosphate deficiency is ~1 mmol/kg body weight and, while only about 11 percent of patients have hypophosphatemia at diagnosis, once therapy is instituted, virtually all patients become profoundly hypophosphatemic. Although there are no controlled studies documenting the absolute benefits of phosphate replacement with respect to survival, a number of theoretical considerations, not the least of which is the decreased erythrocyte 2,3-DPG and its effect on tissue oxygen delivery, suggest that it may be beneficial to partially replace the phosphate deficit. This can be conveniently accomplished by using a balanced potassium phosphate solution, simultaneously replacing both potassium and phosphate deficiencies.

Insulin Therapy

The past decade has seen a renewed interest in the insulin therapy of diabetic ketoacidosis. The reports published during the 1940s had emphasized the need for large pharmacologic doses of insulin, which were claimed to have resulted in a lower mortality. It was assumed that insulin resistance was a common feature and that large doses of insulin were needed to overcome it. During this time, some reports did appear attesting to the efficiency of lower insulin doses, but they were largely ignored. However, after performing studies on insulin kinetics and gaining a better understanding of insulin action, a number of reports appeared in the early and mid-1970s describing the therapeutic effectiveness of small doses of insulin in the treatment of diabetic ketoacidosis. Since that time, these initial studies have been confirmed at many centers and the use of various low-dose insulin regimens is now widely accepted.[34,35]

The data from various studies have shown that the blood glucose falls at a fairly constant and predictable rate, averaging 75 to 100 mg/dl/hr and reaching a concentration of 200 to 300 mg/dl after ~4 to 6 hours of therapy whether high- or low-dose insulin regimens are employed. (In the presence of infection, the rate of decline in the blood glucose concentration may be reduced by about 50 percent.) It is hardly surprising that any route of insulin delivery (subcutaneous, intramuscular, or intravenous) that results in a physiologic plasma insulin concentration will be effective in the treatment of most cases of diabetic ketoacidosis. When large pharmacologic concentrations of insulin are present, late hypoglycemia and hypokalemia are said to be more common potential dangers, but this is hard to substantiate with any degree of confidence. An analysis of the literature shows that the low-dose intravenous and intramuscular regimens appear to be equally effective when comparing resolution of hyperglycemia and acidosis. It is perhaps not advisable (at least initially) to use the intramuscular route in patients with severe extracellular fluid volume contraction and acidosis, as insulin absorption may be irregular.[34,35]

We favor the use of continuous intravenous insulin infusion because a constant plasma concentration is rapidly achieved and the residual effect is short lived after the infusion is stopped, so that there is less risk of late hypoglycemia or hypokalemia. The insulin may be given either with an infusion pump or with an ordinary drip set. It is axiomatic that one must ensure that the infusion is working properly. The problems of infusion using glassware or plastic have probably been overemphasized. It appears to be sufficient to flush 50 to 100 ml of the insulin-containing solution through the infusion apparatus in order to minimize further insulin binding. Alternatively, 1 percent albumin or even 0.5 to 1 ml of the patient's own blood may be drawn into the syringe if an infusion pump is being used. It should be remembered that the residual effect of intravenous insulin is short lived, so that when the infusion is stopped after the diabetic ketoacidosis is corrected, other sources of insulin must be administered to prevent the reappearance of the condition.

Our recommendation is to use an intravenous bolus of insulin initially (0.1 U/kg body wt) followed by the continuous intravenous infusion of an equal amount of insulin per hour. If no response is achieved in 2 hours, we double the hourly dosage. Depending on the initial severity of diabetic ketoacidosis, such rates are usually maintained for 8 to 12 hours, then decreased progressively by half, but rarely to below 1 U/hr in adults.

The low-dose intermittent intramuscular insulin regimen is a simple and equally effective alternative. Extracellular fluid volume replacement is essential in order to ensure optimal absorption of insulin. We recommend an intravenous priming dose of regular insulin (0.1 U/kg) and 10 units intramuscurlarly each hour thereafter, with progressive decrements as with intravenous insulin. The insulin dosage may have to be adjusted should the biological response be inadequate. The successful results with low-dose insulin regimens suggest that the problem of insulin resistance has been overemphasized. Of the potential causes for this resistance, anti-insulin hormones, acidemia, antibodies, circulating antagonists, hypothermia, and lipid metabolites, only the counterregulatory hormones are probably of major clinical and practical significance, particularly when stimulated by infection. This should be borne in mind, and the insulin dosages can be adjusted appropriately.

The clinical reassessment should continue until the patient's mental status has cleared, the extracellular fluid volume has been replenished, the blood pressure is normal, the acid–base status is near normal, and the serum ketones and unmeasured anions have fallen significantly. Oral intake can be gradually resumed once the biochemical and clinical (especially central nervous system) manifestations of diabetic ketoacidosis have been largely reversed assuming that there are no gastrointestinal problems (e.g., vomiting and ileus).

Bicarbonate Therapy

One must weigh the possible benefits and pitfalls to bicarbonate therapy. Advantages have been said to occur because of improved effects of catecholamines on myocardial contractility and vasoconstriction. Acidemia per se may also contribute to peripheral vasodilatation and central nervous system depression. In addition, acidemia can lead to insulin resistance in two possible ways: (1) by decreasing the affinity of insulin receptors for insulin, and (2) by decreasing the number of insulin receptors. On the other hand, there are potential problems with bicarbonate therapy, especially if not given with extreme care. Bicarbonate therapy can lead to hypokalemia, impaired tissue oxygenation due to a leftward shift in the oxygen–hemoglobin dissociation curve (see also discussion of the complication of cerebral edema), as well as a possible sodium overload, but this is unlikely in diabetic ketoacidosis. Two other problems are usually mentioned, a fall in the pH of cerebrospinal fluid due to a Pco_2 rise and rebound metabolic alkalosis; these are probably more of theoretical than practical concern, as the former has little documented evidence to support it as a major problem in diabetic ketoacidosis and the latter can be avoided in the absence of a coexisting potassium or chloride deficit or significant renal failure.

The balance of evidence seems to favor the use of sodium bicarbonate therapy in four major circumstances: (1) a bicarbonate concentration <5 to 10 mEq/liter; (2) a blood Pco_2 that is not appropriately reduced, resulting in severe acidemia (in this circumstance, attention should also be focused on improving ventilation); (3) the failure to reduce acid production with insulin or the presence of another type of acid load; and (4) the presence of significant hypotension with severe acidemia. The quantity of bicarbonate to be administered can be calculated, bearing in mind that there is no need to raise the plasma bicarbonate above 15 mEq/liter as long as there is adequate pulmonary function. To calculate the amount of bicarbonate to be administered, one assumes a bicarbonate distribution in a volume equal to 50 percent of body weight. The load of sodium bicarbonate should be administered over a few hours, one-half initially, and then lesser quantities over time, taking care to monitor the resultant changes in bicarbonate concentration. Should the plasma bicarbonate concentration rise toward 15 mEq/liter, the infusion of exogenous bicarbonate should stop. One should also monitor the plasma potassium concentration carefully to avoid hypokalemia and its sequellae. Finally, if a patient is unable to generate sufficient bicarbonate because of renal disease, bicarbonate must be given along with oral intake.

Precipitating Event

Concurrent with the treatment of diabetic ketoacidosis, it is necessary to treat any precipitating event or accompanying illness. If this approach to therapy is followed, one should be able to minimize greatly the mortality associated with diabetic ketoacidosis.

COMPLICATIONS OBSERVED DURING THERAPY

Problems that complicate therapy include insulin resistance, hypokalemia, hypoglycemia, and relapse into ketoacidosis. In addition, alterations in central nervous system function particularly secondary to cerebral edema, and thrombotic events have received recent attention. The former group of complications have been discussed above.

Cerebral Edema

In a very small group of patients, especially those in the younger age range who appear to be recovering from diabetic ketoacidosis, the clinical course takes a turn for the worse about 10 hours after the onset of usual therapy. At this time, the blood biochemistry results are returning toward normal, but the patient may begin to show drowsiness, become irritable and less rational, and exhibit a disordered state of consciousness. The cause of this constellation of findings, termed cerebral edema, remains obscure. Pathologic examination of the brain of patients who have died with this condition reveals the findings associated with cerebral edema—mainly gross swelling due to accumulation of fluid in the interstitial space, capillary endothelial swelling, and cellular infiltration in the perivascular area. There is usually no evidence of parenchymal cell swelling.[28,29]

Several hypotheses have been advanced to explain this constellation of findings.[31] The most popular theory is that the brain dysfunction is due to a water shift into brain cells because of a more rapid lowering of glucose in the extracellular fluid than the brain glucose concentration.

Another theory involves the production by brain of undetermined solute, or idiogenic osmoles, during hyperglycemic states. In laboratory animals with hyperglycemia (plasma glucose >450 mg/dl) for at least 4 hours, brain volume is normal. The maintenance of normal brain volume in the presence of extracellular hyperosmolality may be due in part to the generation by brain of idiogenic osmoles.[30] When plasma glucose is rapidly lowered with insulin, brain osmolality may not fall as fast as that of plasma. In addition, when plasma glucose is <250 to 300 mg/dl, there may be additional insulin-stimulated transport of potassium into brain cells. This can further increase brain osmolality in the presence of a declining plasma osmolality. The production of cerebral edema generally does not occur in both patients[32] and laboratory animals[30] if insulin is stopped when plasma glucose is ~250 to 300 mg/dl. However, we find both these explanations to be less than complete for several reasons: (1) the maximum difference between blood vs brain glucose concentrations occurs within the first 4 to 6 hours, whereas the syndrome becomes prominent many hours later; (2) when measured, the cerebrospinal fluid and blood glucose concentrations differ by only 100 or 200 mg/dl (5 to 11 mOsm/kg) when symptoms are prominent[32]; (3) the pathologic picture is not consistent with the shift of water from the extracellular fluid into brain cells; and (4) the syndrome appears to be less common in patients recovering from nonketotic coma, where the fall in blood glucose concentration may be even more dramatic.[31]

It has been suggested that other glucose derivatives (sorbitol and fructose) might accumulate in brain cells and cause a water shift, but these compounds, although increased, are not of sufficient magnitude to be responsible for quantitative water shifts.[30] Other hypotheses include a paradoxical cerebrospinal fluid acidosis due to a rapid elevation of the extracellular fluid, but not the cerebrospinal fluid bicarbonate concentration together with a raised P_{CO_2} in both compartments. However, the temporal relationships do not support this hypothesis either. While the mechanism must remain theoretical, it is possible that the combination of the fall in 2,3-DPG in the erythrocytes (due to the phosphate depletion) together with the expected rise in blood pH cause a significant increase in affinity of hemoglobin for oxygen such that oxygen delivery becomes inadequate to meet the local demands of the brain tissue. Furthermore, if the extracellular fluid volume has not beeen fully restored, cerebral blood flow could be compromised. Autopsy findings in patients with cerebral edema as a consequence of diabetic ketoacidosis are in keeping with this hypothesis.

Thrombotic Events

Arterial thromboses are well recognized complications of hyperosmolar states, particularly nonketotic coma, but they are seen in diabetic ketoacidosis as well. Not only does the patient have a contracted extracellular fluid volume, probably with a decreased cardiac output secondary to the acidosis, but in addition the patient has increased platelet aggregation, increased Factor VIII and fibrinogen levels, as well as decreased fibrinolysis. Disseminated intravascular coagulation has also been reported in diabetic ketoacidosis, although the precise cause is not well understood. The treatment of choice for this complication continues to be heparin. Whether it should be used prophylactically in severe diabetic ketoacidosis remains a moot point.

Other Complications

Another complication seen on rare occasions is the temporary retention of large quantities of sodium during and after successful treatment of diabetic ketoacidosis. The precise mechanism involved is not entirely clear, although it may be partially due to the known antinatriuretic effects of insulin.[9]

APPENDIX: OUTLINE OF THERAPY

1. SALINE (WILL VARY WITH SEVERITY AND DURATION OF DIABETIC KETOACIDOSIS). Initial replacement fluid should be isotonic saline:
~2 liters in first 2 hours.*
3 liters in first 6 hours (2 to 6 liters)
6 liters in first 12 hours (3 to 9 liters)

It is important to correct hypotension and restore tissue perfusion; therefore use isotonic (0.9 percent) saline initially. If plasma sodium concentration is >145 mEq/liter, may use hypotonic (0.45 percent) saline. Calculate expected extracellular fluid volume deficit and titrate fluid replacement according to the jugular or central venous pressure and clinical assessment. Continue isotonic saline (or hypotonic saline) until blood sugar is 250 mg/dl; then change to 5 percent dextrose in water.

* The first liter may be given in 30 minutes.

2. POTASSIUM. Add potassium in the form of potassium chloride with some buffered potassium phosphate at rate of 20 to 40 mmol/hr. Withhold potassium if serum potassium is >5 mEq/liter. When urine output is established and blood sugar falling, give 10 mEq potassium/hr if plasma potassium is 5 to 6 mEq/liter, 20 mEq potassium/hr if plasma potassium is 4 to 5 mEq/liter, 30 mEq potassium/hr if plasma potassium is 3.0 to 4.0 mEq/liter, and 40 to 60 mEq potassium/hr if plasma potassium is <3.0 mEq/liter. Use ECG as well as plasma potassium concentration to monitor rate of potassium replacement. Give potassium phosphate at rate of 5 mmol/hr, not to exceed a rate of 50 mmol in 8 hours.

3. BICARBONATE. If bicarbonate concentration is <5 to 10 mEq/liter, the patient will require at least 100 mEq $NaHCO_3$. If the bicarbonate concentration is <5 mEq/liter, >200 mEq $NaHCO_3$ will probably be required. It should be kept in mind that the readily available solutions are hypertonic and additional water may be necessary if the patient is hyperosmolar. Potassium chloride may be necessary to prevent hypokalemia.

4. INSULIN (use only regular insulin).

Intravenous Regimen. Give stat dose of 0.1 to 0.15 U/kg IV, then a similar dose hourly (in isotonic saline, ~0.1 to 0.15 U/kg), using syringe pump or calibrated infusion set. Blood (0.5 to 1.0 ml) may be drawn back into the syringe of a syringe pump, or 50 to 100 ml of the insulin/saline solution may be run through infusion set and discarded before connecting to patient. If no response to IV insulin in 2 hours, double the infusion rate.

Intramuscular Regimen. Give 0.1 to 0.15 U/kg IM as priming dose, then a similar dose every hour. If no change in plasma glucose after 2 hours, change to IV regimen. Do not use this route initially if tissue perfusion is very poor and the patient is hypotensive.

With successful therapy, the blood sugar will fall at ~75 to 100 mg/dl/hr. On average, a glucose concentration of 200 to 300 mg/dl is achieved after 6 to 10 hours. At this time change IV to 5 percent dextrose in water and continue regular insulin either 2 or 4 hourly by IM or SC route until patient is eating again, at which time longer acting insulins may be reinstituted.

5. ADDITIONAL MEASURES.

1. Give antibiotics early if evidence of infection is present. Consider their use if invasive procedures are performed.
2. Give oxygen if Po_2 is <80 mmHg when the patient is breathing room air. Appropriate measures should be taken if respiratory failure is present.
3. Consider low-dose heparin in the unconscious severely hyperosmolar patient (≥380 mosm/liter) and in the elderly.
4. Ensure adequate oral potassium and phosphate replacement continues after the acute episode of diabetic ketoacidosis corrected.

REFERENCES

1. Wolman SL, Fields ALA, Cheema-Dhadli S, et al: Protein conversion to glucose: An evaluation of the quantitative aspects. J Parent Nutr 4:487, 1980
2. Halperin ML, Goldstein MB, Jungas RL, Stinehaugh BJ: Biochemistry and physiology of ammonium excretion. In DW Seldin, G Giebisch (eds): Physiology and Pathology of Electrolyte Metabolism. Raven Press, New York, 1984
3. Denton RM, Halestrap AP: Regulation of pyruvate metabolism in mammalian tissues. Essays Biochem 15:37, 1979
4. Halperin ML, Goldstein M, Richardson R, et al: Quantitative aspects of hyperglycemia in the diabetic: A theoretical approach. Clin Invest Med 2:127, 1980
5. Roscoe JM, Halperin ML, Rolleston FS, et al: Hyperglycemia-induced hyponatremia: Metabolic considerations in calculation of serum sodium depression. Can Med Assoc J 112:452, 1975
6. Pollock AS, Arieff AI: Abnormalities of cell volume regulation and their functional consequences. Am J Physiol 239:F195, 1980
7. Phelps KR, Lieberman RL, Oh MS, et al: Pathophysiology of the syndrome of hyporeninemic hypoaldosteronism. Metabolism 29:186, 1980
8. Schambelan M, Sebastian A: Hyporeninemic hypoaldosteronism. Adv Intern Med 24:385, 1979
9. DeFronzo RA: The effect of insulin on renal sodium metabolism: A review with clinical implications. Diabetologia 21:165, 1981
10. Fraley DS, Adler S: Isohydric regulation of plasma potasium by bicarbonate in the rat. Kidney Int 9:333, 1976
11. Tobin RB: Varying role of extracellular electrolytes in metabolic acidosis and alkalosis. Am J Physiol 195:685, 1958
12. Oster JR, Perez GO, Vaamonde CA: Relationship between blood pH and potassium and phosphorus during acute metabolic acidosis. Am J Physiol 235:F345, 1978
13. Halperin ML, Bear R, Goldstein MB, et al: Interpretation of the serum potassium concentration in metabolic acidosis. Clin Invest Med 2:55, 1979
14. McGarry JD, Foster DW: Diabetic ketoacidosis. p. 185. In Rifkin H, Raskin B (eds): Diabetes Mellitus. Vol. 5. American Diabetes Association, New York, 1981
15. Arieff AI, Carroll HJ: Hyperosmolar nonketotic coma with hyperglycemia: Abnormalities of lipid and carbohydrate metabolism. Metabolism 20:529, 1971
16. Arieff AI, Carroll HJ: Nonketotic hyperosmolar coma with hyperglycemia: Clinical features, pathophysiology, renal function, acid–base balance, plasma–cerebrospinal fluid equilibria and the effects of therapy in 37 cases. Medicine (Baltimore) 51:73, 1972
17. Marliss EB, Ohman JL, Aoki TT, et al: Altered redox state obscuring ketoacidosis in diabetic patients with lactic acidosis. N Engl J Med 283:978, 1970
18. Swan RC, Pitts RF: Neutralization of infused acid by nephrectomized dogs. J Clin Invest 34:205, 1955

19. Halperin ML, Bear RA, Hannaford M, et al: Selected aspects of the pathophysiology of metabolic acidosis in diabetes mellitus. Diabetes 30:781, 1981
20. Pichette C, Bercovici M, Goldstein MB, et al: Elevation of the blood lactate concentration by alkali therapy without requiring additional lactic acid accumulation: Theoretical considerations. Crit Care Med 5:323, 1982
21. Oh MS, Banerji MA, Carroll HJ: The mechanism of hyperchloremic acidosis during the recovery phase of diabetic ketoacidosis. Diabetes 30:310, 1981
22. Sajo IM, Goldstein MB, Sonnenberg H, et al: Sites of ammonia addition to tubular fluid in rats with chronic metabolic acidosis. Kidney Int 20:353, 1981
23. Arieff AI, Leach W, Park R, et al: Systemic effects of $NaHCO_3$ in experimental lactic acidosis in dogs. Am J Physiol 242:F586, 1982
24. Fields ALA, Wolman SL, Halperin ML: Chronic lactic acidosis in a patient with cancer: Therapy and metabolic consequences. Cancer 47:2026, 1981
25. Assan R, Souchal B, Aubert P, et al: Nonketotic comas in diabetics. Presse Med 77:787, 1969
26. Gerich JE, Martin MM, Recant L: Clinical and metabolic characteristics of hyperosmolar, nonketotic coma. Diabetes 20:228, 1971
27. Feig RU, McCurdy DK: The hypertonic state. N Engl J Med 297:1444, 1977
28. Dillon ES, Riggs HE, Dyer WW: Cerebral lesions in uncomplicated fatal diabetic acidosis. Am J Med Sci 192:360, 1936
29. Young E, Bradley RF: Cerebral edema with irreversible coma in severe diabetic ketoacidosis. N Engl J Med 276:665, 1967
30. Arieff AI, Kleeman CR: Cerebral edema in diabetic comas. II. Effects of hyperosmolality, hyperglycemia and insulin in diabetic rabbits. J Clin Endocrinol Metab 38:1057, 1974
31. Guisado R, Arieff AI: Neurological manifestations of diabetic comas: Correlation with biochemical alterations in the brain. Metabolism 24:665, 1975
32. Arieff AI, Carroll HJ: Cerebral edema and depression of sensorium in nonketotic hyperosmolar coma. Diabetes 23:525, 1974
33. Gabow PA, Keahny WD, Fennessey PV, Goodman SI et al: Diagnostic importance of an increased serum anion gap. N Engl J Med 303:854, 1980
34. Padilla AJ, Loeb JN: "Low-dose" versus "high-dose" insulin regimens in the management of uncontrolled diabetes. Am J Med 63:843, 1977
35. Carroll P, Matz R: Uncontrolled diabetes mellitus in adults: Experience in treating diabetic ketoacidosis and hyperosmolar nonketotic coma with low-dose insulin and a uniform treatment regimen. Diabetes Care 6:579, 1983

21

Effects of Water, Acid–Base, and Electrolyte Disorders on the Central Nervous System

Allen I. Arieff

Abnormalities of water, electrolyte, and acid–base balance may lead to a condition known in general terms as metabolic encephalopathy. The term generally indicates a severe disturbance of sensorium that is not due to a structural lesion such as tumor, vascular accident, trauma, or infection of the central nervous system. Causes of metabolic encephalopathy include liver failure, uremia, diabetic ketoacidosis, hypoxia, hypercapnia, and either elevated or decreased blood levels of glucose, sodium, calcium, phosphate, or hydrogen ion. Also included are many exogenous intoxications, such as barbiturates, ethanol, narcotics, general anesthetics, and other miscellaneous intoxicants. Coma may result from metabolic encephalopathy, and this coma is generally reversible with correction of the underlying abnormality.

There are both similarities and differences between structural and metabolic coma. The clinical manifestations may overlap substantially, but the prognosis is substantially different. In a recent international study of 500 patients with nontraumatic coma, Levy and associates[1] evaluated the prognosis on the basis of neurologic evaluation. Depending on the cause of coma, early neurologic status, and the presence or absence for up to 7 days of corneal, papillary, and oculovestibular reflexes, motor response, verbal response, spontaneous eye opening and movement, and oculocephalic and deep tendon reflexes, the prognosis for recovery in patients with nontraumatic coma could be predicted with 99 percent accuracy. However, these findings cannot be extrapolated to patients with metabolic coma. Patients with depressed respiration, absent corneal reflexes, absent deep tendon reflexes, and no response to pain may still make a complete recovery after 6 days of coma induced by barbiturate or glutethimide intoxication.[2] In the study by Levy et al.,[1] only 10 percent of patients had metabolic encephalopathy, and all had hepatic coma. In fact, patients with hepatic encephalopathy had the best overall survival (50 percent) in the series. For other types of metabolic encephalopathy, survival simply cannot be predicted on the basis of neurologic status, because it has not been evaluated. In fact, among 114 hyponatremic patients with depression of sensorium (mean serum Na, 109 mM), a complete neurologic evaluation was reported in fewer than 10 percent of cases.[3,4] Similarly, among large series of patients with diabetic coma, complete neurologic evaluations are rarely reported. Thus, whatever the neurologic status in patients with metabolic coma, a reasonable determinant of prognosis simply cannot be made with our present state of knowledge.

Despite an exhaustive neurochemical literature that deals with the effects of alterations in brain biochemistry, including the effects of electrolyte and acid–base status, much consists of in vitro studies and is appreciated only by neurochemists and those in closely related disciplines. Very little is known to clinicians; thus much information that is potentially of therapeutic and diagnostic importance has not been assimilated into clinical medicine. This chapter reviews the relationship among systemic abnormalities of water, electrolytes, and acid–base metabolism and effects on the central nervous system.

IONIC CONSTITUENTS AND ACID–BASE BALANCE OF NORMAL BRAIN AND CEREBROSPINAL FLUID

Osmotically Active Solute

Unlike extracellular fluid, the principal osmotically active constituents of brain consist of both organic and inorganic solutes. The major inorganic constituents of the brain and their approximate concentrations (mmol/kg wet wt) in the cerebral cortex of mammalian species (rat, cat, dog, human) are Na^+ (50 to 60 mmol/kg), K^+ (85 to 100 mmol/kg), Cl^- (35 to 45 mmol/kg), Ca^{2+} (1 to 2.8 mmol/kg), Mg^{2+} (5 to 6 mmol/kg), and bicarbonate (10 to 2 mmol/kg).[5-7]

It is obvious that the sum of inorganic brain cations far exceeds that of inorganic anions. The total brain cation concentration is ~ 170 mmol/kg wet wt, while anions, including Cl^-, bicarbonate, sulfates, phosphates, and organic acid anions (such as lactate, glutamine, glutamate, and *N*-acetylaspartate) are at most ~ 85 mmol/kg wet wt.[6] The remaining brain intracellular anions are probably polyionic lipids and proteins. Since most brain Cl^- is extracellular, the bulk of intracellular anions are doubtless organic and macromolecular.[6] In addition, there are also minute quantities in the brain of certain trace metals, such as copper, manganese, zinc, iron, tin, aluminum, and rubidium.[6-10]

The actual osmotic activity of any of the aforementioned constituents is not entirely clear. Most Ca^{2+} and Mg^{+2} is probably bound and not osmotically active.[5] The principal intracellular osmotically active cation is K^+, and a substantial portion of intracellular Na^+ is also probably osmotically active.[5,9] The role of organic phosphates in brain osmoregulation also has not been well studied.[11] The osmotic activity in brain of amino acids and other organic acids is uncertain, although these substances appear to play a major role in osmotic adaptation in the cells of many invertebrates[12,13] and amphibians.[14] Those organic intracellular metabolites that are probably osmotically active include glutamate, aspartate, lactate, pyruvate, and alanine.[15]

There is a substantial amount of evidence, both in humans[16-18] and in experimental animals[19-21] that there may be changes in plasma osmolality where the apparent net loss or gain of cellular water and solute does not account for the change in tissue osmolality, assuming that intracellular and extracellular osmolality are in dynamic equilibrium.[22-24] In these instances there may be apparent inactivation of intracellular solute[16,18] or a gain in solute that is not due to commonly measured substances.[20,21,25] This undetermined solute has been called idiogenic osmoles.[19-21] Furthermore, there is a substantial body of evidence suggesting that the brain undergoes osmotic adaptation to hyperosmolar states in a manner distinctly different from that in other tissues. For example, in birds and mammals, muscle and nucleated red blood cells may adapt to hyperosmolar states by loss of water and gain in cation,[19,20,26] while brain adapts primarily by de novo generation of solute by as yet unexplained mechanisms.[19,21,27] However, apparently these mechanisms are not activated immediately; as a result, overly rapid induction of either hyperosmolality or hypoosmolality may be lethal.[4,28,29] Furthermore, the adaptive mechanisms may in themselves provoke functional derangements in the brain. Chronically hyperosmolar or hypoosmolar patients or experimental animals are generally symptomatic and may have depression of sensorium.[25]

Acid–Base Status of Brain and Cerebrospinal Fluid

A substantial number of studies have dealt with the acid–base status of brain and cerebrospinal fluid. Those dealing with the cerebrospinal fluid are generally far less controversial because of the ready applicability of commonly used techniques for direct measurement of gases in cerebrospinal fluid.[30,31] The steady-state relationships between acid–base components in arterial blood versus cisternal cerebrospinal fluid in humans are shown in Figure 21–1. In general, bicarbonate concentration is similar in blood and cerebrospinal fluid (~ 24 mmol/liter). The arterial pH (~ 7.40) is higher than in cerebrospinal fluid (~ 7.32) because P_{CO_2} in cerebrospinal fluid (~ 48 mm Hg) is higher than that in blood (~ 40 mm Hg).

The cerebrospinal fluid protein concentration (~ 40 mg/dl) is minute compared with that in plasma (~ 7 g/dl). However, despite this apparent inferior buffering capacity, the pH of cerebrospinal fluid remains remarkably constant despite substantial changes in arterial pH. In those conditions characterized by acute alterations in systemic P_{CO_2}, such as respiratory alkalosis and acidosis, acute alterations in pH and P_{CO_2} of cerebrospinal fluid take place that are directionally similar to those in arterial blood.[31,32] However, the changes in cerebrospinal fluid pH are initially smaller than those in arterial blood, and within 1 hour, compensatory mechanisms have been initiated.[33]

In acute respiratory alkalosis, there is an increase in the cerebrospinal fluid concentrations of both lactate and other, as yet unidentified organic acids,[7,34,35,36] which results in a decrease of cerebrospinal fluid pH toward normal.[37] This compensation is nearly complete after 4 to 6 hours. With an arterial pH of 7.5 to 7.6, the simultaneously determined

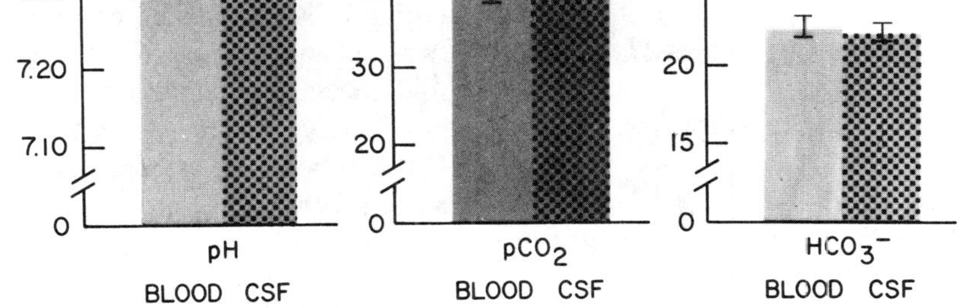

Fig. 21–1. Relationship between the acid–base balance in arterial blood versus cisternal cerebrospinal fluid (CSF) in human subjects. (Data summarized from Katzman R, Pappius HM: Acid–base balance in the cerebrospinal fluid. p. 224. In Katzman R, Pappius HM (eds): Brain Electrolytes and Fluid Metabolism. © 1983. The Williams & Wilkins Co., Baltimore, 1973.)

intracellular pH (pH_i) of brain will rise from 7.05 to above 7.2 after 1 hour with arterial P_{CO_2} below 25 mm Hg, but after 2 to 5 hours, it has returned to normal values. The changes are similar in four different regions of the brain.[36]

In acute respiratory acidosis (arterial P_{CO_2} > 80 mm Hg), there is initially a significant decline in pH of cerebrospinal fluid. Within 1 to 2 hours, bicarbonate concentration of cerebrospinal fluid begins to rise,[7,33,38] but compensation is only minimal after 4 to 6 hours.[7,38] By contrast, although pH_i of brain falls from 7.05 to 6.88 after 1 hour of hypercapnia, it has returned to normal after 3 hours of sustained hypercapnia.[7]

The findings in brain are in marked contrast to those of other tissues. In the liver, changes of extracellular pH over a range of 7.05 to 7.65 have no effect on hepatic pH_i.[39] However, changes in extracellular pH result in corresponding changes of skeletal muscle pH_i.[7,40]

In acute metabolic disturbances of acid–base balance, effects on pH in cerebrospinal fluid are only minimal. When arterial pH was lowered from 7.40 to 7.18 by infusion of HCl, there was no significant alteration in pH of cerebrospinal fluid.[38] Similarly, when $NaHCO_3$ was infused to increase arterial pH from 7.40 to 7.53, the pH of cerebrospinal fluid was unaltered.[38] It appears that neither bicarbonate nor hydrogen ion can readily cross the blood–cerebrospinal fluid barrier, but this barrier is readily permeable to CO_2.

Cerebrospinal Fluid Electrolytes

SODIUM (Na^+)

Cerebrospinal fluid is different from plasma in several important aspects. Since cerebrospinal fluid is essentially protein free and has no cells, the unmeasured anion, that is, the difference between measured cations and measured anions, is close to zero. In general, the cerebrospinal fluid concentrations of (Na^+) + (K^+) are similar to the concentrations of (Cl^-) + (HCO_3). There is considerable variation among mammalian species, but in general the Na^+ concentration in cerebrospinal fluid is similar to that of plasma. However, when Na^+ is expressed as millimoles per kilogram water its concentration is higher in plasma than in cerebrospinal fluid.[41] Because of the osmotic equilibrium between plasma and cerebrospinal fluid, changes in cerebrospinal fluid Na^+ concentration generally parallel those of plasma.

POTASSIUM (K^+)

In contrast to Na^+, the cerebrospinal fluid concentration of K^+ is relatively constant, being essentially independent of the plasma K^+ concentration. In human subjects, the K^+ concentration in cerebrospinal fluid remained at ~ 3.0 mEq/liter despite variations of plasma K^+ between 3.4 to 5.8 mEq/liter.[41] In experimental animals, cerebrospinal fluid K^+ did not change despite marked variation in plasma K^+ induced by either K^+ loading or K^+ depletion.[42] However, in some patients with severe hypokalemia (plasma $K^+ < 2$ mEq/liter), cerebrospinal fluid K^+ concentrations as low as 2.4 to 2.6 mEq/liter have been described.[41] In studies published since 1954, the cerebrospinal fluid K^+ in 56 normal human subjects ± SD has been found to be 2.89 ± 0.26 mEq/liter.[41] In the goat, rabbit, dog, and cat, K^+ concentration in cisternal cerebrospinal fluid has a range of only 2.52 to 2.98 mEq/liter.[41] At least two mechanisms serve to maintain cerebrospinal fluid concentration of K^+ in this narrow range: (1) a carrier-mediated transport of K^+ across the choroid plexus from blood into the cerebrospinal fluid, and (2) exchange of CSF K^+ with brain K^+. Although the evidence is not conclusive, both mechanisms probably require active transport processes.

CALCIUM (Ca^{2+})

In virtually all mammalian species, the Ca^{2+} concentration in cerebrospinal fluid is 2 to 3 mEq/liter. Calcium is secreted by the choroid plexus into the cerebrospinal fluid. Since protein concentration in cerebrospinal fluid is minimal, virtually all Ca^{2+} in cerebrospinal fluid is ionized and is not protein bound. It has long been suggested that the Ca^{2+} concentration in cerebrospinal fluid is similar to that of ionized Ca^{2+} in plasma. However, using modern methodology to measure Ca^{2+}, the plasma-ionized Ca^{2+} concentration is still found to be consistently greater than that in cerebrospinal fluid.[43] However, there is also a potential difference between cerebrospinal fluid and plasma of ~ 5 mV.[44] When this electrochemical gradient is taken into account, there is electrochemical equilibrium for Ca^{2+} between cerebrospinal fluid and plasma in normal human subjects. However, it is still most unlikely that cerebrospinal fluid and plasma-ionized Ca^{2+} are in equilibrium. When plasma Ca^{2+} is altered by Ca^{2+} infusion, parathyroidectomy, parathyroid hormone administration, EDTA, uremia, or vitamin D intoxication, there is little if any change in the Ca^{2+} in cerebrospinal fluid.[41,45,46] Therefore, the bulk of evidence suggests that Ca^{2+} in cerebrospinal fluid is maintained by active secretory processes at the choroid plexus and is not related to plasma-ionized Ca^{2+} levels.

MAGNESIUM (Mg^{2+})

The Mg^{2+} level in cerebrospinal fluid of human subjects is slightly higher than that of plasma. In studies of 1033 patients, Mg^{2+} in cerebrospinal fluid was 2.41 mEq/liter, while that in plasma was 1.82 mEq/liter.[41] The consistency of a higher level of Mg in cerebrospinal fluid than in plasma suggests that there must be active secretion of Mg^{2+} into cerebrospinal fluid, probably at the choroid plexus. Intravenous infusion of $MgSO_4$ to elevate plasma Mg^{2+} levels results in a small rise of Mg concentration in cerebrospinal fluid at very high plasma levels. Elevations in plasma Mg^{2+} of 27 to 700 percent result in a rise of Mg in cerebrospinal fluid of only 20 to 25 percent.[41,47] In animals with renal failure, a 30 percent rise in plasma Mg^{2+} did not affect cerebrospinal fluid concentration of Mg^{2+}.[46] However, a Mg^{2+}-deficient diet did result in a small decrement of cerebrospinal fluid concentration of Mg^{2+} in rabbits.[48] In patients with hypomagnesemia (serum Mg^{2+} < 2.14mEq/liter), Mg^{2+} in cerebrospinal fluid is below normal values.[49]

CHARACTERISTICS OF THE BLOOD-BRAIN BARRIER

Brain Extracellular Space

In general, extracellular space is thought of as that fluid compartment outside the cells. In practice, however, the extracellular space is defined as that fluid compartment that is available for the distribution of a particular marker. The extracellular space is determined at the ratio of distribution of the marker in the tissue to its distribution in a reference fluid that is considered to represent extracellular fluid.[50] If plasma is used as the extracellular fluid, it must be corrected for the Donnan effect. This concept is especially difficult when applied to the brain. There is essentially a dual circulation of fluids about the brain (both blood and cerebrospinal fluid). The vast bulk of evidence suggests that the cerebrospinal fluid is identical with, and a continuation of, the extracellular fluid of the brain.[50-52] The measurement of extracellular space assumes that the marker has equilibrated between tissue and extracellular fluid. In the case of the brain, there is a tendency for any substance entering the brain via the blood to be siphoned off into the cerebrospinal fluid, so that equilibration may not be reached. There is a similar tendency for any substance administered via the cerebrospinal fluid to be siphoned off via the bloodstream. Collectively, these tendencies are known as the sink action of cerebrospinal fluid.[53] In addition, several extracellular markers, such as thiocynate and sulfate, are actively removed from the cerebrospinal fluid by active transport systems at the choroid plexus.[51] To attain the equilibrium conditions between cerebrospinal fluid and brain necessary to determine the extracellular space, the same concentration of extracellular marker must be present in both plasma water and cerebrospinal fluid. This can be attained by simultaneous administration of the extracellular marker in these two compartments.[51] Several different in vivo techniques have been employed.[7,54,55]

A number of different markers have been used to determine the brain extracellular space.[50,51] In addition, brain extracellular space has also been estimated by electron microscopy, tissue diffusion profiles, and measurement of cortical electrical impedance.[51] When brain extracellular space is appropriately determined in mammalian cerebral cortex by any of the aforementioned techniques, the range is from 15 to 25 percent, with a mean value of about 20 percent.[51] Segments of the extracellular space appear to be in free communication only with the bloodstream and other parts only with the cerebrospinal fluid.[55]

Anatomy of the Blood–Brain Barrier

When a nonmetabolizable, nontoxic substance is administered via the bloodstream such that steady-state conditions are maintained for several hours, it will achieve a similar volume of distribution throughout most cell systems. Examples of such substances include inulin, sulfate, salicylic acid, antipyrine, and urea. However, for a given time interval (up to 4 hours), none of the aforementioned will achieve a concentration in the brain as high as its concentration in other tissues such as liver or muscle.[56] This selective behavior of the brain, whereby passage of certain substances out of the blood is restricted, has been called the blood–brain barrier.[57-59] Several factors have been shown to influence the rate of passage of a substance from blood to brain. These include the K_a, configuration, molecular size, charge, and lipid solubility. Lipid-soluble substances penetrate the blood–brain barrier much more rapidly than do non-lipid-soluble substances. For example, one of the reasons that thiopental and amobarbital are more rapid acting barbiturates than phenobarbital is because of their greater lipid solubility. For weak acids and bases, the partition parameter determines their entry in the brain—weak acids tend to be excluded and weak bases concentrated.[60]

The anatomic delineation of the blood–brain barrier is complex and has been described in great detail.[56,61] It will be briefly reviewed here. The principal components of the blood–brain barrier are the brain capillaries, the astrocytic processes (end-feet processes), the thick brain capillary basement membrane, and the thick cell wall (Fig. 21–2). In contrast to capillaries elsewhere in the body, the brain capillary basement membranes function as an epithelial sheet. Brain capillaries are made up of a single layer of endothelial cells, with a dense cytoplasm containing few vesicles. In contrast to other capillaries, brain endothelial cells are connected by tight junctions that act to form a continuous cell layer. A basement membrane surrounds the cells; this is in turn covered by the glial cells, the astrocytic processes of which cover about 85 percent of the capillary surface.[56,61] The intracerebral arterioles and venules are also covered by continuous endothelial cell layers with tight junctions. Both the astrocytic end-feet processes that surround the capillaries, in addition to the thick neuronal cell walls, probably constitute the bulk of the blood–brain barrier. The thick lipid cell wall would tend to exclude those small molecules that pass out of cerebral capillaries but that are not lipid soluble.

UREMIA

Among patients with renal failure, there have been impressive modifications of both the duration and quality of life as a result of dialysis, renal transplantation, and improved medical management. However, patients who have renal failure continue to manifest a variety of neurologic disorders. Patients

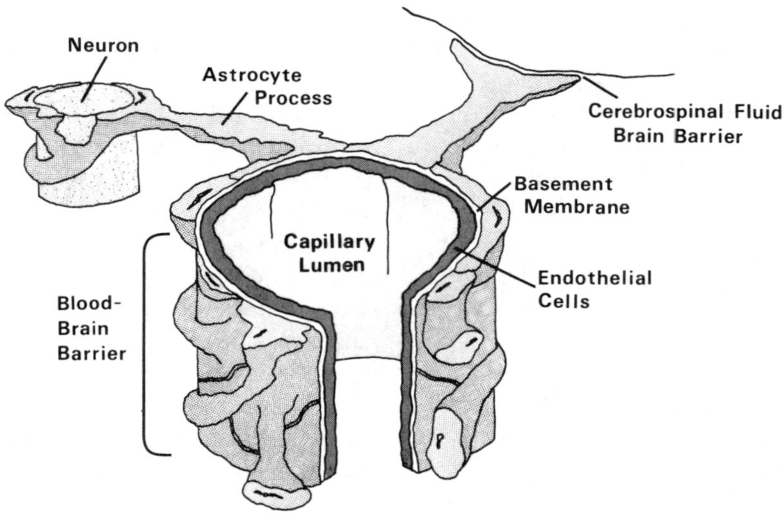

Fig. 21–2. Diagrammatic representation of the blood–brain barrier. The principal components are the astrocytic foot processes, endothelial cells with tight junctions, and a thick capillary basement membrane. The cerebrospinal fluid (CSF)–brain barrier consists primarily of choroid plexus and ependyma. (Original drawing by Bob Surface of Medical Research Graphics, San Francisco, CA.)

with chronic renal failure who have not yet received dialytic therapy may develop a symptom complex progressing from mild sensorial clouding to delirium and coma, with tremor, asterixis, multifocal myoclonus, and seizures. Even after the institution of otherwise adequate maintenance dialysis therapy, patients may continue to be afflicted with more subtle nervous system dysfunction, including impaired mentation, generalized weakness, and peripheral neuropathy. The central nervous system disorders of both untreated renal failure and that persisting in spite of dialysis are referred to as uremic encephalopathy. The dialytic treatment of end-stage renal disease has itself been associated with the emergence of two distinct new disorders of the central nervous system: dialysis disequilibrium and dialysis dementia. The dialysis disequilibrium syndrome is a consequence of the initiation of dialysis therapy in some patients. Dialysis dementia is a progressive generally fatal encephalopathy that affects patients on chronic hemodialysis. This disease may also be a complication of nondialytic therapy for renal failure.

In addition to the foregoing neurologic diseases specifically related to uremia and/or dialysis, a number of other neurologic disorders occur with increased frequency in patients who have end-stage renal disease and are being treated with chronic hemodialysis. Subdural hematoma is an important consideration in patients on hemodialysis who present with sensorial clouding or focal neurologic signs. Electrolyte disorders, vitamin deficiencies, drug intoxication, hypertensive encephalopathy, and acute trace element intoxication must be considered with any altered mental state. Renal transplantation is associated with a variety of nervous system infections and neoplasms, such as reticulum cell sarcoma.

Uremic Encephalopathy

In general, most clinical abnormalities associated with the uremic syndrome are due, at least in part, to disordered function of the nervous system. They involve the organism as a whole, rather than particular organs, and as such reflect the integrated aspects of the central nervous system. A fundamental problem facing nephrologists today is how to assess the adequacy of dialysis. It has been proposed that the "central nervous system provides a linkage of relevance between the chemical lesions, uremic toxins, and abnormal metabolic transactions of renal failure on the one hand, and the clinical, symptomatic lesions on the other."[62] Full rehabilitation of patients cannot be expected without full reversal of the central nervous system dysfunction.

The central nervous system manifestations of uremia include a continuum of signs and symptoms characteristic of many metabolic encephalopathies.[63] The earliest symptoms generally reflect sensorial clouding and may include loss of recent memory and impaired ability to concentrate, with depression, delusions, and slurring of speech. The clinical characteristics of renal failure often fluctuate from day to day in any given patient, so that intervals of lucidity may be intermixed with periods of apathy, confusion or obtundation. Action tremor, asterixis, multifocal myoclonus, and tetany may develop as uremia progresses.

The seizures and coma formerly associated with advanced renal failure are seldom seen with current modes of therapy, notably the early institution of dialysis. The clinical manifestations of acute renal failure do not differ in kind from those seen in chronic renal failure, but tend to be more severe, occur at lower levels of BUN, and in a more fulminant manner. The neurologic manifestations of uremia are generally similar, whatever the underlying renal disease, with the exception of systemic diseases that affect the nervous system directly, such as vasculitis or amyloidosis, and possibly in patients whose renal failure is due to diabetes mellitus or primary hyperparathyroidism.

Acute Renal Failure

The clinical manifestations of acute renal failure have been studied in two large patient series.[64,65] Aberration of mental status was noted as an early and sensitive index of neurologic disorder, with lassitude and lethargy passing rapidly into disorientation and confusion. Fixed attitudes, torpor, and other signs of toxic psychosis were common. When the uremia was untreated and allowed to progress, coma often supervened. Among these patients, cranial nerve signs were common, although usually transient. Both nystagmus and mild facial asymmetries were common. Visual fields remained normal in most patients, papilledema was not observed, and optic fundi were normal. Seven of 13 patients had dysarthria and difficulty in protruding the tongue past the lips. Diffuse weakness was always present. Idiomuscular response to percussion fluctuated from normal to reduced. Fasciculations were often present. Marked variation of deep tendon reflexes was noted in almost all patients, often in an asymmetric pattern. Progression to hyperreflexia with unsustained clonus at the patella or ankle was common.

Electroencephalograms (EEGs) have been evaluated in more than 40 patients with acute renal failure.[64,65] The EEGs of all patients were grossly abnormal when the diagnosis of renal failure was first established. In 16 patients the percentage of EEG power less than 5 Hz, which is a standard measurement of the percentage of EEG power devoted to abnormal (delta) slow-wave activity, was more than 20 times the normal value. The EEG was also abnormal with regard to at least two other parameters of the EEG: the percentage of EEG frequencies above 9 Hz and below 5 Hz. These EEG changes were not affected by dialysis, but returned to normal with recovery of renal function. Similar findings are present in experimental animals with renal failure.[46] The EEG tends to worsen both during and for several hours after hemodialysis.[66-68] When patients with renal failure are placed on dialysis, there is an initial period (up to 6 months) in which the EEG may suggest deterioration in the patient's condition; after this period, the EEG findings tend to approach normal values in patients who continue to be treated with chronic dialysis.[69]

Chronic Renal Failure

The neurologic manifestations reported with chronic renal failure have included virtually all observable clinical abnormalities.[70,71] Patients with chronic renal failure may develop a sense of sluggishness; easy fatigue on exertion; insomnia and daytime drowsiness; cutaneous itching; decreased appetite; impaired ability to focus attention, perform mental arithmetic, or express ideas in more than simple language; erratic memory; slurred speech; vague headaches; waning sexual interest and potency; restlessness; emotional irritability and withdrawal; nausea and vomiting; hypothermia; and sensations of coldness. There may also be paranoid and compulsive personality changes, bizarre behavior, anxiety, disorientation, confusion, hallucinations, ataxia, transient mono-, di-, or hemiplegias, aphagia, partial deafness, and vertigo, all of which may be mixed with occasional episodes of alertness.

The EEG findings in patients with chronic renal failure are milder than those observed in patients with acute renal failure. Several investigations have shown good correlation between the percentage of EEG frequencies and power below 7 Hz and the decline of renal function as estimated by serum creatinine[62] (Fig. 21–3). As in acute renal failure, after dialysis is started, there may be an initial period of clinical stabilization during which the EEG findings deteriorate (up to 6 months), after which it then tends to approach normal values.[62,72] However, still greater improvement is seen after renal transplantation.[62,73] Patients with chronic renal failure demonstrate a generalized slowing of background frequencies, loss of normal alpha rhythm, a shift in both the percentage of EEG frequencies, and power from higher (9 Hz) to lower (7 Hz) frequencies, and an increase in the burst index. Although these findings are nonspecific, there may also be a myoclonic response to photostimulation at different frequencies, which may be more specific for uremia.[62,63,70] Central nervous system dysfunction in uremia can also be quantitated by cognition-dependent performance measures. The cognitive functions known to be impaired in uremia include sustained attention, selective attention, speed of decision making, short-term memory, and mental manipulation of symbols.[62] The choice reaction time test is probably the most useful of those employed. This test measures sustained attention as well as speed of decision making. Although wide individual differences tend to obscure the significance of dialysis or transplantation on going results, a striking improvement may be seen in individual azotemic patients being treated with dialysis and then undergoing renal transplantation.

The causes of the EEG abnormalities ob-

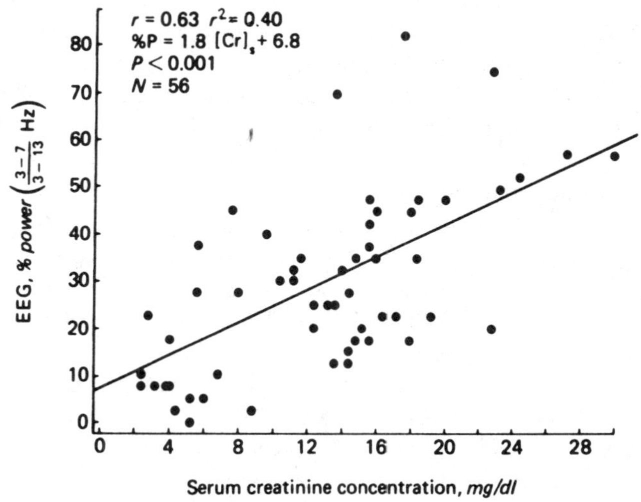

Fig. 21–3. Percentage of slow-wave-associated (3- to 7-Hz) EEG power plotted against concurrent serum creatinine concentrations in 56 azotemic patients with chronic renal failure before onset of maintenance hemodialysis. (Reprinted from Kidney International. Teschan PE, Ginn HE, Bourne JR, et al: Quantitative indices of clinical uremia. Kidney Int 15:676, 1979.)

served in uremic patients are unclear, but there is evidence that a significant common denominator may involve an effect of parathyroid hormone on brain.[46,65,74,75] In experimental animals with acute or chronic renal failure, many of the EEG abnormalities can be shown to be related to a direct effect of parathyroid hormone on brain, leading to an elevated brain content of Ca^{2+}.[46] Studies in patients with either acute or chronic renal failure suggest a similar pathogenesis.[65]

In patients with acute renal failure, the EEG is abnormal within 48 hours of the onset of renal failure[65] and is generally not affected by dialysis[64,66] over a period of up to 3 weeks. During this interval, patients with acute renal failure have been shown to have elevated levels of parathyroid hormone in plasma.[76] Several months after return of renal function, plasma parathyroid hormone levels are normal. Although there are doubtless a multitude of factors contributing to uremic encephalopathy, many investigators have shown no correlation between encephalopathy and any of the commonly measured indicators of renal failure (BUN, creatinine, bicarbonate, pH, potassium).[64–66,75,76] Thus, parathyroid hormone may function as a major uremic toxin.

Biochemical Changes in Brain

To determine the possible causes of the EEG abnormalities and clinical symptoms observed in patients with either acute or chronic renal failure, biochemical studies have been carried out in the brain of patients and laboratory animals. Most of these studies have been done in animals with acute renal failure. Measurements have included brain intracellular pH and concentrations of Na^+, K^+, Cl^-, Al^{3+}, Ca^{2+}, Mg^{2+}, urea, adenine nucleotides (creatine phosphate, ATP, ADP, AMP), lactate, and (Na^+ +K^+)-activated adenosine triphosphatase (ATPase). In patients with acute renal failure, content of H_2O, K^+ and Mg^{2+} is normal, while Na^+ is modestly decreased and Al^{3+} slightly elevated. However, cerebral cortex Ca^{2+} content is almost twice the normal value.[65,74,77] Similar findings have been observed in dogs with acute renal failure.[45,46,78] Permeability of uremic brain in rats to inert molecules, such as inulin and sucrose, is increased. Entry into the brain of Na^+ is impaired, while that of K^+ is increased. The permeability of brain to weak acids, such as sulfate, penicillin, and dimethadione, is normal to low.[79,80]

Alterations of cerebral metabolism that might be related to the aforementioned changes in permeability have also been studied in animals. In the brain of rats with acute renal failure, creatine phosphate, ATP, and glucose were increased, but there were corresponding decreases in AMP, ADP, and lactate. Total brain adenine nucleotide content and (Na^+ + K^+)-activated ATPase were normal to low. The uremic brain used less ATP and thus failed to produce ADP, AMP, and lactate at normal rates. There was a corresponding decrease in the brains metabolic rate, along with elevated glucose and low lactate levels.[81] Recent studies, employing more rapid tissue fixation of dog brain, have shown that creatine-phosphate, ATP and glucose were normal, indicating a normal brain energy reserve.[81a] The brain energy charge was also normal, as was the redox state. Taken together, these studies suggest that there is decreased energy consumption by uremic brain, which probably results from decreased demand for energy, rather than limited supply.[81,81a] Other studies of uremic brain have shown a decrease in cerebral oxygen consumption.[82] Patients with chronic renal insufficiency, (that is, glomerular filtration rate $<$20 ml/min) have decreased brain uptake of glutamine and increased ammonia uptake. The relevance of these findings, in terms of neurotransmitters or other brain function, is unknown.[83]

In animals with either acute or chronic renal failure, both urea concentration and osmolality are similar in brain, cerebrospinal fluid, and plasma. The solute content of brain in animals with acute renal failure is such that essentially all of the increase in brain osmolality is due to an increase of brain urea concentration. However, in animals with chronic renal failure, about one-half the increase in brain osmolality is due to the presence of undetermined solute (idiogenic osmoles) with the other half due to an increase of urea concentration.[14]

In dogs with chronic renal failure, brain content of Na^+, K^+, Cl^-, and water is not different from control values. Similarly, the extracellular space was not different from that of control values.[14] Calcium content was measured in eight parts of the brain in dogs with chronic renal failure for 4 months. Calcium was normal in the subcortical white matter, pons, medulla, cerebellum, thalamus, and caudate nucleus. However, as shown in Figure 21–4, calcium was about 60 percent above control values in both cortical gray matter and hypothalamus. Magnesium content was normal in all eight parts of the brain, as was water content.

In animals that have acute renal failure and metabolic acidosis, the pH_i of brain, and of skeletal muscle as well, is normal [80] (Fig. 21–5). In dogs with chronic renal failure intracellular pH is normal in brain, liver, and skeletal muscle[14] (Fig. 21–6). In patients with renal failure, intracellular pH has been reported to be normal in both skeletal muscle and leukocytes, as well as in the whole body[80,84–87] (Fig. 21–7). The pH of cerebrospinal fluid has also been shown to be normal in both patients and laboratory animals with renal failure.[68,80,88] Thus, despite the presence of extracellular metabolic acidemia in either acute or chronic renal failure, the pH is normal in brain, liver, and skeletal muscle.

Preliminary studies have been carried out in subcellular particles from brain of rats with acute renal failure. In cerebral mitochondria from rats with acute renal failure (BUN = 250 mg/dl), the intramitochondrial pH (pHim) was normal, as were oxygen consumption and stimulation with ADP.[88a] In normal rats, the oxygen consumption, stimulation with ADP and pHim were not acutely altered by several potential "uremic neurotoxins," including tin, aluminum, and parathyroid hormone.[88a] In synaptosomes from cerebral cortex of uremic rats, the uptake of radioactive sodium ($^{22}Na^+$) was similar in normal versus uremic animals. However, veratridine-stimulated sodium uptake was significantly increased in the uremic rats[88b] compared to con-

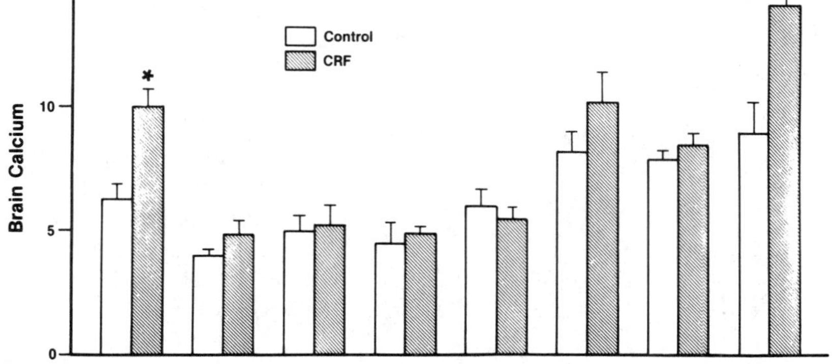

Fig. 21–4. Brain calcium content in eight areas of the brain in dogs with chronic renal failure (CRF) for 4 months. Brain calcium is significantly increased in cerebral cortical gray matter and hypothalamus. (*$p = 0.01$; control $N = 9$). (Reprinted from Kidney International. Mahoney CA, Arieff AI: Central and peripheral nervous system effects of chronic renal failure. Kidney Int 24:170, 1983.)

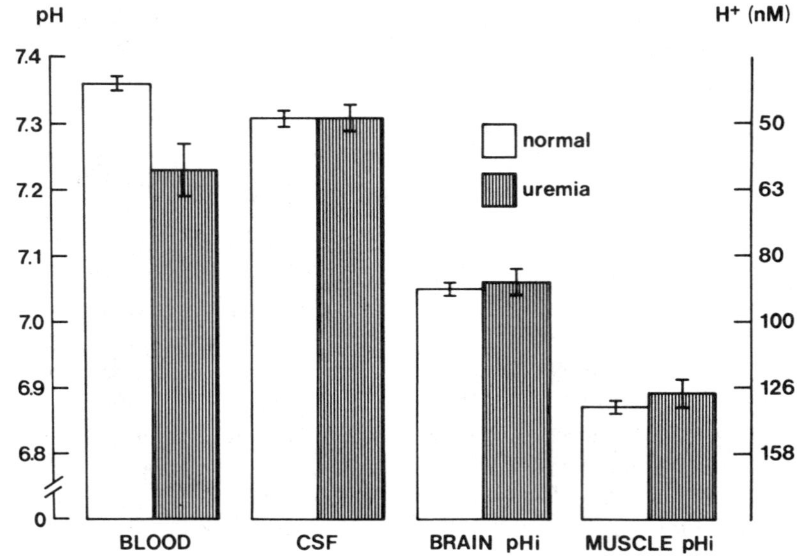

Fig. 21–5. pH of arterial blood and cerebrospinal fluid (CSF) and the intracellular pH (pH_i) in brain (cerebral cortex) and skeletal muscle. In animals with uremia (serum creatinine 11.8 ± 0.4 mg/dl) there was a significant fall in arterial pH. However, there was no change in pH of CSF or in pH_i of brain or muscle. (From Arieff AI, Guisado R, Massry SG, et al: Central nervous system pH in uremia and the effects of hemodialysis. J Clin Invest 58:306, 1976. By permission of the American Society for Clinical Investigation.)

trol animals. The abnormal sodium uptake was not due to a uremic milieu, but probably to an alteration in synaptosomal function induced by the uremic state. The abnormality probably involved the Na-K ATPase pump.[88b]

Pathology

Pathologic studies of brain have been reported in more than 400 patients dying with chronic renal failure.[84] Subdural hemorrhages

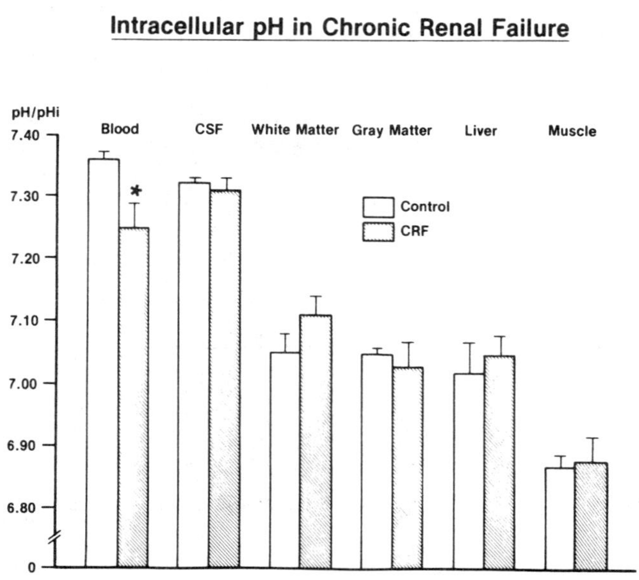

Fig. 21–6. Effects of 4 months of chronic renal failure (CRF) on the intracellular pH (pH_i). In dogs with CRF, the arterial pH is significantly below control values. However, pH_i is normal in brain white and gray matter, liver, and skeletal muscle. Asterisk (*) $p = 0.01$; control $N = 9$; CRF $N = 8$. (Reprinted from Kidney International. Mahoney CA, Arieff AI: Central and peripheral nervous system effects of chronic renal failure. Kidney Int 24:170, 1983.)

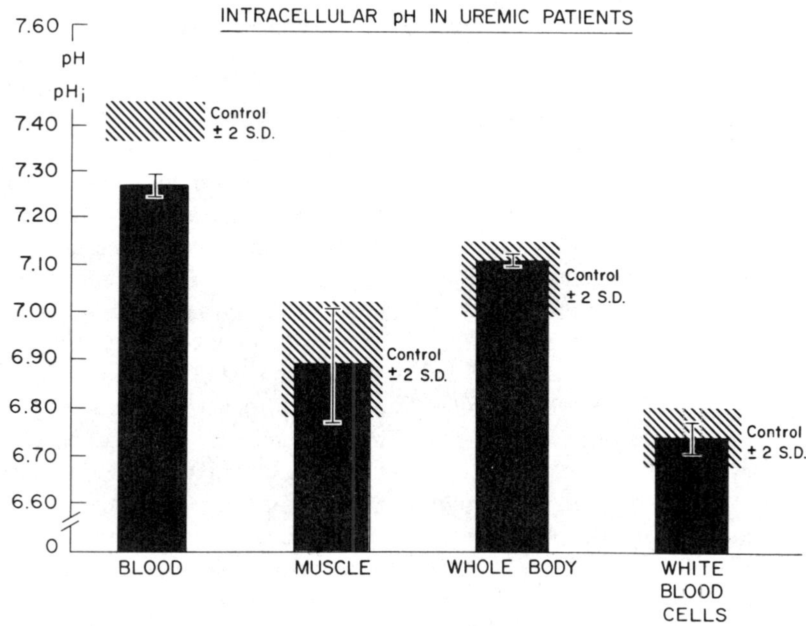

Fig. 21–7. Arterial pH compared with intracellular pH (pH_i) in skeletal muscle, whole body, and white blood cells. Although there is a significant extracellular acidemia, pH_i is normal in muscle, whole body, and white blood cells. Reproduced from Arieff AI: Neurological complications of uremia. p. 2306. In Brenner BM, Rector FC Jr (eds): The Kidney. WB Saunders, Philadelphia, 1981.)

used to be very common in dialyzed subjects, being reported in about 1 to 3 percent of autopsied uremic patients before 1974. In addition, intracerebral hemorrhages were reported to be present in about 6 percent of dialysis patients who expired, but these data are colored by the fact that many patients were receiving oral anticoagulants. Histologic changes in brain are probably nonspecific. Cerebral edema is not present in the brain of patients or laboratory animals with chronic renal failure by either biochemical or histologic criteria. Generalized but variable neuronal degeneration is often present but is inconsistent as to location. Among patients dying of uremia per se, there is some necrosis of the granular layer of the cerebral cortex. Small intracerebral hemorrhages and necrotic foci are seen in about 10 percent of uremic patients. Focal glial proliferation is found in about 2 percent of uremic patients. In general, changes in brain of patients who died with chronic renal failure are probably nonspecific and related more to any concomitant underlying disease state.[89–91]

Although a multitude of factors contribute to uremic encephalopathy, many investigators have shown no correlation between encephalopathy and any of the commonly measured indicators of renal failure. In recent years, there has been considerable discussion of the possible role of parathyroid hormone as a uremic toxin. In particular, a substantial amount of evidence suggests that there are toxic effects of parathyroid hormone on the central nervous system. The evidence for neurotoxicity of parathyroid hormone in both humans and laboratory animals will now be reviewed.

ROLE OF PARATHYROID HORMONE

In patients dying with acute or chronic renal failure, the calcium content in brain cerebral cortex is significantly elevated[65,74] (Fig.

21–8). Dogs with acute or chronic renal failure show increases in brain gray matter calcium and EEG changes similar to those seen in humans with renal failure.[45,46] In dogs, both the EEG and brain calcium abnormalities can be prevented by parathyroidectomy. Conversely, these abnormalities can be reproduced by administration of parathyroid hormone to normal animals, but not by elevation of the (calcium) (phosphate) product nor by hypercalcemia induced by vitamin D intoxication. Thus parathyroid hormone appears essential in producing central nervous system manifestations in the dog model of uremia.

Parathyroid hormone is known to have central nervous system effects even in humans with normal renal function. Neuropsychiatric symptoms are now reported to be among the most frequent manifestations of primary hyperparathyroidism.[91] Patients with primary hyperparathyroidism also have EEG changes similar to those observed in patients with acute renal failure.[65,74] The common denominator appears to be elevated parathyroid hormone. In patients with acute renal failure, the EEG is abnormal within 18 hours of the onset of renal failure and is generally not affected by dialysis for periods of up to 8 weeks[65] (Fig. 21–9). During this interval, patients with acute renal failure have been shown to have elevated levels of parathyroid hormone in plasma. In patients with either primary or secondary hyperparathyroidism, parathyroidectomy results in an improvement of both EEG and psychological testing, suggesting a direct effect of parathyroid hormone on the central nervous system.[74] Similarly, dialysis results in a decrement of brain (cerebral cortex) calcium toward normal in both patients and laboratory animals with renal failure, concomitant with improvement of the EEG.[45,46,74] In uremic patients, both EEG changes and psychological abnormalities are improved by parathyroidectomy or medical suppression of parathyroid hormone.[74,74a] Parathyroid hormone and/or a high brain calcium content are probably responsible, at least in part, for many of the encephalopathic manifestations of renal failure.

The mechanism by which parathyroid hormone might disturb central nervous system function is unclear. The increased calcium content in such diverse tissues as skin, cornea, blood vessels, brain, and heart in patients with hyperparathyroidism suggests that parathyroid hormone may somehow facilitate the entry of Ca^{2+} into such tissues. The finding of increased calcium in the brain of both dogs and patients with chronic renal disease and secondary hyperparathyroidism is consistent

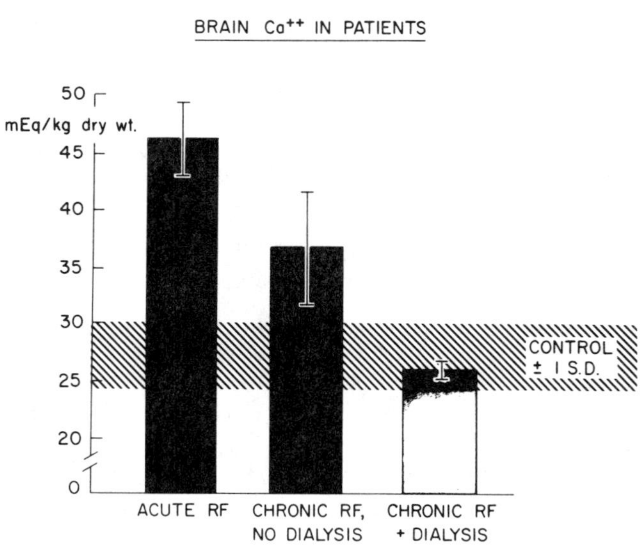

Fig. 21–8. The brain (cerebral cortex) content of calcium (Ca^{2+}) in patients who had acute renal failure, those with chronic renal failure treated with dialysis, or patients with end-stage chronic renal failure treated for at least 2 years with hemodialysis. Brain Ca^{2+} content is significantly greater than control values in patients who had acute renal failure ($p < 0.001$) or chronic renal failure not treated with dialysis ($p < 0.03$). However, in patients treated with dialysis, brain Ca^{2+} content is normal. RF, renal failure. Data are means ± SE. (Data summarized from Arieff AI: Neurological complications of uremia. p. 2306. In Brenner BM, Rector FC Jr (eds): The Kidney. WB Saunders, Philadelphia, 1981.)

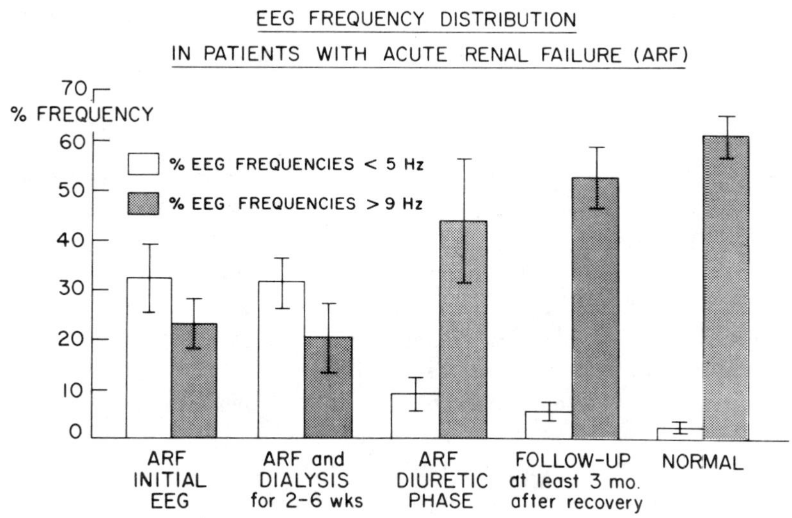

Fig. 21–9. Percentage of EEG frequencies below 5 Hz and above 9 Hz. Normal values are on the right. Patients with acute renal failure (ARF) have significant changes in both those frequencies above 9 Hz and those below 5 Hz. These changes are unaffected by dialysis but become normal with return of renal function. Data from 16 patients with ARF. Data are mean ± SE. (Reprinted from Cooper JD, Lazarowitz VC, Arieff AI: Neurodiagnostic abnormalities in patients with acute renal failure. J Clin Invest 61:1448, 1978. By permission of the American Society for Clinical Investigation.)

with the possibility that part of the central nervous system dysfunction and EEG abnormalities found in acute or chronic renal failure may be due in part to a parathyroid hormone-mediated increase in brain calcium. Calcium is essential for the function of a large number of intracellular enzyme systems, and an increased brain calcium content could disrupt cerebral function by interfering with any of them. It is also possible that parathyroid hormone itself may have a detrimental effect on the central nervous system.

OTHER UREMIC TOXINS

Of a long list of proposed uremic toxins, none has been shown to correlate better than creatinine clearance with any manifestations of uremia.[84] A pathophysiologic role in the central nervous system dysfunction of uremia has been clearly established thus far only for parathyroid hormone, although aluminum may also be important.[10] Pathologic and histologic examinations have generally shown minor nonspecific abnormalities. However, there is a notable lack of ultrastructural investigations of the central nervous system in uremia. Neither brain edema nor intracellular acidosis occurs. The functional significance of the altered brain permeability, decreased brain sodium, and presence of idiogenic osmoles is uncertain. The low turnover rate of high-energy phosphates seen in rats with acute renal failure and the decreased cerebral oxygen consumption may as easily be a result as a cause of the uremic state. The role of neurotransmitters and other peptide hormones in uremia are additional areas in need of further study.

Complications of Therapy of Uremia

DIALYSIS DISEQUILIBRIUM SYNDROME

In patients with chronic renal failure, any of several central nervous system disorders may occur. These disorders seem to occur as a consequence of the dialytic therapy and include dialysis disequlibrium. Dialysis disequilibrium syndrome is a clinical syndrome that occurs in patients being treated with hemodialysis. The syndrome has been described since about 1962[92] and may include headache, nausea, emesis, blurring of vision, muscular twitching, disorientation, hypertension, tremors, and seizures. The EEG may be abnormal,[93] but this has been disputed.[94] More recently, the syndrome of dialysis disequilibrium has been expanded to include milder symptoms, such as muscle cramps, anorexia, restlessness, and dizziness.[95-97] Although dialysis disequilibrium has been reported among all age groups, it is more common among younger patients, particularly the pediatric age group.[8] The syndrome is most often associated with rapid hemodialyis of patients with acute renal failure, but it also has been reported after maintenance hemodialysis of patients with chronic renal failure.[99]

In its mildest and perhaps most common form, dialysis disequilibrium may be manifested by no more than restlessness and severe headache, which may occur during or soon after hemodialysis.[100] These symptoms may be followed by nausea and vomiting, often accompanied by blood pressure elevation. The symptoms may be accompanied by disorientation and tremors, which may progress to siezures, with or without cardiac arrhythmias.[101] Seizures have usually been of the grand mal type.[76,102] Focal seizures have been observed, but these are often due to preexisting focal neurologic disease.[76] Most patients will recover from these symptoms, but recovery may take several days, at which time dialysis may again be necessary.

There has been much debate about the pathogenesis of dialysis disequilibrium. In early studies on patients treated with hemodialysis, a consistent elevation in cerebrospinal fluid pressure was observed.[103] In a few patients who died with, but probably not of, dialysis disequilibrium, the presence of brain edema was demonstrated.[104-106] It has therefore been suggested that brain edema is a major factor underlying the pathogenesis of dialysis disequilibrium. Early clinical investigation in patients with dialysis disequilibrium included evaluation of pressure and composition of the cerebrospinal fluid. In patients with dialysis disequilibrium, findings included a persistent elevation of cerebrospinal fluid pressure and levels of urea that were higher in cerebrospinal fluid than in blood.[92] These findings led to the early formulation that cerebral edema was responsible for most of the manifestations of dialysis disequilibrium.

The presence of brain edema in some patients with dialysis disequilibrium, along with the observation that in patients undergoing rapid hemodialysis, urea levels are higher in cerebrospinal fluid than in blood, led to formulation of the reverse urea hypothesis. Simply put, the reverse urea effect assumes that concentrations of urea are similar in plasma, cerebrospinal fluid, and brain tissue water. With rapid hemodialysis, it is further assumed that clearance of urea will be more rapid from brain. This assumption stems from the observed slower clearance of urea from cerebrospinal fluid than from plasma[92] in patients undergoing rapid dialysis. The decrement of plasma urea leads to a fall in plasma osmolality. It was postulated that, with a slower clearance of urea from brain, osmolality of brain tissue remained elevated above that of plasma, leading to a net movement of water from plasma into brain, with resultant cerebral edema. However, the reverse urea hypothesis was not supported by experimental investigations. Although in uremic laboratory dogs subjected to rapid dialysis, urea levels in cerebrospinal fluid are consistently higher than those of plasma, it appears that the rate of clearance of urea from the brain during hemodialysis essentially parallels that of plasma. After rapid hemodialysis of acutely uremic dogs, brain urea concentration was only about 6 mmol/kg H_2O higher than that of plasma.[78,107] Furthermore, the urea gradient from brain to plasma was similar whether brain edema was present or not. Pappius and co-workers found a slightly higher urea gradient from brain to plasma (~ 12 mmol/kg H_2O), but their animals, in addition to being uremic, had also been infused with urea intravenously. Thus actual analysis of brain tissue in uremic animals treated with rapid hemodialysis has revealed no significant difference between urea concentration of plasma and brain.

Along with the delayed clearance of urea from the cerebrospinal fluid, there was also evidence for paradoxical acidemia of cerebrospinal fluid in both patients and laboratory animals with dialysis disequilibrium. Cowie and co-workers[88] found that in some patients treated with rapid hemodialysis, there is a fall in pH of the cerebrospinal fluid despite a rise in the arterial pH. A similar fall in pH of cerebrospinal fluid occurs after rapid hemodialysis of experimental animals with acute renal failure[80] (Fig. 21–10). The decrement of pH in cerebrospinal fluid may be a major factor in the pathogenesis of dialysis disequilibrium. A fall in pH of cerebrospinal fluid may actually reflect a concomitant drop in brain intracellular pH.

There is a postulated mechanism whereby correction of arterial pH can lead to a paradoxical decline in pH of the cerebrospinal fluid.[30] It is known that CO_2 readily diffuses across the blood–brain barrier, while bicarbonate does so much more slowly. Thus, in a steady state of metabolic acidosis, both P_{CO_2} and HCO_3^- will be similar in cerebrospinal fluid and plasma. If arterial pH is then rapidly brought up to normal with intravenous infusion of HCO_3^-, the concentration of HCO_3^- in cerebrospinal fluid will remain lower than that of blood. As plasma pH is normalized, hyperventilation will subside, and the arterial P_{CO_2} will rise toward normal levels. The increased arterial P_{CO_2} will result in a rapid diffusion of CO_2 into the cerebrospinal fluid. Thus, in the cerebrospinal fluid, there will be a normal to high P_{CO_2} with a low HCO_3^- concentration, while in plasma, both HCO_3^- and P_{CO_2} will be normal. Hence, pH will be nor-

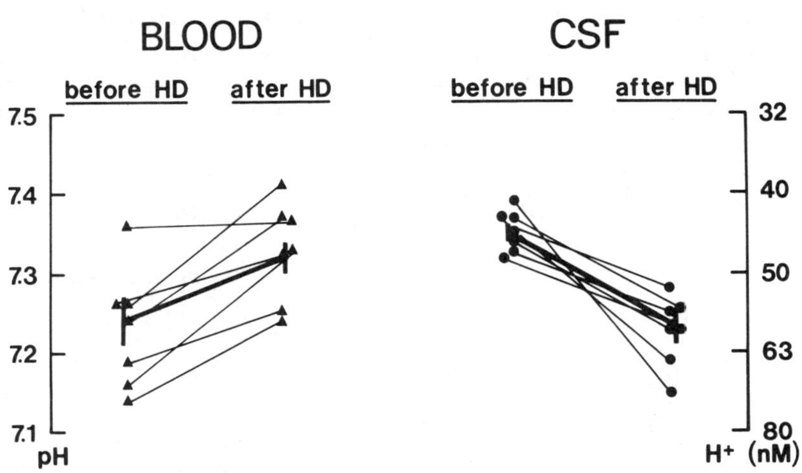

Fig. 21–10. Changes in arterial blood and cerebrospinal fluid (CSF) during rapid hemodialysis (HD). During HD, the blood pH increases from 7.22 ± 0.02 to 7.31 ± 0.01, while bicarbonate rises from 13.7 ± 1.0 to 17.7 ± 0.7 mmol/liter. The simultaneously determined pH in CSF falls from 7.33 ± 0.02 to 7.19 ± 0.02, while CSF bicarbonate falls from 18.9 ± 1.1 to 15.4 ± 0.5 mmol/liter. There was no change in arterial blood P_{CO_2}. Heavy lines are mean ± SE, while each thin line represents a single dog studied before and after rapid HD. (From Arieff AI, Guisado R, Massry SG, et al: Central nervous system pH in uremia and the effects of hemodialysis. J Clin Invest 58:306, 1976. By permission of the American Society for Clinical Investigation.)

mal in blood, but low in cerebrospinal fluid. Such a sequence may occur after correction of arterial pH in patients with cholera or diabetic ketoacidosis but is not usually of clinical significance. However, available evidence, both in patients with chronic renal failure[108] and in uremic dogs,[78] strongly suggests that such a sequence of events does not occur either during or after hemodialysis. In patients maintained with chronic hemodialysis, the arterial P_{CO_2} does not increase either at the end of dialysis or in the interdialytic period thereafter.[108] Furthermore, in animals with acute renal failure treated with rapid hemodialysis, dialysis disequilibrium occurs in the absence of any change in arterial P_{CO_2}.[78] Also, in patients treated with rapid hemodialysis, no difference in the P_{CO_2} or bicarbonate of either plasma or lumbar cerebrospinal fluid was found whether dialysis disequilibrium was present or not.[68,88,109] It is possible that the observed decrement of pH in cerebrospinal fluid observed after rapid dialysis is related to the intravenous influx of bicarbonate (from bicarbonate precursors, such as acetate), which occurs during dialysis. After bicarbonate infusion in dogs with metabolic (lactic) acidosis, there is a substantial increase in mixed venous, but not arterial, P_{CO_2}, which leads to a decrement in pH_i of liver and red cells.[110] Such a sequence may occur during rapid hemodialysis as well. However, most of the decrement in pH of cerebrospinal fluid observed during rapid dialysis is not due to an increase of P_{CO_2} in cerebrospinal fluid but rather to a fall in cerebrospinal fluid bicarbonate.[78] The fall in cerebrospinal fluid bicarbonate is not due to an increment of lactate in cerebrospinal fluid, but rather to the presence of organic acid anions, the identity of which has not yet been determined.

Along with the decrement in pH of cerebrospinal fluid, there is an observed decrease in the pH_i of brain. In dogs with acute renal failure, pH_i is normal in brain and skeletal muscle (Fig. 21–5). After rapid dialysis, there is no change in the pH_i of muscle, but a significant decrement is observed in the pH_i of cerebral cortical gray matter (Fig 21–11).

The increased H^+ ion activity in brain is accompanied by an increase of brain osmole content, which secondarily results in an increase of brain water. The cerebral edema that thus occurs is probably the cause of the observed clinical manifestations of DDS. The presence of postdialysis brain swelling has recently been documented by CAT scan in patients with chronic renal failure.[111] The source of the increased brain H^+ ion is not known, but it may be due to hypoxia, decreased cerebral blood flow, or increased cerebral lactate production. Cerebral hypoxia is unlikely, as the P_{O_2} in cerebrospinal fluid was normal and P_{O_2} of cerebrospinal fluid was similar to that of brain. Furthermore, cerebral hypoxia should lead to increased brain lactate, and

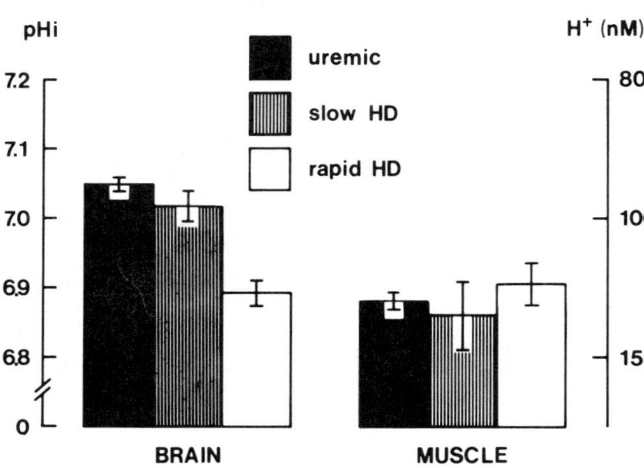

Fig. 21–11. The intracellular pH (pH_i) of brain (cerebral cortex) in normal dogs, uremic dogs treated with rapid hemodialysis (RHD). After rapid hemodialysis, there is a significant decline in the pH of brain. (From Arieff AI, Guisado R, Massry SG, et al: Central nervous system pH in uremia and the effects of hemodialysis. J Clin Invest 58:306, 1976. By permission of the American Society for Clinical Investigation.)

such a phenomenon did not occur.[80] Similarly, decreased cerebral blood flow probably did not occur, as such a circumstance should lead to a fall in Po_2 of cerebrospinal fluid, and an increase in brain and cerebrospinal fluid lactate. In animals treated with rapid hemodialysis, brain and cerebrospinal fluid lactate are normal. Although the exact biochemical sequence leading to an increase in brain H^+ ion is not known, rapid hemodialysis of uremic animals may lead to an increase in brain organic acid(s). In both mammals and amphibians in which abrupt increases in extracellular osmolality are induced, brain content of amino acids increases.[112,113] The presence in brain of strong organic acid(s) would tend to increase osmolality by at least two mechanisms: First, intracellularly bound Na^+ and K^+ ions (as occurs in the hemoglobin molecule), which are osmotically inactive when bound to intracellular protein, may become osmotically active when displaced from protein anions by a H^+ ion. Second, production of increased quantities of organic acids per se could raise brain osmolality. Although the precise mechanism is unclear, rapid dialysis can somehow lead to increased brain osmolality, cerebral edema, and dialysis disequlibrium.

The clinical manifestations of dialysis disequilibrium have been summarized in Table 21–1. For convenience, they have been divided into major and minor symptoms. Mild forms of dialysis disequilibrium may be manifested as no more than restlessness and severe headache, which may occur during or soon after hemodialysis. This is commonly followed by nausea and vomiting, often accompanied by blood pressure elevation. These symptoms may be accompanied by disorientation and tremors. Seizures and cardiac arrhythmias have been reported but are uncommon. When observed, the seizures have usually been of the grand mal type, although focal tremors have been observed. The symptoms are usually self-limited but recovery may take several days. In some instances the seizures may lead to coma. It appears that the modern methods of dialysis have altered the clinical picture of dialysis disequilibrium. Most reports of seizures, coma, and death appeared before 1970. The symptoms of dialysis disequilbrium as reported during the last decade (1973–1983) have generally been mild, consisting of nausea, weakness, headache, fatigue, and muscle cramps. It is also unclear whether any patient ever actually died from dialysis disequilibrium per se or from other associated neurologic complications of dialysis, such as acute stroke, subdural hematoma, subarachnoid hemorrhage, or hyponatremia.[114–117]

Table 21–1. Major and Minor Symptoms and Laboratory Findings Associated with Dialysis Disequilibrium Syndrome

Minor symptoms
Headache
Nausea
Emesis
Muscle cramping
Restlessness
Fatigue
Major symptoms
Muscle tremor
Blurring of vision
Hypertension
Disorientation
Syncope
Seizures (focal or grand mal)
Cardiac arrhythmias
Laboratory findings
No consistent abnormalities

Patients who have renal failure and are being treated with dialysis may exhibit the aforementioned symptoms of headache, nausea, emesis, muscle cramps, and seizure activity because of causes other than dialysis disequilibrium. A differential diagnosis of such patients is shown in Table 21–2. Recently, the diagnosis of dialysis disequilibrium has become a repository for a number of disorders that can occur in patients with renal failure and may affect the central nervous system. It should be stressed that the diagnosis of dialysis disequilibrium should be one of exclusion.

The management of dialysis disequilibrium can be divided into preventive modalities and therapeutic maneuvers. In several studies, this syndrome has been treated by addition of osmotically active solute (glucose, glycerol, al-

Table 21–2. Differential Diagnosis of Dialysis Disequilibrium Syndrome

Copper intoxication
Subdural hematoma
Uremia per se
Nonketotic hyperosmolar coma with hyperglycemia
Cerebral embolus secondary to shunt clotting
Acute cerebrovascular accident
Dialysis dementia
Cardiac arrhythmia
Depletion syndrome
Malnutrition of fluid proportioning system
Excessive ultrafiltration with hypotension and seizures
Hypoglycemia
Wernicke's encephalopathy
Hyperparathyroidism with hypercalcemia (serum Ca >12 mg/dl)
Malignant hypertension
Hyponatremia (serum Na^+ <125 mEq/liter)
Nickel intoxication

bumin, urea, fructose, NaCl, mannitol) to the dialysate, or by substitution of sodium bicarbonate for sodium lactate (or acetate) in the dialysate.[95–97,103,118,119] The purpose of such maneuvers has been to minimize rapid alterations in plasma osmolality or bicarbonate during dialysis. In uremic animals undergoing rapid hemodialysis, addition of glycerol or mannitol to dialysate prevents many of the manifestations of experimental dialysis disequilibrium.[118] Studies on uremic patients undergoing hemodialysis with either glycerol, NaCl, or mannitol added to the dialysate suggest that these agents often improve symptoms that may be associated with dialysis disequilibrium.[95–97,103,119,120] However, the aforementioned studies as well as most others in which osmotically active solute was added to the dialysate were carried out on stable chronic dialysis patients.[95–97,103] Additional studies are needed in patients with acute renal failure, or in those with chronic renal failure undergoing their initial few hemodialysis treatments. Evaluation of the efficacy or prevention of dialysis disequilibrium by addition of solutes to the dialysate must await these additional investigations.

A new technique called pure ultrafiltration has recently been developed. By this technique, the patient is subjected to ultrafiltration without dialysis. The net result is loss of fluid without the patient undergoing dialysis. This procedure can then be followed by conventional dialysis without ultrafiltration. Ultrafiltration results in net fluid loss without a fall in blood pressure, while dialysis without ultrafiltration results in less cardiovascular instability. It has been reported that patient discomfort is minimized by this procedure. The role of ultrafiltration followed by dialysis in the prevention of dialysis disequilibrium is currently being evaluated.

The technique of chronic ambulatory peritoneal dialysis is currently in worldwide use. By this technique, patients undergo continuous low-volume peritoneal dialysis for as long as 24 hr/day. The technique appears to minimize patient discomfort. Symptoms of dialysis disequilibrium have not been reported in patients undergoing chronic ambulatory peritoneal.

In both human subjects and experimental animals, the occurrence of dialysis disequilibrium in patients with acute renal failure can best be prevented by use of slow dialysis, that is, low blood flow rates and short dialysis times (< 4 hours) at frequent intervals (every 1 to 2 days). Until additional therapy becomes available, dialysis disequilibrium can probably be best prevented by employing short, frequent dialyses at low blood flow rates in those patients who are most likely to develop dialysis disequilibrium.

DIALYSIS DEMENTIA

Dialysis dementia, also known as dialysis encephalopathy, is a progressive, frequently fatal neurologic disease first described in the early 1970s. The disease is seen almost exclusively in patients being treated with chronic hemodialysis. Although the early literature focused on the distinctive neurologic findings,[121] more recent reports from both Europe and the United States have suggested that some forms of dialysis dementia may be a part of a multisystem disease that includes encephalopathy, osteomalacic bone disease, proximal myopathy, and anemia.[122-126]

Etiology of this syndrome remains controversial. Although an increase in brain aluminum content has been strongly implicated in some cases of dialysis dementia, the evidence is less convincing in others. Dialysis dementia most likely represents a syndrome complex that is the final common pathway for a variety of etiologic agents. At this stage of our knowledge it seems useful to subdivide dialysis dementia into three categories: (1) an epidemic form related to contamination of the dialysate, probably with aluminum; (2) sporadic cases in which aluminum intoxication is less likely to be a contributory factor; and (3) dementia associated with congenital or early childhood renal disease. This entity has been reported in several children who were never dialyzed or exposed to aluminum compounds. These early childhood cases may represent developmental neurologic defects resulting from exposure of the growing brain to a uremic environment.[127]

The initial reports in 1972–1973 were soon followed by reports throughout the world.[84] The initial patients all had the endemic form and had been on chronic hemodialysis for more than 2 years before the onset of symptoms. Early manifestations consisted of a mixed dysarthria–apraxia of speech with slurring, stuttering, and hesitancy. Personality changes, including psychoses, led to dementia, myoclonus, and seizures. Symptoms initially were intermittent and were often worse during dialysis, but generally became constant. In most cases, the disease progressed to death within 6 months.[128] Speech disturbances were found in 90 percent of patients, affective disorders culminating in dementia in 80 percent, motor disturbances in 75 percent, and convulsions in 60 to 90 percent. In contrast to this fairly distinct clinical picture, brain histology has been normal or nonspecific.

Early in the disease, the EEG shows multifocal bursts of high-amplitude delta activity with spikes and sharp waves, intermixed with runs of more normal-appearing background activity. These EEG abnormalities may precede overt clinical symptoms by 6 months. As the disease progresses, the normal background activity also deteriorates to slow frequencies.[125,128] The EEG has been said to be pathognomonic, but a similar pattern may also be seen in other metabolic encephalopathies. The diagnosis depends on the presence of the typical clinical picture and is confirmed by the characteristic EEG pattern.

Aluminum intoxication was first implicated in this disorder by Alfrey and colleagues in 1976.[10] Aluminum content of gray matter was elevated to 11 times the normal value in patients with dialysis dementia, versus an increase three times normal in patients on chronic hemodialysis without dialysis dementia. Aluminum content was also increased in bone and other soft tissue. Oral phosphate binders containing aluminum were originally suspected as the source of the aluminum, that is, $Al(OH)_3$ and $Al_2(CO_3)_2$.

The source of the increased aluminum content in brain is controversial. Significant absorption of oral aluminum can occur in patients with chronic renal failure, but the weight of evidence is against oral aluminum as the major source. The use of such compounds has been almost universal, yet many cases of dialysis dementia have occurred in an almost epidemic form with striking geographic clusters. Instead, epidemiologic studies have shown a strong association between aluminum in the water used to prepare dialysate and both the epidemic form of dialysis encephalopathy and fracturing dialysis osteodystrophy. In a survey by the European Dialysis and Transplant Association, 92 percent of patients with dialysis encephalopathy had used untreated or softened water, as opposed to 6 percent who had used deionized water.[129] The strongest evidence that aluminum may be directly responsible for dialysis dementia comes from an outbreak in Eindhoven, Holland.[122] Although two dialysis units there used the same untreated municipal water supply and the same dialysate concentrate, one unit had six cases of dialysis dementia in a 9-month period, while the sister unit was unaffected. A corroding aluminum anode in the water-heating system of the affected unit was found to be adding aluminum to the dialysate.

Even low levels of aluminum in the dialysate will result in a net retention of aluminum in the body. Aluminum transferred across the dialyzer binds to a nondialyzable plasma constituent, resulting in higher levels in plasma than in the dialysate. It has been estimated that a dialysate aluminum concentration of only 70 μg/liter results in a minimum positive aluminum balance of 300 μg/day.[131] Significant amounts of aluminum are also absorbed from the gastrointestinal tract after oral administration of aluminum hydroxide. Since aluminum is normally excreted by the kidney, this can lead to significant aluminum retention in patients with renal insufficiency.

Serum aluminum levels generally reflect dialysate aluminum levels, so that most investigators have not found them useful in separating patients with dialysis dementia from other patients dialyzed in the same center. Most workers have found that brain aluminum is elevated in dialysis dementia, but it has been questioned whether high brain aluminum content is the cause of neurotoxicity rather than a chance association. Although some investigators were able to show a good separation between brain cortical gray matter aluminum in hemodialyzed patients with and without dialysis encephalopathy, other investigators have noted considerable overlap.[84,130,132,133] Surprisingly, brain aluminum levels are higher in patients with chronic renal failure not yet on dialysis than in their dialyzed counterparts. Elevated brain aluminum levels are also seen in patients with hepatic encephalopathy and metastatic cancer, although these levels are generally lower than in patients with dialysis encephalopathy[77] (Fig. 21–12). There is no obvious threshold level for brain aluminum that determines toxicity. In general, though, levels above 15 mg/kg dry weight are associated with the encephalopathy, while levels below 5 mg/kg are not.

Deionization of the water used to prepare dialysate has recently been employed as a pre-

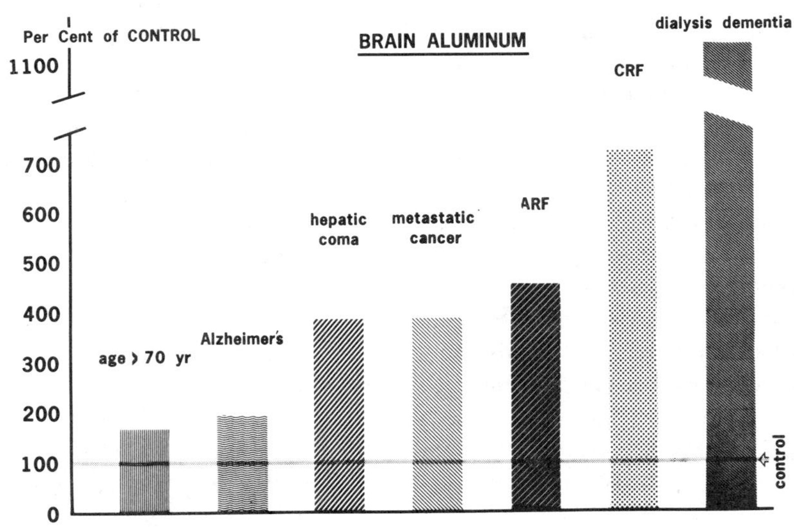

Fig. 21–12. Brain (gray matter) aluminum (Al^{3+}) content in normal patients, renal failure patients, and those who had either hepatic coma or metastatic cancer. The brain Al^{3+} is significantly above normal in patients with hepatic coma as well as those with metastatic cancer. Asterisk (*) signifies $p = 0.01$ as compared with control. Data are present as means ± SE.

ventive measure.[122,123,128,130] However, deionization may be beneficial by removing any number of other agents. Other trace elements may be present in water that can result in central nervous system toxicity. Such elements include cadmium, mercury, lead, manganese, copper, nickel, thallium, boron, and tin.[134] Among these potentially neurotoxic elements no one has measured brain content of cadmium, mercury, nickel, thallium, vanadium, or boron. Manganese was found to be increased in cortical white matter in the eight encephalopathic patients in whom it was measured.[135] These patients also had elevated aluminum levels in gray matter. Copper, zinc, and iron levels were normal. It is important to realize that tin was initially found to be elevated in brain of patients with dialysis dementia, before aluminum had been routinely measured.[132] Tin still is not currently measured in tissue and may prove to correlate with dementia better than aluminum, especially in sporadic cases. A number of trace metals may potentially leach into the dialysate water from the plumbing system after the deionizer, including aluminum, nickel, cadmium, tin, and manganese.

Most of the controversy over the etiology of dialysis dementia has involved sporadic cases. Dialysate aluminum levels are not always elevated, the use of aluminum phosphate binders is no different than in unaffected patients, and brain aluminum levels in patients with dialysis dementia may overlap with those of unaffected patients. There are very few studies on the etiology of these sporadic cases. The largest group of sporadic cases has been reported from Nashville.[136] The incidence of dialysis dementia in the area is 5 percent, despite the use of deionized water for dialysate with aluminum levels of below 5 μg/liter. Bone disease was not clinically apparent in this group. Serum aluminum levels in the encephalopathic group were three to four times higher than in other dialyzed patients despite equivalent prescribed doses of aluminum-containing phosphate binders.[137] These results suggest greater absorption and/or retention of aluminum in this group of encephalopathic patients. No other metals were measured in the Nashville study.

Despite these unresolved questions, most outbreaks of the epidemic form of dialysis dementia have been associated with high levels of aluminum in the dialysate. Lowering the dialysate aluminum to levels below 20 μg/liter, usually by deionization, appears to prevent the onset of the disease in patients newly begun on dialysis. New cases may continue to appear involving those previously exposed to the high aluminum dialysate, although the course is milder and mortality is somewhat decreased.[130] In patients with overt disease, eliminating the source of aluminum has resulted in improvement in some[130,136] but not all patients.[124] Transportation has generally not been helpful in patients with advanced disease. Diazepam or clonazepam are useful in controlling seizure activity associated with the disease, but such treatment becomes ineffective later on and does not alter the final outcome.[130,136]

Treatment of sporadic cases, in which the etiology is not clear, is more difficult. Every effort should be made to identify a treatable cause. Dialysis dementia must be differentiated from other metabolic encephalopathies, such as hypercalcemia and hypophosphatemia, hyperparathyroidism, acute heavy metal intoxication, drug intoxication (notably the long-acting sedatives), and structural neurologic lesions, such as subdural hematoma (Table 21–3). Because of the low incidence, the uncertain etiology, and the poor correlation of plasma with tissue aluminum levels, screening tests have generally not been employed. However, in the European experience, a high incidence of bone disease occurred after a shorter exposure to high aluminum dialysate than was required to produce encephalopathy. Thus screening EEGs and a neurologic examination with emphasis on speech disturbances might be useful in the early detection of encephalopathy in patients with typical osteomalacic bone disease.

There is not sufficient evidence to warrant

Table 21–3. Differential Diagnosis of Dialysis Dementia

Metabolic encephalopathies
Hypercalcemia
Hypophosphatemia
Hypoglycemia
Hyperosmolarity
Hyponatremia
Overt uremia
Drug intoxications
Trace element intoxications (manganese, mercury, lead, nickel, thallium, boron, vanadium, chromium, tin, cadmium)
Hyperparathyroidism
Hypertensive encephalopathy
Dialysis disequilibrium
Structural lesions
Subdural hematoma
Normal pressure hydroencephalus
Stroke

abandoning the general use of oral aluminum gels as phosphate binders. No equally effective substitute is available. Patients would risk severe secondary hyperparathyroidism, a disease of known etiology and high incidence, in an attempt to prevent a disease of low incidence that may not be related to oral aluminum. In contrast, the evidence is quite strong that high aluminum dialysate is associated with a substantial risk of encephalopathy and osteodystrophy. Water should be purified so that dialysate contains no more than 20 μg/liter aluminum, and preferably less than 1μg/liter. Deionization of dialysate aluminum levels should be performed if cases of encephalopathy or osteomalacia are suspected.

HYPONATREMIA

Classification

Hyponatremia is probably the most common electrolyte abnormality seen in a general hospital population. Commonly seen in association with many different systemic disease states, hyponatremia is almost always the result of dilution—either acute or chronic—and total body water may be either high, low, or normal. The pathophysiology of the different types of hyponatremia has been discussed in several review articles,[138,139] and complete lists of the causes of hyponatremia often span several pages. In general, the causes of hyponatremia fall into four major groups, depending on both the patient's volume status and the underlying causes. The causes are detailed in Table 21–4. In the case of extracellular fluid volume depletion, losses of fluid can be either (1) renal of (2) extrarenal. Hyponatremia can then occur when the patient ingests hypotonic fluid. If the extracellular fluid volume is normal or only modesty decreased, hyponatremia is probably related to either (3) hormone deficiency (hypothyroidism, Addison's disease), (4) hormone excess (antidiuretic hormone), (5) drugs that inhibit the ability of the kidney to excrete water, or (6) postsurgical nonosmotic stimuli to retain water. If the extracellular fluid volume is expanded, hyponatremia is usually associated with (7) hepatic cirrhosis, nephrotic syndrome, or congestive heart failure, or (8) acute or chronic renal failure. In a more simplistic sense, hyponatremia is almost always associated with dilution, as it is

Table 21–4. Causes of Hyponatremia

Depletion of extracellular fluid volume
Renal fluid loss with replacement by hypotonic fluid
Extrarenal fluid loss with replacement by hypotonic fluid
Extracellular fluid volume near normal
Hormone deficiency
Addison's disease
Hypothyroidism
Hormone excess (inappropriate secretion of antidiuretic hormone)
Drugs that limit the ability of the kidney to excrete water
Postsurgical nonosmotic stimuli to retain water
Extracellular fluid volume expanded
Effective arterial volume decreased
Hepatic cirrhosis
Nephrotic syndrome
Congestive heart failure
Renal failure
Acute water intoxication
Extracellular fluid volume status uncertain
Chronic renal failure with renal salt wasting
Obstructive uropathy
Interstitial nephropathy
"Cerebral" salt-wasting syndrome
Idiosyncratic reaction to thiazide or thiazide-like diuretics

nearly impossible to lose body fluid (such as urine, diarrhea, emesis) which is hypertonic with respect to the plasma sodium. Acute water intoxication (9) is an extreme case of dilution, in which there is administration of water (usually as intravenous 280 mM glucose in water) when the ability of the kidney to excrete water is impaired. Finally, renal sodium wasting (10) is a potential cause of hyponatremia, but such cases are probably rare. In a syndrome associated with thiazide or thiazidelike diuretics, hyponatremia is probably largely due to loss of Na^+ in the urine. Several other syndromes of hyponatremia are secondary to renal Na^+ wasting as well.

Salt-Wasting Syndromes

In most instances, hyponatremia occurs as a result of dilution of extracellular sodium rather than because of loss of sodium in the urine. When hyponatremia occurs predominantly as a result of loss of sodium in the urine, the condition is known as salt-wasting syndrome. Hyponatremia due to salt-wasting syndromes has been reported episodically at least since the time of Claude Bernard in 1858. The entity was reemphasized by Welt and associates[140] in 1952, and there have since been a number of reported cases. In general, the syndromes of hyponatremia due to excessive loss of sodium in the urine can be classified into four categories: (1) salt-losing nephropathy in patients with chronic renal failure[141]; (2) syndrome of inappropriate secretion of ADH[142] (SIADH); (3) "cerebral salt wasting"[143]; and (4) idiosyncratic reaction to thiazide or thiazidelike diuretics.[144]

In most instances, patients with renal salt wasting and hyponatremia will have chronic renal failure due to interstitial disease[145-147] or obstructive uropathy.[141] Most have had BUN in excess of 150 mg/dl (54 mM), and virtually all such patients would currently be treated with maintenance dialysis therapy. In addition, even with conservative nondialytic management, many could be brought into sodium balance if a low-sodium diet were gradually instituted (see Chapter 14).[148]

Contrary to popular belief, patients with chronic renal failure secondary to polycystic renal disease do not appear to have renal salt wasting.[149] Another large group of salt-wasting hyponatremic patients most likely had the syndrome of inappropriate secretion of antidiuretic hormone (SIADH) at a time when the diagnosis was not fully appreciated.[140,150,151] The patients had all the clinical hallmarks of SIADH and did not have volume contraction, hypotension, or azotemia. After the syndrome of SIADH had been well defined,[142] such cases were seldom reported.

The third group is potentially the most interesting, as they may represent a still poorly understood syndrome called cerebral salt wasting.[140,143,152,153,153a,153b] Such patients have many characteristics of SIADH, but in addition they exhibit several manifestations that are clearly not due to an excess of antidiuretic hormone. Renal function is normal. Most such patients have cerebral lesions (meningitis, brain tumor, stroke), from which the name of the syndrome comes. These patients are unable to conserve sodium on a low-sodium diet and can become hypotensive on a salt-restricted diet. With volume expansion, urine salt loss is accelerated. These patients do not respond normally to mineralocorticoid administration. Successful therapy has involved either severe volume restriction or a combination of high sodium intake plus large does of mineralocorticoid.

The aldosterone–renin axis of such patients has not been studied, nor have antidiuretic hormone levels been measured. In single cases, antidiuretic hormone like activity was found to be elevated[143] and plasma levels of renin and aldosterone were normal,[153b] as was the plasma cortisol.[153b] Clinically, these patients behave as if they had both SIADH and a distal tubular lesion with a form of pseudohypoaldosteronism. More studies are needed to define the lesion in such patients. The condition is rare, with less than 10 well-documented cases.[140,143,152,153] The renal lesion associated with cerebral hyponatremia has been described in only a single case.[153b] In this patient, there was focal loss of about 70 percent of distal tubules, with replacement by fibroconnective tissue. In other distal tubules, there were degenerative changes, with no evidence of interstitial inflammatory disease. To our knowledge, no other patient with this disorder has been subjected to renal biopsy.

There is a syndrome of hyponatremia associated with thiazide or thiazidelike diuretics and renal Na^+ loss.[144] Most such patients have been elderly and have presented with nausea, malaise, and emesis. Only a very small percentage of all patients taking such diuretics will develop hyponatremia. When hyponatremia is present, the concentration of ($Na^+ + K^+$) in urine exceeds that of plasma, and urine osmolality is hypertonic to that of plasma. Although the syndrome has recently been reemphasized because of the propensity to cause permanent neurologic damage, many previous reports may not have been appreciated because of diagnostic confusion with SIADH.[154-156] These patients differ from those with SIADH in that when the diuretic is discontinued, they are able to dilute the urine and excrete a water load normally.

Symptoms of Acute Hyponatremia

The symptoms of acute hyponatremia are dependent on the etiology, magnitude, and acuteness of the condition. In general, symptoms of sustained hyponatremia attributable to a combination of Na^+ depletion and water ingestion[157] differ markedly from those accompanying acute water intoxication. The symptoms of water intoxication are related to both the extent of the fall in serum Na^+ as well as the rapidity with which serum Na^+ is lowered. The causes of such symptoms are discussed in Chapter 23.

Neurologic manifestations of acute water intoxication are usually not observed until plasma Na^+ has fallen below 125 mM[4,158] and may include nausea, emesis, muscular twitching, grand mal seizures, and coma. Acute (less than 24 hours) water intoxication (plasma Na^+ $<$ 125mM) carries a mortality above 50 percent[4,159,160] with a substantial morbidity (usually brain damage). However, when plasma Na^+ is slowly (several days to several weeks) lowered to 125 mM or less by salt depletion and water ingestion, patients are usually less symptomatic.[157,159,160]

In experimental animals with acute water intoxication, coma and seizures may be seen when serum Na^+ is acutely lowered to levels of ~120 mM over a period of 2 hours.[159] When serum Na^+ is reduced to 120 mM over 2 to 3 days, many animals are asymptomatic, but more profound hyponatremia (serum Na^+, $\leq$ 110 mM usually results in varying degrees of paralysis, lethargy, coma, and seizures.[4,159,161] Thus, both in patients and in experimental animals, the neurologic manifestations seem to correlate grossly both with the degree of hyponatremia and with the rapidity of the fall in serum Na^+.

Symptoms of Chronic Hyponatremia

Patients with chronic hyponatremia usually have less fulminant symptoms and a lower morbidity and mortality. In a classic experiment, patients were maintained for 11 days on a salt-free diet, with frequent exposure to high ambient temperature designed to cause excessive perspiration combined with a high water intake.[162] Mean serum Na^+ concentration fell from 147 to 131 mM All these subjects experienced constant thirst, impaired sensation of taste, and anorexia, and several experienced muscle cramps. All had a feeling of general exhaustion, with dyspnea on exertion and dulling of sensorium. Other studies have shown that in patients with a greater depression of serum Na^+ (120 to 130 mM), symptoms of nausea, emesis, and abdominal cramps may occur.[157,158] With even more severe hyponatremia ($<$115 mM), subjects may manifest weakness, lethargy, restlessness, confusion, delirium, and impaired mentation.[4] In addition, muscle twitching is often present, and convulsions may occur. Many other neurologic abnormalities have been reported in patients with chronic hyponatremia, including focal weakness, hemiparesis, ataxia, and Babinski sign.[4,157,160] Patients with chronic hyponatremia may also have organic brain syndrome and cognitive impairment, but depression, overt psychosis, and anxiety are rare.[160a]

Chronic hyponatremia is common in patients with any of several edematous states, including congestive heart failure, nephrotic syndrome, renal insufficiency, or liver failure, in which both total body water and Na^+ are increased.[163] Chronic hyponatremia is also frequently seen in patients with the syndrome of SIADH, which may be caused by various tumors, a number of central nervous system diseases, or lung disease. Among hospitalized patients, an inappropriate ADH-like syndrome is commonly seen with the administration of various drugs, including oral hypoglycemics, tricyclic antidepressant agents, anticancer agents, diuretics, clofibrate, and morphinelike analgesics (see ref. 164 and Chapter 24 for a detailed list of drugs). Chronic hyponatremia may also be seen in patients with salt-losing states, such as salt-losing renal disease, excessive sweating, Addison's disease, and gastrointestinal electrolyte loss,[165] and has also been reported in patients ingesting massive quantities of beer.[160] Finally, evidence has been presented recently that suggests a lowered cerebral threshold for antidiuretic hormone release in certain chronically ill patients. These patients apparently have reset osmostats, manifested as sustained hyponatremia in the face of intact ability to excrete free water.[166]

Chronic hyponatremia in children is less frequent, although acute water intoxication with seizures and altered sensorium has been reported. Inappropriate antidiuretic hormone syndromes are seen in children[167] as well as adults. In addition, in a recent study of growth-retarded infants[168] 28 percent had hyponatremia, which was frequently asymptomatic. These infants appeared to have an unexplained high renal loss of sodium and in addition were given inadequate electrolyte replacement in their feedings.

In unselected hyponatremic patients, the degree of hyponatremia does not always correlate with the severity of symptoms.[254] Patients with serum Na^+ of 115 mM may be asymptomatic, while others whose Na^+ is 120 mM may present in frank coma. The mental status of 65 consecutive hospitalized hyponatremic patients whose plasma Na^+ was $\leq$128 mM is plotted against plasma Na^+ in Fig 21–13. There is generally a good correlation, albeit considerable overlap. Similar findings have been reported by others,[157] in which some patients with serum Na^+ of 108 to 132 mM had severe neurologic manifestations and others with Na^+ of 117 to 133 mM were asymptomatic. In general, however, when plasma Na^+ is below 120 mM, most patients have some depression of sensorium and may experience seizures (Fig. 21–13).

Electroencephalographic Changes

Electroencephalographic abnormalities in hyponatremia are common but are also nonspecific.[169] The most common changes are a loss of normal alpha wave activity with irregular discharges of high-amplitude slow- (4 to 7 Hz) wave activity.[170] These changes are more obvious over the posterior than the anterior portion of the head, and they tend to be more severe with lower levels of serum Na^+. In most cases, EEG changes returned to normal after correction of the hyponatremia.[161,170,171]

Pathology

Very few pathologic studies of the brain of patients who died of hyponatremia have been reported. In the first of the published

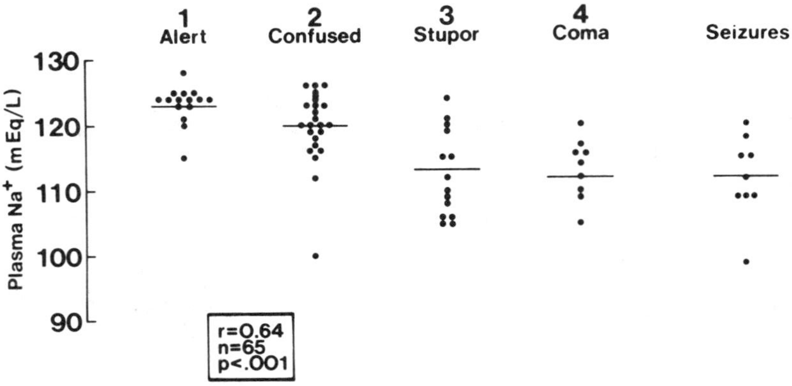

Fig. 21–13. Relationship between plasma Na^+ concentration and depression of sensorium in 65 patients with plasma Na^+ of $\leq$128 mEq/liter. It can be seen that although there is a highly significant overall correlation, substantial overlap among groups of patients is present. All patients who had seizures had plasma Na^+ of <121 mEq/liter. (From Arieff AI, Llach F, Massry SG: Neurological manifestations and morbidity of hyponatremia: Correlation with brain water and electrolytes. Medicine (Baltimore) 55:121, 1976. © 1976. The Williams and Wilkins Co., Baltimore.)

cases, a patient who had absorbed 9000 ml of tap water was studied 1 hour after death.[172] Although not actually measured, the calculated serum Na^+ was <110 mM. Examination of the cranial contents revealed obliteration of the subarachnoid space. The cerebral gyri were flattened, sulci were largely obliterated, there was uniform enlargement of the brain in all directions, and the ventricles were reduced in size. Microscopic examination showed increased vacuolization and swelling of supportive (glial) structures, with cellular swelling apparently confined to white matter. An additional postmortem examination in a patient who died of acute water intoxication revealed gross brain edema with both uncal and tonsillar herniation.[173] In one other patient who had died 3 weeks after an episode of acute water intoxication, no cerebral edema was present.[169]

Several investigators have studied the effects of acute water intoxication on brain in experimental animals. In general, all have found that there is considerably less swelling in the brain than in other tissues (liver, muscle) studied.[161,174,175] Edema is present in both gray and white matter of brain,[161,176] although more so in white matter.[177] The blood–brain barrier is judged to be generally intact in water-intoxicated animals (no penetration into brain of parenterally administered trypan blue).[176]

Microscopic examination of cellular swelling appears to be confined to astrocytes, with sparing of neuronal elements.[176,178] Phase microscopy of brain in water-intoxicated rats[178] revealed mild perivascular glial swelling with severe swelling of astrocytes. Electron microscopic evaluation showed no damage to cytoplasmic organelles, intact mitochondria, and normal tight junctions. There was no evidence of damage to neurons or oligodendrocytes, and the extracellular space was enlarged.

Effects on Brain Water and Electrolytes

Brain water and electrolyte content in hyponatremic animals has been evaluated by a number of different laboratories. Several different animal species have been used, and different degrees of hyponatremia were achieved. The increase in brain water content seems to be greatest in animals with acute hyponatremia (1 to 4 hours) (Fig. 21–14). During

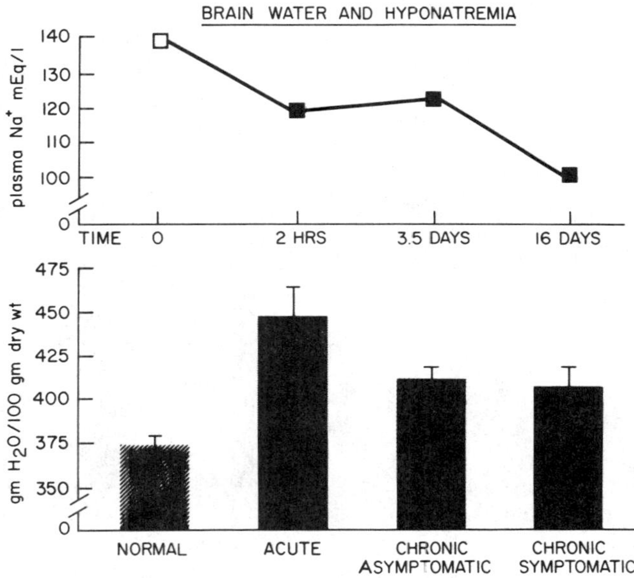

Fig. 21–14. Brain water in normal rabbits, and three groups of hyponatremic animals. In animals in which plasma Na^+ is lowered to 119 mEq/liter in 2 hours, brain water is 17 percent above normal values. When plasma Na^+ is lowered more gradually over 3½ to 16 days, brain water is increased only 7 percent. There is no difference in brain water when symptomatic and asymptomatic chronically hyponatremic animals are compared. (From Arieff AI, Llach F, Massay SG: Neurological manifestations and morbidity of hyponatremia: correlation with brain water and electrolytes. Medicine (Baltimore) 55:121–129, 1976.)

chronic hyponatremia, however, the increase in brain water content is lower than that predicted by the extent of the hyponatremia and also lower than that seen in other tissues.[161,174]

Thus it appears that the actual increase in brain water content in response to hyponatremia is somehow limited by various mechanisms (Fig. 21–14). Brain electrolyte content (mmol/kg dry weight) is minimally decreased in animals made hyponatremic over a period of 1 to 2 hours (Fig. 21–15). When hyponatremia is induced over long periods of time, there is a significant fall in brain content of Na^+, K^+, and Cl^- (Fig. 21–15). The fall in brain content of Na^+ and K^+ in animals with chronic hyponatremia is generally proportional to the fall in serum Na^+ level, although there is also a decrease in brain amino acid content.[179] The principal mechanism limiting the extent of brain swelling in response to prolonged hyponatremia would appear to be the observed decrement in brain electrolyte content, cheifly Na^+ and K^+. This is further substantiated by the decline in brain osmolality observed in hyponatremic animals.[159] Brain osmolality is significantly higher than that of serum in animals made acutely hyponatremic (2 hours). When similar degrees of hyponatremia are induced over a period of several days, brain osmolality falls progressively, eventually reaching levels similar to plasma.[159] Thus, the fall in brain osmolality limits the extent of water gain by brain, by reducing the osmotic gradient induced by the acute fall in serum Na^+.

The change in brain composition that is of greatest order of magnitude in animals with acute hyponatremia is an increase in brain water content, whereas in chronic hyponatremia there is a lesser gain in brain water, but a significant fall in both Na^+ and K^+ content. Several observers have suggested that the encephalopathy associated with hyponatremia may be related to the decrease in brain K^+ seen in experimental animals.[161,175] There is some evidence suggesting that the degree of encephalopathy in acutely hyponatremic rats does not correlate either with the serum Na^+ level or with the brain content of Na^+ or K^+.[161] In acutely water-intoxicated rats, the effects of hyponatremia on brain function appeared to be related to brain edema per se, which occurred before the brain was able to undergo compensatory changes to adapt to the fall in serum Na^+. In animals with chronic hyponatremia, however, significant decrements in brain content of both Na^+ and K^+ were present.

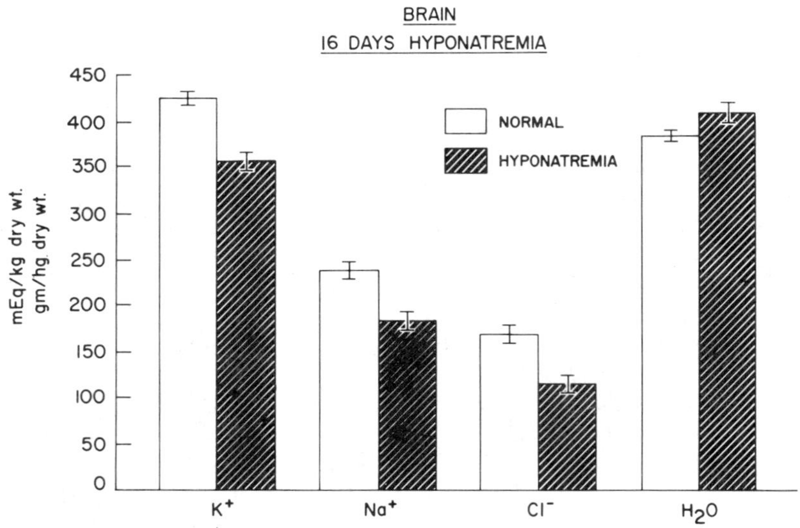

Fig. 21–15. Brain content of Na^+, K^+, Cl^- and water in normal animals and in rabbits with hyponatremia of 16 days' duration (plasma Na^+ 99 mEq/liter). It can be seen that in the hyponatremic animals, brain water content is 7 percent above normal and that brain content of Na^+, K^+, and Cl^- is 17 to 37 percent below normal values. The loss of electrolytes by brain prevented a more substantial gain in brain water. Shaded bars represent hyponatremic animals, and brackets are mean ± SE. (From Arieff AI, Llach F, Massry SG: Neurological manifestations and morbidity of hyponatremia: Correlation with brain water and electrolytes. Medicine (Baltimore) 55:121, 1976. © 1976. The Williams and Wilkins Co., Baltimore.)

Recently, transport systems for both the release and reuptake of neurotransmitter amino acids have been shown to exist in the synaptosomes of brain and spinal cord.[180] A Na^+ gradient is assumed to be one of the major sources of energy for transport of such metabolites against a concentration gradient.[181] In the brain and spinal cord synaptosomes, the neurotransmitter amino acid transport systems are almost totally Na^+ dependent,[180,182] and amino acid uptake in brain slices is largely inhibited by the absence of Na^+.[183]

Hyponatremia, then, may affect brain function by any of several mechanisms. Initially, the symptoms of acute hyponatremia are probably due to brain swelling, with a secondary increase of intracranial pressure. With more prolonged hyponatremia (more than 3 to 4 hours), the brain becomes depleted of both Na^+ and K^+, thereby limiting the increase in brain cell volume. The loss of brain Na^+ may result in both inhibition in brain energy metabolism and interference with neurotransmitter amino acid release at the synaptic level. These changes may affect brain function and may in part be responsible for the encephalopathy of hyponatremia.

Thus, survival in acute hyponatremia depends on the ability of the brain to lower its intracellular osmolality by extruding electrolytes, rather than by gaining water, the latter of which can lead to brain swelling and herniation.[159] In patients with protracted hyponatremia, then, it can be assumed that the brain cell content of Na^+, K^+, and Cl^- is low and that brain water is modestly elevated. The possible effects of any therapy must be evaluated against such a background.

Experimentally, the brain, in contrast to other tissues, does not behave as a perfect osmometer. In both hyper- and hypoosmolar states, the brain will gain or lose less water than will other tissues, such as skeletal muscle.[175] In fact, an osmotic gradient of at least 30 mOsm/kg between plasma and brain appears to be necessary to promote an acute net loss or gain of water from the brain.[184] Treatment of hyponatremia with either water restriction or infusion of 154 mM NaCl would therefore not be expected to have much of an acute effect by shrinking an already swollen brain. When confronted with a patient who has acute hyponatremia, brain edema and threatened herniation, these principles must be considered.

Treatment of Hyponatremia

Any discussion of the therapy of hyponatremia must include the underlying cause, as well as the duration, of the hyponatremia. In many types of hyponatremia, therapy must be primarily directed at the underlying disease state. Even with very low levels of plasma sodium, patients who have volume expansion associated with hepatic cirrhosis, congestive heart failure or nephrotic syndrome will probably not derive benefit from treatment with hypertonic NaCl. In such patients, there is probably a primary stimulus for renal retention of sodium and water.[185] Patients with extrarenal losses of fluid (diarrhea, emesis, third space) may respond with elevations of plasma antidiuretic hormone. When such persons then ingest hypotonic fluid, they may retain water and develop hyponatremia. Such a sequence frequently occurs after surgery, and affected patients may benefit from treatment with hypertonic NaCl.[186-188] In clinical practice, hyponatremia is frequently observed after surgery. Increased antidiuretic hormone activity may be due to volume depletion secondary to blood loss as well as to various combinations of emesis, nasogastric suction, prior diuretic administration, and decreased dietary Na^+ intake, or other nonosmotic stimuli, such as pain, anxiety, or fear. When postsurgical patients are given predominantly hypotonic fluids, hyponatremia may occur, which may result in substantial morbidity and mortality.[172,186,187] Another group of patients in whom acute symptomatic hyponatremia may develop are those with the syndrome of inappropriate secretion of antidiuretic hormone, who ingest or are given large quantities of water.[189] Such patients are often symptomatic from their hyponatremia, and therapy with hypertonic NaCl must be considered.

In patients who have hormone deficiencies that may predispose to hyponatremia (hypothyroidism, adrenal insufficiency), treatment should be directed primarily at the underlying disorder.[190] If the hyponatremia is symptomatic, NaCl should be administered along with the appropriate replacement hormone, since the plasma Na^+ is rarely below 125 mM, and therapy with hypertonic NaCl is rarely required.

A vast number of pharmacologic agents interfere with the ability of the kidney to excrete a water load. Included are large numbers of sedatives, hypnotics, analgesics, oral hypoglycemic agents, tranquilizers, antipsychotic agents, narcotics, and antineoplastic drugs. Hyponatremia associated with these agents may be acute, is often symptomatic, and may require treatment with hypertonic NaCl. Hyponatremia in association with these drugs occurs when patients ingest (or are given) water in excess of the ability of the kidney to excrete it. Such a sequence is actually quite common among psychotic patients who are taking some of the above agents.[192-194] Severe water intoxication may also occur in psychotic persons who are not taking such drugs.[195-198]

CRITERIA FOR TREATMENT OF HYPONATREMIA

In general there are four classes of patients in whom the decision to treat hyponatremia rapidly or slowly must be made: (1) the patient who has the syndrome of inappropriate secretion of antidiuretic hormone and has symptomatic hyponatremia; (2) the patient who has symptomatic hyponatremia secondary to water intoxication and either has substantial psychosis[194,197,198] or is taking drugs that limit the ability of the kidney to excrete water[164] or both; (3) postsurgical patients who have symptomatic hyponatremia, usually due to nonosmotic stimuli to antidiuretic hormone secretion[199] combined with administration of free water[3,186-188,191]; and (4) elderly patients who are taking thiazide or thiazidelike diuretics and who manifest an idiosyncratic reaction that leads to symptomatic hyponatremia.[144] Such patients develop nausea and emesis and lose both Na^+ and K^+ in the urine such that the hyponatremia is largely due to urinary loss of cation. They may also ingest large quantities of water.[154-156,191,200] It is recognizable that in virtually any patient with symptomatic hyponatremia, therapy with hypertonic NaCl may have to be considered. Nonetheless, the aforementioned four groups will encompass most such patients encountered in clinical practice.

It should be emphasized that even in the four classes of patients mentioned, hyponatremia per se is not in and of itself a reason to treat with hypertonic NaCl. Patients with serum sodium below 125 mM who are asymptomatic generally do well when treated with water restriction or intravenous 154 mM NaCl.[159] However, patients who are symptomatic and have serum Na^+ below 120 mM should probably be treated with hypertonic NaCl. The reasons for this therapy will be elucidated.

The treatment of symptomatic hyponatremia has undergone cyclic oscillations over the past 70 years between hypertonic NaCl versus no treatment (i.e., water restriction).[201] Recently it has been suggested that treatment of symptomatic hyponatremia with hypertonic NaCl may lead to a rare neurologic disorder called central pontine myelinolysis. A description of central pontine myelinolysis, its presumed pathogenesis, and any possible relationship to hyponatremia may shed some light on this association.

RELATIONSHIP BETWEEN HYPONATREMIA OR ITS CORRECTION AND CENTRAL PONTINE MYELINOLYSIS

Clinical Studies

Central pontine myelinolysis was probably first described in 1959,[202] in patients who were both alcoholic and malnourished. The lesion involved the center of the basis pontis and often extended from mid-brain to nerves of the lower pons. Most medullary sheaths were destroyed within the area of the lesion. The destruction of myelin involved all tracts, regardless of site of origin, termination, or function. In contrast to the complete destruction of myelin, however, the axis cylinders, nerve cells, and blood vessels were relatively well preserved. For detailed descriptions of the pathology, the reader is referred to several reviews.[202-204] Apparently, there are a large number of reported cases in which extrapontine lesions are present that differ from those lesions present in the pons.[205] Extrapontine demyelinating lesions are frequently anoxic in nature and may not be related to central pontine myelinolysis. The clinical characteristics among patients with documented central pontine myelinolysis are variable and may be minimal to absent.[206-208] In the original description,[202] patients had flaccid quadriplegia, facial weakness, inability to speak and swallow, and impaired response to painful stimuli. Facial and tongue weakness were thought to be a pseudobulbar phenomenon. The symptoms apparently vary according to the extent of the lesion, and in some cases, small lesions in the mid-pons may give rise to minimal symptomatology.[206] More than 170 cases have been described. At least 60 percent have a history of alcoholism, and the remainder have a variety of severe debilitating medical illness, including cancer, lymphoma, leukemia, sepsis, and severe malnutrition. An association with hyponatremia has been noted by several investigators, but this association is by no means universal.[205] In reviews of 172 patients with central pontine myelinolysis, only 43 patients (25 percent) had hyponatremia (serum sodium <128 mM).[207,208] Thus, most patients with central pontine myelinolysis do not have hyponatremia. It must be mentioned that many patients with central pontine myelinolysis have had underlying disease, such as cirrhosis, which are also commonly associated with hyponatremia. Of the 110 cases reviewed by Messert,[208a] six actually had hypernatremia.

It has also been suggested that central pontine myelinolysis may be somehow associated with the overly rapid treatment of hyponatremia.[204,208b,209] Data in humans that might suggest such a relationship are limited. In reviews of 162 patients with central pontine myelinolysis,[9,32] although 2 percent had hyponatremia, only four (2 percent) had a history of rapid correction of hyponatremia. In another study,[204] two patients had their serum Na^+ elevated from a mean of 100 to 131 mM over 3½ days, a rate of correction that is actually quite slow.[3,159,188,189,191] Furthermore, both patients had plasma Na^+ of 100 mM. Data from several laboratories show that in either rabbits, dogs, or rats with serum Na^+ below 110 mM, the mortality is 60 to 85 percent.[210-212] Norenberg and associates[209] reviewed the records of 12 patients with central pontine myelinolysis as well as a control group who also had hyponatremia but were treated with hypertonic NaCl. Among the 13 patients who actually had hyponatremia and were corrected with hypertonic NaCl (seven with central pontine myelinolysis; six without central pontine myelinolysis), the time required to raise serum Na^+ above 128 mM did not differ. Thus, the evidence that overly rapid correction of hyponatremia might have led to the central pontine myelinolysis observed in these patients is minimal. However, the study suggests that elevation of serum Na^+ in alcoholic/malnourished patients to hypernatremic levels may predispose to central pontine myelinolysis.

In summary, central pontine myelinolysis is a demyelinating lesion of the pons that was initially described in alcoholic and/or malnourished persons.[202] Subsequently, it has been described in more than 170 patients, virtually all of whom either had some chronic debilitating medical illness, were malnourished, were chronic alcoholics, or had some combination thereof. The symptoms of central pontine myelinolysis range from a fulminant neurologic picture with quadriplegia, inability to swallow, and other pseudobulbar phenomena,[202,204] to an almost asymptomatic clinical picture with incidental findings at autopsy.[206-208] A positive clinical diagnosis is very difficult, with a diagnostic accuracy that may be as low as 2 percent.[207] A distinct minority of patients with central pontine myelinolysis have had hyponatremia,[207,208,208a,208b] many have in fact been hypernatremic,[208,209] and fewer than 4 percent have had overly rapid correction of hyponatremia with hypertonic NaCl. Thus, in clinical studies available at this time, the association between central pontine myelinolysis and either hyponatremia or its therapy must be regarded as suspect but unproved. The actual diagnosis of central pontine myelinolysis has in the past been made only by postmortem examination. Recently, several cases have been diagnosed by computed tomography (CT) scan of the pons.[212a,212b] Nuclear magnetic resonance may be a still more valuable tool in the future.

Animal Studies

Several studies in laboratory animals have investigated the relationships among hyponatremia, its therapy, and the possible development of central pontine myelinolysis. In one study, Kleinschmidt-DeMasters and Norenberg[213] made rats acutely hyponatremic with subcutaneous vasopressin (10 units/kg) and intraperitoneal 140 mM glucose (5 percent body weight). Mean serum Na^+ ($\pm$ SD) fell from 139 ± 3 to 106 ± 12 mM. Animals were then given 1000 mM NaCl (20 ml/kg) twice in 24 hours, and the survivors were killed after 8 to 10 days. Mean serum Na^+ rose from 106 to 152 mM in about 25 hours. During this interval, the rats lost 26 percent of body weight. Control animals were also made hyponatremic (plasma Na^+, 100 ± 4 mM) and self-corrected to 136 ± 24 mM in 5 days. Demyelinating lesions were found only in rats treated with hypertonic (5.8 percent) NaCl. The lesions did not occur in the pons, but did occur in eight other parts of the brain.

In evaluating the aforementioned study, it must be pointed out that rats that developed demyelinating lesion were "corrected" to grossly hypernatremic levels (152 mM), while controls were only corrected to 136 mM. Also, the substantial weight loss (26 percent of body weight) indicates marked cachexia and a possible predilection to develop central pontine myelinolysis. In a preliminary study,[210] hyponatremic rats (serum Na^+, 110 mM) had their serum Na increased to 132 mM with hypertonic NaCl. None developed central pontine myelinolysis. Thus, it appears that elevation of serum Na^+ to hypernatremic levels against a background of cachexia may lead to central pontine myelinolysis, while correction to 130 to 140 mM does not.[210]

In another study, Laureno[212] produced hyponatremia (serum Na^+ 120 mM) in mongrel dogs (mean weight 16 kg) with vasopressin in oil (2.5 to 3.1 units/kg) and 2000 ml (13 percent body weight) of intraperitoneal water daily. Four days of such a regimen produced a mortality of 63 percent. Sixteen dogs received 514 mM NaCl over 6 hours with water restriction. Five dogs showed neurologic improvement and did not have central pontine myelinolysis, while five deteriorated neurologically and had either central pontine myelinolysis (four dogs) or extrapontine myelinolysis (one dog). There are several rather striking differences, in that before therapy, the four dogs that developed central pontine myelinolysis had a serum Na^+ of 100 ± 4 mM, while the six without central pontine myelinolysis had serum Na^+ of 121 ± 14 mM (p, <0.05). Five of six dogs with myelinolysis were "corrected" to hypertonic (serum Na^+ 142 to 157 mM) levels.

Overall, these animal studies suggest that elevation of very low plasma Na^+ (<105 mM) to hypernatremic levels (>140 mM) with hypertonic NaCl, when superimposed on a background of malnutrition, may induce demyelinating lesions. How such studies relate to more modest correction of plasma Na^+ to subnormal levels (~ 130 mM) is unclear.

Clinical Outcome of Treatment

EFFECTS OF ALCOHOLISM/ MALNUTRITION AND MORTALITY

In considering general concepts for the treatment of symptomatic hyponatremia, certain principles seem pertinent. It must be borne in mind that alcoholic/cachetic subjects probably represent a special case. If one reviews the bulk of the literature for patients with symptomatic hyponatremia and serum Na^+ of ≤ 120 mM, there are at least 144 cases reported in 29 articles.[4] Of these patients, 36 had either chronic alcoholism, malnutrition, or cachexia, with a mean ($\pm$ SD) serum Na^+ of 109 ± 8 mM. The other 108 patients had essentially the same serum Na^+ of 110 ± 8 mM. However, mortality in the alcoholic/cachetic subjects was 67 percent, essentially double that in the other patients (Fig. 21–16). If one considers only the mortality of severe hyponatremia (serum $Na^+ < 106$ mM), this is 86 percent in alcoholic subjects, versus only 66 percent in all patients. Thus, alcoholic/cachetic subjects have a hyponatremia-associated mortality that increases substantially more with lower values of serum Na^+ than does that in other patients (Figs. 21–16 and 21–17).

In general, then, relatively healthy patients with symptomatic hyponatremia (serum Na of ≤ 120 mM) have a mortality of about 33 percent without consideration of therapy. Overall, subjects who have alcoholism/cachexia have a mortality of about 68 percent

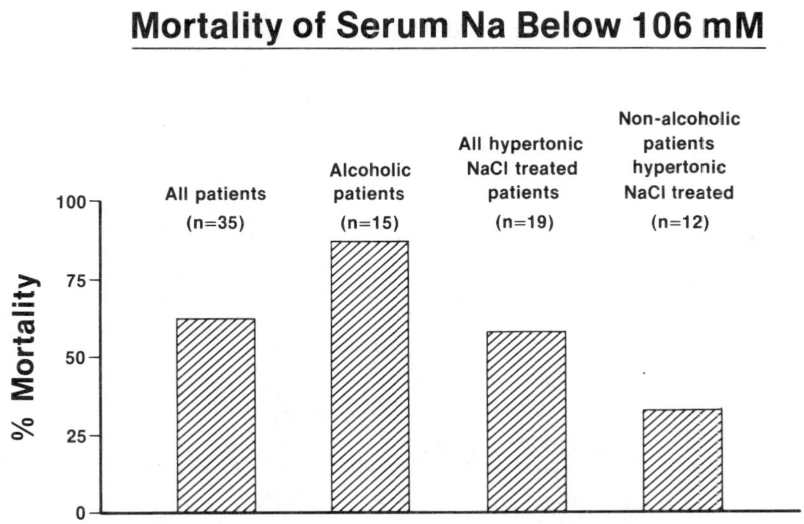

Fig. 21–16. Mortality for patients whose serum sodium (Na) was ≤105 mM. Overall mortality was 63 percent, but among alcoholic/cachetic subjects the mortality was 87 percent. Among relatively healthy subjects who were not alcoholic/cachetic, who did not have debilitating medical illness, and who were treated with hypertonic NaCl, the mortality was 33 percent. (Data from Dubois GD, Arieff AI: Symptomatic hyponatremia: The case for rapid correction. In Narins R (ed): Controversies in Nephrology and Hypertension. Churchill Livingstone, New York, 1984, references 3, 4, 5, 7, 9, 14, 17, 22, 23, 26, 29, 34, 37, 38, 42, 44, 47, 50, 55 cited therein.)

with mean plasma Na of 109 ± 8 mM, and this increases to about 86 percent with plasma Na of ≤105 mM. Any effects of therapy must be considered against such a background (Figs. 21–16 and 21–17).

MORTALITY OF SEVERE HYPONATREMIA AND EFFECTS OF TREATMENT

With all the foregoing in mind, the case for slow versus rapid correction of hyponatremia will now be considered. In general, many physicians do not employ hypertonic NaCl to treat symptomatic hyponatremia because of the presumed hazards of circulatory overload. It should be pointed out that this may be more of a theoretical hazard than a real one; few if any cases of circulatory overload complicating the treatment of hyponatremia have ever been reported. It would appear that one of the major arguments for slow correction of symptomatic hyponatremia is the possible development of central pontine myelinolysis. Although a possible association between hyponatremia and central pontine myelinolysis had been suggested in the 1960s (see refs. 3,5,6,7,9 in ref. 207), a report by Tomlinson et al.[204] strongly suggested that hypertonic (514 mM) NaCl given to a hyponatremic patient might somehow cause central pontine myelinolysis. Their report described two women in their mid-50s, both of whom had nausea and vomiting for 1½ to 3 weeks, a gradual onset of diminished sensorium, and a serum Na^+ of 100 mM. Both patients had their plasma Na^+ eventually corrected to a mean of 140 mM, neither ever regained consciousness, and at autopsy both were found to have had central pontine myelinolysis. As shown in Figure 21–17, among all patients with serum Na^+ below 106 mM, the overall mortality is 63 percent, whatever the therapy.

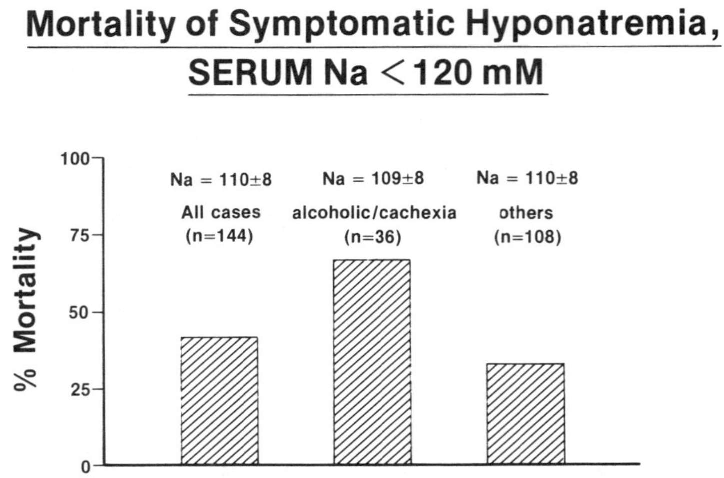

Fig. 21–17. Overall mortality for patients with symptomatic hyponatremia whose serum Na was ≤120 mM. In 114 cases from 29 articles, mean serum Na was 109 mM. Of these patients, 36 had either alcoholism or other debilitating medical illness, and their mean serum Na was 109 mM. The mortality was 67 percent in alcoholic/cachetic subjects, versus only 33 percent in the other patients. (Data from Dubois GD, Arieff AI: Symptomatic hyponatremia: The case for rapid correction. In Narins R (ed): Controversies in Nephrology and Hypertension. Churchill Livingstone, New York, 1984, references 3, 5–9, 12, 14, 17, 20, 22, 22a, 23, 26, 29, 32, 34, 36–38, 42, 44, 45, 47, 50, 52, 53, 55 cited therein.)

Perhaps more significant, few if any patients who were not alcoholic and/or malnourished have developed autopsy-proved central pontine myelinolysis, even though they were rapidly treated with hypertonic NaCl (see refs. 4,5,17,22,23,26,29,37,38,44,55 in ref. 4). In light of the aforementioned, there appears to be little rationale for thinking that in man, rapid treatment of a serum Na^+ of ≤105 mM with hypertonic NaCl may lead to central pontine myelinolysis, as long as the serum Na^+ is not elevated to hypernatremic levels. Rather, survival is rare unless treatment with hypertonic NaCl is rapidly instituted, while in alcoholic subjects whose serum Na^+ is ≤105 mM, the overall mortality is 86 percent whatever the therapy.[207-209,214-216] Thus, a major factor that determines survival in patients with plasma Na^+ < 106 mM is the existence of alcoholism and/or malnutrition. It may be that severe hyponatremia superimposed on a background of debilitating medical illness makes the occurrence of central pontine myelinolysis more likely. It does appear, however, that elevation of plasma Na^+ to hypernatremic levels (>140 mM) in alcoholic/malnourished subjects may lead to central pontine myelinolysis.[204,209]

RAPID TREATMENT OF SYMPTOMATIC HYPONATREMIA, PAST AND PRESENT

Having ascertained that rapid correction of severe (plasma Na^+ of ⩽105 mM) hyponatremia to ~130 mM probably does not lead to central pontine myelinolysis and may well be necessary for survival, we will now examine the case for rapid correction of less severe symptomatic hyponatremia. The definition of slow versus rapid correction of hyponatremia has been somewhat arbitrary. If one examines five large series of hyponatremic nonalcoholic patients published in 1973–1982, there are 30 well-studied patients with symptomatic hyponatremia and plasma Na^+ (± SD) of 111 ±

8 mM.[144,159,189,191,194] In these five studies, plasma Na^+ was increased by a mean rate of 1.9 ± 0.6 mmol/liter per hr, and correction was halted when plasma Na was 123 to 135 mM, with a mean correction to 130 mM. The survival among these 30 patients was 93 percent (Fig. 21–18). None manifested any symptoms of central pontine myelinolysis. If one then examines the older literature for the 15-year period 1951–1965, there are at least 35 well-studied patients in seven series.[3,158,169,186-188,198] Plasma Na^+ (± SD) was 109 ± 11 mM and none of the patients were noted to have conditions that predisposed to central pontine myelinolysis. Among patients treated with hypertonic NaCl from 1951 to 1965, survival was 87 percent overall, which compares favorably with the 93 percent survival recorded in 1973–1982 (Fig. 21–18). Good records are available on the rate of correction for 13 patients in six series,[3,158,169,186,187,198] whose survival was 85 percent, virtually the same as in the group as a whole. The mean rate of increase in serum Na^+ was 2.0 ± 1.7 mmol/liter per hr for the time required to increase (± SD) serum Na^+ from 109 ± 11 to 130 mM. No patient manifested symptoms suggestive of central pontine myelinolysis. Thus, rapid correction of symptomatic hyponatremia with hypertonic NaCl at a rate of 2 mmol/liter per hr resulted in a survival of 85 to 93 percent in two different eras (1961–1965 and 1973–1982). Such data provide overwhelming evidence that rapid correction of symptomatic hyponatremia in nonalcoholic patients (serum Na^+ 84 to 120 mM) to 130 mM does not per se result in central pontine myelinolysis.

SLOW TREATMENT OF HYPONATREMIA

For the 30 patients with symptomatic hyponatremia in 1973–1982 who were corrected rapidly, the mean ± SD rate of correction

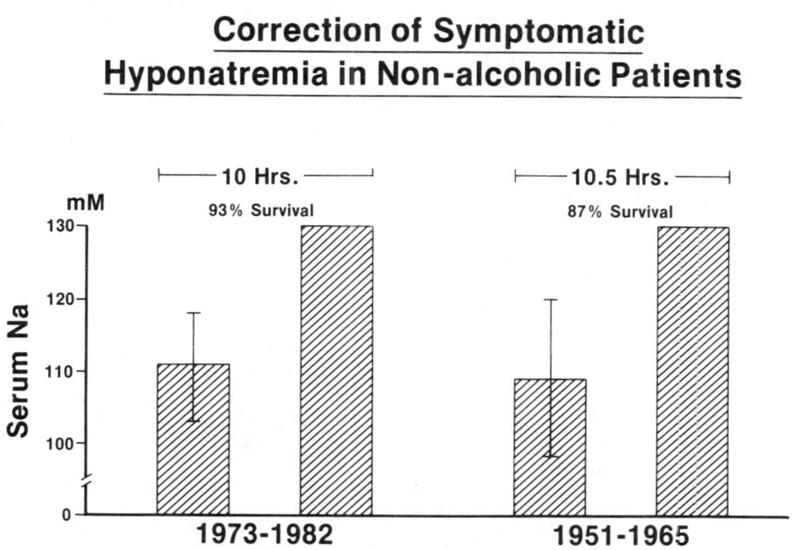

Fig. 21–18. Survival of symptomatic hyponatremia (serum of ≤120 mM among patients treated with hypertonic NaCl in two different periods: 1973–1982 and 1951–1965. Among all patients so treated, the mean rate of increase in serum Na was 2 mmol/hr. Patients with a history of alcoholism/cachexia are not included. Overall survival for all patients excedes 90 percent, and no patient developed central pontine myelinolysis. (Data from Dubois GD, Arieff AI: Symptomatic hyponatremia: The case for rapid correction. In Narins R (ed): Controversies in Nephrology and Hypertension. Churchill Livingstone, New York, 1984, references 3–6, 20, 26, 29, 38, 44, 53, 55 cited therein.)

was 0.7 to 3.4 mmol/liter-hr. Using these figures, we will arbitrarily define slow correction of hyponatremia as a rate of ≤0.6 mmol/liter per hr. Applying such criteria, there were 32 patients in six series[144,159,204,209,217] having a mean (± SD) plasma Na^+ of 111 ± 6 mM. Six of 32 were alcoholic and all had central pontine myelinolysis at autopsy. The overall mortality was 50 percent and among the 26 patients who were not alcoholic, the mortality was 42 percent. In Figure 21–19, we have compared the mortality in nonalcoholic patients studied over the same decade (1973–1982) who had identical serum Na^+ (111 mM) and were treated either rapidly (1.9 ± 0.7 mmol/liter per hr) or slowly (< 0.7 mmol/liter per hr). The survival is 93 percent in the rapid-treated group, versus 58 percent in those with slow treatment. Central pontine myelinolysis occurred only in alcoholic/malnourished subjects.

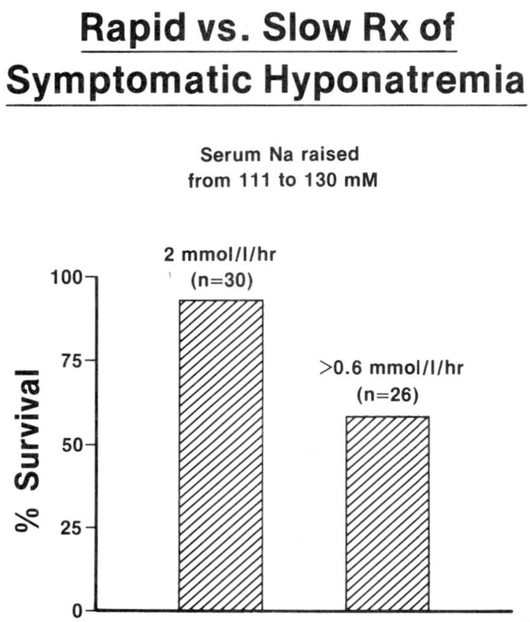

Fig. 21–19. Mortality of symptomatic (serum Na of ≤120 mM) among patients who were treated rapidly (i.e., with hypertonic NaCl such that serum Na was increased at a mean rate of 2 mmol/liter-hr), as compared with patients who were treated slowly (i.e., with fluid restriction, isotonic NaCl, or small quantities of hypertonic NaCl) such that serum Na was increased at a rate of <0.6 mmol/liter-hr. In some of the slowly treated patients, serum Na was never increased above 128 mM. See text for an explanation of the derivation of the rates for rapid versus slow correction. (Data from Dubois GD, Arieff AI: Symptomatic hyponatremia: The case for rapid correction. In Narins R (ed): Controversies in Nephrology and Hypertension. Churchill Livingstone, New York, 1984, references 6, 26, 29, 44, 53, 55, for rapid correction and references 3, 4, 34, 36, 45, 47 for slow correction, cited therein.)

SUMMARY

The data serve to define slow versus rapid treatment of hyponatremia in symptomatic patients who have (1) plasma Na^+ below 120 mM and (2) symptomatic hyponatremia due to any of four general categories, including: syndrome of inappropriate secretion of antidiuretic hormone; acute water intoxication associated with psychosis or certain drugs; postsurgical patients with water intoxication; thiazide or thiazidelike diuretics. Alcoholic or malnourished subjects with symptomatic hyponatremia seem to represent a special case. The mortality among such patients is high, and probably bears little relationship to the therapy. As shown in Figures 21–17 through 21–19, rapid treatment of symptomatic hyponatremia appears to offer the best hope for patient survival.

In general, then, the treatment of symptomatic hyponatremia (serum Na^+ of ≤120 mM) can be summarized. The principles apply only to the four conditions previously enumerated. Such patients should be treated with hypertonic (514 mM) NaCl at a rate of infusion such that plasma Na^+ is raised at a rate of 2 mmol/liter per hr until a serum Na^+ of 125 to 130 mM is achieved. At this time hypertonic NaCl should be discontinued. This regimen may have to be modified in patients with severe renal or cardiac disease. Because of the possible dangers of central pontine myelinolysis, the serum Na^+ should never be increased to hypertonic levels, and indeed should probably not be elevated acutely above 135 mM.

In patients who have symptomatic hyponatremia and have the syndrome of inappropriate secretion of antidiuretic hormone, plasma Na^+ should be raised at the same rate using a combination of 514 mM NaCl and intravenous furosemide. Such a regimen has been shown to increase survival in patients with symptomatic hyponatremia from an overall value of 58 percent to a value above 95 percent and has not been shown to produce central pontine myelinolysis in either patients or laboratory animals.

HYPERNATREMIA

A number of medical conditions are commonly associated with hypernatremia, the preponderance of which are quite different in children versus adults (Table 21–5). In infants, gastroenteritis with diarrhea is the most common cause,[218,220-222] while in elderly persons hypernatremia is often associated with infirmity and inability to obtain water freely, leading to gradual dessication.[219] Small children may also become hypernatremic after accidental administration of a high-solute load, particularly accidental substitution of sodium chloride for sugar in preparation of formula[223,224] or improper dilution of concentrated formulas.[225]

Other causes of hypernatremia include nasogastric hyperalimentation, nonketotic hyperosmolar coma, acute renal failure, renal tubular damage, dialysis, dehydration secondary to elevated ambient temperature, pituitary or renal diabetes insipidus, seawater ingestion, and hyperadrenocorticoid states. A number of central nervous system lesions have been reported to cause hypernatremia. These have been reviewed elsewhere.[25,160,218-220] Generally, diabetes insipidus is associated with hypernatremia only under circumstances in which the patient is unable to obtain water freely or when the lesion responsible for the diabetes insipidus results in a decrease in thirst. There may also be a whole new class of hypernatremic patients who have not been previously diagnosed. Excessive administration of hypertonic solutions of $NaHCO_3$ to critically ill patients suffering cardiac arrest was associated with a dangerously elevated plasma osmolality (377 ± 7 mOsm/kg) in 12 patients, none of whom survived.[226] Similarly, administration of large quantities of $NaHCO_3$ to newborn infants has been associated with hypernatremia and intracranial hemorrhage, with a mortality of 71 percent.[227] Severe hypernatremia has also been observed in patients inadvertently receiving intravenous hypertonic NaCl for therapeutic abortion[228] and may also occur in patients with lactic acidosis who receive large quantities of intravenous $NaHCO_3$.[229]

Neurologic symptoms are among the most prominent manifestations of hypernatremia in

Table 21–5. Etiologies of Hypernatremia in Adults

Infirmity with inability to obtain water
Stroke
Chronic illness
Other causes for alteration of sensorium
Dehydration secondary to hot climate
Hyperalimentation with osmotic diuresis
Oral
Intravenous
Renal water loss
Diabetes insipidus
Chronic renal failure
Dialysis
Proportioning system malfunction
Osmotic loss of water
Steroid hypersecretion
Conn's syndrome
Cushing's syndrome
Excessive hypertonic intravenous sodium solutions ($NaHCO_3$ or NaCl)
Lactic acidosis
Cardiac arrest
Therapeutic abortion (accidental intravenous hypertonic NaCl)
Central nervous system lesions
Hypothalamus
Subcommissural organ
Pineal gland
Supraopticohypophyseal tract
Essential hypernatremia
Extrarenal Water Loss
Febrile illness
Diarrhea
Osmotic
Infectious

patients at both extremes of age, and they frequently alert the physician to the possible existence of a hypernatremic state. In children most cases of hypernatremia are associated with readily reversible underlying systemic illnesses, and it appears that neurologic damage is the primary cause of mortality and morbidity.[230-234] In adults, by contrast, hypernatremia is frequently associated with a grave underlying systemic disorder. It is thus easy to attribute mortality and morbidity to the hypernatremia per se, although neurologic manifestations are nearly always present.[160,235] In addition to the variations in the neurologic manifestations of hypernatremia that may be seen with age, the eventual mortality and morbidity also seem to vary with the rapidity with which the hypernatremic state is attained.

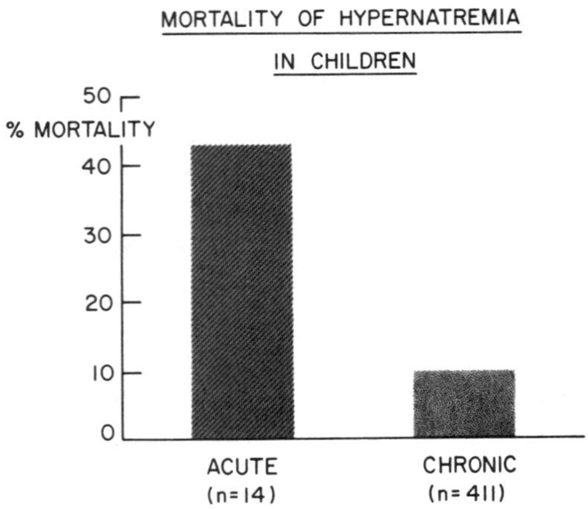

Fig. 21–20. Comparison of the published mortality in children who became hypernatremic (serum Na^+ >100 mEq/liter) over a few hours with that of children who became hypernatremic over several days. (From Covey CM, Arieff AI: Disorders of sodium and water metabolism and their effects on the central nervous system. p. 212. In Brenner BM, Stein JH (eds): Contemporary Issues in Nephrology. Vol. 1. Churchill Livingstone, New York, 1978.)

Symptoms

In children, the mortality of acute hypernatremia (plasma Na^+ above 160 mM for less than 24 hours) exceeds 40 percent, and it is above 10 percent when the hypernatremia develops over a period of several days (Fig. 21–20). Most children who present with chronic (more than 48 hours) hypernatremia have had gastroenteritis with diarrhea.[232,233] It appears that these children became gradually dehydrated over a number of days.[232] A second large group of children have had infections that have resulted in fever with tachypnea.[221,231] Other causes of hypernatremia in the pediatric age group are far less common.[160] Hypernatremic children often manifest a characteristic clinical picture described elsewhere.[221,236] About 67 percent of such patients have symptoms referable to the central nervous system. Most of these children have marked irritability and often emit a high-pitched cry. Depression of sensorium is characteristically present, which varies from moderate lethargy to frank coma. Normal muscle tone is the rule, but many patients have varying degrees of increased muscle tone, and some develop frank seizure activity.[221,232] Meningeal signs are not usually present on admission. The most frequent abnormality found on lumbar puncture is an elevated cerebrospinal fluid protein concentration, without pleocytosis.[236] Although most of these patients are not diabetic, many are hypoglycemic and may also have hyperkalemia, metabolic acidosis, and hypocalcemia.[232,236,237] Seizures are not commonly observed in patients with chronic hypernatremia, but after therapy is begun up to 40 percent may exhibit seizure activity.[230] A similar sequence is observed in hypernatremic rabbits whose serum Na^+ is rapidly lowered to normal with intravenous 140 mM (5 percent) glucose in water.[238]

Both mortality and morbidity of children with chronic hypernatremia are substantial. The mortality in different series is between 10 and 71 percent (Fig. 21–20), and morbidity is very high. Among 100 patients studied by Macauley and Watson,[234] eight sustained brain damage, one had tetraplegia, and seven were either retarded, hyperkinetic, or clumsy. Among 32 hypernatremic patients who were successfully treated and then followed up for 8 years, one was monoplegic, two had seizure disorders, and eight had abnormal EEG findings.[230]

In infants with acute hypernatremia, the most commonly observed symptoms are emesis, fever, and labored respiration. Spasticity may be observed, grand mal seizures occur in almost all patients, and coma is frequent.[233] Neurologic abnormalities, such as hemiparesis and Babinski sign, are common. Both morbidity and mortality are imposing. In the Binghamton, New York, salt-poisoning episode, 14 infants in a hospital nursery were accidently given formula containing 739 to 1170 mEq of NaCl per liter.[224] Of the 14 infants, 11 had symptoms that included muscular twitching or frank convulsions, vomiting, and respiratory distress. The mean serum Na^+ in the 14 patients was 199 mM. These acutely hypernatremic infants displayed signs of avid thirst until they were quite ill. Fever was common in older infants, although not in neonates. Mortality rate was formidable (43 percent) (Fig. 21–20), although one infant with a peak serum Na^+ of 274 mEq/liter survived with treatment. Among seven other children with dehydration and hypernatremia, all survived, but six of the seven had severe brain damage.[239]

Acute hypernatremia is less common than chronic hypernatremia in adults and is generally a result of acute solute loading when it does occur. It has been reported with the accidental introduction of hypertonic NaCl into maternal circulation during therapeutic abortion[228,240] and with the use of NaCl as an emetic.[218] Particularly fulminant symptoms have occurred with malfunction of either hemodialysis or peritoneal dialysis proportioning systems.[241,242] Hot climate has caused an acute rise in serum Na^+ over a few hours.[243] Acute hypernatremia can occur in patients with heat stroke,[244] in those who drown in seawater (which has a Na^+ content of 450 to 500 mM), and has also been described in at least one retarded adult who ingested massive quantities of table salt.[245] Acute hypernatremia is probably not uncommon among patients who are resuscitated after cardiac arrest after having been given large amounts of intravenous $NaHCO_3$.[226]

Typically, hypernatremia in adults occurs as a chronic process wherein the symptoms are obscured by those of other concomitant diseases, which are often of a catastrophic nature.[160,219,235,246] Because of these associated medical conditions, the presenting symptoms are usually not attributable to hypernatremia per se. The sensation of thirst, often intense, may not be verbalized because affected patients frequently have depression of sensorium. The physical signs commonly associated with dehydration, such as altered skin turgor and sunken eye sockets, may not be apparent because of the usual signs of aging. Lethargy, stupor, or coma may be present to varying degrees. Muscle irritability and convulsions have been reported[236,247] but are unusual, and it may be difficult to separate effects of hyperosmolality from those of therapy.

Symptoms similar to those observed in patient have been produced in experimental animals with acute hypernatremia. In rabbits infused with 1000 mM NaCl, severe central nervous system symptoms began to appear when plasma osmolality had reached 350 mOsm/kg. Initially the animals became alternately restless and lethargic, and they went on to develop nystagmus and ataxia, muscular twitching, and trembling. Stupor ensued. Many died of respiratory failure, in most cases at a plasma osmolality of ~430 mOsm/kg[28,29] (Fig. 21–21). A similar picture has been observed in kittens made hypernatremic by intraperitoneal injection with hypertonic NaCl[20] and in animals with hyperosmolar states achieved by infusion of similar osmotic loads of sucrose or mannitol.[29]

Electroencephalographic Changes

In experimental animals, hyperosmolality results in a progressive slowing of background EEG frequencies, but no spikes or paroxysmal

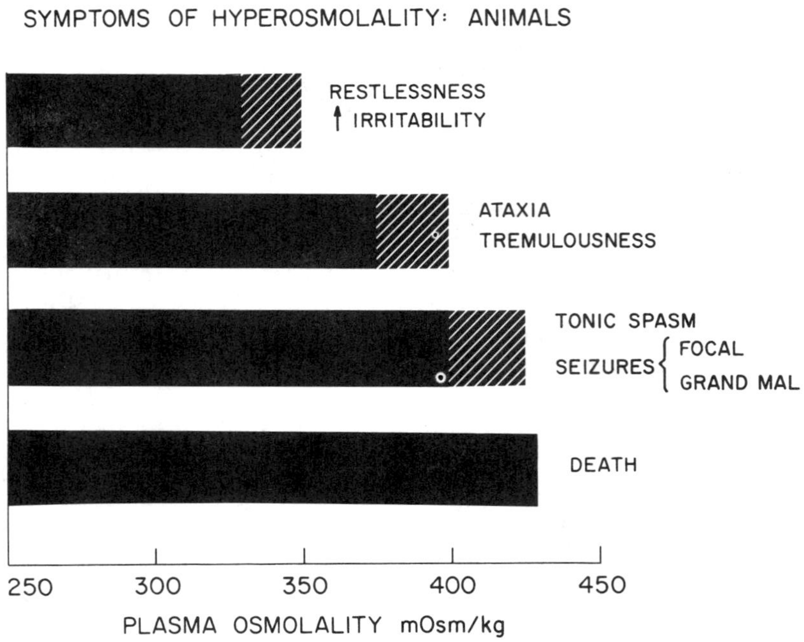

Fig. 21–21. Effects of acute hyperosmolality on symptomatology in experimental animals. Crosshatched areas represent the range of plasma osmolality for each group of manifestations. (From Arieff AI, Guisado R, Lazarowitz VC: Pathophysiology of hyperosmolar states. p. 227. In Disturbances in Body Fluid Osmolality. American Physiological Society, Bethesda, Md., 1977.)

discharges are seen even in the presence of paroxysmal jerking of the body.[28,29,248] These changes suggest alterations at different levels of the nervous system, and probably of spinal cord or peripheral nerve trunks as well, since the paroxysmal jerks and tonic contractions do not disappear after spinal cord or sciatic nerve section.[28]

Other EEG abnormalities are observed at the time that symptoms of hyperosmolality become manifest. There is a generalized reduction in voltage, a disappearance of fast activity, and the appearance of bursts of 4 to 5/sec spindlelike activity. There is gradual progression to 1 to 3/sec high-voltage waves, with cessation of EEG activity at the time of respiratory arrest.[29] The EEG changes appear to be reversible with correction of plasma osmolality to normal.[29]

Electroencephalograms obtained in patients with hypernatremia have generally been normal. However, the EEGs of 10 of 52 hypernatremic children studied by Brick[232] showed a decrease in amplitude similar to that observed in experimental animals, with generalized slowing of the background rhythm. All but two had returned to normal within 2 to 40 days after treatment. The two persistently abnormal EEGs showed typical seizure discharges.

Anatomic Changes in the Brain

In acute hypernatremia, as fluid from the intracellular space moves into the extracellular compartment to establish osmotic equilibrium, the cells initially lose volume.[248] In the brain, this loss of volume may put mechanical traction on delicate cerebral vessels to produce vascular damage.[20]

Autopsies performed on children who died from acute salt poisoning have provided much of our information about the anatomic lesions produced in humans by acute hypernatremia.[233] In these children, there is evidence of widespread cerebrovascular damage. Capillaries and veins are markedly congested, with subcortical parenchymous hemorrhage and subarachnoid bleeding. Venous thromboses, sometimes leading to infarction, and occlusion of major venous sinuses have been observed. Although cerebral edema has been noted in some patients, it is more likely the result of overly rapid rehydration therapy rather than of the hypernatremia per se.

The anatomic brain damage produced by acute hyperosmolality has also been studied in experimental animals. Shrunken grossly dehydrated brains, engorged vessels, and petechial hemorrhages were observed in rabbits made hyperosmolar (mean plasma osmolality of 396 mOsm/kg) by the infusion of 1000 mM NaCl, with a 76 percent mortality. Similar findings were observed in kittens made hypernatremic by intraperitoneal injection of hypertonic saline or sodium bicarbonate. At necropsy 85 percent of the animals had subdural hemorrhage with xanthrochromia of the cerebrospinal fluid, and 7 percent had subdural hematoma.[20]

Similar findings of hemorrhage and congested cerebral vessels have been observed in children dying of chronic hypernatremia.[24] In chronically hypernatremic animals, dehydration and vascular congestion are present,[179] although changes are usually not seen.[248]

Effects of Hypernatremia on Brain Water and Electrolytes

The effects of acute and chronic hypernatremia on brain water and electrolytes in experimental animals are summarized in Figure 21–22, which shows results obtained by several different investigators working with different animal species. In animals with acute hypernatremia (mean serum Na^+, 178 mM) of less than 3 hours' duration there is an abrupt decrease in brain water and a rise in intracellular Na^+ and Cl^- concentration. Potassium con-

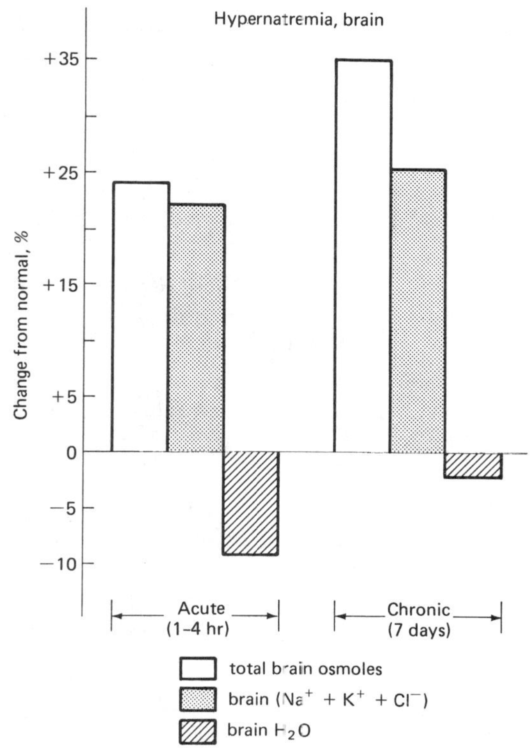

Fig. 21–22. Changes in brain osmol content (mOsm/kg dry weight), brain content of $Na^+ + K^+ + Cl^-$ (mmol/kg dry weight), and brain water content (g H_2O per 100 g dry weight) in animals with experimental hypernatremia. Brain osmolality has been estimated by assuming osmolality of plasma and brain to be equal in a steady state. In animals with acute hypernatremia (1 to 4 hours), brain osmolality increases due to both a loss in water and a gain in solute. Brain water content is 9 percent below control values. Brain osmol content is increased by 24 percent above normal values, with virtually all of the increases in Na^+, K^+, and Cl^-. In chronically hypernatremic animals, brain osmolality is also elevated, but most of the increase is due to a gain in brain solute. Brain water content is similar to normal values. Brain osmol content is 35 percent above control levels; most of the increase is not accounted for by changes in brain content of Na^+, K^+, Cl^-, but is due to undetermined solute (idiogenic osmols). (Reprinted from Arieff AI, Guisado R: Effects on the central nervous system of hypernatremic and hyponatremic states. Kidney Int 10:104, 1976, with permission.)

tent increases minimally.[48] Acutely, the increase in measured intracellular osmolality of the brain can essentially be all accounted for by the observed increases in measured brain electrolyte (Na^+, K^+, Cl^-) concentration.

After several days of sustained hypernatremia, however, brain water content is almost normal.[248] In rabbits that have been hypernatremic (mean serum Na^+, 173 mM) for 7 days, brain water content is normal, in spite of the fact that in these same animals there is still a marked loss of intracellular water in muscle tissue. However, in mice with 4 days of hypernatremia, brain water content remains low.[249] Total brain Na^+ and Cl^- remain elevated in both mice and rabbits, but the increase in measured electrolytes (Na^+, K^+, Cl^-) is not sufficient to account for all of the measured increase in brain osmolality (Fig. 21–22). In other words, there is the appearance of unmeasured solute, which accounts for about 60 percent of the increase in brain intracellular osmolality in chronically (4 to 7 days) hypernatremic animals. The solute (idiogenic osmoles) begins to appear after several hours of hypernatremia and is as yet uncharacterized. In several different laboratories[179,248-250] a rise in intracellular amino acids (glutamine, alanine, asparate, glutamate) has been observed in the brains of chronically hypernatremic animals and appears to contribute at least in part to the rise in brain osmolality. Similar findings have been reported in hypernatremic brain studied in vitro.[251] Other possible mechanisms might include the disassociation of intracellular protein–salt complexes, the action of hydrolytic enzymes in lysozymes activated by hyperosmolality, or some changes in intracellular metabolism leading to accumulation in brain of other low-molecular-weight substances.[236,252] Thus, it appears that the brain may have adaptive mechanisms not found in other body tissues[253] that serve to defend cellular volume. By the generation of idiogenic osmoles the brain is able to achieve osmotic equilibrium with plasma by internal adaptive mechanisms that serve to minimize the loss of brain water.

In the teleologic sense, it would appear advantageous to maintain a normal cerebral cellular volume in the face of changes in plasma osmolality. Abrupt shrinkage of the brain could lead to tearing of cerebral vessels and meninges, with subsequent subdural hemorrhage, as has been described in patients and animals with acute hypernatremia.[236] Thus, from a clinical standpoint, the ability of the brain to generate idiogenic osmoles to maintain cellular volume intact is beneficial to survival. In this sense, it is of interest that the brains of some vertebrates that live parts of their lives in both saltwater and freshwater environments appear to have the ability to adapt to the changing osmotic environment by altering intracellular amino acid content.[12,13,112]

Mortality

The mortality of chronic hypernatremia in children ranges from 7 percent to 29 percent and is summarized in Figure 21–20. Mortality in children with acute hypernatremia averages 43 percent, and about two-thirds of survivors have neurologic sequelae[160] (Fig. 21–20). Because of associated medical conditions that in themselves carry grave prognoses, it is much more difficult to assess the morbidity and mortality of chronic hypernatremia in adults. Figure 21–23 summarizes the experience in the literature for adults with sustained (over 48 hours) hypernatremia (serum Na^+ >160 mM). When one recalls that included in this table are such serious underlying conditions as resuscitation from cardiac arrest, nonketotic hyperosmolar coma and acute stroke with dehydration, it is not surprising that it is associated with a 60 percent mortality. However, from the experience in children, who generally are without chronic underlying disease, it is highly probable that hypernatremia per se adds considerably to the mortality and morbidity of the underlying condition.

Therapy

Hypernatremia is associated with a significant mortality, both in infants and in elderly persons (Figs. 21–20 and 21–23). The problem is of considerable magnitude in both age groups. In studies from several different medical centers, the reported incidence of severe hypernatremia exceeds one patient per hospital per month in the elderly[25] with a slightly higher incidence in children.[25,160] Despite the magnitude of the problem, there is a paucity of hard data available on the quantitative aspects of severe hypernatremia. It has been shown in patients and experimental animals that hyperosmolality per se is potentially lethal (Figs. 21–20 to 21–23). However, overly rapid treatment of hypernatremia by infusion by hypotonic solutions can cause seizures and cerebral edema, which may also be lethal.[226,228,238,240,242] Furthermore, acute hypernatremia secondary to infusion of either hypertonic NaCl or $NaHCO_3$ can lead to abrupt shrinkage of the brain, with tearing of cerebral vessels and subarachnoid or subdural hemorrhage.[224,226–228,245]

Most investigators agree that patients with hypernatremic dehydration should be treated with fluid that provides free water in excess of electrolytes. In both children and adults, fluid therapy is usually calculated so as to be administered over a period of about 48 hours.[218,221] Despite such recommendations, few data in humans or animals are available as to the ideal rate of fluid administration. Fatal cases of cerebral edema, as well as permanent brain damage, have occurred when hypernatremia was completely corrected within 24 hours,[230,232,242] while seizures with cerebral edema occur in more than 50 percent of hypernatremic rabbits when plasma Na^+ is reduced from 185 to 142 mM in 4 hours.[238] The aforementioned studies highlight the dangers of overly rapid correction of hypernatremia. However, they also point out the sparseness of data pertaining to the rate at which one can safely lower plasma Na^+ in hypernatremic states. Currently accepted

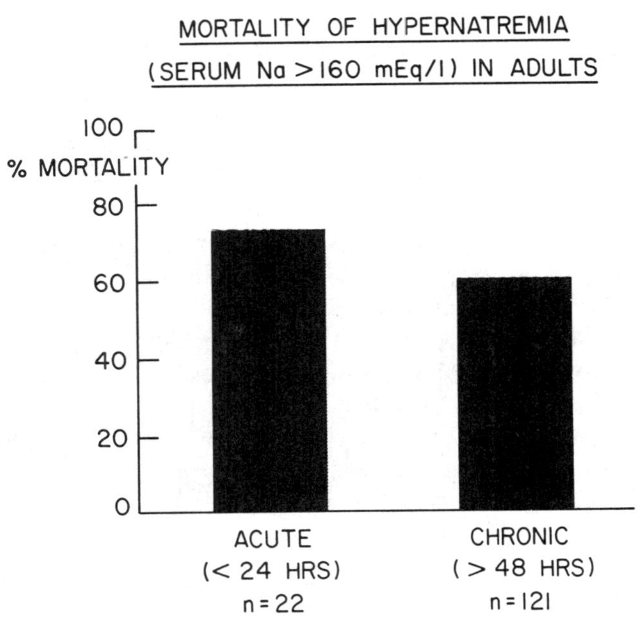

Fig. 21–23. Comparison of published mortality of acute and chronic hypernatremia for adults. When one considers that adults with hypernatremia resulting from such grave conditions as stroke with dehydration, lactic acidosis, resuscitation from cardiac arrest, and hyperglycemic nonketotic coma comprise the bulk of published cases, it is not surprising that eventual mortality is formidable. (From Covey CM, Arieff AI: Disorders of sodium and water metabolism and their effects on the central nervous system. p. 212. In Brenner BM, Stein JH (eds): Contemporary Issues in Nephrology. Vol. 1. Churchill Livingstone, New York, 1978.)

therapeutic regimens for treating hypernatremia in adults or children have recently been reviewed.[160,218,221] On the basis of our present knowledge, recommendations for treatment of chronic hypernatremia in adults, when the hypernatremia is primarily due to water loss, are as follows[160]:

1. If there is evidence of circulatory collapse, the patient should receive initial resuscitation with colloid, such as plasma or a plasma substitute, rapidly enough to correct shock and stabilize the circulatory system.
2. Severe acidosis should be treated. However, because the rapid administration of sodium bicarbonate will aggravate the hypernatremia, under most circumstances moderate acidosis (pH >7.15) should not be corrected immediately. An arterial pH of >7.15 does not appear to depress cardiac output.[254]
3. Fluid deficit should be estimated[160] and the deficit given over a 48-hour period, aiming for a decrement in serum osmolality of approximately 2 mOsm/liter per hr. Maintenance fluids, which include replacement of urinary losses, are given in addition to the deficit.
4. Hypotonic fluid should be administered. In adults, there are few data that would lead one to favor one fluid over another. If the patient has a moderate acidosis, $NaHCO_3$ may be added to the solution, with a proportional reduction in NaCl concentration. The usual replacement fluid will be either 280 mM glucose or 77 mM NaCl.
5. Plasma electrolytes should be monitored at frequent intervals, usually about every 2 hours. It should be stressed that most adult patients with hypernatremia have serious underlying systemic illness, such as stroke, infection, or head trauma. Many such patients appear to die of their underlying illness, rather than of hypernatremia per se. Vigorous attention should be given to the therapy of associated medical conditions, thus reducing morbidity and mortality from the hypernatremia as well.
6. If the hypernatremia is secondary to excessive loss of other body fluids, the replacement fluid should be similar to the fluid actually lost. An estimate of electrolyte concentration of body fluids can be obtained from Table 21–6.

PHOSPHATE DEPLETION

The clinical syndrome of phosphate depletion was originally described in six patients who were either normal or hypothyroid and who had taken magnesium-aluminum hydroxide for up to 130 days. Patients manifested symptoms of weakness, bone pain, anorexia, and malaise concommitant with serum phosphorus of ≤ 1 mg/dl. Symptoms rapidly reversed with phosphate repletion.[255] In a patient with chronic renal failure treated with hemodialysis, $Al(OH)_3$ treatment resulted in a decline of serum phosphorus to 0.7 mg/dl. Symptoms of nausea, depression, emesis, anorexia, and weakness occurred, which improved with elevation of serum phosphorus.[256]

Several review articles have enumerated the multitude of clinical manifestations that may accompany phosphate depletion/hypophosphatemia.[257,258] Similarly, the clinical causes and associations with hypophosphatemia are numerous and varied.[258] Particular organ systems affected by hypophosphatemia include the neuromuscular hematologic (red cells, white cells, and platelets), hepatic, skeletal, muscular, and central nervous system[258] as well as the heart.[259,260] In this section, only the central nervous system manifestations of phosphate depletion are discussed. Other effects of phosphate depletion are discussed in Chapter 12.

Any discussion of the central nervous system effects of phosphate depletion is complicated by the fact that most patients also have multiple abnormalities of electrolytes, nutrition, and acid–base status. In particular, many phosphate-depleted patients also have low plasma levels of sodium, magnesium, calcium, and potassium, in addition to phosphate.

Table 21–6. Electrolyte Content of Body Fluids

Fluid	Na^+ (mEq/liter)	K^+ (mEq/liter)	Cl^- (mEq/liter)	HCO_3^- (mEq/liter)
Plasma				
Mean	140	4.5	102	26
Normal range	137–143	3.5–5.0	98–106	22–30
Saliva				
Mean	33	20	34	—
Normal range	20–46	16–23	24–44	
Gastric juice				
Mean	60	9	84	0
Normal range	30–90	4.3–12	52–124	
Bile				
Mean	149	4.9	101	45
Normal range	120–170	3–12	80–120	30–50
Pancreatic juice				
Mean	141	4.6	77	92
Normal range	113–153	2.6–7.4	54–95	70–110
Small bowel				
Mean	105	5.1	99	50
Normal range	72–158	3.5–6.8	70–127	20–40
Ileal fluid				
Mean	129	11.2	116	29
Normal range	90–140	6–30	82–125	25–30
Cecal fluid				
Mean	80	21	48	22
Normal range	50–116	11–28	35–70	15–30
Cerebrospinal fluid				
Mean	141	2.9	127	23
Normal range	135–147	2.5–3.4	116–132	21–25
Sweat				
Mean	45	4.5	58	0
Normal range	18–97	1–15	18–97	
Aqueous humor				
Mean	143	4.7	108	—
Normal range	142–145	—	106–110	

Source: Reproduced with permission from Arieff AI: Principles of parenteral therapy. p. 567. In Maxwell MH, Kleeman CR (eds): Clinical Disorders of Fluid and Electrolyte Metabolism. © 1972. McGraw-Hill, New York, 1972. Used with the permission of the McGraw-Hill Book Company.

Many are also alcoholic, cachectic, and severely malnourished. The symptoms are similar to those of other metabolic encephalopathies and include weakness, confusion, obtundation, and focal seizures. Coma may occur. This syndrome has been most commonly observed in alcoholic subjects whose serum phosphate was lowered with infusion of glucose and/or amino acids. The interrelationship between symptoms of phosphate depletion and those of other associated electrolyte abnormalities is discussed in Chapter 23.

Clinical Studies

Travis and associates[261] described eight patients who were being treated with glucose/protein solutions intravenously. Hypophosphatemia developed, along with paresthesias and obtundation in some patients. Those with obtundation had marked shifts in the affinity of hemoglobin for oxygen, so that P50 was reduced and tissue oxygen delivery may have been decreased. Those patients with obtundation also had diffuse slowing of the EEG. It has been suggested that many of the clinical manifestations of phosphate depletion may be secondary to decreased blood 2,3-diphosphoglycerate levels, with decreased delivery of oxygen to tissues.[261,262]

Other studies in patients generally report on the effects of acute hypophosphatemia after hyperalimentation. Silvis and Paragas[263] described three starving patients in whom profound hypophosphatemia developed (serum phosphate 0.3 mg/dl) after parenteral hyperalimentation. In all three patients muscular weakness developed; two had seizures and coma and one died. Furlan and associates[264] described two patients with malnutrition associated with chronic gastrointestinal disease. Both were treated with intravenous hyperalimentation, and serum phosphate levels fell below 0.5 mg/dl. Both developed sensory loss, cranial nerve palsies, and respiratory insufficiency secondary to muscular weakness. Both recovered after phosphate repletion.

Animal Studies

Few animal studies have evaluated the effects of phosphate depletion/hypophosphatemia on the central nervous system. In most instances, hypophosphatemia has been achieved by parenteral hyperalimentation, but in two studies effects of dietary phosphate depletion were examined. In those studies dogs were placed on at least 6 weeks of a diet containing virtually no phosphorus but adequate in vitamins, minerals, calories, protein, fat, and carbohydrate. Despite plasma phosphate below 0.8 mg/dl induced by dietary phosphate depletion, no neurologic abnormalities were observed in these dogs.[265,266] Thus, pure hypophosphatemia due to dietary phosphate depletion probably, in and of itself, does not result in neurologic abnormalities.

More revealing have been the effects of acute hypophosphatemia, often combined with starvation/malnutrition. Jacob and coworkers[267] studied dogs that were initially starved (30 percent loss of body weight) and then given intravenous glucose/amino acid solutions such that serum phosphate fell below 0.5 mg/dl in less than 2 days. Many of these dogs developed ataxia and coma, some resulting in death. Brain edema was allegedly observed, with a reported 40 percent increase in brain water. In preliminary studies both in our laboratory and in others, the presence of seizures was confirmed in such animals, but not the brain edema.[266,268] Other abnormalities in these hyperalimented dogs included platelet dysfunction, thrombocytopenia, anemia, infection, and hemorrhage. In an earlier study, Silvis and Paragas[269] found that starved hyperalimented dogs had a mean survival of only 5.4 days with a mean plasma phosphate below 0.5 mg/dl. The mortality was not improved by adding phosphate to the infusion. Derr and Zieve[268] infused starved rats with glucose/amino acid solutions. Coma, seizures, and death occurred in more than one-half the animals that were starved and hyperalimented. Brain edema was never present, and in fact most animals had cerebral dehydration, usually associated with hyperosmolality and hyperglycemia. In those rats in which coma and death resulted, blood glucose exceeded 1100 mg/dl and plasma osmolality exceeded 470 mOsm/liter.

Summary

From the available literature, a neurologic syndrome is associated with hyperalimentation/hypophosphatemia, but probably only in starved/malnourished humans and animals. The exact pathophysiology is unclear, but it may relate to a sequence synthesized by Woods et al.[270] and Farber.[271] Both ATP and inorganic phosphate (P_i) are essential in stabilizing AMP and the total adenine nucleotide content of tissue. They inhibit the enzymes that can cause irreversible degradation of AMP. In phosphate-depleted states, tissue levels of both P_i and ATP are probably diminished. Although not yet studied in brain, this is probably true for red blood cells and heart[256,261,272] and may also be true for brain.[267] ATP inhibits 5-nucleotidase and P_i inhibits AMP deaminase and to some extent, 5-nucleotidase. When inhibition of AMP deaminase is ineffective (due to phosphate depletion), the concentration of inosinic acid (IMP) increases, and both AMP and IMP undergo dephosphorylation with formation of adenosine and inosine, and eventually hypoxanthine, uric acid, and allantoin. Such a sequence could result in tissue necrosis. Infusion of glucose/amino acids to a starved phosphate-depleted animal (or patient) would create a demand for phosphate (for protein synthesis and glucose metabolism) that could not be met. This could lead to the sequence just described in liver, which probably occurs in skeletal muscle as well.[273]

DIABETIC COMA

Coma as a complication of diabetes mellitus, has been described for more than 100 years.[274] In the context that the term coma is usually applied when referring to diabetic patients, the term is a misnomer. Most of these patients do have some depression of sensorium, which usually takes the form of impaired response to verbal or painful stimuli, but many patients are alert and responsive and are therefore not comatose. In the strict sense, one should not diagnose diabetic coma unless there is at least some depression of sensorium, usually to a state of obtundation.[275,276] Obtundation can be defined as a state of dull indifference in which increased stimulation is required to evoke a response.[270] If one excludes stroke, at least four syndromes of metabolic derangements associated with diabetes can be classified as diabetic coma: (1) diabetic ketoacidosis, (2) nonketotic hyperosmolar coma with hyperglycemia (nonketotic coma), (3) hypoglycemia, and (4) lactic acidosis. There is an abundance of clinical descriptions of these entities (see Chapter 20). Although there has been much fruitful investigative work on the biochemical derangements characterizing these clinical entities, the actual cause of coma is not known in any of them.

Diabetic Ketoacidosis

Diabetic ketoacidosis is a metabolic abnormality characterized by hyperglycemia (blood glucose <250 mg/dl) and metabolic acidosis arterial pH <7.25 and/or plasma bicarbonate <16 mM due to hyperketonemia (plasma acetoacetate + β-hydroxybutyrate >7 mmol/liter) (plasma acetest 2 + at a 1:1 dilution), with depression of sensorium to at least a state of obtundation. The disorder is most common among juvenile or growth-onset diabetic patients.

The pathogenesis of diabetic ketoacidosis has been adequately reviewed elsewhere.[277,278-282] Despite more than 100 years of clinical and experimental investigation, the pathogenesis of coma in this disorder has not been elucidated. Several important theories will be briefly reviewed.

KETONEMIA

There have been many suggestions that hyperketonemia per se may be important in the genesis of coma in patients with diabetic ketoacidosis. The only experimental studies that relate to this problem were performed before 1940, and they have not yet been confirmed. It has been reported that in rabbits, infusion of either acetoacetate acid or sodium acetoacetate resulted in coma.[283] Under similar circumstances, infusion of either β-hydroxybutyrate or sodium β-hydroxybutyrate did not result in coma, although some of these animals had unexplained deaths.[283] Infusion of HCl to achieve a similar plasma bicarbonate as was obtained with β-hydroxybutyric acid infusion did not result in coma. These studies suggest that acetoacetate may somehow affect cerebral function in a way such that coma results. Studies by Kety and co-workers[284] in patients with ketoacidosis are somewhat supportive of this concept in that they demonstrate a continuing fall in cerebral utilization of oxygen with increasing plasma ketone levels. Furthermore, the brain can probably metabolize β-hydroxybutyrate to γ-hydroxybutyrate, a substance that acts as an anesthetic agent.[285] Thus, hyperketonemia may impair cerebral oxygen utilization and also have an anesthetic effect, both of which may contribute to depression of sensorium.

METABOLIC ACIDOSIS

Metabolic acidosis is probably not an important cause of coma in ketoacidotic subjects. Acidosis per se is usually not associated with coma in patients with a variety of systemic diseases, such as uremia, cholera,[30,286] and hypercapnia.[287,288] Furthermore, infusion or ingestion of acid (HCl or NH_4Cl) to induce acute metabolic acidemia does not cause coma in laboratory animals[283-287] or human subjects.[30,290]

There has been some evidence suggesting that depression of sensorium correlates not with arterial pH, but rather with the pH of cerebrospinal fluid.[30] However, subsequent investigation has failed to confirm these earlier impressions. There was no apparent relationship between depression of sensorium and pH of cerebrospinal fluid in patients with nonketotic coma,[275] in subjects with cholera who were treated with $NaHCO_3$,[286] or in patients with ketoacidosis who received intravenous $NaHCO_3$.[291,292] In the latter two groups of patients, despite the fact that pH of cerebrospinal fluid fell after administration of intravenous $NaHCO_3$, there was actually an improvement in sensorium. It is thus most likely that intracellular pH of brain, rather than pH of cerebrospinal fluid, actually correlates with depression of sensorium. Since there is a generally poor correlation between pH of cerebrospinal fluid versus brain intracellular pH,[7,31,293-295] especially in metabolic disorders, it may be that in the earlier studies,[30] conditions were such that brain intracellular pH and pH in cerebrospinal fluid had undergone similar changes.

In rats with diabetic ketoacidosis, brain intracellular pH is probably normal, as is lactate concentration.[296,297] The cerebrospinal fluid pH is also usually normal in patients with ketoacidosis.[292,298] Thus, it is unlikely that brain intracellular pH is depressed in ketoacidotic subjects. However, in patients with severe acidemia (pH <7.00), there is probably a decrement in brain intracellular pH. Such cerebral intracellular acidosis can impair the conversion of glucose 6-phosphate to pyruvate by inhibition of phosphofructokinase in brain.[299] Subsequently, Krebs cycle inhibition could then lead to coma.

CEREBRAL HYPOXIA

Hypoxia is a well-known cause of coma.[276] Patients with ketoacidosis have several abnormalities that might theoretically predispose to hypoxia, such as hyperviscosity of the blood[300] and decreased cerebral oxygen consumption.[284] If hypoxia were severe, there could be a fall in brain intracellular pH due to increased brain lactate, as well as a decrease in brain high-energy phosphate compounds. Neither sequence is likely to occur. In animals with ketoacidosis, brain intracellular pH and lactate are probably normal. Total brain adenine nucleotides are also normal.[296,297] If the action of Na^+–K^+-ATPase in brain were impaired, there should be increases in brain Na^+ and decreases in K^+. Preliminary studies in animals do not support this hypothesis. Thus, at the present time there are no data to support an important role for cerebral hypoxia in the pathogenesis of coma associated with ketoacidosis.

HYPEROSMOLALITY

It has been demonstrated that hyperosmolality per se can induce coma in laboratory animals,[248] and extracellular hyperosmolality is probably an important cause of coma in ketoacidotic patients. Other factors may be equally important. Many patients with high plasma osmolality are alert, while those with lower levels of extracellular osmolality may be comatose.[301] In both patients and laboratory animals, it appears that plasma osmolality must exceed 340 mOsm/kg before there is depression of sensorium.[248,275,298] In 438 ketoacidotic patients with coma, the mean plasma osmolality was only 322 mOsm/kg.[302] Overall, however, there is a significant correlation between depression of sensorium and extracellular osmolality (Fig. 21–24). Thus, hyperosmolality probably contributes to depression of sensorium at levels in excess of 340 mOsm/kg,[29] but it is not the only factor.

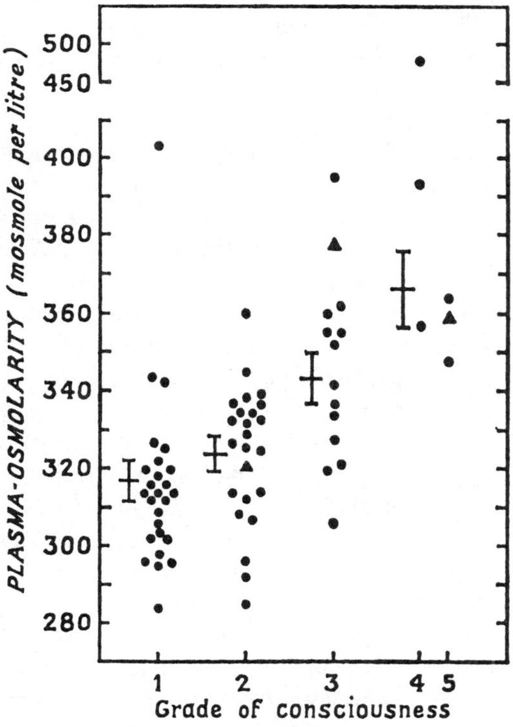

Fig. 21–24. Relationship between state of consciousness and plasma osmolality (calculated) in 70 patients with diabetic ketoacidosis. Increasing numbers on abscissa denote increasing depression of sensorium. (From Fulop M, Tannenbaum H, Dreyer N: Ketotic hyperosmolar coma. Lancet 2:635, 1973.)

OTHER FACTORS

Intravascular deposition of fibrin has been demonstrated in brains of some patients dying with ketoacidotic coma. The fibrin deposition was associated with ischemic tissue damage.[303] Studies of the coagulation system in these patients demonstrated thrombocytopenia with advanced elevated plasma fibrinogen levels. The hypothesis has been put forth that cerebral intravascular coagulation, by occluding small vessels and producing local ischemia, may play a major role in production of coma in ketoacidotic patients. However, such cerebral intravascular fibrin deposition[304] is probably not a major or consistent abnormality. In all probability, coma in diabetic ketoacidosis is caused by a number of factors acting in combination. There is hyperviscosity of the blood and impaired cerebral oxygen utilization. The brain probably sustains some direct effect of acetoacetate, and perhaps of β-hydroxybutyrate as well, which tends to produce coma. During diabetic ketoacidosis, about one-half of the brain's source of energy may come from ketones, hence ketone metabolites probably accumulate in the brain. It also may be that certain metabolites of glucose (fructose 6-phosphate, glocuse 6-phosphate, citrate, acetyl-CoA), which accumulate in the brain of ketoacidotic animals, manifest central nervous system toxicity. Hyperosmolality is present to varying degrees in all patients with diabetic ketoacidosis, and may play some role in depression of sensorium. Disseminated intravascular coagulation appears to be present in some patients with diabetic ketoacidosis. Such a coagulopathy could result in localized areas of cerebral hypoperfusion, which may accelerate depression of sensorium. Finally, many patients with diabetic ketoacidosis have severe associated medical conditions, such as sepsis, myocardial infarction, and pneumonia. These diseases may in themselves lead to depression of sensorium. The multiplicity of factors undoubtedly accounts for the fact that no single variable, such as arterial pH, plasma ketone levels, pH of cerebrospinal fluid or blood glucose concentration can consistently be correlated with depression of sensorium. The best correlation is still that with plasma osmolality.

Nonketotic Coma

Rather than being two distinct entities, diabetic ketoacidosis and nonketotic coma actually represent a continuum, with many patients having biochemical characteristics of both. However, in most patients the primary problem is either hyperosmolality with dehydration or metabolic acidemia. Nonketotic hyperosmolar coma with hyperglycemia (nonketotic coma) is characterized by hyperglycemia (plasma glucose >600 mg/dl) and hyperosmolality (plasma osmolality >350 mOsm/kg) without significant ketonemia (plasma acetest below 2+ at a 1:1 dilution) with depression of sensorium to at least a stupor.[305] The pathogenesis of nonketotic coma has been extensively studied; in all probability it represents a heterogeneous entity. There is interplay between free fatty acid mobilization and metabolism, insulin secretion, growth hormone, dehydration, and hyperosmolality. These various pathogenetic features have been discussed elsewhere,[277,302,305] (see Chapter 20).

NEUROLOGIC MANIFESTATIONS

Neurologic manifestations are prominent in patients with nonketotic coma. About 36 percent of patients are diagnosed initially as having an acute stroke,[305] with about 27 percent exhibiting either hemiparesis or Babinski sign. About 0 to 15 percent of patients with nonketotic coma present with seizures.[305-309] The seizures are usually of a focal nature, although some grand mal seizures and myoclonus are frequent,[306,307,309] as are other focal neurologic findings. The seizures are often resistant to conventional anticonvulsant therapy.[307,308]

Focal neurologic changes have included aphasia, homonymous hemianopsia, hemisensory defects, hemiparesis, hyperreflexia, and both simple and complex visual hallucinations. In general, most of the aforementioned changes are reversible after correction of the metabolic abnormalities. Evidence of brainstem dysfunction in the form of the tonic eye deviation and nystagmus has also been reported, suggesting at least occasional involvement of the vestibular system. A variety of autonomic nervous system changes, such as hyperpnea and hypertension, may also be observed. This variety of neurologic changes in patients with nonketotic coma cannot be explained by a single structural lesion, but rather appears to represent a widespread functional disturbance that may affect any level of the nervous system.[306,309]

The multiplicity of neurologic involvement often suggests the presence of acute cerebral parenchymal damage, but CT scans, cerebral angiography, and neuropathologic examinations usually fail to disclose structural abnormalities that correlate with the clinical observations. Furthermore, in surviving patients, the prompt resolution of the neurologic deficit without presistent sequelae suggests that acute vascular accidents or other structural lesions are an unlikely explanation for the clinical findings. The mean age of patients presenting with nonketotic coma is about 62 years, and many have some sort of preceding cerebrovascular abnormality. It is possible that localized areas of vascular insufficiency may render certain neuronal groups more sensitive to the metabolic changes of nonketotic coma, resulting in transient functional neurologic changes. A similar phenomenon has been observed in experimental animals allowed to recover from hemiparesis induced by unilateral cerebral artery ligation.[310] When acute hyperosmolality is induced in these animals, there is the reappearance of neurologic deficits which correspond functionally to the anatomic areas of the brain previously subjected to the acute vascular insult.

SEIZURE ACTIVITY AND BIOCHEMICAL CHANGES

The mechanisms by which hyperosmolality may induce neuronal discharges leading to seizure activity are not well known. In the clinical situation, seizure activity is very rare in ketoacidotic patients[301] but is present in about 15 percent of those patients with nonketotic coma.[30,306] Thus, hyperketonemia may in some manner suppress the effects of hyperosmolality on the central nervous system. In both ketoacidosis and nonketotic coma, there is probably some suppression of Krebs cycle activity in the brain. In ketoacidosis in the rat, there is accumulation of citrate in the brain.[296] In addition, hyperosmolality per se can inhibit Krebs cycle activity.[29] With Krebs cycle inhibition, the energy supply of the brain may be met, at least in part, by metabolism of ketones, lactate, glutamate, and perhaps other amino acids as well.[311,312] In particular, γ-aminobutyric acid (GABA) is found in high concentrations only in nervous tissue.[313,314] GABA has been shown to be a cortical depressant, raising the seizure threshold.[315] In the brain, GABA can be metabolized to succinate via the GABA shunt, which is an alternative to the Krebs cycle for the conversion of α-ketoglutarate to succinate.[316] The GABA shunt can provide up to 40 percent of the brain's energy requirement under certain circumstances.[316] Thus, in patients with nonketotic coma, it may be that increased metabolism of GABA lowers the seizure threshold.[317] Conversely, in ketoacidotic animals, brain tissue levels of GABA are normal,[318] which may account in part for the absence of seizures.

EFFECTS OF HYPERGLYCEMIA ON THE BRAIN

Depression of sensorium in patients with either ketoacidosis or nonketotic coma has been found to correlate with extracellular hyperosmolality (Figs. 21–24 and 21–25), but not with hyperglycemia, or with pH of either blood or cerebrospinal fluid.[275,291,292,298] The mechanisms by which hyperosmolality can induce coma are unclear. There is a general impression that hyperglycemia, as is the case with some acute hyperosmolar states,[248] should cause cerebral dehydration. However, evidence both in patients and in laboratory animals with hyperglycemia suggests that this is not the case. Patients dying with nonketotic coma have not been reported to show evidence of cerebral dehydration. In fact, among 14 patients who died with nonketotic coma, postmortem examination of the brain showed no evidence of cerebral dehydration,[305,319–325] and several had cerebral edema.[319,323,324]

IDIOGENIC OSMOLES

In laboratory animals, rapid elevation of plasma glucose by infusion of 2.87 M glucose (1 ml/min) caused cerebral dehydration and death in 60 to 90 minutes.[325] However, when plasma glucose in rabbits is elevated to ~61 mM (1100 mg/dl) in 1 hour, the sequence of events in brain is different.[19] After 1 to 2 hours of hyperglycemia, there is an initial decrease in brain water content (Fig. 21–26). However, when plasma glucose is then maintained at ~1100 mg/dl for 4 to 6 hours, brain water content returns to normal values. By comparison, under similar circumstances skeletal muscle water content falls significantly after 2 hours and remains depressed (Fig. 21–26). The secondary increase of brain water to normal values is accompanied by an increase in brain osmole content such that brain and plasma osmolality are similar. This increase in brain osmole content is only partially accounted for by changes in brain content of measured solute-glucose, lactate, sorbitol, myosinitol, urea, Na^+, K^+, or Cl^-—the remainder consisting of idiogenic osmoles (Fig. 21–27).

The generation of idiogenic osmoles during hyperglycemia thus enables the brain to

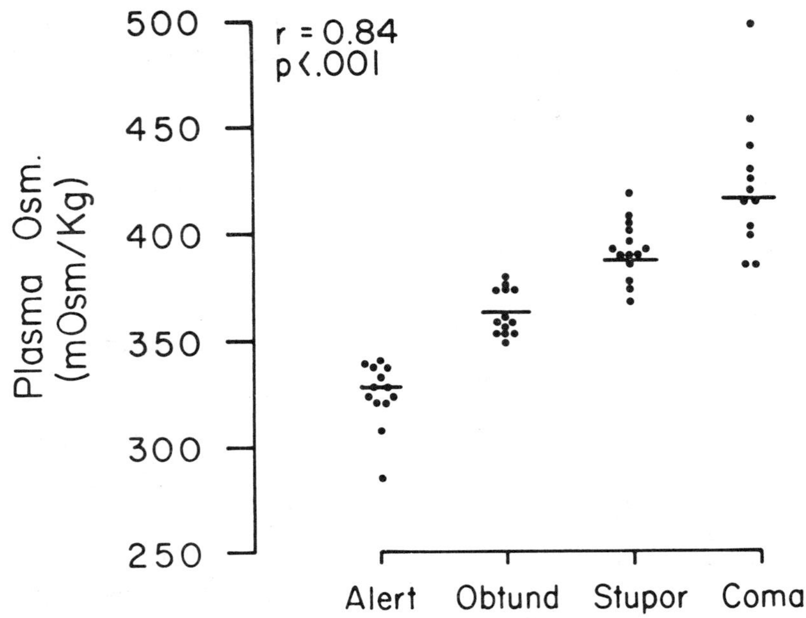

Fig. 21–25. Relationship between depression of sensorium and plasma osmolality (Osm) is 53 patients with blood glucose >600 mg/dl, but without ketoacidosis. In calculating the correlation coefficient *r*, alertness was counted as 1, obtundation (obtund) as 2, stupor as 3, and coma as 4. For each group, plasma osmolality is significantly different from that of the adjacent group(s) $p < 0.01$. (From Arieff AI, Carroll HJ: Cerebral edema and depression of sensorium in nonketotic hyperosmolar coma. Diabetes 23:525, 1974. Reproduced with permission from the American Diabetes Association, Inc.)

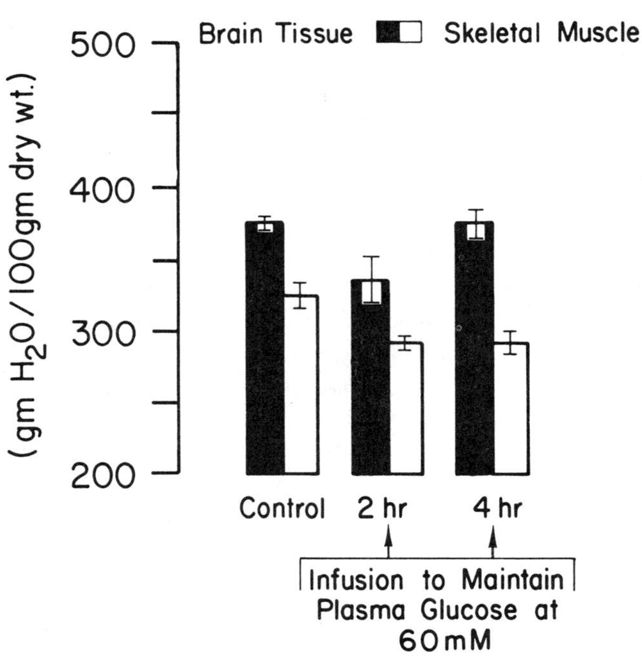

Fig. 21–26. Brain and muscle water content. After 2 hours of hyperglycemia, there is a loss of about 10 percent in both brain and muscle water content. After 4 hours of hyperglycemia, the brain water content is the same as in controls, but muscle water content remains low. (From Guisado R, Arieff AI: Neurological manifestations of diabetic comas: Correlation with biochemical alterations in the brain. Metabolism 24:665, 1975. © 1975 The Williams and Wilkins Co., Baltimore.)

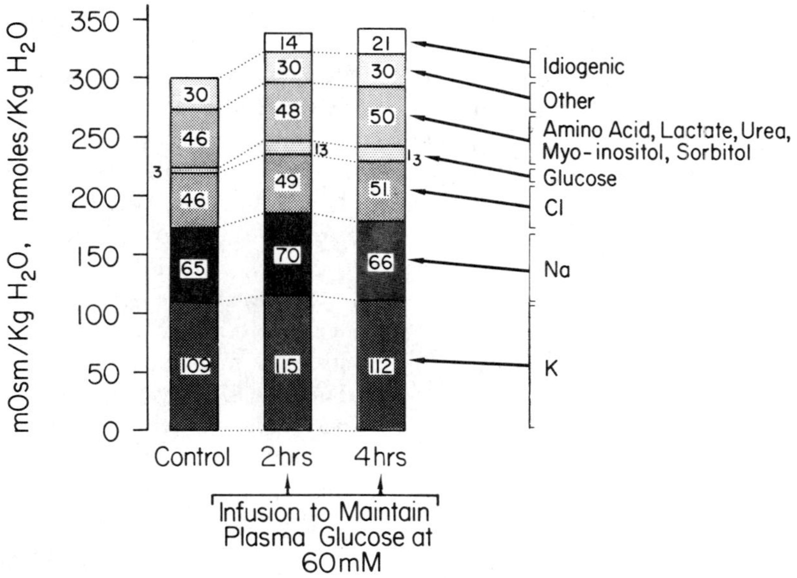

Fig. 21–27. Comparison of effects on brain solute composition of 1 to 4 hours of hyperglycemia. After 1 hour of glucose infusion, virtually all the increase in brain solute is due to increase in concentration of glucose and electrolytes. After 2 to 4 hours of hyperglycemia, about one-half the increase in brain solute is due to presence of undetermined solute. (From Arieff AI, Guisado R, Lazarowitz VC: Pathophysiology of hyperosmolar states. p. 227. In Disturbances in Body Fluid Osmolality. American Physiological Society, Bethesda, Md., 1977.)

achieve osmotic equilibrium with plasma despite a lesser loss of water and/or gain in solute than would be expected if the brain were a more perfect osmometer. Such a mechanism is probably homeostatic, permitting the brain to maintain its intracellular volume and inorganic solute concentration within the normal range at a time when plasma osmolality is markedly elevated. In animals with experimental nonketotic coma, generation of idiogenic osmoles by brain appears to be a response to hyperglycemia rather than to hyperosmolality per se. When plasma osmolality is elevated to similar levels (~350 mOsm/kg) over a 4- to 6-hour period by infusion of either mannitol or glycerol,[326,327] essentially all of the increase in brain osmolality is due to loss of water by brain, with a subsequent increase in brain concentration of Na^+, K^+, and Cl^-. The identity of the idiogenic osmoles in brain has not been established at this time.

OTHER BIOCHEMICAL CHANGES IN BRAIN

Several possible explanations have been advanced to explain the adaptive processes of the brain to hyperglycemia. Some have suggested that the brain might synthesize fructose, sorbitol, or myosinitol in quantities such that brain intracellular osmolality would be increased by levels similar to that of plasma.[328,329] Other workers have suggested that glucose might enter brain cells to achieve intracellular concentrations of sufficient magnitude to equalize plasma and brain osmolalities.[323] However, these theories have not been validated by experimental evidence. During hyperglycemic states in laboratory animals, brain glucose concentration has been only about 20 to 30 percent that of plasma glucose.[19] The theories concerning possible generation of fructose, myosinitol, or sorbitol by brain were based on findings of increased levels of sorbitol in cerebrospinal fluid during hyperglycemic states. However, during hyperglycemic states in laboratory animals, sorbitol in brain has never been present in osmotically significant amounts.[19,309]

OSMOTIC ADAPTATION

Although the identity of the idiogenic osmoles in brain is unknown, they may represent changes in the intracellular binding of cations (Na^+ and K^+). At least 20 percent of brain K^+ and Na^+ are normally nonexchangeable[5] and thus probably osmotically inactive. Various types of osmotic stress can alter the brain intracellular binding of Na^+ and K^+ in vitro.[9] Also hyperosmolality induced by intravenous infusion of NaCl decreases the amount of bound Na^+ and K^+ in brain[248] in vivo. Although the effects of brain have not yet been directly evaluated, an intracellular acidosis can increase cellular osmolality in other cells, such as red blood cells,[33] by displacement of bound K^+ ion with H^+ ion. Such a phenomenon may occur in cerebral cortex as well.

Thus, the adaptation of brain to hyperglycemic states depends on the interaction of several factors that may occur within the brain, including dehydration, some gain in measured solute, and generation of idiogenic osmoles. The net effect on brain volume will be based on the rapidity, duration, and degree of the hyperglycemia, as well as various characteristics of individual patients.

EFFECTS OF ACUTE RESPIRATORY DISTURBANCES

The clinical manifestations of acute respiratory disorders have been well described in Chapters 8 and 23. It is well known that respiratory alkalosis, acidosis and hypoxia all can have profound effects on the central nervous system.

Respiratory Acidosis

Respiratory acidosis is frequently associated with depression of sensorium as manifested by lethargy, stupor, or obtundation.[331] Coma may supervene with substantial degrees of CO_2 retention (arterial P_{CO_2} >60 mm Hg). The quantification of symptoms that are referable to CO_2 retention is complicated by the fact that "pure" hypercapnia is rare without concomitant hypoxia. Patients with chronic obstructive pulmonary disease or bronchial asthma usually have hypoxia when they are hypercapnic. Nonetheless, by examining separately the effects on the central nervous system of hypoxia and hypercapnia, it should be possible to ascertain some of the effects of each.

With the induction of acute hypercapnia (P_{CO_2}, 80 to 90 mm Hg) without hypoxia (arterial P_{O_2} >70 mm Hg), there are similar decrements in pH of both arterial blood and cerebrospinal fluid.[31,332] There is thus no barrier to the penetration of CO_2 into the cerebrospinal fluid.[31] However, largely because of an increase in cerebral blood flow, the P_{CO_2} in cerebrospinal fluid will rise relatively less than arterial P_{CO_2}, resulting in a smaller decline of pH in cerebrospinal fluid.[333] Within 1 hour after the P_{CO_2} is elevated, there is a gradual rise in the bicarbonate concentration in cerebrospinal fluid, such that pH of cerebrospinal fluid begins to rise toward normal values. These changes precede any alterations in arterial bicarbonate concentration. After 3 hours with arterial P_{CO_2} maintained >80 mm Hg, the cerebrospinal fluid bicarbonate has risen (in the dog) by ~5 mM. However, after 6 hours of hypercapnia, the pH of cerebrospinal fluid is still significantly below normal values.[31,334] After 1 day of hypercapnia, pH in cerebrospinal fluid is normal, while cerebrospinal fluid bicarbonate is 35 mM, which is significantly above normal. However, arterial pH is still acidotic, demonstrating the lag between systemic compensation by the kidneys versus cerebrospinal fluid compensatory via transport across the choroid plexus.[334] The renal compensatory mechanisms for respiratory acidosis are discussed in Chapter 8. The increased bicarbonate concentration in cerebrospinal fluid is secreted by the choroid plexus. Although it is not entirely clear whether hypercapnia or cerebrospinal fluid acidemia is the stimulus for increased secretion of bicarbonate, it is clear that bicarbonate is formed at the choroid plexus and transported against a concentration gradient into the cerebrospinal fluid. The process is carbonic anhydrase dependent and can be largely blocked by the action of acetazolamide.[31]

The compensatory mechanisms of brain in animals with acute respiratory acidosis are more rapid than those in blood or cerebrospinal fluid. With acute hypercapnia (P_{CO_2}, 80 to 90 mm Hg) in the dog, arterial pH falls from 7.36 to 7.07 in 1 hour while the simultaneously measured pH_i in brain (cerebral cortex) is 6.90, as compared with a normal value of 7.06. However, after only 30 to 60 minutes of hypercapnia, the calculated cerebral cortex bicarbonate concentration has increased to 57 percent above the normal value.[7,335] After 3 hours of hypercapnia, with no change in arterial pH, brain pH_i has returned to normal values. The brain bicarbonate is now 24.4 mEq/kg H_2O (normal value 11.3 mEq/kg H_2O). Within 3 hours with both arterial and cerebrospinal fluid P_{CO_2} maintained at ~85 mm Hg, brain was able to normalize its pH_i by generating bicarbonate.

The means by which the brain restores its pH_i to normal during respiratory acidosis are complex. There is substantial generation of bicarbonate in brain, most of which takes place within the first 30 minutes.[335] The mechanisms by which the brain generates bicarbonate are unclear, although they are probably not secondary to the action of carbonic anhydrase, as acetazolamide does not block brain bicarbonate generation.[336] There are, however, several other means by which the brain might generate bicarbonate. Numerous reactions of the brain produce CO_2, particularly those involving decarboxylation. There could be direct hydroxylation of gaseous CO_2 to bicarbonate, as occurs in some elasmobranch fish.[337] Other CO_2-producing reactions in brain include metabolism of glucose via the Krebs (tricarboxylic acid) cycle and conversion of glutamic acid to γ-aminobutyric acid.[339] Furthermore, most of these reactions are intimately linked to glucose metabolism, since glutamic acid is produced via the Krebs cycle, and pyruvate, a product of the metabolism of glucose via the Embden–Meyehof pathway (glycolysis), is a precursor of most amino acids found in brain. Several steps in the metabolism of glucose are pH dependent, and it is quite possible that intracellular acidosis might shift equilibria to favor certain CO_2-producing reactions.[338]

There also appears to be a fixed amount of nonbicarbonate buffer in brain, which is equivalent to ~33 mmole buffer per kilogram brain tissue.[340] After the initial 2 to 3 hours of hypercapnia, there is a marked upward shift in the brain CO_2 dissociation curve,[334] so that brain buffering capacity increases with increasing P_{CO_2}. There is also probably increased conversion of glutamic acid to α-ketoglutamic acid, with liberation of NH_3.[341] The metabolism of glutamic acid could remove a potential source of H^+ ion, while increased production of NH_3 could buffer additional H^+ ion by conversion to NH_4^+.[341] Thus, buffering by the brain in respiratory acidosis is the result of many complex interacting factors.

Respiratory Alkalosis

Respiratory alkalosis is frequently observed in patients with several systemic disease states, which include bronchial asthma, hepatic cirrhosis, salicylate intoxication, hypoxia, sepsis, and certain lesions of the brain. In these conditions, the related symptoms are usually those of the underlying disorder rather than of the alkalosis per se. Modest acute respiratory alkalosis may be accompanied by only mild symptoms, such as paresthesias and dizziness. However, more severe alkalosis (pH, 7.52 to 7.65) in patients with respiratory insufficiency and hypoxia can result in a symptom complex of hypotension, seizures, asterixis, myoclonus, and coma.[342]

The arterial P_{CO_2} is one of the primary regulators of cerebral blood flow,[343] but there is also an effect of brain extracellular pH.[344] Hypocapnia is a potential cerebral vasoconstrictor. This effect is utilized clinically during anesthesia, where hyperventilation (to induce hypocapnia) can effectively decrease intracranial volume and relieve cerebral swelling.[345] By contrast, both hypercapnia and hypoxia are potent cerebral vasodilators.[344]

With acute hypocapnia in experimental animals, there is an initial rise in the brain pH.[7,36,340,346] Almost immediately, there is a decline in brain bicarbonate concentration concomitant with a rise in brain concentration of lactate.[7,36,347,348] Within 2 hours, with arterial P_{CO_2} maintained <20 mm Hg brain pH_i has returned to control values. The return of brain pH_i to normal occurs concomitant with the fall of brain bicarbonate, which in turn is almost stoichiometric with the increase in lactate.[7,36,340,342,347] There is also a rise of lactate and fall in bicarbonate in cerebrospinal fluid, but the cerebrospinal fluid lactate is not high enough to account for the observed decline in cerebrospinal fluid bicarbonate.[7,349,350]

In addition to the rise in brain lactate, there is also a change in the brain CO_2 dissociation curve[334,346] such that brain buffering capacity is decreased. There is probably a significant decrement in brain concentration of ATP and ADP, but not of phosphocreatine.[36,347] The decrease in brain buffering capacity did not relate with the finding that there were no alterations in brain concentration of glutamic acid, glutamine, or NH_3.[332] Thus, although brain buffering capacity is decreased during hypocapnia, the biochemical mechanisms are not known.

Therefore, within 2 hours of the onset of respiratory alkalosis, the brain, after an initial rise in pH_i, has restored its pH_i to normal. This is accomplished primarily by cerebral vasoconstriction, leading to a reduction in cerebral blood flow and increased anaerobic metabolism,[344,351] with an increase in brain lactate, and eventually to a fall in brain bicarbonate.[7,36,340,347] The aforementioned sequence appears to represent the brain's primary response to acute respiratory alkalosis.

EFFECTS OF ACUTE METABOLIC ACID–BASE DISTURBANCES

In contrast to respiratory abnormalities, relatively little investigation has been carried out on the effects of metabolic disorders of acid–base metabolism on the central nervous system.

Metabolic Acidosis

Metabolic acidosis has been induced in laboratory animals by means of HCl or NH_4Cl infusion.[352,353] In some animals, with an arterial pH of 7.06 and plasma bicarbonate of 6 mM, the brain pH_i fell by 0.29 pH units, with no change in the brain extracellular space.[353] In other studies, however, metabolic acidosis in rats (NH_4Cl injection; arterial pH 7.31) had no effect on brain pH_i or bicarbonate concentration.[80] In rats with diabetic ketoacidosis (plasma ketones 9.5 mmol/liter), there was no change in brain pH_i.[296] Thus, it appears that metabolic acidosis has a small and inconsistent effect on brain pH_i.

Metabolic Alkalosis

Metabolic alkalosis has been produced in hypocapnic rats and dogs by the infusion of $NaHCO_3$.[352-354] In rats with arterial pH of 7.80 (P_{CO_2} 16 mm Hg; bicarbonate 25 mM), there were increases in brain lactate and pyruvate concentrations, with an increase in the lactate:pyruvate ratio from 16 to 24.[354] There was no significant change in brain pH_i as compared with normal values. In normocapnic dogs and rats, when arterial pH was raised to 7.52 to 7.71 by $NaHCO_3$ infusion (plasma bicarbonate 34 mM), there was no significant change in brain ATP, ADP, AMP, or phosphocreatine.[343] Therefore, in experimental animals, sustained metabolic alkalosis (arterial pH of 7.52 to 7.80) has essentially no effect on brain pH_i, there is only a minimal rise in brain lactate concentration, and there is no obvious change in brain bicarbonate.[352-354]

ACKNOWLEDGMENTS

This work was supported by grants AM-28127 and AM-18350 from the Public Health Service, National Institutes of Health; by a grant from the Kroc Foundation; and by the Research Service of the Veterans Administration. The studies cited were done in colaboration with the following: C. R. Kleeman, A. Kerian, G. Guisado, V. C. Lazarowitz, S. G. Massry, F. Llach, J. Cooper, C. Covey, M. Cogan, R. Park, C. Mahoney, G. Dubois, W. Leach, P. Sarnacki, and C. Fraser.

The support of Doctors T. Reed, J. Kirsch, D. Newman, M. Taylor, M. Papadakis, and M. Carmichael is gratefully acknowledged.

REFERENCES

1. Levy DE, Bates D, Caronna JJ, et al: Prognosis in nontraumatic coma. Ann Intern Med 94:293, 1981
2. Arieff AI, Friedman EA: Coma following non-narcotic drug overdosage: Management of 208 adult patients. Am J Med Sci 266:405, 1973
3. Bartholomew LG, Scholz DA: Reversible postoperative neurological symptoms: Report of five cases secondary to water intoxication and sodium depletion. JAMA 162:22, 1956
4. Dubois GD, Arieff AI: Symptomatic hyponatremia: The case for rapid correction. In Narins R (ed): Controversies in Nephrology and Hypertension. Churchill Livingstone, New York, 1984
5. Katzman R, Pappius HM: Brain ions. p. 111. In Brain Electrolytes and Fluid Metabolism. Williams & Wilkins, Baltimore, 1973
6. Tower TB: Inorganic constituents. p. 1. In Lajtha A (ed): Handbook of Neurochemistry. I. Chemical Architecture of the Nervous System. Plenum Press, New York, 1969
7. Arieff AI, Kerian SG, Massry SG, et al: Intracellular pH of brain: Alterations in acute respiratory acidosis and alkalosis. Am J Physiol 230:804, 1976
8. Smythe WR, Alfrey AC, Craswell PW, et al: Trace element abnormalities in chronic uremia. Ann Intern Med 96:302, 1982
9. Hanig RC, Aprison MH: Determination of calcium, copper, iron, magnesium, manganese, potassium, zinc and chloride in several brain areas. Anal Biochem 21:169, 1967
10. Alfrey AC, LeGendre GR, Kaehny WD: The dialysis encephalopathy syndrome: Possible aluminum intoxication. N Engl J Med 294:184, 1976
11. Bessman SP: Osmotic implications of changes in metabolic intermediates in the brain. Proc Am Soc Neurochem 7:103, 1976
12. Florkin M, Schoffeniels E: Isosmotic intracellular regulation. p. 89. In Florkin M, Schoffeniels E (eds): Molecular Approaches to Ecology. Academic Press, New York, 1969
13. Forster RP, Goldstein L: Intracellular osmoregulatory role of amino acids and urea in marine elasmobranchs. Am J Physiol 230:925, 1976
14. Mahoney CA, Arieff AI: Central and peripheral nervous system effects of chronic renal failure. Kidney Int 24:170, 1983
15. Rapoport SI: Permeability and osmotic properties of the blood brain barrier: Osmotic edema. p. 118. In Rapoport S (ed): Blood Brain Barrier in Physiology and Medicine. Raven Press, New York, 1976
16. Carroll HJ, Gotterer R, Altshuler B: Exchangeable sodium, body potassium, and body water in previously edematous cardiac patients; evidence for osmotic inactivation of cation. Circulation 32:185, 1965
17. Welt LG, Orloff DM, Kydd DM, et al: An example of cellular hyperosmolarity. J Clin Invest 29:935, 1950
18. Elkinton JR, Winkler AE, Danowski TS: Inactive cell base and the measurement of changes in cell water. Yale J Biol Med 17:383, 1944
19. Arieff AI, Kleeman CR: Studies on mecha-

nisms of cerebral edema in diabetic comas: Effects of hyperglycemia and rapid lowering of plasma glucose in normal rabbits. J Clin Invest 52:571, 1973

20. Finberg L, Luttrell C, Redd H: Pathogenesis of lesions in the nervous system in hypernatremic states: Experimental studies of gross anatomic changes and alterations of chemical composition of the tissues. Pediatrics 23:46, 1959
21. McDowell ME, Wolf AV, Steer A: Osmotic volumes of distribution: Idiogenic changes in osmotic pressure associated with administration of hypertonic solutions. Am J Physiol 180:545, 1955
22. Appelboom JWT, Brodsky WA, Tuttle WS, et al: The freezing point depression of mammalian tissues after sudden heating in boiling distilled water. J Gen Physiol 41:1153, 1958
23. Arieff AI, Kleeman A, Keushkerian A, et al: Brain tissue osmolality: Method of determination and variations in hyper- and hypo osmolar states. J Lab Clin Med 79:334, 1972
24. Maffly RH, Leaf A: The potential of water in mammalian tissues. J Gen Physiol 42:1257, 1959
25. Arieff AI, Guisado R: Effects on the central nervous system of hypernatremic and hypotremic states. Kidney Int 10:104, 1976
26. Kregenow FM: The response of erythrocytes to hypertonic media. J Gen Physiol 58:396, 1971
27. Baxter CF, Thurston JH, Arieff AI, et al: Organic molecules in the osmotic regulation of nervous tissue. Proc Am Soc Neurochem 7:14, 1976
28. Dodge PR, Sotos JF, Gomstrop I, et al: Neurophysiologic disturbances in hypertonic dehydration. Trans Am Neurol Assoc 87:33, 1962
29. Sotos JF, Dodge PR, Meara P, et al: Studies in experimental hypertonicity. I. Pathogenesis of the clinical syndrome, biochemical abnormalities and cause of death. Pediatrics 26:925, 1960
30. Posner JB, Plum F: Spinal fluid pH and neurologic symptoms in systemic acidosis. N Engl J Med 277:605, 1967
31. Katzman R, Pappius HM: Acid–base balance in the cerebrospinal fluid. p. 224. In Katzman R, Pappius HM (eds): Brain Electrolytes and Fluid Metabolism. Williams & Wilkins, Baltimore, 1973
32. Davson H: The cerebrospinal fluid. p. 714. In Davson H (ed): A Textbook of General Physiology. 4th Ed. Williams & Wilkins, Baltimore, 1970
33. Lee JE, Posner JB, Plum F: Buffering capacity of cerebrospinal fluid in acute respiratory acidosis in dogs. Am J Physiol 217:1035, 1969
34. Plum F, Posner JB: Blood and cerebrospinal fluid lactate during hyperventilation. Am J Physiol 212:864, 1967
35. Wichser J, Kazemi H: CSF Bicarbonate regulation in respiratory acidosis and alkalosis. J Appl Physiol 38:504, 1975
36. Pelligrino DA, Musch TI, Dempsey JA: Interregional differences in brain intracellular pH and water compartmentation during acute normoxic and hypoxic hypocapnia in the anesthetized dog. Brain Res 214:387, 1981
37. Hornbein TF, Pavlin EG: Distribution of H^+ and HCO_3^- between CSF and blood during respiratory alkalosis in dogs. Am J Physiol 228:1149, 1975
38. Pavlin EG, Hornbein TF: Distribution of H^+ and HCO_3^- between CSF and blood during respiratory acidosis in dogs. Am J Physiol 228:1145, 1975
39. Park R, Leach W, Arieff AI: Determination of the liver intracellular pH in vivo and its homeostasis in acute acidosis and alkalosis. Am J Physiol 236:F240, 1979
40. Waddell WJ, Butler TC: Calculation of intracellular pH from the distribution of 5, 5-dimethyl-2, 4-oxazolidinedione (DMO). Application to skeletal muscle of the dog. J Clin Invest 38:720, 1959
41. Katzman R, Pappius HM: Cerebrospinal fluid ions. p. 75. In Katzman R, Pappius HM (eds): Brain Electrolytes and Fluid Metabolism. Williams & Wilkins, Baltimore, 1973
42. Bradbury MWB, Kleeman CR: Stability of the potassium concentrations of cerebrospinal fluid and brain. Am J Physiol 213:519, 1967
43. Ames A, Sakanoue M, Endo S: Na, K, Ca, Mg, and Cl concentrations in choroid plexus fluid and cisternal fluid compared with

plasma ultrafiltrate. J Neurophysiol 27:672, 1964
44. Held D, Fencl V, Papenheimer JR: Electrical potential of cerebrospinal fluid. J Neurophysiol 27:942, 1964
45. Arieff AI, Massry SG: Calcium metabolism of brain in acute renal failure: Effects of uremia, hemodialysis and parathyroid hormone. J Clin Invest 53:387, 1974
46. Guisado R, Arieff AI, Massry SG: Changes in electroencephalograms in acute uremia: Effects of parathyroid hormone and brain electrolytes. J Clin Invest 55:738, 1975
47. Oppelt WW, MacIntyre I, Rall DR: Magnesium exchange between blood and cerebrospinal fluid. Am J Physiol 205:959, 1963
48. Bradbury MWB, Kleeman CR, Bagdoyan H, et al: The calcium and magnesium content of skeletal muscle, brain, and cerebrospinal fluid as determined by atomic absorption flame photometry. J Lab Clin Med 71:884, 1968
49. Woodbury J, Lyons K, Carretta R, et al: Fluid and serum levels of magnesium zinc, and calcium in man. Neurology (NY) 18:700, 1968
50. Davson H: The extracellular space of brain and cord. p. 107. In Davson H (ed): Physiology of the Cerebrospinal Fluid. J & A Churchill, London, 1968
51. Katzman R, Pappius HM: Fluid compartments. p. 33. In Katzman R, Pappius HM (eds): Brain Electrolytes and Fluid Metabolism. Williams & Wilkins, Baltimore, 1973
52. Brightman MW, Shivers RR, Prescott L: Morphology of the walls around fluid compartments in nervous tissue. pp. 3–32. In Cserr HF, Fenstermacher JD, Fencl V (eds): Fluid Environment of the Brain. Academic Press, New York, 1975
53. Oldendorf WH, Davson H: Brain extracellular space and the sink action of the CSF. Arch Neurol 17:196, 1967
54. Bourke RS, Greenberg ES, Tower DB: Variation of cerebral cortex fluid spaces in vivo as a function of species brain size. Am J Physiol 208:682, 1965
55. Levin E, Arieff AI, Kleeman CR: Evidence of different compartments in the brain for extracellular markers. Am J Physiol 221:1319, 1971
56. Crone C: Properties of the blood brain barrier with special emphasis on glucose. p. 3. In Cserr HF, Fenstermacher JD, Fencl V (eds): Fluid Environment of the Brain. Academic Press, New York, 1975
57. Ehrlich P: Das Sauerstoff-Bedurfinis des Organismus, Eine Farbenanaltyische Studie, pp. 69–72, Berlin, 1885
58. Lewandowsky M: Aur Lehre Von Der Cerebrospinalflussigkeit. Z Klin Med 40:480, 1900
59. Goldman EE: Die Aussere und Innere Sekretion des Gesunden und Gesunden und Kranken Organismus im Lichte der "Vitalen Farbung." Beitr Z Klin Chir 64:192, 1909
60. Rapoport SI: Regulation of drug entry into the nervous system. p. 153. In Rapoport S (ed): Blood Brain Barrier in Physiology and Medicine. Raven Press, New York, 1976
61. Rapoport S: I. Sites and functions of the blood-brain barrier. p. 43. In Rapoport S (ed): Blood Brain Barrier in Physiology and Medicine. Raven Press, New York, 1976
62. Teschan PE, Ginn HE, Bourne JR, et al: Quantitative indices of clinical uremia. Kidney Int 15:676, 1979
63. Raskin NH, Fishman RS: Neurologic disorders in renal failure. N Engl J Med 294:143, 1976
64. Locke SJ, Merrill JP, Tyler HR: Neurological complications of acute uremia. Arch Intern Med 108:75, 1961
65. Cooper JD, Lazarowitz VC, Arieff AI: Neurodiagnostic abnormalities in patients with acute renal failure. J Clin Invest 61:1448, 1978
66. Kiley J, Hines O: Electroencephalographic evaluation of uremia. Arch Intern Med 116:67, 1965
67. Kennedy AC, Linton AI, Renfrew S, et al: The pathogenesis and prevention of cerebral dysfunction during dialysis. Lancet 1:790, 1964
68. Hampers CL, Doak PB, Callaghan MN, et al: The electroencephalogram and spinal fluid during hemodialysis. Arch Intern Med 118:340, 1966
69. Kiley JE, Woodruff MW, Pratt KL: Evaluation of encephalopathy by EEG frequency analysis in chronic dialysis patients. Clin Nephrol 5:245, 1976
70. Raskin NH, Fishman RA: Neurologic disor-

ders in renal failure. N Engl J Med 294:143, 1976
71. Teschan PE, Ginn HE: The nervous system. p. 3. In Massry SG, Sellers AL (eds): Clinical Aspects of Uremia and Dialysis. Charles C Thomas, Springfield, IL, 1976
72. Kiley J, Hines O: Electroencephalographic evaluation of uremia. Arch Intern Med 116:67, 1965
73. Kiley JE, Woodruff MW, Pratt KL: Evaluation of encephalopathy by EEG frequency analysis in chronic dialysis patients. Clin Nephrol 5:245, 1976
74. Cogan M, Covey C, Arieff AI, et al: Central nervous system manifestations of hyperparathyroidism. Am J Med 65:963, 1978
74a. Goldstein DA, Feinstein EI, Chiu LA, et al: The relationship between the abnormalities in EEG and blood levels of parathyroid hormone in dialysis patients. J Clin Endocrinol Metabol 51:130, 1980
75. Hagstam KE: EEG frequency content related to chemical blood parameters in chronic uremia. Scand J Urol Nephrol 7(suppl 1):1, 1971
76. Tyler HR: Neurologic disorders in renal failure. Am J Med 44:734, 1968
76. Massry SG, Arieff AI, Coburn JW, et al: Divalent ion metabolism in patients with acute renal failure: Studies on the mechanism of hypocalcemia. Kidney Int 5:437, 1974
77. Arieff AI, Cooper JD, Armstrong D, et al: Dementia renal failure and brain aluminum. Ann Intern Med 90:741, 1979
78. Arieff AI, Massry SG, Barrientos A, et al: Brain Water and electrolyte metabolism in uremia: Effects of slow and rapid hemodialysis. Kidney Int 4:177, 1973
79. Fishman RA: Permeability changes in experimental uremic encephalopathy. Arch Intern Med 126:835, 1970
80. Arieff AI, Guisado R, Massry SG, et al: Central nervous system pH in uremia and the effects of hemodialysis. J Clin Invest 58:306, 1976
81. Van den Noort S, Eckel RE, Brine K, et al: Brain metabolism in uremic and adenosine-infused rats. J Clin Invest 47:2133, 1968
81a. Mahoney CA, Sarnacki P, Arieff AI: Uremic encephalopathy: Role of brain energy metabolism. Amer J Physiol: Renal, Fluid Elect Physiol 246:(in press), 1984
82. Scheinberg D: Effects of uremia on cerebral blood flow and metabolism. Neurology (NY) 4:101, 1954
83. Deferrari G, Garibotto G, Robaudo C, et al: Brain metabolism of amino acids and ammonia in patients with chronic renal insufficiency. Kidney Int 20:505, 1981
84. Arieff AI: Neurological complications of uremia. p. 2306. In Brenner BM, Rector FC Jr (eds): The Kidney. WB Saunders, Philadelphia, 1981
85. Maschio G, Bazzato G, Bertaglia E, et al: Intracellular pH and electrolyte content of skeletal muscle in patients with chronic renal acidosis. Nephron 7:481, 1970
86. Levin GE, Baron DN: Leukocyte intracellular pH in patients with the metabolic acidosis of renal failure. Clin Sci Mol Med 52:325, 1977
87. Tizianello A, De Ferrari G, Gurreri G, et al: Effects of metabolic alkalosis, metabolic acidosis and uraemia on whole-body intracellular pH in man. Clin Sci Mol Med 52:125, 1977
88. Cowie J, Lambie AT, Robson JS: The influence of extracorporeal dialysis on the acid–base composition of blood and cerebrospinal fluid. Clin Sci 23:397, 1962
88a. Arieff AI, Fraser C, Leach W: Cerebral mitochondrial function in uremia: Effects of aluminum, tin and PTH. Clin Res 32:439A, 1984
88b. Fraser CL, Sarnacki P, Arieff AI: Altered Na transport in brain of uremic rats: Relation to neurotransmission in uremia? Clin Res 32:532A, 1984
89. Olsen S: The brain in uremia. Acta Psychiatr Scand 36 (suppl 156):1, 1961
90. Rotter W, Roettger, P: Comparative pathologic–anatomic study of cases of chronic global renal insufficiency with and without hemodialysis. Clin Nephrol 1:257, 1974
91. Burks JS, Alfrey AC, Huddlestone J, et al: A fatal encephalopathy in chronic haemodialysis patients. Lancet 1:764, 1976
92. Kennedy AC, Linton AL, Eaton JC: Urea levels in cerebrospinal fluid after hemodialysis. Lancet 1:410, 1962
93. Kennedy AC, Linton AL, Luke RG, et al: Electroencephalographic changes during hemodialysis. Lancet 1:408, 1963
94. Kiley JE, Woodruff MW, Pratt KL: Evalua-

tion of encephalopathy by EEG frequency analysis in chronic dialysis patients. Clin Nephrol 5:245, 1976
95. Rodrigo F, Shideman J, McHugh R, et al: Osmolality changes during hemodialysis. Ann Intern Med 86:554, 1977
96. Van Stone JC, Carey J, Meyer R, et al: Hemodialysis with glycerol containing dialysate. ASAIO J 2:119, 1979
97. Pagel MD, Ahmad S, Vizzo JE, et al: Acetate and bicarbonate fluctuations and acetate intolerance during dialysis. Kidney Int 21:513, 1982
98. Grushkin CM, Korsch B, Fine RN: Hemodialysis in small children. JAMA 221:869, 1972
99. Porte FK, Johnson WJ, Klass DW: Prevention of dialysis disequilibrium syndrome by use of high sodium concentration in the dialysate. Kidney Int 3:327, 1973
100. Fukusige M, Tado O, Matsuki S, et al: Hemodialysis with kill-type artificial kidney: Clinical study on disequilibrium syndrome. Acta Urol Jpn 17:89, 1971
101. Mawdsley C: Neurological complications of hemodialysis. Proc R Soc Med 65:871, 1972
102. deC Peterson H, Swanson AG: Acute encephalopathy occurring during hemodialysis. Arch Intern Med 113:877, 1964
103. Kennedy AC, Luke RG, Linton AL: Dialysis disequilibrium syndrome. p. 66. In Shaldon S, Cook GC (eds): Acute Renal Failure. Blackwell, London, 1964
104. Kretchmar LH, Green WM, Waterhouse CW, et al: Repeated hemodialysis in chronic uremia. JAMA 184:1030, 1963
105. Rosen SM, O'Connor K, Shaldon S: Hemodialysis disequilibrium. Br Med J 2:672, 1964
106. Peterson HdeC, Swanson AG: Acute encephalopathy occurring during hemodialysis. Arch Intern Med 113:877, 1964
107. Pappius HM, Dossetor JB: The effects of rapid hemodialysis on brain tissues and cerebrospinal fluid of dogs. Can J Physiol Pharmacol 45:129, 1967
108. Rosenbaum BJ, Coburn JW, Shinaberger JH, et al: Acid–base status during the interdialytic period in patients maintained with chronic hemodialysis. Ann Intern Med 71:1105, 1969
109. Pauli HG, Vorburger C, Reubi F: Chronic derangements of cerebrospinal fluid acid–base components in man. J Appl Physiol 17:993, 1962
110. Arieff AI, Leach W, Park R, et al: Systemic effects of $NaHCO_3$ in experimental lactic acidosis in dogs. Am J Physiol 242:F586, 1982
111. Greca G, Dettori P, Biasoli S, et al: Brain density studies during dialysis. Lancet 2:582, 1980
112. Baxter CF, Baldwin RA: A functional role for amino acids in the adaption of tissues from the nervous system to alterations in environmental osmolality. p. 599. In Fonnum F (ed): Amino Acids as Chemical Transmitters. Plenum, New York, 1978
113. Baxter CF, Ortiz CL: Amino acids and the maintenance of osmotic equilibrium in brain tissue. Life Sci 5:2321, 1966
114. Siddiqui JY, Fitz AE, Lawton RL, et al: Causes of death in patients receiving long-term hemodialysis. JAMA 212:1350, 1970
115. Tallal A, Halbrook H, Barbour BH, et al: Subdural hematoma associated with long-term hemodialysis for chronic renal disease. JAMA 212:1847, 1970
116. Weber DL, Reagan T, Leeds M: Intracerebral hemorrhage during hemodialysis. NY J Med 72:1853, 1972
117. Leonard CD, Weil C, Scribner BH: Subdural hematomas in patients undergoing hemodialysis. Lancet 2:239, 1969
118. Arieff AI, Lazarowitz VC, Guisado R: Experimental dialysis disequilibrium syndrome: Prevention with glycerol. Kidney Int 14:270, 1978
119. Rosen RA, Lazarowitz VC, Arieff AI: Dialysis disequilibrium syndrome: Prevention with glycerol. Kidney Int 14:683, 1978
120. Porte FK, Johnson WJ, Klass DW: Prevention of dialysis disequilibrium syndrome by use of high sodium concentration in the dialysate. Kidney Int 3:327, 1973
121. Alfrey AC, Mishell JM, Burks J, et al: Syndrome of dyspraxia and multifocal seizures associated with chronic hemodialysis. Trans Am Soc Artif Intern Organs 18:257, 1972
122. Flendrig JA, Kruis H, Das HA: Aluminum and dialysis dementia. Lancet 1:1235, 1976
123. Ward MK, Feest TG, Ellis HA, et al: Osteomalacic dialysis osteodystrophy: Evidence for a water-borne aetiological agent, probably aluminum. Lancet 1:841, 1978
124. Wing AJ: Dialysis dementia in Europe: Re-

port from the registration committee of the EDTA. Lancet 2:190, 1980
125. Pierides AM, Edwards WG, Cullum UX, et al: Hemodialysis encephalopathy with osteomalacic fractures and muscle weakness. Kidney Int 18:115, 1980
126. Prior JC, Cameron EC, Knickerbocker WJ, et al: Dialysis encephalopathy and osteomalacic bone disease. Am J Med 72:33, 1982
127. Rotundo A, Nevins TE, Lipton M, et al: Progressive encephalopathy in children with chronic renal insufficiency in infancy. Kidney Int 21:486, 1982
128. Dunea G, Mahurkar SD, Mamdami B, et al: Role of aluminum in dialysis dementia. Ann Intern Med 88:502, 1978
129. Parkinson IS, Ward MK, Feest TG, et al: Fracturing dialysis osteodystrophy and dialysis encephalopathy. Lancet 1:406, 1979
130. Berkseth RO, Shapiro FL: An epidemic of dialysis encephalopathy and exposure to high aluminum dialysate. p. 42. In Schrier GE, Winchester JF (eds): Controversies in Nephrology. Georgetown University Press, Georgetown, MD, 1980
131. Kaehney WD, Alfrey AC, Holman RE, et al: Aluminum transfer during hemodialysis. Kidney Int, 12:361, 1977
132. Alfrey AC, LeGendre GR, Kaehney WD: The dialysis encephalopathy syndrome: Possible aluminum intoxication. N Engl J Med 294:184, 1976
133. McDermott JR, Smith AI, Ward MK, et al: Brain aluminum concentration in dialysis encephalopathy. Lancet 1:901, 1978
134. Weiss B: The behavioral toxicology of metals. Fed Proc 37:22, 1978
135. Cartier F, Allain P, Gary J, et al: Progressive myoclonic encephalopathy in dialysis patients. Nouv Presse Med 7:97, 1978
136. Dewberry FL, McKinney TD, Stone WJ: The dialysis dementia syndrome: Report of fourteen cases and review of the literature. Am Soc Artif Intern Organs J 3:102, 1980
137. McKinney TD, Sprague SM, Hourani MR, et al: Parathyroid hormone mediated aluminum deposition and egress in the rat. Kidney Int 17:40, 1980
138. Weitzman R, Kleeman CR: Water metabolism and the neurohypophyseal hormones: Hypoosmolar syndromes. p. 6154. In Maxwell MH, Kleeman CR (eds): Clinical Disorders of Fluid and Electrolyte Metabolism. McGraw-Hill, New York, 1980
139. Schrier RW, Berl T: Disorders of water metabolism. p. 1. In Schrier RW (eds): Renal and Electrolyte Disorders. 2nd Ed. Little, Brown, Boston, 1980
140. Welt LG, Seldin DW, Nelson WP, et al: Role of the central nervous system in metabolism of electrolytes and water. Arch Intern Med 90:355, 1952
141. Abu-Asha H, Ibrahim A, Salif AM, et al: Sodium-losing nephropathy. J Urol 121:8, 1979
142. Bartter FC, Scwartz WB: The syndrome of inappropriate secretion of antidiuretic hormone. Am J Med 42:790, 1967
143. Epstein FH, Levitin H, Glaser G, et al: Cerebral hyponatremia. N Engl J Med 265:513, 1961
144. Ashraf N, Locksley R, Arieff AI: Thiazide-induced hyponatremia associated with death or neurological damage in outpatients. Am J Med 70:1163, 1981
145. Levere AH, Wesson LG: Salt-losing nephritis. N Engl J Med 255:373, 1956
146. Hughes JM: Salt-losing nephritis. Arch Intern Med 114:190, 1964
147. Polak A: Sodium depletion in chronic renal failure. J R Coll Physicians Lond, 5:333, 1971
148. Danovitch GM, Bourgoignie JJ, Bricker NS: Reversibility of the "salt-losing" tendency of chronic renal failure. N Engl J Med 296:15, 1977
149. Maldonado MM, Yium JJ, Suki WN, et al: Electrolyte excretion in polycystic kidney disease: Interrelationship between sodium, calcium, magnesium, and phosphate. J Lab Clin Med 90:1066, 1977
150. Schwartz WB, Tassel D, Bartter FC: Further observations on hyponatremia and renal sodium loss probably resulting from inappropriate secretion of antidiuretic hormone. N Engl J Med 262:743, 1960
151. Goldberg M, Handler JS: Hyponatremia and renal wasting of sodium in patients with malfunction of the central nervous system. N Engl J Med 263:1037, 1960
152. Peters JP, Welt LG, Simes EAH, et al: A salt wasting syndrome associated with cere-

bral disease. Trans Assoc Am Physicians 63:57, 1950
153. Cort JH: Cerebral salt wasting. Lancet 1:752, 1954
153a. Oster JR, Perez GO, Larios O, et al: Cerebral salt wasting in a man with carcinomatous meningitis. Arch Intern Med 143:2187, 1983
153b. Al-Mufti H, Arieff AI: Hyponatremia due to cerebral salt wasting syndrome: A combined cerebral and distal tubular lesion. Am J Med 1984 (in press)
154. Conger JD, McIntyre JA, Jacoby WJ: Central pontine myelinolysis associated with inappropriate antidiuretic hormone secretion. Am J Med 47:813, 1969
155. Beresford HR: Polydipsia, hydrochlorothiazide and water intoxication. JAMA 214:879, 1970
156. Fichman MP, Vorherr H, Kleeman CR, et al: Diuretic-induced hyponatremia. Ann Intern Med 75:853, 1971
157. Stormont JM, Westerhouse C: The genesis of hyponatremia associated with marked overhydration and water intoxication. Circulation 24:191, 1961
158. Swanson AG, Iseri OA: Acute encephalopathy due to water intoxication. N Engl J Med 258:831, 1958
159. Arieff AI, Llach F, Massry SG: Neurological manifestations and morbidity of hyponatremia: Correlation with brain water and electrolytes. Medicine (Baltimore) 55:121, 1976
160. Covey CM, Arieff AI: Disorders of sodium and water metabolism and their effects on the central nervous system. p. 212. In Brenner BM, Stein JH (eds): Contemporary Issues in Nephrology. Vol. 1. Churchill Livingstone, New York, 1978
160a. Gehi MM, Rosenthal RH, Fizette NB, et al: Psychiatric manifestations of hyponatremia. Psychosomatics 22:739, 1981
161. Rymer MM, Fishman RA: Protective adaptation of brain to water intoxication. Arch Neurol 28:49, 1973
162. McCance RA: Experimental sodium chloride deficiency in man. Proc R Soc Biol 119:245, 1936
163. Edelman IS, Leibman J, O'Meara MP, et al: Interrelations between serum sodium concentration, serum osmolarity and total exchangeable sodium, total exchangeable potassium and total body water. J Clin Invest 37:1236, 1958
164. Miller M, Moses A: Drug-induced states of impaired water excretion. Kidney Int 10:96, 1976
165. Fuisz RE: Hyponatremia Medicine (Baltimore) 42:149, 1963
166. DeFronzo R, Goldberg M, Agus ZS: Normal diluting capacity in hyponatremic patients. Ann Intern Med 84:538, 1976
167. Varavithya W, Hellerstein S: Acute symptomatic hyponatremia. J Pediatr 71:269, 1967
168. Day G, Radde I, Balfe JW, et al: Electrolyte abnormalities in very low birthweight infants. Pediatr Res 10:522, 1976
169. Lipsmeyer E, Ackerman GL: Irreversible brain damage after water intoxication. JAMA 196:286, 1966
170. Pampiglione G: The effect of metabolic disorderson brain activity. J R Coll Phycns Lond, 7:347, 1973
171. DeTroyer A, Demanet JC: Clinical, biological, and pathogenic features of the syndrome of inappropriate secretion of antidiuretic hormone. Q J Med 45:521, 1976
172. Helwig FC, Schultz CB, Curry DE: Water intoxication: report of a fatal case with clinical, pathological and experimental studies. JAMA 104:1569, 1935
173. Raskind M: Psychosis, polydipsia, and water intoxication: Report of a fatal case. Arch Gen Psychiatry 30:112, 1974
174. Holliday MA, Kalayci MN, Harrah J: Factors that limit brain volume changes in response to acute and sustained hyper- and hypo-natremia. J Clin Invest 47:1916, 1968
175. Dila CJ, Pappius HM: Cerebral water and electrolytes: An experimental model of inappropriate secretion of antidiuretic hormone. Arch Neurol 26:85, 1972
176. Wasterlain CG, Posner JB: Cerebral edema in water intoxication. I. Clinical and chemical observations. Arch Neurol 19:71, 1968
177. Herschkowitz N, McGillivray B, Cumings TN: Biochemical and electrophysiological studies in experimental cerebral edema. Brain 88:557, 1965
178. Wasterlain CG, Torack RM: Cerebral edema in water intoxication. II. An ultrastructural study. Arch Neurol 19:79, 1968
179. Thurston JH, Hauhart RE, Jones EM, et

al: Effects of salt and water loading on carbohydrate and energy metabolism and levels of selected amino acids in the brain of young mice. J Neurochem 24:953, 1975
180. Bennett JP, Logan WJ, Snyder SH: Amino acids as central nervous transmitters: The influence of ions, amino acids analogues, and ontogeny on transport systems for L-glutamic and L-asparatic acids and glycine into central nervous synaptosomes of the rat. J Neurochem 21:1533, 1973
181. Schultz SG, Currant PF: Coupled transport of sodium and organic solute. Physiol Rev 50:637, 1970
182. Lajtha A, Sershen H: Inhibition of amino acid uptake by the absence of sodium in slices of brain. J Neurochem 11:77, 1975
183. Lajtha AL, Maker HS, Clarke DD: Metabolism and transport of carbohydrates and amino acids. p. 348. In Siegel GJ, Albers RW, Agranoff BW, et al (eds); Basic Neurochemistry, 3rd Ed. Little, Brown, Boston, 1981
184. Stern EW, Coxon RV: Osmolality of brain tissue and its relation to brain bulk. Am J Physiol 204:1, 1964
185. Levinsky NG: Refractory ascites in cirrhosis. Kidney Int 14:93, 1978
186. Zimmerman B, Wangensteen OH: Observations on water intoxication in surgical patients. Surgery 31:654, 1952
187. Wynn V, Rob CG: Water intoxication. Lancet 1:587, 1954
188. Scott JC, Welch JS, Berman IB: Water intoxication and sodium depletion in surgical patients. Obstet Gynecol 26:168, 1965
189. Hantman D, Rossier B, Zohlman, R, et al: Rapid correction of hyponatremia in the syndrome of inappropriate secretion of antidiuretic hormone. Ann Intern Med 78:870, 1973
190. Macaron C, Famuyiwa O: Hyponatremia of hypothyroidism. Arch Intern Med 138:820, 1978
191. Ayus JC, Olivero JJ, Frommer JP: Rapid correction of severe hyponatremia with intravenous saline solution. Am J Med 72:43, 1982
192. Cadnapaphornchai P, Taher S, McDonald FD: Syndrome of inappropriate antidiuretic hormone secretion in chronic schizophrenia. Kidney Int 14:647, 1978
193. Hariprasad MK, Eisinger RP, Padmanabhan CS, et al: Reset osmostat associated with hyponatremia and dementia in psychotic patients. Kidney Int 14:653, 1978
194. Rosenbaum JF, Rothman JS, Murray GB: Psychosis and water intoxication. J Clin Psychiatry 40:287, 1979
195. Rendell M, McGrane D, Cuesta M: Fatal compulsive water drinking. JAMA 240:2557, 1978
196. Wright R: Overdosing on water. Newsweek March 14, 46, 1977
197. Dubovsky SL, Grabon S, Berl T, et al: Syndrome of inappropriate secretion of antidiuretic hormone with exacerbated psychosis. Ann Intern Med 79:551, 1973
198. Langgard H, Smith WO: Self-induced water intoxication without predisposing illness. N Engl J Med 266:378, 1962
199. Schrier RW, Berl T: Nonosmolar factors affecting renal water excretion. N Engl J Med 292:81, 1975
200. Kennedy, RM, Early LE: Profound hyponatremia resulting from a thiazide-induced decrease in urniary diluting capacity in a patient with primary polydipsia. N Engl J Med 202:1185, 1970
201. Mengoli LR: Excerpts from the history of postoperative fluid therapy. Am J Surg 121:311, 1971
202. Adams RD, Victor M, Mancall EL: Central pontine myelinolysis: A hitherto undescribed disease occurring in alcoholic and malnourished patients. Arch Neurol Psychiatry 81:154, 1959
203. Schneck SA: Central pontine myelinolysis. p. 859. In Minckler J (ed): Pathology of the Nervous System. McGraw-Hill, New York, 1976
204. Tomlinson BE, Pierides AM, and Bradley WG: Central pontine myelinolysis. Q J Med 65:373, 1976
205. Wright DC, Laureno R, Victor M: Pontine and extrapontine myelinolysis. Brain 102:361, 1979
206. Tihen WS: Central pontine myelinolysis and Rosenthal fibers of the brainstem. Neurology (NY) 22:710, 1972
207. Goebel HH, Herman-Ben Zur P: Central pontine myelinolysis: A clinical and pathological study of 10 cases. Brain 95:495, 1972
208. Chason JL, Landers JW, Gonzalez JE: Cen-

tral pontine myelinolysis. J Neurol Neurosurg Psychiatry 27:317, 1964

208a. Messert B, Orrison WW, Hawkins MJ, et al: Central pontine myelinolysis. Neurology (NY) 147, 1979

208b. Brucar PJ, Norenberg MD, Yarnell PR: Hyponatremia and central pontine myelinolysis. Neurology (NY) 27:223, 1977

209. Norenberg MD, Leslie KO, Robertson AS: Association between rise in serum sodium and central pontine myelinolysis. Ann Neurol 11:128, 1982

210. Ayus JC, Krothapalli R, Pace E, et al: Safety of rapid correction of severe hyponatremia in Sprague-Dawley rats. Kidney Int 23:117, 1983

211. Dubois GD, Leach W, Arieff AI: Central pontine myelinolysis and hyponatremia. Clin Res 31:98A, 1983

212. Laureno R: Central pontine myelinolysis following rapid correction of hyponatremia. Ann Neurol 13:232, 1983

212a. Thompson DS, Hutton JT, Stears JC, et al: Computerized tomography in the diagnosis of central and extrapontine myelinolysis. Arch Neurol 38:243, 1981

212b. Gross SG, Bell RD: Central pontine myelinolysis and rapid correction of hyponatremia. Texas Med 78:59, 1982

213. Kleinschmidt-DeMasters BK, Norenberg MD: Rapid correction of hyponatremia and demyelination: Relation to central pontine myelinolysis. Science 211:1068, 1981

214. Berry K, Olszewski J: Central pontine myelinolysis: A case report. Neurology (NY) 13:531, 1963

215. Hilden T, Svendsen TL: Electrolyte disturbances in beer drinkers. Lancet 2:245, 1975

216. Demanet JC, Bennyns M, Stevens-Recmans C: Coma due to water intoxication in beer drinkers. Lancet 2:1115, 1971

217. Telfer RB, Miller EM: Central pontine myelinolysis following hyponatremia, demonstrated by computerized tomography. Ann Neurol 6:455, 1979

218. Ross EJ, Christie SBM: Hypernatremia. Medicine (Baltimore) 48:441, 1969

219. Zierler KL: Hyperosmolarity in adults: A critical review. J Chron Dis 7:1, 1958

220. Park R, Guisado R, Arieff AI. Nutrient deficiencies in man and animals: Water p. 363. In Rechcigl M (ed): In CRC Handbook for Nutrition and Food: Section E: Nutritional Disorders. Vol. II. CRC Press, Boca Raton, FL, 1978

221. Finberg L: Hypernatremic (hypertonic) dehydration in infants. N Engl J Med 289:196, 1973

222. Rapoport S: Hyperosmolarity and hyperelectrolytemia in pathological conditions of childhood. Am J Dis Child 74:682, 1947

223. Elton NW, Elton WJ, Nazareno JP: Pathology of acute salt poisoning in infants. Am J Clin Pathol 39:252, 1963

224. Finberg L, Kiley J, Luttrell CN: Mass accidental salt poisoning in infancy: A study of a hospital disaster. JAMA 184:187, 1963

225. Colle E Ayoub E, Raile R: Hypertonic dehydration (hypernatremia) role of feedings high in solutes. Pediatrics 22:5, 1958

226. Mattar JA, Well MH, Shubin H, et al: Cardiac arrest in the critically ill. Am J Med 56:162, 1974

227. Simmons MA, Adcock EW, Bard H, et al: Hypernatremia and intracranial hemorrhage in neonates. N Engl J Med 291:6, 1974

228. DeVillota ED, Cavanilles JM, Stein L, et al: Hyperosmolar crisis following infusion of hypertonic sodium chloride for purposes of therapeutic abortion. Am J Med 55:116, 1973

229. Park R, Arieff AI: Lactic acidosis: Current concepts. In Schade DS (ed): Clinics in Endocrinology and Metabolism. Vol. 12, No. 2. WB Saunders, Philadelphia, 1983

230. Morris-Jones PH, Houston IB, Evans RC: Prognosis of the neurological complications of acute hypernatremia. Lancet 2:1385, 1967

231. Banister A, Siddiqi S, Hatcher GW: Treatment of hypernatremia dehydration in infancy. Arch Dis Child 50:179, 1975

232. Bruck E, Abal G, Aceto T: Pathogenesis and pathophysiology of hypertonic dehydration with diarrhea. Am J Dis Child 115:122, 1968

233. Finberg L: Pathogenesis of lesions in the nervous system in hypernatremic states. I. Clinical observations of Infants. Pediatrics 23:40, 1959

234. Macauley D, Watson M: Hypernatremia as a cause of brain damage. Arch Dis Child 42:485, 1967

235. Knowles HC: Hypernatremia. Metabolism 5:508, 1956

236. Katzman R, Pappius HM: Hypernatremia

and hyperosmolarity. p. 278. In Katzman R, Pappius HM (eds): Brain Electrolytes and Fluid Metabolism. Williams & Wilkins, Baltimore, 1973

237. Stevenson, RE, Bowyer FP: Hyperglycemia with hyperosmolar dehydration in non diabetic infants. J Pediatr 77:818, 1970
238. Hogan G, Dodge PR, Gill SR, et al: Pathogenesis of seizures occurring during restoration of plasma tonicity to normal in animals previously chronically hypernatremic. Pediatrics 43:54, 1969

238a. Arieff AI: Principles of parenteral therapy. p. 567. In Maxwell MH, Kleeman CR (eds): Clinical Disorders of Fluid and Electrolyte Metabolism. McGraw-Hill, New York, 1972

239. Finberg L, Harrison HE: Hypernatremia in infants: An evaluation of the clinical and biochemical findings accompanying this state. Pediatrics 16:1, 1955
240. Cameron JM, Dayan AD: Association of brain damage with therapeutic abortion induced by amniotic fluid replacement: Report of two cases. Br Med J 1:1010, 1966
241. Bluemle LW: Current status of chronic hemodialysis. Am J Med 44:749, 1968
242. Smith RJ, Block MR, Arieff AI, et al: Hypernatremic hyperosmolar coma complicating chronic peritoneal dialysis. Proc Clin Dialysis Transplant Forum 4:96, 1974
243. Toor M, Wertheimer E, Massry S, et al: Development and correction of hypernatremia during a two hour hike at 42°C at Sodom. Hasefuah. 57:244, 1959
244. Levine JA, Heatstroke in the aged. Am J Med 47:25, 1977
245. Johnston JG, Robertson WO: Fatal ingestion of table salt by an adult. Western J Med 126:141, 1977
246. Nellis GF: The Hyperosmolar Non-ketoacidotic Diabetic Syndrome: A Clinical Study. Drukkerij Van Dendrenen BV, Groningen, Amsterdam, 1975
247. Sparacio RR, Anziska HS, Schutta HS: Hypernatremia and chorea: A report of two cases. Neurology (NY) 26:46, 1976
248. Arieff AI, Guisado R, Lazarowitz VC: Pathophysiology of hyperosmolar states. p. 227. In Andreoli TE, Grantham JJ, Rector FC (eds): Disturbances in Body Fluid Osmolality. Bethesda, Md, American Physiological Society, 1977
249. Thurston JH, Hauhart RE, Schulz DW: Effect of chronic hypernatremic rehydration on brain carbohydrate, energy, and amino acid metabolism in weanling mice. J Neurochem 40:240, 1983
250. Lockwood AH: Acute and chronic hyperosmolality: Effects on cerebral amino acids and energy metabolism. Arch Neurol 32:62, 1975
251. Chan PH, Fishman RA: Elevation of rat brain amino acids, ammonia and idiogenic osmoles induced by hyperosmolality. Brain Res 161(2):293, 1979
252. Fishman RA: Cell Volume, pumps, and neurologic function: Brain's adaptation to osmotic stress. p. 159. In Plum F (ed): Brain Dysfunction in Metabolic Disorders. Raven Press, New York, 1974
253. Kregenow FM: The response of duck erythrocytes to hypertonic media. J Gen Physiol 58:396, 1971
254. Wildenthal K, Mierzwiak DS, Myers RW, et al: Effects of acute lactic acidosis on left venticular performance. Am J Physiol 214:1352, 1968
255. Lotz M, Zisman E, Bartter FC: Evidence for a phosphorus-depletion syndrome in man. N Engl J Med 278:409, 1968
256. Lichtman MA, Miller DR, Freeman RB: Erythrocyte adenosine triphosphate depletion during hypophosphatemia in a uremic subject. N Engl J Med 280:240, 1969
257. Fitzgerald FT: Hypophosphatemia. West J Med 122:482, 1975
258. Knochel JP: The pathophysiology and clinical characteristics of severe hypophosphatemia. Arch Intern Med 137:203, 1977
259. Darsee JR, Nutter DO: Reversible severe congestive cardiomyopathy in three cases of hypophosphatemia. Ann Intern Med 89:867, 1978
260. Fuller TJ, Nichols WW, Brenner BJ, et al: Reversible depression in myocardial performance in dogs with experimental phosphorus deficiency. J Clin Invest 62:1194, 1978
261. Travis SF, Sugerman HJ, Ruberg RL, et al: Alterations of red-cell glycolytic intermediates and oxygen transport as a consequence of hypophosphatemia in patients receiving intravenous hyperalimentation. N Engl J Med 285:763, 1971
262. Bellingham AJ, Detter JC, Lenfant C: Regulatory mechanisms of hemoglobin-oxygen affinity in acidosis and alkalosis. J Clin Invest 50:700, 1971

263. Silvis SE, Paragas PD, Jr: Paresthesias, weakness, seizures, and hypophosphatemia in patients receiving hyperalimentation. Gastroenterology 62:513, 1972
264. Furlan AJ, Hanson M, Cooperman A, et al: Acute areflexic paralysis. Arch Neurol 32:706, 1975
265. Gold LW, Massry SG, Arieff AI, et al: Renal bicarbonate wasting during phosphate depletion: A possible cause of altered acid–base homeostasis in hyperparathyroidism. J Clin Invest 52:2556, 1973
266. Rosen R, Leach W, Arieff AI: Neurologic manifestations of hyperalimentation and hypophosphatemia. Neurology (NY) 28:389, 1978
267. Jacob HS, Yawata Y, Craddock P, et al: Hyperalimentation hypophosphatemia: Hematologic–neurologic dysfunction due to ATP depletion. Trans Assoc Am Physicians 63:143, 1973
268. Derr RF, Zieve L: Weakness, neuropathy and coma following total parenteral nutrition in underfed or starved rats: Relationship to blood hyperosmolality and brain water loss. J Lab Clin Med 92:521, 1978
269. Silvis SE, Paragas PV Jr: Fatal hyperalimentation syndrome. Animal studies. J Lab Clin Med 78:918, 1971
270. Woods HF, Eggleston LV, Krebs HA: The cause of hepatic accumulation of fructose 1-phosphate on fructose loading. Biochem J 119:501, 1970
271. Farber E: ATP and cell integrity. Fed Proc 32:1534, 1973
272. Brautbar N, Bacyznski R, Carpenter C, et al: Impaired energy metabolism in rat myocardium during phosphate depletion. Am J Physiol 242:F699, 1982
273. Knochel JP, Barcenas C, Cotton JR, et al: Hypophosphatemia and rhabdomyolysis. J Clin Invest 62:1240, 1978
274. Editorial: Ketones and coma. N Engl J Med 284:328, 1971
275. Arieff AI, Carroll HJ: Cerebral edema and depression of sensorium in nonketotic hyperosmolar coma. Diabetes 23:525, 1974
276. Plum F, Posner JB: Metabolic brain diseases causing coma. p. 132. In Plum F, Posner JB (eds): Diagnosis of Stupor and Coma. FA Davis, Philadelphia, 1966
277. Gerich JE, Martin MM, Recant L: Clinical and metabolic characteristics of hyperosmolar nonketotic coma. Diabetes 20:228, 1971
278. Martin HE, Smith K, Wilson ML: The fluid and electrolyte therapy of severe diabetic acidosis and ketosis. A study of twenty nine episodes (twenty six patients). Am J Med 24:376, 1958
279. McGarry JD, Foster DW: Regulation of ketogenesis and clinical aspects of ketotic state. Metabolism 21:471, 1972
280. Wieland O: Diabetic acidosis: Biochemical aspects. p. 533. In Liebel BS, Wrenshall GA (eds): On the Nature and Treatment of Diabetes. Excerpta Medica Foundation, New York, 1965
281. McGarry JD, Foster DW: Ketogenesis and its regulation. Am J Med 61:9, 1976
282. Felig P: Diabetic ketoacidosis. N Engl J Med 290:1360, 1974
283. Schneider R, Droller H: Relative importance of ketosis and acidosis in production of diabetic coma. Q J Exp Physiol 28:323, 1938
284. Kety SS, Polis BD, Nadler CS, et al: The blood flow and oxygen consumption of the human brain in diabetic acidosis and coma. J Clin Invest 27:500, 1948
285. Guisado R, Arieff AI: Neurological manifestations of diabetic comas: Correlation with biochemical alterations in the brain. Metabolism 24:665, 1975
286. Pierce NF, Fedson DS, Brigham KL, et al: Relation of ventilation during base deficit to acid–base values in blood and spinal fluid. J Appl Physiol 30:677, 1971
287. Dufano M, Ishikawa S: Hypercapnia: Mental changes and extrapulmonary complications. Ann Intern Med 63:829, 1965
288. Huang YH, Mogenson GJ: Differential effects of central and hypothalamic lesions on food and water intake. Exp Neurol 43:276, 1974
289. Pitts RF, Alexander RS: The nature of the renal tubular mechanism for acidifying the urine. Am J Physiol 144:239, 1945
290. Pitts RF, Lotspeich WD, Schiess WA, et al: The renal regulation of acid–base metabolism in man. I. The nature of the mechanism for acidifying the urine. J Clin Invest 27:48, 1948
291. Assal JP, Aoki TT, Manzano FM, et al: Metabolic effects of sodium bicarbonate in management of diabetic ketoacidosis. Diabetes 23:405, 1974
292. Ohman JL, Marliss EB, Aoki TT, et al: The

cerebrospinal fluid in diabetic ketoacidosis. N Engl J Med 284:283, 1971
293. Siesjo BK: The regulation of cerebrospinal fluid pH. Kidney Int 1:360, 1972
294. Siesjo BK, Kjallquist A: A new theory for the regulation of the extracellular pH in the brain. Scand J Clin Lab Invest 24:1, 1969
295. Kjallquist A, Nardini M, Siesjo BK: The regulation of extra- and intracellular acid–base parameters in the rat brain during hyper-and hypocapnia. Acta Physiol Scand 76:485, 1969
296. Ruderman NB, Ross PS, Berger M, et al: Regulation of glucose and ketone-body metabolism in brain of anesthetized rats. Biochem J 138:1, 1974
297. Blackshear PJ, Alberti KGMM: Experimental diabetic ketoacidosis. Biochem J 138:107, 1974
298. Fulop M, Tannenbaum H, Dreyer N: Ketotic hyperosmolar coma. Lancet 2:635, 1973
299. Folbergrova J, MacMillan V, Siejo BK: The effect of hypercapnic acidosis upon some glycolytic and Krebs cycle associated intermediates in the rat brain. J Neurochem 19:2507, 1972
300. Reubi FC: Glomerular infiltration rate, renal blood flow and blood viscosity during and after diabetic coma. Circ Res 1:410, 1953
301. Nabarro JDN: Hyperosmolar non-ketotic coma. p. 551. Lievbel BS, Wrenshall GA (eds): On the Nature and Treatment of Diabetes. Excerpta Medica Foundation, New York, 1965
302. Foster DW: Insulin deficiency and hyperosmolar coma. Adv Intern Med 19:159, 1974
303. Timperly WR, Preston FE, Ward JD: Cerebral intravascular coagulation in diabetic acidosis. Lancet 1:952, 1974
304. Anderson JM, Machin GA, McKinlay I, et al: Diabetic ketoacidosis and intracerebral thrombosis. Lancet 1:1341, 1974
305. Arieff AI, Carroll HJ: Nonketotic hyperosmolar coma with hyperglycemia: Clinical features, pathophysiology, renal function, acid–base balance, plasma–cerebrospinal fuid equilibrium and the effects of therapy in 37 cases. Medicine, (Baltimore) 51:73, 1972
306. Macarrio M: Neurological dysfunction associated with non-ketotic hyperglycemia. Arch Neurol 19:525, 1968
307. Macarrio M, Messis CP, Vastola EF: Focal seizures as a manifestation of hyperglycemia without ketoacidosis. Neurology (NY) 15:195, 1965
308. Daniels JC, Chokroverty S, Barron KD: Anacidotic hyperglycemia and focal seizures. Arch Intern Med 124:701, 1969
309. Guisado R, Arieff AI: Neurological manifestations of diabetic comas; Correlation with biochemical alterations in the brain. Metabolism 24:665, 1975
310. Posner JB, Swanson AG, Plum F: Acid–base balance in cerebrospinal fluid. Arch Neurol 12:479, 1965
311. Marks V, Rose C: Cerebral metabolism and hypoglycemia. p. 52. In Marks V, Rose C (eds): Hypoglycemia. Blackwell, Oxford, 1965
312. Stone WE, Tews JK, Whisler KE, et al: Incorporation of carbon from glucose into cerebral amino acids, proteins and lipids, and alterations during recovery from hypoglycemia. J Neurochem 19:321, 1972
313. Himwich WA, Agrawal HC: Amino acids: Free amino acid pool of central nervous system. p. 33. In Lajtha A (ed): Handbook of Neurochemistry. Plenum, New York, 1969
314. Roberts E, Rothstein M, Baxter CF: Some metabolic studies of gamma-aminobutyric acid. Proc Soc Exp Biol Med 97:796, 1958
315. Hayashi T: Inhibition and excitation due to GABA in the central nervous system. Nature 182:1076, 1958
316. Baxter CD: The nature of gamma-aminobutyric acid. p. 289. In Lajtha A (ed): Handbook of Neurochemistry. Vol. 3. Metabolic Reactions in the Nervous System. Plenum, New York, 1970
317. Curtis DR, Watkins JC: The pharmacology of amino acids related to gamma-aminobutyric acid. Pharmacol Rev 17:347, 1965
318. Flock V, Tyce GM, Owen CA Jr: Glucose metabolism in brains of diabetic rats. Endocrinology 85:428, 1969
319. Rubin HM, Kramer R, Drash A: Hyperosmolality complicating diabetes mellitus in childhood. J Pediatr 74:177, 1969
320. DiBenedetto RJ, Crocco JA, Soscia JL: Hyperglycemic nonketotic coma. Arch Intern Med 116:74, 1965
321. Halmos PB, Nelson JK, Lowry RC: Hyperosmolar non-ketoacidotic coma in diabetes. Lancet 1:675, 1966
322. Jackson WPU, Forman R: Hyperosmolar

non-ketotic diabetic coma. Diabetes 15:714, 1966

323. Fernandez JP, McGinn JT, Hoffman RS: Cerebral edema from blood-brain glucose differences complicating peritoneal dialysis second membrane syndrome. NY State J Med 68:677, 1968
324. Hayes TM, Woods CJ: Unexpected death during treatment of uncomplicated diabetic ketoacidosis. Br Med J 4:32, 1968
325. VanHarreveld A, Hooper NK, Cusick JT: Brain electrolytes and cortical impedance. Am J Physiol 201:139, 1961
326. Guisado R, Arieff AI, Massry SG: Effects of glycerol infusion on brain water and electrolytes. Am J Physiol 227:865, 1974
327. Arieff AI, Kleeman CR: Cerebral edema in diabetic comas. II. Effects of hyperosmolality, hyperglycemia and insulin in diabetic rabbits. J Clin Endocrinol Metab 38:1057, 1974
328. Clements RS Jr, Prockop LD, Winegrad AI: Acute cerebral edema during treatment of hyperglycaemia. Lancet 2:384, 1968
329. Prockop LD: Hyperglycemia, polyol accumulation, and increased intracranial pressure. Arch Neurol 25:126, 1971
330. Davson H: Ionic equilibrium, bioelectric potentials, and active transport. p. 550. In Davson H (ed): A Textbook of General Physiology. Williams & Wilkins, Baltimore, 1970
331. Refsum HE: Relationship between state of consciousness and arterial hypoxemia and hypercapnia in patients with pulmonary insufficiency breathing air. Clin Sci 25:361, 1963.
332. Pavlin EG, Hornbein TF: Distribution of H^+ and HCO_3^- between CSF and blood during metabolic acidosis in dogs. Am J Physiol 228:1134, 1975
333. Fencl V, Vale JR, Broch JA: Respiration and cerebral blood flow in metabolic alkalosis and acidosis in humans. J Appl Physiol 27:67, 1969
334. Kazemi H, Shannon DC, Carvallo-Gil E: Brain CO_2 buffering capacity in respiratory acidosis and alkalosis. J Appl Physiol 22:241, 1967
335. Ponten U: Consecutive acid–base change in blood, brain tissue and cerebrospinal fluid during respiratory acidosis and baseosis. Acta Neurol Scand 42:455, 1966
336. Kjallquist M, Nardini M, Siejso BK: The effect of acetazolamide upon tissue concentrations of bicarbonate, lactate, and pyruvate in the rat brain. Acta Physiol Scand 77:241, 1969
337. Maren TH: Bicarbonate formation in cerebrospinal fluid: Role in sodium transport and pH regulation. Am J Physiol 222:885, 1972
338. Roberts E, Kuriyama K: Biochemical–physiological correlations in studies of the gamma-aminobutyric acid system. Brain Res 8:1, 1968
339. Pollay M: Transport mechanisms in the choroid plexus. Fed Proc 33:2064, 1974
340. Ponten U: Acid–base changes in rat brain tissue during acute respiratory acidosis and baseosis. Acta Physiol Scand 68:152, 1966
341. Kazemi H, Shore NS, Shih VE, et al: Brain organic buffers in respiratory acidosis and alkalosis. J Appl Physiol 34:478, 1973
342. Kilburn KH: Shock, seizures and coma with alkalosis during mechanical ventilation. Ann Intern Med 65:977, 1966
343. Severinghaus JW, Lassen N: Step hypocapnia to separate arterial from tissue pCO_2 in the regulation of cerebral blood flow. Circ Res 20:272, 1967
344. Caronna JJ, Plum F, Siesjo BK: POC_2 gradients between blood and CSF in rat during alterations of acid-base balance. Am J Physiol 227:1173, 1974
345. Shenkin HA, Bouzarth WF: Clinical methods of reducing intracranial pressure. N Engl J Med 282:1465, 1970
346. Roos A: Intracellular pH and buffering power of rat brain. Am J Physiol 221:176, 1971
347. Granhohm L, Siejso BK: The effects of hypercapnia and hypocapnia upon the cerebrospinal fluid lactate and pyruvate concentrations and upon the lactate, pyruvate, ATP, ADP, phosphocreatine and creatine concentrations of cat brain tissue. Acta Physiol Scand 75:257, 1969
348. Leusen I, Demeester G: Lactate and pyruvate in the brain of rats during hyperventilation. Arch Intern Physiol Biochim 74:25, 1966
349. VanVaerenbergh PJJ, Demeester G, Leusen I: Lactate in cerebrospinal fluid during hyperventilation. Arch Intern Physiol Biochim 73:738, 1965
350. Nara Y, Geha AS, Baue AE: Blood and cere-

bral lactate metabolism during sustained hyperventilation in anesthetized intact dogs. Surgery 69:940, 1971

351. Gotoh F, Meyer JS, Takagi Y: Cerebral effects of hyperventilation in man. Arch Neurol 12:410, 1965
352. Siejso BK, Ponten U: Acid–base changes in the brain in nonrespiratory acidosis and alkalosis. Exp Brain Res 2:176, 1966
353. Kibler RF, O'Neill RP, Robin ED: Intracellular acid–base relations of dog brain with reference to the brain extracellular volume. J Clin Invest 43:431, 1964
354. Granholm L, Siejso BK: The effect of combined respiratory and nonrespiratory alkalosis on energy metabolites and acid–base parameters in the rat brain. Acta Physiol Scand 81:307, 1971

22

Fluid and Electrolyte Metabolism in Normal and Abnormal Pregnancy

Marshall D. Lindheimer
Adrian I. Katz

Definition of normal volume homeostasis in gestation continues to be disputed. Two decades ago salt was condemned, gravidas were told to avoid it, and prophylactic diuretics were often prescribed. Lately, pregnant women have been considered subtle sodium wasters, supplemental salt has been advocated as a means of avoiding preeclampsia,[1] and volume expansion is recommended by some in the treatment of acute hypertension near term.[2,3] A third view is that renal handling of sodium is identical in pregnant and nonpregnant women and that therapy to reduce blood pressure and edema should be the same in both.[4,5] In this chapter we review renal and humoral alterations during normal pregnancy, as well as how these changes influence salt metabolism, water handling, proton excretion, and blood pressure. We also discuss volume homeostasis during abnormal gestation, with emphasis on preeclampsia.

WEIGHT GAIN IN NORMAL PREGNANCY

Mean weight gain of healthy primigravidas eating without restriction is 12.5 kg, whereas that of multiparous women is ~1 kg less; most of this gain (≃9.5 kg) occurs after the 20th gestational week.[6,7] The distribution of weight added during pregnancy, discussed in detail by Hytten,[7] is summarized in Table 22–1. Of interest is that not all the increase can be accounted for by products of conception, by tissues directly concerned with reproduction, or in total body water and that ~3 kg of the added weight is believed to represent increments in maternal fat stores.[7-9] (The value of 12.5 kg reported in this British study is the gain experienced by gravidas manifesting no edema or leg edema only. Hytten and colleagues[6,7] also found that 15 percent of normal pregnant women developed generalized edema. Their weight gain averaged 14.5 kg, of which 4.9 kg was due to increases in extracellular–extravascular compartments.)

The value of 12.5 kg is considerably greater than averages reported during the 1920s. It is now apparent, however, that the earlier studies were not comparable because investigators manipulated diets, included results from abnormal gestations, and used data from women observed for periods shorter than the final two trimesters. What is more surprising is that in the past, and even at present, many practitioners tended to regard published averages as upper limits of permissible weight gain,

Table 22–1. Analysis of Weight Gain

Tissues and Fluids Accounted for	Increase in Weight (g) 10 wk	20 wk	30 wk	40 wk
Fetus	5	300	1,500	3,400
Placenta	20	170	430	650
Amniotic fluid	30	350	750	800
Uterus	140	320	600	970
Mammary gland	45	180	360	405
Blood	100	600	1,300	1,250
Extracellular extravascular fluid	0	30	80	1,680
Total	340	1,950	5,020	9,155
Total weight gained	650	4,000	8,500	12,500
Weight not accounted for	310	2,050	3,480	3,345

[a] Source: Modified from Hytten FE, Weight gain in pregnancy. In Hytten FE, Chamerlain, eds. Clinical Physiology in Obstetrics. Oxford, Blackwell, Scientific Publications, 1980.

disregarding the fact that there is a plus as well as a minus to deviations about a mean. Many gravidas have therefore been admonished for excessive weight gain, and their salt or calorie intake, or both, has been needlessly restricted. It is emphasized that some women gain little weight, while others gain twice the average, and the gestation may proceed uneventfully in both.

ALTERATIONS IN FLUID VOLUMES

Increments in total body water and extracellular fluid of mother and fetus have been measured by a variety of techniques, including D_2O, antipyrine, thiocyanate, bromide, radiosodium, and mannitol. Table 22–2 summarizes some of the published data for total body water and extracellular volume during pregnancy. Investigators using antipyrine found increments exceeding weight gain, obviously erroneous overestimates, while with one exception values obtained using deuterium oxide are quite consistent from one report to another. Especially commendable are the serial studies of Hytten, Pipe, and their colleagues,[9,14] who noted increases of 7.7 and 7.2 liters, respectively, from the 10th through the 38th weeks.

The gains in extracellular fluid during pregnancy range from 3 to 7 liters. The accuracy of these measurements, however, elicits considerable concern. Ranges are wide in individual reports, there is often little correspondence in those subjects in whom both extracellular and total body water were measured simultaneously, and unaccountable and often large fluctuations occur during pregnancy. It is also apparent that the effect of gestation on the behavior of extracellular tracers has been poorly evaluated. For instance sucrose and mannitol traverse the placenta slowly and inulin probably not at all. Thiocyanate that enters the cell and normally overestimates extracellular volume also equilibrates slowly with the fetal space. Radiosodium and bromide are the tracers that equilibrate most rapidly with amniotic fluid, but the former marker also exchanges slowly with bone sodium. Obviously more research is necessary before firm conclusions can be drawn.

As with water-free weight gain (Table 22–1), investigators cannot account for the distribution of all the fluid they measure and speculate that the properties of the ground substance in connective tissue may be altered in pregnancy. Fekete[25] observed that the ability of the skin and subcutaneous tissues to absorb water from solutions of varying content is greater in pregnant women than in nonpregnant women. The absorbed water was released

Table 22–2. Increases in Total Body and Extracellular Water in Pregnancy

Investigators	Subjects	Tracer	Basis of Change	Mean Increment (liters)
		Total Body Water		
Seitchik and Alper[8]	4	Antipyrine	Late pregnancy compared with 6–7 wk postpartum	12.6
Flanagan et al.[10]	17	Antipyrine	Wk 12–17 and 35–50 compared (data only partially serial)	10.2
Hutchinson et al.[11]	4	D_2O	Wk 36–38 and 1 wk postpartum compared	5.7
McCartney et al.[12]	5	D_2O	Wk 37–39 and 1 wk postpartum compared (gain estimated from bar graph, Fig. 22–1	6.8
Seitchik et al.[13]	21	D_2O	Serial measurement (×5): early pregnancy through wk 37–40	3.1[a]
Hytten et al.[14]	93	D_2O	Studied serially at 10, 20, 30, 38 wk and 6–7 wk postpartum:	
			Gain during gestation	7.7
			Wk 38 vs postpartum	8.5
Seitchik[15]	27	D_2O	Derived from cross-sectional data in 126 nonpregnant gravid and postpartum subjects	7.6[a]
Emerson et al.[16]	5	D_2O	Wk 16–20 and term compared	5.2
Pipe et al.[9]	27	D_2O	Serial study wk 10–14, 24–28, 36–38, and postpartum:	
			Gain during pregnancy	7.2
			Wk 36–38 vs postpartum	7.3
		Extracellular Water		
Chesley[17]	442	Thiocyanate	Both serial and cross-sectional	6.3
Chesley and Boog[18]	16	Thiocyanate	Before labor and 6 wk postpartum compared	6.1
Caton et al.[19]	10	Thiocyanate	Term and 4 wk postpartum compared	5.5
Cariati and Centaro[20]	19	Thiocyanate	Term subjects compared with their theoretical nonpregnant value	6.1
Röttger[21]	44	Thiocyanate	Cross-sectional study:	
			Early gestation vs term	6.9
			Term vs 9 days postpartum	4.3
Freidberg[22]	7	Thiocyanate	1st trimester vs term	6.6[b]
Flanagan et al.[10]	13	Thiocyanate	Partially serial: wk 19–22 and 34–40 compared	4.5
Hytten[7]	—	Thiocyanate	Unpublished results; details not given	6.0
Freidman et al.[23]	31	Bromide	Term subjects vs 15 controls	4.0
McCartney et al.[12]	5	Radiosodium[c]	Wk 37–39 compared with 1 wk postpartum (gain estimated from bar graph, their Fig. 1)	5.0

[a] Dilution of D_2O measured in urine.

[b] This investigator estimated maternal gain only as 4.4 liters; thus, with fetal total, totals 6.6 liters.

[c] See also Plentl and Gray,[24] as several workers have measured radiosodium spaces as percentage weight at term, without calculating gain.

when the tissues were treated with hyaluronidase. Other workers[26,27] subsequently noted that gestation and/or estrogen influence hydration of mucopolysaccharide ground substance; Robertson,[28,29] surprised when he failed to find an obvious relationship between edema and the level of colloid osmotic pressure in a group of gravidas, speculated that a good deal of the physiologic edema seen in many normal pregnancies may be due to estrogen-induced hydration of the ground substance. The relevance of this speculation lies both in the fact that such "complexed" fluid may be poorly mobilized by diuretics and in the possibility that alterations in interstitial compliance, which can conceivably influence blood pressure, may be mediated through humorally induced changes in mucopolysaccharides.[30] Certainly this area, too, should be explored further.

Table 22–1 also shows that the fluid gained during pregnancy is not only stored in the products of conception, but in the maternal extracellular spaces as well. This physiologic hypervolemia is due to increases in both plasma and interstitial volumes.

Both Evans blue dye and radioiodinated serum albumin have been used in studies of plasma volume during gestation. Hytten and Leitch[31] as well as Chesley[32] have reviewed the literature concerning these measurements, which includes more than 30 publications (see table 1.1 in ref. 31). Initially it was claimed that plasma volume, which increases approximately 50 percent during pregnancy, reached a peak by the 30th gestational week, declining slowly toward term. It is now apparent, however, that such decreases were in error and attributable to the fact that late in pregnancy the indicator may not attain complete mixing within 10 minutes if the subject is positioned in a supine or sitting position.[33] More recently, two serial studies[34,35] comprising 152 women and in which the gravidas were positioned in lateral recumbency have established that the increments begin in the first trimester, accelerate in the second, peak near gestational week 32, and remain elevated until term (Fig. 22–1). While the average gain in plasma volume of most gravidas regardless of their initial size is 1200 ml, larger increments may occur when there are multiple fetuses.[36,37] Failure of plasma volume to increase appropriately has been correlated with lower birth weight and/or poor reproduction by several investigators.[38-43]

Whereas the increments in plasma volume occur primarily during the first two trimesters, increases in maternal interstitial volume are greatest in the final trimester. Of note, however, is the fact that in pregnancy, the volume receptors sense such substantial gains in intravascular and interstitial fluids as normal, and when salt restriction or diuretic therapy limits this hypervolemia, the maternal response is similar to that of salt-depleted, nonpregnant subjects.

SODIUM HOMEOSTASIS

During pregnancy there is a cumulative retention of ~950 mEq of sodium distributed between the products of conception and the maternal extracellular volume (Table 22–3). This gain, accumulated over 9 months, is gradual; even during late pregnancy, the period of most rapid gain, the quantity retained is usually too small to be detected by conventional balance techniques. Since renal sodium handling is the prime determinant of volume homeostasis, it is appropriate to consider how hormonal and hemodynamic changes that occur during normal gestation might influence urinary sodium excretion.

Factors Tending to Promote Renal Excretion of Sodium

INCREASED GLOMERULAR FILTRATION

Marked alterations in renal hemodynamics occur during gestation, as both glomerular filtration rate and renal plasma flow increase up to 30 to 50 percent above prepregnancy

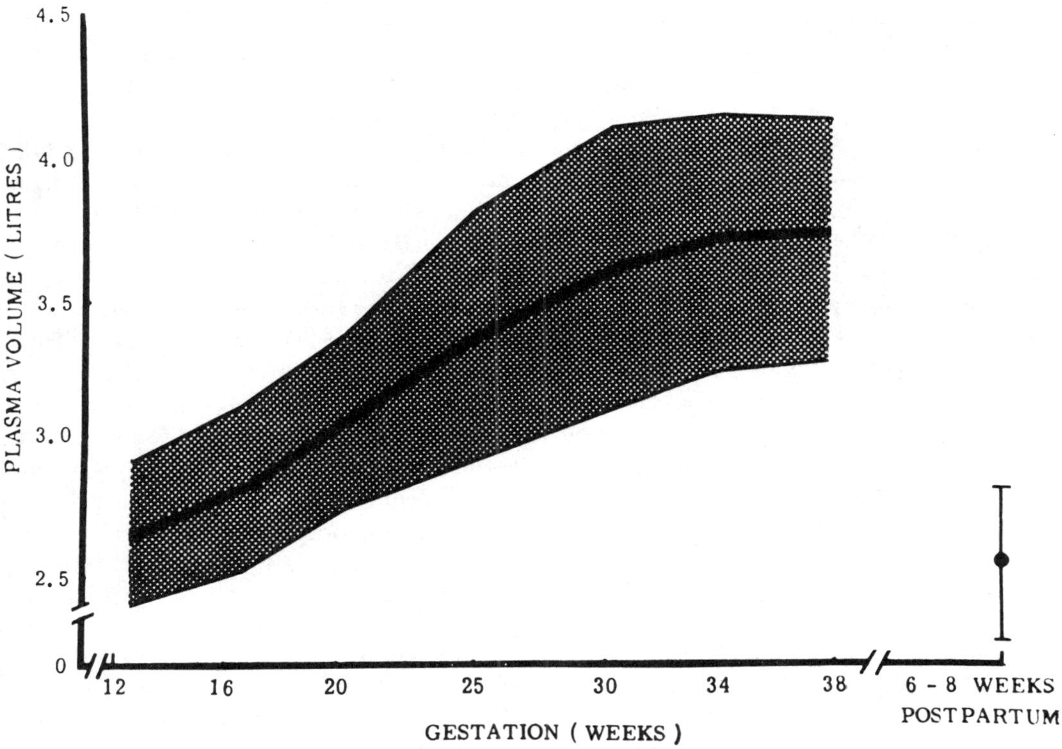

Fig. 22–1. Serial study of mean plasma volume during normal pregnancy. Bar and shaded area, ±1 SD. (From Pirani BBK, Campbell DM, MacGillivray I: Plasma volume in normal first pregnancy. Br J Obstet Gynaecol 78:406, 1971.)

levels.[43-45] Significant increments in 24-hour creatinine clearances are apparent 4 weeks after conception, peak 9 to 11 weeks later, and are then sustained through the 36th gestational week, after which a small decrease may occur.[46-48] The increment in glomerular filtration rate means that the kidneys receive an additional filtered load of 5000 to 10,000 mEq sodium daily. Obviously this increased filtration is accompanied by parallel increments in tubular reabsorption; otherwise, massive sodium depletion would quickly ensue. This ability of the kidney to adjust to increments in reabsorption—glomerular-tubular balance—is not peculiar to pregnancy, for it occurs in both human subjects and experimental animals when glomerular filtration rate is acutely or chronically increased by a variety of maneuvers. The mechanisms whereby these changes take place are not completely understood. In the case of the gravida, the adaptive increment in tubular reabsorption not only equals the large increase in filtered load, but an additional 2 to 6 mEq sodium is reabsorbed

Table 22–3. Storage of Minerals During Pregnancy[a]

Storage Site	Sodium (mEq)	Potassium (mEq)	Calcium (g)
Fetus	290	154	28.00
Placenta	57	42	0.65
Amniotic fluid	100	3	Negligible
Uterus	80	50	0.22
Breasts	35	35	0.06
Plasma	140	4	0.12
Red cells	5	24	0.38
Interstitial fluid	240	8	0.25
Total	947	320	29.68

[a] Source: Hytten FE, Leitch I: The Physiology of Human Pregnancy. 2nd Ed. Blackwell, Oxford, 1971.

daily for fetal and maternal stores. This increase in tubular sodium reabsorption represents the largest renal adjustment during pregnancy.

In pregnant rats glomerular filtration rate increases, and the increment is said to parallel that in plasma volume.[49] Such parallelism, however, is less obvious in humans. The increase in filtered sodium during rodent gestation is paralleled by a proportionate rise in renal microsomal Na–K-ATPase, suggesting that this enzyme may play a role in the enhanced sodium reabsorption of pregnancy.[50] The relevance of this latter observation is unknown, but it is of interest that several diuretics inhibit Na–K-ATPase.[51]

HUMORAL AGENTS

The concentration of several potentially natriuretic hormones rises during pregnancy. Progesterone inhibits the sodium-retaining effects of infused mineralocorticoids in adrenalectomized nonpregnant subjects and may also have a direct inhibitory effect on the reabsorption of filtrate in the proximal tubule.[52] In pregnancy, levels of this hormone increase manyfold compared with those measured during the luteal phase of the menstrual cycle.[53–60] Arginine vasopressin levels have also been noted to increase during gestation by one group of investigators,[61] but not by another group.[62] While in experimental animals pharmacologic doses of arginine vasopressin may be natriuretic and inhibit sodium reabsorption at both proximal and distal nephron sites, it is unclear whether this hormone influences salt excretion in nonpregnant animals or in humans when administered in physiologic doses. Still, Torres et al.[63] have reported that nonpressor doses of arginine vasopressin increase both sodium and urate excretion in gravidas. The effect on the natriuretic system of oxytocin, which increases markedly during pregnancy, is unclear. Also, the roles of circulating neurophysins, melanocyte stimulating hormone, and vasodilating prostaglandins, the levels of which may also increase ingestation, are obscure, but all these hormones may be natriuretic at least under certain circumstances (reviewed in ref. 64).

Finally, no discussion of the effect of salt-losing hormones on the kidney is complete without allusion to natriuretic hormone. Since 1961, renal physiologists have devoted considerable effort to elucidating the nature of a natriuretic factor distinct from changes in glomerular filtration rate or mineralocorticoid activity. Whether this factor is a salt-losing hormone or the natriuresis is produced by alterations of intrarenal physical factors had remained controversial for many years, but more recent evidence has suggested that it is in fact a humoral agent of low molecular weight that may work in part by inhibiting the membrane Na–K-ATPase. At least one group of investigators claims to be able to assay the hormone in biologic fluids.[65–68] Furthermore, the natriuretic hormone is now thought by some to be a significant determinant of sodium excretion in uremic patients, to play a role in the pathogenesis of certain hypertensive states, and to be absent in certain edematous diseases[68] (see also Chapters 2 and 14).

Lindheimer and Weston[69] evaluated the role of natriuretic factors in pregnant women. Hypotonic saline infusions were given to mineralocorticoid-treated, maximally hydrated subjects, a technique that permits localization of events to various regions of the nephron from the analysis of changes in water and solute excretion. The alterations in fractional urine flows, free water generation, and sodium clearances observed were consistent with the hypothesis that volume expansion inhibited proximal tubular sodium reabsorption in these gravidas, but that most of the increment in sodium delivery was reabsorbed at more distal sites. In these experiments glomerular filtration rate increased substantially, and the natriuresis that occurred could have been explained by the concomitant increase in filtered sodium, as well as by alteration in tubular reabsorption. Thus, although the study demonstrated the presence of tubular factors different from aldosterone in human pregnancy, it did not elucidate their role in renal sodium handling.

Little or no research has focused on natriuretic hormone in pregnancy since this report[69] appeared more than a decade ago. The possibility that such a hormone exists has been given new impetus by a radioimmunoassay that is relatively easy to perform.[66] These findings may stimulate new interest in the role of natriuretic hormone in normal and abnormal pregnancies.

PHYSICAL FACTORS

Decrements in plasma albumin concentration and renal vascular resistance as well as an increase in renal plasma flow during pregnancy are all factors that could enhance sodium excretion.[31,64] There is disagreement in the literature as to whether filtration fraction rises or falls during gestation,[43-45] but if the latter is correct, this would lead to decrements in postglomerular oncotic pressure, which in turn would decrease tubular sodium reabsorption. All these potentially natriuretic effects, however, may be opposed by a small decrease in arterial pressure, such as observed during normal pregnancy.

Factors Tending to Enhance Sodium Reabsorption

HUMORAL AGENTS

Production of several antinatriuretic hormones also increases substantially during gestation. The humoral agents that have been studied in greatest detail are aldosterone and desoxycorticosterone.

Aldosterone

The secretory rate, plasma concentration, and excretion of aldosterone and its metabolites are all elevated in normal pregnancy, the values often exceeding those measured in patients with primary aldosteronism[4,58,60,61,70-86] (Fig. 22–2). These changes have been viewed by some as balancing the increases in filtered sodium and progesterone production, while other investigators regard the augmented aldosterone levels as excessive and consider volume homeostasis in pregnant women similar to that of volunteers with experimentally produced chronic volume expansion or of patients with primary aldosteronism. A corollary to this latter view is that increased aldosterone production may be an epiphenomenon secondary to the high levels of angiotensin II that accompany normal pregnancy.

The concept that aldosterone secretion increases in order to balance the increments in glomerular filtration rate and/or progesterone production is based on the following reasoning. Filtration rate increases 50 percent, and if glomerulotubular balance is maintained constant in the proximal tubule, as the results of micropuncture experiments in pregnant rats suggest,[87,88] more sodium will reach aldosterone-sensitive parts of the distal nephron. Compensatory increments occur and prevent sodium wasting. Since progesterone is a competitive inhibitor of aldosterone at these nephron sites, even greater than usual amounts of the hormone must be secreted in order to prevent sodium loss. In this respect, early investigators noted (with one exception[78]) correlations between pregnanediol and aldosterone secretion[72] and excretion[75] in gravidas. More recently, both aldosterone and progesterone were shown to increase sequentially throughout gestation.[58,60,80,82] Also, injection of progesterone into women with intact placentas but dead fetuses resulted in increased urinary aldosterone.[89]

The contrary opinion, that aldosterone levels in pregnancy may be excessive, was derived from the following observations. In nonpregnant subjects the sodium retention induced by continued administration of mineralocorticoids usually ceases in 1 week (after ~400 mEq sodium has been retained and weight has increased 2 to 3 kg) and sodium balance

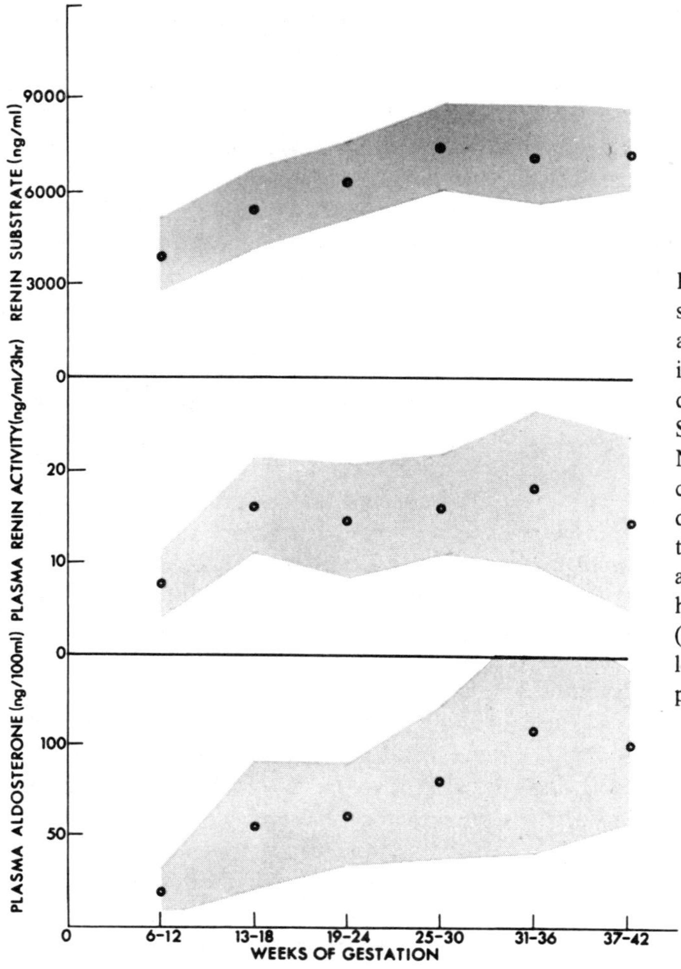

Fig. 22–2. Sequential changes in renin substrate concentration, plasma renin activity, and plasma aldosterone levels in normotensive pregnancy. Circles indicate mean values, shaded areas ±1 SD. (From Weinberger MH, Kramer, NJ, Petersen LP, et al: Sequential changes in the renin–angiotensin–aldosterone systems and plasma progesterone concentration in normal and abnormal pregnancy. p. 263. In Lindheimer MD, Katz AI, Zuspan FP (eds): Hypertension in Pregnancy. Wiley, New York, 1976. Reprinted by permission of John Wiley & Sons, Inc.)

is regained—the renal escape phenomenon. After this new steady state is achieved, additional doses of the mineralocorticoid do not cause further sodium retention. Results from earlier studies seem to demonstrate that mineralocorticoids[90,91] or adrenocorticotropic hormone (ACTH)[92] do not induce sodium retention in pregnant women; such data are compatible with the view that the increased secretion of aldosterone during pregnancy actually exceeds physiologic requirements and that the escape mechanism was already operative. In addition, the maternal physiologic hypervolemia approximates, and at times exceeds, that observed in subjects whose extracellular fluid volume has been expanded by mineralocorticoids. Finally, in the near-term pregnant rat sodium balance does not appear to be aldosterone related.[93]

Neither of the above formulations appears sufficient to explain the alterations in aldosterone metabolism that occur in gestation. In nonpregnant subjects aldosterone-dependent sodium reabsorption amounts to less than 2 percent of their filtered load. By contrast, the daily increment in filtered sodium during pregnancy ranges between 5000 and 10,000 mEq. Aldosterone-stimulated sodium retention is clearly inadequate to balance this increased load appreciably.

Progesterone administered to normal volunteers increases aldosterone excretion,[94-97] but even when administered doses resemble secretion rates in pregnancy, increments are less than those observed during normal gestation. Furthermore, the increases in urinary aldosterone seem to correlate with progesterone-induced volume contraction.[98] Watanabe et al.[89] studied women in whom the fetus had died but was still in utero. Aldosterone secretion had fallen toward levels measured in nonpregnant subjects but increased again after progesterone was administered. Salt balance, however, was not measured.

There are data suggesting that aldosterone levels in pregnancy are not excessive. Secretion, excretion, and blood levels of the hormone change appropriately and in a manner similar to that seen in nonpregnant subjects when extracellular fluid volume is altered either by varying sodium intake[4,75-77,99-103] (Fig. 22–3) or by postural maneuvers,[100,104,105] as well as by administration of diuretics[106-108] or mineralocorticoids.[109] In fact, although baseline levels are already high, sodium restriction leads to marked increases in aldosterone secretion, blood levels, and excretion, and these increments surpass those seen when nonpregnant subjects are similarly restricted (Fig. 22–3). Relatively small doses of mineralocorticoids produce salt retention in pregnant women ingesting carefully supervised constant diets[109] in contrast to the earlier observations in the literature described above, which had suggested that the renal tubule was relatively insensitive to aldosterone during pregnancy. Patterns of solute and water excretion in acutely expanded women resemble those of normal nonpregnant subjects[69] and differ from those observed in volunteers with chronically expanded volume and in patients with primary aldosteronism. Finally, heparinoid, an inhibitor of aldosterone biosynthesis, produces a natriuresis in pregnant women considerably

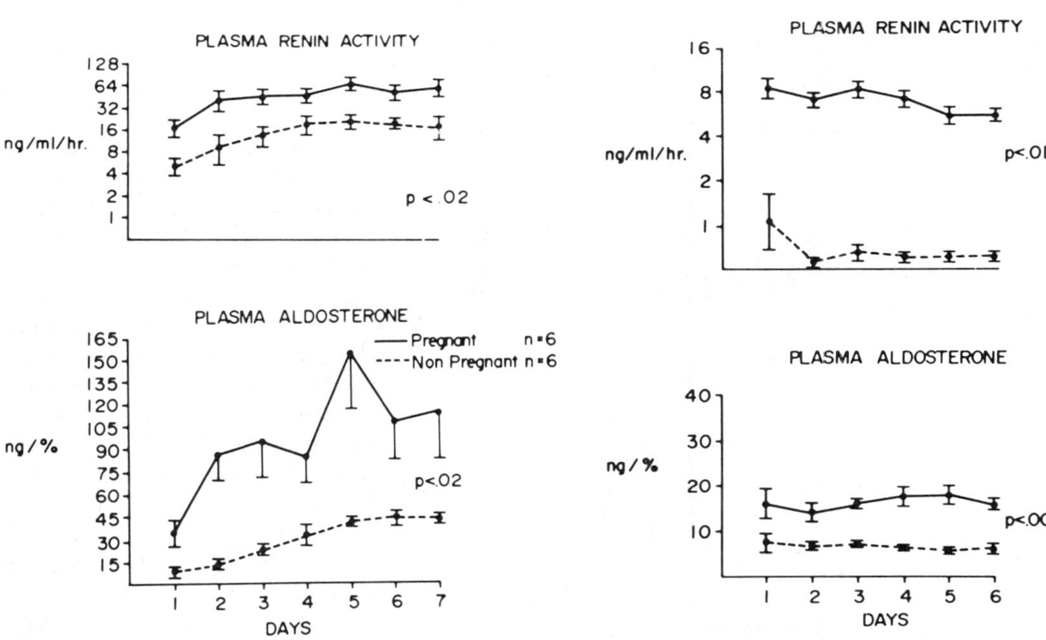

Fig. 22–3. Plasma renin activity and aldosterone levels in six third-trimester and six nongravid women ingesting diets containing 10 mEq/day of sodium (left), and 300 mEq/day of sodium (right). Both renin activity and aldosterone levels are higher in the gravida at each level of salt intake. Note that aldosterone rises to strikingly high levels with sodium restriction, while a diet containing 300 mEq sodium suppressed neither renin nor aldosterone in the pregnant women. (Adapted from Bay WH, Ferris TF: Factors controlling plasma renin and aldosterone in pregnancy. Hypertension 1:410, 1979. By permission of the American Heart Association, Inc.)

before aldosterone excretion decreases to levels near those measured in nonpregnant subjects.[110]

Representative experiments from two studies[109,110] designed to elucidate the role of augmented aldosterone secretion are illustrated in Figures 22–4 and 22–5. In the first study, mineralocorticoid activity was increased by administering exogenous corticoids.[109] Desoxycorticosterone acetate (DOCA) administered during the third trimester caused a substantial decline in urinary sodium excretion that was sustained throughout treatment, and aldosterone excretion decreased from 126 to 28 μg/24 hr. This decline in excretion is the expected result if the aldosterone secretory mechanism is not autonomous but is volume sensitive. After stopping DOCA administration, a natriuresis ensued that did not subside until the ninth day of the recovery period, coinciding with the return of aldosterone excretion to its high pretreatment value.

In another study[110] aldosterone excretion was decreased without concomitant volume expansion by administering heparinoid (RO1-8307), which inhibits aldosterone secretion by undefined mechanisms. Baseline aldosterone excretion in the gravida depicted in Figure 22–5 exceded 200 μg/24 hr despite a daily sodium intake of 120 mEq. Heparinoid administration was started and aldosterone excretion began to decrease on the third day of treatment and continued to decline during the next 5 days, remaining depressed until discontinuance of therapy. Natriuresis commenced during day 3 of heparinoid therapy while aldosterone excretion, although reduced, was still

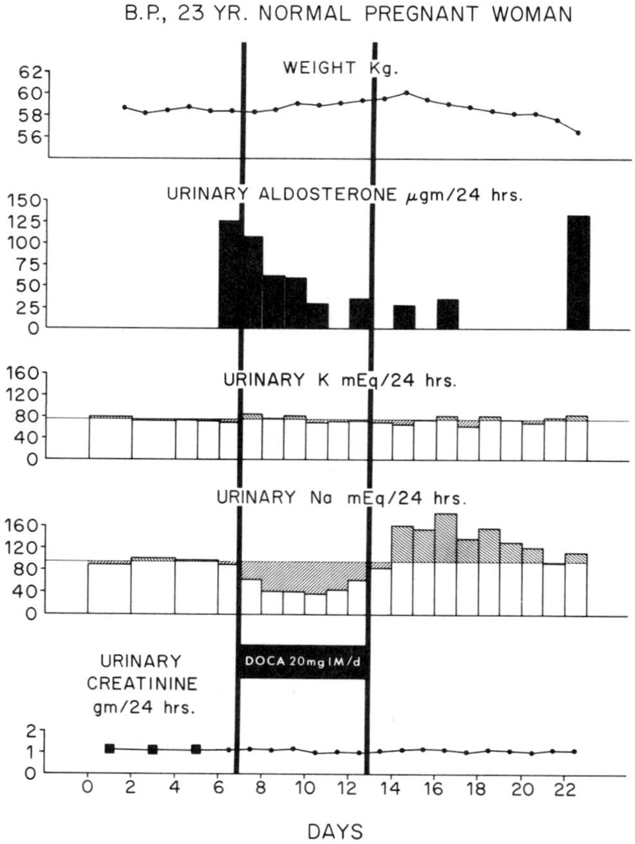

Fig. 22–4. Effect of desoxycorticosterone acetate in a normal pregnant woman. Heavy vertical lines separate treatment periods. Horizontal lines for urinary sodium and potassium are arithmetic averages of pretreatment values. Wider bars denote excretion rates per 24 hours in 48-hour urine collection. All other excretion rates were determined in 24-hour urine collections. (From Ehrlich EN, Lindheimer MD: Effect of administered mineralocorticoids on ACTH in pregnant women. Attenuation of kaliuretic influence of mineralocorticoids during pregnancy. J Clin Invest 51:1301, 1972. By permission of the American Society for Clinical Investigation.)

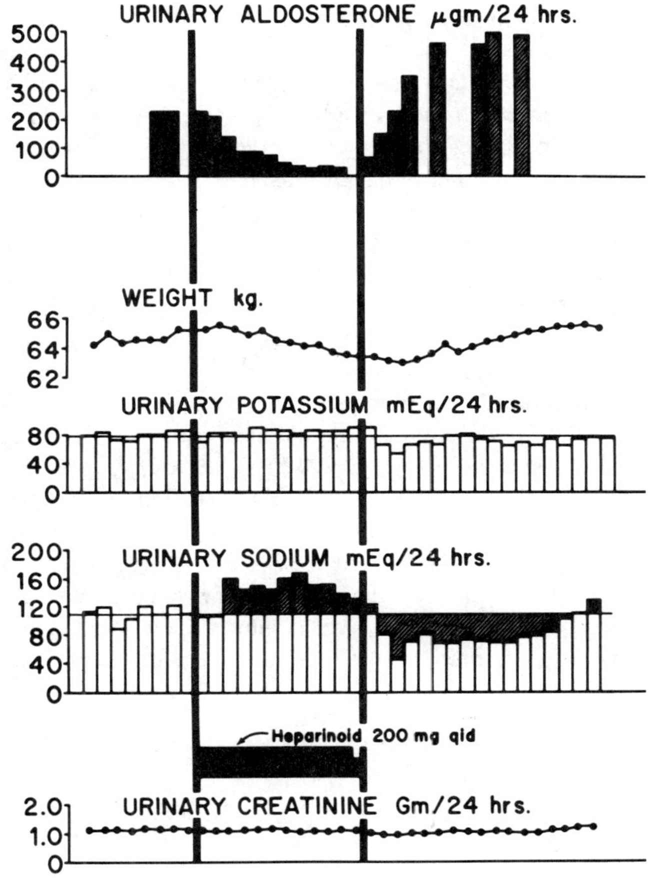

Fig. 22–5. Effect of an inhibitor of aldosterone synthesis (heparinoid) in a normotensive 21-year-old pregnant woman. See description in Figure 22–4. (From Ehrlich EN: Heparinoid-induced inhibition of aldosterone secretion in pregnant women: The role of augmented aldosterone secretion in sodium conservation during normal pregnancy. Am J Obstet Gynecol 109:963, 1971.)

well above normal nonpregnant values. During the recovery period, sodium loss abated as urinary aldosterone increased toward control levels. Aldosterone excretion then surpassed baseline excretion and a period of positive sodium balanced ensued, presumably recouping the salt lost during protracted heparinoid therapy.

In summary, it appears that changes in aldosterone production are not excessive but serve a homeostatic function in pregnancy as they do in nonpregnant subjects. Although circulating levels of aldosterone are high, production of the hormone remains responsive to physiologic demands. In fact, in the presence of sodium depletion, the increase in aldosterone secretion can be striking, whereas with volume expansion, hormonal levels and excretion decrease, albeit sluggishly.* Thus, elevated aldosterone, far from causing excessive sodium retention, could even represent a compensatory response to suboptimal increases in sodium content and extracellular fluid volume.

* It is also possible that aldosterone receptors decrease or are altered during gestation and that this is a partial cause of the elevated levels. That this may be so is suggested by the fact that volume expansion with DOCA or high-sodium diet does not completely suppress aldosterone levels in gravidas to the extent seen in nongravid subjects (Figs. 22–3 and 22–4), differences that cannot be explained by alterations in hormonal protein binding during pregnancy. Also, the availability of lymphocyte receptors to another adrenal hormone, cortisol, may be decreased in gravid women.[111]

Desoxycorticosterone

Secretion of the potent mineralocorticoid desoxycorticosterone (DOC) is greatly increased during gestation, as reflected in elevated levels of plasma DOC, its free index, plasma DOC-SO_4, and increases in urinary free DOC excretion, as well as in the urinary metabolite tetrahydrodesoxycorticosterone.[61,83,84,112–118] In the single instance in which DOC production has been measured using a urinary metabolite isotope dilution method, the production rate near term was more than 40 times greater than that measured 3 days postpartum (8000 μg/24 hr vs 174 μg/24 hr).[112] Originally it was hypothesized that much of this DOC came from a fetal source,[118,119] but the current view is that most of the DOC in the maternal compartment arises by extraadrenal 21-hydroxylation of circulating progesterone.[120,121] In this respect, activity of the enzyme responsible for 21-hydroxylation of progesterone to DOC may be enhanced when estrogen levels are increased,[122] as they are in gestation, and steroid 21-hydroxylase activity, which is present in human kidneys, has been found to be greater in the kidney of a pregnant woman.[123]

Sequential measurements of plasma DOC demonstrate a continuous rise throughout normal gestation, with the most dramatic increments occurring in the third trimester[61,83,84,116] (Fig. 22–6). It should be noted that similar sequential patterns have been described for aldosterone, progesterone, and estradiol and that such correlations are not infrequently cited in discussions concerning renal salt balance. However, whereas aldosterone is very loosely bound to plasma proteins so that rising plasma concentrations with advancing pregnancy presumably result in comparable increments in the biologically ac-

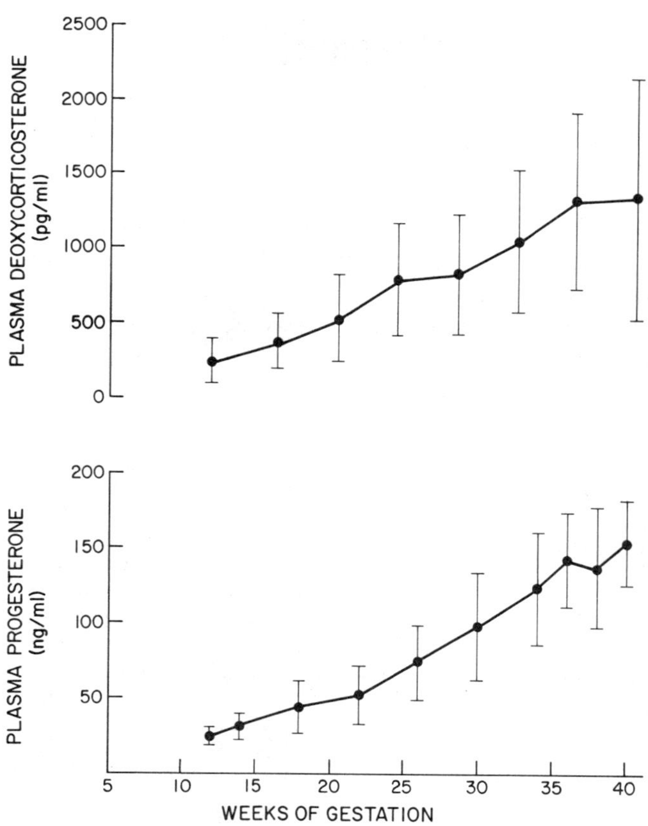

Fig. 22–6. Plasma desoxycorticosterone (top) and progesterone (bottom) levels throughout normal pregnancy. Note continuous increase to term. (Adapted from Parker CJ Jr, Everett RB, Quirk JG Jr, et al: Hormone production during pregnancy in the primigravid patient: Plasma levels of progesterone and 5α pregnane-3,20-dione throughout pregnancy of normal women and women who develop pregnancy-induced hypertension. Am J Obstet Gynecol 135:778, 1979; and II. Parker, CR Jr, Everett RB, Whalley PJ, et al: Plasma concentrations of deoxycorticosterone throughout pregnancy in normal women and in women who developed pregnancy-induced hypertension. Am J Obstet Gynecol 138:627, 1980.)

tive free steroid (this is also suggested by marked concomitant increases of aldosterone metabolites in the urine), each of the other hormones is bound to carrier protein, cortisol-binding globulin in the case of DOC and progesterone, and sex steroid-binding globulin with respect to estradiol. Since concentrations of these globulins also rise during gestation, it is not clear whether the increments in total plasma concentration of these hormones arc accounted for by the simultaneous increase in the carrier protein or whether the biologically free moiety also rises above nonpregnant levels. The situation is even more complex in the case of DOC, which is bound to cortisol-binding globulin with an avidity similar to cortisol and probably greater than progesterone, and alterations in the concentrations of one or both of the latter hormones may also influence the levels of plasma free DOC. Nolten and colleagues[119] addressed these problems by measuring both the free DOC index, which accurately reflects differences in the concentration of the unbound hormone, as well as urinary free DOC excretion. Both were elevated in late pregnancy, the latter markedly so, (that is, 1100 ng/24 hr compared with 90 ng/24 hr in nonpregnant controls).

Problems that may arise when investigators analyze plasma levels of total DOC and attempt to correlate their findings with alterations in sodium balance are illustrated in a series of studies undertaken by Nolten and Ehrlich in collaboration with our group. When the effects of prolonged administration of ACTH were studied in third-trimester women, cumulative sodium retention occurred, attributed in part to enhanced DOC secretion. This is because the high baseline rate of urinary tetrahydrodesoxycorticosterone (THDOC) excretion characteristic of gestation increased sharply during treatment, but aldosterone was depressed.[113] In later studies, however, elevated plasma DOC in third-trimester women not only was unresponsive to changes in salt intake, but surprisingly failed to respond to either ACTH or dexamethasone administration, whereas plasma cortisol rose and fell in the expected manner.[115,124] These studies suggested that DOC may be unresponsive to volume changes and could be pathogenic in certain abnormal salt-retaining states during pregnancy. The apparent discrepancy between responses of urinary THDOC and plasma DOC to ACTH was reconciled by a study in third-trimester women that took into consideration binding interactions of DOC and cortisol with plasma cortisol-binding globulin, and demonstrated that although total plasma DOC was unchanged, the free DOC concentration rose significantly during ACTH administration.[115,124] This was due to displacement of DOC from cortisol-binding globulin by the ACTH-induced increment in cortisol, and since the concentration of the free moiety is quite small compared with the bound concentration, the alterations took place without an apparent change in the level of total DOC. The increase in this free and biologically active DOC could therefore account for the ACTH-induced salt retention; it would also be available for hepatic metabolism to THDOC, thereby accounting for the increased urinary excretion of this metabolite. These observations support the now obvious fact that conclusions about total DOC concentration may be misleading and underscore the need to use measurements that reflect the free steroid fraction, particularly in pregnancy, where increased quantities of circulating cortisol and progestins compete for binding sites on elevated cortisol-binding globulin levels. The results described also have implications beyond the original scope of the study, as they identify an additional mechanism aside from those regulating secretion whereby biologic activity of steroids, specifically those involved with volume regulation, may be modulated.

The role of the augmented free DOC levels in pregnancy is obscure, and the metabolism of DOC during gestation is also poorly understood. Circulating DOC-SO_4, almost undetectable in nonpregnant subjects, is markedly elevated in pregnancy.[118,121] Since DOC sulfurylated in the liver is immediately excreted into the bile, the bulk of plasma DOC-SO_4 measured in gravidas must be formed elsewhere. Nolten and Ehrlich[119] have speculated that this extrahepatic conversion of DOC to DOC-SO_4 may be important to normal volume homeostasis and blood pressure control in gestation and that decrements in conversion may occur in diseases such as preeclampsia. Casey and MacDonald[121] further suggest that sulfurylation of DOC occurs in the kidney, an important end organ of the hormone's action. They note that C_{21} hydroxysteroid sulfotransferase, the putative enzyme in the conversion reaction, is present in the fetal but absent in the adult kidney. These workers further speculate that pregnancy may induce activity in the maternal kidney, and if sulfotransferase activity were not induced to optimal levels (i.e., during a first pregnancy) the intracellular concentration of DOC formed from progesterone in the renal cells would be excessive and could act in situ to effect the salt retention characteristic of preeclampsia. These hypotheses are obviously speculative; however, if confirmed, they would demonstrate that DOC plays an important role in volume regulation during pregnancy.[125]

Other Hormones

The production and blood levels of estrogens, a group of hormones known to induce sodium retention,[52,126] increase during pregnancy.[60,127] The precise mechanism of their antinatriuretic actions, discussed elsewhere,[52,64] is not entirely clear, but part of the sodium-retaining effect of estrogens may be mediated through stimulation of the renin–angiotensin–aldosterone system. In this respect, at least one-half the marked increase in renin activity of pregnant women has been attributed to estrogen-induced increments in renin substrate.[60,128,129] Also, as noted, high levels of estrogens may enhance the extraadrenal 21-hydroxylase activity and thereby increase the conversion of natriuretic progesterone to the salt-retaining hormone DOC.[122]

The role in sodium metabolism during pregnancy of several hormones with potentially antinatriuretic activity remains to be elucidated. These include prolactin, placental lactogen, growth hormone, ACTH, and cortisol. The latter hormone, the total and free levels of which[55,130,131] increase in pregnancy, has always been considered only mildly antinatriuretic, however, we have already mentioned that elevated cortisol will displace the potent mineralocorticoid DOC from cortisol-binding globulin. On the other hand, urinary free cortisol is often directly correlated with sodium excretion,[99,105,115] suggesting that cortisol may be involved in the natriuretic system. Catecholamines may also affect sodium excretion either directly, via sympathetic innervation of the kidney, or indirectly by their hemodynamic effects. Plasma levels and urinary excretion of epinephrine and norepinephrine are either unchanged or slightly decreased,[132–136] but urine dopamine, which may be natriuretic, was found to be elevated in one study.[137]

Finally, the excretion of urinary 18-hydroxycorticosterone increases during pregnancy,[86] but blood levels appear unchanged.[117] Currently, however, there is uncertainty as to whether 18-hydroxycorticosterone, an aldosterone precursor, is itself a potent mineralocorticoid or has only minimal salt-retaining action.

RENIN–ANGIOTENSIN SYSTEM

Angiotensin II can be natriuretic or antinatriuretic, depending on experimental circumstances, but in nongravid women its contribution to volume homeostasis relates to its role in the control of aldosterone secretion. Plasma renin activity, concentration, and substrate as well as angiotensin II levels increase markedly in pregnancy, and normal gravidas are resistant to the pressor and renal effects of infused angiotensin[4,58,60,61,81,101,102,105,107,128,129,138–145] (Fig. 22–2). (See also refs. 43, 50, and 146 for extensive discussions of the renin–angiotensin system in pregnancy.) Besides the kidneys, the gravid uterus also produces considerable quantities of renin, although its contribution to the circulating levels of the hormone is currently unknown (reviewed in refs. 50 and 146). In addition, very high levels of renin are present in amniotic fluid. There is also evidence that renin and its substrate may have different kinetic characteristics in pregnant subjects and that much of the renin present in the blood and amniotic fluid is a high-molecular-weight form, most of which is inactive.[50,146] Of further interest is the observation that while progestins and estrogen enhance circulating angiotensin concentrations, they decrease plasma renin concentration, presumably due to feedback inhibition of renin secretion by elevated angiotensin II levels. This is not the case in pregnancy, as renin concentration remains increased throughout gestation despite elevated levels of circulating angiotensin.

Whether the changes in the renin–angiotensin system during pregnancy result from or cause alterations in volume homeostasis is unclear. Baseline renin activity, already elevated despite renal hyperemia and physiological hypervolemia, is further increased by sodium restriction[4,101,102,129] (Fig. 22–3) or by assumption of a supine or upright posture[105,129,147–149] and is decreased by volume loading.[4,100,101,129] In these circumstances, the changes correlated directly with those of plasma or urinary aldosterone.[4,100,101,105,150] Similarly, Wilson and colleagues,[60] who studied 69 gravidas sequentially throughout gestation, noted significant correlations between renin activity and both plasma and urinary aldosterone. However, other investigators[58,151,152] have been unable to find such correlations and have hypothesized that the renin–angiotensin system is not a major determinant of aldosterone secretion during pregnancy.

Finally, it has been suggested that the enhanced renin secretion may be secondary to increments in the production of vasodilating prostaglandins during gestation.[4,5] The uterus is a rich source of both prostaglandin E_2 (PGE_2) and prostacyclin, and increased synthesis of these lipid hormones may take place in the endothelium of the gravida's blood vessels.[153,154] In this respect, increased quantities of both PGE_2 and metabolites of prostacyclin have been measured in both plasma and urine of normotensive gravidas.[4,155–158] The hypothesis advanced is that this general vasodilatation leads to decreased blood pressure and to dilated vascular volume during pregnancy. The latter, or the increased prostacyclin levels themselves, lead to compensatory stimulation of the renin–angiotensin system, which can explain why there is increased angiotensin and aldosterone levels despite the absolute hypervolemia of gestation (i.e., the "effective volume" is still sensed as suboptimal), as well as increased renal perfusion—a direct prostaglandin effect. This hypothesis is supported in part by the observation that saralasin, an angiotensin inhibitor, decreases the blood pressure of certain pregnant animals, but not in nonpregnant animals of the same species[159–162] and that ingestion of indomethacin, a cyclooxygenase inhibitor, by normal pregnant women increases their angiotensin sensitivity to values similar to those measured in nonpregnant subjects.[163] On the other hand, increased levels of vasodilatory prostaglandins are not a universal observation in pregnancy, and some investigators have noted that plasma PGE or circulating metabolites of prostacyclin increase only in mid- or late gestation,[156,157,164] considerably after increases in renin, aldosterone, and vascular volume have already occurred. Also, 1 Sar 8 Ile angiotensin, an angiotensin II antagonist, failed to alter the blood pressure of four normotensive pregnant women.[165]

PHYSICAL FACTORS

Maternal posture may strongly influence sodium excretion during pregnancy. Two other factors that should be taken into account are the antinatriuretic potential of elevations in ureteral pressure (in the upright or supine position) and the newly formed uterine vasculature, which has been likened to an arteriovenous shunt.

Upright posture decreases sodium excretion in nonpregnant subjects, and the antinatriuretic effects of this position may be exaggerated in pregnancy.[104] Furthermore, in late gestation merely turning from a lateral to a supine position also results in decreased sodium excretion.[69,166-168] In one study[166] this decrement still occurred when thick wall catheters were inserted into the ureter, thus excluding ureteral compression by the enlarged uterus as an explanation. Lindheimer and Weston[69] characterized the supine antinatriuresis further by demonstrating that this effect occurs despite considerable volume loading, and independent of large doses of mineralocorticoids or increased glomerular filtration rate and renal plasma flow. These workers also adduced data suggesting that the antinatriuretic effect of supine posture was mediated in part by an increased fractional reabsorption of filtrate in the proximal nephron. Subsequently, Lindheimer and colleagues[105] performed metabolic balance studies in which gravidas eating a constant diet were kept in bed positioned in lateral recumbency for 2 or 3 days, after which they were up and about or sitting during the day, and slept supine on a head-up tilted bed at night. These women, all in their third trimester of pregnancy, remained in positive sodium balance throughout this period and excreted the retained salt during a final recovery day when they were again positioned in lateral recumbency. In parallel experiments using the same protocol, gravidas were pretreated with DOCA, and although the concomitant expansion abolished the increment of aldosterone that occurs with assumption of an upright posture, acute and chronic sodium retention still occurred.[169] Such data underscore the potent antinatriuretic effects of posture. Even though these studies were designed to obtain functional data concerning postural maneuvers and obviously did not resemble the physiologic circumstances ordinarily confronting most gravidas, the results observed are applicable to volume homeostasis in pregnant women. During the supine upright period, sodium retention was accompanied by weight gain and occasional mild ankle swelling, but was otherwise well tolerated. There was no occurrence of either hypertension or qualitative proteinuria. In essence, the authors provoked symptomless and well-tolerated weight gain that appeared and disappeared rapidly. In the past such rapid increases in weight would alarm physicians who attributed them to complications such as imminent preeclampsia. However, here we see that changes in activity pattern (i.e., hours of upright posture) alone may lead to readily reversible weight gains and do not necessarily signal a pathologic condition. Finally, bed rest in the lateral recumbent position is helpful in the rare instances in which a diuretic appears necessary.

Postural influences may also be responsible for alterations in circadian solute and water excretion observed in some gravidas. Recumbent pregnant women display rhythmic behavior of urine flow and creatinine clearance, as well as aldosterone and electrolyte excretion, which are similar to those of nonpregnant subjects (i.e., daytime peaks and nighttime nadirs).[170-173] However, ambulation results in more striking changes in the pregnant than in the nonpregnant state, with excretory peaks frequently occurring at night.[173] Parboosingh and Doig[174,175] noted, however, that nighttime excretion of sodium and solute-free water is greatest in the first trimester, when postural effects of pregnancy are minimal, and suggest that humoral rather than mechanical causes are responsible for these changes.

Maternal posture may also play a role in determining salt excretion by its influence on ureteral pressure. The calyces, renal pelves, and ureters are normally markedly dilated during pregnancy. The role of both humoral and obstructive factors in the etiology of this dilatation is detailed elsewhere.[64] Of interest is the finding by Rubi and Sala[176] of a marked increase in intraureteral pressure in third-trimester gravidas in the supine or standing position; they also found this pressure to decrease significantly when the obstructive influence of the gravid uterus was removed by placing subjects in the lateral decubitus or knee–chest position, or by cesarean delivery of the fetus. Graded ureteral obstruction decreases sodium excretion in dogs, an effect that is a direct function of the elevated pressure, since the decrement in urinary sodium occurs in the absence of discernible decreases in glomerular filtration rate.[177,178] It is tempting to speculate that during pregnancy part of the antinatriuretic effects of the supine and upright positions may be mediated by the transient or sustained increments in ureteral pressure associated with these postures.

Finally, the uteroplacental circulation has been likened to an arteriovenous shunt.[179,180] In both human subjects and experimental animals the creation of arteriovenous shunts causes sodium retention via alterations in aldosterone secretion, or by direct renal tubular effects.[181,182]

Effects of Acute and Chronic Sodium Loads

Whether gravidas are sodium losers or retainers could be verified experimentally in studies designed to test their ability to excrete infused saline. Unfortunately, with but few exceptions,[100,183] most investigators studied normotensive and hypertensive gravid women only, but not nonpregnant subjects.[184–187] There are also methodologic problems, for the women were usually positioned on their backs during the study, a position that is antinatriuretic in gravid but not in nonpregnant subjects. Dietary salt seems to have been controlled before the test in only one study,[187] a significant limitation, since most reports were performed during a period when salt restriction during pregnancy was fashionable. In one carefully conducted study Chesley et al.[183] examined the effects of hypertonic saline in both third-trimester women and in nonpregnant controls and observed similar sodium excretion in both groups. On the other hand, Weinberger et al.[100] noted that gravidas infused with 2 liters saline excreted less of the load over a period of 4 hours than did nongravid controls. In all other reports, the gravidas appeared to excrete sodium as well as nonpregnant subjects, despite the fact that in most of these studies the pregnant women were positioned on their backs during the test. Such data suggest that gravidas excrete sodium loads at least as well as do nonpregnant women. A similar conclusion can be drawn from animal studies, as term pregnant rats excrete acute sodium loads as well as, or better than, virgin littermate controls.[188,189]

The above conclusions do not necessarily apply to more chronic homeostatic mechanisms. Results of available metabolic balance studies conflict in that some investigators suggest that gravidas have difficulty conserving sodium and may even manifest signs of volume depletion when dietary salt content is too low,[187,190] while others state that sodium balance is achieved similarly in pregnant and nonpregnant subjects.[4] However, the concensus seems to be that gravid subjects are unable to conserve sodium on a low-sodium diet. In the study by Bay and Ferris,[4] dietary restriction to 10 mEq/day should have revealed discernible differences between pregnant and control subjects favoring the gravidas. This is because in late gestation there is daily positive balance of 3–6 mEq. However, the pregnant women excreted in fact 1 to 2 mEq more; they not only failed to gain the usual 0.45 to 0.9 kg (1 to 2 lb) of weight expected during a 7-day period late in pregnancy, but actually lost an average of 1 kg during the study. In addition, plasma aldosterone increased to markedly high levels even for gravidas (Fig. 22–3). Thus the data of Bay and Ferris[4] fail to demonstrate convincingly their conclusions that salt balance in pregnant and nonpregnant subjects is similar, but probably support the concept that some gravidas have a slow renal leak and may cope poorly with rigid salt restriction. When these gravidas do cope, however, balance is achieved by stressing compensatory mechanisms, such as steroid production.

POTASSIUM HOMEOSTASIS

Potassium may play a role in volume control via its influence on the renin–angiotensin–aldosterone system and by controlling vascular reactivity. Theoretically, one might expect pregnant women to waste potassium in their urine, primarily because gravidas who eat and excrete normal quantities of sodium have high blood levels of aldosterone and other potent mineralocorticoids. However, instead of losing potassium, there is a cumulative retention of ~350 mEq of this cation, most of which is stored in the fetal space as well as in the organs of reproduction (Table 22–3). Moreover, in striking contrast to nonpregnant subjects, gravidas are resistant to the kaliuresis provoked by the combination of exogenous mineralocorticoids and a high-sodium diet (Fig. 22–4). This ability to conserve potassium in the face of high concentrations of potent mineralocorticoids such as aldosterone and DOC and the delivery to distal nephron sites of substantial quantities of sodium has been ascribed to the increased levels of progesterone that also occurs during pregnancy.[109]

Data supporting the progesterone hypothesis are illustrated in Figure 22–7. In this study intramuscular desoxycorticosterone acetate, 20 mg/day, was administered to a normal male consuming a constant diet containing 240 mEq sodium daily. Transient sodium retention occurred followed by urinary escape, as evidenced by a return to control values. A kaliuresis appeared on the first day of desoxycorticosterone administration, in contrast to the effects of desoxycorticosterone in the pregnant women depicted in Figure 22–4, which was sustained until progesterone was administered. While continuing the desoxycorticosterone therapy, 100 mg/day of intramuscular progesterone was added to the treatment regimen. Potassium excretion decreased markedly, while urinary sodium changed but

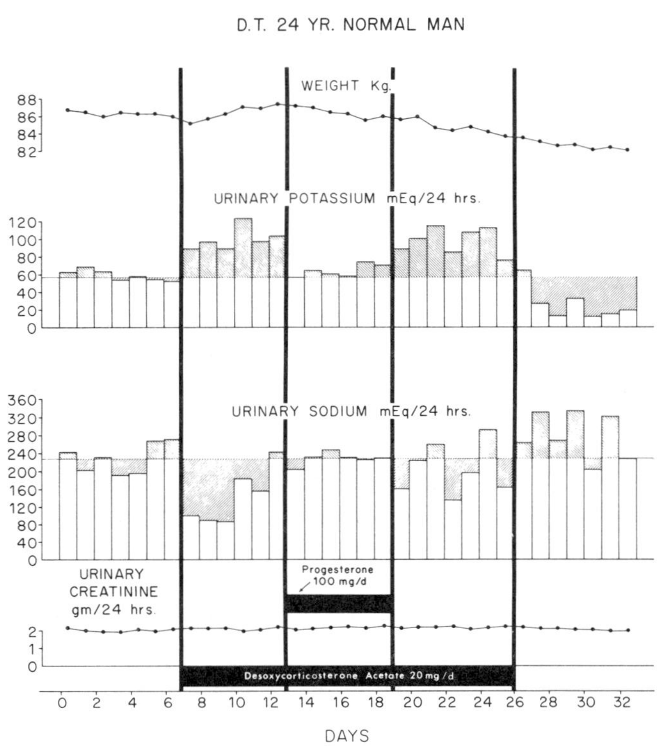

Fig. 22–7. Effect of progesterone administered intramuscularly to a 24-year-old normal male volunteer during continuous treatment with intramuscular desoxycorticosterone acetate. See description in Figure 24–4. (From Ehrlich EN, Lindheimer MD: Effect of administered mineralocorticoids on ACTH in pregnant women. Attenuation of kaliuretic influence of mineralocorticoids during pregnancy. J Clin Invest 51:1301, 1972. By permission of the American Society for Clinical Investigation.)

little. In essence, the experiment simulated two conditions seen in normal gestation: (1) extracellular volume was increased owing to the initial phase of mineralocorticoid-induced salt retention, and (2) with progesterone administration there was no kaliuresis even though plasma mineralocorticoids were high, and the subject excreted abundant sodium in the urine, having already experienced the mineralocorticoid escape phenomenon.

Resistance to the kaliuretic effects of steroids may benefit pregnant women with certain potassium-losing diseases. For example, the excessive renal potassium loss and hypokalemia characteristic of primary aldosteronism and Bartter's syndrome may be ameliorated by gestation.[191,192] Furthermore, if the pregnancy milieu resists kaliuretic stimuli, one might speculate that women with underlying disorders that impair their ability to excrete infused potassium may be jeopardized by gestation as may be the case, for example, in gravidas with sickle cell anemia.

Patients with sickle cell hemoglobin have a specific potassium-excretory defect independent of the angiotensin–aldosterone system, and presumably related to their nephropathy.[193] However, nonpregnant subjects with sickle cell disease are usually normokalemic as long as renal function remains normal; only by sophisticated testing (i.e., potassium or sodium sulfate infusions and furosemide administration) is the secretory defect revealed. Hyperkalemia does not occur until moderate renal insufficiency is present, and at this point in the natural history of the nephropathy potassium levels are noted to be increased out of proportion to the level of azotemia. In pregnancy, however, we have seen transient hyperkalemia in several gravidas with sickle cell hemoglobin whose renal function was normal or only minimally decreased. (D.A. Richardson, A.I. Katz, and M.D. Lindheimer unpublished observations).

CASE STUDY. The patient was a 26-year-old nullipara with sickle cell hemoglobin. Her first-trimester blood pressure was 100/60 mm Hg; urine was protein free. Dyspnea, epigastric pain, nausea, vomiting, and headaches developed during gestational week 24. On admission, blood pressure was 150/110 mm Hg, and there was 3+ proteinuria and a reticulocytosis of 24 percent. A diagnosis of sickle cell crisis was made, and after an exchange transfusion and hydration her symptoms improved and blood pressure became normal.

Figure 22–8 shows the subsequent course of this patient until delivery by cesarean section of a healthy 1040-g boy, who survived. Note that massive proteinuria occurred; the patient's blood pressure was labile, but renal function was well maintained. Since she was nephrotic, a high-protein diet was prescribed, presumably one rich in potassium. Hyperkalemia developed with values ranging from 5.7 to 6.3 mEq/liter. After delivery, a vena cavagram was normal, and a renal biopsy demonstrated sickle cell nephropathy only. One year postpartum, potassium levels were normal, and her urine was protein free.

We have further noted that gravidas with sickle cell disease tend to have lower aldosterone levels than do those of pregnant women with AA hemoglobin (D.A. Richardson, A.I. Katz, and M.D. Lindheimer, unpublished observations). Thus one might speculate that this renal secretory defect combined with the elevated progesterone levels that accompany gestation make these women susceptible to hyperkalemia when challenged with the extra potassium in high-protein diets or in transfused blood, or when they develop renal insufficiency of a degree that would not ordinarily provoke hyperkalemia in nongravid subjects with sickle cell disease.

WATER HANDLING IN PREGNANCY

Plasma osmolality (P_{osm}) decreases during normal gestation to values that average 8 to 10 mOsm/kg below that of nonpregnant women.[28,194-197] This decrement starts shortly after conception, becomes statistically significant during gestational week 5, and reaches

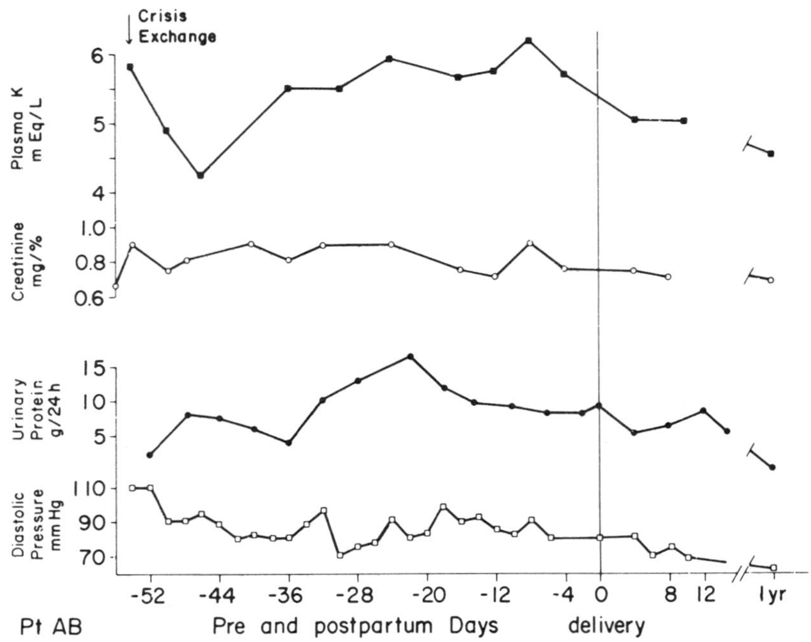

Fig. 22–8. Clinical course of a gravida with sickle cell nephropathy who developed a crisis and hypertension followed by nephrotic proteinuria. Note the persistence of hyperkalemia despite preserved renal function, attributed in part to a high-protein–high-potassium diet administered when she manifested heavy proteinuria. One year postpartum her plasma potassium level was normal. (From DA Richardson, AI Katz and MD Lindheimer, unpublished observations.)

a plateau by the tenth week of pregnancy, after which the decline is sustained until term (Fig. 22–9). Only about 1.5 mOsm/kg of this decrease is due to decrements in urea levels, most of the fall resulting from a decline in plasma sodium and its attendant anion (Fig. 22–9). Thus pregnancy is characterized by a true decrease in effective plasma osmolality.

If similar decreases in P_{osm} were to occur in a nonpregnant subject, secretion of antidiuretic hormone would cease and a large, continuous water diuresis similar to that of patients with diabetes insipidus would ensue. However, pregnant women maintain their P_{osm}, and water loading or fluid restriction leads to appropriate dilution and concentration of their urine. Such data suggest that osmoregulation is altered during pregnancy. Indeed, we have reported that the osmotic thresholds for both vasopressin secretion and thirst decrease by ~10 mOsm/kg each during gestation in both humans and rodents[62,198,199] (Fig. 22–10). It should be stressed that parallel declines in the osmotic thresholds for vasopressin release and thirst are required in order to maintain the new steady-state plasma osmolality (P_{osm}) within a narrow range. For example, P_{osm} will rise despite maximal antidiuretic hormone secretion if the subject is not stimulated to drink more than usual amounts at a lower level of body tonicity. Conversely, considerable polydipsia would be required to maintain any given level of P_{osm} in the absence of vasopressin secretion.

The ability to excrete water is also altered in normal gestation. During pregnancy merely changing from lying on one's side to a supine position markedly decreases urine flow, and quiet standing may be more antidiuretic in pregnant than in nongravid subjects.[69,104,166–168,200–202] This effect of supine posture can occur in at least some patients without incre-

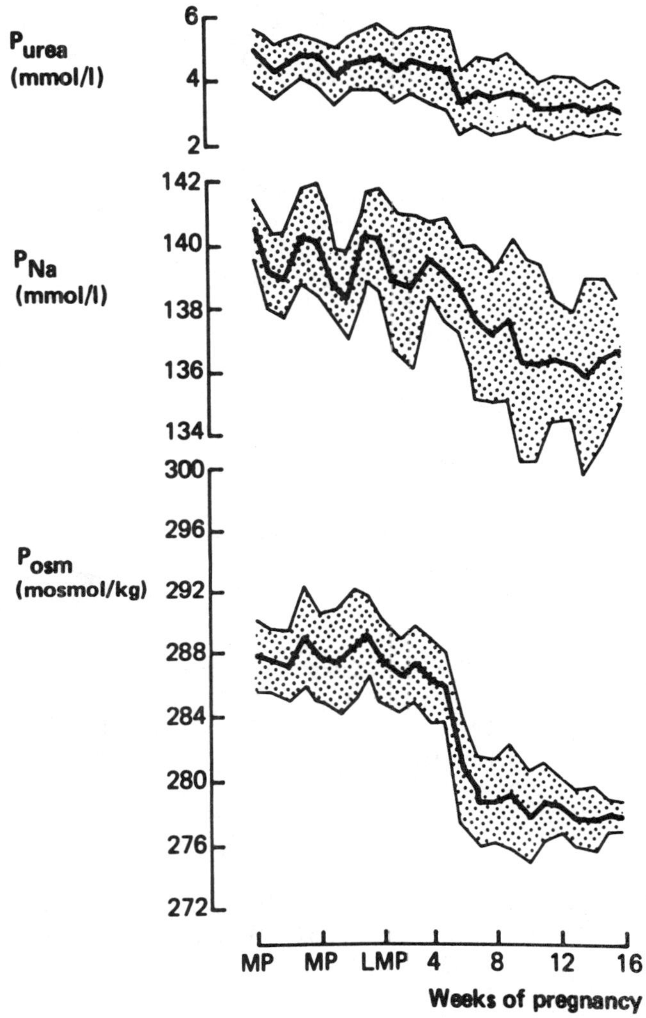

Fig. 22–9. Plasma osmolality (P_{osm}), sodium (P_{Na}), and urea (P_{urea}) measured at weekly intervals from before conception through the first trimester in nine gravidas, all of whom had a successful obstetric outcome. Solid line is the mean; stippled area, ±1 SD. MP, Menstrual period; LMP, last menstrual period. (From Davison JM, Valloton MB, Lindheimer MD: Plasma osmolality and urinary concentration and dilution during and after pregnancy. Evidence that lateral recumbency inhibits maximal urinary concentrating ability. Br J Obstet Gynaecol 88:472, 1981.)

ments in antidiuretic hormone levels, since it has been observed in a patient with diabetes insipidus.[203] In one combined crossed-sectional serial investigation in which the volunteers were studied in a sitting position, the women excreted water loads faster in early pregnancy, but considerably slower near term compared with nonpregnant controls.[204] It should be noted, however, that these nonosmotic effects on water handling are not sufficient, by themselves, to explain the decline in P_{osm} during gestation. No single position is maintained all day; in addition, the posturally induced antidiuresis rarely retards urine flow sufficiently to maintain the chronically reduced P_{osm}, and thus the decreased plasma serum sodium levels[196,197,205,206] observed in pregnancy.

Little is known about nonosmotic factors controlling vasopressin secretion in pregnancy, but in the nongravid human volume is an important determinant of antidiuretic hormone release.[207] Hypovolemia stimulates, while increments in intravascular volume may blunt, hormone secretion. In gestation absolute blood volume increases markedly, but just how the "effective volume" is sensed is a subject of considerable speculation. In this respect it is of interest that the pregnant rat, which also experiences a 40 to 50 percent increase

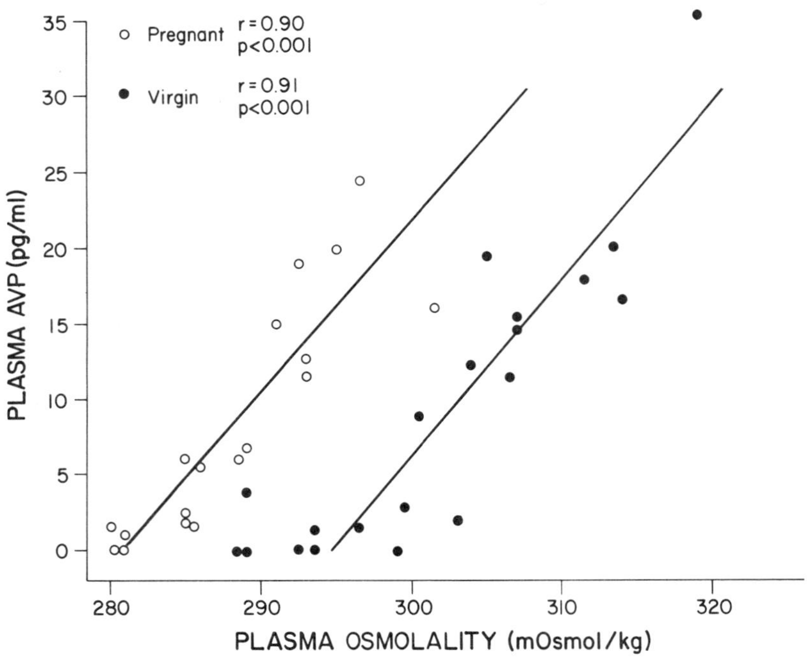

Fig. 22–10. Relationship between plasma osmolality and plasma AVP when the blood tonicity of rats was acutely altered by intraperitoneal injections of saline solutions, ranging from 200 to 1200 mOsm/kg. Each symbol represents one animal. Open circles show gravid ($r = 0.90$; $p < 0.001$) and solid circles show control ($r = 0.91$; $p < 0.001$) animals. Note the parallel regression lines; in the pregnant animal this line intersects the x axis (the apparent threshold for AVP secretion) ~11 mOsm/kg below that derived from the virgin animals. (From Durr JA, Stamoutsos BA, Lindheimer MD: Osmoregulation in pregnancy: Evidence for resetting of the threshold for vasopressin secretion during gestation. J Clin Invest 68:337, 1981. By permission of the American Society for Clinical Investigation.)

in plasma volume near term, resets its volume-sensing vasopressin secretory mechanisms in such a fashion that the increased total blood volume is sensed as normal.[208]

It is a fascinating paradox that although plasma vasopressin levels are normal[62] or even increased[61] in gestation, and while gravidas have little trouble in concentrating their urine, an enzyme in the blood of pregnant women, presumably of placental origin, inactivates vasopressin and oxytocin.[209,210] Activity of this aminopeptidase, also labeled vasopressinase and oxytocinase, is greatest at term, when pregnant women may excrete ingested water less efficiently. There are conflicting reports as to whether pregnant women are resistant to the renal actions of injected Pitressin[63,211–213] or whether gravidas with central diabetes insipidus require more replacement therapy to maintain water balance, although the body of evidence seems to support the latter view.[214] For instance, in reviewing reports of pregnancy in 79 women with central diabetes insipidus, Hime and Richardson[214] noted that the diagnosis was established by modern criteria in only 26 cases. The disease worsened in 13 of these women, was unchanged in five, but surprisingly improved in four; there were no data relevant to the course of gestation in the remaining four women. However, even if resistance to exogenous vasopressin were convincingly proved, it could be due to factors other than the circulating vasopressinase. For example, there could be an increased volume of distribution or metabolic clearance of the hormone, the latter due perhaps to the greater renal and hepatic blood flow, or there might be increments in prostaglandin production and other humoral changes that might blunt the renal effects of vasopressin. In this respect, resistance to exogenous vasopressin has been noted in gravid goats and rats, species that produce no vasopressinase.[215,216]

Urinary Concentration and Dilution

Theoretically, alterations in renal hemodynamics that accompany gestation should be expected to compromise maximal concentrating and diluting ability because of the large increments in filtered solute per nephron. Table 22–4 summarizes nine reports (only three of which included nonpregnant controls) where U_{max} was determined after overnight dehydration, administration of vasopressin or its analogue, or a combination of these maneuvers.[197,217–224] Maximal osmolality appears slightly lower in the gravidas, but obviously more data are necessary to confirm this. More important, U_{max} in pregnant women is sufficiently high, and the difference from nonpregnant controls is too small, to be of any biological significance.

There is little substantive information on the diluting capacity of pregnant women, despite recurring statements in the literature that gravidas lose their ability to handle water loads as pregnancy progresses.[204,225] We have measured minimal urine osmolality during sustained maximal diuresis in normal gravidas noting that their U_{osm} (25 to 88 mOsm/Kg) were in the range considered normal for nonpregnant subjects. Davison and colleagues[197] observed that minimal values in six women who underwent loading in the third trimester were similar to those measured 8 to 10 weeks postpartum.

In the report cited above, urine diluting ability was tested with the patients in lateral recumbency, the authors being aware that supine posture may interfere with the attainment of minimal osmolal concentration (or maximum free water generation) during gestation. Serendipitously they also made the observation that while lateral recumbency is the required position for prenatal measurement of most renal functional parameters, this posture interferes with tests of concentration. U_{max} actually fell in patients dehydrated 12 hours when they assumed a lateral decubitus position for an additional 3 hours, but increased when the test was repeated with the subjects

Table 22–4. Urinary Concentrating Ability in Pregnant Women

	Maximum $U_{Osm}^{a,b}$ (mOsm/kg)		
Investigators	Nonpregnant	Pregnant	Dehydration Time (hr)
Kaitz[217]	—	935 ± 118 (30)	24
McCartney et al.[218]	—	910 ± 113 (7)	20
Norden and Tuttle[219]	—	942 ± 207 (24)	24
Reeves and Brumfitt[221]	—	75% > 850 (33)	21
Williams et al.[222]	1,052 ± 92 (20)	930 ± 95 (45)	24
Norden et al.[223]	—	899 ± 133 (75)	16, then Pitressin injected
Davison et al.[197]	854 ± 107 (6)	752 ± 110 (6)	17
Hutchon et al.[224]	1,141 ± 223 (7)	826 ± 223 (8)	15
Hutchon et al.[224]	1,109 ± 225 (7)	932 ± 169 (27)	Received Desmopressin (DDAVP) without dehydration

[a] mean ± SD.
[b] Numbers in parentheses represent number of subjects.

sitting quietly. This observation may be explained by fluid mobilization from the extremities during bed rest, which results in either volume suppression of antidiuretic hormone release or in a mild osmotic diuresis. Such observations demonstrate the importance of upright posture, such as quiet sitting, when tests of maximum urine concentration ability are performed in pregnancy, and illustrate another reason why the data summarized in Table 22–4 are still inconclusive.

Alterations During Abnormal Gestation

Oliguria often accompanies preeclampsia and, not surprisingly, such patients have been shown to have a decreased capacity to excrete water loads.[226] Furthermore, the antidiuretic effects of posture may be more pronounced in hypertensive or preeclamptic subjects.[202,227] Vasopressin levels were no different than those of normal gravidas in one report,[61] but the sensitivity of the concentrating mechanism to the hormone and the ability of vasopressin secretion to be suppressed by water loading during preeclampsia remain to be established.

It should be noted that most of the early literature devoted to abnormalities in water handling in pregnancy is incomplete, having predated the development of sensitive and specific radioimmunoassays for arginine vasopressin; only recently have investigators developed reliable techniques that ensure that the vasopressinase in maternal plasma is immediately inactivated when blood samples are drawn. Both obstacles have now been eliminated, and soon more may be known regarding certain uncommon syndromes complicating gestation, such as transient central (J.M. Davison, personal communication) and nephrogenic diabetes insipidus of pregnancy. We have recently studied two women who developed florid diabetes insipidus in the third trimester, one associated with preeclampsia, whose disease subsided approximately 1 week postpartum. Neither had evidence of obstructive uropathy, and their urine remained hypotonic and unresponsive to exogenous vasopressin despite markedly elevated P_{osm}. Plasma vasopressin measured in one patient was high in relationship to the very dilute urine (Barron, Cohen, Emmanuel, Lindheimer, and Robertson, unpublished results).

Renal Regulation of Acid Excretion

Acid–base metabolism is altered during normal pregnancy. Blood levels of hydrogen ions decrease by 2 to 4 nmol/liter early in gestation, a decrement that is sustained throughout pregnancy.[228-233] Thus arterial, or arterialized capillary, blood pH is usually 7.42 to 7.44 in pregnant compared with 7.38 to 7.40 in nonpregnant women. This mild alkalemia is believed to be respiratory in origin, since gravidas normally hyperventilate and arterial P_{CO_2} decreases from a mean of 39 mm Hg when nonpregnant to 31 mm Hg during gestation.[231,234,235] Simultaneously, plasma bicarbonate levels decrease by ~4 mEq, so that values from 18 to 22 mEq/liter should be considered normal.

Not many studies have been done of renal reclamation and regeneration of bicarbonate during pregnancy. Lim et al.[231] infused 300 to 500 mEq of hypertonic bicarbonate into women in the third trimester. The bicarbonate titration curve from this study is depicted in Figure 22–11. Despite large filtered loads of bicarbonate, reabsorption continued to increase, and even when plasma levels reached 31 mEq/liter, the points remained close to the line of complete reabsorption. Since pregnant women are hypocapnic and have increased extracellular volumes, which should lead to an exaggerated splay in the titration curve and/or a decrease in apparent T_m, these results were not anticipated. A small but persistent bicarbonate leak occurred at lower plasma bicarbonate concentrations in preg-

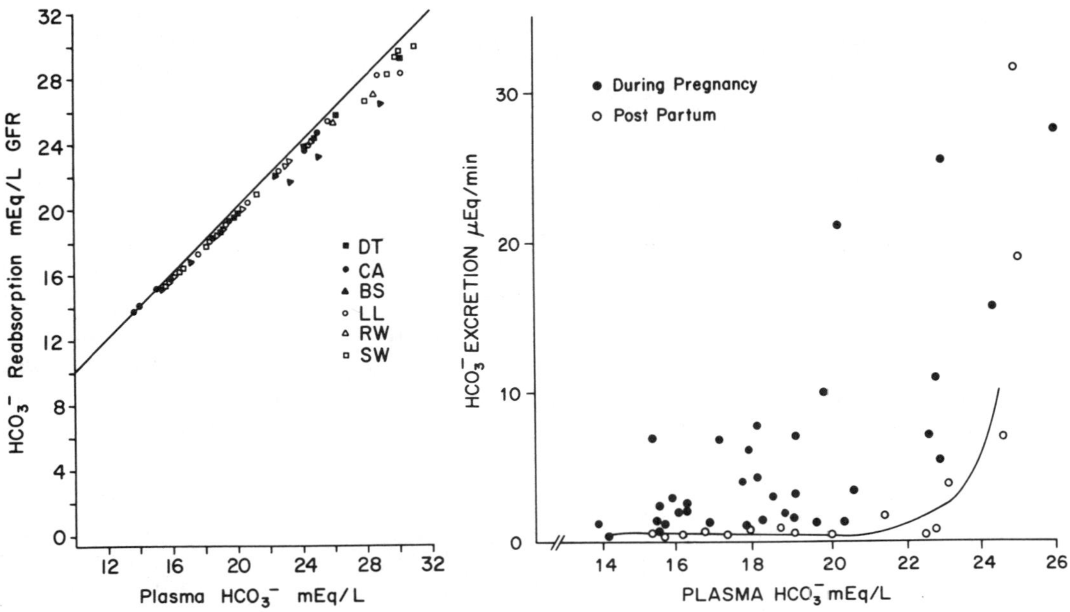

Fig. 22–11. (Left) Bicarbonate titration curves in six third-trimester women before and after slow infusion of 5 percent $NaHCO_3$ solution. In subject BS, who displays the widest splay, the infusion inadvertently ran faster for a period of 20 to 30 minutes. (Right) Bicarbonate excretion as a function of plasma HCO_3 concentration in gravid women (solid circles) and in two women who were restudied after delivery (open circles). T_{HCO_3} is lower in the pregnant subjects (mean 18.9 mEq/liter), but even when suppressed the bicarbonaturia is still trivial. (From Lim VJ, Katz AI, Lindheimer MD. Acid base regulation in pregnancy. Am J Physiol. 231:1764, 1976.

nant women than in the same women postpartum (Fig. 22–11). This slight bicarbonaturia was occasionally present at plasma bicarbonate concentrations as low as 15 to 16 mEq/liter.

Administration of NH_4Cl to pregnant women results in urinary acidification of at least a similar magnitude to that of similarly tested nonpregnant subjects.[231,232,236] It is of interest that the decrement in urine pH as well as the increases in titratable acid and ammonium excretion occur even though the blood pH decreases only slightly from 7.44 to 7.40. Thus, substantial bicarbonate regeneration can be demonstrated at blood pH values higher than in nonpregnant women, and in fact regeneration begins when values are still alkaline compared with the nonpregnant state. Finally, distal hydrogen secretory capacity, as measured by the increment in urinary P_{CO_2} tension during the bicarbonaturia evoked by the bicarbonate infusions, appeared to be intact during pregnancy.[231]

Acid–base parameters have been measured during gestations complicated by hypertension.[232,236-238] Values for pH, P_{CO_2}, plasma bicarbonate, and the effects of chronic NH_4Cl loading are similar to those measured during normal pregnancy. One investigator noted decreased ability to excrete ammonia after acute acid loading, but the decrement was small and of little clinical significance.[232]

In summary, the kidney's capacity to secrete protons appears unchanged by pregnancy, but steady-state plasma bicarbonate and P_{CO_2} levels are lower than in nonpregnant women. These values are altered little in preeclampsia.

HYPERTENSIVE COMPLICATIONS OF PREGNANCY*

Hypertension during gestation remains a major cause of mortality and morbidity in both mother and fetus. This section briefly reviews the hypertensive disorders of gestation focusing on preeclampsia. The management of hypertension in pregnancy is detailed by us and by others elsewhere;[43,239-241] the present discussion is limited to recent controversies concerning the use of antihypertensive agents as well as volume loading in the treatment of preeclampsia.

Alterations of Blood Pressure in Pregnancy

Blood pressure recordings have been part of prenatal care since the introduction of the sphygmomanometer, but precise data on frequency distribution of blood pressures have appeared only recently. Mean blood pressure decreases early in gestation, and by mid-trimester diastolic levels are often 10 mm Hg less than postpartum measurements. Blood pressure then increases, gradually approaching prepregnancy values near term. Since cardiac output rises rapidly during the first trimester[31] and remains relatively constant thereafter, the decrement in pressure is due to a marked decrease in peripheral vascular resistance. This is greatest in the uterine vasculature, which eventually develops into a large low-resistance shunt, but other organ systems, including the kidney and skin, participate in the generalized vasodilatation of pregnancy. For instance, renal plasma flow increases an average of 35 percent, and the increments in blood flow to the skin occasionally lead to the appearance of vascular spiders during pregnancy. The slow rise in blood pressure toward nonpregnant levels that follows the mid-trimester nadir is also of interest, because it demonstrates that increasing vasoconstrictor tone is a feature of late pregnancy, both in women who remain normotensive, as well as in those who develop preeclampsia.

Observation of a physiologic decrement in blood pressure during pregnancy raises the question of the upper limits of normal blood pressure during gestation and whether these limits differ from those in nonpregnant populations in this respect. The results of two large epidemiologic surveys are revealing. Page and Christianson[242] analyzed blood pressure results from 12,954 gravidas. They noted that perinatal mortality increased significantly when mean arterial pressure exceeded 90 mm Hg in mid-trimester and 95 mm Hg in late pregnancy. Friedman and Neff[243] analyzed data from 38,636 women and noted that fetal loss rose abruptly when diastolic levels were greater than 84 mm Hg at any period of gestation. In essence, fetal outcome is threatened by levels of maternal blood pressure within the range generally considered normal (by most) in nonpregnant populations. Therefore, we consider diastolic levels of 75 mm Hg in the second and 85 mm Hg in the third trimester as the upper limits of normal. (Actually, fetal risks are not only dependent on the degree of hypertension, but on its cause as well. This finding is suggested in these same surveys, in which gestational outcome in borderline or mildly hypertensive gravidas becomes markedly poorer if qualitative proteinuria is present, implying preeclampsia or glomerular disease as the etiology of the hypertension.)

The cause of the decrease in peripheral vascular resistance is obscure. Levels of estrogen and progesterone which may relax smooth muscle, are increased, but as noted these increments are most marked in the latter half of gestation, while the decrement in peripheral resistance is maximal early in pregnancy. The possible role of increased vasodilatory prostaglandins in producing vascular resistance to the increased levels of circulating angiotensin II during gestation has already been alluded

* References cited in this section, with rare exceptions, are restricted to material relating to fluid and electrolyte metabolism. Additional sources can be found in several detailed reviews (refs. 5,43,45,64,238,239,241).

to, and little is known about catecholamine metabolism during pregnancy. While most investigators focus on hormonal imbalances that may cause hypertension in pregnancy, the opposite is also possible. In this respect, the authors are aware of a gravida in whom severe symptomatic postural hypotension developed during pregnancy that was resistant to treatment with mineralocorticoids and sodium loading. The problem disappeared after delivery.

Classification of Hypertension in Pregnancy[43,64,241]

The literature dealing with high blood pressure in pregnancy is confusing largely because it may be difficult to distinguish clinically between preeclampsia, essential or secondary hypertension, renal disease, and combinations of these separate entities. For instance, normal blood pressure early in pregnancy does not necessarily differentiate preeclampsia from essential hypertension, since women with the latter disease experience an early gestational decrement in blood pressure to normal values. In addition, an accelerated phase of essential hypertension, which is actually a rare event in pregnancy, as well as certain forms of renal disease such as glomerulonephritis, lupus erythematosus, and pheochromocytoma, may all mimic preeclampsia. These diagnostic problems are best illustrated in reports in which the etiology of hypertension complicating pregnancy has been determined by renal biopsy (cited in refs. 239 and 244). Of particular interest is a study in which an academic nephrologist and an obstetrician recorded their impression before biopsy, and an accurate diagnosis was made on clinical grounds in only 58 percent of the patients.[245] Such studies also indicate that a diagnosis of pure preeclampsia is often erroneous when the patient is a multigravida and underscore the problems inherent in interpreting the literature when diagnosis is based on clinical criteria alone; most suspect are those series in which most patients described as preeclamptic or toxemic are multiparous.

There is also confusion concerning the nomenclature and classification of diseases that cause high blood pressure in pregnancy. Of the many classifications proposed, the one set forth by the American College of Obstetricians and Gynecologists Committee on Terminology appears to us to be both simple and useful. The hypertensive disorders of pregnancy are divided into four categories.

PREECLAMPSIA–ECLAMPSIA

This hypertensive disorder, peculiar to pregnancy, is associated with proteinuria, edema, and at times coagulation abnormalities. It occurs primarily in nulliparas, usually after their 20th gestational week and often near term. When the disease progresses to a convulsive phase, it is termed eclampsia. Attempts to categorize this disease as mild or severe should be discouraged, and all patients suspected of having preeclampsia should be hospitalized. This is because women with seemingly mild disease, for instance a young gravida with a blood pressure of 140/90 mm Hg and minimal proteinuria, can suddenly convulse, a dangerous event if she is an outpatient.

In the past, enormous importance was given to excessive weight gain and edema, a characteristic of more than 70 percent of women manifesting preeclampsia. However, these signs also occur in many normotensive gravidas, and therefore it is not surprising that in the large epidemiologic survey analyzed by Friedman and Neff[243] neither edema nor maternal weight gain alone could be correlated with poor fetal outcome.

CHRONIC HYPERTENSION

Most women in this category have essential hypertension, but in some the increased pressure is secondary to a variety of conditions, including preexisting renal parenchymal disease, renal artery stenosis, coarctation of the aorta, primary hyperaldosteronism, renin-secreting tumors, and pheochromocytoma. Presence of hypertensive retinopathy and the knowledge that hypertension was present before the pregnancy or before the 20th gestational week aids in the diagnosis, with the exception of uncommon instances of early preeclampsia in patients with hydatidiform disease, fetal hydrops, and perhaps renal parenchymal disease.

Hypertensive patients—primary or secondary—are more susceptible to superimposed preeclampsia than are normotensive gravidas, and their course and prognosis are usually unaffected by pregnancy. The exception to this outcome is those with pheochromocytoma, in which maternal mortality in undiagnosed cases approaches 50 percent. Considering the catastrophic outcome in pregnancies complicated by undiagnosed pheochromocytoma and the therapeutic success that follow prepartum diagnosis of this disease, measurement of plasma and urinary catecholamines or of vanillylmandelic acid excretion is indicated in all hypertensive pregnant patients.

CHRONIC HYPERTENSION WITH SUPERIMPOSED PREECLAMPSIA

This condition is often overdiagnosed. Some use this classification for all chronic hypertensives and patients with known renal disease whose blood pressure suddenly increases during the third trimester, while others require that increments in proteinuria also be present. In this respect, a recent survey of pregnancy in women with underlying parenchymal renal disease is of interest. Superimposed preeclampsia was diagnosed on clinical grounds in 12 patients and eclampsia in one, but postpartum renal biopsies revealed that the glomerular lesions characteristic of preeclampsia were present in only seven gravidas, including the one who had convulsed.[246]

In our experience hypertensive women with superimposed preeclampsia are often multiparas, and their disease may present quite early in the last trimester. If their gestations are permitted to continue, many manifest extremes of hypertension, heavy proteinuria, coagulation abnormalities, oliguria, and decreasing renal function, and the fetus often succumbs. Chesley[43] has claimed that if these patients conceive again there is a strong possibility that this acute syndrome will recur.

LATE, TRANSIENT, OR GESTATIONAL HYPERTENSION

These women develop hypertension alone, late in pregnancy or in the immediate puerpuerium, but their blood pressure returns to normal by postpartum day 10. If the patient is nulliparous, it may be difficult to distinguish this disease from preeclampsia. Most of the women with late hypertension will have high blood pressure again in subsequent gestations, an entity that was once labeled recurrent toxemia. It is probable that patients with this disease represent a population destined to develop essential hypertension later in life, analogous to women with gestational hyperglycemia who eventually become frank diabetics. Finally, the word "gestational" was included with "late" and "transient" in describing this category because the term gestational hypertension is extensively used in the current literature. However, since preeclampsia is also a gestational disease, we believe the terms "late" and "transient" hypertension more appropriate. This is especially true, since the pregnancy prognosis of women in this fourth group is much more favorable than that of patients with preeclampsia.

Pathophysiology of Preeclampsia[43,240,241]

HYPERTENSION

The blood pressure rise in preeclampsia usually occurs late in pregnancy. However, midterm blood pressures, while normal, are in fact higher in many (but not all) women who later manifest hypertension near term than in gravidas who remain normotensive throughout gestation. Studies of remote hypertension in such patients suggest that pregnant women whose diastolic levels at midterm are "normal," but that measure 70 mm Hg or more, often develop frank hypertension near term and belong to two populations: women who are actual or potential hypertensives (the latter having experienced the physiologic decrement of early pregnancy), and gravidas who are destined to manifest preeclampsia and whose peripheral vascular tone may be inappropriately elevated quite early in gestation.

Hypertension in preeclampsia often shows an interesting reversal of the circadian blood pressure rhythms that normally occur in pregnant and in nonpregnant women, that is, morning peaks and nighttime nadirs. In preeclampsia the rhythm may be abolished or even reversed, the highest pressures occurring at night.

The rise in blood pressure in preeclampsia is typically labile because of an intense vascular sensitivity to endogenous pressor peptides and amines. Whereas normal pregnant women are quite resistant to the pressor effects of infused angiotensin, those destined to develop preeclampsia manifest increased pressor responsiveness to this peptide many weeks before any clinical signs of the disease.[142] In women with chronic essential hypertension, sensitivity to infused angiotensin also increases before the development of superimposed preeclampsia.[247] In this respect there are discrepancies in the literature dealing with the renin–angiotensin system in preeclampsia. Some report decreased renin concentration, renin activity, and angiotensin levels in this disease compared with normal pregnancy, while others have noted increments in both plasma renin activity and circulating angiotensin II in preeclampsia.[58,61,64,146,239,240,241] One must keep in mind, however, that even at lower concentrations these pressor substances probably play a pathogenetic role, if the exquisite sensitivity of the vasculature is taken into account. Nevertheless, some observations argue against a role of angiotensin II in the pathogenesis of hypertension in preeclampsia. The antagonist 1 Sar 8 Ile angiotensin failed to lower the blood pressure in preeclamptics, and both saralasin and converting enzyme inhibitor (SQ 20881) were ineffective when administered shortly after delivery to preeclamptic patients whose blood pressure had remained elevated.[165,248,249] Finally, although renin substrate levels are similar in normotensive gravidas and preeclamptics, that of the latter group contains a greater percentage of a high-molecular-weight angiotensinogen however, the meaning of this difference is presently obscure.[145]

Other humoral substances implicated in the pathogenesis or maintenance of high blood pressure in preeclampsia, including catecholamines, prolactin, and vasopressin, are discussed elsewhere.[43,240,241] There is controversy as to whether norepinephrine levels rise, but the vasculature of preeclamptics is more sensitive to the pressor effects of this amine. The literature also abounds with references to unknown humoral substances said to be important in the pathophysiology of preeclampsia, but most of these reports are unconfirmed.

Most recently, investigators have turned their attention to the vasodilating prostaglandins, proposing that an impaired ability of the uterus or blood vessels to synthesize these lipids, or an increase in their inactivation, may cause hypertension because of an imbalance between circulating pressor substances (e.g., angiotensin) and the counteracting effects of prostaglandins E or I on vascular smooth muscle. Another attractive feature of this hypothesis is the fact that an appropriate balance between vascular prostacyclin and platelet thromboxane synthesis is considered important for normal clotting. Thus deficient prostaglandin I production may be linked to the coagulation problems that may accompany preeclampsia.

In keeping with the prostaglandin deficiency theory are the following observations: (1) prostaglandin inhibition increases blood pressure in pregnant animals; (2) ingestion of aspirin or indomethacin, both cyclooxygenase inhibitors, decreases the vascular resistance of normotensive gravidas to infused angiotensin to levels seen in preeclampsia; (3) prostaglandin levels may be decreased in the placenta, decidua, chorion, and amnion of women with preeclampsia; (4) urinary excretion of both PGE and prostacyclin decreases in this disease; and (5) prostacyclin generation is decreased, despite increased levels of its stimulating factor, in the maternal and fetal vessels of such patients.[5,154,158,250-255]

The Kidney and Volume Homeostasis

The effects of preeclampsia on the kidney include a morphologic lesion in the glomerulus characterized by intracapillary swelling (glomerular endotheliosis), functional changes in renal hemodynamics, abnormal protein excretion, and alterations in the tubular handling of urate as well as sodium.

Both glomerular filtration rate and renal plasma flow decrease, and since the decrement in glomerular filtration rate is greater, the filtration fraction falls. The drop in glomerular filtration rate is approximately 25 percent in most cases, but on occasion may progress to renal failure.[43,45,64]

Abnormal proteinuria almost always accompanies preeclampsia. The proteinuria may be minimal, moderate, or severe (i.e., in the nephrotic range) and is nonselective.[45,64] Nephrotic syndrome deserves emphasis, for in the past heavy proteinuria was believed to be uncommon in preeclampsia and, when it did occur, it was considered to indicate a severe form of the disease. It is now apparent that preeclampsia is the most common cause of nephrotic syndrome in pregnancy and that the diagnosis may be overlooked if one fails to consider diastolic levels between 80 to 90 mm Hg abnormal in these patients.[244]

The tubular handling of urate is altered in preeclampsia. Uric acid clearance decreases. The decrement may occur earlier and may be more profound than that in glomerular filtration rate, so that the urate:inulin (or urate:creatinine) clearance ratio is decreased as well. This results in a rise in plasma uric acid levels, which may help in distinguishing preeclampsia from other hypertensive complications of gestation. The level of hyperuricemia correlates directly with the decrement in plasma volume that occurs in preeclampsia, and indirectly with plasma renin activity.[256]

SODIUM RETENTION AND EDEMA

Edema alone imparts no adverse prognosis to reproductive outcome, and fetal size may even be greater in such patients.[6,7,243] Nevertheless, rapid weight gain and generalized edema are features of preeclampsia, and the ability to excrete sodium is usually impaired in the preeclamptic patient. The degree of impairment varies, and in clinical practice these women frequently are able to tolerate dietary sodium in excess of 100 mEq/day. If given diuretics or rigidly salt-restricted diets they may manifest signs of salt depletion.[190,257-259] Furthermore, the disease can occur without fluid retention, in which case it is often more severe.[43] Even when edema is present, plasma volume is decreased, compared with normal pregnancy, and hemoconcentration occurs.[35,42,43]

The cause of sodium retention in certain women with preeclampsia is obscure. The decrease in glomerular filtration, in general to levels comparable to or still above those in nongravid women, seems insufficient to explain it. Aldosterone levels in early and midpregnancy are similar to those in women destined to develop third-trimester hypertension as compared with those who remain normotensive throughout gestation,[82] while production, plasma concentrations, and urinary excretion of the hormone actually decrease when preeclampsia occurs.[58,61,73,85,89,117,260]

The metabolism of other hormones that influence sodium excretion has scarcely been evaluated in preeclampsia; when it has been studied, the results thus far are contradictory or inconclusive. Moreover, most investigators have simply measured circulating levels of these humoral agents without attempting to relate the values to the patient's salt balance or weight gain. The significance of blood levels and urinary excretion of these hormones cannot be interpreted properly unless they are related to the subject's volume status as well as to the sensitivity of her renal receptors.

It was once hypothesized that decrements in the production of progesterone, a vasodilating hormone with natriuretic actions, might be one reason why salt is abnormally retained in preeclampsia.[75] Several investigators later noted that circulating levels of progesterone are unaltered in this disease.[57-59] More recently, however, it has even been the suggestion that extraadrenal conversion of this hormone to the potent mineralocorticoid desoxycorticosterone may be accelerated in preeclampsia.[125]

Although plasma desoxycorticosterone levels have been reported to be either decreased[61,119] or unchanged[112,117] in preeclampsia, circulating levels of hormone are probably high in relationship to the patient's extracellular volume. Finally, prolactin, which may both increase sodium retention and affect vascular reactivity, has been reported to be either decreased, normal, or elevated in preeclampsia.[261-267]

EFFECT OF ACUTE AND CHRONIC SODIUM LOADS

The "salt tolerance test," used initially in Germany and popularized in this country by Dieckmann and colleagues,[184] was once used as a means of diagnosing preeclampsia. In a number of investigations, preeclamptic women were either unable to concentrate the urine sodium normally, had decreased sodium excretory rates, or excreted a smaller percentage of the total infused load compared with normotensive gravidas.[183,185-187] However, in these studies hypertonic solutions were infused and/or the women were lying supine. This could have introduced methodologic errors that would be more significant in preeclampsia, because antidiuretic hormone (released by hypertonic solution) is more vasoactive,[268,269] and supine posture more antinatriuretic[227] in preeclamptic than in normal gravidas.

Nonpregnant hypertensives respond to saline loading with an exaggerated natriuresis when compared with normal controls. In pregnant subjects with essential hypertension, however, the data are conflicting. Dieckmann, Chesley, and their respective colleagues[183,184] as well as Lindheimer and Katz[270] noted that pregnant hypertensives excreted quantities of sodium equal to or less than those of normotensive pregnant women. In contrast, Sarles et al.[187] demonstrated an increased excretory response in pregnant women with essential hypertension. This latter study is unique, however, in that diagnosis had been established by renal biopsy and the women who manifested an exaggerated natriuresis all had evidence of nephrosclerosis in their kidneys.

Controversies Concerning Volume Loading in the Management of Preeclampsia

The decrement in plasma volume accompanied by salt retention in preeclampsia is the basis of a major controversy in the management of the disease. Some investigators believe the decreased intravascular volume is the primary event that may be responsible for the rise in blood pressure in preeclampsia, that is, placental hypoperfusion may induce release of a pressor substance from the uterus, or relative hypovolemia may result in excessive instead of compensatory secretion of catecholamines. This naturally leads to recommendation of volume expansion, an approach rejected by traditional hypertension experts. They believe that decrements in volume are secondary to vasoconstriction as well as to the effects of the hypertension on renal sodium excretion, the so-called pressure natriuresis. Since cardiac output is often unchanged or increased in preeclampsia[43,45,271,272] while myocardial performance is compromised, these authorities warn that treatment with volume expanders is dangerous and may lead to aggravation of the hypertension as well as pulmonary edema. Consequently, they advocate use of vasodilating drugs and diuretics. Data in the literature currently favor the first view, for it appears that in preeclampsia the decrease in plasma volume precedes the occurrence of hypertension[35,43] and that the central venous pressure is low and varies inversely with the severity of the blood pressure elevation.[273]

One of the studies quoted most by those who believe that decreased volume is a primary event in preeclampsia is that done in 1958 by Robinson,[1] who conducted a prospective analysis of 2019 unselected pregnancies. One group of women were instructed to consume a diet relatively low in sodium, while another group were told to add large amounts of salt to their meals. Robinson[1] observed that the incidence of toxemia, recurrent toxemia, placental infarcts, and a number of complications associated with delivery was significantly higher in the low-salt group. In addition, salt was added to the diets of several women who had developed hypertension and, as shown in Figure 22–12, blood pressure was shown to decrease. Unfortunately, this trial was conducted under field conditions; no attempts were made to verify whether the women had actually consumed the prescribed diets or to collect 24-hour urines and measure sodium excretion. To date, however, no reports have appeared that either confirm or refute these observations, while several investigators have

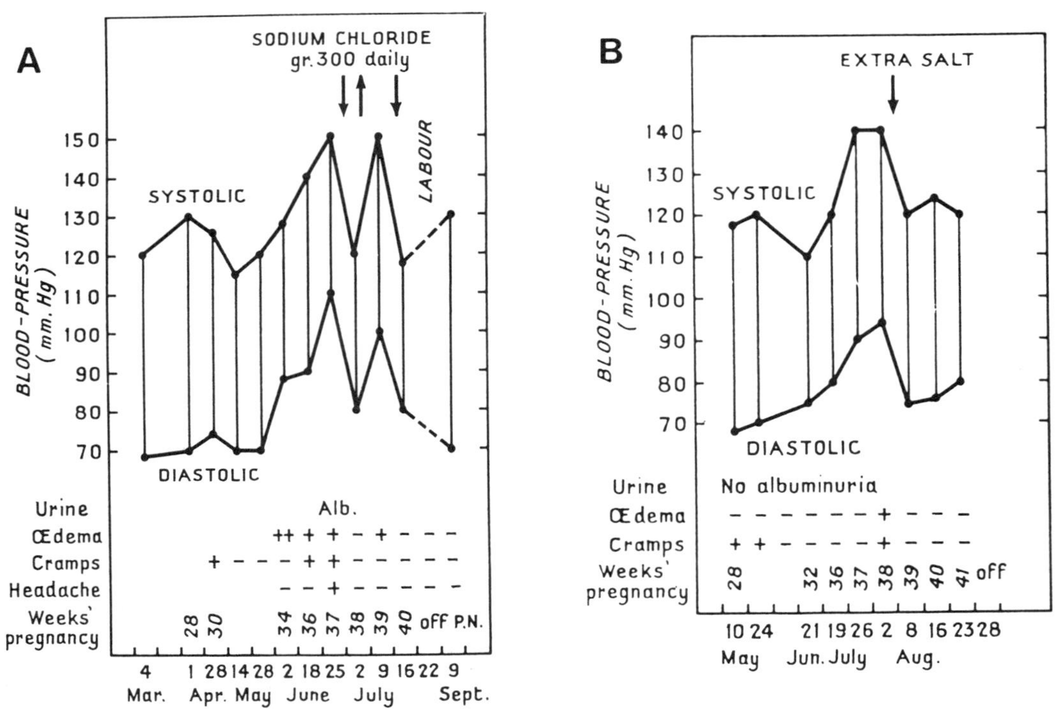

Fig. 22–12. Effect of manipulating dietary sodium intake in two gravidas who developed hypertension in pregnancy. (A) Increasing salt intake (downward arrow) was followed by a decrement in blood pressure, while decreasing dietary sodium (upward arrow) was followed by hypertension and headaches. (B) This patient's blood pressure decreased and edema disappeared when extra salt was added to the diet. PN, postnatal. (From Robinson M: Salt in pregnancy. Lancet 1:178, 1958.)

claimed that many preeclamptics tolerate normal or increased sodium in their diets without signs that their condition is deteriorating.[274-277]

Recently, several investigators have recommended loading with parenteral fluids such as albumin as a treatment modality in preeclampsia.[2,3] The use of such therapy has been prompted by observations that preeclamptic women may have low central venous pressure and occasionally manifest postpartum vascular collapse.[257] This concept is not new, as periodic reports of treating hypertensive gravidas with albumin solutions, with plasma expanders such as dextran or with salt loading abound in the literature.[43] In reviewing available documentation presented by authors who have used volume expansion to treat preeclampsia, we find their data equivocal and unconvincing. The ongoing experience of Gallery et al.[3] is one exception.

Gallery and co-workers studied hospitalized hypertensive gravidas whose blood pressure remained elevated despite 48 hours of bed rest. Plasma volume and extracellular spaces were measured with Evans blue dye and mannitol, respectively; the patients then received 500 ml of a commercial stable protein substitute intravenously over a 15- to 20-minute period. Rapid decreases in both systolic and distolic pressure occurred, from 143/101 to 126/86 mm Hg, and persisted for about 48 hours (Fig. 22–13). Remeasurement of intravascular and extracellular compartments demonstrated that the decrement in pressure was accompanied by restoration of an initially low plasma

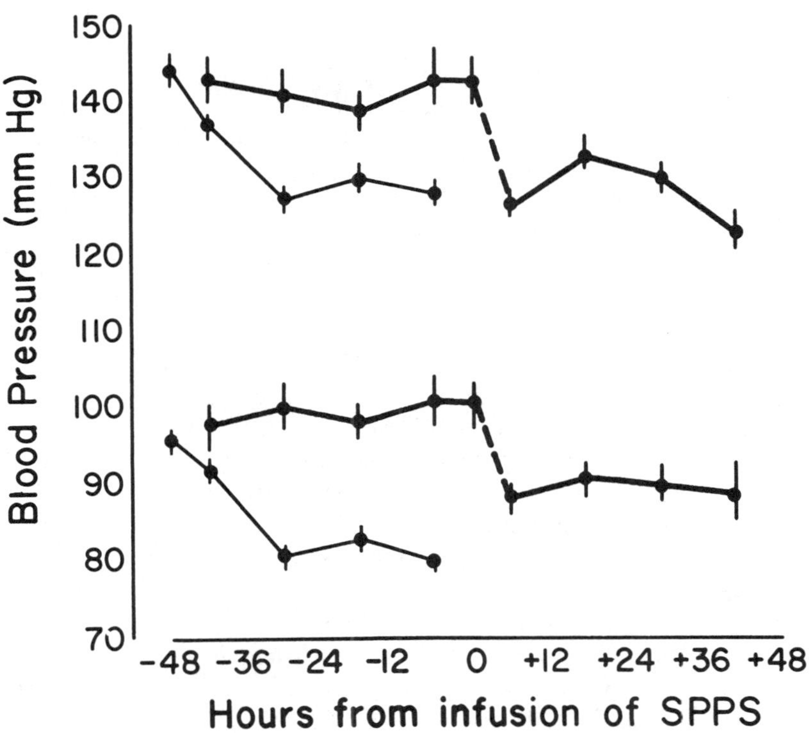

Fig. 22–13. Effect of bed rest and a rapid infusion of plasma protein substitute on the systolic and diastolic blood pressure in women with pregnancy-induced hypertension. Thick line represents treated women. Thin line represents course of patients whose blood pressure declined with rest alone. (From Gallery EDM, Delprado W, Györy AZ: Antihypertensive effect of plasma volume expansion in pregnancy-associated hypertension. Aust NZ J Med 11:20, 1981.)

volume in these subjects to values more normal for pregnancy, the increment in intravascular volume being due to mobilization of fluid from the interstitial space. Gallery et al.[3] acknowledge the possibility that the decrement in pressure may be due to contamination of the plasma protein infusate with vasodilatory peptides such as bradykinin, but believe that if such were the case the decreases in blood pressure would be transient, whereas their observations show persistent decreases in blood pressure. These studies are still in progress.

While the results of these elegant studies are impressive, it should be noted that most of the patients had only moderate disease. Myocardial performance may be compromised in severe preeclampsia. If volume expansion, especially with saline, were to further sensitize these patients' vasculature to endogenous angiotensin and catecholamines, such therapy could conceivably aggravate their hypertension and possibly induce pulmonary or brain edema, complications known to occur in preeclampsia.[43,278,279] In sum, it is prudent to withhold plasma expansion in preeclamptics until a great deal more of carefully collected data are available for analysis.

Diuretics

In marked contrast to those who recommend volume expansion in the management of preeclamptics is the view that these patients should be treated with diuretic agents. In fact, diuretics have not only been prescribed to treat preeclampsia, but also to prevent it, to alleviate excessive weight gain, and to mobilize asymptomatic edema. In several detailed reviews on the use and abuse of diuretics, especially the benzothiadiazides, in pregnancy the authors (cited in refs. 43 and 45) have concurred that saluretic therapy does more harm than good during gestation. Nevertheless, recent texts[5,280] still claim that diuretic therapy is important in the management of the hypertensive disorders of pregnancy and that loop diuretics are an important adjunct treatment (e.g., in combination with diazpoxide) in controlling severe hypertension late in gestation, especially during acute emergencies.

Prophylactic thiazide therapy has been reported to reduce the incidence of preeclampsia in certain susceptible populations, but these claims could not be confirmed.[43] In fact, more recent information derived from a large epidemiologic survey suggests that diuretics given to pregnant patients who have neither hypertension nor renal disease—presumably women with gestational edema or abnormal weight gain—may increase perinatal mortality and are associated with an increase in complications during labor.[281]

Saluretic drugs are successful in mobilizing edema fluid, but it is unclear as to whether such treatment will favorably influence the course of preeclampsia. in fact, there is anecdotal evidence that some fulminant instances of this syndrome occur in "dry" preeclamptics[43]

Diuretics are not without risk. Complications in the mother include pancreatitis, volume contraction, alkalosis, decreased carbohydrate tolerance, electrolyte problems such as severe hypokalemia, and death, while complications in the neonate include arrhythmias, thrombocytopenia, hyponatremia, and perhaps intrauterine growth retardation.

Thiazides decrease the abnormal vascular reactivity to angiotensin II characteristic of preeclampsia. However, these drugs also reduce the metabolic and placental clearance of dehydroepiandrosterone sulfate, which is considered by some to reflect a decrease in the fetoplacental circulation or function.

It remains to be established whether the normal increment in maternal extracellular volume is required for optimal uteroplacental perfusion. One report demonstrated that diuretics limited the physiologic hypervolemia in normotensive women who subsequently delivered infants of lower weight than did in the control group.[282] It should also be noted that in preeclampsia, where intravascular volume is already decreased, administration of diuretics has been accompanied by signs of serious fluid and electrolyte depletion in prepartum women as well as hypotension and shock after delivery.[43,257-259]

Cardiac output has alternatively been described as decreased, unchanged, and increased in preeclampsia. Recently reports describing the intrapartum monitoring of severe preeclamptics using the Swan-Ganz catheter have shown that these extremely hypertensive patients have increased cardiac output combined with low pulmonary wedge pressures, a pattern that suggests a hyperdynamic hypovolemic state.[271,272] Since placental perfusion is already decreased in these women and cardiac compensation is already maximal, further volume depletion could conceivably lead to decreases in cardiac output and placental perfusion.

Because diuretic agents have yet to be proved beneficial, while the risks associated with their use are substantial, there are few unequivocal indications for diuretic therapy during gestation. The only patients for whom we prescribe saluretics without hesitation are pregnant women with heart disease.

In conclusion, it is fair to say that sodium restriction is being condemned in 1984 almost with the same fervor with which it had been advocated two decades ago. We are now aware that asymptomatic edema is normal in pregnancy. It is also clear that many preeclamptics do not deteriorate when their dietary sodium is liberalized. However, there are still many gaps in our knowledge, and until they are filled, the pregnant woman should be allowed to salt her food to taste. If the physician feels compelled to treat asymptomatic edema, bed rest with the patient positioned in lateral recumbency usually results in effective diuresis; if preeclampsia is suspected, hospital observation is preferable to diuretic therapy.

ACKNOWLEDGMENTS

We thank Ms. C. Regovic for her excellent secretarial assistance. Some of the authors' own work cited was supported by grants from the National Institutes of Health (HD 05572 and RR55), the American Heart Association, and the Mother Aid Research Fund of The Chicago Lying-in Hospital.

REFERENCES

1. Robinson M: Salt in pregnancy. Lancet 1:178, 1958
2. Cloeren SE, Lippert TH, Hinselmann M: Hypovolemia in toxemia of pregnancy: Plasma expander therapy with surveillance of central venous pressure. Arch Gynaekol 215:123, 1973
3. Gallery EDM, Delprado W, Györy AZ: Antihypertensive effect of plasma volume expansion in pregnancy-associated hypertension. Aust NZJ Med 11:20, 1981
4. Bay WH, Ferris TF: Factors controlling plasma renin and aldosterone in pregnancy. Hypertension 1:410, 1979
5. Ferris TF: Toxemia and hypertension. p. 1. Renal diseases. p. 235. In Burrow GN, Ferris TF (eds): Medical Complications During Pregnancy. 2nd Ed. WB Saunders, Philadelphia, 1982
6. Thomson AM, Billewicz WZ: Clinical significance of weight trends during pregnancy. Br Med J 1:243, 1957
7. Hytten FE: Weight gain in pregnancy. p. 193. In Hytten FE, Chamberlain G (eds): Clinical Physiology in Obstetrics. Blackwell, Oxford, 1980
8. Seitchik J, Alper C: The estimation of changes in body composition in normal pregnancy by measurement of body water. Am J Obstet Gynecol 71:1165, 1956
9. Pipe NG, Halliday D, Edmonds CJ, et al: Changes in fat-free mass, and body water in human normal pregnancy. Br J Obstet Gynaecol 86:929, 1979
10. Flanagan B, Muldowney FP, Cannon PJ: The relationships of circulating red cell mass, basal oxygen consumption and lean body mass during normal human pregnancy. Clin Sci 30:439, 1966
11. Hutchinson DL, Plentl AA, Taylor HC: The total body water and water turnover in pregnancy studied with deuterium oxide as isotopic tracer. J Clin Invest 33:235, 1954

12. McCartney CP, Pottinger RE, Harrod JP: Alterations in body composition during pregnancy. Am J Obstet Gynecol 77:1038, 1959
13. Seitchik J, Alper C, Szutka A: Changes in body composition during pregnancy. Ann NY Acad Sci 110:821, 1963
14. Hytten FE, Thomson AM, Taggart N: Total body water in normal pregnancy. J Obstet Gynaecol Br Commonw 73:553, 1966
15. Seitchik J: Total body water and total body density of pregnant woman. Obstet Gynecol 29:155, 1967
16. Emerson K, Poindexter EL, Kothari M: Changes in total body composition during normal and diabetic pregnancy. Obstet Gynecol 45:505, 1975
17. Chesley LC: A study of extracellular water changes in pregnancy. Surg Gynecol Obstet 76:589, 1943
18. Chesley LC, Boog JM: Changes in extracellular fluid at delivery and in the puerperium. Surg Gynecol Obstet 77:261, 1943
19. Caton WL, Roby CC, Reid DC, et al: Plasma volume and extracellular fluid volume during pregnancy and the puerperium. Am J Obstet Gynecol 57:471, 1949
20. Cariati A, Centaro A: Compartamento e volutazione del volume dei liquidi in gravidanza. Riv Obstet Ginecol 7:476, 1952
21. Röttger H: Über den Wasserhaushalt in der physiologischen und toxischen. Schwangerschaft. I. Der Wasserhaushalt in der physiologischen Schwangerschaft. Arch Gynaekol 184:59, 1953
22. Friedberg V: Untersuchungen über die Wasser-und Elektrolytverteilung in der normalen und pathologischen Schwangerschaft. Zentralbl Gynaekol 80:159, 1958
23. Friedman MM, Goodfriend MJ, Berlin PF, et al: Extracellular fluid in normal pregnancy. Am J Obstet Gynecol 61:609, 1951
24. Plentl AA, Gray MJ: Total body water, sodium space, and total exchangeable sodium in normal and toxemic pregnant women. Am J Obstet Gynaekol 78:472, 1959
25. Fekete S: The significance of mucopolysaccharides in the pathogenesis of toxemias of pregnancy. Acta Med Acad Sci Hung 5:293, 1954
26. Reinits KG: The acid mucopolysaccharides of the sexual skin of apes and monkeys. Biochem J 74:27, 1960
27. Langgard H, Hvidberg E: The composition of oedema fluid provoked by oestradiol and acute inflammatory oedema fluid. J Reprod Fertil (Suppl) 9:37, 1969
28. Robertson EG: Oedema in normal pregnancy. J Reprod Fert (Suppl) 91:27, 1969
29. Robertson EG: Water metabolism. Clin Obstet Gynaecol 2:431, 1975
30. Lucas J, Floyer MA: Changes in body fluid distribution and interstitial tissue compliance during the development and reversal of experimental hypertension. Clin Sci Mol Med 47:1, 1974
31. Hytten FE, Leitch I: The Physiology of Human Pregnancy. 2nd Ed. Blackwell, Oxford, 1971
32. Chesley LC: Plasma and red cell volumes during pregnancy. Am J Obstet Gynecol 112:440, 1972
33. Chesley LC, Duffus GM: Posture and apparent plasma volume in late pregnancy. Br J Obstet Gynaecol 78:406, 1971
34. Pirani BBK, Campbell DM, MacGillivray I: Plasma volume in normal first pregnancy. Br J Obstet Gynaecol 80:884, 1973
35. Gallery EDM, Hunyor SM, Györy AZ: Plasma volume contraction: a significant factor in both pregnancy-associated hypertension (preeclampsia) and chronic hypertension in pregnancy. QJ Med 192:593, 1979
36. Rovinsky JJ, Jaffin H: Cardiovascular hemodynamics in pregnancy. I. Blood and plasma volume in multiple pregnancy. Am J Obstet Gynecol 93:1, 1965
37. Fullerton WT, Hytten FE, Klopper AI, et al: A case of quadruplet pregnancy. Br J Obstet Gynaecol 72:791, 1965
38. Gibson HG: Plasma volume and glomerular filtration rate in pregnancy and their relationship to differences in fetal growth. J Obstet Gynaecol Br Commonw 80:1067, 1973
39. Duffus GM, MacGillivray I, Dennis KJ: The relationship between baby weight and changes in maternal weight, total body water, plasma volume, electrolytes and proteins, and urinary estriol excretion. Br J Obstet Gynaecol 78:97, 1971
40. Arias F: Expansion of intravascular volume and fetal outcome in patients with chronic

hypertension and pregnancy. Am J Obstet Gynecol 123:610, 1975

41. Soffronoff EC, Kaufmann BM, Connaughton JF: Intravascular volume determinations and fetal outcome in hypertensive diseases of pregnancy. Am J Obstet Gynecol 127:4, 1977
42. Sibai BM, Abdella TN, Anderson GD, et al: Plasma volume determination in pregnancies complicated by chronic hypertension and intrauterine fetal demise. Obstet Gynecol 60:174, 1982
43. Chesley LC: Hypertensive Disorders in Pregnancy. Appleton-Century-Crofts, E. Norwalk, CT, 1978
44. Davison JM, Dunlop W: Renal hemodynamics and tubular function in normal pregnancy. Kidney Int 18:152, 1980
45. Lindheimer MD, Katz AI: The renal response to pregnancy. p. 1762. In Brenner BM, Rector FC Jr (eds); WB Saunders, Philadelphia, 1981
46. Davison JM, Hytten FE: Glomerular filtration during and after pregnancy. J Obstet Gynaecol Br Commonw 81:588, 1974
47. Davison JM, Noble MCB: Serial changes in 24 hour creatinine clearance during normal menstrual cycles and the first trimester of pregnancy Br J Obstet Gynaecol 88:10, 1981
48. Davison JM, Dunlop W, Ezimokhai: 24 hour creatinine clearances during the third trimester of normal pregnancy. Br J Obstet Gynaecol 87:106, 1980
49. Baylis C: The mechanism of the increase in glomerular filtration rate in the twelve-day pregnant rat. J Physiol (Lond) 305:405, 1980
50. Lindheimer MD, Katz AI: Kidney function in the pregnant rat. J Lab Clin Med 78:633, 1971
51. Katz AI, Epstein FH: Physiologic role of sodium-potassium-activated adenosine triphosphate in the transport of cations across biologic membranes. N Engl J Med 278:253, 1968
52. Katz AI, Lindheimer MD: Actions of hormones on the kidney. Annu Rev Physiol 39:97, 1977
53. Pearlman WH: Progesterone in normal pregnancy. Biochem J 67:1, 1957
54. Short RV, Eton B: Progesterone in peripheral blood of pregnant women. J Endocrinol 18:418, 1959
55. Rosenthal HE, Slaunwhite WJ Jr, Sandberg AA: Transcortin: A corticosteroid-binding protein of plasma X. Cortisol and progesterone interplay and unbound levels of these steroids in pregnancy. J Clin Endocrinol Metab 29:352, 1969
56. Lin TJ, Lin SL, Erlenmeyer F, et al: Progesterone production rates during the third trimester of pregnancy in normal women, diabetic women, and women with abnormal glucose tolerance. J Clin Endocrinol Metab 34:287, 1972
57. Lindberg BS, Nilsson BA, Johansson EDB: Plasma progesterone levels in normal and abnormal pregnancy. Acta Obstet Gynecol Scand 53:329, 1974
58. Weinberger MH, Kramer NJ, Petersen LP, et al: Sequential changes in the renin–angiotensin–aldosterone systems and plasma progesterone concentration in normal and abnormal human pregnancy. p. 263. In Lindheimer MD, Katz AI, Zuspan FP (eds): Hypertension in Pregnancy. Wiley, New York, 1976
59. Parker CJ Jr, Everett RB, Quirk JG Jr et al: Hormone production during pregnancy in the primigravid patient: Plasma levels of progesterone and 5a-pregnane-3, 20-dione throughout pregnancy of normal women and women who develop pregnancy induced hypertension. Am J Obstet Gynecol 135:778, 1979
60. Wilson M, Morgani AA, Zervoudakis J, et al: Blood pressure, the renin–aldosterone system and sex steroids throughout normal pregnancy. Am J Med 68:97, 1980
61. Weir RJ, Doig A, Fraser R, et al: Studies of the renin–angiotensin–aldosterone system, cortisol DOC, and ADH in normal and hypertensive pregnancy. p. 251. In Lindheimer MD, Katz AI, Zuspan FP (eds): Hypertension in Pregnancy. Wiley, New York, 1976
62. Davison JM, Gilmore EA, Dürr T. et al: Altered osmotic thresholds for vasopressin secretion and thirst in human pregnancy. Clin J Physiol, in press.
63. Torres C, Schewitz LJ, Pollak VE: The effect of small amounts of antidiuretic hormone on sodium and urate excretion in pregnancy. Am J Obstet Gynecol 94:546, 1966
64. Lindheimer MD, Katz AI: Kidney Function

and Disease in Pregnancy. Lea and Febiger, Philadelphia, 1977
65. deWardner HE: Natriuretic hormone. Clin Sci Mol Med 53:1, 1977
66. Gruber KA, Whitaker JM, Buckalew VM Jr: Endogenous digitalis-like substance in plasma of volume expanded dogs. Nature 287:743, 1980
67. deWardner HE: The natriuretic hormone: Recent developments. Clin Sci 63:415, 1982
68. Bricker NS: Sodium homeostasis in chronic renal disease. Kidney Int 21:886, 1982
69. Lindheimer MD, Weston PV: Effect of hypotonic expansion on sodium, water and urea excretion in late pregnancy. The influence of posture on these results. J Clin Invest 48:947, 1969
70. Venning EH, Singer B, Simpson GA: Adrenocortical function in toxemia of pregnancy. Am J Obstet Gynecol 67:542, 1954
71. Martin JD, Mills IH: Aldosterone excretion in normal and toxemic pregnancies. Br Med J 2:571, 1956
72. Jones KM, Lloyd-Jones R, Riondel A, et al: Aldosterone excretion and metabolism in normal men, women, and in pregnancy. Acta Endocrinol (Copenh) 30:321, 1959
73. Kumar D, Feltham LAW, Gornall AG: Aldosterone excretion and tissue electrolytes in normal pregnancy and preeclampsia. Lancet 1:541, 1959
74. Tait JF, Little B, Tait SAS, et al: The metabolic clearance rate of aldosterone in pregnant and nonpregnant subjects estimated by both single-injection and constant-infusion methods. J Clin Invest 41:2093, 1962
75. Ehrlich EN, Laves M, Lugibihil K, et al: Progesterone–aldosterone interrelationships in pregnancy. J Lab Clin Med 59:588, 1962
76. Stark G: Zum Abbau und der Bildung des Aldosterone bei Nichtschwangeren und Schwangeren. Arch Gynecol 197:484, 1962
77. Watanabe M, Meeker CI, Gray MJ, et al: Secretion rate of aldosterone in normal pregnancy. J Clin Invest 42:1619, 1963
78. Thomas JP, Flynn TG: Adrenal function in normal pregnancy and toxaemia. Clin Sci 26:69, 1964
79. Tait JF, Little B: The metabolism of orally and intravenously administered labeled aldosterone in pregnant subjects. J Clin Invest 47:2423, 1968
80 Ledoux F, Genest J, Nowacznski W, et al: Plasma progesterone and aldosterone in pregnancy. Can Med Assoc J 112:943, 1975
81. Lammintausta R, Erkkola R: Renin–angiotensin–aldosterone system and sodium in normal pregnancy: A longitudinal study. Acta Obstet Gynecol Scand 56:221, 1977
82. Smeaton TC, Anderson GJ, Fulton IS: Study of aldosterone levels in plasma during pregnancy. J Clin Endocrinol Metab 44:1, 1977
83. Nolten WE, Lindheimer MD, Oparil S, et al: Desoxycorticosterone in normal pregnancy I. Sequential studies of the secretory patterns of desoxycorticosterone, aldosterone and cortisol. Am J Obstet Gynecol 132:414, 1978
84. Wintour EM, Coghlan JP, Oddie CJ, et al: A sequential study of adrenocorticosteroid level in human pregnancy. Clin Exp Pharmacol Physiol 5:399, 1978
85. Hubl W, Büchner M, Bellée H, et al: Study of plasma aldosterone in normal pregnancy, in pre-eclamptic women and in cord plasma of newborns. Endokrinologie 73:162, 1979
86. Bauknecht H, Vecsei P, Endres H, et al: Urinary free 18-hydroxycorticosterone, plasma aldosterone and urinary aldosterone metabolites in normal pregnancy. Am J Obstet Gynecol 144:28, 1982
87. Alexander EA, Churchill S, Bengele HH: Renal hemodynamics and volume homeostasis during pregnancy in the rat. Kidney Int 18:173, 1980
88. Bishop JHV, Green R: Effect of pregnancy on glucose reabsorption by the proximal convoluted tubule in the rat. J Physiol (Lond) 319:271, 1981
89. Watanabe M, Meeker CI, Gray MJ, et al: Aldosterone secretion rates in abnormal pregnancy. J Clin Endocrinol Metab 25: 1665, 1965
90. Assali NS, Clark LC, Sobel EH: Studies on toxemia of pregnancy: Effect of desoxycorticosterone acetate (DCA) on hemodynamics and electrolyte excretion in normal pregnant women. J Clin Endocrinol Metab 13:1030, 1957
91. Stark G, Derra M: Der Einfluss hoher Aldosterone auf die Electrolytausscheidung bei gesunden Schwangeren. Arch Gynecol 200:715, 1965
92. Assali NS, Surjemoto R: Studies on toxemia

of pregnancy: Effects of corticotropic hormone (ACTH) on hemodynamics and excretion of electrolytes of normal pregnant women. Metab Clin Exp 3:303, 1954
93. Churchill S, Bengele HH, Melby JC, et al: Role of aldosterone in sodium retention or pregnancy in the rat. Am J Physiol 240: R175, 1981
94. Laidlaw JC, Ruse JL, Gornall AG: The influence of estrogen and progesterone on aldosterone excretion. J Clin Endocrinol Metab 22:161, 1962
95. Oelkers W, Schoneschofer M, Blumel A: Effects of progesterone and four synthetic progestagens on sodium balance and the renin–aldosterone system in man. J Clin Endocrinol Metab 39:882, 1974
96. Crane MG, Harris JJ: Effects of estrogens and gestagens on the renin–aldosterone system. p. 100. In Fregly MJ, Fregly MS (eds): Oral Contraceptives and High Blood Pressure. Dolphin Press, Gainesville, FL, 1974
97. Oparil S, Ehrlich EN, Lindheimer MD: Effects of progesterone on renal sodium handling in man. Relation to aldosterone excretion and plasma renin activity. Clin Sci Mol Med 49:139, 1975
98. Crane MG, Harris JJ: Effect of estrogens and gestagens on exchangeable sodium. p. 159. In Fregly MJ, Fregly MS (eds): Oral Contraceptives and High Blood Pressure. Dolphin Press, Gainesville, FL, 1974
99. Ehrlich EN: Reciprocal variations in urinary cortisol and aldosterone in response to increased salt intake in humans. J Clin Endocrinol Metab 26:1160, 1966
100. Weinberger MH, Kramer NJ, Grim CE, et al: The effect of posture and saline loading on plasma renin activity and aldosterone concentration in pregnant, non-pregnant and estrogen treated women. J Clin Endocrinol Metab 44:69, 1977
101. Becker RA, Hayashi RH, Franks RC, et al: Effects of positional change and sodium balance on the renin-angiotensin system, big renin and prostaglandins in normal pregnancy. J Clin Endocrinol Metab 46:467, 1978
102. Oliver WJ, Neel JV, Crekin RJ, et al: Hormonal adaptation of the stress imposed on sodium balance by pregnancy and lactation in the Yanomama Indians, a culture without salt. Circulation 63:110, 1981
103. Gray MJ, Munro AB, Sims EA, et al: Regulation of sodium and total body water metabolism in pregnancy. Am J Obstet Gynecol 89:760, 1964
104. Assali NS, Dignam WJ, Dasgupta K: Renal function in human pregnancy. II. Effects of venous pooling on renal hemodynamics and water electrolytes and aldosterone excretion during normal pregnancy. J Lab Clin Med 54:394, 1959
105. Lindheimer MD, del Greco F, Ehrlich EN: Postural effects on Na and steroid excretion, and serum renin activity during pregnancy. J Appl Physiol 35:343, 1973
106. Ehrlich EN: Reciprocal variations in urinary cortisol and aldosterone in response to the sodium-depleting influence of hydrochlorothiazide and ethacrynic acid in humans. J Clin Endocrinol Metab 27:836, 1967
107. Lammintausta R, Erkkola R, Eronen M: Effect of chlorthiazide treatment on renin-aldosterone system during pregnancy. Acta Obstet Gynecol Scand 57:389, 1978
108. Beitins IA, Bayard F, Levitsky L, et al: Plasma aldosterone concentration at delivery and during the newborn period. J Clin Invest 51:386, 1972
109. Ehrlich EN, Lindheimer MD: Effect of administered mineralocorticoids on ACTH in pregnant women. Attenuation of kaliuretic influence of mineralocorticoids during pregnancy. J Clin Invest 51:1301, 1972
110. Ehrlich EN: Heparinoid-induced inhibition of aldosterone secretion in pregnant women: The role of augmented aldosterone secretion in sodium conservation during normal pregnancy. Am J Obstet Gynecol 109:963, 1971
111. Nolten WE, Lindheimer MD, Oparil S, et al: Secretory patterns and altered tissue binding of cortisol in pregnancy. Clin Res 26:493A, 1978 (abst.)
112. Brown RD, Strott CA, Liddle GW: Plasma deoxycorticosterone in normal and abnormal pregnancy. J Clin Endocrinol Metab 35:736, 1972
113. Ehrlich EN, Biglieri EG, Lindheimer MD: ACTH-induced sodium retention in pregnancy. Role of deoxycorticosterone and corticosterone. J Clin Endocrinol Metab 38:701, 1974
114. Sippell WG, Becker H, Versmold HT, et al: Longitudinal studies of plasma aldosterone,

corticosterone, deoxycorticosterone, 17-hydroxyprogesterone, cortisol and cortisone determined simultaneously in mother and child at birth and during the early neonatal period. I. spontaneous delivery. J Clin Endocrinol Metab 46:971, 1978
115. Nolten WE, Lindheimer MD, Oparil S, et al: Desoxycorticosterone in normal pregnancy. II. Cortisol-dependent fluctuations in free plasma deoxycorticosterone. Am J Obstet Gynecol 133:644, 1979
116. Parker CR Jr, Everett RB, Whalley, PJ, et al: Hormone production in pregnancy in the primigravida. II. Plasma concentrations of deoxycorticosterone throughout pregnancy in normal women and in women who developed pregnancy induced hypertension. Am J Obstet Gynecol 138:626, 1980
117. Den K, Tomita M, Miuake Y, et al: Studies of maternal and fetal 11-deoxycorticosterone, corticosterone, 18-hydroxycorticosterone and aldosterone in normal and toxemic pregnancy. Endocrinol Jpn 27:703, 1980
118. Nolten WE, Holt LH, Rueckert PA: Desoxycorticosterone in normal pregnancy. III. Evidence of a fetal source of desoxycorticosterone. Am J Obstet Gynecol 139:477, 1980
119. Nolten WE, Ehrlich EN: Sodium and mineralocorticoids in normal pregnancy. Kidney Int 18:162, 1980
120. Winkel CA, Milewich L, Parker R Jr, et al: Conversion of plasma progesterone to deoxycorticosterone in men, nonpregnant and pregnant women, and adrenalectomized subjects. Evidence for steroid 21-hydroxylase activity in nonadrenal tissues. J Clin Invest 66:803, 1980
121. Casey ML, MacDonald PC: Metabolism of deoxycorticosterone and deoxycorticosterone sulfate in men and women. J Clin Invest 70:312, 1982
122. MacDonald PC, Cutrer S, MacDonald SC, et al: Regulation of extraadrenal steroid 21-hydroxylase activity: Increased conversion of plasma progesterone to deoxycorticosterone during estrogen treatment of women pregnant with a dead fetus. J Clin Invest 69:469, 1982
123. Winkel CA, Simpson ER, Milewich L, et al: Deoxycorticosterone (DOC) biosynthesis in human kidney: Potential for the formation of a potent mineralocorticoid in its site of action. Proc Natl Acad Sci (USA) 77:7069, 1980
124. Ehrlich EN, Nolten WE, Oparil S, et al: Mineralocorticoids in normal pregnancy. p. 189. In Lindheimer MD, Katz AI, Zuspan FP (eds): Hypertension in Pregnancy. Wiley, New York, 1976
125. Winkel CA, Casey ML Guerami A, et al: Ratio of plasma deoxycorticosterone (DOC) levels to plasma progesterone (P) levels in pregnant women who did or did not develop pregnancy-induced hypertension (PIH). p. 185. In Abstracts to the 30th Annual Meeting of the Society for Gynecological Investigation, 1983
126. Dignam WS, Voskian J, Assali NS: Effect of estrogens on renal hemodynamics and excretion of electrolytes in human subjects. J Clin Endocrinol Metab 16:1032, 1956
127. DeHertogh R, Thomas K, Bietlot Y, et al: Plasma levels of unconjugated estrone, estradiol, estriol and HCS throughout pregnancy in normal women. J Clin Endocrinol Metab 40:93, 1975
128. Helmer OM, Judson WE: Influence of high renin substrate levels on renin–angiotensin system in pregnancy. J Clin Endocrinol Metab 99:9, 1967
129. Hsueh WA, Leutcher JA, Carlson EJ, et al: Changes in active and inactive renin in pregnancy. J Clin Endocrinol Metab 54:1010, 1982
130. O'Connell M, Welsh GW III: Unbound plasma cortisol in pregnant and Enovid E-treated women as determined by ultrafiltration. J Clin Endocrinol Metab 29:563, 1969
131. Nolten WE, Rueckert PA, Lindheimer MD, et al: A simple method for determining the free cortisol index in plasma: Measurements in human pregnancy. J Lab Clin Med 93:146, 1979
132. Zuspan FP: Urinary excretion of epinephrine and norepinephrine during pregnancy. J Clin Endocrinol Metab 30:357, 1970
133. Lederman RR, McCann DS, Work B Jr, et al: Endogenous plasma epinephrine and norepinephrine in last trimester of pregnancy and labor. Am J Obstet Gynecol 129:5, 1977
134. Poland ML, Lucas CP: Plasma epinephrine and norepinephrine in normotensive and pregnancy-induced hypertensive pregnancies. p. 161. In Bonnar J, MacGillivray I,

Symonds EM (eds): Pregnancy Hypertension. MTP Press, Lancaster, England, 1980
135. Tunbridge RDG, Donnai P: Plasma noradrenaline in normal pregnancy and in hypertension of late pregnancy. Br J Obstet Gynaecol 88:105, 1981
136. Pedersen EB, Rasmussen AB, Christiensen NJ, et al: Plasma noradrenaline and adrenaline in preeclampsia, essential hypertension and normotensive pregnant control subjects. Acta Endocrinol (Copenh) 99:594, 1982
137. Perkins CM, Hancock KW, Cope GF, et al: Urine dopamine in normal primigravid pregnancy and women taking oral contraceptives. Clin Sci 61:423, 1981
138. Brown JJ, Davis DL, Doak PB, et al: Plasma renin in normal pregnancy. Lancet 2:900, 1963
139. Abdul-Karim R, Assali NS: Pressor response to angiotensin in pregnant and nonpregnant women. Am J Obstet Gynecol 82:246, 1961
140. Chesley LC, Wynn RM, Silverman NI: Renal effects of angiotensin II infusions in normotensive pregnant and nonpregnant women. Circ Res 13:232, 1963
141. Chesley LC, Talledo E, Bohler CS, et al: Vascular reactivity to angiotensin II and norepinephrine in pregnant and nonpregnant women. Am J Obstet Gynecol 91:837, 1965
142. Gant NF, Daley GL, Chand S, et al: A study of angiotensin II pressor response throughout primigravid pregnancy. J Clin Invest 52:2682, 1973
143. Gordon DB, Sachin IN: Chromatographic separation of multiple renin substrates in women. Effect of pregnancy and oral contraceptives. Proc Soc Exp Biol Med 156:461, 1977
144. Gordon DB, Sachin IN: Simultaneous measurements of PRA, PRC and PRR and the relationship of renin reaction rate to renin substrate concentration. Clin Exp Hypertens 2:65, 1980
145. Tewksbury DA, Dart RA: High molecular weight angiotensinogen levels in hypertensive pregnant women. Hypertension 4:729, 1982
146. Symonds EM: The renin–angiotensin system in pregnancy. Obstet Gynecol Annu 10:45, 1981
147. Boonshaft B, O'Connell JMB, Hays JM, et al: Serum renin activity during normal pregnancy. Effect of alterations of posture and sodium intake. J Clin Endocrinol Metab 28:1641, 1968
148. Weinberger MH, Peterson LP, Herr MJ, et al: The effect of supine and lateral recumbency on plasma renin activity during pregnancy. J Clin Endocrinol Metab 36:991, 1973
149. Brandes JM, Abramovici H, Katz M, et al: The effect of postural changes on plasma renin activity during normal and pathologic pregnancies. Obstet Gynecol 52:530, 1978
150. Vallotton MB, Davison JM, Riondel AM, et al: Response of the renin–aldosterone system and antidiuretic hormone to oral water loading and hypertonic saline infusion during and after pregnancy. Clin Exp Hypertens B1:385, 1982
151. Weir RJ, Paintin DB, Brown JJ, et al: A serial study in pregnancy of plasma concentrations of renin, corticosteroids, electrolytes and proteins and of haematocrit and plasma volume. Br J Obstet Gynaecol 78:590, 1971
152. Weir RJ, Brown JJ, Fraser R, et al: Relationship between plasma renin, renin substrate, angiotensin II, aldosterone and electrolytes in normal pregnancy. J Clin Endocrinol Metab 40:108, 1975
153. Gerber JG, Payne NA, Murphy RC, et al: Prostacyclin produced by the pregnant uterus in the dog may act as a circulating vasodepressor substance. J Clin Invest 67:632, 1981
154. Pregnancy and the arachidonic-acid cascade. (Editorial.) Lancet 1:997, 1982
155. Meese CO, Fischer C, Hoffman LH, et al: Assessment of uterine and renal prostaglandin synthesis in pregnancy by gas chromatography–mass spectometry. INSERM 91:167, 1979
156. Lewis PJ, Boylan P, Friedman LA, et al: Prostacyclin in pregnancy. Br Med J 1:1581, 1980
157. Bolton PJ, Jagee M, Myatt L, et al: Maternal plasma 6-oxo-prostaglandin and $F_{1\alpha}$ levels. Br J Obstet Gynaecol 88:1101, 1981
158. Goodman RP, Killam RP, Brash AR, et al: Prostacyclin production during pregnancy. Comparison of production during normal pregnancy and pregnancy complicated by hypertension. Am J Obstet Gynecol 142:817, 1982
159. Ferris TF, Venuto RC, Bay WH: Studies

of the uterine circulation in the pregnant rabbit. p. 351. In Lindheimer MD, Katz AI, Zuspan FP (eds): Hypertension in Pregnancy. Wiley, New York, 1976
160. Douglas BH: The rat as a model for preeclampsia. p. 441. In Lindheimer MD, Katz AI, Zuspan FP (eds): Hypertension in Pregnancy. Wiley, New York, 1976
161. Broughton-Pipkin F, O'Brien PMS: Effect of the specific angiotensin antagonist (Sar) (Ala^8) angiotensin II on blood pressure of the renin–angiotensin system in conscious pregnant ewe and fetus. Am J Obstet Gynecol 132:7, 1978
162. Fowler WL Jr, Johnson JA, Kurz KD, et al: Role of the renin–angiotensin system in maintaining arterial pressure in conscious pregnant rats. Endocrinology 109:290, 1981
163. Everett RB, Worley RJ, MacDonald PC, et al: Effect of prostaglandin synthetase inhibitors on pressor response to antiotensin II in human pregnancy. J Clin Endocrinol Metab 1007, 1978
164. Whalen JB, Clancey CJ, Farley DB, et al: Plasma prostaglandins in pregnancy. Obstet Gynecol 51:52, 1978
165. Saruta T, Nakamura R, Nagahama S, et al: Effects of an angiotensin II analogue on blood pressure, renin, and aldosterone in women on oral contraceptives and toxemia. Gynecol Obstet Invest 12:11, 1981
166. Pritchard JA, Barnes AC, Bright RH: The effect of supine posture on renal function in near-term pregnant women. J Clin Invest 34:777, 1955
167. Chesley LC, Sloan DM: The effect of posture on renal function in late pregnancy. Am J Obstet Gynecol 89:754, 1964
168. Lindheimer MD: Further characterization of the influence of supine posture on renal function in late pregnancy. Effect of rapid saline infusion on renal sodium, water, and uric metabolism. Gynecol Invest 1:69, 1970
169. Ehrlich EN, Oparil S, Lindheimer MD: Role of augmented aldosterone secretion in regulation of volume homeostasis in pregnancy. p. 274. In Fregly MJ, Fregly MS (eds): Oral Contraceptives and High Blood Pressure. Gainesville, FL, Dolphin Press, 1974
170. Pystynen P, Pankama P: Diurnal variations in urine excretion, and sodium and potassium excretion in healthy and toxaemic women in late pregnancy. Acta Obstet Gynecol Scand 44:408, 1965
171. Horska S, Vedra B: Diurnal variations of glomerular filtration and renal handling of electrolytes in normal and toxemia pregnancies. Am J Obstet Gynecol 90:285, 1964
172. Lindheimer MD, Roux J: Role of posture in sodium, water, and potassium homeostasis of an abnormal pregnancy. Metabolism 619, 1970
173. Kalousek G, Hlavacek C, Nedoss B, et al: Circadian rhythms of creatinine and electrolyte excretion in healthy pregnant women. Am J Obstet Gynecol 103:856, 1969
174. Parboosingh J, Doig A: Renal nyctohemoral excretion patterns of water and solutes in normal pregnancy. Am J Obstet Gynecol 116:609, 1973
175. Parboosingh J, Doig A: Studies of nocturia of normal pregnancy. Br J Obstet Gynaecol 80:888, 1973
176. Rubi RA, Sala NL: Ureteral function in pregnant women. III. Effect of different positions and fetal delivery upon ureteral tonus. Am J Obstet Gynecol 101:230, 1968
177. Fulop M, Brazeau P: Increased ureteral back pressure enhances renal tubular reabsorption. J Clin Invest 49:2315, 1970
178. Suki WN, Guthrie AG, Martinez-Maldonado M, et al: Effects of ureteral pressure elevation on renal hemodynamics and urine concentration. Am J Physiol 220:38, 1971
179. Burwell CS: The placenta as a modified arteriovenous fistula, considered in relation to circulatory adjustments to pregnancy. Am J Med Sci 195:1, 1938
180. Heckel GP, Tobin CE: Arteriovenous shunts in the myometrium. Am J Obstet Gnyecol 71:199, 1956
181. Epstein FH, Post RS, McDowell ME: The effect of arteriovenous fistula on renal hemodynamics and electrolyte excretion. J Clin Invest 32:233, 1953
182. Mandin H: Mechanism of natriuresis after closure of chronic arteriovenous fistula on renal hemodynamics and electrolyte excretion. J Clin Invest 52:2225, 1973
183. Chesley LC, Valenti C, Rein H: Excretion of sodium loads by nonpregnant, and pregnant normal, hypertensive and preeclamptic women. Metabolism 7:575, 1958
184. Dieckmann WJ: The Toxemias of Preg-

nancy. 2nd Ed. CV Mosby, St. Louis, 1952
185. Dieckmann WJ, Pottinger RE, Rynkiewicz LM: Etiology of preeclampsia–eclampsia. Sodium chloride test for the diagnosis of preeclampsia. Am J Obstet Gynecol 63:783, 1952
186. Wilson JR, Williams JM Jr. Hayashi TT: Hypertonic saline infusions for the differential diagnosis of the toxemias of pregnancy. Am J Obstet Gynecol 73:30, 1957
187. Sarles HE, Hill SS, LeBlanc AL, et al: Sodium excretion patterns during and following intravenous sodium chloride loads in normal and hypertensive pregnancies. Am J Obstet Gynecol 102:1, 1968
188. Katz AI, Lindheimer MD: Renal handling of acute sodium loads in pregnancy. Am J Physiol 225:696, 1973
189. Lindheimer MD, Katz AI, Koeppen BM, et al: Kidney function and sodium handling in the pregnant spontaneously hypertensive rat. Hypertension 5:498, 1983
190. Schewitz LJ: Hypertension and renal disease in pregnancy. Med Clin North Am 55:47, 1971
191. Biglieri EG, Slaton PE: Pregnancy and primary aldosteronism. J Clin Endocrinol Metab 27:1628, 1967
192. Klaus D, Klumpp F: Einfluss der Schwangershaft auf das Bartter-Syndrome. Klin Wochenschr 49:1280, 1971
193. DeFronzo RA, Taufield PA, Black H, et al: Impaired renal tubular potassium secretion in sickle cell disease. Ann Intern Med 90:310, 1979
194. Hytten FE: Physiological changes in early pregnancy. Br J Obstet Gynaecol 75:1193, 1968
195. Robertson EG, Cheyne GA: Plasma biochemistry in relation to oedema of pregnancy. Br J Obstet Gynaecol 79:769, 1972
196. MacDonald HN, Good W: Changes in plasma sodium, potassium and chloride concentrations in pregnancy and the puerperium with plasma and serum osmolality. Br J Obstet Gynaecol 78:798, 1971
197. Davison JM, Vallotton MB, Lindheimer MD: Plasma osmolality and urinary concentration and dilution during and after pregnancy: Evidence that lateral recumbency inhibits maximal urinary concentrating ability. Br J Obstet Gynaecol 88:472, 1981
198. Durr JA, Stamoutsos BA, Lindheimer MD: Osmoregulation in pregnancy: Evidence for resetting of the threshold for vasopressin secretion during gestation. J Clin Invest 68:337, 1981
199. Durr JA, Stamoutsos BA, Barron WM, et al: Osmoregulation in the pregnant Brattleboro rat. An NY Acad Sci 394:481, 1982
200. Walker EW, McManus M, Janney JC: Kidney function in pregnancy. II. Effects of posture and diuresis. Proc Soc Exp Biol Med 31:392, 1934
201. Hendricks CH, Barnes AC: Effect of supine posture on urinary output in pregnancy. Am J Obstet Gynecol 69:1225, 1955
202. Klopper A: Changes in renal function in late pregnancy. Lancet 2:565, 1964
203. Whalley PJ, Roberts AD Jr, Pritchard JA: The effects of posture on renal function during pregnancy in a patient with diabetes insipidus. J Lab Clin Med 58:867, 1961
204. Hytten FE, Klopper AI: Response to a water load in pregnancy. Br J Obstet Gynecol 70:811, 1963
205. Newman RL: Serum electrolytes in pregnancy, partuition and puerperium. Obstet Gynecol 10:51, 1957
206. Herbinger UW, Wichman H: Die extrazellulären und intraerythrozytären Elektrolyte während der zweiten Schwangerschafthälfte. Gynaecologia (Basel) 163:1, 1967
207. Schrier RW, Berl T, Anderson RJ: Osmotic and nonosmotic control of vasopressin release. Am J Physiol 236:F321, 1979
208. Barron WM, Stamoutsos BA, Lindheimer MD: Role of volume in the regulation of vasopressin secretion during pregnancy in the rat. J Clin Invest, in press
209. Tuppy H: The influence of enzymes on neurohypophysial hormones. p. 67. Handbuch der Experimentellen Pharmakologie. Vol 23: Neurohypophysial Hormones and Similar Peptides. Springer-Verlag, Berlin, 1968
210. Rosenbloom AA, Sach J, Fisher DA: The circulating vasopressinase of pregnancy: Species comparison and radioimmunoassay. Am J Obstet Gynecol 121:316, 1975
211. Roth K, Slater S: Inactivation of vasopressin during pregnancy. Am J Obstet Gynecol 83:1325, 1962
212. Vorherr H, Friedberg V: Uber die Wirkung von Adiuretin auf die Diurese in der Schwan-

gerschaft. Klin Wochenschr 42:201, 1964
213. Kleeman CR, Vorherr H: Water metabolism and neurohypohyseal hormones. p. 1479. In Bondy PK, Rosenberg LE (eds): Duncan's Disease of Metabolism. 7th Ed. WB Saunders, Philadelphia, 1974
214. Hime MC, Richardson JA: Diabetes insipidus and pregnancy. Case report, incidence and review of the literature. Obstet Gynecol Surv 33:375, 1978
215. Stamoutsos BA, Barron WM, Lindheimer MD: Effect of gestation on osmoregulation in the homozygous Brattleboro rat with diabetes insipidus. Clin Res 30:363A, 1982 (Abst.)
216. Olsson K, Benlamlih S, Dahlborn K, et al: Effects of water deprivation and hyperhydration in pregnant and lactating goats. Acta Physiol Scand 115:361, 1982
217. Kaitz AL: Urinary concentrating ability in pregnant women with asymptomatic bacteriuria. J Clin Invest 40:1331, 1961
218. McCartney CP, Spargo B, Lorincz AB, et al: Renal structure and function in pregnant patients with acute hypertension, osmolar concentration. Am J Obstet Gynecol 90:579, 1964
219. Norden CW, Tuttle EP Jr: Impairment of urinary concentrating ability in pregnant women with asymptomatic bacteriuria. P. 73. In Kass EH (ed): Progress in Pyelonephritis. FA Davis, Philadelphia, 1965
220. Elder HA, Kass EH: Renal function in bacteriuria of pregnancy: Its relationship to prematurity, acute pyelonephritis, and excessive weight gain. P. 81. In Kass EH (ed): Progress in Pyelonephritis. FA Davis, Philadelphia, 1965
221. Reeves DS, Brumfitt W: Localization of urinary tract infection. A comparative study of methods. P. 53. In O'Grady F, Brumfitt W (eds): Urinary Tract Infection. Proceedings of the First National Symposium. Oxford University Press, London, 1968
222. Williams GL, Campbell H, Davies KJ: Urinary concentrating ability in women with asymptomatic bacteriuria in pregnancy. Br Med J 3:212, 1969
223. Norden CW, Levy PS, Kass EH: Predictive effect of urinary concentrating ability and hemagglutinating antibody titer upon response to antimicrobial therapy in bacteriuria of pregnancy. J Infect Dis 121:588, 1970
224. Hutchon DJR, Van Zijl JAWM, Campbell-Brown BM, et al: Desmopressin as a test of urinary concentrating ability in pregnancy. J Obstet Gynecol 2:206, 1982
225. Janney JC, Walker EW: Kidney function in pregnancy. I. Water diuresis in normal pregnancy. JAMA 99:2078, 1932
226. McManus MA, Riley GA, Janney JC: Water diuresis in the toxemias of pregnancy. Am J Obstet Gynecol 28:524, 1934
227. Redd J, Mosey LM, Langford HG: Effect of posture upon sodium excretion in preeclampsia. Am J Obstet Gynecol 100:343, 1968
228. Sjöstedt S: Acid–base balance of arterial blood during pregnancy, at delivery, and in the puerpuerium. Am J Obstet Gynecol 84:775, 1962
229. Seed EA, Battaglia FC, Hellegers AE: Effect of pregnancy on the pH, PCO_2, and bicarbonate concentrations of peripheral venous blood. Am J Obstet Gynecol 88:1086, 1964
230. Lucius H, Gahlenbeck H, Kleine HO, et al: Respiratory functions, buffer system, and electrolyte concentrations of blood during human pregnancy. Respir Physiol 9:311, 1970
231. Lim VS, Katz AI, Lindheimer MD: Acid–base regulation in pregnancy. Am J Physiol 231:1764–70, 1976
232. Gallery EDM, Györy AZ: Urinary concentration, acid excretion, and acid–base status in normal pregnancy: Alterations in pregnancy-associated hypertension. Am J Obstet Gynecol 135:27, 1979
233. Fadel HE, Northop G, Missenheimer R, et al: Normal pregnancy: A model of sustained respiratory alkalosis. J Perinat Med 3:195, 1979
234. Boutourline-Young H, Boutourline-Young E: Alveolar carbon dioxide levels in pregnant parturient and lactating subjects. Br J Obstet Gynaecol 63:509, 1956
235. Lyons HA, Antonio R: The sensitivity of the respiratory center in pregnancy and after the administration of progesterone. Trans Assoc Am Physicians 72:173, 1959
236. Assali NS, Herzig D, Singh BP: Renal response to ammonium chloride acidosis in normal and toxemic pregnancies. J Appl Physiol 7:367, 1955

237. Fadel HE, Northop H, Misenheimer R, et al: Acid–base parameters in pre-eclamptic and diabetic pregnancies. Maternal blood and amniotic fluid studies. J Perinat Med 202, 1979
238. Templeton AA, Kelman GR: Arterial blood gases in preeclampsia. Br J Obstet Gynaecol 84:290, 1977
239. Gant NF, Worley RJ: Hypertension in Pregnancy; Concepts and Management. Appleton-Century-Crofts, E. Norwalk, CT, 1980
240. Lindheimer MD, Katz AI: Pathophysiology of preeclampsia. Annu Rev Med 32:273, 1981
241. Lindheimer MD, Katz AI: Hypertension and pregnancy. In Genest J, Kuchel O, Hamet P, et al (eds): Hypertension: Physiopathology and Treatment. McGraw-Book, New York, 1983, P. 889
242. Page EW, Christianson R: The impact of mean arterial blood pressure in middle trimester upon the outcome of pregnancy. Am J Obstet Gynecol 125:740, 1976
243. Friedman EA, Neff RK: Pregnancy Hypertension, a Systematic Evaluation of Clinical Criteria. PSG, Littleton, MA, 1977
244. Fisher KA, Luger A, Spargo BH, et al: Hypertension in pregnancy: Clinical–pathological correlations and late prognosis. Medicine (Baltimore) 60:267, 1981
245. Pollak VE, Nettles JB: The kidney in toxemia of pregnancy: A clinical and pathological study based on renal biopsies. Medicine (Baltimore) 39:469, 1960
246. Katz AI, Davison JM, Hayslett JP, et al: Pregnancy in women with kidney disease. Kidney Int 18:192, 1980
247. Gant NF, Jiminez JM, Whalley P, et al: A prospective study of angiotensin II pressor responsiveness in pregnancies complicated by chronic essential hypertension. Am J Obstet Gynecol 127:369, 1977
248. Broughton-Pipkin F, Oats JJN, Symonds EM: The effect of a specific AII antagonist (saralasin) on blood pressure in the immediate puerpuerium. P. 75. In Bonnar J, MacGillivray I, Symonds EM (eds): Pregnancy Hypertension. MTP Press, Lancaster, England, 1980
249. Sullivan JM, Palmer EJ, Schoenberger AA, et al: Rats TE, SQ 20881: Effect on eclamptic–preeclamptic women with postpartum hypertension. Am J Obstet Gynecol 131:707, 1978
250. Terragno NA, Terragno DA: The role of prostaglandins in the control of uterine blood flow. P. 392. In Lindheimer MD, Katz AI, Zuspan FP (eds): Hypertension in Pregnancy. Wiley, New York, 1976
251. Pedersen EB, Christensen NJ, Christensen P, et al: Preeclampsia—a state of prostaglandin deficiency? Urinary prostaglandin excretion, the renin–aldosterone system, and circulating catecholamines in preeclampsia. Hypertension 5:105, 1983
252. Demers LM, Gabbe SG: Placental prostaglandin levels in preeclampsia. Am J Obstet Gynecol 137, 1976
253. Robinson JS, Redman CWG, Clover L, et al: The concentrations of prostaglandins E and F, 13-14-dehydro-15 oxo-prostaglandin F and thromboxane B_2 in tissue obtained from women with and without preeclampsia. Prostaglandins Med 3:223, 1979
254. Remuzzi G, Marchesi D, Zoja C, et al: Reduced umbilical and placental vascular prostacyclin in severe pre-eclampsia. Prostaglandins 20:105, 1980
255. Remuzzi G, Zoja C, Marchesi D, et al: Plasmatic regulation of vascular prostacyclin in pregnancy. Br Med J 282:512, 1981
256. Beaufils M, Uzan S, DonSimoni R, et al: Metabolism of uric acid in normal and pathologic pregnancy. Contrib Nephrol 132, 1981
257. Tatum HJ, Mule JG: Puerpueral vasomotor collapse in patients with toxemia: A new concept of the etiology and a rational plan of treatment. Am J Obstet Gynecol 71:492, 1956
258. Mule JG, Tatum HJ, Sawyer RE: "Nitrogenous retention" in patients with toxemia of pregnancy—an unusual complication of salt restriction. Am J Obstet Gynecol 74:526, 1957
259. Palomaki J, Lindheimer MD: Sodium depletion simulating deterioration in a toxemic pregnancy. N Engl J Med 282:88, 1970
260. VandeWiele R, Gurpide E, Kelly WG, et al: The secretory rate of progesterone and aldosterone in normal and abnormal pregnancy. Acta Endocrinol (Copenh) 35:[Suppl 51]:159, 1960
261. Redman CWG, Bonnar J, Beilin LJ, et al:

Prolactin in hypertensive pregnancy. Br Med J 1.304, 1975

262. Dubowitz L, Strong F, Hawkins DF, et al: Toxaemia of pregnancy and prolactin. Br Med J 2:445, 1975
263. Biswas S, Rodeck CH: Plasma prolactin levels during pregnancy. Br J Obstet Gynaecol 83:683, 1976
264. Sadovsky E, Weinstein D, BenDavid M, et al: Serum prolactin in normal and pathologic pregnancy. Obstet Gynecol 50:559, 1977
265. Ho-Yuen B, Cannon W, Woolley S, et al: Maternal plasma and amniotic fluid prolactin levels in normal and hypertensive pregnancy. Br J Obstet Gynaecol 85:293, 1978
266. Jenkins DM, Perry LA: Plasma prolactin in pregnancy-induced hypertension in pregnancy. p. 261. In Bonnar J, MacGillivray I, Symonds EM (eds): Pregnancy Hypertension. MTP Press, Lancaster, England, 1980
267. Ranta T, Stenman U-H, Unnerus H-A, et al: Maternal plasma prolactin levels in preeclampsia. Obstet Gynecol 55:428, 1980
268. Dieckmann WJ, Michel H: Vascular–renal effects of posterior pituitary extracts in pregnant women. Am J Obstet Gynecol 33:131, 1937
269. Schokaert JA, Lambillon J. Un nouveau test permettant le diagnostique précoce et différential des preéclamptiques. Brux Med 17:1468, 1937
270. Lindheimer MD, Katz AI: Effects of hypotonic expansion on sodium and water excretion in hypertensive non-preeclamptic gravidas. Am J Obstet Gynecol 111:1053, 1971
271. Benedetti TJ, Cotton DB, Read JC, et al: Hemodynamic observations in severe preeclampsia with a flow-directed pulmonary artery catheter. Am J Obstet Gynecol 136:465, 1980
272. Rafferty TD, Berkowitz RL: Hemodynamics in patients with severe toxemia during labor and delivery. Am J Obstet Gynecol 138:263, 1980
273. Joyce TH III, Debnath KS, Baker EA: Preeclampsia—relationship of CVP and epidural analgesia. Anesthesiology 51:S297, 1979 (Abst.)
274. Zuspan FP, Bell JD: Variable salt-loading during pregnancy with preeclampsia. Obstet Gynecol 18:530, 1961
275. Mengert WF, Tacchi DA: Pregnancy toxemia and sodium chlorida. A preliminary report. Am J Obstet Gynecol 81:601, 1961
276. Bower D: The influence of dietary salt intake on pre-eclampsia. Br J Obstet Gynaecol 71:123, 1964
277. Foote RG, Lundbrook AP: The use of liberal diets in pre-eclamptic toxemia and essential hypertension of pregnancy. NZ J Med 77:242, 1973
278. Benedetti TJ, Quilligan EJ: Cerebral edema in severe pregnancy-induced hypertension. Am J Obstet Gynecol 137:860, 1980
279. Beeson JH, Duda EE: Computed axial tomography scan demonstration of cerebral edema in eclampsia preceded by blindness. Obstet Gynecol 60:529, 1982
280. Finnerty FA Jr: Hypertension and pregnancy. p. 866. In Genest J, Koiw E, Kuchel O (eds): Hypertension. 1st Ed. McGraw-Hill, New York, 1977
281. Christianson R, Page EW: Diuretic drugs and pregnancy. Obstet Gynecol 48:647, 1976

SECTION III

Special Considerations

23

Clinical Manifestations of Electrolyte Disorders

Gary D. Dubois
Allen I. Arieff

Electrolyte disorders can produce numerous clinical manifestations that may result in considerable morbidity and even mortality. However, most such manifestations are reversible if appropriate treatment is instituted. This chapter is organized by clinical manifestations rather than by specific electrolyte disorders. Each section discusses which electrolyte disorders may cause a given manifestation and gives information on incidence, associated findings, clinical effects of treatment, and pathophysiology. Manifestations are arranged under five major headings: (1) neuromuscular and neuropsychiatric; (2) cardiovascular, (3) gastrointestinal, (4) hematologic, and (5) hormonal and metabolic. Tables provide quick reviews of the various etiologies for these major manifestations.

This discussion is designed to heighten the index of suspicion of undiagnosed disorders and to aid in assessing the clinical significance of undetected biochemical abnormalities. Early diagnosis and correction are important in limiting the morbidity and mortality from these disorders, many of which are exacerbated by other forms of medical and nutritional treatment. Our fundamental understanding of the actual pathogenesis of the clinical abnormalities associated with water, electrolyte, and acid–base disorders is still largely incomplete, especially concerning unrecognized manifestations, aspects of pathophysiology, and optimal approaches to treatment. Due to the breadth of topics covered, references are largely limited to key studies and reviews. These do not always represent the original observations, but are chosen for their accessibility, breadth, and ability to cite the more complete literature.

NEUROMUSCULAR AND NEUROPSYCHIATRIC MANIFESTATIONS

Seizures

Exitable tissues such as the nervous system are sensitive to changes in the intracellular and extracellular ionic environment. Clinically such changes can produce many of the neuropsychiatric and cardiovascular manifestations of electrolyte disorders. Seizure activity is an example of increased excitability in the central nervous system and is a common manifestation of a number of electrolyte disor-

Table 23–1. Seizure Potential of Electrolyte Disorders[a]

Electrolyte Disorder	Presence of Seizures
Acidosis	−
Alkalosis	+
Hypernatremia	+[b]
Hyperglycemia	+[c,d]
Severe hyponatremia	+
Hypocalcemia	+
Hypercalcemia	±
Hypomagnesemia	+
Hypophosphatemia	+
Hyperkalemia	−

[a] −, no association; +, common association; ±, uncommon association.
[b] Especially during treatment.
[c] With elevated serum osmolality.
[d] Very often focal.

ders (see Table 23–1). Laboratory investigation should be undertaken to diagnose such disorders, since in most patients the convulsive tendency will be completely and permanently reversed during or after correction of the electrolyte disorder. In addition, such seizures are normally refractory to the usual medical regimens used to control seizure disorders.

Multiple mechanisms are probably involved in the pathophysiology of seizure initiation. It is presumed, however, that the final common pathway involves increased excitability in certain nerve cells and networks. Rapid firing of such networks can spread throughout the brain to produce generalized seizures or only spread locally to produce focal seizures.

Neuromuscular irritability has been loosely expressed in terms of extracellular cation concentrations as a proportional relationship:

$$\text{Neuromuscular irritability} = \frac{F\,(\mathrm{K}^+)}{(\mathrm{Na}^+)/(\mathrm{Ca})\,(\mathrm{H}^+)}$$

where F equals a proportionality factor.[1] There is much physiologic evidence supporting alterations in nerve cell and axon excitability with changes in the extracellular concentrations of these cations. However, more detailed studies of the effects of concentration and osmolality changes on synaptic junctions, on spread of seizure activity, and on networks of inhibitory as well as excitatory nerve cells are needed to explain seizure pathophysiology more fully. Individuals with preexisting primary seizure disorders can experience increased frequency and severity of convulsive attacks when an electrolyte disorder is superimposed. In the past, hyponatremia induced by water loading was used as a challenge test to unmask latent primary epilepsy. In some patients, old neurologic lesions such as strokes serve as the latent focus for seizure activity. Electrolyte and osmolality disorders can unmask such foci leading to focal or generalized seizures. In addition, severe electrolyte disorders are capable of producing seizures in subjects without prior or concurrent nervous system illness. Some of the specific disorders will now be discussed.

ALKALOSIS AND ACIDOSIS

Alkalosis increases neural excitability and tends to precipitate seizures in patients with primary epilepsy. Acute respiratory alkalosis produced by hyperventilation is often utilized during electroencephalography (EEG) to stimulate seizure foci. Severe alkalosis (pH near 7.6) can produce seizures in patients who do not have a prior history of epilepsy. Such alkalosis is usually produced by a combination of respiratory and metabolic alkalosis components. Such seizures are usually reversed by permitting one or both components to be corrected.

Patients with chronic respiratory failure (hypercarbia with compensatory metabolic alkalosis) are especially susceptible to seizures, coma, and death during rapid correction of the hypercarbia.[2–4] Such seizures are often heralded by increasing confusion, asterixis, and myoclonic jerks. Most patients have an arterial pH of 7.55 or greater, although occasional patients manifest the syndrome with less alkalosis. Correction of the hypercarbia permits the severe metabolic alkalosis to be expressed as rising extracellular pH. This can easily be achieved by the use of modern mechanical ventilation and should be avoided by careful follow-up of blood gases after initiation of therapy.

The kidneys may require a few days to execute the excess bicarbonate and correct the metabolic alkalosis. Meantime, dead space can be added to the ventilator to allow P_{CO_2} to remain elevated sufficiently to avoid severe alkalosis and precipitation of this often fatal syndrome.[2]

Experimental studies of hypercarbia demonstrate a profound decrease in cerebral blood flow after correction of hypercarbia over a few minutes. The decrease in cerebral blood flow was enhanced by coexistent metabolic alkalosis and appeared to cause cerebral ischemia.[5] Attempts to reverse this neurologic syndrome have included reinstitution of hypercarbia, as well as administration of acetazolamide to augment cerebral blood flow[6] and to hasten renal bicarbonate excretion. Hypoxia should be fully corrected. There is no evidence that Diamox (acetazolamide) should be used prophylactically, nor has there been any clinical trial for its use in the syndrome, since the syndrome can be avoided by prudent use of the ventilator.

Most patients undergoing correction of hypercarbia require volume and chloride repletion to permit renal correction of metabolic alkalosis. A urine chloride excretion of >30 mEq/day, off diuretics indicates an adequate chloride intake.[7] In addition, large amounts of potassium are required due to the enhanced excretion of potassium that accompanies the bicarbonate diuresis.[8] Complete correction of metabolic alkalosis is often not necessary in chronic lung disease patients, since mild hypercarbia may persist after the patient has been weaned off the mechanical ventilator.

In contrast to alkalosis, acidosis does not appear to produce seizure activity, although tremors, jerking of extremities, and clonic movements are often noted in patients with hypercapnia.[9,10] Severe acidosis ($pH < 7.1$) and hypercapnia have both been observed experimentally to decrease neuronal excitability.[11-13]

HYPERNATREMIA AND HYPEROSMOLAR STATES

Seizures frequently occur before and especially during treatment of hyperosmolar states such as hypernatremia and nonketotic hyperglycemia. Patients become most symptomatic when serum sodium is above 160 mmol/liter or the osmolality exceeds 350 mOsm/kg.

Chronic hypernatremia in adults seldom causes seizures.[14] Adult patients with acute hypernatremia may manifest neurologic alterations, but these patients often have other catastrophic illness that could have caused the neurologic alterations (see Chapter 21).

Hypernatremia in infants is commonly associated with seizures and has been studied in two basic etiologic subgroups: (1) infants with severe dehydration, usually due to gastroenteritis or diarrhea[15,16]; and (2) infants without dehydration but with acute salt poisoning.[17,18] Both groups manifest variable degrees of lethargy, stupor, and coma, which are interspersed with episodes of hyperirritability and a shrill cry. Muscle twitching and seizures are noted in both groups; however, each group has distinct clinical components.

Infants with gastroenteritis, diarrhea and/or fever can become severely dehydrated. Symptomatic infants often manifest hypernatremia with serum Na of 160 mmol/liter (range 151 to 188 mmol/liter), severe acidosis (pH near 7.1), and prerenal azotemia.[19-21] In this group, seizures seldom occur until treatment has been initiated; they are usually generalized rather than focal and most often occur during the first 24 hours of treatment. The occurrence of seizures is quite variable, ranging from zero to two-thirds of infants in different series. Factors thought to be relevant are the initial degree of electrolyte imbalance,[20] presence of significant azotemia,[20,22] and acidosis.[19] Exclusion of febrile patients lowers the incidence of seizures.[21] Dehydrated infants manifest a very high incidence of hyperpyrexia, which cannot always be documented as attributable to infection.

In addition, the rate of correction of the

hypernatremia[21] is a significant factor. Recent attempts have been made to quantitate the rate of correction that provides the fewest seizures during treatment. Infants who seized were found to have a decrease in serum sodium of ~1 mmol/liter-hr compared with those groups not experiencing seizures who averaged a fall in serum sodium below 0.6 mmol/liter-hr.[21] The rate of correction of azotemia and acidosis does not appear to be as significant as the correction of hypernatremia, although infants with initial significant azotemia were more likely to manifest seizures.[19,20]

Salt poisoning has been studied during the accidental poisoning of infants given formula containing NaCl instead of sugar.[17,18] Fourteen infants became severely hypernatremic (mean serum Na 199 mmol/liter), over just 3 or 4 days. In contrast to infants with dehydration, these infants experienced generalized seizures and coma before the initiation of their treatment to correct the hypernatremia. Mortality was high (43 percent), although the survivors appeared to return to normal neurologic function. Autopsy revealed intracranial bleeding, petechial hemorrhages, and vascular thrombosis of a greater degree than that noted in infants with dehydration-induced hypernatremia.

Such early symptomatology and high mortality in the salt-poisoned infants could have been primarily due to the greater severity of hypernatremia as compared with dehydrated infants (mean serum Na 199 mmol/liter vs 160 mmol/liter). However, the salt-poisoned infants also had a more acute form of hypernatremia. Animal studies[23] suggest that this may be the crucial difference, since the brain can adjust to hypermolality if adequate time is allowed to generate idiogenic osmoles.[24] This same process can cause brain edema in the patient with chronic hypernatremia if the hypernatremia is corrected faster than the brain can dispose of the idiogenic osmoles (see Chapter 21).

Hyperosmolality due to the combined effect of increased extracellular electrolytes plus severe hyperglycemia can produce coma and focal or generalized seizures.[25-27] The clinical setting is usually one of nonketotic hyperglycemia rather than of ketoacidosis. Up to 25 percent of these patients experience seizures, 75 percent of which are focal in nature. Symptomatic patients usually manifest blood glucose levels of 33 to 66 mmol/liter (600 to 1200 mg/dl) and elevated serum osmolality ranging from 350 to 400 mOsm/kg. Continuous focal seizures have been observed as the presenting sign in 6 percent of patients with nonketotic hyperglycemia.[27a] These focal seizures may continue for up to 6 days and may be limited to one anatomic area, such as an upper extremity. This restriction to one limb or neurologic area suggests that there is a single focus, possibly a structural lesion caused by previous injury. This focus may be more susceptible to stimulation by hyperosmolality.[25,26] Such seizures are generally refractory to treatment with antiepileptic medications, but can be controlled by lowering the osmolality and blood glucose levels.[25] In both hypernatremia and hyperglycemia, the brain manufactures idiogenic osmoles, but in hyperglycemia, they can apparently dissipate more quickly. Readjustment is faster during treatment of hyperglycemia, making brain edema less common and speed of correction less a factor than for hypernatremia.

HYPONATREMIA

Acute hyponatremia (less than 12 hours to develop) and subacute hyponatremia (less than 48 hours and greater than 12 hours to develop) are probably the most common cause of seizures due to electrolyte disorders. Such a rapid progression of hyponatremia is usually due to increased water intake either by tap water enemas, hypotonic intravenous therapy or occasionally, by self-induced water intoxication. In conjunction with a decreased ability of the kidney to excrete water (e.g., elevated antidiuretic hormone, antidiuretic medications, renal failure) the water load can lead to a rapid decrement of serum sodium. Seizures resulting from a slow (greater than 3 days) fall in serum sodium below 100 mmol/liter are quite rare, even in the presence of other neurologic manifestation of hyponatremia.

Hyponatremia-related seizures are almost always generalized in nature, although they may occur during treatment, most often seizures decrease in frequency as serum sodium rises. Patients with primary seizure disorders manifest increased frequency of seizures if hyponatremia is induced.[27]

Review of the literature reveals at least 23 patients with acute hyponatremia and 24 patients with subacute hyponatremia.[28-38] Eleven of 23 patients (49 percent) with acute hyponatremia seized during their clinical courses. The mean serum sodium level for the two groups was not significantly different (with seizure, 107 mmol/liter; without seizure, 112 mmol/liter). Of the 24 patients with subacute hyponatremia, 19 (79 percent) had at least one seizure. The mean serum sodium was the same for patients with and without seizures (113 mmol/liter).

Hyponatremia—whether acute or chronic—can lead to alterations in the level of consciousness. Confusion, lethargy, stupor, and rarely coma usually precede the onset of seizures. Despite the early alterations in level of consciousness, the onset of a seizure is often the factor that precipitates a medical investigation. The onset of seizures is usually associated with further decline in level of consciousness. Of 31 patients who seized, 24 (77 percent) lapsed into stupor or coma immediately afterward, and their level of consciousness did not improve until correction of hyponatremia was well under way (hours to days). Four of 31 patients who seized awoke in a confused or lethargic state after the postictal period. Two patients had stupor or coma before the onset of seizures. Most patients with chronic hyponatremia and many patients with acute or subacute hyponatremia will progress to stupor or coma without seizure activity. Usually their serum sodium levels are below 120 mmol/liter.

The occurrence of seizures is often associated with a decline in the level of consciousness, but the presence of neither seizures nor coma can predict outcome of treatment. Multiple other neurologic signs often transiently come and go during hyponatremia and its correction.

CALCIUM METABOLISM DISORDERS

Seizures often occur in association with hypocalcemia due to hypoparathyroidism.[14,39-41] During acute hypocalcemia, the onset of tetany usually precedes the onset of seizures. Therefore, most patients receive calcium supplementation before manifesting seizures. In infants, and occasionally in adults, tetany may mimic seizures. Serum calcium levels should be measured in patients who manifest seizure activity. Hypocalcemic seizures are usually generalized with loss of consciousness but are more abortive than the seizures of primary epilepsy.[14] Focal, psychomotor, and petit mal seizures, as well as status epilepticus, have occasionally been observed.[41] Seizures in chronic hypocalcemic patients are usually refractory to the usual anticonvulsant medications but often will decrease in frequency or disappear with chronic calcium and vitamin D treatment.[42] Acute administration of intravenous calcium may acutely decrease seizure activity, but chronic EEG changes may take weeks to months to approach normal. In addition, patients with primary epilepsy who develop hypocalcemia, such as from chronic phenylhydantoin use, may experience increased frequency and intensity of convulsions despite taking their previously effective anticonvulsant medications.[42]

Hypercalcemia only rarely causes convulsions, with most reported cases being children whose chronic seizure frequency decreased after reversal of hypercalcemia.[43-46] One should not assume that seizures in adults with hypercalcemia are primarily due to the hypercalcemia.[47]

Hypocalcemia decreases excitability in mammalian neurons.[14,48] Axonal membrane potentials begin to oscillate, and neurons spontaneously produce bursts of activity (chalazonitis). Hypercalcemia stabilizes membrane and nerve cell activity. Despite severe hypercalcemia or hypocalcemia, brain calcium levels remain close to normal unless hypercalcemia is due to hyperparathyroidism. The cause of the alterations in central nervous system function is not clear. Changes in local ionized and intracellular calcium as well as plasma parathyroid hormone levels may play significant roles but await further study.

Magnesium depletion with hypomagnesemia can increase seizure activity.[14,49,50] The clinical settings include severe malnutrition, alcoholic withdrawal, and neonatal hypocalcemia. Many of these patients have additional conditions that predispose to convulsions. Hypocalcemia, alkalosis, and delirium tremens all may contribute, in conjunction with hypomagnesemia, to increase the susceptibility to seizure activity. Correction of hypocalcemia alone without correction of hypomagnesemia may not abolish seizures or tetany.

Among alcoholics undergoing withdrawal, those patients manifesting seizures generally have lower serum magnesium levels and a greater seizure potential as measured by photomyoclonus.[50] Patients were most susceptible during episodes in which both respiratory alkalosis and hypomagnesemia were severe. The serum magnesium levels are often normal on admission and then fall during delirium tremens. Patients usually demonstrate tremors and hyperreflexia before the onset of seizures.

Lethargy, Stupor, and Coma

Electrolyte disorders are extremely common causes of lethargy and stupor, although they represent only about 5 percent of all cases of nontraumatic coma.[55] Lethargy and stupor are usually readily reversed by correction of the electrolyte imbalance. If persistent, then other causes of the disordered sensorium should be searched for. Prognostic indicators of recovery have not been analyzed for coma due to electrolyte disorders,[55] and clinical examination cannot always be relied on to distinguish between structural lesions and metabolic causes. The discovery of an abnormal serum laboratory value often tends to curtail neurologic diagnostic workups. Thus structural lesions may be missed.

As with other forms of metabolic encephalopathy, patients usually manifest a stepwise clinical progression of symptoms. Changes in cognitive function, awareness, and attention are noticed first. The patient is disoriented, confused, or unable to remember. In some cases a coarse tremor and asterixis is noted. The patient may progress to stupor and then to coma. Not uncommonly in electrolyte disorders, myoclonus and seizures accompany alterations in consciousness. Stuporous patients often become comatose after undergoing a seizure. Unlike the transitory postictal state seen in primary epilepsy, this depression of consciousness persists until diagnosis and treatment bring about correction of the electrolyte disorder—hypernatremia, hyponatremia respiratory acidosis, metabolic acidosis, severe metabolic alkalosis, hypophosphatemia, hyperglycemia, and hypoglycemia are important examples. Nonmetabolic causes for protracted unresponsiveness to stimuli (greater than 30 minutes) include (1) status epilepticus, (2) elderly patients with old cerebrovascular accident scars, and (3) when the seizures are produced by a cerebral structural lesion.[56]

Focal neurologic signs can be noted in conjunction with electrolyte disorders but are often transitory and usually do not fit into the patterns associated with a single brain structural lesion. The clinical course depends on the rate of progression and severity of the electrolyte disorder. The patient may manifest confusion, stupor, seizure, and coma over just a few hours or in an insidiously slow manner over days.

Brain chemical composition, both intracel-

Table 23–2. Etiologies of Lethargy, Stupor, and Coma[a]

Electrolyte Disorder	Lethargy	Stupor	Coma
Hypernatremia	+	+	+
Hyponatremia	+	+	+
Hyperkalemia	−	−	−
Hypokalemia	+	−	−
Hypercalcemia	+	+	+
Hypocalcemia	+	±	−
Hypermagnesemia	+	−	(±)[c]
Hypomagnesemia	+[b]	−	−
Respiratory acidosis	+	+	+
Metabolic acidosis	+	+	+[d]
Respiratory alkalosis	+	−	−
Metabolic alkalosis	+	+	+[e]
Hypophosphatemia	+	+	+
Hyperglycemia	+	+	+
Hypoglycemia	+	+	+

[a] −, no association; +, common association; ±, rare association.
[b] Apathy, confusion, inattention.
[c] Clinical coma secondary to respiratory paralysis, hypoxia, and hypotension.
[d] Rare with simple acidosis (see text).
[e] Only if severe alkalosis or posthypercapnic alkalosis.

lular and extracellular, is tightly regulated, permitting the brain to maintain its basic composition despite significant change in systemic concentrations of cations and anions. Table 23–2 lists the disorders that cause a decline in level of consciousness.

HYPEROSMOLALITY–HYPERNATREMIA AND HYPERGLYCEMIA

Hypernatremia is well known to be associated with lethargy, stupor, and coma in infants whose disorder is acute or chronic.[57] When arousable, these infants may give forth a shrill, characteristic cry. Typically infants are lethargic with intermittent episodes of irritability,[57,58] and they develop seizures and a decline in level of consciousness if treated too rapidly with hypotonic fluids. Residual neurologic deficits are common.[20,58]

Adult hypernatremia may also be associated with lethargy, stupor, and coma, although careful quantitation of manifestations with severity and etiology of hypernatremia has not yet been reported. Often, stupor or coma due to other causes prevents the patient from obtaining water and thus produces hypernatremia. The pathophysiology of brain adaptation to hyperosmolality and its effects on treatment are discussed in Chapter 21.

Severe hyperglycemia is a well-documented cause of lethargy, stupor, and coma.[25] Coma is usually noted when blood osmolality exceeds 350 mOsm/kg.[27] Level of consciousness correlates well with degree of hyperosmolality. Coma can usually be reversed by lowering the serum osmolality and rehydrating the patient.

HYPONATREMIA

Acute and chronic hyponatremia can lead to alteration in level of consciousness. Confusion, lethargy, and stupor progressively appear, depending largely on both the rate and magnitude of the decrement in serum sodium. Coma occurs only rarely before the onset of seizures.[28-37] The onset of seizures is usually associated with further decline in consciousness. Of 31 patients who seized, 24 (77 percent) lapsed into stupor or coma immediately afterward, and the level of consciousness did not improve until correction of hyponatremia was well under way (hours to days). Only two patients manifested stupor or coma before seizing. Serum sodium levels were usually below 115 mmol/liter in those with seizure, stupor, and coma. Most patients had experienced acute (onset of 12 hours) or subacute (less than 48 hours) hyponatremia, which provokes more dramatic manifestations than does chronic hyponatremia. The occurrence of neurologic manifestations in association with hyponatremia correlates with a higher mortality when compared with asymptomatic patients. However, neurologic findings of seizure, stupor, and coma have not been found to predict outcome of treatment within the symptomatic group; other more detailed examinations to predict outcome have not been undertaken for hyponatremic coma.[55]

POTASSIUM DISORDERS

Hypokalemia rarely causes lethargy and somnolence.[59,60] Hyperkalemia is not known to cause lethargy, stupor, or coma. The brain appears to regulate its extracellular potassium concentrations avidly, probably allowing the brain to continue functioning at systemic levels of hyperkalemia that lead to paralysis and cardiac asystole.[60a] Potassium placed directly on the cerebral cortex produces "spreading depression" with temporary loss of cortical function.

CALCIUM DISORDERS

Hypocalcemia may cause mild diffuse encephalopathy and, if severe, it can occasionally lead to lethargy and stupor.[56] Coma is very rare, although due to the tendency toward tetany and seizures, patients occasionally present with postictal changes in consciousness.

Hypercalcemia can produce the typical progressive decline in level of consciousness noted for metabolic encephalopathies. Most patients manifest diffuse signs of mild encephalopathy such as confusion, disorientation, and lethargy. Patients predisposed to abrupt rises in serum calcium (hypercalemic crisis), such as those with neoplasm or dehydration, will often progress to stupor and even coma with serum calcium levels above 3.5 mmol/liter (14 mg/dl). The severity of such changes in consciousness is quite variable from one patient to another.[61,56] Hypercalcemic crisis, if left untreated, can rapidly lead to acute renal failure and obtundation.

The pathophysiology of the effects of hypercalcemia on brain function is not entirely clear. As with other cations, the brain appears to be somewhat protected from the effects of fluctuations in serum calcium concentration.[63] Electroencephalographic changes have been described[64-66] but do not always correlate well with the degree of hypercalcemia or the extent of mental status change. EEG findings may take weeks to resolve after correction of systemic hypercalcemia.[66a]

MAGNESIUM DISORDERS

Magnesium depletion has not been associated with stupor or coma even after the seizures commonly associated with severe depletion.[49,67] Patients are noted to be excited, tremulous, and hallucinating. They may intermittently appear lethargic, detached, and unable to sustain attention.[68,69] During chronic experimental magnesium depletion, symptomatic patients manifested apathy, but hypocalcemia and hypokalemia were also present.[51]

In the past hypermagnesemia was used as an anesthetic and was thought to depress central nervous system function. More recently, however, hypermagnesemia has been found merely to paralyze, giving the appearance of coma, but with awareness and sensations intact.[70-72] These studies were done under controlled conditions, in which respiratory failure and severe hypotension could be avoided. Very high serum magnesium levels were obtained (7.5 mmol/liter or 15 mEq/liter) without true loss of consciousness.

Clinical hypermagnesemia is a more complicated problem, usually involving patients with renal failure, a group predisposed to magnesium toxicity. Patients with moderate elevation of serum magnesium (above 2.5 mmol/liter) may demonstrate drowsiness, mild lethargy, slurred speech, and ataxic gait, but not stupor or coma. Patients with elevation of serum magnesium above 2.5 mmol/liter usually become areflexic, paralyzed, and hypotensive, may develop respiratory failure, and are observed to be in flaccid coma.[71] Serum magnesium levels range from 2.7 to 4.55 mmol/liter.

Currently there is not sufficient information to decide whether clinical magnesium toxicity can cause true coma. If it does, however, it is probably by the secondary mechanisms of hypoxia and hypotension. Characteristics of clinical hypermagnesemia that do not favor a direct depression of brain functions include the following: (1) there is no progression through stupor and coma; (2) although lethargy occurs, confusion and cognitive defects are not reported early in the course; and (3) paralysis, hypotension, and respiratory depression precede the comalike state.

ACID–BASE DISORDERS

The brain can rapidly adjust to fluctuations in hydrogen ion and bicarbonate concentrations but is less adept at compensating for changes in carbon dioxide tension. Compensation is best for metabolic acidosis, fair for respiratory and metabolic alkalosis, and poor for respiratory acidosis. Failure to compensate or exceeding the ability of the brain to compensate usually results in a decline in brain function.

Thus, all acid–base disorders can potentially affect the brain; however, due to compensation, most of these disorders do not produce clinical symptoms. Only respiratory acidosis routinely produces stupor and coma. Most forms of metabolic acidosis by themselves rarely cause coma. Respiratory alkalosis usually produces only confusion and lightheadedness. Severe alkalosis or posthypercapnic alkalosis can cause significant stupor and coma.

RESPIRATORY ACIDOSIS

Patients with acute respiratory failure who manifest respiratory acidosis and hypoxia are found to have a high incidence of lethargy and stupor when arterial P_{CO_2} tension exceeds 60 mm Hg and oxygen tension falls below 55 mm Hg.[9] The slower the rise in carbon dioxide tension, the more time for brain adaptation and the less dramatic are the patients' symptoms. Some of these patients progress to coma if hypoventilation increases, which occasionally occurs with unassisted oxygen therapy. Kilburn observed that in patients with similar degrees of hypoxia, coma best correlated with the severity of acidosis and hypercarbia of >88 mm Hg.[10] Of seven patients who were comatose, only two manifested seizures as well. Coma seldom occurs in hypercapnic patients who breathe room air, since air hunger keeps their hypercarbia from going too high. Hypoxemia will intervene before coma from hypercarbia occurs.

Carbon dioxide readily passes through the blood–brain barrier and across cell membranes. Since bicarbonate is largely excluded by these barriers, brain cells must compensate for rapid shifts in carbon dioxide tension. To a considerable degree, brain intracellular pH can compensate within a few hours to a new level of hypercarbia. This ability can be exceeded under experimental conditions.[73] Likewise, brain extracellular fluids (cerebrospinal fluid) are found to have increasingly high bicarbonate concentrations as hypercarbia progresses. Failure to keep pace with the hypercarbia-induced acidosis is thought to allow brain cells to become acidotic, resulting in stupor and coma.[56]

METABOLIC ACIDOSIS

Simple metabolic acidosis rarely produces coma. Patients may experience delirium, lethargy, or mild stupor. The brain can buffer itself well against metabolic acidosis. When these buffers fail, however, brain and cerebrospinal fluid pH fall progressively and this lowered pH correlates with decline in consciousness to stupor or coma.[74] This has not been clinically useful because cerebrospinal fluid pH lags behind true brain pH. The factors that cause a patient's brain to fail to compensate are not understood, but are probably multifactorial.

Patients with diabetic ketoacidosis, nonketotic hyperosmolar coma, and toxic ingestions of aspirin, methanol, or ethylene glycol can manifest severe alterations in consciousness. The pathophysiology varies and is not limited to brain acidosis alone.

Diabetic ketoacidosis usually produces lethargy or stupor, but fewer than 10 percent of patients manifest true coma. The pathophysiology is not understood, but hyperosmolality, cerebral hypoxia, and cerebral edema may play a role. At our present level of knowledge, coma in patients with diabetic ketoacidosis correlates best with the plasma osmolality[75] and to some extent with plasma levels of acetoacetic acid.[75a,75b] Hyperosmolar coma due to nonketotic hyperglycemia is discussed under hyperosmolar states (Chapter 20). Unlike the situation in ketoacidosis, the degree of depression of sensorium in patients with nonketotic hyperosmolar coma correlates very well with the level of plasma osmolality, but not with hyperglycemia or arterial pH.[76]

Treatment of metabolic acidosis with bicarbonate may actually woresen brain intracellular acidosis. Hypoventilation leads to an increase in the systemic carbon dioxide levels and, by diffusing into the cerebrospinal fluid and brain, produces a more severe intracellular acidosis.[74]

ALKALOSIS

Acute respiratory alkalosis produces cerebral vasoconstriction and a marked decline in cerebral blood flow. As a result, confusion and lethargy may occur. These effects are transient and, despite continued hyperventilation, do not progress to stupor or coma.[56]

Severe hyperbicarbonatemia (>50 mmol/liter) is often associated with confusion, lethargy, stupor, and rarely coma.[76a] These patients can be divided into two main etiologic groups. (1) patients with hypercapnea; and (2) patients who have progressively become alkalotic due to other metabolic situations, such as hyperaldosteronism and gastric suction.

Posthypercapneic patients demonstrate a substantial degree of symptomatology, often manifesting anxiety, confusion, myoclonus, seizures, and coma.[2-4] Experimental studies reveal that the cerebral vessels are hypersensitized by hyperbicarbonatemia. Therefore, a decrease in arterial carbon dioxide levels in the presence of hyperbicarbonatemia produces severe reductions in cerebral blood flow.[5] Coma can sometimes be reversed by allowing a rise in arterial carbon dioxide tension by lowering minute ventilation. Mechanical ventilation may have to be slowed for hours to days to permit renal bicarbonate excretion to reduce the hyperbicarbonatemia. It may also be necessary to provide sufficient chloride, sodium, and potassium.[76a]

A second group of patients have severe metabolic alkalosis without a history of respiratory failure. They may demonstrate agitation, delirium, and lethargy, but only rarely stupor and coma. These manifestations usually reverse within a few days of correction of alkalosis. The pathophysiology of these findings is less understood than those of the previous syndrome.[76a]

Mild hypoxemia may be a contributing factor; although these patients are not in respiratory failure, they may hypoventilate due to the severity of their alkalosis.[77,78] Arterial Po_2 levels may be 60 mm Hg, and many patients also have some degree of volume contraction and hypocalcemia. Surprisingly, patients with primary aldosteronism have not been reported to have alterations in their levels of consciousness despite severely elevated levels of serum bicarbonate.[76a]

PHOSPHATE DEPLETION WITH HYPOPHOSPHATEMIA

Severe hypophosphatemia (<0.323 mmol/liter or <1 mg/dl) induced in malnourished or alcoholic patients by hyperalimentation can result in stupor or coma,[54,79,80] while some patients may experience grand mal seizures.[53] The syndrome is unlike delirium tremens in that patients initially manifest weakness, tingling, and numbness of the extremities and circumoral regions. In addition, they do not have hallucinations.

The pathophysiology of these central nervous system effects is not yet known.[54] A decrease in oxygen delivery to the brain, due to altered P50 of hemoglobin, has been suggested to play a role.[79] Alterations in brain energy metabolism have not yet been demonstrated. (See also Chapter 21).

Electroencephalography

The EEG has been studied in a number of water, electrolyte, and acid–base abnormalities including uremia, phosphate depletion, hyponatremia, hypernatremia, hyperglycemia and hypoglycemia, hypercalcemia and hypocalcemia, and hepatic encephalopathy. Some of these findings have been reviewed.[81] Although there are many new and sophisticated techniques for evaluation of the EEG, most clinical neurologists and internists are only familiar with the classic techniques of power spectrum and frequency analysis as described almost 40 years ago.[82,83] In general, normal frequencies are usually above 9 Hz, and abnormal frequencies below 7 or 5 Hz. In abnormal EEGs associated with metabolic encephalopathies, there is a shift in both the frequency distribution and the power spectrum to those frequencies below 7 or 5 Hz.

In general, at our present state of knowledge, it is not possible to differentiate one metabolic encephalopathy from another on the basis of the EEG alone. However, it is often possible to differentiate structural from metabolic causes of coma. In structural lesions, the EEG will often have localizing features, which can help pinpoint a discrete anatomic lesion. In metabolic encephalopathies, the EEG usually shows a generalized disturbance and is similar in all leads. In hepatic encephalopathy, the EEG findings are said to be characteristic[84] and in dialysis dementia, they are said to be highly specific.[85] Of all the aforementioned metabolic disorders in which the EEG has been evaluated, the changes of uremia have been by far the most extensively studied. These are summarized in Chapter 21.

Myoclonus, Fasciculations, and Cramps

MYOCLONUS

Myoclonic jerks or myoclonus are abrupt, shocklike, observable muscle contractions. They are irregular in occurrence, amplitude, and distribution. Unlike seizures, these contractions are asynchronous, and, unlike cramps, or tetany, they are not sustained. A set of muscles may contract simultaneously and partially move a limb or the trunk. At the other extreme, just a small part of one muscle may contract, mimicking a fasciculation. Sensory stimulation, such as touch, sound, or flickering lights, may exacerbate myoclonus. Repeated stimuli in some conditions may recruit further contractions and can end in a seizure. See Table 23–3 for etiologies of myoclonus, fasciculations, and cramps.

Table 23–3. Etiologies of Myoclonus, Fasciculations, and Cramps

Electrolyte Disorder	Myoclonus	Fasciculations	Cramps
Hypernatremia	+	−	+
Hyponatremia	+	+	+
Hyperkalemia	−	+	−[c]
Hypokalemia	−	+	+[d]
Hypercalcemia	−	−	−
Hypocalcemia	−	+	+[d]
Hypermagnesemia	−	−	−
Hypomagnesemia	+	+	+[d]
Respiratory acidosis	+	−	−
Metabolic acidosis	−	−	−
Respiratory alkalosis	−	−	+[d]
Metaboic alkalosis	+[b]	−	+[d]
Hypophosphatemia	−	−	−

[a] −, no association; +, common association; ±, uncommon association.
[b] Due to rapid correction of respiratory acidosis.
[c] Cramps noted in familial hyperkalemic periodic paralysis.
[d] Cramps may be due to coexistent tetany.

Myoclonus is often associated with severe respiratory acidosis, in which it may become severe and sustained, resulting in seizures.[10] The myoclonus tends to be worse if the patient is hypoxic as well as hypercapnic. The tendency toward myoclonus usually decreases with correction of the respiratory acidosis, but may reappear if the correction is too rapid and produces metabolic alkalosis. Encephalopathy, myoclonus, and seizures may then occur.[3] Myoclonus is also commonly associated with acute or chronic hyponatremia[30,31,86] and is less commonly related to magnesium deficiency[49] and hyperosmolar states such as hypernatremia[87] and nonketotic hyperosmolar coma.[25]

Myoclonus can be a general finding in certain metabolic encephalopathies. In addition to the etiologies listed above, uremic and anoxic encephalopathy as well as high-dose penicillin toxicity can cause myoclonus.[56] The pathophysiology of myoclonus is not well understood. It involves abnormal discharges of groups of motor neurons. Cortical, cerebellar, brainstem, and spinal cord dysfunction have all been suggested as possible origins of the phenomena.

FASCICULATIONS

Fasciculations are small, abrupt contractions noted to occur in a larger muscle. Like myoclonus, the contraction is fleeting, but unlike myoclonus the contraction always remains small, about the size of one motor unit. Each motor unit is made up of a group of nerve fibers, all of which are jointly innervated by one motor neuron. Spontaneous firing of that motor neuron produces a rapid twitch of its motor unit. Fasciculations indicate a diseased motor neuron but do not necessarily mean that the muscle fibers are denervated. Denervation produces fibrillations on the electromyogram.

Fasciculations are said to occur with hyponatremia, hyperkalemia, hypokalemia, hypocalcemia, hypomagnesemia, and hypophosphatemia[88,89] (see Table 23–3). Some of these observations are likely to have been episodes of myoclonus, and the subject needs more clarification with electromyographic studies. Nevertheless, the muscle twitching often vanishes after correction of these electrolyte disorders and does not necessarily represent permanent or progressive neurologic disease.

CRAMPS

Muscle cramps are spasmotic, involuntary, painful contractions that last for longer than a few seconds and are therefore too long to be fasciculations, myoclonic jerks, tremors, or chorea.[90] They are commonly noted to occur with electrolyte disorders, which may produce isolated cramps or cramps as a part of tetany. Hypernatremia with dehydration commonly causes cramps, particularly when it follows hard exercise in heat with only water as replacement.[88]

Muscle Weakness and Paralysis

Many electrolyte disorders can produce muscle weakness;[88] a few can produce paralysis as well (Table 23–4). The weakness and paralysis are generally rapidly reversible with correction of the electrolyte disorder. Exceptions include myopathic changes and rhabdomyolysis, which require muscle tissue repair. In addition, permanent brain damage from hyponatremia or hypernatremia can produce weakness or paralysis, or both.

The pathophysiology of weakness and paralysis is complex and multifactorial. Voluntary movement requires function of the cerebral cortex, descending motor tracts, lower motor neuron, peripheral nerve, neuromuscular junction, and finally the muscle itself. Electrolyte disorders often act at multiple sites along these pathways, and for many of the disorders the pathophysiology is only partially understood. The following discussion is a simplification of the known pathophysiology.

Table 23–4. Etiologies of Muscle Weakness and Paralysis[a]

Electrolyte Disorder	Muscle Weakness	Paralysis
Hypernatremia	+	−
Hyponatremia	+	+
Hyperkalemia	+	+
Hypokalemia	+	+
Hypercalcemia	+	−
Hypocalcemia	+	−
Hypermagnesemia	+	+
Hypomagnesemia	+	−
Respiratory acidosis	−	−
Metabolic acidosis	−	−
Respiratory alkalosis	+	−
Metabolic alkalosis	+	−
Hypophosphatemia	+	+

[a] −, no association; +, common association.

Potassium depletion and hyperparathyroidism act mainly on the muscle, producing myopathy.[88] Under certain circumstances, hypokalemia and hypophosphatemia can cause further muscle damage by rhabdomyolysis, Hyperkalemia, potassium depletion, and hypercalcemia effect muscle electrophysiology and neuromuscular transmission. Hypocalcemia, alkalosis, and magnesium depletion produce hyperirritability of nerve and muscle membranes, creating weakness and tetany. Hypermagnesemia interrupts neuromuscular transmission at the neuromuscular junction and increases the excitation threshold for nerve axons.[71] Acute hyponatremia directly effects the muscle, producing cramps and fasciculations, but weakness and paralysis are probably due to effects on the central nervous system and commonly present as hemiparesis. Chronic hyponatremia also occasionally causes hemiparesis.

POTASSIUM DISORDERS

Four disorders of potassium metabolism can give rise to weakness and paralysis. These include hypokalemic myopathy, hyperkalemia, and the familial diseases, namely, hyperkalemic, hypokalemic and normokalemic periodic paralysis.

HYPOKALEMIA AND POTASSIUM DEPLETION

Potassium depletion and the associated hypokalemia produce muscle weakness and paralysis by a number of effects on the muscle and its blood supply.[88] The pathophysiology will not be discussed in detail, but four main types of defects have been noted: (1) electrochemical and ion-transport abnormalities involving changes in intracellular electrolytes and membrane potentials, (2) impaired muscle blood flow with exercise, (3) metabolic abnormalities including impaired glycogen synthesis and storage and (4) muscle necrosis (rhabdomyolysis) when the muscles are exercised.[88]

Although the degree of hypokalemia does not always correlate with the degree of total body potassium depletion, serum potassium levels usually correlate well with onset and severity of weakness. Patients with serum potassium of 3 to 3.5 mmol/liter rarely complain of muscle weakness, and clinically detectable weakness is rare. Weakness is usually observed when serum potassium is below 2.5 mmol/liter, and there may be serum elevations of muscle enzymes. Below 2 mmol/liter, exercise can precipitate rhabdomyolysis, and paralysis is observed.[88,91,92] Hypokalemic weakness is an important symptom in that it usually, but not always, precedes the onset of paralysis. The progression to paralysis can be insidious or can occur suddenly with little or no change in serum potassium level. Proximal limb muscles are most affected, usually progressing in an ascending manner from lower to upper extremities.

Weakness and paralysis can be rapidly reversed toward normal within a few hours of potassium repletion. Residual weakness may occur if rhabdomyolysis has occurred. Potassium repletion must be carefully monitored and can produce tetany. The etiology of this event is unclear, but there is often an accompanying hypocalcemia; treatment with calcium will often reverse the tetany.

HYPERKALEMIA

Hyperkalemia, as does hypokalemia, can produce an ascending weakness and paralysis of the proximal limb muscles. Respiratory muscles may be involved, but cerebration and cranial nerve function are usually spared. Unlike hypokalemia, progression to paralysis is related to further changes in serum potassium. Paralysis often occurs with serum potassium levels of ≥ 6.8 mmol/liter. Life-threatening cardiac arrhythmias usually occur before complete paralysis occurs. Electrocardiogram changes are usually present providing a rapid diagnosis of hyperkalemia. Calcium should be administered to provide some degree of cardiac protection while specific treatment to reduce the hyperkalemia is under way. It should be remembered that rapid infusion of glucose without insulin can suddenly raise serum potassium even higher in diabetic patients with hypoaldosteronism (type IV renal tubular acidosis). Acetylcholinesterase inhibitors do not reverse hyperkalemic paralysis as they do for patients with paralysis due to myasthenia gravis and hypermagnesemia.[71,93]

FAMILIAL PERIODIC PARALYSIS

Patients with familial periodic paralysis manifest weakness and paralysis episodically, accompanied by (1) an acute rise in serum potassium (hyperkalemic form), (2) an acute decrease in serum potassium (hypokalemic form), or (3) rarely no change in serum potassium (normokalemic form). A given family usually manifests only the hypokalemic form or a combination of the hyperkalemic, normokalemic forms. Hyperthyroidism can cause a reversible disorder that is subtype of the hypokalemic periodic paralysis. Paralysis occasionally provokes respiratory failure.

Attacks of paralysis are provoked by a variety of stimuli that depend on the specific disorder, but include rest after exercise, sleep, a high intake of carbohydrate, and oral potassium loads.[94] Preexisting hyperkalemia exacerbates the hyperkalemic form and sometimes will decrease the severity of the hypokalemic form. Likewise, preexisting hypokalemia exacerbates the hypokalemic form, and the use of diuretics to lower serum potassium may decrease attacks in the hyperkalemic form. Acute reversal of hyperkalemia or hypokalemia during an attack is usually associated with restoration of muscle power. However, the alterations in serum potassium concentrations are not solely responsible for paralysis, but are themselves a by-product of metabolic and membrane conductance changes. Interestingly, acetazolamide has proved effective for the treatment of both hyperkalemic and hypokalemic periodic paralysis. For a comprehensive review, see ref. 95.

PHOSPHATE DEPLETION AND HYPOPHOSPHATEMIA

Clinical phosphate depletion can occur in the setting of malnutrition of calories, minerals, and vitamins. Muscle weakness is often present, and mild myopathic changes can be observed on muscle biopsy. Experimental isolated phosphate depletion demonstrates that the lack of phosphate in the absence of malnutrition is sufficient to produce muscle weakness.[96,97] Proximal limb weakness is typical, and muscles may become tender and painful. Hyperreflexia can be noted, and cranial nerve muscles are seldom involved. Clinically, the severity of weakness and myopathy varies with the underlying etiology of the chronic phosphate depletion.[97] The serum phosphorus concentration is often normal or only moderately decreased despite total body phosphate depletion.

Continued phosphate restriction in association with heightened metabolic stress, such as exertion, fever, or increased calorie intake, will acutely produce hypophosphatemia and exacerbate weakness even to the point of paralysis and respiratory failure.[53,98-100] In the absence of chronic phosphate depletion, acute hypophosphatemia must be severe (serum phosphorus $<$0.33 mmol/liter, or 1 mg/dl) to produce such symptoms as muscle weakness. Unlike chronic phosphate depletion, acute weakness due to acute hypophosphatemia can involve proximal and distal muscle groups, produce hyporeflexia and areflexia instead of hyperreflexia, and can affect cranial nerve muscles, causing ptosis and problems with mastication.[97] Electromyographic evidence supports a neurogenic component to the pathophysiology as well as some degree of myopathic component.

Muscle damage due to rhabdomyolysis can occur with hypophosphatemia in three clinical settings: (1) during treatment of alcohol withdrawal; (2) during the treatment of starvation with hyperalimentation or refeedings; and (3) during the treatment of diabetic ketoacidosis.[88] Are three groups usually present to the hospital with normal or elevated serum phosphorus concentrations, which then decrease dramatically both with progression of the illness and with treatment. Severe acute hypophosphatemia induced in normal persons has not caused rhabdomyolysis.

Experimental phosphate depletion produces cellular metabolic derangements that limit energy production and reduce the pool of high-energy storage molecules.[88] In agreement with clinical observations, however, severe additional stresses such as exercise or hyperalimentation are required to produce observable metabolic changes and rhabdomyolysis in animals.

MAGNESIUM

Hypermagnesemia suppresses impulse transmission across the neuromuscular junction by decreasing acetylcholine release, postsynaptic membrane responsiveness, and the amplitude of the motor end-plate potential.[71] Weakness and decrease in muscle stretch reflexes occur at serum levels of 2 to 2.5 mmol/liter and paralysis and areflexia at 3.5 to 5 mmol/liter.[101-103] These effects are partially reversed by phytostigmine, an anticholinesterase drug, and demonstrate the importance of the hypermagnesemia effect on the neuromuscular junction. Parenteral calcium will also aid in the reversal of the neuromuscular effects of hypermagnesemia. Most patients with severe hypermagnesemia have some degree of renal insufficiency as well, so that dialysis may also be required to lower serum magnesium levels.

Hypomagnesemia causes increased neuromuscular irritability and can produce excess responses to stimuli, hyperreflexia, weakness, and tetany. These effects are often made worse by the presence of coexistent hypocalcemia and hypokalemia. Muscle power may be affected by changes in muscle electrolyte composition, which involve elevation of muscle calcium, sodium, and chloride with a decline in muscle magnesium, potassium, and phosphorus.[88] Repletion of only one or two electrolyte deficiencies rather than all three—magnesium, calcium, potassium—provides partial but not full recovery of neuromuscular function. There have been no clinical reports of rhabdomyolysis in the setting of isolated hypomagnesemia, although magnesium depletion often is present in alcoholics or malnourished patients who may manifest rhabdomyolysis.

HYPONATREMIA

The weakness and occasional paralysis noted in patients with hyponatremia are usually associated with a progressive decline in central nervous system function. Patients initially complain of weakness and muscle cramps. Myoclonic jerks can often be observed. Weakness may be focal in nature, and hemiparesis is not an uncommon presentation. The patient may develop lethargy or stupor, which can be followed by seizures with flaccid paralysis and sustained coma.[29,30,34] These manifestations can often be reversed by correction of the hyponatremia. However, those patients with severe serum sodium below 120 mM in addition to symptomatology have both a high morbidity and a high mortality.

During their clinical course, hyponatremic patients may manifest a transient array of neurologic signs that include hyporeflexia, Babinski sign, anisocoria, sluggish papillary responses, hemiparesis, and quadriparesis. Clinical improvement is usually associated with abrupt cessation of myoclonic jerks, the return of semipurposeful movements and a lightening of the stupor or coma. Structural brain lesions can cause similar but sustained neurologic manifestations and must be considered in the differential diagnosis.

Chronic hyponatremia can cause weakness, lethargy, and occasionally stupor, coma, and seizures. The pathophysiology of muscle weakness in hyponatremic persons is not understood. Lower motor neuron and muscle symptoms occur (cramps, fasciculations), but higher central nervous system manifestations are also evident (e.g., myoclonus, seizures, coma).

CALCIUM AND PARATHYROID HORMONE

Chronic hypocalcemia, with and without hypoparathyroidism, can produce muscle cramps, intermittent tetany, and mild weakness; paralysis and myopathic changes do not occur.[88] However, hypocalcemia can be associated with vitamin D deficiency, which does cause significant muscle weakness. Infants with rickets and adults with osteomalacia often manifest severe proximal limb muscle weakness with hypotonia.[105] The hypocalcemia in this condition is usually mild and cannot account for the abnormalities of muscle function. The weakness resolves with vitamin D repletion.

Hypercalcemia, regardless of etiology, usually causes a moderate generalized weakness and fatigue without paralysis. Hypercalcemia itself does not appear to cause myopathic changes or rhabdomyolysis. However, there is currently much interest in the mechanisms by which calcium enters the diseased muscle cell by transport systems and alterations in membrane integrity. A rise in the normally low intracellular calcium concentration is thought to participate in rhabdomyolysis, which can be seen with either hypokalemic, hypophosphatemic, or alcoholic myopathy.[88]

Primary and secondary hyperparathyroidism may be associated with mild to severe proximal limb weakness, which can lead to limitation of activity.[88,106] Patients may complain of muscular aches and pains, as well as difficulty climbing stairs and getting out of chairs. Lower extremity weakness usually precedes upper extremity symptoms. Serum calcium levels do not correlate well with the degree of weakness.[107]

Muscle biopsy reveals atrophy of fibers, with the type II muscle fibers being the most extensively involved, suggesting a neuropathic lesion with possible elevations.[107] However, fasciculations are not observed clinically, except in the tongue, in patients with primary hyperparathyroidism. Electromyographic find ings have been interpreted to support either myopathy or neuropathic patterns.[88,107] Weakness improves significantly within days to weeks after correction of hyperparathyroidism, but return of full muscle power may be postponed until the reversal of atrophy.[106]

Muscle Stretch Reflexes

Alteration of the muscle stretch reflexes occurs in a number of electrolyte disorders (see Table 23–5). Decreased reflex action (i.e., hyporeflexia and areflexia) is due to either decreased nerve conduction, decreased muscle strength, decreased transmission at the neuromuscular junction, or decreased activity of the lower neuron. Heightened reflex action (i.e., hyperreflexia) is produced by decreased upper motor neuron function, heightened muscle contractibility, or increased neuromuscular junction transmission. A specific electrolyte disorder often affects multiple sites along the reflex arc pathway and thus can produce variable clinical manifestations. For example, hyponatremia can cause fluctuating neurologic signs with transient hyperreflexia one minute and hyporeflexia the next. Many patients present with neurologic signs consistent with structural brain lesions such as stroke or tumor, but these neurologic signs usually resolve with correction of the electrolyte disorder.

Areflexia is uncommon but can occur with severe muscle weakness or paralysis. Causes include severe hyperkalemia, hypokalemic myopathy, hypophosphatemic myopathy, severe hypermagnesemia, and hyponatremia. Hyporeflexia is commonly noted to occur in patients with hypokalemia, hyperkalemia, acute hypophosphatemia, hyponatremia, hypermagnesemia, or severe hypercapnia. For

Table 23–5. Muscle Stretch Reflexes[a]

Electrolyte Disorder	Hyperreflexia	Hyporeflexia	Areflexia
Hyperkalemia	+[b]	+	+
Hypokalemia	±	+	+
Hyponatremia	+	+	+
Hypernatremia	+	?	−
Hypomagnesemia	+	−	−
Hypermagnesemia	−	+	+
Hypocalcemia	+	−	−
Hypercalcemia	+	−	−
Hypophosphatemia	+[c]	+[d]	+[d]
Respiratory acidosis	+[e]	+[f]	−
Respiratory alkalosis	+	−	−

[a] −, no association; +, common association; ±, uncommon association.
[b] Early hyperkalemia.
[c] Chronic phosphate depletion.
[d] Acute hypophosphatemia.
[e] Moderate hypercapnia.
[f] Severe hypercapnia.

etiologies that act by producing muscle weakness, such as hypokalemic and hypophosphatemic myopathy, reflexes may be observed as long as there is muscle strength. Paralysis may occur suddenly and unexpectedly even though reflexes are present. If neuromuscular electrophysiology is altered, such as in hyperkalemia or hypermagnesemia, diminished reflexes are an important warning sign of impending paralysis. Reflexes are usually lost at magnesium levels of 2 to 2.5 mmol/liter. Potassium levels are more variable, depending on the rate of rise in concentration, but at levels above 7 mmol/liter muscle paralysis usually occurs.

Hyperreflexia is noted to occur in conditions of heightened neuromuscular irritability. Such conditions often cause tetany and include hypocalcemia, hypomagnesemia, and respiratory alkalosis. Hyperreflexia has also been observed with hyperkalemia, hypercalcemia,[88] hypophosphatemia,[97] mild to moderate hypercapnia, hypernatremia, and hyponatremia. Hyperreflexia generally resolves with correction of the electrolyte disorder.

Abnormal Reflexes

Certain electrolyte disorders are initially overlooked because they produce abnormal reflexes and other focal neurologic signs. Extensor-toe signs can be observed, often in association with paresis, hyperreflexia, or coma, and may suggest structural neurologic disease, such as stroke or tumor. Hyponatremia, nonketotic hyperosmolar hyperglycemia,[27] hypophosphatemia, and hypercapnia[108] are such disorders. Pupils may not react normally. Careful neurologic examination often indicates that the findings are not typical of one structural neurologic lesion, thereby suggesting a metabolic etiology.

Sensory Changes

Paresthesias are the most common sensory change noted. Disorders causing tetany may also cause tingling in hands and circumoral regions (alkalosis, hypocalcemia, hypomagnesemia, and hypokalemia). In addition, more generalized paresthesias are noted in about 10 percent of patients with hypercalcemia[109] and rarely in hyperkalemia and are one of the earliest signs of acute symptomatic hypophosphatemia[53,79,96] The pathophysiology of paresthesias has not been fully investigated, but for disorders causing tetany it is assumed to be due to hyperexcitability of sensory neurons.

Occasionally sensory loss occurs with paresthesias progressing to numbness followed by anesthesia. This may occur in conjunction with tetany and with acute hypophosphatemia. The sensation of light touch is most severely affected, but decreased sensations of pain, position, and vibration have also been recorded.[93,110] Hypermagnesemia does not cause anesthesia as was once thought.[71] It merely prevents the subject from reporting sensations by causing paralysis.

Rarely the special senses are heightened or suppressed by electrolyte disorders. McCance studied hyponatremia in volunteers and observed a loss of taste, which quickly reversed with salt.[112] Auditory hyperacusis is associated with magnesium depletion,[113] while decreased auditory acuity accompanies hypercalcemia.[114,115] Hypercalcemia also can produce refractive changes in the eye,[116] while chronic hypoparathyroidism often creates lenticular cataracts. Olfactory paresthesias have been noted in addisonian patients with hyperkalemia.[93]

Headache

Chronic headaches are occasionally due to chronic electrolyte disorders such as chronic respiratory acidosis, hypercalcemia, and hyponatremia. Respiratory failure with acidosis and hypoxia is commonly accompanied by headache.[10,108] The headaches are described as dull, throbbing occipital pain with radiation to behind the eyes. They are often worse at night and on awakening.[108] Some patients with respiratory acidosis have increased intracranial pressure and papilledema due to cerebral

Table 23–6. Cause of Headache, Papilledema, Nystagmus, and Asterixis

Clinical Manifestations	Etiology
Headache	Chronic hypercalcemia Acute and chronic hypercapnia Acute and chronic hyponatremia
Papilledema	Acute and chronic hypercapnia Chronic hypocalcemia Hyponatremia (rare)
Nystagmus	Magnesium depletion Central pontine myelinolysis
Asterixis	Acute and chronic hypercapnia Rapid correction of hypercapnia with metabolic alkalosis ?Hyponatremia ?Magnesium depletion

vasodilation. The increased intracranial pressure has been postulated to produce the headaches, although measurements of cerebospinal fluid pressure have not correlated well with the occurrence of headache.[10]

A review of a number of series of hypercalcemic patients with primary hyperparathyroidism reveals that 5 to 50 percent manifest chronic headache that usually improves after surgical correction of the hyperparathyroidism.[117,118] The headaches are dull, continuous, and generalized. A few patients with hypercalcemia due to other etiologies manifest headaches as well (Table 23–6).

Papilledema

Papilledema is commonly associated with acute or chronic hypercapnia, chronic hypocalcemia, and rarely hyponatremia (Table 23–6). Blurring of optic disks to frank papilledema can be seen with severe hypercapnia,[108] which may occur without abnormal elevation in cerebrospinal fluid pressure. It is presumed to be mainly due to vasodilation of retinal vessels and resolves with correction of the hypercapnia. In contrast, papilledema due to chronic hypocalcemia is related to increased intracranial pressure,[39,40] is usually mild, and correlates with cerebrospinal fluid pressure. It is thought that there is an increased production of cerebrospinal fluid, which is reversed by correction of serum calcium levels back to normal.[97]

Nystagmus

Vertical (downbeat) nystagmus and occasionally horizontal nystagmus have been reported in four patients with severe magnesium depletion and coexistent malnutrition.[69,122] All four patients had a history of small bowel resection that had predisposed them to malnutrition and unusually severe hypomagnesemia (0.11 to 0.05 mmol/liter). Nystagmus was noted in primary gaze as well as upward and downward positions. Patients complained of diplopia and of jumping eyes (oscillopsia). In addition, other signs of magnesium depletion such as tetany, muscle weakness, dysphagia, and mental status changes were observed. Magnesium repletion did not correct nystagmus, which persisted for 2 weeks to several months. Other neurologic manifestations corrected rapidly with magnesium repletion, including possible pseudobular signs such as dysphagia and positive Babinski. It is not clear whether hypomagnesemia unmasks a nutritional brain lesion or whether it directly participates in formation of lesions leading to nystagmus (Table 23–6).

ASTERIXIS

Asterixis[123] is most commonly associated with uremic or hepatic encephalopathy. In addition, it often accompanies acute and chronic hypercapnia.[10] Asterixis has not been clearly linked with other electrolyte disorders, although it has occasionally been observed in the setting of magnesium depletion[124] (Table 23–6).

TETANY

The tetany syndrome is characterized by paresthesias, carpal–pedal spasms, and generalized muscle twitchings and may progress to focal or generalized seizures.[125] Muscle spasms can produce laryngeal stridor leading to asyphyxiation. Individuals who are near the threshold for tetany, but who require an added stimulus to manifest tetany, are said to have latent tetany. Hyperventilation (alkalosis), percussion of peripheral nerves (facial nerve, Chvostek's sign), and limb ischemia (Trousseau's sign), are used to elicit latent tetany.

Hypocalcemia[14] and alkalosis[126] are well-recognized causes of tetany. Severe potassium depletion can produce latent tetany,[7,8] although the associated muscle weakness can mask manifestations of tetany. In addition, alkalosis, hypomagnesemia, and hypocalcemia often complicate potassium depletion and these increase the tendency for tetany to occur.[129,130] Hypomagnesemia in conjunction with hypocalcemia[51,67] produces tetany. Hypomagnesemia alone, but usually in the setting of corrected hypocalcemia,[49,131] can produce latent and overt tetany. The tendency to manifest tetany increases with the coexistence of multiple etiologic factors; for example, patients with severe hypocalcemia and acidosis can be asymptomatic or manifest only latent tetany. However, if acidosis is reversed by respiratory alkalosis or metabolic alkalosis, the patient will often manifest overt tetany.

Primary neuromuscular disease can rarely produce pseudotetany, even though electrolyte disorders have been ruled out by laboratory testing.[132,133] These patients also must be differentiated from a rare group of patients without neurologic disease, but who exhibit latent and overt tetany with normal serum electrolyte values. They are said to have normocalcemic tetany, and they possibly have latent hypoparathyroidism.[134,135]

Studies of the pathophysiology of tetany suggest that the peripheral nerve axon and/or the motor end plate are the sites affected, rather than the central nervous system.[14,125] The use of local anesthesia to block peripheral nerve conduction does not stop tetany. However, blockade at the motor end plate by curare terminates tetany in dogs.[40] Calcium ions are required for normal acetycholine release at the neuromuscular junction, but the mechanisms by which hypocalcemia produces tetany are unclear. Alkalosis, potassium depletion and hypomagnesemia may directly alter neuromuscular excitability, but also could interact with calcium in an additive manner in producing tetany. For example, alkalosis decreases the concentration of ionized calcium by increasing the binding of calcium ions to anionic sites.

Fever

Fever usually signals a systematic inflammatory response, often in response to infection. However, occasionally fever is produced by an electrolyte disorder. Whereas moderately severe hypercalcemia does not cause fever, hypercalcemic crisis can produce fever along with nausea, vomiting, weakness, lethargy, dehydration, hypertension, and tachycardia.[136]

Acute hypernatremia is often associated with fever in children.[57,138] However, most often such patients have an initial febrile illness, such as gastroenteritis, that then leads to dehydration and hypernatremia. Infants without infection who have hypernatremia due to salt poisoning manifest fever.[139] Patients with nonketotic hyperosmolar coma often are febrile, but concomitant infection is almost always present. The clinician should never assume that fever is due to the electrolyte disorder alone.

Hypoventilation and Hyperventilation

The physiology of respiration is complex and highly regulated. Oxygenation, acid–base status, mental state, and muscle function are among the principal factors involved. Electrolyte disorders often contribute to the pathophysiology of hyperventilation. For in-depth discussion, see refs. 140 and 141.

Hypoventilation occurs as compensation for

metabolic alkalosis via chemoreceptor mechanisms. The hypoventilation is roughly proportional to the degree of hyperbicarbonatemia.[76a] In rare instances, severe metabolic alkalosis suppresses respiration sufficiently to cause hypoxia and hypercapnia.[77,78] Hypoventilation also occurs due to weakness of the respiratory muscles,[108] which may be due to hypokalemic[88] or hypophosphatemic myopathy,[99] to paralysis from hyperkalemia or hypermagnesemia,[71,142] or to familial hypokalemic periodic paralysis.

Hyperventilation usually occurs as compensation for metabolic acidosis. The time course and degree of compensation, which have been carefully studied in volunteers and in critically ill patients, are proportional to the degree of acidosis.[74,143,144]

Cerebellar and Extrapyramidal Signs

ATAXIA

Ataxia is a rare finding in electrolyte disorders that may occur in patients with hypophospatemia,[54] hypercalcemia,[118] or hyponatremia.[145a] Alcoholics commonly manifest ataxia and occasionally have magnesium depletion as well. Alcoholic withdrawal, tremors, and hyperreflexia are exacerbated by coexistent hypomagnesemia. However, a correlation between the severity of ataxia and magnesium depletion has not been reported.

EXTRAPYRAMIDAL SIGNS

Chorea and rigidity are only rarely associated with electrolyte imbalance. Choreathetoid movements have been most commonly associated with chronic hypocalcemia due to idiopathic hypoparathyroidism.[40] Such movements are not always improved by treatment of the hypocalcemia, suggesting a permanent structural lesion. In addition, some patients are noted to have calcifications in the basal ganglia, red suggesting a pathophysiologic role for structural lesions.

Transient chorea has been associated with both hypernatremia and magnesium depletion.[87,88,124] Four patients with hypernatremia have been observed to manifest chorea during or after treatment,[87,146] two of whom were children with salt poisoning.

Muscle rigidity can be due to extrapyramidal system disease or to increased muscle tone or hypertonia. Hyponatremia, hypernatremia, and hypocalcemia[145] all have been noted to produce muscle rigidity. Hypertonia is probably the primary cause for such rigidity except in the case of chronic hypocalcemia.

Neuropsychiatric Manifestations of Electrolyte Disorders

As clinicians, we strive to label observed behavior and to use those labels to suggest causality, prognosis, and treatment. We often attribute a patient's behavioral aberrations to personality quirks, "intensive care psychosis," and the like. But we must remember to examine the possibility that a given behavioral aberration might reflect an electrolyte disorder, which is treatable and usually reversible, and which, if overlooked, can produce serious consequences.

Little is known about the pathophysiology of behavioral aberrations as they relate to the electrolyte disorders. One cannot assume that similar manifestations have similar pathophysiologies. In addition, previous psychiatric backgrounds and concurrent conditions may play important roles in the way in which a given patient responds to a given electrolyte disorder. Thus, a particular electrolyte disorder can be assigned only to a general behavioral pattern, not to a specific behavior.

Despite recent attempts to standardize psychiatric terminology (Diagnostic and Statistical Manual, Mental Disorders (DMS I–III) American Psychiatric Assoc. 1952, 1968, 1978) designed to aid investigators in defining behaviors and syndromes, the observations re-

Table 23–7. Psychiatric Manifestations of Electrolyte Disorders

Manifestations	Etiologies
Apathy, lassitude, and depression	Hyperglycemia, chronic hyponatremia, metabolic alkalosis, hypercalcemia, hypocalcemia, hypercapnia, magnesium and potassium depletion
Cognitive defects	Hyponatremia, hypernatremia, hypocalcemia, hypercalcemia, magnesium and phosphate depletion, hypercapnia, hypocapnia, and rarely potassium depletion
Hallucinations	
Visual and auditory	Magnesium depletion, hypercalcemia, hypocalcemia, hypocapnia, and potassium depletion
Visual only	Hypernatremia

ported in the literature have not yet been reinterpreted and are beyond the scope of this chapter. The following psychiatric manifestations have been grouped into five categories of signs and symptoms, on the basis of clinical usefulness:

1. Apathy, lassitude, and depression (Table 23–7)
2. Confusion, delirium, and psychosis (Table 23–8)
3. States of arousal (e.g., irritability, anxiety, and danger) as well as emotional lability (see Table 23–9)
4. Cognitive defects (e.g., decreased memory, decreased ability to concentrate or to perform mental tasks (Table 23–7)
5. Auditory and visual hallucinations, as distinct from psychosis (Table 23–7)

Alexander[145a] recently published a monograph that reviews the clinical knowledge available concerning psychiatric manifestations of electrolyte disorders.

APATHY, LASSITUDE, AND DEPRESSION

The etiology of apathy, lassitude, and depression may be situational, it may be primary, or it may be secondary to electrolyte and other systemic disorders. Disorders of calcium metabolism most commonly produce states of depression. Hypercapnia,[9,147] depletion of magnesium[51,148,149] or potassium,[60,150] as well as chronic hyponatremia[151] are occasionally associated with apathy, lassitude, and depression. The disorders of calcium metabolism bear further discussion.

Table 23–8. Confusion, Delirium, and Psychosis

Reported Associations			
Confusion	Delirium	Psychosis	Electrolyte Disorder
+	?	?	Hypernatremia
+	+	+	Hyponatremia
?	?	?	Hyperkalemia
+	±	+	Hypokalemia
+	+	+	Hypercalcemia
?	+	+	Hypocalcemia
?	?	?	Hypermagnesemia
+	±	±	Hypomagnesemia
+	+	±	Respiratory acidosis
+	?	?	Respiratory alkalosis
+	?	?	Metabolic alkalosis
+	+	?	Phosphate depletion

[a] −, no association; +, common association; ±, uncommon association; ?, information not available.

Table 23–9. States of Arousal Associated with Electrolyte Disorders

Type of Arousal	Disorders
Anxiety	Hypocalcemia, hypercalcemia, magnesium and phosphate depletion, respiratory acidosis, alkalosis
Restlessness	Hyponatremia, magnesium depletion
Irritability	Hyponatremia, hypernatremia in infants, hypo- and hypercalcemia, magnesium and phosphate depletion, respiratory acidosis
Aggressiveness	Hypo- and hypercalcemia, magnesium depletion
Anger	Hypercalcemia, magnesium depletion
Insomnia	Magnesium depletion

Hypercalcemia and Hypocalcemia

Hypercalcemia commonly causes neuropsychiatric disturbances of which depression is the most frequent presentation. Twenty to 50 percent of patients with hypercalcemia due to primary hyperparathyroidism are found to have depression or other psychiatric problems.[61,152–156] The spectrum runs from asymptomatic, to lassitude, to depression, to depressive psychosis, and to catatonic stupor. Petersen[61] observed that most patients manifest a neurasthenic personality during the period in which they are hypercalcemic. A few patients become psychotic and are noted to have extremely elevated serum calcium levels (>4 mmol/liter). Neither primary nor secondary hyperparathyroidism necessarily results in hypercalcemia. Some of these patients are normocalcemic but manifest mental symptoms very similar to those of hypercalcemic patients, suggesting that excess parathyroid hormone may cause neurotoxicity separate from the effects of hypercalcemia. Regardless of the etiology, mental symptoms due to hypercalcemia are usually rapidly reversed by corrective treatment.[157–159]

Hypocalcemia also can cause depression, but less often than does hypercalcemia. In addition, hypocalcemia can produce depression often accompanied by agitation and irritability. Correction of hypocalcemia via oral supplements and vitamin D analogues can dramatically reduce depressive symptoms, especially if the hypocalcemia is not of recent onset. Follow-up of patients who have had neck surgery reveals a group who probably have parathyroid insufficiency.[160] About one-half of this group complained of neuropsychiatric changes such as lassitude and depression. Many patients were found to improve with calcium supplementation.[161]

CONFUSION, DELIRIUM, AND PSYCHOSIS

Electrolyte disorders have been reported to cause confusion, delirium, and psychosis. Delirium is characterized by a cloudy state of consciousness, decreased attention span, misperception, and disordered thought and sleep patterns (DMS III). Onset is often rapid and acute, with electrolyte disorders being a prominent etiology, along with other metabolic and toxic excephalopathies. Psychosis is similar to delirium in that thought content and organization are disrupted; however, psychosis may have systemitized delusions, a chronic course, alterations in effect, and less global cognitive impairment. These distinctions are not easily made, and definitions in the past have been less clear cut. Therefore, terminology of past literature does not hold strictly to current definitions. Table 23–8 lists the reported associations of confusion, delirium, and psychosis with the various electrolyte disorders.

Certain electrolyte disorders are well known to present with psychiatric manifestations that can mimic primary psychiatric illness. These disorders include hyponatremia,[161–163] hypercalcemia,[61,117,154] hypocalcemia,[48,164,165] and chronic respiratory acidosis.[9,10] Other disorders are more commonly associated with serious medical illness and may also develop during ongoing care for such illness. These disorders more commonly cause confusion and delirium rather than psychosis. Included among such disorders are acute water intoxication,[57] postparathyroidectomy-induced hypocalcemia,[48] hypophosphatemia,[53,79,111,166] hypomagnesemia,[69,148,149] severe hypokalemia,[59,60,150] and severe alkalosis complicating the rapid correction of hypercapnia.[2,3] Disorders that seem to be limited to mild confusion include chronic hypernatremia in adults, hyperventilation syndrome (respiratory alkalosis), and uncomplicated matabolic alkalosis.

STATES OF AROUSAL

Electrolyte disorders occasionally produce arousal that may manifest predominantly as anxiety, restlessness, irritability, aggressiveness, or anger (see Table 23–10). Emotions may be quite labile, with patients being quiet and inattentive, followed by periods of agitation.

As with other manifestations of electrolyte disorders, the causality is suggested by disappearance of the manifestation after correction of the disorder. Many patients responding to electrolyte imbalance with psychiatric manifestations have a psychiatric history, suggesting that latent psychiatric problems may predispose patients to these types of manifestations.

COGNITIVE FUNCTIONS

A person's ability to think, to solve problems, to concentrate on a task, and to remember constitute cognitive functions. These abilities are easily impaired by neurologic and systemic illness, such as electrolyte disorders (see Table 23–7). A change in cognitive function is often the initial manifestation of electrolyte disorders.

Hyponatremia and Hypernatremia

Dullness of mental process,[151] memory loss, and decreased ability to perform simple tasks have been noted in patients with acute or

Table 23–10. Effects of Electrolyte Disorders on the Systemic Arterial System

Electrolyte Disorder	Experimental Observation[a]	Pressor Reactivity[b]	Clinical Observation[c]
Respiratory acidosis	VD	D	NC
Metabolic acidosis	VD	D	NC or D
Respiratory alkalosis	VC	I	NC,[d] D[e]
Metabolic alkalosis	VD	D	NC
Hyperkalemia	VD	D	D
Hypokalemia	VC	I,[f] D[g]	?[h]
Hypercalcemia	VC	NC	I
Hypocalcemia	VD	D	D
Hypomagnesemia	VC	I	I
Hypermagnesemia	VD	D	D
Hypochloremia	VC	I	NC
Hyperphosphatemia	VD[i]	?	?

[a] VD, vasodilation, or VC, vasoconstriction, as observed in isolated arterial segments.
[b] I, increased, D, decreased, or NC, no change, as observed in isolated vessel reactivity to norepinephrine.
[c] I, increased, D, decreased, or NC, no change, as observed in clinically observed blood pressure.
[d] Awake humans.
[e] Anesthetized humans.
[f] Initially.
[g] Sustained hypokalemia.
[h] Determined by etiology of hypokalemia.
[i] VD of muscle and brain arteries.

chronic hyponatremia. Acute hyponatremia associated with water intoxication produces cognitive impairment, but neurologic manifestations often progress rapidly to seizures and coma. Intellectual impairment is not always reversible with correction of hyponatremia.[28,37]

Hypernatremia appears to have a less profound effect on cognitive function than does hyponatremia. Decreased memory and impaired thinking are observed as late symptoms.[167] The old and very young are more susceptible to symptomatic hypernatremia. Hypernatremia, especially in infants, may lead to permanent cognitive impairment.

Calcium Disorders

Both acute and chronic hypocalcemia are frequent causes of impaired mentation. Postsurgical hypocalcemia can produce reversible acute organic brain syndrome with memory impairment.[164] Chronic forms of hypocalcemia, especially in children, can cause progressive mental impairment and dementia.[164,168] These manifestations are usually only slightly reversible with correction of the hypocalcemia.

Hypercalcemia of any etiology can impair mental function. Recent memory is affected more than is distant memory.[155] These patients demonstrate inattention and decreased ability to concentrate.[165,169]

Magnesium, Phosphate, and Potassium Depletion

Patients with magnesium depletion may experience disorientation, memory loss, and confabulation.[68] Experimental magnesium depletion has not been noted to induce cognitive impairment.[51] Phosphate depletion has similar effects.[165,166] Unlike the two preceding disorders, potassium depletion has only rarely been associated with cognitive impairment;[150] exclusion of other coexistent etiologies has not been documented.

Respiratory Alkalosis and Acidosis

Hyperventilation (respiratory alkalosis) can result in inability to concentrate and perform simple tasks. Patients with chronic hyperventilation syndrome may also manifest concentration and memory impairment.[171] Mild respiratory alkalosis (P_{CO_2} of 20 to 30 mm Hg) usually produces only decreased awareness.

Acute respiratory acidosis can produce lethargy and subsequently coma. These patients manifest decreased attention and become incoherent early in their course. Chronic hypercapnia is better tolerated, however, and these patients may have long-standing neuropsychiatric symptoms without dramatic changes in level of consciousness. Intracellular acidosis, increased cerebral blood flow, and increased intracranial pressure all may contribute to the pathophysiology.[86,108] In addition, hypoxia often accompanies hypercapnia and exacerbates the cognitive impairment.

AUDITORY AND VISUAL HALLUCINATIONS

Hallucinations are usually experienced in the setting of delirium or psychosis. The person sees or hears images and sounds that do not exist. Hypomagnesemia with magnesium depletion is the most common electrolyte disorder associated with hallucinations (see Table 23–7). Up to 50 percent of hypomagnesemic patients manifest auditory or visual hallucinations;[68] however, alcoholism probably contributes to the etiology of hallucinations in many of these patients. It has been postulated that hypomagnesemia exacerbates the neuropsychiatric manifestations of alcohol withdrawal, while magnesium repletion can prevent or improve such manifestations.[172]

Acute severe changes in serum calcium can also produce auditory and visual hallucinations. Hypercalcemic crisis (>4.0 mmol/liter) and postoperative hypocalcemia are the clinical settings most likely to produce hallucinations.[48,61,155,156]

Hallucinations are rarely associated with hypokalemia[59,60] and respiratory alkalosis.[173] Although neuropsychiatric manifestations are prominent in the clinical presentation of hyponatremia, respiratory acidosis, or hypophosphatemia, the presence of hallucinations in these disorders has not been emphasized.[166]

CARDIOVASCULAR MANIFESTATIONS

Vascular Smooth Muscle Function and Blood Pressure

Changes in extracellular ion concentration can produce alterations in vascular smooth muscle tone, which may then lead to vasoconstriction. In addition to this direct effect on muscle tone, vascular reactivity to neural and humoral regulation can be altered by changes in such ion concentrations. Reflex mechanisms usually intervene and adjust for changes in vascular tone such that blood pressure remains near normal in most electrolyte disorders. However, if cardiovascular reflex and cardiac output are affected as well, blood pressure and tissue perfusion can be significantly increased or decreased. Table 23–10 summarizes the predominant vascular changes that are noted clinically and experimentally.

Research has progressed from the in vitro study of isolated arterial segments to the examination of microcirculatory changes in intact animals. The regulation of circulation has multiple levels of control and involves systemic asjustments via neural and humoral pathways, as well as local blood flow changes governed by various mediators, such as metabolic by-products, prostaglandins, and bradykinins. Most vascular beds are found to autoregulate blood flow relative to the metabolic demands of the tissue served. This autoregulation involves complex pathophysiology but is partly explained by changes in extracellular potassium and proton concentrations.

A great amount of variation exists between the degree and type of vascular response, depending on the size of vessel studied, the species under investigation, and the organ from which the vessel arises. Veins have been studied much less than arteries but appear to be less reactive to electrolyte changes. It is uniformly noted, however, that most changes in ionic concentration lead only to transient alterations in vascular tone. Thus, calcium infusion will only raise blood pressure transiently and then become ineffective. Sustained elevations above that of plasma magnesium have been used to produce vasodilation and control of hypertension in patients with eclampsia. Specific electrolyte disorders will be discussed, including a review of what is known concerning the response of the coronary circulation.

An acute rise in extracellular potassium above 5 mmol/liter decreases vascular tone and allows increased blood flow through most systemic vascular beds.[174,175] This response is graded and is proportional to the magnitude of change in potassium concentration. This vasodilation is more sustained and is enhanced by first exposing the vessel to hypokalemia. Hypokalemia down to 1 mmol/liter increases vascular tone.[176] Such changes are quite transient, especially the response to hyperkalemia, and last only a few minutes before vascular tone returns to normal. In addition, these changes are modest compared with vascular changes seen with norepinephrine-induced vasoconstriction or with exercise hyperemia. Hyperkalemia also reduces the vascular reactivity of most vessels to acetylcholine or to norepinephrine. Hypokalemia initially produces increased reactivity to norepinephrine but, if sustained, eventually leads to less than normal reactivity.

It has long been speculated that minute-to-minute changes in extracellular potassium are involved in autoregulation of blood flow. It appears that the initial phases of exercise hyperemia are in part modulated by a rapid release of potassium from muscle cells.[175] Tissues undergoing metabolic stress, such as ischemic myocardium or the brain with seizure activity, have increased extracellular potassium, which may lead to vasodilation.

The cerebral circulation appears to be especially sensitive to increased potassium. Pial arteries are easily vasodilated by local administration of potassium. Cortical blood flow is always in a dynamic flux proportional to the neural activity taking place in that region.[177] Extracellular potassium concentration is elevated in such areas of increased activity, as are many other metabolic products, such as carbon dioxide.

Clinically, acute hyperkalemia may precipitate cardiovascular collapse, which has been mainly attributed to cardiac arrest after depression of cardiac conduction. Hemorrhage or endotoxemia exacerbates hyperkalemia, provoking a vicious circle of vasodilation. Hypermagnesemia appears to have a similar effect in shock states. Intravenous calcium can cause a transient reversal of some of the vascular effects of hyperkalemia in a manner similar to its cardiac effect.

Chronic hypokalemia and hypertension are frequently noted to coexist in the same patient. Although this may be due to primary hyperaldosteronism or Cushing's disease, more commonly hypokalemia results from the use of diuretics. However, epidemiologic studies in untreated hypertensive populations reveal some patients with a mild hypokalemia. It is not yet known whether this contributes to the elevated peripheral vascular resistance noted in these patients.[175]

ACIDOSIS AND ALKALOSIS

Both acidosis and alkalosis can have a profound effect on circulation due to cardiac, pulmonary, and vascular sites of action. Because carbon dioxide itself also has a profound effect on the vascular tree, the effects of these disorders must be divided into respiratory and metabolic acidosis, as well as respiratory and metabolic alkalosis. In general, respiratory acidosis, metabolic acidosis, or metabolic alkalosis can cause arterial vasodilation, while respiratory alkalosis usually provokes vasoconstriction.

Acute hypercapnia (respiratory acidosis) promotes both cerebral and systemic vasodilation. The patient will feel warm, with flushed skin, bounding pulse, and diaphoresis. Hypercapnia stimulates a sympathetic nervous system response with a rise in cardiac output, permitting blood pressure to remain normal. These responses may be modified in the patient with coexistent hypoxemia, congestive heart failure, or beta-adrenergic blockade.[108] Cerebral vessels are more reactive to changes in blood CO_2 concentrations than are the other systemic vascular beds and have been the most extensively studied. It is still unclear whether alterations in P_{CO_2} or extracellular pH are most significant.[178]

Patients with chronic hypercapnia may have clinical signs of increased intracranial pressure, such as headache and papilledema. It is postulated that these changes are due to the cerebral vasodilation that occurs with hypercapnia.[108]

Respiratory alkalosis or hypocapnia acutely produces vasoconstriction of skin, intestine, kidney, and cerebral arterioles[171] without alteration in blood pressure. However, in anesthethetized patients and animals respiratory alkalosis may provoke severe hypotension.[179] Chronic hypocapnia, due to high altitude, for example, can produce a series of hemodynamic changes involving multiple cardiac and vascular adjustments in which hypoxia plays a role as well.

Metabolic acidosis produces arterial vasodilation, which may exacerbate hemorrhagic and endotoxic shock. Both respiratory and metabolic acidosis reduce vascular reactivity to norepinephrine stimulation,[178] and thus may contribute to the course of irreversible shock. Although metabolic acidosis causes arterial vasodilation, the venous circulation appears to vasoconstrict both after exercise and in severe acidosis (7.0 to 7.2 pH units). This may predispose to pulmonary congestion even when only small amounts of fluid are administered to such patients. Cholera patients have been studied with right heart cathetherization.[180-182] These subjects had high filling pressures and high cardiac outputs corrected by administration of alkali. Interestingly, many of these patients were volume depleted, and bedside evaluations had suggested that they would be able to tolerate substantial fluid administration. Metabolic alkalosis has been noted to produce vasodilation.[76,183] Posthypercapnia-induced metabolic alkalosis is an especially important exception. Rapid correction of hypercapnia with resultant respiratory and metabolic alkalosis often produces severe cerebral vasoconstriction, leading to confusion, seizures, coma, and death.[2-4] Experimental studies in dogs suggest that cerebral blood flow falls sufficiently enough to produce cerebral hypoxia.[5]

HYPOCALCEMIA AND HYPERCALCEMIA

Likewise, calcium lowered in perfusion solutions passing through intact vascular beds results in a reduction in pressure and a decrease in vascular resistance. In addition, epinephrine and norepinephrine have fewer vasoconstrictive effects in the presence of hypocalcemia.[184] Calcium channel blockers provoke a similar series of changes in vascular beds.[185,186] Different segments of the arterial vascular bed have different degress of dependency on calcium for their norepinephrine activity. The smallest pre- and postcapillary resistance vessels are the most dependent on adequate calcium to elicit contraction when stimulated by norepinephrine. The larger arteries and arterioles are less affected by hypocalcemia.[187]

Clinical hypotension attributed to hypocalcemia is a rare event, although phosphate infusion can produce a sudden drop in serum calcium levels with a subsequent drop in blood pressure.[188] Hypocalcemic patients may be dependent on humoral mechanisms to support their blood pressure.[189]

Hypercalcemia increases vascular smooth muscle tension,[186] producing vasoconstriction, increased vascular resistance, and occasionally increased blood pressure.[190,191] This has been shown in intact animal studies, which demonstrate a slight rise in systemic vascular resistance when serum calcium is elevated.[192-194] The change is only slight due to cardiovascular reflexes that readjust the acute changes induced by hypercalcemia. Transient clinical hypertension has been noted in renal failure patients in whom hypercalcemia was induced by dialysis or calcium infusion.[195,196] Many patients with hypercalcemia due to primary hyperparathyroidism are hypertensive.[197-200]

MAGNESIUM DEPLETION AND HYPERMAGNESEMIA

Acute reductions in serum magnesium below normal (0.7 to 1.2 mmol/liter) produce increased vascular tension, vasoconstriction, and increased peripheral vascular resistance. In addition, vasoconstriction stimulated by norepinephrine, angiotensin, acetylcholine, or serotonin is augmented by hypomagnesemia.[201] Hypertension is therefore associated with acute hypomagnesemia, but whether this effect continues in sustained hypomagnesemia is controversial. Chronic hypomagnesemia is noted to coexist with hypertension in patients with alcoholism, atherosclerosis, eclampsia, diabetes mellitus, and essential hypertension.[202] Magnesium depletion studies in human subjects and animals demonstrate mild increases in blood pressure and peripheral vascular resistance.[202-204]

Hypermagnesemia produces vasodilation and hypotension by both direct and indirect mechanisms.[71,201] Vasodilation is a direct effect of reduced vascular smooth muscle tone, while indirectly, there may be a decrease in the vascular response to humoral pressor substances, which may alter both central and peripheral nervous system regulation of the circulation. Infusions of magnesium cause variable decreases in blood pressure when serum levels reach 1 to 2.5 mmol/liter; above these levels, hypotension and shock are common.

Clinical hypermagnesemia is induced either by therapeutic infusions of magnesium, as for eclamptic patients, or by certain antacids taken by patients with renal insufficiency, particularly after excessive loads of magnesium. Patients from both groups are known to manifest severe hypotension[142,205] that may be refractory to pressor agents. Hypotension can be transiently improved by intravenous administration of calcium. If renal function is normal and intravenous magnesium is halted, the magnesium levels generally fall rapidly, resulting in a rise in blood pressure. However, if renal insufficiency is present, patients may require dialysis to lower serum magnesium levels and reverse hypotension. Hemodialysis has improved blood pressure within 30 minutes,[142] while peritoneal dialysis has generally produced a much slower recovery.[205] An elevated serum magnesium level, usually above 2.5 mmol/liter (5 mEq/liter) should be present in order to suggest hypermagnesemia as the etiology of refractory hypotension. Shock due to other etiologies, such as hemorrhage or tissue trauma, can produce hypermagnesemia.[201,206] However, serum magnesium seldom increases to $>$ 2 mmol/liter when due to hemorrhagic or traumatic shock. In patients with refractory hypotension and renal failure, correction with dialysis is indicated if serum magnesium levels exceed 2.5 mmol/liter.

Hyponatremia and Hypernatremia

There is little clinical or experimental evidence that hyponatremia or hypernatremia can affect vascular tone or blood pressure. Hypernatremia due to dehydration is associated with hypotension and shock, but this is thought to be related to hypovolemia rather than to hyperosmolality. Likewise, patients with hyponatremia usually have normal blood pressure unless hypovolemia is present as well.

HYPOCHLOREMIA AND HYPERPHOSPHATEMIA

Alterations in vascular tone and reactivity (by anion effects) have not been studied as extensively as cation effects. It appears that changing cation concentrations have more dramatic effects and more known clinical relevance. Experimental studies, however, demonstrate that chloride and phosphate may participate in the physiology of blood flow regulation.[207]

Acute reductions in serum chloride concentration with substitution by other anions (other than bicarbonate) appear to produce vasoconstriction and increased reactivity to norepinephrine. Although most organ beds have not been studied, the cerebral vessels appear to be the most sensitive to changes in chloride concentration. Betz and associates[208,209] demonstrated a decrease in cat pial vessel diameter during in vivo microperfusion. Clinically hypochloremia is not an isolated electrolyte disorder, and its role in blood pressure regulation in states of salt depletion, metabolic alkalosis, and anion gap metabolic acidosis has yet to be delineated.

Hyperphosphatemia has been found to produce vasodilation in muscle, and during exercise venous phosphate concentrations rise. Therefore, an acute rise in phosphate concentration has been postulated to be one factor in the complex process of exercise hyperemia.[207] The decrease in ionized calcium that accompanies acute rises in serum phosphate may play a significant role in the observed vasodilation.

CORONARY CIRCULATION

The role of cations in altering the coronary circulation has recently come under increasing study, especially in view of the new class of drugs used to block calcium channels. Although clinical information remains scanty, experimental studies of isolated coronary ar-

Table 23–11. Effect of Electrolyte Disorders on the Coronary Arterial System: Experimental Findings

Disorder	Vascular Response[a]
Respiratory acidosis	VD
Metabolic acidosis	VD
Respiratory alkalosis	VC
Metabolic alkalosis	VC
Hyperkalemia	VD
Hypokalemia	?
Hypercalcemia	VC
Hypocalcemia	VD
Hypomagnesemia	VC
Hypermagnesemia	VD

[a] VD, vasodilation, or VC, vasoconstriction, as observed in isolated animal coronary artery segments.

teries, isolated perfused hearts, and intact animals suggest the effects listed in Table 23–11.

Calcium entry into vascular smooth muscle plays a key role in bringing about contraction and vasoconstriction.[210] Hypercalcemia has not been clinically associated with angina. Calcium channel blockers, like hypocalcemia, produce coronary vasodilation. This effect can be partially reversed by raising the extracellular calcium concentration.[186]

Respiratory alkalosis, metabolic alkalosis, and hypomagnesemia appear to produce coronary vasoconstriction clinically. It was noted that patients with Prinzmetal's angina often have episodes of arterial spasm in association with hyperventilation and respiratory alkalosis.[211-213] Subsequently infusions to produce acute metabolic alkalosis were also found to decrease coronary blood flow.[211] However, patients with classic angina and documented coronary artery disease did not manifest angina or decrease coronary blood flow during hyperventilation.[214]

Myocardial Performance

The pumping intensity of the heart is modified by numerous factors such as heart rate, filling and emptying pressures (preload and afterload), and the action of endogenous and exogenous ionotropic agents. Electrolyte disorders can alter myocardial performance in experimental and clinical situations. Animal models include isolated papillary muscle, isolated perfused heart, or intact animal studies. Studies on human subjects use both invasive and noninvasive cardiac measurements.

Direct effects on the myocardium are best studied in denervated hormone-free systems such as the isolated muscle and heart. In addition, electrolyte disorders have a more pronounced effect on such a system. Intact animal studies demonstrate compensatory changes that occur within the cardiovascular system. Studies on human subjects are less specific but provide the most clinically useful information.

The impact of electrolyte disorders at several levels of study is summarized in Table 23–12. Hypocalcemia, hypophosphatemia, and acidosis can result in decreased myocardial performance clinically only when these disorders are severe.

HYPOCALCEMIA

Experimental studies have documented the importance of calcium ions in the contraction of cardiac muscle. Acute elevations of calcium augment cardiac contractility, while acute reductions in calcium decrease cardiac contractility.[215] Hypocalcemia is not usually associated with clinical heart failure, although about 25 cases of reversible hypocalcemic heart failure can be found in the literature.

A review of 19 such patients demonstrates three age groups: (1) neonates, (2) children aged 8 to 14 years, and (3) adults aged 19 to 76 years (average age 40 years). The most common etiology of hypocalcemia in these patients was idiopathic or postsurgical hypoparathyroidism. Patients who met the following criteria: (all but one case) were reported on: (1) no other cause for cardiac failure was found, (2) patients improved with calcium and vitamin D therapy, (3) standard forms of heart failure treatment had failed, and (4) follow-

Table 23–12. Effects of Electrolyte Disorders on Myocardial Contractility

Electrolyte Disorder	Clinical[a] Observation	Isolated[a] Heart or Muscle	Intact[a] Animal
Acidosis	DC	DC	IC,[b] DC[c]
Alkalosis	?	IC	IC
Hyperkalemia	?	DC	—
Hypokalemia	?	IC	—
Hypercalcemia	IC[d]	IC	—
Hypocalcemia	DC[e]	DC	—
Hypomagnesemia	?	—	—
Hypophosphatemia	DC	DC	DC

[a] DC, decreased contractility, IC, increased contractility, or (?) unknown effects.
[b] Early in acidosis.
[c] Late in severe acidosis.
[d] Acute but not sustained increase in contractility.
[e] In both acute and chronic hypocalcemic states.

up on maintenance therapy did not detect clinical heart disease.[216-218].

The average nadir of serum calcium concentration at the time of cardiac failure was 1.27 mmol/liter, or 5.1 mg/dl, for the entire group of patients. Neonates manifested heart failure with less severe hypocalcemia, average 1.5 mmol/liter, as compared with children, average 0.875 mmol/liter, and adults, average 1.175 mmol/liter. The total serum protein and albumin concentrations, when provided, were normal. Ionized calcium levels were not performed. Serum phosphorus levels were generally elevated, with an average value of 2.74 mmol/liter, or 8.5 mg/dl. No patient had azotemia. In four of seven patients for whom serum magnesium determinations were done, the values were below normal. These patients also received magnesium treatment in conjunction with calcium and vitamin D.

Most hypocalcemic patients became symptomatic with overt tetany before hypocalcemia was severe enough to produce cardiac failure. Tetany, which usually initiates treatment of hypocalcemia, was overt in seven of 13 subjects, while four patients manifested latent tetany (positive Chvosteks' or Trousseau's sign). Cardiac failure is apparently a rare manifestation of hypocalcemia. When present, it is refractory to standard heart failure treatment but is readily reversible with calcium and vitamin D therapy and magnesium when depletion is present.

HYPOPHOSPHATEMIA

Recent clinical and experimental evidence suggests that severe hypophosphatemia can impair myocardial performance.[219,220] One patient study involved seven critically ill patients who had hypophosphatemia in addition to other serious medical problems.[219] The mean serum phosphorus was 0.31 mmol/liter and improvement in myocardial performance was noted during phosphate repletion. In dogs with experimental phosphate depletion, overt cardiac failure did not occur, but there was a substantial decline in several indices of cardiac contractility.[220]

ACIDOSIS

Severe respiratory or metabolic acidosis can cause a decrease in myocardial performance,[221,222] although there is wide individual variation in the reported severity of acidosis. Some patients with acidosis will not manifest any signs of cardiac failure while others with similar blood pH will present with cardiac failure and even shock. Acidosis of various etiologies but with similar depression of arterial pH may result in different degrees of myocardial depression (see Chapter 9). Studies in preparations of isolated heart muscle and isolated perfused hearts reveal that a decrease in cardiac muscle contractility can be demonstrated with arterial pH below 7.2. These studies demonstrate that there is direct action of acidosis on myocardial tissue, which is capable of depressing myocardial performance. However, in vivo intact animal studies reveal important modifications in this in vitro effect. Intact animals often manifest an increase in cardiac contractility in the initial phases of acidosis that may persist down to a pH of 7.1. However, with arterial pH near pH 6.9, experimental animals usually have severe reductions in contractility and myocardial performance[222,223] and cardiovascular collapse may occur suddenly.

As acidosis progresses sympathetic nerve activity increases and the adrenal glands release catecholamines into the bloodstream. This response is partly due to cardiovascular reflexes, but also is due to an effect of acidosis to stimulate release of catecholamines directly from both adrenal glands and nerve terminals. The catecholamines in turn stimulate cardiac beta-adrenergic receptors, which tends to increase contractility back toward normal. Beta-adrenergic blockade prevents this increase in contractility. Intact animals with beta-adrenergic blockade may develop cardiac failure at a similar degree of acidosis as has been shown to decrease contractility in studies on isolated heart muscle.[224] It has been suggested that patients on medications causing beta-adrenergic blockade may be more susceptible to myocardial depression by acidosis, but this has not yet been studied. The compensatory ionotropic action of catecholamines appears to allow the heart to tolerate a greater degree of acidosis than would be possible in isolated heart muscle preparations.

Experimental studies suggest that as acidosis progresses in severity the myocardium becomes increasingly resistant to the effect of beta-adrenergic stimulation. The loss of stimulation correlates well with the decline in myocardial performance that usually occurs at arterial pH values below 7.0.[223,225] As beta-adrenergic effectiveness decreases, cholinergic influiences predominate, producing bradycardia and further reduction in myocardial performance. In addition, acidosis produces vasodilation, which further contributes to the cardiovascular collapse.

The clinician is occasionally faced with an acidotic patient with irreversible shock, who is resistant to both endogenous and exogenous ionotropic agents. Attempts to reverse this resistance to ionotropic stimulation have been largely empirical. Treatment of metabolic acidosis with bicarbonate may not be beneficial. Recent studies have shown that myocardial performance may actually worsen in dogs with different forms of metabolic acidosis who are treated with $NaHCO_3$.[226,226a] However, some improvement was achieved in earlier studies,[224,225] in which responses to injections of norepinephrine and epinephrine on contratile force where found to be more effective after correction of acidosis with bicarbonate or with the buffer THAM (2-amine,2-hydroxymethyl-1,3-propanediol). THAM, which can penetrate cells, had more effect than bicarbonate which primarily buffers the extracellular space.

The etiology of acidosis also contributes to the differing effects of acidosis on the myocardium. Clinical diabetic ketoacidosis and uremic acidosis have less effect on myocardial performance than some forms of lactic acidosis. The pathophysiology of these differences is no doubt quite complex and include the factors discussed above. In addition, alterations of intracellular pH and intracellular metabolism probably play an important role in determining whether a certain type of acidosis depresses myocardial performance (see Chapters 6 and 7).

HYPERMAGNESEMIA

Hypermagnesemia does not appear to directly alter cardiac contractility, but a decline in myocardial performance could participate in the hypotension which can occur with hypermagnesemia.[71] Human experimental studies on the effects of intravenous magnesium sulfate revealed that administration by continuous infusion (30 to 50 mg/min) did not adversely effect cardiac performance. However, when a bolus of magnesium sulfate (7.5 g) was administered over 30 seconds there was a decrease in myocardial performance as measured by systolic time intervals.[227]

POTASSIUM DEPLETION

Chronic potassium depletion has been shown to produce pathological changes in animal myocardial tissue. The clinical significance of potassium depletion on myocardial performance is unclear.[7] Patients with congestive heart failure are at risk of potassium depletion due to secondary hyperaldosteronism and to treatment with digoxin and diuretics. Although clinical exacerbation of heart failure by potassium depletion has not been documented, patients who have potassium depletion should probably be treated due to their propensity for arrhythmias.

ECG Changes

P WAVE AMPLITUDE

Hyperkalemia is the only electrolyte disorder that has been clearly demonstrated to affect the P wave of the electrocardiogram (ECG). Atrial conduction slows with a rise in serum potassium level, producing a widening and lowering in height of the P wave. Such changes may be noted with serum potassium levels of $\geq$ 7 mmol/liter. The P wave amplitude continues to decrease as serum potassium rises, eventually leading to the disappearance of the P wave with atrial arrest.[228] Decreased P wave amplitude can also be noted in uremic patients with hypermagnesemia, but these patients often have coexistent hyperkalemia[101] (Chapter 13).

P-R INTERVAL AND ATRIOVENTRICULAR BLOCK

The P-R interval of the ECG can be lengthened by hyperkalemia, hypercalcemia, severe hypermagnesemia, hypokalemia, and sustained magnesium deficiency. The P-R interval is determined by the conduction velocity through the atria, atrioventricular (AV) node, and bundle of His. Electrolyte disorders do not significantly speed the conduction velocity and therefore do not clinically shorten the P-R interval; however, they can produce various degrees of atrioventricular block (AV block) (Chapter 13), (See Table 23–13.)

Both hyperkalemia and hypokalemia can slow conduction velocity, but to different degrees. The effect of hypokalemia is small, producing only a slight increase in the P-R interval that seldom exceeds the normal limit of 0.20 seconds. When at its severest, the P wave can be found along the downslope of the preceding large U wave.[229] In contrast, hyperkalemia has a dual effect on conduction velocity. At plasma level 6 to 6.5 mmol/liter, conduction velocity increases. At levels near or above 7.5 mmol/liter, velocity decreases, progressing to first-degree AV block. Clinical hyperkalemia seldom causes second- or third-degree block. The exception to this observation is the patient who manifests a higher-grade AV block in association with rapid intravenous potassium administration or with coexistent digitalis toxicity.[230]

Digitalis and hyperkalemia have additive effects on conduction velocity and together increase the likelihood of AV block. At the same time, a rise in serum potassium in the digitalis-toxic patient can suppress dangerous ventricular ectopy. Fortunately, there is a margin of safety between suppressing ectopy and producing complete heart block.[230] Close cardiac monitoring is imperative during intravenous potassium therapy. Theoretically, intravenous potassium loads given to digitalized patients can elevate serum potassium to a greater extent than ordinarily expected. This would be due to inhibition of normal potassium transport into cells by cardiac glycoside.

Table 23–13. ECG Manifestations of Electrolyte Disorders: P-Wave, P-R Interval, and Atrioventricular Block

P-Wave Amplitude

Hyperkalemia
Reduction or disappearance of P wave

P-R Lengthened by the Following Disorders
Hyperkalemia
Hypercalcemia
Severe hypermagnesemia
Hypokalemia
Sustained magnesium deficiency

Clinical Associations of Atrioventricular Block with Electrolyte Disorders[a]

	Heart Block		
Disorder	1st-Degree	2nd-Degree	3rd-Degree
Hyperkalemia	+	±	±
Hypokalemia	±	−	−
Hypercalcemia	+	±[b]	−
Hypocalcemia[c]	−	−	−
Hypermagnesemia	+	+	+
Magnesium depletion	±	−	−

[a] +, Common associaion; ±, uncommon association; −, no association.
[b] One case report.
[c] Can exacerbate effects of hyperkalemia.

Hypercalcemia can occasionally produce first-degree AV block, but usually the P-R interval lengthens only slightly to remain within the upper limit of normal (0.2 seconds). It is not clear whether hypercalcemia can produce second-degree AV block, although one such case (serum calcium of 15.3 mg/dl) has been reported.[231]

Hypocalcemia does not ordinarily produce changes in the P-R interval. However, if conduction velocity is decreased for other reasons, such as hyperkalemia, it can decrease still further with hypocalcemia. Uremic patients often manifest the combination of hyperkalemia and hypocalcemia.

Hypermagnesemia when below 5 mEq/liter produces little change in the ECG. When levels of 5 to 10 mEq/liter are reached, experimentally induced acute hypermagnesemia decreases conduction velocity and lengthens the P-R interval. First- and second-degree AV block, as well as sinoatrial (SA) block, have been reported. Complete heart block can occur with levels of magnesium exceeding 15 mEq/liter.[232]

Prolongation of the P-R interval occurs in association with sustained magnesium depletion. It is currently thought that intracellular and extracellular potassium depletion, which often accompanies magnesium depletion, is the main etiologic factor producing P-R prolongation.[233] In animals, P-R interval changes are not seen until potassium depletion is allowed to occur.[234,235] In humans, correction of magnesium depletion without potassium repletion does not always reverse prolongation of the P-R interval.[51]

QRS WIDTH, HEIGHT, AND VENTRICULAR CONDUCTION

Electrolyte disorders can affect the QRS width, height, and configuration. As with the P-R interval, most of these changes can be attributed to altered conduction through myocardial tissue. Disorders that affect the QRS interval are listed in Table 23–14.

Hyperkalemia and severe hypermagnesemia can produce QRS widening beyond the nor-

Table 23–14. ECG Manifestations of the Electrolyte Disorders: QRS Width and Ventricular Conduction[a]

Electrolyte Disorder	QRS Widening[b]	Bundle Branch Block[c]
Hyperkalemia	+	+
Hypokalemia	±	–
Hypercalcemia	±	–
Hypocalcemia	–[d]	–
Hypermagnesemia	+	±
Magnesium depletion	±[e]	–

[a] +, common association; ±, uncommon association; –, no association.
[b] QRS widening not exceeding 0.12 seconds.
[c] QRS widening exceeding 0.12 seconds (may not have a typical form).
[d] QRS narrows, but not clinically noticeable.
[e] Early magnesium deficiency.

mal limit of 0.12 seconds. Severe hypokalemia, early magnesium depletion, and hypercalcemia produce widening on serial ECGs, but the maximum QRS width usually remains within the normal limit of 0.12 seconds.

Hyperkalemia begins to affect the QRS width when serum concentrations of 6 to 7 mmol/liter are reached. As potassium concentrations rise, the ventricular conduction slows, further producing very wide QRS complexes. With serum potassium levels of 8 to 9 mmol/liter, the QRS and T waves merge to form a sine-wave pattern. This pattern precedes the onset of ventricular fibrillation or asystole and requires urgent treatment. If the T waves are of opposite polarity to the widened QRS complex, the pattern will mimic ventricular tachycardia.[229]

The effects of hyperkalemia on the conduction system are usually uniform throughout the ventricles. Therefore, widening of both the initial and terminal portions of QRS occurs. In addition, QRS widening is usually noted diffusely across limb and chest leads. Slowed ventricular conduction is manifested by numerous changes in QRS form. Severely hyperkalemic patients manifest combinations of right and left axis deviation, anterior and posterior fascicular blocks, with or without right or left bundle branch block. In a review of 18 such patients in the literature, 15 were found to have serum potassium concentrations in excess of 7.5 mmol/liter.[236-240] Uniform widening of the QRS interval produces a typical bundle branch block pattern, with widening of both the initial and terminal portions of the QRS.[228]

As with other ECG manifestations of hyperkalemia, it is expected that coexistent hyponatremia, acidosis, hypocalcemia, and possibly hypermagnesemia can augment hyperkalemic effects. Therefore, more serious manifestations can be observed for any given serum potassium concentration.[228,229]

Severe hypermagnesemia in the range of 2.5 to 5 mmol/liter can produce widening of the QRS interval up to ~ 0.12 seconds.[232] Uremic patients with hypermagnesemia have been noted to have widening of the QRS at serum magnesium levels below 4 mmol/liter. One patient manifested a bundle branch block pattern with a serum magnesium level of 3.7 mmol/liter and serum potassium level of 5.0 mmol/liter. This pattern reverted to normal with correction of the hypermagnesemia, while serum potassium remained unchanged.[241] Serum magnesium exceeding 7.5 mmol/liter can produce complete heart block.

Magnesium depletion is not consistently associated with ECG changes. Some patients with prolonged magnesium depletion accompanied by hypokalemia and hypocalcemia manifest widening of the QRS complex. On the other hand, experimental magnesium depletion in human subjects failed to demonstrate any change in the QRS.[51] Animal studies of early magnesium depletion, before the onset of hypokalemia, demonstrate a slight widening of QRS,[235] but such is not always observed.[234]

Changes in QRS height or voltage are an uncommon manifestation of electrolyte disorders. Severe potassium deficiency causes a slight increase in QRS height. Interestingly, intravenous administration of saline or potassium will lower the QRS back to normal.[242] Magnesium depletion occasionally produces low QRS complexes that revert to normal with magnesium repletion.

Q-T INTERVAL

The Q-T interval can be shortened or lengthened by electrolyte disorders (Table 23–15). Hyperkalemia and hypercalcemia shorten the Q-T interval, while hypocalcemia, and possibly magnesium depletion, can lengthen it. The Q-T interval normally varies with changes in heart rate, necessitating a correction by using the R-R interval and the formula

$$\text{Q-Tc} = \text{Q-T}/(\text{R-R})$$

In addition, myocardial disease and certain drugs can produce changes in the Q-T interval. Therefore, most studies have attempted to exclude these factors. There are three methods of measuring the Q-T interval with respect to the T wave: (1) to the onset of the T wave, designated the Q-oTc interval; (2) to the apex (Q-aTc; and (3) to the end of the T wave (Q-Tc).

Hyperkalemia speeds the rate of ventricular repolarization, producing a shortening of the Q-Tc interval. A significant change begins to occur with serum potassium levels of 5.5 to 6 mmol/liter. With more severe hyperkalemia (8 to 9 mmol/liter), this process continues until in conjunction with a widening QRS, the T wave and QRS merge into a sine-wave pattern. The sine-wave pattern mimics ventricular fibrillation and must be treated immediately, since it tends to progress to ventricular fibrillation or asystole. Intravenous calcium is probably the initial treatment of choice. Principles of treatment of hyperkalemia are discussed in Chapter 9.

Hypercalcemia also speeds the rate of ventricular repolarization and shortens the Q-T intervals. If other conditions that affect the Q-T interval are excluded, the degree of hypercalcemia correlates well with change in Q-T interval. The best correlation is for serum levels of calcium between 2.75 to 4.0 mmol/liter, or 11 to 16 mg/dl. Correlation also varies with the method of measurement used. The Q-aTc (apex) method provides the best results until severe hypercalcemia (4 mmol/liter, or 16 mg/dl) is reached.[243] A widening of the T wave occurs when serum calcium is above 4 mmol/liter or 16 mg/dl. Successful treatment of the hypercalcemia tends to return the Q-T interval back toward normal.[229]

Hypocalcemia is the major electrolyte disorder one should suspect when analyzing a prolonged Q-T interval. Ventricular repolarization is delayed, producing a lengthening of the Q-Tc interval up to 140 percent of normal.

The clinician must watch for changes induced by hypokalemia that can mimic Q-T prolongation. Hypokalemia does not significantly lengthen the Q-Tc interval, but increased U wave height can fool the observer if the Q-U interval is mistaken for a Q-Tc interval. Since hypocalcemia does not normally cause a Q-Tc interval in excess of 140 percent of normal, inclusion of a U wave should be suspected for Q-Tc measurements that exceed the limits produced by hypocalcemia. The S-T segment provides a clue to which disorder is present. Hypokalemia usually produces S-T segment depression, whereas hypocalcemia does not change the normal isoelectric S-T segment.

Patients with both hypokalemia and hypocalcemia may manifest S-T segment depression, Q-Tc prolongation, diminished T wave height, and prominent U waves. Hypocalcemia does not alter the Q-U interval; therefore, the T wave can merge with the prominent U waves produced by hypokalemia. Raising the serum calcim level shortens the Q-Tc interval and separates the T wave from the U wave.

Prolongation of the Q-Tc interval has not been consistently observed in the setting of magnesium depletion. Chronic studies of magnesium-depleted subjects[51] do demonstrate a slightly prolonged Q-Tc interval, but this change is most consistent with the effect of hypocalcemia also present in these patients. Animal studies also suggest that Q-Tc changes are most likely due to the associated hypocalcemia.

The effect of hypermagnesemia on the Q-T interval is unclear. Although magnesium levels of 5 to 10 mEq/liter are said to lengthen Q-Tc intervals, this has only been documented

Table 23–15. ECG Manifestations of the Electrolyte Disorders: Q-Tc Interval and S-T Segment

Q-Tc Interval	
Disorders that shorten Q-Tc	Disorders that lengthen Q-Tc
Hyperkalemia	Hypocalcemia
Hypercalcemia	
	Pseudo-lengthening due to U wave
	Hypokalemia
	Severe magnesium depletion

S-T Segment[a]	
Depression	Elevation
+ Hyperkalemia	± Hyperkalemia (rarely)
+ Hypokalemia	
± Early magnesium depletion	
± Hypermagnesemia[b]	
± Alkalosis	
± Hypernatremia	
± Respiratory acidosis	
− Hypocalcemia	
− Hypercalcemia	

[a] +, common association; ±, uncommon association; −, no association.
[b] Noted in uremic patients.

in uremic patients who also have coexistent hypocalcemia.[232,245]

S-T SEGMENT ELEVATION AND DEPRESSION

Elevation and depression of the S-T segment are most commonly produced by myocardial ischemia and injury, but also by certain electrolyte disorders (Table 23–15). Electrolyte disorders may also produce ECG changes, which are similar in all leads, as compared with ischemic-related changes, which affect leads specific for a given area of myocardium. Depression of the S-T segment may be noted with either hyperkalemia, hypokalemia, respiratory acidosis, or magnesium deficiency. Elevation of the S-T segment is an occasional manifestation of hyperkalemia. Moderately advanced hyperkalemia usually causes mild S-T segment depression, which occurs in association with QRS widening. Rarely S-T segment elevation that mimics pericarditis may occur. If a QS wave is also present, produced by interventricular conduction delay, the ECG can closely mimic an acute myocardial infarction.[229]

Hypokalemia initially causes changes in the T wave and U wave. As hypokalemia pro gresses in severity (2.0 to 2.83 mmol/liter, S-T segment depression in excess of 0.5 mm is observed.[242] Other abnormalities such as hypernatremia, alkalosis, or experimental respiratory acidosis (produced by inhalation of 30 percent carbon dioxide) may be associated with S-T segment depression as well.

Magnesium depletion is occasionally associated with S-T segment depression. Potassium depletion may occur in the later stages of magnesium depletion and is likely to be the major etiologic factor causing S-T segment depression. However, in some animal studies of early magnesium depletion, S-T depression was observed before serum potassium levels fell. The separate effects of intracellular potassium versus magnesium depletion require further investigation.[51,229,235]

T WAVE

The T wave represents the summary of electrical voltage of fibers during their repolarization at the end of each ventricular contraction. This process is dramatically affected by both the extracellular potassium concentration and the ratio of intracellular to extracellular potassium concentrations.[247] Thus hyperkalemia and hypokalemia are the most common and most dramatic disorders affecting the T wave. In addition, alterations in other electrolyte concentrations can alter T wave form (Table 23–16).

Even slight rises in serum potassium (5.5 to 6 mEq/liter) can produce dramatic effects on T waves by increasing the rate of ventricular repolarization. As the rate of repolarization increases, the T waves becomes more narrow, symmetric, and peaked. The amplitude usually increases, but may remain normal. The more acute the changes in serum potassium, the more pronounced are the ECG changes. Therefore, patients with chronic hyperkalemia may have normal or only mild ECG changes.

Table 23–16. ECG Manifestations of the Electrolyte Disorders: T Wave and U Wave[a]

Peaked T Waves	
+	Hyperkalemia
+	Hypocalcemia
±	Early magnesium deficiency
?	Hypermagnesemia in uremic patients (? hyperkalemia)
−	Acidosis, but may exacerbate hyperkalemic changes
−	Hyponatremia, but may exacerbate hyperkalemic changes
Flattened T Waves	
+	Hypokalemia
±	Alkalosis
±	Sustained magnesium deficiency (? potassium deficiency)
U Waves	
+	Hypokalemia
±	Hypomagnesemia (during refeeding without magnesium)

[a] +, common association; ±, uncommon association; −, no association; ?, questionable association.

It has been postulated that intracellular potassium rises with chronic hyperkalemia. This would return the intracellular to extracellular concentration ratio back toward normal, reducing the electrophysiologic effects of chronic hyperkalemia. This theory has yet to be investigated fully for most excitable tissues in states of chronic hyperkalemia. Acidosis and hyponatremia alone have no effect on T wave form, but when coupled with hyperkalemia these conditions may enhance the ECG changes of hyperkalemia.

At higher serum potassium levels (8 to 9 mEq/liter), the T waves merge with the widened QRS complex to produce a sine-wave pattern that precedes the onset of ventricular fibrillation and asystole.

Hypocalcemia mimics hyperkalemia by producing a peaking of the T wave. These two disorders often occur together in the uremic patient and, especially in the acutely ill patient, they may produce serious cardiac problems. Nonelectrolyte causes of peaked T waves include tachycardia, subendocardial infarction, and massive cerebrovascular accident.[229] The T wave changes of hyperkalemia may be masked by coexisting left ventricular hypertrophy or by digitalis therapy.[229]

The effect of magnesium depletion and excess on T wave form is not clear. Uremic patients with hypermagnesemia have been reported to have peaked T waves, but the role of hyperkalemia appears to be a significant additive factor.[71,101] Clinically, hypomagnesemia may not be associated with any ECG changes. Those changes that have been observed are usually attributed to the accompanying hypokalemia and/or hypocalcemia.[51,248] Tall peaked T waves have been noted in the ECGs of malnourished children who were refed without adequate magnesium repletion.[249] Before the initiation of feeding, these patients manifested low, flat T waves. The pathophysiology of peaked T waves in early magnesium depletion is unknown, but an interesting possibility[235] suggests that despite normal serum potassium levels, intracellular potassium depletion may be producing a relative hyperkalemia. Alcoholic patients often manifest hypomagnesemia and, in addition, may have alterations in T waves.[248,250] The role of magnesium depletion in these changes is unclear.

Studies in laboratory animals are somewhat at variance with the clinical data. In experimental animals with magnesium depletion, reproducible ECG changes are observed. In early magnesium depletion, before a fall in serum potassium, tall, peaked T waves can be seen. These T waves are not narrow, as seen in hyperkalemia.[235,251] Sustained magnesium depletion is usually accompanied by hypokalemia and potassium depletion. Experimental and clinical studies demonstrate flattened T waves[234,248,252] that were reversed best with potassium supplementation.

Flattening of the T wave and increase in U wave height are associated with hypokalemia. Ventricular repolarization is slowed, producing less summation of signals from each fiber. T waves become broader and flatter. As hypokalemia progresses, the T wave amplitude decreases and the U wave amplitude increases.

The normal U wave amplitude is 5 to 50 percent as high as the associated T wave. When U wave amplitude exceeds that of the T wave, hypokalemia should be suspected. These changes are best seen in leads II and III and in the mid-precordial leads. Prominent U waves may also be seen with bradycardia, hypertension, or left ventricular hypertrophy, as well as with the use of quinidine, procainamide, or certain phenothiazines.

The correlation between the degree of hypokalemia versus ECG changes is good. For example, Surawicz et al.[242] found T wave, U wave, or S-T segment changes in 10 percent of patients with serum potassium levels between 3.0 and 3.5 mEq/liter. For the range of 2.7 to 3.0 mEq/liter, 35 percent had ECG changes, and for < 2.7 mEq/liter, 78 percent had abnormalities on ECG. It has been suggested that alkalosis and hypernatremia may aggravate the ECG effects of hypokalemia.[247]

Hypercalcemia has little effect on T wave form, except at levels above 16 mg/dl, at which T waves may widen.[247]

Arrhythmias

Electrolyte disorders can either produce arrhythmias or modify arrhythmias produced by other etiologies, such as heart disease or digitalis toxicity. Clinical studies usually report the frequency of arrhythmia per patient or the incidence of an arrhythmia in compared populations. Electrolyte disorders and their effects on arrhythmias are summarized in Table 23–17.

BRADYCARDIA

Sinus bradycardia is known to occur with moderate hypermagnesemia and with severe acidosis. As magnesium levels rise, a transient increase in heart rate is noted, followed by bradycardia at levels as low as 2.25 mmol/liter, or 4.5 mEq/liter.[232] Acidosis also usually causes an initial tachycardia, which is thought to be due to release of catecholamines. Near pH 7.1, however, the myocardium becomes resistant to catecholamine stimulation, and vagal-like influence predominates. There is some evidence that acetylcholinesterase is inhibited at this pH level, enhancing vagal stimulation.[183] Hyperkalemia and hypercalcemia are noted to cause bradycardia only in instances of rapid rises in serum levels by intravenous administration.[229,230] In addition, a rapid change from hypokalemia to normokalemia can induce bradycardia.

ATRIAL ARRHYTHMIAS

The incidence and number of premature atrial contractions are increased by both hypokalemia and hyperkalemia.[230] Hypokalemic patients, with or without known heart disease, are found to have a higher incidence of prema-

Table 23–17. Arrhythmias Associated with Electrolyte Disorders[a]

Arrhythmias	Hypokalemia	Hyperkalemia	Acidosis	Alkalosis	Hypercalcemia	Hypocalcemia	Hypermagnesemia	Hypomagnesemia
Bradycardia		I	I		I		I	
Premature atrial contractions	I	I						
Atrial tachycardia	I		?	I				?
Junctional rhythm	I	I						
Asystolic arrest		I					I	
Premature ventricular contraction	I	I	?	?	I			I
Ventricular tachycardia and fibrillation	I		I	I	I	?		I
Premature ventricular contractions[b]	I			?			I	I
Ventricular tachycardia and fibrillation[b]	I			I			I	I
Conduction block[c]	D	I					I	
Atrial and ventricular ectopy[c]	I	D	D	I	I	D	D	I

[a] I, increased occurrence of arrhythmia; D, decreased occurrence of arrhythmia; ?, questionable association.
[b] With acute myocardial infarction.
[c] With digitalis.

ture atrial contractions when compared with normokalemic patients.[62]

Magnesium depletion has not been clearly demonstrated to be a primary cause of cardiac arrhythmias.[248,255,256] It increases the risk of supraventricular arrhythmias for patients on digitalis or for patients who have suffered an acute myocardial infarct. Intracellular and extracellular potassium depletion often accompany magnesium depletion and contribute to the production of arrhythmias. Parenteral magnesium is a useful treatment for supraventricular arrhythmias, whether serum magnesium levels are decreased or not. Thus, the reversal of an arrhythmia with magnesium treatment does not prove that magnesium depletion is the major cause of the arrhythmia.

Alkalosis predisposes patients to supraventricular arrhythmias in normal volunteers. Case reports usually involve critically ill patients with respiratory failure who receive overly zealous mechanical ventilation.[257,258] Risk factors do not include preexisting heart disease, unless patients are digitalized. Arrhythmias usually occur when arterial pH exceeds 7.55, and correction of the alkalosis often allows return to normal sinus rhythm. Such arrhythmias are usually refractory to antiarrhythmic medications unless the alkalosis is also treated.

Junctional rhythms evolve from situations of conduction block and are therefore seen with severe hypokalemia or rapidly induced hyperkalemia.[230] Asystolic arrest is due to severe depression of atrioventricular and intraventricular conduction. This may occur in conjunction with either rapid rises in serum potassium or with severe hypermagnesemia.[71,230] Magnesium levels above 8 mmol/liter are usually required to produce asystolic arrest, whereas patients will experience respiratory muscle paralysis at considerably lower levels.

VENTRICULAR ARRHYTHMIAS

Ventricular arrhythmias involve premature ventricular contractions (PVCs), ventricular tachycardia, and ventricular fibrillation. Hypokalemia is the most important electrolyte disorder which is associated with ventricular arrhythmias. Even slight reductions in serum potassium levels are associated with a greater frequency of PVCs and with a higher risk of ventricular tachycardia and ventricular fibrillation.[62,230] In addition, hypomagnesemic patients with normal serum potassium levels also appear to have increased frequency of PVCs and ventricular tachycardia.[259,260]

Hypokalemia and hypomagnesemia may both prolong repolarization and lengthen the Q-T interval, which can produce repolarization alternans.[260] This appears on the ECG as alternation in amplitude or polarity of the T wave and U wave without any change in QRS complex. Episodes of repolarization alternans can herald or follow ventricular arrhythmias and occur in settings of severe Q-T prolongation of multifactorial origin.[260]

Hyperkalemia up to serum levels of ~6 mmol/liter may produce increased automaticity and more frequent PVCs, especially if the serum potassium level has risen quickly.[230] Clinical hypocalcemia or hypercalcemia alone will only rarely produce ventricular arrhythmias, although these conditions can exacerbate arrhythmias produced by other cases.[229,260,261,262]

Severe metabolic acidosis, with arterial pH of~ 7.0, will increase the risk of ventricular tachycardia and ventricular fibrillation. Animal studies consistently demonstrate lowering of the ventricular fibrillation threshold in the presence of metabolic acidosis.[144,262] Clinical respiratory failure is often associated with ventricular arrhythmias, even though animal studies do not demonstrate lowering of the ventricular fibrillation threshold with respiratory acidosis.[108,263] Therefore, because of this discrepancy, it is uncertain whether respiratory acidosis is an important etiologic factor in the arrhythmias associated with respiratory failure. Alkalosis is also occasionally associated with ventricular arrhythmias, especially in the setting of overly rapid treatment of respiratory failure.[257,258] When cardiac arrhythmia is associated with an underlying acid–base disorder, the arrhythmia is often resistant to antiarrhythmic medications until the acid–base disorder has been corrected.

ARRHYTHMIAS AND MYOCARDIAL INFARCTION

The risk of cardiac arrhythmias markedly increases in the setting of acute myocardial infarction. Electrolyte disorders can exacerbate this tendency. For example, patients with acute myocardial infarction who have hypokalemia upon initial evaluation have a greatly increased frequency of PVCs, ventricular tachycardia, and ventricular fibrillation during their hospital course.[264,265] Patients with acute myocardial infarction who also have hypomagnesemia have an increased frequency of PVCs, ventricular tachycardia, and ventricular fibrillation.[266] Diuretic and digitalis treatment predispose patients to potassium and magnesium depletion. Monitoring and maintaining serum potassium in the normal range is recognized as an important adjunct in the treatment of patients with myocardial infarction. Magnesium therapy suppresses certain arrhythmias even when serum magnesium levels are normal, but its role in arrhythmia therapy in this setting requires further study.

Severe respiratory alkalosis, with arterial pH above 7.6, can exacerbate the supraventricular and ventricular arrhythmias associated with myocardial infarction. Such arrhythmias may be resistant to antiarrhythmic drugs, but will often respond to reduction of pH back toward normal values.[257]

ARRHYTHMIAS AND DIGITALIS

Both the therapeutic and toxic effects of digitalis can be modified by disorders of electrolyte and acid–base metabolism. In particular, changes in serum potassium concentration have the most significant effects on cardiac performance in digitalized patients, but changes in serum magnesium, calcium, and pH can also alter digitalis effects.

Digitalis augments myocardial contractility and slows electrical conduction. With digitalis toxicity, patients may manifest an increased frequency of PVCs, a decreased PVC coupling interval, a decreased refractory period, and an increased risk of ventricular tachycardia. As toxicity progresses, atrioventricular conduction is slowed to the point where there may be production of second- and third-degree AV block. Paroxysmal atrial tachycardia and AV junctional tachycardia are also commonly observed.

The presence of hypokalemia may intensify the tendency of digitalis to produce ectopic beats and arrhythmias. On the other hand, mild hyperkalemia may suppress digitalis-induced ectopia, but at higher serum potassium levels it can actually enhance the conduction block due to digitalis. Fortunately, there is a margin of safety. The cautious administration of potassium can act to suppress arrhythmias before complete heart block occurs.[230] Constant cardiac monitoring is recommended, however.

Magnesium depletion with or without hypokalemia can enhance many of the arrhythmias associated with digitalis toxicity.[248, 256, 259] Administration of magnesium generally decreases arrhythmias associated with digitalis toxicity, whether hypomagnesemia is present or not. However, since severe hypermagnesemia can actually enhance conduction block, parenteral magnesium should be given gradually, and not as a bolus. As with potassium therapy, continuous cardiac monitoring is required.

Hypocalcemia reduces both the therapeutic and toxic effects of digitalis.[229,230] Calcium chelating agents have been used successfully to treat experimental and clinical digitalis toxicity. Hypercalcemia is suspected of increasing digitalis toxicity, but this possibility requires clinical confirmation.[230]

The effects of acidosis and alkalosis in the digitalized patient remains unclear. Experimental studies suggest that acidosis is protective, while alkalosis increases digitalis toxicity. Correction of acidosis and alkalosis can alter serum potassium levels, but not always in predictable ways.[267,268] Therefore, in order to minimize digitalis toxicity, serum potassium should be monitored and maintained in the normal or slightly high range during changes in arterial pH.

GASTROINTESTINAL MANIFESTATIONS

Anorexia

Anorexia is a common symptom of many disease conditions in humans, including several disorders of water, electrolyte, and acid–base metabolism. The pathophysiology of anorexia has not been well studied, but effects on both the central nervous system and gastrointestinal tract are probably important. Anorexia is one of the earliest manifestations of hyponatremia, a disorder that may substantially involve the central nervous system. Severe but reversible anorexia is a common manifestation in a high percentage of patients with either magnesium depletion (70 percent) or phosphate depletion (50–100 percent).[51,96,269] Loss of appetite was a symptom in 17 percent to 37 percent of patients who had hypercalcemia due to primary hyperparathyroidism.[61,109] Additional etiologies of anorexia include chronic metabolic acidosis and hypocalcemia.

Nausea and Vomiting

Nausea and vomiting are common symptoms of many different electrolyte disorders. Both acute hypernatremia and acute hyponatremia commonly cause nausea and vomiting. These symptoms generally do not occur when the serum sodium has not fallen to less than 128 mEq/liter but this is also in large part dependent on how quickly the serum levels fall. At the other end of the scale, serum sodium above 150 mEq/liter is also commonly associated with nausea and vomiting, particularly in children.

Hypomagnesemia experimentally produced in human subjects has been shown frequently to cause nausea and vomiting.[51] On the other hand, hypermagnesemia as studied in human subjects and animals almost uniformly causes nausea and vomiting with serum levels greater than 10 mEq/liter, and occasionally with serum levels between 3 and 10 mEq/liter.[101,270]

Hypercalcemia is commonly associated with nausea and vomiting. Such symptoms may be found in 80 percent of patients in hyperparathyroid crisis,[271] whereas milder forms of primary hyperparathyroidism produce these symptoms in fewer than 25 percent of patients.[61,109] In laboratory animals, hypophosphatemia alone (serum phosphate <1 mg/dl) does not induce symptoms.[271a,271b] Clinical hypophosphatemia without hypercalcemia seldom causes nausea and vomiting.

Dysphagia

Although rarely noted with hyperparathyroidism, dysphagia, often appears to be due to the effect of a mass lesion in the neck rather than to hypercalcemia.[155,271,272] At least three cases of reversible dysphagia associated with magnesium deficiency have been reported.[69,273] Esophageal motility in one of these patients was decreased during upper gastrointestinal x-ray examination, but returned to normal after magnesium repletion.

Constipation

Constipation is often associated with hypercalcemia and hypokalemia. Hypokalemia is a well-recognized clinical cause of decreased gut motility and can lead to constipation and paralytic ileus.

Hypercalcemia frequently produces constipation, with about one-third of patients with primary hyperparathyroidism complaining of this symptom.[61,109,271] The pathophysiology of constipation due to hypercalcemia is unknown. Speculations as to its origin include changes in smooth muscle tone, as well as changes in both autonomic and intrinsic neural activity. Another, but less likely, explanation is that the constipation is secondary to the dehydration and decreased food intake associated with hypercalcemia.

Paralytic Ileus

Hypokalemia and potassium depletion are well-recognized but not well-documented causes of clinical hypomotility and paralytic ileus. Abdominal distention, nausea, vomiting, and constipation can accompany the hypomotility state. Experimental studies in potassium-depleted rats and dogs have demonstrated decreased motility with normal muscle tone in the bowel. However, as potassium stores are further depleted, muscle tone also decreases, leading to dilation of bowel segments.[274] These animal studies explain in part, why gastric atony and megacolon occur in severely potassium-depleted patients.[275]

The participation of hypermagnesemia and hypomagnesemia in the pathophysiology of paralytic ileus is unclear.[51,89] In a case report of one patient with experimentally induced magnesium deficiency, in whom ileus developed with a serum magnesium of 0.65 mEq/liter, the serum potassium was not available, hence the role of hypokalemia could not be assessed. After magnesium repletion, motility improved, but during a repeat study in this same patient, no ileus was observed.

Experimental hypermagnesemia is known to decrease autonomic input to the gastrointestinal tract. Although nausea and vomiting can occur with serum magnesium levels >6 mEq/liter, ileus has only been reported in infants. In a study of two newborn infants born to eclamptic women who had received magnesium therapy, both were found to have hyporeflexia, hypoactive bowel sounds, and abdominal distention,[276] with a mean serum magnesium level of 7.2 mEq/liter. These infants failed to pass meconium stools and therefore required enemas. Both recovered normal bowel motility after reduction in serum magnesium and removal of meconium plugs.

Diarrhea and Streatorrhea

Hypocalcemia is associated with a number of gastrointestinal manifestations, many of which are more pronounced when the hypocalcemia is due to either hypoparathyroidism or pseudohypoparathyroidism. Diarrhea and steatorrhea are the most commonly reported gastrointestinal manifestations associated with hypocalcemia,[277,278] although a few cases of constipation, ileus, and megacolon have been observed.[275,279] Such patients frequently show decreased bowel motility, as shown by barium contrast studies. These facts are consistent with many physiologic studies demonstrating that decreased intestinal tone may cause either diarrhea or constipation. Malabsorption and steatorrhea can be demonstrated in some hypocalcemic patients. However, malabsorption itself, regardless of the etiology, can cause hypocalcemia, which may worsen the steatorrhea. Thus the principal electrolyte abnormalities associated with diarrhea and steatorrhea are often multiple and interrelated. Barium contrast studies in patients with hypocalcemia due to hypoparathyroidism may reveal distended bowel loops and loss of normal mucosal folds, which resemble the changes seen in sprue. Mucosal biopsies occasionally reveal areas of atrophy in these patients. Gluten-free diets usually do not improve gastrointestinal symptoms, but correction of hypocalcemia with calcium and vitamin D may produce symptomatic improvement.

Abdominal Pain

Abdominal pain may occur in hypokalemic states or may be associated with hypercalcemia. Cramping and abdominal distention can be produced by paralytic ileus accompanying severe hypokalemia. The abdominal pain associated with hypercalcemia may involve peptic ulcer disease, pancreatitis, and other unknown factors. Given a broad population with hyperparathyroidism and hypercalcemia, abdominal pain will occur in 15 to 30 percent of patients. Up to one-half these patients will have associated peptic ulcer disease,[109] while another 7 to 10 percent will have pancreatitis. Patients presenting with the fulminant symptoms of hyperparathyroid crisis will have more prominent gastrointestinal symptoms. Abdominal pain or tenderness to palpation was found in 15 to 48 percent of such patients, while nausea and vomiting occurred in 80 percent. Symptoms usually resolved with parathyroidectomy and reduction in serum calcium.[272]

Acid Production

Gastric acid production may be acutely stimulated by oral or intravenous calcium, while acute reductions in serum calcium decrease gastric acid production. Thus, it is not surprising that achlorhydria has been found in hypoparathyroid patients in whom serum calcium levels were below 7 mg/dl.

The effect of chronic hypercalcemia on gastric acid secretion and the development of peptic ulcer disease is quite controversial.[280,281] There is probably an increased incidence of peptic ulcer disease (10 to 15 percent) in patients with primary hyperparathyroidism. An additional 15 percent of such patients will have epigastic pain without x-ray evidence of ulcers.[109] Patients with hypercalcemia due to other etiologies are said to develop peptic ulcer disease only rarely, although the evidence is scanty. The pathophysiology of peptic ulcer disease in this setting may be related to increased gastrin levels. Gastrin levels can be stimulated by hypercalcemia in patients with gastrinomas (Zollinger-Ellison syndrome).[280,281] Some patients demonstrate elevated gastric acid production and/or elevated serum gastrin levels that resolve after parathyroidectomy, although such an association is not always present.

Pancreatitis

The incidence of acute and chronic pancreatitis is increased in patients with hypercalcemia of various etiologies, including primary hyperparathyroidism. Pancreatitis may eventually occur in 7 to 10 percent of patients with hyperparathyroidism and in up to 25 to 30 percent of patients presenting with hyperparathyroid crisis. Fifty to 80 percent of patients in crisis demonstrate nausea, vomiting, or abdominal pain.[271] Calcification of the pancreas was visible on x-ray film in 32 percent of all cases of pancreatitis. "Normal" values for serum calcium in patients presenting with pancreatitis should raise the suspicion that hypercalcemia was present before the attack. After resolution of the pancreatitis, serum calcium levels should be rechecked[282,283] and parathyroid hormone levels measured if clinically appropriate.

HEMATOLOGIC MANIFESTATIONS

Hemolysis

Severe hypophosphatemia (serum phosphate below 0.5 mg/dl) is often associated with a reversible hemolytic anemia, which has been reported both clinically[284,285] and experimentally in dogs.[286] Red blood cell metabolism is disrupted as phosphate depletion occurs. The cells become more rigid and spherical as their adenosine triphosphate (ATP) levels drop. The spleen then begins to remove such cells, producing microspherocytes in the process.

Lesser degrees of hypophosphatemia may also produce biochemical changes in red blood cell metabolism. As serum phosphorus falls below normal, glycolytic pathways may be somewhat disrupted, reducing cellular ATP and 2,3-diphosphoglycerate (2,3-DPG) levels.[287] It appears that when red cell ATP levels drop below 15 percent of normal, hemolysis is more likely to occur.[284,285] Chromium red cell survival was markedly reduced in such hypophosphatemic patients, but reversed to near normal only 2 days after serum phosphorus concentrations had been restored to the normal range. Red cell ATP levels rose rapidly out of the danger range (above 15 percent of control), but were not restored to normal for 2 weeks.[284] Some biochemical parameters will begin correcting even before phosphate repletion brings serum levels back to normal.

It appears from clinical reports that other factors may aggravate the effects of hypophosphatemia on red cell metabolism and hemolysis. Coexistent acidosis, respiratory alkalosis, magnesium depletion, alcoholism, and septicemia are all suspected of either creating increased cellular energy requirements or exacerbating the defects on ATP production. For a more thorough discussion, see refs. 54 and 288.

Platelet Dysfunction

Platelet dysfunction has been produced experimentally by hyperalimentation induced hypophosphatemia in the malnourished dog.[(286)] These dogs hemorrhaged massively into gut and skin. Impairment of clot refraction, reduced platelet survival, thrombocytopenia, megakaryocytosis and large platelet diameter were noted. Cellular adenosine triphosphate (ATP) levels in platelets were below normal as in the red cells of phosphate depleted subjects. These platelet abnormalities could be prevented by phosphate supplementation and could be reversed by phosphate repletion. After 6 days of severe hypophosphatemia (below 0.5 mg/dl), animals demonstrated skin and gastrointestinal bleeding at autopsy. A decrease in platelet survival could be detected within one day of beginning the hyperalimentation.

The clinical literature does not definitely associate phosphate depletion and bleeding.[54]

However, some patients on hyperalimentation are said to manifest bleeding with hypophosphatemia. The starved, bleeding alcoholic patient, who receives phosphate depleted blood transfusions may be in a clinical situation where platelet dysfunction could become important.(54)

It should be noted that hyperalimentation induced hypophosphatemia provokes both a reduced supply of phosphate and a concomitant accelerated metabolic demand for phosphate. In combination these produce the most dramatic symptomatology.(54)

Leukocyte Dysfunction

Severe phosphate depletion can hamper the functions of leukocytes or polymorphonuclear neutrophils (PMN) to chase, capture and kill bacteria. Craddock and associates(290) have demonstrated a 50 percent decrease in PMN chemotactic, phagocytotic and bactericidal activity in dogs with hyperalimentation induced hypophosphatemia. One patient who was being hyperalimentated demonstrated hypophosphatemia and had white cell dysfunction similar to that mentioned above. As in the experimental situation, these defects were reversible either by *in vivo* phosphate repletion or by adding phosphate and adenosine to *in vitro* studies. Serum phosphorous levels of less than 1 mg/dl were required to lower white cell adenosine triphosphate levels and to produce functional changes in leukocytes. The leukocyte dysfunction is probably clinically important. The number of episodes of infection were compared between hypophosphatemic patients and patients with normal serum concentrations of phosphorus. Thirteen of eighteen hypophosphatemic patients were thought to be infected, while one of ten patients were noted to have infections in the phosphate-replete group.[290] *Salmonella*-infected guinea pigs that were also hypophosphatemic, had an increased mortality versus animals that received phosphate.[291] Dogs with hyperalimentation-induced hypophosphatemia were more likely to die secondary to infections than were phosphate-repleted controls.[284,286] For more details on the pathophysiology of leukocyte dysfunction due to hypophosphatemia, see refs. 54 and 288.

Oxygen–Hemoglobin Affinity

The affinity or binding of oxygen to hemoglobin is altered by a number of clinical conditions, such as acidosis, alkalosis, hypophosphatemia, hypothermia, and fever. Increased affinity for oxygen means that oxygen is bound more tightly to hemoglobin, and for any given concentration of oxygen a greater number of oxygen binding sites of the hemoglobin molecules will be filled with oxygen molecules. In the lung, this facilitates the loading of hemoglobin with oxygen, but in the systemic capillaries it decreases oxygen dissociation and may thereby decrease tissue oxygen delivery. Decreased affinity for oxygen has just the opposite effects.

The percentage of hemoglobin that has oxygen bound to it is called percentage saturation and depends not only on the affinity of hemoglobin for oxygen, but on the oxygen concentration or partial pressure of oxygen (Po_2 in mm Hg) to which the hemoglobin is exposed as well. This relationship is depicted by the oxygen–hemoglobin dissociation curve.[292] For any given oxygen concentration (mmHg), there is a percentage saturation representing the equilibrium between bound oxygen and dissociated free oxygen. The lung capillaries are high in oxygen concentration, thus hemoglobin becomes highly saturated with oxygen. In the systemic capillaries, hemoglobin is exposed to lower oxygen concentrations, and oxygen dissociates until the lower percentage of saturation is reached.

A change in the affinity of hemoglobin for oxygen shifts the oxygen–hemoglobin dissociation curve either to the right or left producing different degrees of saturation for a given oxygen concentration.[292] The oxygen concentration that produces 50 percent saturation of hemoglobin is utilized to quantitate the degree of shift that occurs with a change in affinity. This value is called the P50 and has units of mmHg.[292]

The oxygen affinity for hemoglobin can be altered either by changes in arterial pH, body temperature, or the concentration of 2,3-diphosphoglycerate (2,3-DPG) inside the red blood cell. Affinity is decreased by acidosis, fever, or increased 2,3-DPG concentration in red cells. Decreased affinity produces a shift in the dissociation curve to the right, an increased P50, and less saturation for a given oxygen concentration. It is possible that these changes increase tissue oxygen delivery and could be adaptive in situations of tissue hypoxia. Hemoglobin affinity for oxygen is increased either by alkalosis, hypothermia, or a decreased red cell 2,3-DPG concentration. This produces a leftward shift of the curve, a lower P50, and increased saturation for a given blood oxygen concentration. With increased affinity, it has been postulated that, upon reaching hypoxic tissue, the hemoglobin would less readily release oxygen so that the oxygen delivery to the tissues would decrease. The clinical significance of these changes remains controversial, but it could be of importance in states of anemia, acidosis, shock, and hypoxia.[292]

Changes in pH and temperature affect hemoglobin–oxygen affinity immediately, whereas alterations in 2,3-DPG may require up to several days to become significant. The production of 2,3-DPG in red cells is decreased by acidosis, phosphate depletion, and the storage or banking of blood. Production of 2,3-DPG is increased by alkalosis and hypoxemia. Therefore, acute acidosis produces a right shift in the oxygen–hemoglobin dissociation curve while, if the acidosis is sustained for a few days, 2,3-DPG production drops, thereby bringing the curve back toward the left, usually to a near-normal P50. Similar adjustments occur for alkalosis, returning the curve back toward normal.

Phosphate depletion reduces the activity of the red blood cell glycolytic pathway, thereby reducing the production of 2,3-DPG. Left shifts in the oxygen–hemoglobin curve are well documented in clinical settings of severe hypophosphatemia.[79,289,293] These shifts correlate well with observed reductions in cellular 2,3-DPG levels. Hypophosphatemia for prolonged periods below 0.323 mmol/liter (serum phosphorous below 1 mg/dl) produces a significant change in red cell 2,3-DPG. Phosphate repletion will begin to restore 2,3-DPG production even before the serum phosphorus rises above 0.323 mmol/liter (1 mg/dl).[79] Full correction of 2,3-DPG levels with subsequent return of the oxygen–hemoglobin dissociation curve to normal can require up to 48 hours.[79]

HORMONAL AND METABOLIC MANIFESTATIONS

Changes in hormonal release and action play important roles in the body's ability to respond to environmental and metabolic stresses. With the development of hormone assays and receptor studies, evidence is accumulating that electrolyte disorders produce many alterations in hormonal and metabolic systems. Most of these alterations are adaptive and rise through normal regulatory pathways. Others are produced by a disruption of normal regulation that may not be adaptive.

Hormonal and metabolic regulation is extremely complex, involving numerous steps of modulation and disruption. For example, hormonal synthesis, secretion, delivery, binding, and metabolic breakdown are only a few of the steps involved in a hormonal system. Numerous changes may occur with electrolyte disorders, although the clinical significance of many of these changes is still unclear.

Changes in serum hormone concentrations are the most thoroughly studied aspect of hormonal systems. Hormone levels can decrease or increase due to electrolyte disorders. For example, acidosis provokes a release of norepinephrine from sympathetic nerve terminals. The norepinephrine in turn stimulates the release of glucocorticoids and catecholamines from the adrenal glands as well as renin from the renal juxtaglomerular cells.[183,294] The release of catecholamines is important in sustaining myocardial performance in acidotic states.

Potassium is involved in the release of numerous hormones. Hyperkalemia can cause increased levels of insulin, glucagon, aldosterone, growth hormone, and catecholamines.[7] In addition, in vitro studies demonstrate that hyperkalemia increases the release of ACTH, thyrotropin, and luteinizing hormone.[170] Acute and chronic hyperkalemia suppress plasma renin levels. Potassium depletion produces a decrease in blood levels of insulin, aldosterone, and growth hormone. Further investigations of insulin metabolism reveal that potassium depletion alters the form of insulin that is released. An inactive form, proinsulin, is found to be released in greater quantities, while the release of active insulin is decreased.

Magnesium depletion decreases the release, but not the synthesis, of parathyroid hormone.[295,296] Within minutes of starting magnesium repletion, increased parathyroid hormone release can occur. In addition, elevated blood hormone levels do not necessarily lead to increased hormone efficacy at the target tissue. There are several reasons for this. Hormone receptor number and/or affinity can be altered. In addition, if binding does not occur, the cell may not be able to respond due to uncoupling of the receptor system or altered cellular metabolism. For example, magnesium depletion decreases the action of parathyroid hormone on bone. Normally parathyroid hormone acts to increase release of calcium from bone which helps to correct hypocalcemia. Such failure for the target tissue to respond is part of the etiology of hypocalcemia due to magnesium depletion.[295] Another example is metabolic acidosis, which decreases binding of insulin to cell receptors. Insulin resistance due to acidosis may be explained at least in part on this basis.

Cellular metabolism can be directly altered. Severe hypophosphatemia disrupts cell energy metabolism. Acidosis inhibits gycolysis and probably inhibits gluconeogenesis. Hyperosmolar states stimulate the production in cells of amino acids and other substrates that allow cells to minimize cell volume changes.[24] Magnesium depletion stimulates cholesterol production, resulting in elevated serum cholesterol levels.[202] Further research is required to assess the clinical significance of these and other yet to be discovered changes in hormonal regulation and intracellular metabolism.

REFERENCES

1. Natelson S, Miletich DJ, Seals CF, et al: Clinical biochemistry of epilepsy. I. Nature of the disease and a review of the chemical findings in epilepsy. Clin Chem 25:889, 1979
2. Rotheram EB, Safar P, Robin ED: CNS disorder during mechanical ventilation in chronic pulmonary disease. JAMA 189:993, 1964
3. Kilburn KH: Shock, seizures, and coma with alkalosis during mechancial ventilation. Ann Intern Med 65:977, 1966
4. Faden A: Encephalopathy following treatment of chronic pulmonary failure. Neurology (NY) 26:337, 1976
5. Safar P, Nemoto EM, Severinghaus JW: Pathogenesis of central nervous system disorder during artificial hyperventilation in compensated hypercarbia in dogs. Crit Care Med 1:5, 1973
6. Coteu S, Severinghaus JW, Singer MM: The effect of ventilation and acetazolamide (Diamox) on cerebral blood flow in chronic respiratory acidosis. Anesthesiology 29:203, 1968
7. Cronin RE, Knochel JP: The consequences of potassium deficiency. In Acid–base and Potassium Homeostasis. Brenner BM, Stein JH (eds): Contemporary Issues in Nephrology. Vol. 2. Churchill Livingstone, New York, 1978 p 205
8. Cohen JJ, Gennari FJ, Harrington JT: Disorders of potassium balance. p 908. In Brenner BM, Rector FC Jr (eds): The Kidney. 2nd Ed. WB Saunders, Philadelphia, 1981
9. Sieker HO, Hickam JB: Carbon dioxide intoxication: The clinical syndrome, its etiology and management with particular refer-

ence to the use of mechanical respirators. Medicine (Baltimore) 35:389, 1956
10. Kilburn KH: Neurologic manifestations of respiratory failure. Arch Intern Med 116: 409, 1965
11. Woodbury DM, Rollins LT, Gardner MD, et al: Effects of carbon dioxide on brain excitability and electrolytes. Am J Physiol 192:79, 1958
12. Caspers H, Speckmann EJ: Cerebral Po_2, Pco_2 and pH: changes during convulsive activity and their significance for spontaneous arrest of seizures. Epilepsia 13:699, 1972
13. Bingmann D, Kolde G, Speckman EJ: Effects of elevated Po_2 values in the supernate on the neural activity in hippocampal slices. p. 97. Klee, MR et al (Eds): Physiology and Pharmacology of Epileptogenic Phenomena. Raven Press, New York, 1982
14. Katzman R, Pappins HM: Brain Electrolytes and Fluid Metabolism. Williams & Wilkins, Baltimore, 1973
15. Weil WB, Wallace WM: Hypertonic dehydration in infancy. Pediatrics 17:171, 1956
16. Finberg L: Pathogenesis of lesions in the nervous system in its hypernatremic states. I. Clinical observations in infants. Pediatrics 23:40, 1959
17. Elton NW, Elton WJ, Nazareno JP: Pathology of acute salt poisoning in infants. Am J Clin Pathol 39:252, 1963
18. Finberg L, Kiley J, Luttrell CN: Mass accident salt poisoning in infancy. JAMA 184:187, 1963
19. Bruck E, Abal G, Aceto TJ: Pathogenesis and pathophysiology of hypertonic dehydration with diarrhea. Am J Dis Child 115:122, 1968
20. Morris-Jones PH, Hanston IB, Evans RC: Prognosis of the neurological complications of acute hypernatremia. Lancet 2:1385, 1967
21. Kahn A, Brachet E, Blum D: Controlled fall in natremia and risk of seizures in hypertonic dehydration. Intensive Care Med 5:27, 1979
22. Stephenson JBP: Uraemia as a determinant of convulsions in acute infantile hypernatremia. Arch Dis Child 46:676, 1971
23. Pollock AS, Arieff AI: Abnormalities of cell volume regulation and their functional significances. Am J Physiol 239:F195, 1980
24. Arieff AI, Guisado R, Lazarowitz UC: The pathophysiology of hyperosmolar states. p. 227. In Andreoli TE, Grantham JJ, Rector FC Jr (eds): Disturbances in Body Fluid Osmolality. American Physiological Society, Bethesda, MD, 1977
25. Maccario M: Neurological dysfunction associated with nonketotic hyperglycemia. Arch Neurol 19:525, 1968
26. Daniels JC, Chokroverty S, Barron KD: Anacidotic hyperglycemia and focal seizures. Arch Intern Med 124:701, 1969
27. Arieff AI, Carroll HJ: Nonketotic hyperosmolar coma with hyperglycemia: Clinical features, pathophysiology, renal function, acid–base balance, plasma–cerebrospinal fluid equilibria and the effects of therapy in 37 cases. Medicine (Baltimore) 51:73, 1972
27a. Singh BM, Gupta DR, Strobos RJ: Nonketotic hyperglycemia and epilepsia partialis continua. Arch Neurol 29:187, 1973
28. Zimmermann B, Wangensteen OH: Observations on water intoxication in surgical patients. Surgery 31:654, 1952
29. Wynn V, Rob CG: Water intoxication. Differential diagnosis of the hypotonic syndromes. Lancet 1:587, 1954
30. Bartholomew LG, Scholz DA: Reversible postoperative neurological symptoms. JAMA 162:22, 1956
31. Swanson AG, Iseri OA: Acute encephalopathy due to water intoxication. N Engl J Med 258:831, 1958
32. Carter NW, Rector FC, Jr, Seldin DW: Hyponatremia in cerebral disease resulting from the inappropriate secretion of antidiuretic hormone. N Engl J Med 264:67, 1961
33. Whalley PJ, Pritchard JA: Oxytocin and water intoxication. JAMA 186:601, 1963
34. Lipsmeyer E, Ackerman GI: Irreversible brain damage after water intoxication. JAMA 196:286, 1966
35. Hantman D, Rossier B, Zohlman R, et al: Rapid correction of hyponatremia in the syndrome of inappropriate secretion of antidiuretic hormone. Ann Intern Med 78:870, 1973
36. Still JA Jr, Modell JH: Acute water intoxication during transurethral resection of the prostate, using glycine solution for irrigation. Anesthesiology 38:98, 1973
37. Arieff AI, Llach F, Massry SG: Neurological manifestations and morbidity of hyponatre-

mia: Correlation with brain water and electrolytes. Medicine (Baltimore) 55:121, 1976
38. Ayus JC, Olivero JJ, Frommer JP: Rapid correction of severe hyponatremia and intravenous hypertonic saline solution. Am J Med 72:43, 1982
39. Grant DK: Papilloedema and fits in hypoparathyroidism with a report of three cases. Q J Med 22:243, 1953
40. Sugar O: Central neurological complication of hypoparathyroidism. Arch Neurol Psychiatry 70:86, 1953
41. Vignaendra V, Frank AO, Lim CL: Absence status in a patient with hypocalcemia. Electroencephalogr. Clin Neurophysiol 43:429, 1977
42. Gupta MM, Grover DN: Hypocalcaemia and convulsions. Postgrad Med J 53:330, 1977
43. Albright F, Burnett CH, Cope O, et al: Acute atrophy of bone (osteoporosis) simulating hyperparathyroidism. J Clin Endocrinol Metab 1:711, 1941
44. Dodd K, Graubarth H, Rapoport S: Hypercalcemia, nephropathy and encephalopathy following immobilization. Pediatrics 6:124, 1950
45. Beare JM, Millar JH: Epileptiform fits during calciferol therapy. Lancet 260:884, 1951
46. Harmon M: Parathyroid adenoma in a child: Report of case presenting as central nervous system disease and complicated by magnesium deficiency. Am J Dis Child 91:313, 1956
47. Bauermeister DE, Jenning ER, Cruse DR, et al: Hypercalcemia with seizures—a clinical paradox. JAMA 201:146, 1967
48. Mikkelsen EJ, Reider AA: Post-parathyroidectomy psychosis: Clincal and research implications. J Clin Psychiatry 40:352, 1979
49. Fishman RA: Neurological aspects of magnesium metabolism. Arch Neurol 12:562, 1965
50. Wolfe SM, Victor M: The relationship of hypomagnesemia and alkalosis to alcohol withdrawal symptoms. Ann NY Acad Sci 162:973, 1969
51. Shils ME: Experimental human magnesium depletion. Medicine (Baltimore) 48:61, 1969
52. Chutkow JG, Grabow JD: Clinical and chemical correlations in magnesium-deprivation encephalopathy of young rats. Am J Physiol 223:1407, 1972
53. Silvis SE, Paragas PD: Paresthesias, weakness, seizures, and hypophosphatemia in patients receiving hyperalimentation. Gastroenterology 62:513, 1972
54. Knochel JP: The pathophysiology and clinical characteristics of severe hypophosphatemia. Arch Intern Med 137:203, 1977
55. Levy DE, Bates D, Caronna JJ, et al: Prognosis in nontraumatic coma. Ann Intern Med 94:293, 1981
56. Plum F, Posner JB: The Diagnosis of Stupor and Coma. 3rd Ed. FA Davis, Philadelphia, 1982
57. Covey CM, Arieff AI: Disorders of sodium and water metabolism and their effects on the central nervous system. p. 212. In Brenner BM, Stein JH (eds): Contemporary Issues in Nephrology. Churchill Livingstone, New York, 1978
58. Macaulay D, Watson M: Hypernatremia in infants as a cause of brain damage. Arch Dis Child 42:485, 1967
59. Elman R, Shatz BA, Keating RE, et al: Intracellular and extracellular potassium deficits in surgical patients. Ann Surg 136:111, 1952
60. Bradbury MW: Electrolyte disorders and the brain. p. 1023. In Maxwell MH, Kleinman CR (eds): Clinical Disorders of Fluid and Electrolyte Metabolism. McGraw-Hill, New York, 1972
60a. Bradbury MWB, Kleeman CR: Stability of the potassium content of cerebrospinal fluid and brain. Amer J Physiol 213:519, 1967
61. Petersen P: Psychiatric disorders in primary hyperparathyroidism. J Clin Endocrinol Metab 28:1491, 1968
62. Davidson S, Surawicz B: Ectopic beats and atrioventricular conduction disturbances in patients with hypopotassemia. Arch Intern Med 120:280, 1967
63. Carman JS, Jimerson DC, Post RM: Electrolyte changes associated with shifts in affective states. p. 277. In Alexander PE (ed): Electrolytes and Neuropsychiatric Disorders. SP Books, New York, 1981
64. Kurtz D: The EEG in parathyroid dysfunction. p. 77. In Remond A (ed): Handbook of Electroencephalography and Clinical

Neurophysiology. Elsevier, Amsterdam, 1976

65. Allen EM, Singer FR: Electroencephalographic abnormalities in hypercalcemia. Neurology (New York) 20:15, 1970
66. Cohn R, Sode J: The EEG in hypercalcemia. Neurology (New York) 21:154, 1971
66a. Cogan MG, Covey CM, Arieff AI, et al: Central nervous system manifestations of hyperparathyroidism. Am J Med 65:963, 1978
67. Hanna S, MacIntyre I, Harrison M, et al: The syndrome of magnesium deficiency in man. Lancet 1:172, 1960
68. Hall RC, Joffe JR: Hypomagnesemia and psychiatric symptoms. JAMA 224:1749, 1973
69. Hamed IA, Lindeman RD: Dysphagia and vertical nystagmus in magnesium deficiency. Ann Intern Med 89:222, 1978
70. Somjen G, Hilmy M, Stephen CR: Failure to anesthetize human subjects by intravenous administration of magnesium sulfate. J Pharmacol Exp Ther 154:652, 1966
71. Randall RE, Cohen MD, Spray CC Jr, et al: Hypermagnesemia in renal failure. Ann Intern Med 61:73, 1967
72. Mordes JP, Wacker WEC: Excess magnesium. Pharmacol Rev 29:273, 1978
73. Arieff AI, Kerian A, Massry SG, et al: Intracellular pH of brain: Alterations in acute respiratory acidosis and alkalosis. Am J Physiol 230:804, 1976
74. Posner JB, Plum F: Spinal-fluid pH and neurological symptoms in systemic acidosis. N Engl J Med 277:605, 1967
75. Fulop M: The ventilatory response in severe metabolic acidosis. Clin Sci Mol Med 50:367, 1976
75a. Dodds EC, Robertson JD: The relation of aceto-acetic acid to diabetic coma and the cause of death. Lancet 1:852, 1930
75b. Lazarowitz VC, Arieff AI: Ketoacidosis and coma. Clin Res 26:420A, 1978
76. Arieff AI, Carroll HJ: Cerebral edema and depression of sensorium in nonketotic hyperosmolar coma. Diabetes 23:525, 1974
76a. Harrington JT, Kassirer JP: Metabolic alkalosis. p. 227. In Cohen JJ, Kassirer JP (eds): Acid–Base. Little, Brown, Boston, 1982
77. Oliva PB: Severe alveolar hypoventilation in a patient with metabolic alkalosis. Am J Med 52:817, 1972
78. Shear L, Brandman IS: Hypoxia and hypercapnia caused by respiratory compensation for metabolic alkalosis. Am Rev Respir Dis 107:836, 1973
79. Travis S, Sugerman HJ, Ruberg RL, et al: Alterations of red-cell glycolytic intermediates and oxygen transport as a consequence of hypophosphatemia in patients receiving intravenous hyperalimentation. N Engl J Med 285:763, 1971
80. Prins JS, Schrijver H, Staghouwer JM: Hyperalimentation, hypophosphatemia and coma. Lancet 1:1253, 1973
81. Pampiglione G: The effect of metabolic disorders on brain activity. J Roy Coll Physicians (Lond) 7:347, 1973
82. Laidlaw J: The application in general medical conditions of a visual method of assessing and representing generalized electroencephalographic abnormalities. J Neurol Neurosurg Psychiatry 22:69, 1959
83. Engel GL, Romano J, Ferris EB, et al: A simple method of determining frequency spectra in the electroencephalogram: Observations on physiological variations in glucose, oxygen, protein and acid–base balance on the normal electroencephalogram. Arch Neurol Psychiatry 51:134, 1944
84. Losowsky MS, Scott BB: Hepatic encephalopathy. Br Med J 3:279, 1973
85. Arieff AI, Cooper JD, Armstrong D, et al: Dementia, renal failure and brain aluminum. Ann Intern Med 90:741, 1979
86. Arieff AI, Schmidt RW: Fluid and electrolyte disorders and the central nervous system. p. 1409. In Maxwell MH, Kleeman CR (eds): Clinical Disorders of Fluid and Electrolyte Metabolism. 3rd Ed. McGraw-Hill, New York, 1980
87. Sparacio RR, Anziska B, Chutta HS: Hypernatremia and chorea: A report of two cases. Neurology (New York) 26:46, 1976
88. Knochel JP: Neuromuscular manifestations of electrolyte disorders. Am J Med 72:521, 1982
89. Shils ME: Experimental human magnesium depletion. I. Clinical observations and blood chemistry alterations. Am J Clin Nutr 15:133, 1964
90. Layzer RB, Rowland LP: Cramps. N Engl J Med 285:31, 1971
91. Conn JW, Knopf RF, Nesbit RM: Primary

aldosteronism: Present evaluation of its clinical characteristics and of the results of surgery. p. 327. In Baulien EE, Robel P (eds): Aldosterone. Blackwell, Oxford, 1964
92. Jensen OB, Mosdal C, Reske-Nielsen E: Hypokalemic myopathy during treatment with diuretics. Acta Neurol Scand 55:465, 1977
93. Pollen RH, Williams RH: Hyperkalemic neuromyopathy in Addison's disease. N Engl J Med 263:273, 1960
94. Pearson CM, Kalyanaraman K: The periodic paralysis: Hyperkalemic periodic paralysis. p. 1192. In Stanbury JB, Wyngaarden JB, Fredickson DS (eds): The Metabolic Basis of Inherited Disease. 3rd Ed. McGraw-Hill, New York, 1972
95. Buruma OJS, Schipperheyn JJ: Periodic paralysis. p. 147. In Vinken PJ, Bruyn GW (eds): Handbook of Clinical Nephrology. Elsevier/North-Holland Amsterdam, 1979
96. Lotz M, Zisman E, Bartter FC: Evidence for a phosphorus-depletion syndrome in man. N Engl J Med 278:409, 1968
97. Parfitt AM, Leerekoper M: Clinical disorders of calcium, phosphorus, and magnesium metabolism. p. 947. In Maxwell MH, Kleeman CR (eds): Clinical Disorders of Fluid and Electrolyte Metabolism. 3rd Ed. McGraw-Hill, New York, 1980
98. Weintraub MI: Hypophosphatemia mimicking acute Guillain-Barré Strohl syndrome: A complication of parenteral hyperalimentation. JAMA 235:1040, 1976
99. Newman JH, Neff TA, Ziporin P: Acute respiratory failure associated with hypophosphatemia. N Engl J Med 296:1101, 1977
100. Furlan AJ, Hanson M, Cooperman A, Farmer RG: Acute areflexic paralysis: Association with hyperalimentation and hypophosphatemia. Arch Neurol 32:706, 1975
101. Randall RE, Cohen MD, Spray CC: Hypermagnesemia in renal failure. Ann Intern Med 61:73, 1964
102. Freeman RM, Lawton RL, Chamberlain MA: Hard-water syndrome. N Engl J Med 276:1113, 1967
103. Aikawa JK: Magnesium: Its Biologic Significance. CRC Press, Boca Raton, FL, 1981
104. Dubois GD, Arieff AI: Symptomatic hyponatremia: The case for rapid correction. In Narins R (ed): Controversies in Nephrology and Hyptertension. Churchill Livingstone, New York, 1984, p 393
105. Aurbach GD, Marx SJ, Spiegel AM: Parathyroid hormone, calcitonin, and the calciferols. p. 922. In Williams RH (ed): Textbook of Endocrinology. 6th Ed. WB Saunders, Philadelphia, 1981
106. Riddick FA: Primary hyperthyroidism. Med Clin North Am 81:871, 1967
107. Patten BM, Bilezikian JP, Mallette LE, et al: Neuromuscular disease in primary hyperparathyroidism. Ann Intern Med 80:182, 1974
108. Madias NE, Cohen JJ: Respiratory acidosis. p. 307. In Cohen JJ, Kassirer JP (eds): Acid–Base. Little, Brown, Boston, 1982
109. Mallette LE, Bilezikian JP, Heath DA, et al: Primary hyperparathyroidism: Clinical and biochemical features. Medicine (Baltimore) 53:127, 1974
110. Bartter FC: The parathyroid gland and its relationship to diseases of the nervous system. J Nerv Ment Dis 32:1, 1953
111. Zeluff GW, Suki WN, Jackson D: Depletion of body phosphate—Ubiquitous, subtle, and dangerous. Heart Lung 6:519, 1977
112. Epstein FH: Signs and symptoms of electrolyte disorders. p. 499. In Maxwell MH, Kleeman CR (eds): Clinical Disorders of Fluid and Electrolyte Metabolism. McGraw-Hill, New York, 1980
113. Smith WO: Magnesium deficiency in the surgical patient. Am J Cardiol 13:667, 1963
114. Hunter D, Turnbull HM: Hyperparathyroidism: Generalized osteitis fibrosa. Br J Surg 19:203, 1931
115. Simpson JA: Aphonia and deafness in hyperparathyroidism. Br Med J 1:494, 1954
116. Warwick OH, Yendt ER, Olin JS: The clinical features of hypercalcemia associated with malignant disease. Can Med Assoc J 85:719, 1961
117. Karpati G, Frame B: Neuropsychiatric disorders in primary hyperparathyroidism: Clinical analysis with review of the literature. Arch Neurol 10:387, 1964
118. Anspach WE, Clifton WM: Hyperparathyroidism in children. Am J Dis Child 58:540, 1939
119. Hines JR, Suker JR: Some unusual manifestations of parathyroid disease. Surg Clin North Am 53:221, 1973

120. Scott JC, Welch JS, Berman IB: Water intoxication and sodium depletion in surgical patients. Obstet Gynecol 26:168, 1965
121. Aurbach GD, Potts JT: The parathyroids. Adv Metab Dis 1:45, 1964
122. Saul RF, Selhorst JB: Downbeat nystagmus with magnesium depletion. Arch Neurol 38:650, 1981
123. DeGowin EL, DeGowin RL: Bedside Diagnostic Examination. 3rd Ed. Macmillan, New York, 1976
124. Smith WO, Hammarsten JF, Eliel LP: The clinical expression of magnesium deficiency. JAMA 174:159, 1960
125. Kugelberg E: Neurologic mechanism for certain phenomena in tetany. Arch Neurol Psychiatry 56:507, 1946
126. Okel BB, Hurst JW: Prolonged hyperventilation in man. Arch Intern Med 108:157, 1961
127. Saltzman HA, Heyman A, Sieker HO: Correlation of clinical and physiologic manifestations of sustained hyperventilation. N Engl J Med 268:1431, 1963
128. Fourman P: Experimental observations on the tetany of potassium deficiency. Lancet 2:525, 1954
129. Whang R, Welt LG: Observations in experimental magnesium depletion. J Clin Invest 42:305, 1963
130. Robson WL, Arbus GS, Balfe JW: Bartter's syndrome: Differentiation into two clinical groups. Am J Dis Child 133:636, 1979
131. Wacker WEC, Moore FD, Ulmer DD, et al: Normocalcemic magnesium deficiency tetany. JAMA 180:161, 1962
132. Partanen VSJ, Soininen H, Saksa M, et al: Electromyographic and nerve conduction findings in a patient with neuromyotonia, normocalcemic tetany and small-cell lung cancer. Acta Neurol Scand 61:216, 1980
133. Simpson JA: The neurological manifestations of idiopathic hypoparathyroidism. Brain 75:76, 1952
134. Dimich A, Bedrossian PB, Wallach S: Hypoparathyroidism: Clinical observations in 34 patients. Arch Intern Med 120:449, 1967
135. Burckhardt P, Tscholl-Ducommun J, Ruedi B: Parathyroid response to EDTA in hypoparathyroidism and in tetany. Acta Endocrinol (Copenh) 94:346, 1980
136. Agus ZS, Goldfarb S, Wasserstein A: Disorders of calcium and phosphate balance. p. 940. In Brenner BM, Rector FC Jr (eds): The Kidney 2nd Ed. Vol. 1. WB Saunders, Philadelphia, 1981
137. Knowles HC Jr: Hypernatremia. Metabolism 5:508, 1956
138. Ross EJ, Christie SBM: Hypernatremia. Medicine (Baltimore) 48:441, 1969
139. Finberg L: Hypernatremic (hypertonic) dehydration in infants. N Engl J Med 289:196, 1973
140. Forster HV, Dempsey JA: Ventilatory adaptations. p. 845. In Hornbein TF (ed): Regulation of Breathing. Part 2. Marcel Dekker, New York, 1981
141. Lahiri S, Gelfand R: Mechanisms of acute ventilatory responses. p. 773. In Hornbein TF (ed): Regulation of Breathing. Part 2. Marcel Dekker, New York, 1981
142. Ferdinandus J, Pederson JA, Whang R: Hypermagnesemia as a cause of refractory hypotension, respiratory depression, and coma. Arch Intern Med 141:669, 1981
143. Ehlers SM, Petzel RA, Brown DC, et al: Ventilatory response in lactic acidosis and diabetic ketoacidosis. Min Elect Metab 3:200, 1980
144. Harrington JT, Cohen JJ. Metabolic acidosis. p. 121. In Cohen JJ, Kassirer JP (eds): Acid–Base. Little, Brown, Boston, 1982
145. Potter JD, Robertson SP, Johnson JD: Magnesium and the regulation of muscle contraction. Fed Proc 40:2653, 1981
145a. Alexander PE (ed): Electrolytes and Neuropsychiatric Disorders. SP Books, New York, 1981
146. Mann TP: Transient choreo-athetosis following hypernatremia. Dev Med Child Neurol 11:637, 1969
147. Refsum HE: Relationship between state of consciousness and arterial hypoxaemia and hypercapnia in patients with pulmonary insufficiency breathing air. Clin Sci 25:361, 1963
148. Welt LG, Gitelman HJ: Disorders of magnesium metabolism. DM 1(5):1, 1965
149. Wacker WEC, Parisi AF: Magnesium metabolism. N Engl J Med 278:658, 1968
150. Mitchell W, Feldman F: Neuropsychiatric aspects of hypokalemia. Can Med Assoc J 98:49, 1968
151. McCance RA: Experimental sodium chlo-

ride deficiency in man. Proc R Soc Lond [Biol] 119:245, 1936
152. Alveryd A, Bostrom H, Wengle B, et al: Indications for surgery in the elderly patient with primary hyperparathyroidism. Acta Chir Scand 142:491, 1976
153. Rookus P, Speelman JJ: Psychiatric disturbances in hyperparathyroidism. Psychiatr Neurochir 64:46, 1961
154. Agras S, Oliveau DC: Primary hyperparathyroidism and psychosis. Can Med Assoc J 91:1366, 1964
155. Aurbach GD, Mallette LE, Patten BM, et al: Hyperparathyroidism: Recent studies. Ann Intern Med 79:566, 1973
156. Hockaday TDR, Keyne WM, McKenzie JK: Catatonic stupor in elderly women with hyperparathyroidism. Br Med J 1:85, 1966
157. Reinfrank RF: primary hyperparathyroidism with depression. Arch Intern Med 108: 606, 1961
158. Anderson J: Psychiatric aspects of primary hyperparathyroidism. Proc R Soc Biol Med 61:1123, 1968
159. Noble P: Depressive illness and hyperparathyroidism. Proc R Soc Med 67:1066, 1974
160. Fourman P, Davis RH, Jones KH, et al: Parathyroid insufficiency after thyroidectomy. Br J Surg 50:608, 1963
161. Fourman P, Rawnsley K, Davis RH, et al: Effect of calcium on mental symptoms in partial parathyroid insufficiency. Lancet 2: 914, 1967
162. Burnell GM, Foster TA: Psychosis with low sodium syndrome. Am J Psychiatry 128: 1313, 1972
163. Gehi MM, Rosenthal RH, Fizette NB, et al: Psychiatric manifestations of hyponatremia. Psychosomatics 22:739, 1981
164. Denko JD, Kaelbling R: The psychiatric aspects of hypoparathyroidism. Acta Psychiatr Scand 38(Suppl 164):1, 1962
165. Jefferson JW, Marshall JR: Neuropsychiatric Features of Medical Disorders. Plenum, New York, 1981
166. Kreisberg RA: Phosphorus deficiency and hypophosphatemia. Hosp Pract 12:121, 1977
167. McCance RA, Young WF: The secretion of urine during dehydration and rehydration. J Physiol (Lond) 102:415, 1944
168. Aurbach GD, Potts JT Jr: The parathyroids. p. 45. In Levine R, Luft R (eds): Advances in Metabolic Disorders. Vol. 1. Academic Press, New York, 45, 1964
169. Lehrer GM, Levitt MF: Neuropsychiatric presentation of hypercalcemia. Mt Sinai J Med 27:10, 1960
170. Knochel JP: Role of glucoregulatory hormones in potassium homeostasis. Kidney Int 1:443, 1977
171. Waites TF: Hyperventilation—chronic and acute. Arch Intern Med 138:1700, 1978
172. Victor M: The role of hypomagnesemia and respiratory alkalosis in the genesis of alcohol-withdrawal symptoms. Ann NY Acad Sci 215:235, 1973
173. Allen TE, Agus B: Hyperventilation leading to hallucinations. Am J Psychiatry 125:632, 1968
174. Haddy FJ, Scott JB, Florio MA, et al: Local vascular effects of hyperkalemia, alkalosis, hypercalcemia, and hypomagnesemia. Am J Physiol 204:202, 1963
175. Haddy FJ: The role of potassium ions in regulating vascular resistance. Adv Microcirc 11:43, 1982
176. Haddy FJ: Potassium deficiency and heart function. J Chron Dis 26:467, 1973
177. Baptista AG: Aspects of cerebral circulation. p. 129. In Himwich HE (ed): Brain Metabolism and Cerebral Disorders. 2nd Ed. Spectrum Publications, New York, 1976
178. Kuschinsky W: Role of hydrogen ions in regulation of cerebral blood flow and other regional flows. Adv Microcirc 11:1, 1982
179. Gennari FJ, Kassirer JP: Respiratory alkalosis. p. 349. In Cohen JJ, Kassirer JP (eds): Acid–Base. Little, Brown, Boston, 1982
180. Harvey RM, Enson Y, Lewis ML, et al: Hemodynamic effects of dehydration and metabolic acidosis in asiatic cholera. Trans Assoc Am Physicians 79:177, 1966
181. Harvey RM, Enson Y, Lewis ML, et al: Hemodynamic studies on cholera. Effects of hypovolemia and acidosis. Circulation 37:709, 1968
182. Greenough WB III, Hirschhorn N, Gordon RS, Jr, et al: Pulmonary oedema associated with acidosis in patients with cholera. Trop Geogr Med 28:86, 1976
183. Mitchell JH, Wildenthal K, Johnson RL Jr: The effects of acid–base disturbances on cardiovascular and pulmonary function. Kidney Int 1:375, 1972

184. Betz E, Enzenross HG, Vlahov V: Interaction of H^+, Na, Ca^{++} in the regulation of local pial vascular resistance. Pfluegers Arch 343:79, 1973
185. Weiss GB: Calcium and contractibility in vascular smooth muscle. p. 71. In Narahas T, Bianchi CP (eds): Advances in General and Cellular Pharmacology. Plenum, New York, 1977
186. Altura BT: Influence of calcium ions on microvascular permeability, contractility and reactivity. Adv Microcirc 11:62, 1982
187. Sutter MC, Hallback M, Jones JV, et al: Contractile responses to noradrenaline: Varying dependence on external calcium of consecutive vascular segments of perfused rat hind quarters. Acta Physiol Scand 99:166, 1977
188. Shackney SE, Hasson J: Precipitons fall in serum calcium, hypotension, and acute renal failure after intravenous phosphate therapy for hypercalcemia. Ann Intern Med 66:906, 1967
189. Zawada EI Jr, Brickman AS, Maxwell MH, et al: Hypertension associated with hyperparathyroidism is not responsive to angiotension blockage. J Clin Endocrinol Metab 50:912, 1980
190. Haddy FJ: Local effect of sodium, calcium and magnesium upon small and large blood vessels of the dog forelimb. Circ Res 8:57, 1960
191. Frohlich ED, Scott JB, Haddy FJ: Effect of cations on resistance and reponsiveness of renal and forelimb vascular beds. Am J Physiol 203:583, 1962
192. Overbeck HW, Molnar JI, Haddy FJ: Resistance to blood flow through the vascular bed of the dog forelimb. Am J Cardiol 7:533, 1961
193. Hinke JAM, Wilson ML, Burnham SC: Calcium and the contractility of arterial smooth muscle. Am J Physiol 106:211, 1964
194. Scheidegger D, Lambertus JD, Schellenberg JC: Role of the systemic vasculature in the hemodynamic response to changes in plasma ionized calcium. Arch Surg 115:206, 1980
195. Weidmann P, Massry SG, Coburn JW, et al: Blood pressure effects of acute hypercalcemia. Ann Intern Med 76:740, 1972
196. Zawada ET Jr, Bennett EP, Stinson JB et al: Serum calcium in blood pressure regulation during dialysis. Arch Intern Med 141:657, 1981
197. Rosenthal FD, Roy S: Hypertension and hyperparathyroidism. Br Med J 4:396, 1972
198. Christenson T, Hellstrom K, Wengle B: Blood pressure in subjects with hypercalcemia and primary hyperparathyroidism detected in a health screening programme. Eur J Clin Invest 7:109, 1977
199. Kleerekoper M, Rao DS, Frame B: Hypercalcemia, hyperparathyroidism and hypertension. Cardiovasc Med 3:1283, 1978
200. Heath H III, Hodgson SF, Kennedy MA: Primary hyperparathyroidism. N Engl J Med 302:189, 1980
201. Altura BM: Magnesium and regulation of contractility of vascular smooth muscle. Adv Microcirc 11:77, 1982
202. Lim P, Jacob E: Magnesium status of alcoholic patients. Metabolism 21:1045, 1972
203. Dagirmanjian R, Goldman H: Magnesium deficiency and distribution of blood in the rat. Am J Physiol 218:1464, 1970
204. Haddy FJ, Scott JB: Mechanism of the acute pressor action of hypokalemia, hypomagnesemia, and hypo-osmolality. Am Heart J 85:655, 1973
205. Mordes JP, Swartz R, Arky RA: Extreme hypermagnesemia as a cause of refractory hypotension. Ann Intern Med 83:657, 1975
206. Valencic F, Dodich BN, Hill OA Jr, et al: Arterial-venous magnesium gradients in hypovolemic shock: An indication of the irreversible state. Proc Soc Exp Biol Med 150:660, 1975
207. Kreye VAW, Ziegler FW: Anions and vascular smooth muscle function. Adv Microcirc 11:114, 1982
208. Betz E, Heuser D: Actions and interactions of cations and anions on pial arteries. p. 71. In Cervos-Navarro J et al. (Eds): Advances in Neurology. Vol. 20. Raven Press, New York, 1978
209. Betz E, Karlitzky G, Heuser D: The effect of pial perivascular chloride on the diameters of small pial arteries. Acta Neurol Scand 56(suppl 64): 390, 1977
210. Fleckenstein A: Specific pharmacology of calcium in myocardial, cardiac pacemakers and vascular smooth muscle. Annu Rev Pharmacol 17:149, 1977
211. Yasne H, Nagao M, Omote S, et al: Coronary

arterial spasm and Prinzmetal's variant form of angina induced by hyperventilation and Tris-buffer infusion. Circulation 58:56, 1978
212. Neill WA, Hattenhauer M: Impairment of myocardial O_2 supply due to hyperventilation. Circulation 52:854, 1975
213. Rowe GG, Castillo CA, Crumpton CA: Effects of hyperventilation on systemic and coronary hemodynamics. Am Heart J 63:67, 1962
214. Wilson JR, Goldberg S, Hirshfeld JW, et al: Effects of respiratory alkalosis on coronary vascular dynamics and myocardial energetics in patients with coronary artery disease. Am Heart J 102:202, 1981
215. Shiner PT, Harris WS, Weissler AM: Effects of acute changes in serum calcium levels on the systolic time intervals in man. Am J Cardiol 24:42, 1969
216. Falko JM, Bush CA, Tzagournis M, et al: Congestive heart failure complicating the hungry bone syndrome. Am J Med Sci 271:85, 1976
217. Giles TD, Iteld BJ, Rives KL: The cardiomyopathy of hypoparathyroidism. Chest 79: 225, 1981
218. Connor TB, Rosen BI, Blaustein MP, et al: Hypocalcemia precipitating congestive heart failure. N Engl J Med 307:869, 1982
219. O'Connor LR, Wheeler WS, Bethune JE. Effect of hypophosphatemia on myocardial performance in man. N Engl J Med 297:901, 1977
220. Fuller TJ, Nichols WW, Brenner BJ, et al: Reversible depression in myocardial performance in dogs with experimental phosphorus deficiency. J Clin Invest 62:1194, 1978
221. Wildenthal K, Mierzwiak DS, Myers RW, et al: Effects of acute lactic acidosis on left ventricular performance. Am J Physiol 214: 1352, 1968
222. Williamson JR, Schaffer SW, Ford C, et al: Contribution of tissue acidosis to ischemic injury in the perfused rat heart. Circulation 33(Suppl 1):13, 1976
223. Anderson MN, Border JR, Mouritzen CV: Acidosis, catecholamines and cardiovascular dynamics: When does acidosis require correction: Ann Surg 166:344, 1967
224. Rocamora JM, Downing SE: Preservation of ventricular function by adrenergic influences during metabolic acidosis in the cat. Circ Res 24:373, 1969
225. Thrower WB, Darby TO, Aldinger EE: Acid–base derangements and myocardial contractility. Arch Surg 82:56, 1961
226. Arieff AI, Leach W, Park R, et al: Systemic effects of $NaHCO_3$ in experimental lactic cidosis in dogs. Am J Physiol 242:F586, 1982
226a. Minot AS, Dodd K, Saunders JM: The acidosis of guanidine intoxication. J Clin Invest 13:917, 1934
227. Critelli G, Ferro G, Peschle C, et al: Myocardial contractility after injection or prolonged infusion of magnesium sulfate. Acta Cardiol 32:65, 1977
228. Surawicz B: Relationship between electrocardiogram and electrolytes. Am Heart J 73:814, 1967
229. VanderArk CR, Ballantyne F III, Reynolds EW Jr: Electrolytes and the electrocardiogram. Cardiovasc Clin 5:270, 1973
230. Fisch C: Electrolytes and the heart. p. 1599. In Hurst JW (ed): The Heart. McGraw-Hill, New York, 1982
231. Crum WD, Till HJ: Hyperparathyroidism with Wenckebach's phenomenon. Am J Cardiol 6:838, 1960
232. Mordes JP, Swartz R, Arky RA: Extreme hypermagnesia as a cause of refractory hypotension. Ann Intern Med 83:657, 1975
233. Watanabe Y, Dreifus LS: Electrophysiological effects of magnesium and its interactions with potassium. Cardiovasc Res 6:79, 1972
234. Wener J, Pintar K, Simon MA, et al: The effects of prolonged hypomagnesemia on the cardiovascular system in young dogs. Am Heart J 67:221, 1964
235. Seta K, Kleiger R, Hellerstein EE, et al: Effect of potassium and magnesium deficiency on the electrocardiogram and plasma electrolytes of purebred beagles. Am J Cardiol 17:516, 1966
236. Pryor R, Blount SG: The clinical significance of true left axis deviation, left intraventricular blocks. Am Heart J 72:391, 1966
237. Ewy GA, Karliner J, Bedynek JL Jr: Electrocardiographic QRS axis shift as a manifestation of hyperkalemia. JAMA 215:429, 1971
238. Punja MM, Scheebaum R, Cohen J: Bifascicular block induced by hyperkalemia. J Electrocardiol 6:71, 1973
239. Cohen HC, Rosen KM, Pick A: Disorders of impulse conduction and impulse formation caused by hyperkalemia in man. Am Heart J 89:501, 1975

240. Bashour T, Hsu I, Gorfinkel HJ, et al: Atrioventricular and intraventricular conduction in hyperkalemia. Am J Cardiol 35:199, 1975
241. Randall RE, Cohen MD, Spray CC: Hypermagnesemia in renal failure. Ann Intern Med 61:73, 1974
242. Surawicz B, Braun HA, Crum WB, et al: Quantitative analysis of the electrocardiographic pattern of hypopotassemia. Circulation 16:750, 1957
243. Bronsky D, Dubin A, Waldstein SS, et al: Calcium and the electrocardiogram. II. The electrocardiographic manifestations of hyperparathyroidism and of marked hypercalcemia. Am J Cardiol 1:833, 1961
244. Ginsberg H, Schwartz KV: Hypercalcemia and complete heart block. Ann Intern Med 79:903, 1973
245. Langer GA: The intrinsic control of myocardial contraction–ionic factors. N Engl J Med 285:1065, 1971
246. MacDonald FM, Simson E: Human ECG during and after inhalation of 30% CO_2. J Appl Physiol 6:304, 1953
247. Kleeman K, Singh BN: Serum electrolytes and the heart. p. 145. In Maxwell MH, Kleeman CR (eds): Clinical Disorders of Fluid and Electrolyte Metabolism. 3rd Ed. McGraw-Hill, New York, 1980
248. Burch GE, Giles TD: The importance of magnesium deficiency in cardiovascular disease. Am Heart J 94:649, 1977
249. Caddell JL: The effect of magnesium therapy on cardiovascular changes in severe protein-calorie malnutrition. Trop Geograph Med 21:33, 1969
250. Evans W: Alcoholic cardiomyopathy. Am Heart J 61:556, 1961
251. Vitale JJ, Hellerstein EE, Nakamura M, et al: Effects of magnesium-deficient diet upon puppies. Circ Res 9:387, 1961
252. Seelig MS: Electrocardiographic patterns of magnesium depletion in alcoholic heart disease. Ann NY Acad Sci 162:902, 1969
253. Ebert PA: Relationship of myocardial potassium content and atrial fibrillation. Circulation 41(Suppl II):137, 1970
254. Olsson SB: Nature of cardiac arrhythmias and electrolyte disturbances. Acta Med Scand (Suppl)647:33, 1981
255. Chadda KD, Lichstein E, Gupta P: Hypomagnesemia and refractory cardiac arrhythmia in a nondigitalized patient. Am J Cardiol 31:98, 1973
256. Iseri LT, Freed J, Bures AR: Magnesium deficiency and cardiac disorders. Am J Med 58:837, 1975
257. Ayres SM, Grace WJ: Inappropriate ventilation and hypoxemia as causes of cardiac arrhythmias. Am J Med 46:495, 1969
258. Lawson NW, Butler GH III, Ray CT: Alkalosis and cardiac arrhythmias. Anesth. Anal 52:951, 1973
259. Dyckner T, Wester PO: Ventricular extrasystoles and intracellular electrolytes before and after potassium and magnesium infusions in patients on diuretic treatment. Am Heart J 97:12, 1979
260. Walter PE: Arrhythmias related to abnormal repolarization. p. 305. In Hurst JW (ed): The Heart. McGraw-Hill, New York, 1979
261. Bronsky D, Dubin A, Waldstein SS, et al: Calcium and the electrocardiogram. II. The electrocardiographic manifestations of hyperparathyroidism and marked hypercalcemia from various etiologies. Am J Cardiol 7:833, 1961
262. Kambara H, Iteld BJ, Phillips J: Hypocalcemia and intractable ventricular fibrillation. Ann Intern Med 86:583, 1977
263. Rogers RM, Spear JF, Moore EN, et al: Vulnerability of canine ventricle to fibrillation during hypoxia and respiratory acidosis. Chest 63:986, 1973
264. Duke M: Thiazide-induced hypokalemia: Association with acute myocardial infarction and ventricular fibrillation. JAMA 239:43, 1978
265. Pick A: Arrhythmias and potassium in man. Am Heart J 72:295, 1966
266. Dyckner T: Serum magnesium in acute myocardial infarction. Acta Med Scand 207:59, 1980
267. Perez GO, Oster JR, Vaamonde CA: Serum potassium concentration in acidemic states. Nephron 27:233, 1981
268. Adrogue HJ, Madias NE: Changes in plasma potassium concentration during acute acid–base disturbances. Am J Med 71:456, 1981
269. Shields HM: Rapid fall of serum phosphorus secondary to antacid therapy. Gastroenterology 75:1137, 1978
270. Rude RK, Singer FR: Magnesium deficiency and excess. Annu Rev Med 32:245, 1981
271. Lemann J, Donatelli AA: Calcium intoxica-

tion due to primary hyperparathyroidism. Ann Intern Med 60:447, 1964
271a. Rosen RA, Leach W, Arieff A: Central nervous system dysfunction and hypophosphatemia. Kidney Int 12:460, 1977
271b. Gold SW, Massry SG, Arieff AI, et al: Renal bicarbonate wasting during phosphate depletion: A possible cause of altered acid–base homeostasis in hyperparathyroidism. J Clin Invest 52:2556, 1973
272. Albright F, Reifenstein EC Jr: The Parathyroid Glands and Metabolic Bone Disease. Williams & Wilkins, Baltimore, 1948
273. Flink EB: Dysphagia in magnesium deficiency. (Editorial.) Ann Intern Med 89:282, 1978
274. Henrikson HW: Effect of potassium deficiency on gastrointestinal motility in rats. Am J Physiol 164:263, 1951
275. Schuster MM: Megacolon in adults. p. 1812. In Sleisenger MH and Fordtran JS (eds): Gastrointestinal Disease. 2nd Ed. WB Saunders, Philadelphia, 1978
276. Sokal MM, Koenigsberger MR, Rose JS, et al: Neonatal hypermagnesemia and the meconium-plug syndrome. N Engl J Med 286:823, 1972
277. Clarkson B, Kowlessar OD, Horwith M, et al: Clinical and metabolic study of a patient with malabsorption and hypoparathyroidism. Metabolism 9:1093, 1960
278. Jackson WPU: Steatorrhea and hypoparathyroidism. (Letter to the editor.) Lancet 1:1086, 1957
279. Snodgrass RW, Mellinkoff SM: Idiopathic hypoparathyroidism with small bowel x-ray features of sprue, without steatorrhea. Am J Dig Dis 7:273, 1962
280. Barreras RF: Calcium and gastric secretion. Gastroenterology 64:1168, 1973
281. Christiansen J: Primary hyperparathyroidism and peptic ulcer disease. Scand J Gastroenterol 9:111, 1974
282. Goebell H: The role of calcium in pancreatic secretion and disease. Acta Hepatogastroenterol (Stuttg) 23:151, 1976
283. Engel JJ, Bischel MD: Acute pancreatitis and kidney disease. Dialy Trans 10:817, 1981
284. Jacob HS, Amsden T: Acute hemolytic anemia with rigid red cells in hypophosphatemia. N Engl J Med 285:1446, 1971
285. Klock JC, Williams HE, Mentzer WC: Hemolytic anemia and somatic cell dysfunction in severe hypophosphatemia. Arch Intern Med 134:360, 1974
286. Yawata Y, Hebbel RP, Silvis S, et al: Blood cell abnormalities complicating the hypophosphatemia of hyperalimentation: Erythrocytes and platelet ATP deficiency associated with hemolytic anemia and bleeding in hyperalimented dogs. J Lab Clin Med 84:643, 1974
287. Lichtman MA, Miller DR, Freeman RB: Erythrocyte adenosine triphosphate depletion during hypophosphatemia in an uremic subject. N Engl J Med 280:240, 1969
288. Fitzgerald F: Hypophosphatemia. Adv Intern Med 23:137, 1978
289. Jacob HS: Severe hypophosphatemia: A previously ignored cause of cellular dysfunction. West J Med 122:501, 1975
290. Craddock PR, Yawata Y, Van Santen L: Acquired phagocyte dysfunction: A complication of the hypohosphatemia of parenteral hyperalimentation. N Engl J Med 290:1403, 1974
291. Garner GB, Heubner PR, O'Dell BL: Dietary phosphorus and salmonellosis in guinea pigs. Proc Am Soc Exp Biol 26:799, 1967
292. Thomas HM, Lefrak SS, Irwin RS, et al: The oxyhemoglobin dissociation curve in health and disease. Role of 2,3-diphosphoglycerate. Am J Med 57:331, 1974
293. Lichtman MA, Miller DR, Cohen J, et al: Reduced red cell glycolysis, 2,3-diphosphoglycerate and adenosine triphosphate concentration, and increased hemoglobin oxygen affinity caused by hypophosphatemia. Ann Intern Med 74:562, 1971
294. Anderson RJ, Rose CE, Berns AS, et al: Mechanism of effect of hypercapnic acidosis on renin secretion in the dog. Am J Physiol 238:F119, 1980
295. Massry SG: Disorders of magnesium metabolism. p. 1639. In Earley LE and Gottschalk CW (eds): Strauss and Welt's Diseases of the Kidney. 3rd Ed Little, Brown, Boston, 1979
296. Levi J, Massry SG, Coburn JW, et al: Hypocalcemia in magnesium depleted dogs. Metabolism 23:323, 1974

24

Drugs and Water Metabolism

Arnold M. Moses
Stanley A. Blumenthal
David H.P. Streeten

Many drugs commonly used in the practice of medicine enhance or inhibit the excretion of free water. These drugs may act either by altering antidiuretic hormone release or its action on the renal tubule. Other drugs may alter water excretion by producing changes in renal function not mediated by antidiuretic hormone. This chapter reviews the clinically important pharmacologic actions of drugs that alter the excretion of free water by actions mediated at least in part via alterations in antidiuretic hormone release.

SULFONYLUREAS

The antidiuretic action of chlorpropamide is like that of antidiuretic hormone, since it usually occurs without a fall in glomerular filtration rate or osmolal clearance. The antidiuretic action of chlorpropamide in patients with diabetes insipidus is proportionate to the patient's ability to liberate antidiuretic hormone in response to dehydration.[1] Additional evidence for the role of endogenous antidiuretic hormone is derived from observations that ethanol and diphenylhydantoin, both inhibitors of antidiuretic hormone release, overcome the antidiuretic action of chlorpropamide.[1,2] The antidiuresis caused by chlorpropamide occurs even in the water-loaded condition[1] and therefore does not occur through a decrease in water intake.

Chlorpropamide has no antidiuretic effect in patients with nephrogenic diabetes insipidus, in the Brattleboro rat,[3] or in the toad bladder in vitro.[4] However, it enhances the action of arginine vasopressin in the toad bladder,[4,5] as well as in rats,[3,6] dogs,[7] and humans.[8,9] A similar augmentation by chlorpropamide occurs in the homozygous Brattleboro rat (di/di) injected with the nonpressor vasopressin analogue 1-desamino-8-D-Arginine vasopressin, also called desmopressin.[10] The latter phenomenon is associated with an enhanced activation of renal medullary adenylate cyclase activity by dDAVP in renal medullary membranes of rats treated with chlorpropamide (Fig. 24–1). The increased adenylate cyclase activity together with an unchanged phosphodiesterase activity results in increased renal medullary cyclic adenosine monophosphate (cAMP) content[10] Fig. 24–2), presumably causing increased hydroosmotic effect of vasopressin. Further studies have demonstrated that in vivo chlorpropamide significantly lowers the Michaelis constant (K_m) for adenosine triphosphate (ATP).[11,12] Since

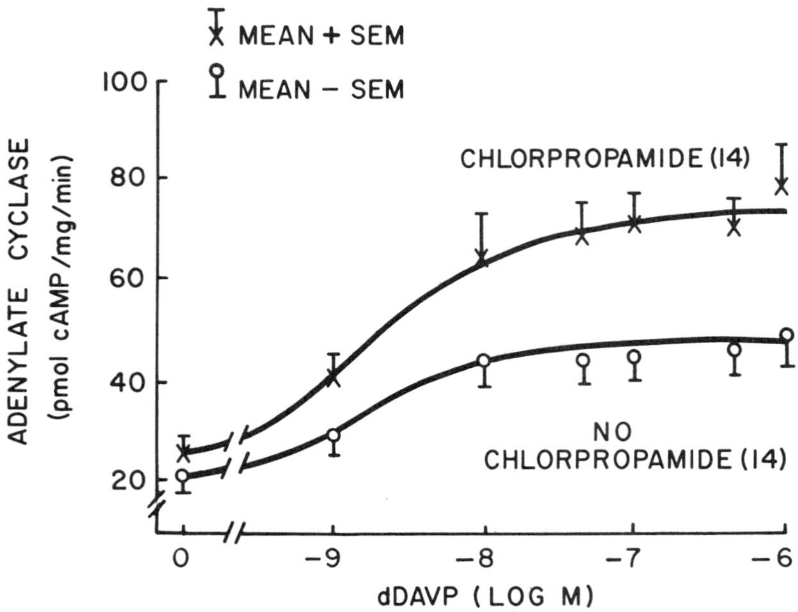

Fig. 24–1. Dose response of adenylate cyclase activity to dDAVP stimulation in renal medullary cell membrane preparations obtained from Brattleboro DI rats, either untreated or treated with chlorpropamide. Enzyme activity was significantly increased by the drug. (From Moses AM, Coulson R: Augmentation by chlorpropamide of dDAVP-induced antidiuresis and stimulation of renal medullary adenylate cyclase and accumulation of cyclic AMP. Endocrinology 106:967, 1980. © 1980 The Williams & Wilkins Co., Baltimore.)

there is a vasopressin-sensitive adenylate cyclase in both the mammalian collecting tubule and the thick ascending limb of the loop of Henle,[13] the effect of in vivo chlorpropamide on enhancing vasopressin-stimulated adenylate cyclase activity and on lowering the K_m for ATP could occur at either or both loci. Preliminary evidence suggests that the chlorpropamide effect on the cAMP response to vasopressin is in the medullary thick ascending limb of the loop of Henle.[14] Such an action might enhance medullary hypertonicity and thus augment the antidiuretic response to vasopressin. Since all these actions were observed only in vivo, they may be indirect, perhaps via a metabolite.

The in vitro addition of chlorpropamide to the toad bladder inhibits vasopressin-stimulated prostaglandin synthesis.[15] This action was proposed as the mechanism for the chlorpropamide-induced enhancement of water flow in response to vasopressin. In contrast, we have shown that the injection of chlorpropamide in rats with diabetes insipidus significantly augments the urinary prostaglandin E_2 (PGE_2) response to dDAVP.[12] Since our experiments indicate that in vivo chlorpropamide augments the responses of both rat renal cAMP and prostaglandin systems to stimulation by dDAVP, and since the biochemical pathways for the cAMP and PGE_2 systems are different, converging only at the hormone receptor site, we believe that in vivo chlorpropamide acts at the receptor of the vasopressin-sensitive part of the tubule to augment the action of vasopressin. A receptor locus of action is supported by the observation that activation of adenylate cyclase by postreceptor stimuli is not altered by in vivo chlorpropamide.[10]

Studies on the isolated perfused kidneys of homozygous Brattleboro rats were conducted

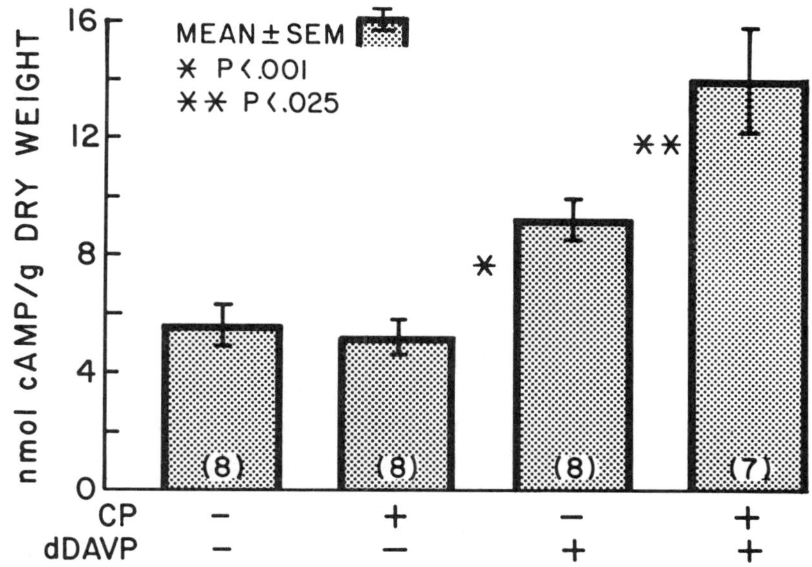

Fig. 24–2. Renal cAMP concentration of isolated perfused Brattleboro rat kidneys in the presence and absence of dDAVP and chlorpropamide. Chlorpropamide treatment alone had no effect, but it significantly enhanced the response to dDAVP. (From Moses AM, Coulson R: Augmentation by chlorpropamide of dDAVP-induced antidiuresis and stimulation of renal medullary adenylate cyclase and accumulation of cyclic AMP. Endocrinology 106:967, 1980. © 1980 The Williams & Wilkins Co., Baltimore.)

to determine whether in vivo chlorpropamide augments the vascular responses to antivasopressin. Chlorpropamide did not augment the vasoconstrictor response to arginine vasopressin and, in fact, the drug interfered with the arginine vasopressin-induced decrease in glomerular filtration rate.[11]

In addition to the overwhelming evidence for the peripheral augmentation of antidiuretic hormone by chlorpropamide, we believe that chlorpropamide stimulates the release of arginine vasopressin. Chlorpropamide increases the amount of radioimmunoassayable arginine vasopressin in the urine of water-loaded patients[8] and bioassayable antidiuretic hormone in the plasma.[16] In contrast, others have found no increase in plasma arginine vasopressin or neurophysin levels during chlorpropamide treatment.[17] Nevertheless, there is indirect evidence for an effect of chlorpropamide on vasopressin release. For instance, tolazamide has a diuretic action in water-loaded normal subjects and cirrhotics,[18] while it augments the action of dDAVP both in patients and in rats with diabetes insipidus. It does not increase urinary AVP excretion in hydrated patients.

Next, a central action is suggested by the observation that damage to the hypothalamic–pituitary axis appears to sensitize humans and rats to the action of chlorpropamide. The effect of chlorpropamide is greater in hydrated patients with diabetes insipidus than in normal subjects[8] (Fig. 24–3), and chlorpropamide exerts a greater antidiuretic action in stalk-sectioned rats than in intact rats.[19] Last, a central mode of action of chlorpropamide is supported by the restoration of normal drinking behavior in patients with hypodipsia.[20]

There are numerous reports of patients with diabetes mellitus, treated with chlorpropamide, in whom water retention and hyponatremia developed.[21–24] Chlorpropamide may even induce symptomatic hyponatremia in patients

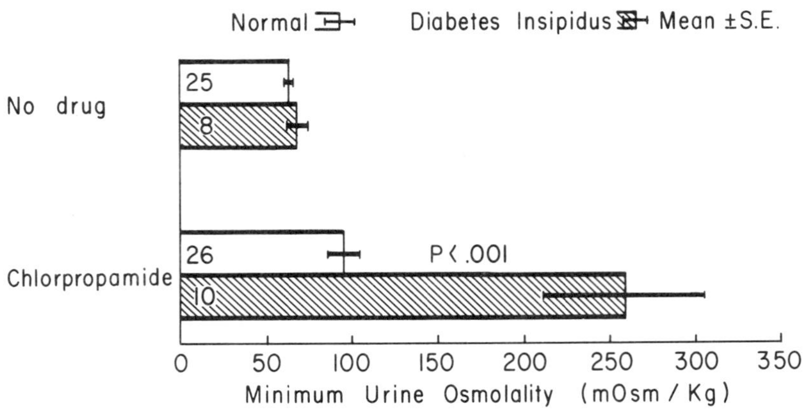

Fig. 24–3. Effect of chlorpropamide on the minimum urine osmolality obtained during a maintained water load in normal subjects and patients with diabetes insipidus. Without drug therapy, both groups diluted equally. On chlorpropamide, the diabetes insipidus patients had a decreased ability to dilute the urine. (From Moses AM, Numann P, Miller N: Mechanism of chlorpropamide-induced antidiuresis in man: Evidence for the release of ADH and enhancement of peripheral action. Metabolism 22:59, 1973. © 1973 The Williams & Wilkins Co., Baltimore.)

with diabetes insipidus.[25,26] Dilutional hyponatremia in patients with diabetes mellitus treated with chlorpropamide, is more frequent when there is an underlying tendency to retain fluids, such as occurs in congestive heart failure or cirrhosis of the liver. Excessive fluid intake and diuretic therapy also aggravate the tendency for dilutional hyponatremia to develop.[26] The antidiuretic action of chlorpropamide is additive to that of carbamazepine[27] and of diuretics, and we can assume additive actions with other water-retaining drugs. The incidence of hyponatremia in chlorpropamide-treated patients with diabetes mellitus has been estimated to be 4 percent[23] to 16 percent.[28] A recent review has disclosed that the syndrome of inappropriate secretion of antidiuretic hormone is more likely to develop in elderly women in whom the dosage of chlorpropamide was recently increased.[29] Davis et al. presented evidence that chlorpropamide is more likely to produce hyponatremia in diabetics whose glucose level is well controlled.[30] The degree of water retention produced by chlorpropamide may be mild and asymptomatic or it can be life threatening. Nocturnal angina pectoris as a consequence of water retention has also been attributed to chlorpropamide.[31]

Tolbutamide usually has no effect on water metabolism. It is ineffective in the treatment of diabetes insipidus. However, dilutional hyponatremia has occasionally been reported in patients treated with tolbutamide for diabetes mellitus.[21,32-35] This is not a frequent or predictable action of the drug.

Several sulfonylurea drugs have diuretic actions in spite of the fact that, like chlorpropamide, they enhance the action of vasopressin. The diuretic sulfonylureas increase the action of vasopressin in the toad bladder.[36] Glyburide[37] and tolazamide increase the antidiuretic action of vasopressin in homozygous Brattleboro rats. There is no evidence that any of these drugs alters vasopressin release. There is evidence, however, that glyburide[37] and glipizide[38] act as proximal tubular diuretics and cause an increase in sodium absorption at the diluting sites of the distal nephron. This action results in increased free water excretion without natriuresis. It should not be surprising that some sulfonylureas have proximal tubular actions, since they are structurally related to acetazolamide, furosemide, and the thiazide diuretics.

Tolazamide, acetohexamide, glyburide, and glipizide increase free water excretion in water-loaded normal subjects.[38,39] Glyburide has a similar action in hydrated patients with diabetes mellitus[39] as well as in patients and in rats with diabetes insipidus.[39,40] In hyponatremic, edematous, cirrhotic patients, tolazamide improves the excretion of a water load.[18] In contrast, Yapp et al. found that glyburide did not have a diuretic action in a patient with the syndrome of inappropriate secretion of antidiuretic hormone (SIADH) of unknown cause.[41] We have evidence that tolazamide interferes with excretion of water in patients with SIADH due to oat cell carcinoma of the lung. Glipizide may have caused SIADH in an elderly diabetic patient.[42] It is apparent that this group of drugs usually but not always exerts a diuretic action. Antidiuresis may result from the augmented action of nonsuppressible circulating vasopressin.

CLOFIBRATE

Clofibrate (chlorphenoxyisobutyrate) has an antidiuretic action both in patients with central diabetes insipidus and in normal subjects[43-46] as well as in normal Long-Evans rats.[43] A chemically similar antilipidemic agent, halophenate, has also been reported to exert antidiuretic action in a patient with central diabetes insipidus.[47] Clofibrate has no intrinsic antidiuretic action. It is ineffective in the homozygous Brattleboro rat,[43,48] and it does not cause water retention in patients with nephrogenic diabetes insipidus.[49,50] The antidiuretic action of clofibrate in patients with diabetes insipidus is proportional to the patient's ability to release AVP during dehydration (Fig. 24–4) and can be overcome by ethanol.[43] These observations support the concept that arginine vasopressin mediates the antidiuretic action of clofibrate.

Clofibrate does not augment the antidiuretic action of antidiuretic hormone in studies using the homozygous Brattleboro rat.[43,51] Nor does clofibrate potentiate the effect of antidiuretic hormone on osmotic water flow across the toad bladder.[52] Clofibrate appears to act by releasing endogenous arginine vasopressin, since it is shown to increase the amount of arginine vasopressin in the urine of hydrated normal subjects[43] (Fig. 24–5).

Although clofibrate causes weight gain in some patients with hyperlipidemia, there are no documented cases of a dilutional hyponatremic state resulting from treatment with this drug. This apparently is due to the relative resistance of normal subjects to the antidiuretic action of clofibrate. The antidiuretic action of clofibrate (2 g/day), like that of chlorpropamide, is more effective in patients with diabetes insipidus than in normal subjects.[43] In addition, it is necessary to administer 6 to 8 g clofibrate daily to produce the picture of SIADH in patients with psychogenic polydipsia.[46] This is three or four times the usual therapeutic dose used in the treatment of diabetes insipidus or hyperlipidemia.

TRICYCLIC COMPOUNDS

Carbamazepine is chemically related to the tricyclic antidepressant drugs, but its pharmacologic actions resemble those of phenytoin. Carbamazepine is the drug of choice in the treatment of trigeminal and glossopharyngeal neuralgia; it also has important anticonvulsant properties. Since the first description of the antidiuretic action of carbamazepine in 1966,[53] the drug has since been shown to have an antidiuretic action in a variety of situations, excluding nephrogenic diabetes insipidus.[49,54] Carbamazepine inhibits the excretion of a water load in normal subjects[55] and in rats.[56] The antidiuresis caused by carbamazepine is inhibited by phenytoin[57] and ethanol[58] and is additive to that of chlorpropamide[27] and clofibrate.[46] Carbamazepine has no intrinsic antidiuretic action,[56] and it does not augment the antidiuretic action of submaximal amounts of antidiuretic hormone in the toad bladder,[56,59] in rats with diabetes insipidus,[56] or

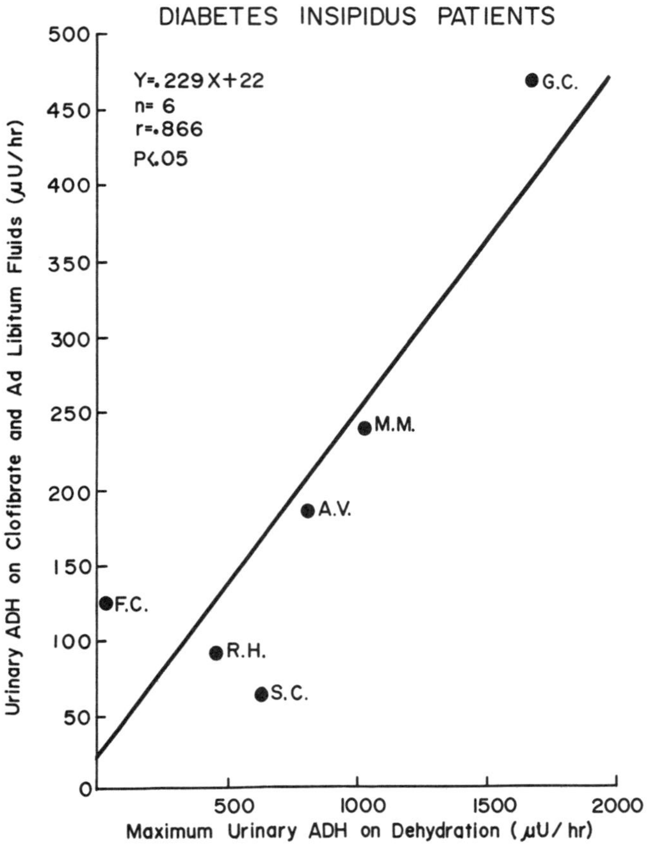

Fig. 24–4. Relationship between the maximum urinary arginine vasopressin (AVP) excretion in six patients with diabetes insipidus during a standardized dehydration procedure and the amount of AVP excreted when they were treated with clofibrate and allowed to drink ad libitum. (From Moses AM, Howanitz J, vanGemert M, et al: Clofibrate-induced antidiuresis. J Clin Invest 52:535, 1973. By permission of the American Society for Clinical Investigation.)

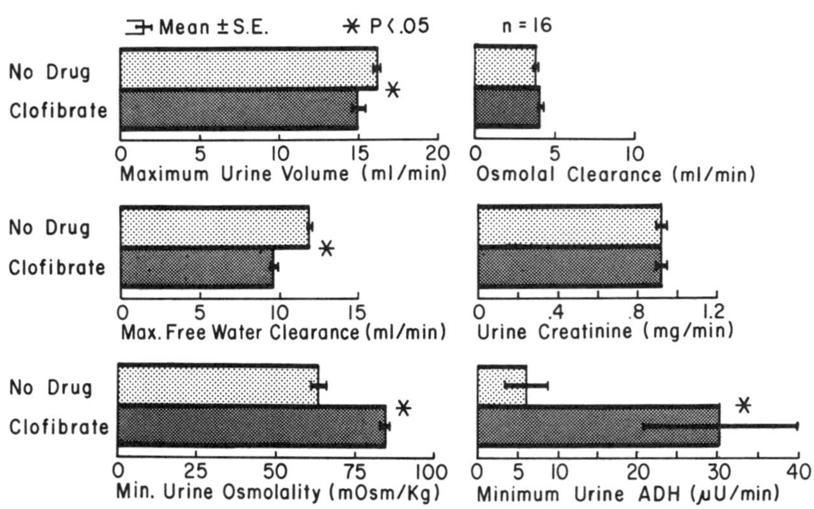

Fig. 24–5. Influence of clofibrate therapy on the ability of 16 normal subjects to excrete a maintained water load. Clofibrate decreased maximum urine volume and free water clearance and increased minimum urine osmolality and arginine vasopressin (AVP). (From Moses AM, Howanitz J, vanGemert M, et al: Clofibrate-induced antidiuresis. J Clin Invest 52:535, 1973. By permission of the American Society for Clinical Investigation.)

dog.[48] Most investigators have found that the drug increases plasma antidiuretic hormone concentrations.[55,60,61] However, increased plasma arginine vasopressin levels have not always been found, even when there was an impaired ability to excrete a water load.[62,63]

Carbamazepine has caused water intoxication in patients being treated for trigeminal neuralgia[57,64,65] or epilepsy.[66] In a survey of 55 neurologic patients being treated with carbamazepine, seven were found to be hyponatremic.[67] Serum sodium inversely correlated with blood levels of the drug, and the hyponatemia occurred primarily in older patients. Henry et al. also noted a strong statistical correlation between hyponatremia and carbamazepine doses greater than 700 mg/day and steady-state carbamazepine serum levels over 8.3 μg/ml.[66] Carbamazepine may induce congestive heart failure,[68] and cardiovascular disease may be a predisposing factor in the development of SIADH.[60,69]

The syndrome of inappropriate secretion of antidiuretic hormone has been reported in patients treated with tricyclic antidepressants, such as amitriptyline (Elavil), thiothixene (Navane), desipramine (Norpramin), and fluphenazine (Prolixin).[70-74] There are no available figures on the incidence of hyponatremia in a large group of patients treated with these agents.

A patient with diabetes insipidus was treated with protriptyline for control of sleep-related symptoms; his diabetes insipidus improved to the extent that he could discontinue his treatment with vasopressin.[75] Although there is no information on the mechanism involved, the tricyclic compounds may eventually be found to release vasopressin, since they act on the central nervous system and are similar in structure to carbamazepine, which apparently does release arginine vasopressin.

Thioridazine (Mellaril) does not induce inappropriate secretion of antidiuretic hormone, but may cause water intoxication by stimulating excessive water intake. Despite a baseline normal urinary diluting capacity, certain psychiatric patients may develop hyponatremia because of nonosmotic stimulation of antidiuretic hormone release, which may lead to inability of the normal kidney to excrete an excessive fluid load.[76,77] Dryness of the mouth caused by the anticholinergic action of this and other tricyclic agents may increase water intake.[78]

ANTIMETABOLITES

The antimetabolite vincristine may produce severe inappropriate secretion of antidiuretic hormone in patients being treated for cancer.[79-81] One case has been reported in which SIADH occurred after a massive overdosage of vincristine.[82] The syndrome is usually recognized 1 or 2 weeks after the onset of treatment and usually subsides about 2 weeks after the drug is discontinued. Elevated plasma concentrations of arginine vasopressin have been found in patients with this syndrome.[83] Recurrent elevations of urinary arginine vasopressin may occur 8 to 10 days after repeated treatment with vincristine.[81] In the latter case recurrent SIADH was prevented by prophylactic fluid restriction. A neurotoxic mechanism is supported by the observation that the addition of vincristine to the incubated rat neurohypophysis causes microscopic changes, including precipitation of microtubules and deposition of crystals in nerve fibers and pituicytes.[84] The syndrome of inappropriate secretion of antidiuretic hormone may also result from therapy with a similar vinca alkaloid, vinblastine, particularly when used in large doses.[85-87]

Cyclophosphamide has produced an antidiuretic hormone-like antidiuresis when injected intravenously into water-loaded patients.[88] One patient, a 5-year-old boy, developed a fatal hyponatremia after high-dose cyclophosphamide therapy.[89] The antidiuresis is related to the urinary excretion of active alkylating metabolites of the drug.[90] These observations in human subjects are in contrast to the finding that the drug causes diuresis in animals.[91] There is one reported case of SIADH induced by cis-dichlorodiammineplatinum II in a patient who had a malignant thymoma.[92] The water-retaining properties of these oncolytic drugs are particularly important because patients so treated are frequently hydrated to prevent the formation of uric acid stones and drug-related cystitis.

DRUGS THAT AFFECT NEUROTRANSMISSION

This section is limited to a discussion of agents reported to alter water excretion in a clinical context. It is not meant to be a discussion of neurotransmitters, which may be involved physiologically or pathophysiologically in the release of vasopressin.

There is confusion as to whether narcotic agents have a clinically significant action on water metabolism, or even whether they alter the release of vasopressin in physiologic experiments. As early as 1944, de Bodo demonstrated that administration of morphine to dogs caused an antidiuresis along with an increased level of circulating antidiuretic substance.[93] Since that time narcotic agents have been reported to induce an antidiuretic effect in various species (see ref. 94). In contrast, studies in rats and human subjects demonstrate an inhibitory effect of morphine on the release of vasopressin. Morphine decreased arginine vasopressin levels in rats when hormone levels were normal or elevated arginine vasopressin levels by increasing plasma osmolality.[95] Morphine anesthesia in humans may not increase plasma arginine vasopressin levels; in fact, the subsequent response to surgical stress may actually be attenuated by the morphine anesthesia.[96] When an antidiuresis has been reported, a tolerance seems to develop, and diuresis subsequently develops during chronic narcotic administration.[97,98] Leedy et al. have demonstrated that the response of plasma arginine vasopressin to the intracerebroventricular administration of morphine is both dose and time dependent.[99] Small doses of morphine inhibit and larger doses first stimulate and subsequently inhibit the release of arginine vasopressin. Studies with narcotic antagonists such as oxilorphan and butorphanol have generally demonstrated an inhibition of vasopressin release, with resultant diuresis[100-102] or elevation of the osmotic threshold for vasopressin release.[103] In contrast, naloxone does not alter basal arginine vasopressin levels in humans.[104]

In vitro studies have not provided a definitive answer to the role of opiates in the release of vasopressin. Weitzman et al. demonstrated that β-endorphin caused the release of vasopressin from the isolated neurohypophysis.[105] However, subsequent studies that were also performed on the isolated rat neurohypophysis have revealed either no effect[106] or an inhibitory effect[107] of opiates on vasopressin release.

The clinical implications of these studies are rather vague. However, prudence should dictate that water balance should be carefully monitored in patients receiving large doses of narcotics, especially in association with other features such as advanced age, disease, stress, and drugs that tend to interfere with free water excretion. There are reports that narcotic antagonists may improve the condition of patients with inappropriate secretion of antidiuretic hormone caused by disease of the central nervous system,[103] but no systematic study of this phenomenon has appeared in the literature.

There is abundent evidence that cholinergic and adrenergic mechanisms are involved in the release of arginine vasopressin, but the clinical connotations at this time are marginal. Burn et al. first noted that smoking or nicotine injection could result in antidiuresis.[108] There is evidence in human subjects[109] and monkeys[110] that these agents increase circulating arginine vasopressin, which presumably accounts for the antidiuresis. Clonidine, an α-adrenergic agonist used in the treatment of hypertension, can increase urine flow in the dog through inhibition of arginine vasopressin release.[111,112] This action appears to result from a direct inhibitory action of clonidine on the central nervous system.[112] Under certain circumstances, however, clonidine may stimulate release of arginine vasopressin, as evidenced in a case report of inappropriate secretion of antidiuretic hormone in a patient treated with clonidine.[113] In laboratory experiments dopamine has been reported to stimulate,[114] inhibit,[115] or be uninvolved[116] in the release of vasopressin. Limited clinical evidence using the dopamine agonist bromocriptine would support a possible stimulatory role of dopamine on arginine vasopressin release. Robinson et al.[117] have reported that bromocriptine enhances the osmotically stimulated rise in plasma arginine vasopressin in normal subjects, and there is a case report of a patient with cirrhosis of the liver in whom profound hyponatremia developed after treatment with bromocriptine.[118] Despite the limited observations on the association of this group of agents with clinically significant alterations in water metabolism, the clinician should remain alert to this possibility.

ETHANOL AND DIPHENYLHYDANTOIN

Ethanol has a well-described diuretic action generally attributed to an inhibition of vasopressin release. When hydrated subjects are given ethanol along with hypertonic saline, the antidiuretic response to the latter is blocked.[119] In dehydrated dogs, ethanol causes the steady-state plasma osmolality to be higher than normal, suggesting that even though ethanol interferes with arginine vasopressin secretion, a sufficiently high plasma osmolality will restimulate the release of arginine vasopressin.[120] This concept is supported by evidence obtained in normal subjects in whom plasma arginine vasopressin levels were decreased by ethanol, more so in younger persons.[121] This pharmacologic action was employed in treating a 31-year-old woman who had inappropriate secretion of antidiuretic hormone from tuberculous meningitis.[122] Several reports present somewhat contrary information. One group was unable to demonstrate that the diuresis induced by ethanol was associated with a suppressed level of plasma vasopressin.[123] Another group demonstrated a high level of plasma arginine vasopressin during a period of ethanol-induced diuresis.[124] These data suggest that suppression of arginine vasopressin release is not the sole determinant of ethanol-induced diuresis.

Diphenylhydantoin inhibits vasopressin release in the dehydrated rat[125] and in the isolated rat neurohypophysis.[126] It causes a diuresis in hydrated normal subjects and in patients with the syndrome of inappropriate secretion of antidiuretic hormone due to disease of the central nervous system[127] or after cranial surgery.[128] It is ineffective when the syndrome is due to bronchogenic carcinoma.[127]

ACKNOWLEDGMENT

This work was supported by VA Research Funds and grant RR-229 from the General Clinical Research Centers Program of the Division of Research Resources, National Institutes of Health.

REFERENCES

1. Miller M, Moses AM: Mechanism of chlorpropamide action in diabetes insipidus. J Clin Endocrinol Metab 30:488, 1970
2. Liberman B, Borges R, Wajchenberg BL: Evidence for a role of antidiuretic hormone (ADH) in the antidiuretic action of chlorpropamide. J Clin Endocrinol Metab 36:894, 1973
3. Miller M, Moses AM: Potentiation of vasopressin action by chlorpropamide in vivo. Endocrinology 86:1024, 1970
4. Ingelfinger JR, Hays RM: Evidence that chlorpropamide and vasopressin share a common site of action. J Clin Endocrinol Metab 29:738, 1969
5. Mendoza SA, Brown CF Jr: Effect of chlorpropamide on osmotic water flow across toad bladder and the response to vasopressin, theophylline and cyclic AMP. J Clin Endocrinol Metab 38:883, 1974

6. Berndt WO, Miller M, Kettyle WM, et al: Potentiation of antidiuretic effect of vasopressin by chlorpropamide. Endocrinology 86:1028, 1970
7. Zweig SM, Ettinger B, Earley LE: Mechanism of antidiuretic action of chlorpropamide in the mammalian kidney. Am J Physiol 221:911, 1971
8. Moses AM, Numann P, Miller M: Mechanism of chlorpropamide-induced antidiuresis in man: Evidence for release of ADH and enhancement of peripheral action. Metabolism 22:59, 1973
9. Murase T, Yoshida S: Mechanism of chlorpropamide action in patients with diabetes insipidus. J Clin Endocrinol Metab 36:174, 1973
10. Moses AM, Coulson R: Augmentation by chlorpropamide of dDAVP-induced antidiuresis and stimulation of renal medullary adenylate cyclase and accumulation of cyclic AMP. Endocrinology 106:967, 1980
11. Moses AM, Fenner R, Schroeder ET, et al: Further studies on the mechanism by which chlorpropamide alters the action of vasopressin. Endocrinology 111:2025, 1982
12. Moses AM, Fenner R, Schroeder ET, et al: Use of the Brattleboro rat in studies of the mechanism by which chlorpropamide enhances the action of vasopressin. Ann NY Acad Sci 394:513, 1982
13. Jard S, Butlen D, Rajerison R, et al: The vasopressin-sensitive adenylate cyclase from the mammalian kidney. p. 211. In Moses AM, Share L (eds): Neurohypophysis. S Karger, Basel 1977
14. Braun-Werness JL, Kusano E, Dousa TP: Action of chlorpropamide (CPMD) on cyclic AMP (cAMP) metabolism in medullary tubules. Program of the 15th Annual Meeting of the American Society of Nephrology, Chicago, December, 1982, 157A
15. Zusman RM, Keiser HR, Handler JS: Inhibition of vasopressin-stimulated prostaglandin E biosynthesis by chlorpropamide in the toad urinary bladder. Mechanism of enhancement of vasopressin-stimulated water flow. J Clin Invest 60:1348, 1977
16. Czakó L, Nagy É, László FA: Effect of chlorpropamide, clofibrate and carbamazepine treatment on the plasma ADH level in diabetes insipidus. p. 40. Proceedings of the Seventh Congress of the Hungarian Society of Endocrinology and Metabolism, Debrecen, 1975
17. Pokracki FJ, Robinson AG, Seif SM: Chlorpropamide effect: Measurement of neurophysin and vasopressin in humans and rats. Metabolism 30:72, 1981
18. Moses AM, Miller M, Streeten DHP: Pathophysiologic and pharmacologic alterations in the release and action of ADH. Metabolism 25:697, 1976
19. Czakó L, Nagy É, László FA: Mechanism of chlorpropamide antidiuresis. Acta Physiol Acad Sci Hung 49:177, 1977
20. Bode HH, Harley BM, Crawford JD: Restoration of normal drinking behavior by chlorpropamide in patients with hypodipsia and diabetes insipidus. Am J Med 51:304, 1971
21. Hagen GA, Frawley TF: Hyponatremia due to sulfonylurea compounds. J Clin Endocrinol Metab 31:570, 1970
22. Garcia M, Miller M, Moses AM: Chlorpropamide-induced water retention in patients with diabetes mellitus. Ann Intern Med 75:549, 1971
23. Weissman PN, Shenkman L, Gregerman RI: Chlorpropamide hyponatremia: Drug-induced inappropriate antidiuretic-hormone activity. N Engl J Med 284:65, 1971
24. Hayes JS, Kaye M: Inappropriate secretion of antidiuretic hormone induced by chlorpropamide. Am J Med Sci 263:137, 1972
25. Cinotti GA, Stirati G, Ruggiero F: Abnormal water retention and symptomatic hyponatremia in idiopathic diabetes insipidus during chlorpropamide therapy. Postgrad Med J 48:107, 1972
26. Piters K: Chlorpropamide-induced hyponatremia. J Clin Endocrinol Metab 43:1085, 1976
27. Radó JP: Combination of carbamazepine and chlorpropamide in the treatment of "hyporesponder" pituitary diabetes insipidus. J Clin Endocrinol Metab 38:1, 1974
28. Martin RJ, Robinson SR: Chlorpropamide-induced hyponatremia. South Med J 69:1524, 1976
29. Tanay A, Firemann Z, Yust I, et al: Chlorpropamide-induced syndrome of inappropriate antidiuretic hormone secretion. J Am Geriatr Soc 29:334, 1981
30. Davis FB, Boh DM, Davis PJ, et al: Factors

moderating the effect of oral sulfonylureas on free water clearance. J Clin Pharmacol 22:97, 1982

31. Strauss CF: Chlorpropamide and angina pectoris. Ann Intern Med 78:454, 1973
32. Luethi A, Studer H: Antidiuretic action of chlorpropamide and tolbutamide. Minn Med 52:33, 1969
33. Gossain VV, Hagen GA, Sugawara M: Drug-induced hyponatremia in psychogenic polydipsia. Postgrad Med J 52:720, 1976
34. Darlow BA: Symptomatic hyponatraemia associated with tolbutamide therapy. Postgrad Med J 53:223, 1977
35. Lichtenberg L, Abraira C: Tolbutamide-associated hyponatremia. JAMA 240:2433, 1978
36. Urakabe S, Shirai D, Ando A, et al: Effect of sulfonylureas on the permeability to water and electrical properties of the urinary bladder of the toad. Jpn Circ J 34:595, 1970
37. Moses AM, van Gemert M, Miller M: Evidence that glyburide-induced diuresis is not mediated by inhibition of ADH. Horm Res 5:359, 1974
38. Preuss HG, Rodelas R, Terlinsky A, et al: Effects of glipizide on water and electrolyte handling in water-loaded humans. Renal Physiol (Basel) 4:173, 1981
39. Moses AM, Howanitz J, Miller M: Diuretic action of three sulfonylurea drugs. Ann Intern Med 78:541, 1973
40. Radó JP, Borbely L, Szende L, et al: Investigation of the diuretic effect of glibenclamide in healthy subjects and in patients with pituitary and nephrogenic diabetes insipidus. Horm Metab Res 6:289, 1974
41. Yap PL, Harrower ADB, Davidson NMcD, et al: Glibenclamide and syndrome of inappropriate secretion of antidiuretic hormone. Br Med J 5:1137, 1977
42. Ducobu J, Dupont P: Hyponatremiée liee à la prise de glipizide. Thérapie 36:597, 1981
43. Moses AM, Howanitz J, vanGemert M, et al: Clofibrate-induced antidiuresis. J Clin Invest 52:535, 1973
44. de Gennes J-L, Bertrand C, Basile B, et al: Première démonstration de l'activité antidiurétique, pharmacologique et thérapeutique du Clofibrate (Atromid-S) dans le diabète insipide pitresso-sensible. CR Acad Sci Paris 269:2607, 1969
45. de Gennes J-L, Desbois J-CI, Marie J: Étude thérapeutique du clofibrate au cours des diabètes insipides pitresso-sensibles de l'enfant. Sem Hop Paris 46:754, 1970
46. Radó JP, Juhos E, Sawinsky I: Dose–response relations in drug-induced inappropriate secretion of ADH: Effects of clofibrate and carbamazepine. Int J Clin Pharmacol 12:315, 1975
47. Gattereau A, Davignon J, Verdy M, et al: Halofenate versus clofibrate in the management of true diabetes insipidus. Can Med Assoc J 110:1275, 1974
48. Bäisset A, Cotonat J, Dumas J-C, et al: Recherches sur l'action antidiurétique de la carbamazépine. Therapie 288:663, 1973
49. Bonnici F: Antidiuretic effect of clofibrate and carbamazepine in diabetes insipidus: Studies on free water clearance and response to a water load. Clin Endocrinol 2:265, 1973
50. László FA, Czakó L: Effect of clofibrate on water metabolism in hypothalamic and ADH-resistant diabetes insipidus. Acta Med Acad Sci Hung 30:139, 1973
51. Uhlich E, Loeschke K, Eigler J, et al: Clofibrate therapy in diabetes insipidus. Klin Wochenschr 49:436, 1971
52. Tarpey MM, Mendoza SA: Effects of clofibrate on water permeability and short-circuit current of toad urinary bladder. J Pharmacol Exp Ther 214:5, 1980
53. Braunhofer J, Zicha L: Eröffnet tegretal neue therapiemöglichkeiten bei bestimmten neurologischen und endokrinen krankheitsbildern? Med Welt 36:1875, 1966
54. Czakó L, László FA: Antidiuretic effect of carbamazepine in diabetes insipidus. Int J Clin Pharmacol 11:58, 1975
55. Kimura T, Matsui K, Sato T, et al: Mechanism of carbamazepine (Tegretol)-induced antidiuresis: Evidence for release of antidiuretic hormone and impaired excretion of a water load. J Clin Endocrinol Metab 38:356, 1974
56. Uhlich E, Loeschke K, Eigler J: Zur antidiuretischen wirkung von carbamazepin bei diabetes insipidus. Klin Wochenschr 50:1127, 1972
57. Sordillo P, Sagransky DM, Mercado R, et al: Carbamazepine-induced syndrome of inappropriate antidiuretic hormone secretion.

Reversal by concomitant phenytoin therapy. Arch Intern Med 138:299, 1978
58. Schaison G, Nathan C, Dreyfus G: Diagnostic et traitements actuels du diabète insipide à propos de dix observations. Sem Hop Paris 49:2825, 1973
59. Meier KE, Mendoza SA: Effects of carbamazepine on the water permeability and short-circuit current of the urinary bladder of the toad and the response to vasopressin, adenosine 3′,5′-cyclic phosphate and theophylline. J Pharmacol Exp Ther 200:95, 1977
60. Smith NJ, Espir MLE, Baylis PH: Raised plasma arginine vasopressin concentration in carbamazepine-induced water intoxication. Br Med J 2:804, 1977
61. Summy-Long JY, Keil LC, Crawford IL: Effect of carbamazepine on salt–water balance, plasma and urine vasopressin in unanesthetized rats. Fed Proc 38:754, 1979
62. Stephens WP, Coe JY, Baylis PH: Plasma arginine vasopressin concentrations and antidiuretic action of carbamazepine. Br Med J 1:1445, 1978
63. Meinders AE, Cejka V, Robertson GL: The antidiuretic action of carbamazepine in man. Clin Sci Mol Med 47:289, 1974
64. Flegel KM, Cole CH: Inappropriate antidiuresis during carbamazepine treatment. Ann Intern Med 87:722, 1977
65. Kato DB: Dilutional hyponatremia and water intoxication during carbamazepine therapy. A case report and review of the literature. Drug Intell Clin Pharm 12:392, 1978
66. Henry DA, Lawson DH, Reavey P, et al: Hyponatraemia during carbamazepine treatment. Br Med J 1:83, 1977
67. O'Hare J, O'Driscoll D, Duggan B, et al: Hyponatraemia and carbamazepine intoxication. Ir J Med Sci 149:10, 1980
68. Terrence CF, Fromm G: Congestive heart failure during carbamazepine therapy. Ann Neurol 8:200, 1980
69. Stephens WP, Espir MLE, Tattersall RB, et al: Water intoxication due to carbamazepine. Br Med J 1:754, 1977
70. Luzecky MH, Burman KD, Schultz ER: The syndrome of inappropriate secretion of antidiuretic hormone associated with amitriptyline administration. South Med J 67:495, 1974
71. Ajlouni K, Kern MW, Tures JF, et al: Thiothixene-induced hyponatremia. Arch Intern Med 134:1103, 1974
72. de Rivera JLG: Inappropriate secretion of antidiuretic hormone from fluphenazine therapy. Ann Intern Med 82:811, 1975
73. Dhar SK, Ramos RR, Minot ND: Inappropriate antidiuresis during desipramine therapy. Arch Intern Med 138:1750, 1978
74. Madhusoodanan S, Osnos R: Amitriptyline-induced hyponatremia—a case report. Mt Sinai J Med 48:431, 1981
75. Clark RW, Schmidt HS, Sotos JF: Reversal of chronic diabetes insipidus during treatment with protriptyline. South Med J 71: 1567, 1978
76. Rao KJ, Miller M, Moses, AM: Water intoxication and thioridazine (Mellaril). Ann Intern Med 82:61, 1975
77. Raskind MA, Orenstein H, Christopher TG: Acute psychosis, increased water ingestion and inappropriate antidiuretic hormone secretion. Am J Psychiatry 132:907, 1975
78. Mendelson WB, Deza PC: Polydipsia, hyponatremia, and seizures in psychotic patients. J Nerv Ment Dis 162:140, 1976
79. Meriwether WD: Vincristine toxicity with hyponatremia and hypochloremia in an adult. Oncology 25:234, 1971
80. Oldham RK, Pomeroy TC: Vincristine-induced syndrome of inappropriate secretion of antidiuretic hormone. South Med J 65: 1010, 1972
81. Stuart MJ, Cuaso C, Miller M, et al: Syndrome of recurrent increased secretion of antidiuretic hormone following multiple doses of vincristine. Blood 45:315, 1975
82. Wakem CJ, Bennett JM: Inappropriate ADH secretion associated with massive vincristine overdosage. Aust NZ J Med 5:266, 1975
83. Robertson GL, Bhoopalam N, Zelkowitz LJ: Vincristine neurotoxicity and abnormal secretion of antidiuretic hormone. Arch Intern Med 132:717, 1973
84. Rufener C, Nordmann J, Rouiller C: Effet de la vincristine sur l'hypophyse postérieure de rat *in vitro.* Neurochirugie 18:137, 1972
85. Ginsberg SJ, Comis RL, Fitzpatrick AV: Vinblastine and inappropriate ADH secretion. N Engl J Med 296:941, 1977
86. Winter SC, Arbus GS: Syndrome of inappropriate secretion of antidiuretic hormone sec-

ondary to vinblastine overdose. Can Med Assoc J 117:1134, 1977
87. Stahel RA, Oelz O: Syndrome of inappropriate ADH secretion secondary to vinblastine. Cancer Chemother Pharmacol 8:253, 1982
88. Steele TH, Serpick AA, Block JB: Antidiuretic response to cyclophosphamide in man. J Pharmacol Exp Ther 185:245, 1973
89. Harlow PJ, DeClerck YA, Shore NA, et al: A fatal case of inappropriate ADH secretion induced by cyclophosphamide therapy. Cancer 44:896, 1979
90. Defronzo RA, Braine H, Colvin OM, et al: Water intoxication in man after cyclophosphamide therapy: Time course and relation to drug activation. Ann Intern Med 78:861, 1973
91. Zedeck MS, Mellet LB, Cafruny EJ: The diuretic effects of cyclophosphamide and nornitrogen mustard: Relationship to antidiuretic hormone. J Pharmacol Exp Ther 153:550, 1966
92. Levin L, Sealy R, Barron J: Syndrome of inappropriate antidiuretic hormone secretion following cis-dichlorodiammineplatinum II in a patient with malignant thymoma. Cancer 50:2279, 1982
93. de Bodo RC: The antidiuretic action of morphine and its mechanism. J Pharmacol Exp Ther 82:74, 1944
94. Van Wimersma Greidanus TB, Van Ree JM, Goedemans HJH, et al: Effects of β-endorphin fragments on plasma levels of vasopressin. Life Sci 29:783, 1981
95. Van Wimersma Greidanus TB, Thody TJ, Verspaget H, et al: Effects of morphine and β-endorphin on basal and elevated plasma levels of α-MSH and vasopressin. Life Sci 24:579, 1979
96. Philbin DM, Coggins CH, Emerson CW, et al: Plasma vasopressin levels and urinary sodium excretion during cardiopulmonary bypass. Comparison of halothane and morphine anesthesia. J Thor Cardiovasc Surg 77:582, 1979
97. Marchand C, Denis G: Diuretic effect of chronic morphine treatment in rats. J Pharmacol Exp Ther 162:331, 1968
98. Inturrisi CE, Fujimoto JM: Studies on the antidiuretic action of morphine in the rat. Eur J Pharmacol 2:301, 1968
99. Leedy A, Aziz LA, Forsling ML, et al: The effect of intracerebroventricular injections of morphine on vasopressin release in the rat. J Physiol (Lond) 311:401, 1981
100. Nutt JG, Jasinski DR: Diuretic action of the narcotic antagonist oxilorphan. Clin Pharmacol Ther 15:361, 1974
101. Miller M: Inhibition of ADH release in the rat by narcotic antagonists. Neuroendocrinology 19:241, 1975
102. Lightman SL, Forsling ML: Evidence for endogenous opioid control of vasopressin release in man. J Clin Endocrinol Metab 50:569, 1980
103. Miller M, Moses AM: Clinical states due to alteration of ADH release and action. p. 153. In Moses AM, Share L (eds): Neurohypophysis. S Karger, Basel, 1977
104. Morley JE, Baranetsky NG, Wingert TD, et al: Endocrine effects of naloxone-induced opiate receptor blockade. J Clin Endocrinol Metab 50:251, 1980
105. Weitzman RE, Fisher DA, Minick S, et al: Beta-endorphin stimulates secretion of arginine vasopressin *in vivo.* Endocrinology 101:1643, 1977
106. Christensen JD, Fjalland B: Lack of effect of opiates on release of vasopressin from isolated rat neurohypophysis. Acta Pharmacol Toxicol 50:113, 1982
107. Iversen LL, Iversen SD, Bloom FE: Opiate receptors influence vasopressin release from nerve terminals in rat neurohypophysis. Nature 284:350, 1980
108. Burn JH, Truelove LH, Burn I: The antidiuretic action of nicotine and of smoking. Br Med J 1:403, 1945
109. Husain MK, Fernando N, Shapiro M, et al: Radioimmunoassay of arginine vasopressin in human plasma. J Clin Endocrinol Metab 37:616, 1973
110. Hayward JN, Pavasuthipaisit K: Vasopressin released by nicotine in the monkey. Neuroendocrinology 21:120, 1976
111. Humphries MH, Reid IA: Suppression of antidiuretic hormone secretion by clonidine in the anesthetized dog. Kidney Int 7:405, 1975
112. Reid IA, Nolan PL, Wolf JA, et al: Suppression of vasopressin secretion by clonidine: Effect of alpha-adrenoceptor antagonists. Endocrinology 104:1403, 1979
113. Burrows AW, Gribbin B: Clonidine-induced

dilutional hyponatremia. Postgrad Med J 55:42, 1979
114. Kimura T, Share L, Wang BC, et al: Central effects of dopamine and bromocriptine on vasopressin release and blood pressure. Neuroendocrinology 33:347, 1981
115. Passo SS, Thornborough JR, Ferris CF: A functional analysis of dopaminergic innervation of the neurohypophysis. Am J Physiol 241:E186, 1981
116. Ball SG, Tree M, Morton JJ, et al: Circulating dopamine: Its effect on the plasma concentrations of catecholamines, renin, angiotensin, aldosterone and vasopressin in the conscious dog. Clin Sci 61:417, 1981
117. Robinson BG, Clifton-Bligh P, Posen S, et al: The effect of bromocriptine on circulating vasopressin. Clin Sci 63:367, 1982
118. Marshall AW, Jakobovits AW, Morgan MY: Bromocriptine-associated hyponatraemia in cirrhosis. Br Med J 285:1534, 1982
119. Kleeman CR, Rubini ME, Lamdin E, et al: Studies on alcohol diuresis. II: The evaluation of ethyl alcohol as an inhibitor of the neurohypophysis. J Clin Invest 34:448, 1955
120. Millerschoen NR, Riggs DS: Homeostatic control of plasma osmolality in the dog and the effect of ethanol. Am J Physiol 217:431, 1969
121. Helderman JH, Vestal RE, Rowe JW, et al: The response of arginine vasopressin to intravenous ethanol and hypertonic saline in man: The impact of aging. J Gerontol 33:39, 1978
122. Ducobu J, Dupont P, Jonckheer J: Inappropriate secretion of ADH corrected by ethanol in tuberculous meningitis. Lancet 1:214, 1981
123. Bearn J, Davies R, Forsling ML: The diuresis induced by ethanol in man is not due to suppression of plasma vasopressin. Clin Sci 63:65p, 1982
124. Linkola JR, Ylikahri R, Fyhrquist F, et al: Plasma vasopressin in ethanol intoxication and hangover. Acta Physiol Scand 104:180, 1978
125. Moses AM, Miller M: Osmotic influences on the release of vasopressin. p. 225. In Greep RO, Astwood EB, Knobil E, et al (eds): Handbook of Physiology. Endocrinology, Sect. 7. Vol. IV. The Pituitary Gland and Its Neuroendocrine Control. Part 1. American Physiological Society, Washington, D.C., 1974
126. Guzek JW, Russell JT, Thorn NA: Inhibition by diphenylhydantoin of vasopressin release from isolated rat neurohypophyses. Acta Pharmacol Toxicol 34:1, 1974
127. Fichman MP, Kleeman CR, Bethune JE: Inhibition of antidiuretic hormone secretion by diphenylhydantoin. Arch Neurol 22:45, 1970
128. Landolt AM: Treatment of acute postoperative inappropriate antidiuretic hormone secretion with diphenylhydantoin. Acta Endocrinol 76:625, 1974

25

Sites of Action and Clinical Uses of Diuretics

Bruce E. Berger
David G. Warnock

The effects of diuretics on the homeostatic systems regulating salt, water, potassium, and acid–base metabolism are multiple and complex. The clinical manifestations and biochemical alterations that diuretics produce, both toxic and therapeutic, are reviewed in this chapter. By emphasizing the tubular sites of action and clinical usefulness of each drug group, diuretic agents can be prescribed with specific physiologic responses in mind. As a result, the therapeutic end point will be clearly defined, specific diuretics will be chosen to achieve that goal, and the predictable side effects of each class of drugs will be anticipated. The most frequent problems that physicians encounter when administering diuretics to patients involve acid–base and fluid–electrolyte disturbances. The medical history can ascertain the duration, type, and reason for diuretic therapy, enable an estimation of fluid and electrolyte balance and lead to an awareness and understanding of other potential interactions. The physical examination serves to determine actual volume status and sodium stores. It also permits assessment of clinical sequellae attendant to the use and overuse of diuretics. The baseline laboratory data obtained will be predicted, in part, by the specific disturbances anticipated. Among the determinations typically necessary are serum electrolytes, blood urea nitrogen (BUN), creatinine, glucose, calcium, phosphorus, magnesium, and osmolarity. Urine determinations include urine analysis, osmolarity, sodium, potassium, chloride, and creatinine. A diuretic screen on a specimen of blood and urine can be performed if surreptitious diuretic abuse is suspected. A common misconception is that creatinine clearance is routinely affected by diuretic administration. Glomerular filtraton rate generally, remains unaffected with diuretic usage. However, the glomerular filtration rate can be reduced with the induction of marked intravascular volume depletion. In certain hyponatremic, edematous patients glomerular filtration rate can be increased as a result of a diuretic-induced increase in renal plasma flow.[1] Although it is difficult to interpret urinary electrolyte concentration during administration of a diuretic, it is important to be aware that electrolyte balance generally occurs with chronic administration of these drugs. Urinary electrolyte determinations at this point will reflect dietary intake.

CARBONIC ANHYDRASE INHIBITORS

Carbonic anhydrase is present in many nephron sites, including cytoplasm, in luminal and basolateral membranes, and in the red cells in the peritubular capillaries. The predominant site is in the proximal tubule, where this enzyme catalyzes the CO_2 hydration/dehydration reactions involved in bicarbonate reabsorption.[2] Inhibitors of carbonic anhydrase cause a sodium bicarbonate diuresis and a reduction in total body bicarbonate stores.

These agents were the forerunners of modern diuretics. Carbonic anhydrase inhibitors are unsubstituted sulfonamide derivatives and were developed when it was noted that bacteriostatic sulfonamides caused hyperchloremic metabolic acidosis with large volumes of alkaline urine. Other sulfonamide diuretics (i.e., thiazides) were then developed so as to separate the natriuretic effect from the effects on bicarbonate handling.

Therapeutic Uses

GLAUCOMA

The aqueous humor contains a high concentration of bicarbonate ion. Inhibition of carbonic anhydrase decreases the rate of aqueous humor formation and thereby decreases intraocular pressure. This effect can be used in the chronic treatment of glaucoma.[3]

URINARY ALKALINIZATION

Uric acid and cystine are relatively insoluble in acid urines. Theoretically, enhanced renal excretion can be achieved by increasing urinary pH with carbonic anhydrase inhibitors. Similarly, renal excretion of weak acids, such as aspirin, is increased by raising the urine pH. These effects are of relatively short duration and require bicarbonate infusion to maintain continuing bicarbonaturia. Maintenance of increased urine flow (through solute or water diuresis) has been shown to be more important than urinary alkalinization in protecting against acute uric acid nephropathy.[4]

REDUCTION OF TOTAL BODY BICARBONATE STORES

Carbonic anhydrase inhibition will cause an acute sodium bicarbonate diuresis as long as the filtered load of bicarbonate exceeds the renal capacity for bicarbonate absorption. This approach can be useful in chronic metabolic alkalosis associated with the use of other diuretic agents. Another example is posthypercapnic metabolic alkalosis; carbonic anhydrase inhibitors can be used to correct this condition if saline administration is ineffective or is contraindicated because of elevated cardiac filling pressures.[5,6]

Although the treatment of choice in chloride-sensitive metabolic alkalosis in NaCl and KCl, severe cor pulmonale or left ventricular dysfunction may render this form of treatment ineffective and potentially detrimental. Thiazides and loop diuretics are frequently associated with metabolic alkalosis in this setting. Gastric aspiration, vomiting, and posthypercapnic metabolic alkalosis may also occur. Furthermore, the normal respiratory response to metabolic alkalosis, that is, an elevation in the arterial P_{CO_2}, will reduce arterial oxygen content. This consequence of the respiratory response to metabolic alkalosis can aggravate preexisting reductions in the arterial P_{O_2}. A carbonic anhydrase inhibitor may be valuable in those patients with metabolic alkalosis or in those who are unable to tolerate or are unresponsive to NaCl and KCl and who also have a primary respiratory alkalosis. In one series, eight patients developed metabolic alkalosis and had an exacerbation of their underlying respiratory disorder; diuretic therapy, alone or in combination with steroid therapy, was the most frequent cause for generating the metabolic alkalosis.[5] Patients were treated with acetazolamide (250 to 500 mg IV or PO) as necessary to ameliorate the alkalosis.

Bear et al.[5] noted that metabolic alkalosis and chronic respiratory acidosis (i.e., a combined acid–base disorder) are not uncommon in the setting of chronic obstructive pulmonary disease. The generation of metabolic alkalosis from intravascular volume depletion and electrolyte loss secondary to diuretic use typically requires 24 to 48 hours to develop. However, metabolic alkalosis can develop rapidly secondary to the institution of vigorous diuretic therapy in patients with chronic lung disease.

It is therefore important to recognize those patients and clinical settings in whom this type of mixed acid–base disorder occurs. It must be emphasized that before acetazolamide therapy is instituted, the patient must demonstrate adequate ventilatory reserve. The use of this agent in patients who are unable to increase their minute ventilation will result in a metabolic acidosis superimposed on their preexisting respiratory acidosis.

ACUTE MOUNTAIN SICKNESS

Weakness, breathlessness, dizziness, and nausea can be seen in healthy people who rapidly ascend above 3000 m and overexert themselves. The symptoms are usually mild and last for a few days. In some patients, rapidly progressing pulmonary or cerebral edema can develop and become life threatening. Acetazolamide is a useful prophylactic agent that increases performance status and decreases overall symptomatology. The normal respiratory alkalosis produced by hypoxemia is attenuated during sleep. The efficacy of acetazolamide in preventing acute mountain sickness is due to acute metabolic acidosis, which stimulates respiration and therefore minimizes the degree of hypoxemia. A recent study proposed the use of acetazolamide (500 mg in a sustained-release form) by mouth at night for five nights at the start of a climb.[7]

HYPERPHOSPHATEMIA

Carbonic anhydrase inhibitors cause phosphaturia[8] and have been used as adjuncts in the treatment of hyperphosphatemia. Hyperphosphatemia can occur when glomerular filtration is reduced, when tubular reabsorption is increased (hypoparathyroidism), or when there is an acute phosphate load as occurs with chemotherapy, rhabdomyolysis, and phosphate laxative abuse.[9]

Treatment of hyperphosphatemia depends on the state of renal function. If renal function is significantly impaired, hemodialysis will be necessary if hyperphosphatemia is severe enough to result in a (calcium) (phosphate) product above 60 or to cause tetany. If renal function is adequate, a brisk infusion of normal saline or an isotonic mixture of saline and sodium bicarbonate (250 to 300 ml/hr) and acetazolamide (500 mg IV every 6 hours) can markedly increase renal phosphate excretion.[10] Serum calcium levels must be determined frequently because of the possibility of inducing tetany.

OTHER USES

Carbonic anhydrase inhibitors have been used as adjuvants for the treatment of epilepsy[11] and in some forms of hyperkalemic[12] and hypokalemic periodic paralysis.[13]

Clinical Toxicities

HYPERCHLOREMIC METABOLIC ACIDOSIS

The development of a non-anion gap metabolic acidosis is the predictable consequence of the chronic reduction of body bicarbonate stores. Bicarbonate wasting will ultimately limit the diuretic efficacy of carbonic anhydrase inhibitors in direct proportion to the overall reduction in filtered load of bicarbonate.

RENAL STONES

Phosphaturia occurs during the bicarbonaturic response to carbonic anhydrase inhibition.[8] Calcium excretion remains normal or is slightly decreased during this acute phase. Prolonged use of these agents results in metabolic acidosis and increased calcium excretion.[14] Renal excretion of solubilizing factors (e.g., citrate) may decline with chronic usage.[15] Calcium phosphate salts are relatively insoluble at alkaline pH values, so renal stone formation and nephrocalcinosis can occur.

RENAL POTASSIUM WASTING

K^+ wasting can be severe, especially during the acute bicarbonaturic stage. This complication may limit the usefulness of carbonic anhydrase inhibitors in treating chronic metabolic alkalosis associated with prior diuretic administration.

OTHER TOXICITIES

Drowsiness and paresthesias are commonly observed with large doses of chronic anhydrase inhibitors. Hypersensitivity reactions (fever, rashes, bone marrow suppression, interstitial nephritis) can occur as well.[16]

CONTRAINDICATIONS

Carbonic anhydrase inhibitors should be avoided in hepatic cirrhosis. Alkalinization of the urine will decrease the urinary trapping of NH_4^+ and may contribute to the development of hepatic encephalopathy because of increased ammonia delivery to the systemic circulation.[17]

THIAZIDES

The thiazide diuretics emerged out of efforts to synthesize more potent carbonic anhydrase inhibitors. Chemical modification of the parent compounds changed the anion composition of the diuresis, resulting in the presence of chloride, rather than bicarbonate, with sodium in the urine. Subsequent work has shown that the benzothiadiazides inhibit NaCl transport independently of any effect on carbonic anhydrase activity. Some members of this group retain significant carbonic anhydrase inhibitory activity, but this effect is not related to the primary mode of action.

Thiazides inhibit NaCl reabsorption in the early segments of the distal tubule. Early clearance studies demonstrated an effect on NaCl reabsorption during excretion of dilute urine in the water-loaded state.[18] This finding suggested that the site of action of the thiazides was at a cortical diluting segment. Furthermore, thiazides had no appreciable effect on urinary concentration. More recent studies have shown that the primary site of action of thiazides is in the distal convoluted tubule and that there is no effect on thick ascending limb function.[19] There may also be an effect on NaCl reabsorption in the late proximal tubule, but this is not observed in the usual clinical setting.[19-21] Any increase in NaCl delivery out of the proximal tubule would be reabsorbed in the uninhibited thick ascending limb of the loop of Henle.

Very little is known about the mechanism by which NaCl transport is inhibited by thiazides. There is a lumen-negative electrical potential difference in the distal convoluted tubule, which is consistent with electrogenic Na^+ reabsorption. In contrast to the collecting tubule system, there does not appear to be any mineralocorticoid-dependent Na^+ transport in the distal convoluted tubule. The mechanism(s) through which the thiazides interact with the NaCl transport system is/are unclear, but these systems can also be shown to be responsive to thiazide analogues. Furthermore, the different actions of thiazides can be separated from each other. Nondiuretic thiazide analogues that block the chloretic effect of chlorothiazide without effecting its carbonic anhydrase inhibitory activity have been synthesized.[22]

An active reabsorptive process for Ca^{2+} in

the distal convoluted tubule is in part modulated by parathyroid hormone. Thiazides augment Ca^{2+} reabsorption at this site.[23] Current evidence suggests that a Na^+/Ca^{2+} countertransport system exists in the basolateral membrane of proximal, and presumably distal convoluted, tubules.[24] It is conceivable that inhibition of Na^+ entry by thiazides may lower cell Na^+ concentration and thereby increase Na^+/Ca^{2+} exchange across the basolateral membrane. As a result, cell Ca^{2+} would fall and Ca^{2+} entry across the luminal membrane would increase. In addition, inhibition of the lumen-negative electrical potential difference by thiazides would favor Ca^{2+} entry across the luminal membrane, and the overall result would be a thiazide-induced increase in Ca^{2+} absorption.

A second mechanism by which thiazides augment Ca^{2+} reabsorption has been attributed to extracellular fluid volume depletion.[25] According to this concept, NaCl diuresis leads to enhanced proximal nephron reabsorption of Na^+ and Ca^{2+}. It was initially thought that this effect required the presence of parathyroid hormone, since hypoparathyroid patients treated with thiazides did not demonstrate an amelioration in their hypercalciuria. However, it was recently demonstrated that hypoparathyroid rats and dogs reduce urinary calcium excretion when treated with thiazides.[25] Furthermore, it has been shown clinically that when hypoparathyroid patients on chlorthalidone are placed on a NaCl-restricted diet and vitamin D therapy is discontinued, urinary calcium excretion will remain low.[26]

Thus, the overall effect of thiazides on calcium excretion appears to be mediated by both a direct effect at the distal convoluted tubule and by salt depletion. The hypocalciuric effect of thiazides may be obscured if volume expansion (e.g., increased dietary salt intake) is superimposed on chronic thiazide therapy.

Evidence has accrued that the thiazide diuretics have extrarenal actions. The first observations were made in hypertensive patients with severe chronic renal failure; oral chlorothiazide had an antihypertensive effect that was not due to an increase in urinary sodium excretion. Plasma K^+ levels decreased and uric acid and BUN concentrations increased, suggesting intracellular ion shifts or perhaps a volume-depleting effect via the gastrointestinal system.[27] Potassium homeostasis has recently been examined in anuric chronic hemodialysis patients.[28] Serum K^+ levels were acutely lower after the oral administration of 15 mg/kg chlorothiazide than after intravenous furosemide or as compared with control periods. The plasma K^+ increased at the end of 6 hours by 0.6 mEq/liter during the control periods, compared with an increase of 0.2 mEq/liter after chlorothiazide. This effect was independent of changes in blood volume, acid–base status, renin–aldosterone activity, or glucose/insulin concentrations in these anuric patients and was therefore presumed to be an extrarenal effect of the thiazide.[28]

Therapeutic Uses

REDUCTION IN EXTRACELLULAR VOLUME

The usual therapeutic end point of diuretic therapy is mobilization of salt and water from interstitial compartments and reduction in the extracellular fluid volume.[29] Thiazide diuretics are often an appropriate choice because of the mild, sustained nature of their diuretic effect. More potent agents, or combinations of agents, may be required if the therapeutic response to thiazides is inadequate.

IDIOPATHIC HYPERCALCIURIA

Thiazide therapy is effective in reducing calcium stone formation in idiopathic hypercalciuria[30] regardless of the underlying disorder (i.e., a primary hyperabsorptive state, primary renal phosphate leak, or primary renal calcium leak). Urinary calcium excretion is reduced nearly 50 percent in stone formers and is reduced in normocalciuric individuals as well.[31] The great majority of patients treated with hydrochlorothiazide (50 to 100 mg/day) become stone free over a 3-year follow-up period.[32] (See also Chapter 10.) The hypocalciuric response appears to be mediated by a relative increase in calcium reabsorption induced by thiazides at the distal tubule.[23] Volume depletion also plays a role, since sodium chloride administration blocks the hypocalciuric response.[33] The beneficial effect of thiazides on calcium stone formation is also apparent in normocalciuric individuals.[33,34]

NEPHROGENIC DIABETES INSIPIDUS

Thiazide diuretics can reduce polyuria and polydipsia in patients who are not responsive to antidiuretic hormone. In responsive patients the urine volume is reduced by 50 percent.[35] The beneficial effect is likely due to plasma volume reduction, with an attendant fall in glomerular filtration rate and enhanced proximal reabsorption of NaCl. Dietary sodium restriction can potentiate the beneficial effects of thiazides on urine volume in this setting.[36] Nephrogenic diabetes insipidus develops in many patients treated with lithium carbonate. Lithium toxicity—whether acute (associated with high levels) or chronic (associated with therapeutic levels)—is usually manifested as a renal tubular dysfunction. In addition to impaired concentration of the urine, a defect in urinary acidification at the distal tubule has been demonstrated.[37] The concentrating defect can persist months after discontinuation of lithium therapy. Thiazide diuretics can ameliorate the lithium-induced polyuria by increasing the fractional reabsorption of sodium in the proximal tubule. This is achieved at the expense of mild sodium depletion. Lithium excretion is intimately related to sodium balance; sodium depletion causes lithium levels to rise, while sodium repletion does the converse.[38] Therefore, to minimize the development of acute lithium toxicity in patients placed on a diuretic, it has been recommended that the dosage of lithium be reduced by one-third to one-half and adjusted thereafter on the basis of serum levels.[39]

TYPE II RENAL TUBULAR ACIDOSIS

This form of renal tubular acidosis, when fully expressed, is manifested by the impaired capacity for reabsorption of bicarbonate, amino acids, glucose, and phosphate (Fanconi syndrome). The result of the urinary loss of bicarbonate is a hyperchloremic metabolic acidosis. A new steady-state level of plasma bicarbonate will develop once the filtered load of bicarbonate no longer exceeds the reabsorptive capacity of the proximal tubule. Amelioration of the degree of bicarbonaturia with a resulting higher plasma bicarbonate concentration can be achieved with thiazides. Depletion of the effective arterial blood volume is necessary in order to achieve enhanced proximal bicarbonate reabsorption.[40] Sodium restriction will enhance the effect, while sodium repletion negates the effect.[41]

Clinical Toxicities

GENERAL EFFECTS

Weakness, fatiguability, and paresthesias occur, similar to the effects of carbonic anhydrase inhibitors. Impotence has also been reported as a side effect of thiazide therapy.[42]

K^+ DEPLETION AND METABOLIC ALKALOSIS

These effects accompany the volume contraction and secondary hyperaldosteronism that occur with diuretic therapy. (These issues are discussed in the section on the K^+-sparing diuretics.)

IMPAIRED CARBOHYDRATE INTOLERANCE

Hyperglycemia and glycosuria may occur in susceptible patients who are overtly diabetic or who have abnormal glucose tolerance tests. The effect is dose related and may be the result of impaired pancreatic release of insulin[43] or of a blockade in peripheral glucose utilization.[44]

HYPERURICEMIA AND HYPERLIPIDEMIA

Serum uric acid levels usually rise when patients are placed on thiazide diuretics.[45] Most patients remain asymptomatic and do not require therapy to lower their uric acid levels. Gout may be precipitated or intensified in susceptible subjects. There is no convincing evidence that hyperuricemia is a cardiovascular risk factor. There are associations between hypertension, hyperuricemia, and hyperlipemia, but it is not clear whether diuretics modify or affect these associations. It is certain that effective antihypertensive therapy reduces the incidence of cardiovascular disease in the hypertensive patient,[46] but the role of diuretic use in treating mild hypertension is controversial.

HYPONATREMIA

Life-threatening hyponatremia can occur in a very small number of patients who have recently begun diuretic therapy.[47] This effect appears to be related to reduction in the diluting capacity of the kidney, and/or a sustained release of antidiuretic hormone. Preexistent polydipsia and negative Na^+ balance may play central roles in the development of acute hyponatremia.[48] In the setting of restricted Na^+ intake with continuing water intake, thiazides will produce an actual decrease in urine volume, hence impaired "free" water generation. The negative sodium balance produced by the thiazides may result in a nonosmolar stimulus for antidiuretic hormone release. Thus, in the clinical setting of liberal water intake and limited sodium ingestion, the administration of a thiazide diuretic can result in hyponatremia through retention of water and acute excretion of Na^+. Diuretic-induced hyponatremia in nonedematous patients has also been ascribed to hypokalemia and total-body K^+ depletion.[49] Correction of potassium depletion appeared to restore serum sodium levels to normal. It was postulated that sodium shifted into cells in order to compensate for depletion of intracellular potassium. Many potential factors may explain thiazide-induced hyponatremia, but restricted Na^+ intake coupled with liberal fluid intake appear to be the most important factors. (See also Chapter 5.)

HYPERCALCEMIA

Although it is well recognized that the administration of thiazides to susceptible individuals will produce hypercalcemia, it is important to realize that serum calcium concentrations may also increase in normal individuals by 0.5 to 1.0 mg/dl.[50] When thiazides are first administered, serum Ca^{2+} may be elevated due to hemoconcentration and increased ionized Ca^{2+}. This effect may persist for several weeks before returning toward normal.

Intravenous chlorothiazide exerts a similar effect on normal subjects. Elevation of ionized and total serum Ca^{2+} concentrations will be noted by 2 hours after thiazide administration and will persist for 2 hours. The intravenous effects of thiazides appear to be dependent on parathyroid hormone, since elevated Ca^{2+} levels are not observed in hypoparathyroid patients.[50]

The administration of thiazides to susceptible individuals will produce a persistent elevation of serum calcium or outright hypercalcemia. Most of these individuals have had parathyroid adenomas; however, hypercalcemia may also be observed in patients on vitamin D therapy for osteoporosis and hypoparathyroidism, in patients with multiple myeloma, or in end-stage renal disease patients with secondary hyperparathyroidism.[51] (See also Chapter 10.)

ALLERGIC REACTIONS

Skin rashes are occasionally seen. Serious allergic reactions are extremely rare, but do include hemolytic anemia, thrombocytopenia, acute pancreatitis, cholestatic jaundice, acute pulmonary edema, and interstitial nephritis.[52,53]

CONTRAINDICATIONS

Thiazides should be used very cautiously in patients with cirrhosis to avoid K^+ depletion and precipitation of hepatic encephalopathy. Renal insufficiency may be intensified by overzealous diuretic use in patients with established renal failure. Digitalis toxicity may become manifest or intensified due to diuretic-induced K^+ depletion.

LOOP AGENTS

These agents inhibit NaCl reabsorption in the thick ascending limb of the loop of Henle. Due to the large NaCl absorptive capacity of this segment, agents that act at this site produce a diuretic effect much greater than that seen with any other diuretic group.

The loop agents are rapidly absorbed and handled by renal secretion as well as glomerular filtration.[54] Diuretic response is usually extremely rapid after intravenous injection. The response to furosemide correlates with its urinary concentration. Defects in the secretory component of its clearance may result from simultaneous administration of agents that compete for proximal tubule secretion (e.g., probenecid, nonsteroidal antiinflammatory agents). Metabolites of ethacrynic acid and furosemide have been identified, but it is not known whether they have any diuretic activity.[55]

These drugs inhibit NaCl transport in the thick ascending limb of the loop of Henle. The effect has been localized to a transport site at the luminal membrane, and probably corresponds to a coupled entry mechanism for Na^+, Cl^-, and possibly K^+. It was formerly thought that an "active" chloride pump was present in the thick ascending limb. The current view favors some sort of coupled NaCl transport system driven by a traditional Na^+–K^+-ATPase in the basolateral membrane.[56] The loop agents inhibit NaCl transport at the luminal membrane NaCl entry step.

The thick ascending limb is thought to play an important role in handling divalent cations. Inhibition of active NaCl transport causes an associated increase in Mg^{2+} and Ca^{2+} excretion.[57] Chronic use of loop agents has been associated with Mg^{2+} wasting and severe hypomagnesemia. Ca^{2+} excretion can be strikingly increased with loop agents and saline infusions, an effect that is of great usefulness in the acute management of hypercalcemia. This effect must be clearly distinguished from the thiazides, which are used to decrease Ca^{2+} excretion.

Loop agents appear to have direct effects on blood flow through several different vascular beds. Furosemide can be shown to increase renal blood flow and to cause a redistribution of blood flow within the renal cortex. The hemodynamic effects appear to involve the renin–angiotensin system and vasodilatory prostaglandins. However, the hemodynamic effects have not been directly linked to the diuretic response. Furosemide and ethacrynic acid have been shown to improve pulmonary congestion and to reduce left ventricular filling pressures as an acute hemodynamic effect before any measurable increase in urinary output occurred.[58,59]

Therapeutic Uses

ACUTE PULMONARY EDEMA

The therapeutic goal is a rapid reduction in extracellular fluid volume and venous return in order to decrease right ventricular filling pressure. An improvement in cardiac function may precede the onset of diuresis. This response is due to an extrarenal hemodynamic response with an increase in venous capacitance[58] and may even be observed in anephric patients.

Some patients with marked acidemia may initially be refractory to the action of diuretics. This may result from (1) decreased renal blood flow (and therefore, decreased filtration and secretion), and (2) competition with accumulated organic anions for secretion at the S_2 segment of the proximal tubule. Improvement in cardiac function with oxygen, morphine, rotating tourniquets, nitrates (and phlebotomy, if necessary), and amelioration of the acidosis with bicarbonate may enhance the efficacy of diuretics in this setting.

REFRACTORY EDEMA

Loop diuretics are used when the patient does not respond to salt restriction and/or less potent agents. Diuresis will ensue as long as interstitial fluid is mobilized without compromising intravascular volume. Loop agents are also useful in patients who have diminished renal function and volume overload.

HYPERCALCEMIA

Loop agents can promote a striking increase in urinary excretion of calcium with a prompt reduction in the serum calcium level. The effect is very useful in the acute treatment of hypercalcemia. Inhibition of thick ascending limb function also causes marked excretion of NaCl, water, K^+, and Mg^{2+}.[57] Extracellular fluid volume depletion must be avoided to ensure a continued diuretic response. In the clinically euvolemic patient, an approach is to infuse 1 to 2 liters of normal saline followed by furosemide (10 to 40 mg) intravenously. Once the diuresis begins, the urine flow rate can be matched with the rate of saline infusion to avoid volume depletion. K^+ and Mg^{2+} may be added to the saline infusion when serum concentrations begin to decrease. Urine electrolyte excretion should be determined in order to guide replacement therapy whenever a prolonged diuresis ensues.

INTOXICATIONS

Various metabolic disorders may respond to increases in urine flow rate. For example, halides seem to be absorbed in the thick ascending limb; loop diuretics are therefore useful in treating bromide, fluoride, and iodide intoxications.[60] Saline must be administered to replace urinary losses of Na^+ and to provide Cl^- so as to avoid extracellular fluid volume depletion. Hyperkalemia is another condition for which renal clearance of K^+ may be increased by the use of loop agents and saline infusion.

HYPERURICEMIA

Loop agents can cause hyperuricemia, presumably due to extracellular volume depletion and enhanced proximal reabsorption. Uricosuric congeners of ethacrynic acid include Indacrinone (MK-196) and tienilic acid (ticrynafen).[60b] These congeners inhibit proximal reabsorption of uric acid, and are, therefore, uricosuric. Serum uric acid levels are diminished, but acute renal insufficiency can result if the urinary load of uric acid increases too rapidly. These agents may be useful in patients with symptomatic hyperuricemia who require diuretic therapy for management of hypertension or congestive heart failure.

Cholestatic jaundice and acute renal failure have occurred with the use of ticrynafen,[61,62] and it is no longer available in the United States.

SYNDROME OF INAPPROPRIATE SECRETION OF ANTIDIURETIC HORMONE

Regardless of the etiology, the chronic inappropriate secretion of antidiuretic hormone (SIADH) can be treated by several means. Since the hallmark of this disorder is the inability of the kidney to excrete dilute urine, the cornerstone of therapy is fluid restriction.[63] Should this prove impractical, due to obligatory fluid intake for nutritional or chemotherapeutic reasons, or because of poor patient compliance, then demeclocycline (600 to 1200 mg/day) or lithium carbonate (600 to 900 mg/day) may be used. Demeclocycline appears to be more efficacious and less toxic than lithium.[64]

Serious side effects observed with lithium include anxiety, confusion, disorientation, paresthesias, and hyporeflexia. These neurologic findings may also be seen with hyponatremia. Therefore, institution of lithium therapy in SIADH may initially appear to worsen the neurologic picture.[64] Demeclocycline is metabolized by the liver and should be used cautiously, if at all, in patients with liver disease.[63] In the hyponatremic cirrhotic patient, demeclocycline can be nephrotoxic and cause a natriuresis that results in progressive prerenal azotemia.[65] Assays for measuring demeclocycline are not routinely available. Serum concentrations can be approximated by measuring serum tetracycline levels with a standard microbiologic assay.[65] The therapeutic endpoint is a serum level of 2 μg/ml. The use of oral furosemide (40 mg/day) and generous dietary sodium intake (~200 mEq sodium per day) was recently reported effective in the long-term management of SIADH.[66] Furosemide inhibits antidiuretic hormone-stimulated concentration of the urine, while the salt intake compensates for the natriuresis produced by furosemide. The choice of therapy for SIADH depends on individual factors of compliance, the severity of hyponatremia, and the availability of continued follow-up care.

The use of high-dose cyclophosphamide ($\geq$50 mg/kg) in chemotherapeutic regimens will predictably result in a state of inappropriate antidiuresis. This response develops between 2 and 12 hours after the administration of cyclophosphamide and persists for 24 hours.[67] The significant reductions in serum sodium concentration and urine flow rate that occur have been associated with symptomatic hyponatremia and volume expansion. The continuous infusion of furosemide (0.05 mg/kg-hr) and saline, starting 8 hours before cyclophosphamide infusion and continuing for 24 hours thereafter, effectively prevents hyponatremia and maintains brisk urine flow rates.[68] Furosemide toxicity or significant side effects have not been observed with this protocol, but potassium replacement is usually required.

ACUTE HYPONATREMIA

Traditionally, a serum sodium concentration below 120 mEq/liter has been regarded as a medical emergency. The rapidity with which hyponatremia develops and the underlying general status of the patient influence the actual level of serum sodium that produces life-threatening complications.[69a] The combined use of furosemide and hypertonic saline has been shown to acutely correct severe hyponatremia in the syndrome of inappropriate secretion of antidiuretic hormone.[47,70] The rapid administration of hypertonic saline can transiently increase the serum sodium concentration. However, this is a short-lived effect and, may occasionally precipitate volume overload. Furosemide is used to produce a natriuresis and to avoid volume overload, as well as to inhibit concentration of the urine. The net effect is the excretion of free water because the urine is more dilute than the hypertonic saline infusate. This method has since been shown to be effective in treating hyponatremia from causes other than the syndrome of inappropriate secretion of antidiuretic hormone. The rapid correction of severe hyponatremia within 24 hours to mild hyponatremic levels (130 mEq/liter) has been shown to be without any sequellae from the treatment.[69a,71] Of critical importance when employing hypertonic saline is the prior assessment of the patient's volume status. Since patients with SIADH usually are in a volume-repleted state, urinary sodium excretion typically approximates sodium intake.[63] Therefore, low urine Na^+ concentration does not always imply a decrease in intravascular volume. In the euvolemic or total-body sodium-expanded patient, diuresis with furosemide can be established before the use of hypertonic saline. The amount of hypertonic saline to be infused per hour is estimated from measurements of hourly urine electrolytes. Furosemide is administered as necessary to maintain a brisk diuresis. The dose must be individually assessed, and potassium and magnesium replacement are usually required. In addition to potassium and magnesium depletion, the use of furosemide incurs the risk of producing volume contraction and metabolic alkalosis. Patients with acute, severe hyponatremia and volume depletion can be treated effectively with normal saline replacement. In these patients with volume depletion, the total sodium deficit and the time required for correction will determine the rate of saline replacement.

Clinical Toxicities

Loop agents have in common with the thiazides an increased delivery of salt and water to more distal segments of the nephron. The predictable consequence of this effect is enhanced renal secretion of K^+ and H^+. The clinical result is hypokalemic metabolic alkalosis, which reflects the potency of the diuretic agent and the extracellular fluid volume status. (These effects are discussed in the section on K^+-sparing diuretics.)

MAGNESIUM AND CALCIUM HANDLING

Magnesium wasting is another predictable consequence of the effects of loop agents on the thick ascending limb.[57] Magnesium wasting can also occur with the thiazide diuretics. Clinically significant hypomagnesemia seems to occur more commonly with chronic use of loop agents.

The serum magnesium level should be measured and appropriate replacement therapy administered, since hypomagnesemia can impair parathyroid hormone secretion and produce end-organ resistance. It should be noted, however, that the serum magnesium level is not an accurate indication of total-body stores; therefore, the magnitude of magnesium depletion is judged, in part, but the clinical circumstances.

Marked magnesium depletion may require 1 to 2 mEq/kg body weight for replacement over the first 24 to 48 hours. It should be kept in mind that despite hypomagnesemia, nearly 50 percent of parenterally administered magnesium sulfate will be excreted in the urine. Magnesium replacement can be given as magnesium sulfate (8.12 mEq magnesium per gram) 16 mEq intramuscularly every 2 to 4 hours. Serum levels should be measured frequently. In the setting of renal failure, the dose is significantly reduced, and serum levels must guide replacement therapy.[72]

Volume status is another factor that can influence divalent cation excretion. Loop agents are known for their hypercalciuric effect, but clinical instances of hypercalcemia have been noted. If the chronic use of loop agents causes volume depletion, resulting in volume contraction, then proximal reabsorption of Ca^{2+} is apparently enhanced, and hypercalcemia will develop. Increased salt intake and/or less potent diuretics are indicated in this condition. If volume depletion is avoided in normal individuals, the hypercalciuric action of loop diuretics does not result in frank hypocalcemia. Ionized and total concentrations of serum Ca^{2+} appear to be maintained by a compensatory increase in parathyroid hormone release.[25] Indeed, hypocalcemia has been observed in hypoparathyroid patients to whom furosemide is administered.[73]

OTOTOXICITY

Ototoxicity is another well-described effect of ethacrynic acid and furosemide.[74-75] Unique to the loop diuretics, ototoxicity, has been ascribed to the drug-induced changes in the electrolyte composition of endolymph. Although ototoxicity associated with the use of ethacrynic acid is rare, permanent deafness can develop. Furosemide-induced ototoxicity usually occurs in patients with coexisting renal disease. The coadministration of other ototoxic drugs, such as ethacrynic acid and aminoglycosides, is not a prerequisite, but it may potentiate the development of ototoxicity. In a recent review of cases reported to the Food and Drug Administration, 8 of 29 cases involved other ototoxic agents.[74] Hearing loss is usually transient (from ½ hour to 24 hour after administration), but permanent hearing loss (which is the rule in ethacrynic acid ototoxicity) can occur. The total intravenous dose of furosemide that can result in deafness has been reported to be as little as 40 mg. Six patients developed deafness with dosages of 200 mg or less. In all cases in which deafness occurred with intravenous furosemide, the rate administered was greater than the recommended 4 mg/min.[74]

CONTRAINDICATIONS

Idiosyncratic and hypersensitivity reactions occur with the use of loop agents. Manifestations of these reactions include myelosuppression, skin rashes, hepatic dysfunction, and paresthesias. Acute allergic interstitial nephritis is well documented. It should be remembered that furosemide is a sulfonamide derivative and may demonstrate cross-reactivity in patients who are sensitive to other sulfonamides, that is, sulfa drugs used for urinary tract infections, carbonic anhydrase inhibitors, and thiazides.[53,76]

COMBINED USE OF LOOP AGENTS AND THIAZIDES

Some patients are refractory to the usual doses of loop agents and are therefore vulnerable to dose-related side effects, such as ototoxicity, if abnormally large amounts of the drugs are administered. Combinations can be used as an alternative approach if it is established that renal blood flow has not been compromised by prior volume depletion.

Thiazides and loop agents can be shown to inhibit NaCl absorption in the proximal tubule.[20,77,78] This effect appears to be independent of any carbonic anhydrase activity of these agents, but requires higher luminal concentrations of the drugs than is achieved with normal clinical use.

The proximal effect of thiazides is not usually appreciated because any increase in NaCl delivery out of the proximal tubule is simply picked up in the next down-stream segment; the thick ascending limb has a large capacity to reabsorb NaCl and probably masks any proximal effect of the thiazides. As a result, the usual clinical response to the thiazides is that associated with the inhibition of NaCl reabsorption in the distal convoluted tubule. A true synergy occurs when thiazides and loop agents are administered together. Both classes may increase NaCl delivery out of the proximal tubule. With inhibition of the thick ascending limb by the loop agents, as well as inhibition of the distal convoluted tubule by the thiazides, the overall result is a profound diuretic effect greater than that achieved with either agent alone.

Therapeutic Uses

Combined thiazide–furosemide therapy can be effective in managing refractory edema resulting from cirrhosis, nephrotic syndrome, and severe cardiac dysfunction. This approach has recently been demonstrated to be efficacious in treating hypertensive azotemic patients with increased plasma volumes. The addition of hydrochlorothiazide, 50 to 100 mg/day, to an average furosemide dose of 360 mg/day resulted in a significant improvement in blood pressure control and decreased plasma volume and weight. Attendant with this response, however, was marked kaluresis and an increase in BUN and creatinine. In four of the eight patients treated with combined therapy this regimen was terminated. In two of the patients, nausea and vomiting consistent with uremia developed. Short-term follow-up of those patients maintained on combination therapy disclosed no improvement in renal function. The degree to which azotemia worsened was related to the preexisting level of azotemia.[79] Thus, although a combined thiazide–furosemide approach is generally efficacious in producing a diuresis, persons with preexisting renal insufficiency (serum creatinine >3.0 mg/dl) are at a high risk of developing worsened renal function. It remains to be seen whether the long-term benefit of better control of the hypertension outweighs the short-term worsening in renal function.

If a patient has not responded to a reasonable dose of furosemide (e.g., 160 to 200 mg), then 5 to 20 mg metolazone or 50 to 100 mg hydrochlorothiazide may be added.[79-81] It is important to realize that since diuretics require tubular secretion and filtration for their action, 80 mg furosemide twice a day is not necessarily equivalent to 160 mg furosemide once a day. A diuretic response to the latter dosage can be observed without a response to the former dosage. This principle is important when administering diuretics to patients with chronic renal insufficiency. In patients with intense Na^+ retention and mild renal insufficiency, the earlier addition of a thiazide diuretic is justified. The underlying principle in this situation is to inhibit NaCl reabsorption at sites distal to the action of the loop diuretics. The lack of efficacy of a loop diuretic in this setting may be due to the distal reabsorption of the furosemide-induced natriuresis rather than to a poor primary effect of furosemide in effecting a natriuresis. In addition to the synergistic effect of loop and thiazide diuretics, this approach will lessen the dose-dependent side effects associated with higher doses of the loop agents.

Clinical Toxicities

Very impressive amounts of fluid can be mobilized in patients who have been refractory to single agents. Routine outpatient use cannot be recommended because of the serious consequences of volume depletion.[82] K^+ wasting is extremely common and requires parenteral K^+ administration with careful monitoring of the fluid and electrolyte status.[80] There is also a potential adverse effect on renal function in patients with preexisting renal insufficiency.

K^+-SPARING DIURETICS

Within the kidney, potassium homeostasis is achieved in the aldosterone-responsive segment of the distal nephron (i.e., the collecting tubule). This region not only functions to reabsorb filtered K^+ that escapes the proximal nephron during K^+ depletion, but also secretes K^+ when there is a surfeit. K^+ secretion in the cortical collecting tubule is influenced, but not solely determined by, the presence of aldosterone. The primary determinant of K^+ secretion is the favorable electrochemical gradient that exists between the tubule cell and the lumen. Increased luminal flow rates, increased Na^+ delivery, and a lumen-oriented negative electrical potential difference act to maintain this gradient. Aldosterone serves to enhance the effects of these factors.[83,84] K^+

secretion is intimately related to Na^+ transport. Increased Na^+ absorption resulting from an increase in distal delivery generates an electrical potential that is oriented lumen negative within the collecting tubule and stimulates K^+ secretion into the lumen. Furthermore, it has been demonstrated that stimulation of the basolateral membrane Na^+–K^+-ATPase is a direct consequence of increased intracellular Na^+ concentration.[85] Aldosterone increases the sodium permeability of the luminal membrane. Increased aldosterone levels allow increased luminal uptake of Na^+, which in turn stimulates the Na^+–K^+-ATPase. Aldosterone may also increase luminal permeability to K^+ and H^+. The overall effect of mineralocorticoids on K^+ secretion is related to the increase in luminal membrane K^+ permeability and enhanced Na^+–K^+-ATPase activity.

Ammoniagenesis has been demonstrated to be coupled to K^+ and H^+ homeostasis. Hypokalemia and/or acidosis stimulates ammonia production.[86]

K^+-sparing diuretics exert their effect by interfering with these determinants of K^+ secretion. Aldosterone antagonists decrease the component of K^+ secretion which is coupled to Na^+ absorption and also inhibits the direct effects of aldosterone on K^+ handling. The nonsteroidal K^+-sparing diuretics, triamterene and amiloride, exert their effects by directly inhibiting Na^+ transport across the luminal membrane of the collecting tubule. As a result, the transepithelial electrical potential is reduced and the luminal membrane is hyperpolarized, reducing one of the factors that normally favors K^+ secretion. The decrease in the Na^+–K^+-ATPase activity resulting from the decrease in intracellular Na^+ concentration combines with the voltage-dependent defect to make the electrochemical gradient less suitable for K^+ secretion.

Therapeutic Uses

The members of the K^+-sparing diuretics antagonize the effects of aldosterone at the cortical collecting tubule. Inhibition may occur by a direct antagonism at the level of cytoplasmic mineralocorticoid receptors (spirolactones including spironolactone and prorenone),[87] by suppression of renin or angiotensin II generation (nonsteroidal antiinflammatory agents, captopril), or by directly inhibiting Na^+ transport by the collecting tubule (triamterene, amiloride).[88] These agents are used during states of mineralocorticoid excess, either due to primary hypersecretion (Conn's syndrome, ectopic adrenocorticotropic hormone production) or to secondary hyperaldosteronism. Amiloride has been used in the treatment of Bartter's syndrome and has been shown to ameliorate the hypokalemia in diverse syndromes associated with renal K^+ wasting.[89] Congestive heart failure, cirrhosis, and the nephrotic syndrome are conditions associated with renal salt retention and diminished effective extracellular volume. Diuretic use contributes to further volume contraction and thereby intensifies secondary hyperaldosteronism. In the setting of enhanced mineralocorticoid secretion and continued delivery of Na^+ and volume to distal nephron sites, renal K^+ wasting occurs due to K^+ secretion at the level of the collecting tubule. K^+-sparing diuretics, either direct or indirect antagonists of aldosterone, are used in this setting to blunt the K^+ secretory response and prevent depletion of the intracellular K^+ stores.

Clinical Toxicities

HYPERKALEMIA AND METABOLIC ACIDOSIS

The K-sparing diuretics inhibit renal K^+ and H^+ secretory systems. Hyperkalemia and mild hyperchloremic metabolic acidosis are dose-related side effects observed when aldosterone antagonists are used as a sole diuretic agent. Spironolactone-induced hyperchloremic acidosis in patients with cirrhosis can be more severe. This may be due to a concomitant respiratory alkalosis, diarrhea, or a renal acidification defect due to cirrhosis.[90] With fixed-dosage combinations, there appears to be a fairly even trade-off, so that both the hypokalemia and metabolic alkalosis due to the thiazide is ameliorated by the aldosterone antagonist. There may be a problem with the bioavailability of some of the fixed-dosage forms so that the thiazide associated side effects may predominate (e.g., metabolic alkalosis, hyponatremia).[91] Spirolactones can act as agonists that stimulate H^+ secretion in model systems.[92] An analogous effect in humans is yet to be recognized clinically.

ENDOCRINE ABNORMALITIES

The synthetic steroidal agents may cause endocrine abnormalities by agonist effects on other steroid-receptor complexes. Gynecomastia and androgenlike side effects have been reported with the use of spironolactone.

TRIAMTERENE NEPHROLITHIASIS

Triamterene-induced nephrolithiasis has been estimated to occur in 1 per 1500 patients taking a triamterene-containing diuretic. Susceptible persons can develop stones within 6 months after initiation of therapy. Of 181 triamterene calculi analyzed, approximately 30 percent were principally triamterene. In the remaining 70 percent, triamterene formed the nidus of the stone or was deposited within the calcium oxalate or uric acid matrix.[93] Individuals with a prior history of renal lithiasis appear to be particularly susceptible.[94]

TRIAMTERENE-INDUCED ACUTE RENAL FAILURE

Reversible nonoliguric acute renal failure has been reported in otherwise healthy subjects administered triamterene and indomethacin.[95] Triamterene, unlike furosemide, hydrochlorothiazide, and spironolactone, increases urinary PGE_2 excretion 10-fold above baseline control. Certain renal prostaglandins have been shown to modulate the vasoconstrictive effects of angiotensin II, thereby maintaining renal blood flow. Thus, the increase in urinary PGE_2 excretion in these susceptible individuals may be an autoregulatory effect by the kidney that resulted from a primary decrease in renal blood flow induced by triamterene. The addition of indomethacin counteracted the adaptive increase in prostaglandin synthesis and thus precipitated acute renal failure.

MISCELLANEOUS

Spironolactone has been reported to induce a mild nonspecific hepatitis when administered to a woman with primary aldosteronism.[96]

CONTRAINDICATIONS

These agents can cause severe, even fatal, hyperkalemia in susceptible patients. Oral K^+ administration should be discontinued if aldosterone antagonists are administered. Patients with chronic renal insufficiency are especially vulnerable in this regard and should not be treated with aldosterone antagonists. Patients with preexistent liver disease may have impaired metabolism of triamterene or spironolactone, so that dosing has to be carefully adjusted. Since triamterene and amiloride directly inhibit Na^+ transport in the collecting tubule, it follows that a diuretic response can even be observed in the absence of endogenous mineralocorticoid activity. However, the absence of the normal compensatory increase in aldosterone predisposes such persons to a greater increase in serum K^+ concentrations.

AGENTS THAT AFFECT H_2O EXCRETION

Antidiuretic hormone acts at the collecting tubule to modulate the concentration of the final urine. Antidiuretic hormone secretion is reduced during hypotonic volume expansion, and large volumes of dilute urine are formed.

During volume contraction and in hypertonic conditions, antidiuretic hormone is secreted and the urine is concentrated by water abstraction.

It is important to appreciate the central role of the thick ascending limb during concentration as well as dilution of the urine. Urinary concentration, modulated by antidiuretic hormone, is driven by the hypertonic medullary interstitium, which is generated by the salt transport out of the thick ascending limb and the countercurrent exchange system. Dilution of the urine requires the same salt transport systems in the thick ascending limb of the loop of Henle in addition to NaCl reabsorption in the distal convoluted tubule (i.e., cortical diluting segment). Therefore, urinary concentration and dilution can be inhibited by loop agents that inhibit salt transport in the thick ascending limb. Thiazides inhibit NaCl transport in segments that dilute the urine but do not seem to contribute to the hypertonic medullary interstitium. Therefore, thiazides inhibit urinary diluting ability, but not the ability to concentrate the urine maximally.

Two major groups need to be specifically considered with respect to the excretion of water: osmotic diuretics and antidiuretic hormone antagonists.

OSMOTIC DIURETICS. Mannitol is an osmotic diuretic that obligates the renal excretion of H_2O.[97] This agent is not readily metabolized and is handled primarily by glomerular filtration, without any important tubular reabsorption or secretion. By definition, osmotic diuretics are poorly absorbed, so they must be given parenterally. If given by mouth, an osmotic diarrhea can result. This effect can be used to potentiate the effects of K^+-binding resins or elimination of various drugs from the gastrointestinal tract in conjunction with activated charcoal.

Osmotic diuretics primarily limit water reabsorption in those segments of the nephron that are freely permeable to water, namely, the proximal tubule, descending limbs of the loop, and collecting tubules. The presence of a nonreabsorbable solute such as mannitol prevents the normal absorption of H_2O by imposing a countervailing osmotic force. As a result, urine volume increases in conjunction with mannitol excretion. This will in turn result in a diminished gradient for NaCl reabsorption in the late proximal and distal nephrons. Mannitol-induced washout of the hypertonic medullary interstitium, secondary to increased blood flow, serves to further diminish the gradient for NaCl reabsorption and thereby potentiates the natriuresis. The magnitude of the natriuresis is determined by the preexisting volume status and renal blood flow. Patients suffering from prerenal azotemia or chronic renal insufficiency will undergo a proportionally greater water than salt diuresis as compared with subjects who are euvolemic or who have normal renal function.

In the presence of maximal water diuresis and maximal antidiuresis, mannitol blunts the magnitude of free-water clearance and osmolar clearance by producing a urine osmolality that approaches isotonicity with plasma. Mannitol has been shown to increase glomerular filtration rate by decreasing systemic oncotic pressure and increasing renal plasma flow secondary to volume expansion.

Acute actions of mannitol infusion also affect the acid–base and electrolyte composition of the blood. Expansion of the extracellular volume at the expense of intracellular dehydration results in a decrease in serum sodium, chloride, and bicarbonate concentrations. This mannitol-associated acidosis appears to be the result of extracellular fluid dilution with bicarbonate-poor intracellular fluid. The long-term consequence of mannitol administration is hypertonic, hyponatremic dehydration.

Potassium homeostasis is altered with mannitol infusion. As a result of water abstraction from the intracellular space in response to the increased osmolality of the extracellular space, potassium shifts occur, probably due to cell volume regulation. This effect is independent of the extracellular fluid pH. The increase in serum potassium is offset by continuing K^+ excretion during the mannitol diuresis.

ANTIDIURETIC HORMONE ANTAGONISTS. ADH antagonists include Li^+ salts and tetracycline derivatives (demeclocycline). Antidiuretic antagonists inhibit the effects of antidiuretic homrone at the collecting tubule. This effect occurs at some step after cAMP generation, since the effects of cAMP can be antagonized by Li^+ salts in various model systems.[38]

Therapeutic Uses

OLIGURIA

Osmotic diuretics are used to increase water excretion in preference to natriuresis. This effect can be used when renal hemodynamics are compromised or when avid Na^+ retention limits the response to conventional agents.[98] Care must be exercised when using mannitol in edematous states. The initial mannitol dose of 12.5 g is repeated up to a daily total of 50 g, depending on the clinical response. This effect can be used to maintain the urine volume and to prevent anuria after a hemolytic reaction or other causes of large pigment loads to the kidney (refer to the section on acute renal failure under nonedematous states in the clinical use of diuretics). Dehydration should be corrected before the administration of mannitol.

INTRACRANIAL HYPERTENSION

Osmotic diuretics reduce total body water more than total body cation content and therefore reduce intracellular volume. This effect is used to reduce intracranial pressure in neurosurgical conditions and to reduce intraocular pressure for ophthalmologic procedures. Occasionally other agents are used, including urea, glycerol, and sucrose. To reduce intracranial pressure or edema, 100 to 150 g mannitol in 500 ml saline is rapidly infused. Mannitol reduction in intracranial hypertension is present within 90 minutes. A mild rebound phenomenon may occur several hours later.[97]

DIALYSIS-RELATED STATES

Patients undergoing hemodialysis may develop muscle cramps or hypotension. The use of mannitol in dialysis-associated hypotension should be reserved for those patients with evidence of increased extracellular fluid (i.e., edema). The typical dose is 6.25 to 12.5 g of 50 percent mannitol, repeated hourly if necessary, with the final dose administered before the last hour of dialysis. Dialysis dysequilibrium syndrome is a disorder that typically occurs in patients undergoing dialysis for acute renal failure or with the initiation of dialysis for chronic renal failure. Although the precise pathophysiologic mechanisms remain to be elucidated, an increase in brain osmolarity, cerebral edema, and a decrease in cerebrospinal fluid pH have been demonstrated. The addition of mannitol or other osmotically active agents to the dialysate have been shown to ameliorate symptoms associated with dialysis dysequilibrium syndrome.[99] Since the rationale of treatment is to minimize rapid shifts in plasma osmolarity, the infusion of mannitol into the intravascular space in a dose calculated to offset the reduction in plasma osmolarity resulting from the clearance of urea should as effective as the addition of mannitol to the dialysate.

MISCELLANEOUS

Intoxication with bromides, barbiturates, and other drugs excreted by the kidney has been treated with mannitol.

SYNDROME OF INAPPROPRIATE SECRETION OF ANTIDIURETIC HORMONE

Antidiuretic hormone antagonists are clinically used to manage inappropriate antidiuretic hormone-secretion syndromes when water restriction has failed to correct the abnormality.[100] Serum levels can be monitored directly from Li^+ therapy, with a serum concentration of 1 mmol/liter as a desirable end point. Demeclocycline levels can be approximated by peak and trough levels for standard tetracycline. While not precisely correct, this approach does permit adjusting the usual dose (900 to 1200 mg/day) to achieve a therapeutic serum level of 2 μg/ml.[65]

Clinical Toxicities

Mannitol rapidly distributes in the extracellular compartment and extracts H_2O from the intracellular compartment. Hyponatremia and expansion of the extracellular fluid volume are the predictable consequences. If resulting urine flow is inadequate, this effect can cause florid pulmonary edema in patients with congestive heart failure. Headache, nausea, and vomiting are commonly observed in patients treated with osmotic diuretics. Hyperkalemia and metabolic acidosis may develop in susceptible persons. Hypernatremia may occur with the chronic administration of mannitol.

The major complications of antidiuretic hormone antagonists relate to their pharmacologic effect. The effect on the syndrome of inappropriate secretion of antidiuretic hormone is to produce a state of tubular unresponsiveness to the homrone (i.e., a nephrogenic diabetes insipidus). Renal concentrating ability is abolished, and severe hypernatremia can result. Careful monitoring of the patient's fluid and electrolyte status is required. The side effects associated with Li^+ therapy include tremulousness, mental obtundation, leukocytosis, acute renal failure, and a renal tubular acidosis. Lithium dosages must be reduced if a patient is taking Li^+ and thiazides at the same time.[39]

CLINICAL USE OF DIURETICS

Edematous States

Salt and water retention with edema formation generally occurs in response to an ineffective arterial blood volume. Diuretic therapy in this setting may lead to further compromise of the effective arterial blood volume, as well as organ hypoperfusion. This sequence of events will then intensify the homeostatic responses that caused salt retention in the first place. On the other hand, judicious use of diuretics can mobilize interstitial edema fluid and restore plasma volume. Therefore, the use of diuretics to mobilize edema requires careful monitoring of the patient's hemodynamic status and an understanding of the pathophysiology of the underlying condition.

CONGESTIVE HEART FAILURE

The primary therapeutic goal is to improve myocardial function by increasing contractility. Mobilization of pulmonary vascular congestion with diuretics may improve oxygenation and thereby improve myocardial function. On the other hand, if cardiac output is being maintained at the expense of high filling pressures, then diuretics may diminish ventricular end-diastolic volumes and thereby impair cardiac output. Afterload reduction (hydralazine, nitroprusside), and inotropic agents are more direct approaches to the underlying problem. Diuretic use in this setting should not supersede these therapeutic modalities.

This issue is especially critical in the setting of right ventricular failure as a result of primary or secondary pulmonary hypertension or right ventricular infarction. The clinical diagnosis of a right ventricular infarct is difficult to make by electrocardiographic means.[101,102] Predominant right ventricular infarction has been estimated to occur in 3 to 5 percent of all acute myocardial infarctions.[102] Right ventricular infarcts may occur in as many as 25 percent of patients with inferior wall infarcts. Right ventricular filling pressures must be maximized to ensure adequate right ventricular output. If the pulmonary artery wedge pressure is not elevated, the dependence of left ventricular filling pressure on right ventricular output will be compromised by diuretic administration.

The same sequence of events underlies right ventricular failure from pulmonary hypertension. Diuretic-induced volume contraction will predictably reduce preload and, thus, severely compromise cardiac output. It is important to keep in mind that the use of diuretics in cor pulmonale or congestive heart failure may result in a mixed acid–base disorder. A diuretic-induced metabolic alkalosis can be superimposed on respiratory acidosis due to cor pulmonale or respiratory alkalosis from left ventricular dysfunction. Finally, diuretic-induced K^+ depletion can seriously increase the risk of digitalis toxicity and may precipitate serious ventricular arrhythmias.[103]

CIRRHOSIS

Elevated hepatic venous outflow pressure, reduced plasma oncotic pressure, and the development of arteriovenous fistulae predispose to the development of ascites and edema. Vigorous diuretic therapy to mobilize ascites can result in marked depletion of the effective arterial plasma volume, hypokalemia, and metabolic alkalosis and contribute to the development of hepatic encephalopathy and the hepatorenal syndrome.[104,105] It must be realized that during rapid diuresis, volume is mobilized from nonascitic compartments. In the presence of edema, less than 1 liter/day of ascites can be mobilized; in the absence of peripheral edema, ascites is poorly mobilized. Diuretic administration in the latter setting will mobilize less than 300 ml of ascites per day. Forced diuresis of more than this amount will lead to intravascular volume contraction and decreased glomerular filtration rate.[106] Rarely does the need exist for more rapid diuresis. Bed rest and sodium restriction can initiate a diuresis, and up to 300 ml of ascites fluid can be mobilized per day. The absolute natriuretic response to ethacrynic acid and chlorothiazide has been shown to be dependent on the preexisting state of sodium balance. Absolute sodium excretion in cirrhotics with ascites treated with ethacrynic acid and chlorothiazide is less than in normal controls on a low-sodium diet.[107] Cirrhotic patients administered these two diuretics under controlled conditions excrete 24 percent of the filtered sodium load, in contrast to 30 percent in normal subjects.[108] These observations coupled with the known sites of action of these diuretics suggest that there is increased fractional reabsorption of sodium in the proximal tubule associated with decreased glomerular filtration rate in cirrhotic patients,[107,108] although increased Na^+ reabsorption in nephron segments distal to the cortical diluting segment cannot be excluded.

Recent studies in nonazotemic cirrhotic patients with ascites and edema, have examined the efficacy of spironolactone alone, furosemide alone and the combination of spironolactone and furosemide in initiating and maintaining a diuresis.[109] Enhanced sodium uptake in the collecting tubule due to secondary hyperaldosteronism compromised the efficacy of furosemide. Less than one-half of cirrhotic patients treated initially with furosemide, in dosages up to 160 mg/day, underwent a natriuresis, which subsequently abated in all but one patient. Serum potassium concentrations fell significantly in the furosemide-responsive group, and interestingly in the furosemide nonresponsive group as well.[109] In the furosemide-nonresponsive group, a kaluresis occurred despite the absence of a natriuresis.

When spironolactone was the initial diuretic, nearly all patients responded to 300 mg/day; one-third of the patients were able to maintain a diuresis without the addition of furosemide. The efficacy of furosemide versus spironolactone and the ultimate dosage of spironolactone was significantly correlated with plasma renin activity and aldosterone levels.[109]

In another study that employed a maximal dose of 400 mg/day spironolactone, fully 75 percent of patients experienced a sustained diuresis. At the same time, nearly 30 percent of the patients who served as controls underwent a spontaneous diuresis within the first week of hospitalization that eventuated in complete resolution of ascites and edema.[110]

In addition to the enhanced and sustained

diuresis seen with spironolactone, potassium homeostasis is maintained. Aldosterone antagonists minimize the kaluresis that occurs with diuretic-induced distal delivery of sodium to an aldosterone-primed collecting tubule. In these two studies,[109,110] the serum potassium concentration increased 0.5 to 1.6 mEq/liter with spironolactone. Whereas furosemide was associated with a 200 percent increase in daily potassium excretion, spironolactone resulted in only a 33 percent increase in potassium excretion. When diuresis was limited to less than 0.5 kg/day, the incidence of encephalopathy, hepatorenal syndrome, and death was identical for the control group and the diuretic group.[110]

Thus, when circumstances dictate the need for diuretic therapy (e.g., compromised ventilatory status or noncompliance to a strict dietary program), spironolactone, with furosemide as required, can effectively produce and maintain a diuresis with minimal serious risks, as long as a daily weight loss is limited to 0.5 kg/day.[111] A recommended approach is to initiate therapy with bed rest, a 1- to 2-g sodium diet, and a 500- to 1500-ml fluid restriction as dictated by the presence of hyponatremia. If a spontaneous diuresis does not ensue, then spironolactone 25 mg every 6 hours is begun. The dose of spironolactone is doubled every 4 days until a diuresis occurs or 400 mg/day is reached. Furosemide 40 mg/day is then added and doubled as necessary every 48 hours. Once a diuresis begins, the dosage(s) of the diuretic(s) can often times be reduced.

NEPHROTIC SYNDROME

Depletion of the effective arterial plasma volume in conjunction with reduced plasma oncotic pressures and increased total-body sodium stores may occur in the nephrotic syndrome and appears to be dependent on the underlying glomerular lesion.[112,113] Reduced effective arterial blood volume can be assessed by evaluating for orthostatic changes in blood pressure and pulse. The efficacy and potential toxicity of the loop and thiazide diuretics require an understanding of the altered intrarenal hemodynamics in the nephrotic syndrome. Proximal tubular reabsorption of sodium is influenced by the peritubular capillary protein concentration. Initial studies with ethacrynic acid and chlorothiazide in patients with the nephrotic syndrome and serum albumin concentrations less than 2 g/dl revealed that 41 percent of the filtered sodium load was excreted, in contrast to 30 percent in normal controls. These findings suggest that sodium retention in the nephrotic syndrome is due to increased sodium reabsorption at distal sites.[112] The potential effectiveness of loop agents was highlighted in a recent study of patients with minimal change disease and varying degrees of renal insufficiency who presented with anasarca and severe hypoalbuminemia.[114] Oliguria was present in nearly every patient, and one-half were hypertensive. In 13 of the 15 patients, the use of furosemide was temporally associated with a diuresis that resulted in improvement or normalization of renal function. This finding was noted irrespective of any subsequent remission of the nephrotic syndrome and proteinuria. The hemodynamic alterations (i.e., decreased glomerular filtration rate and filtration fraction) observed before diuretic administration were ascribed to interstitial edema and increased intrarenal pressures. The low filtration fraction argued against hypoperfusion as a contributing influence to the decreased glomerular filtration rate. Although the data in this report are encouraging, definitive statements concerning the use of furosemide in minimal change disease and renal insufficiency must await prospective controlled studies. Furthermore, acute tubular necrosis has been reported in association with minimal change disease.[115–119] Prudence must therefore be exercised with the vigorous use of diuretics in patients with minimal change disease who present with oliguria, since acute tubular necrosis can result from diuretic-induced intravascular volume depletion.

IDIOPATHIC EDEMA SYNDROME

This disorder is typically seen in women who are being treated with diuretics. It occurs with the use of thiazides as well as loop agents. These patients are often weight conscious and employed in a paraprofessional field. The initial reason for diuretic administration may be obscure. They complain of weight gain, bloating, and edema upon cessation of diuretics.[120-122] The etiology of the edema is believed to be due in part to the diuretic-induced stimulation of the renin–angiotensin system. Both the degree of sodium retention and the weight gain have been found to correlate with preexisting plasma renin activity. Maximum weight gain is usually evident by 10 days after cessation of diuretics, and spontaneous diuresis subsequently ensues. A small percentage of women may require initial sodium restriction to control edema formation.[120-122] In addition to the effect of diuretics, a sudden increase in carbohydrate and sodium intake after a period of fasting is associated with sodium retention. Glucose refeeding has been shown to increase proximal tubule Na^+ reabsorption independent of the state of total-body sodium.[123] The carbohydrate effect is thought to be associated with an increase in circulating catecholamine levels.[124] The mechanisms of salt and water retention have not yet been fully defined in this condition.

Nonedematous States

HYPERTENSION

Moderate salt restriction may be sufficient to control essential hypertension in patients who can comply with this approach.[125] A thiazide diuretic is usually the first drug to be used for treating mild essential hypertension and can produce adequate control in nearly two-thirds of these patients. Careful hemodynamic measurements have demonstrated an initial fall in peripheral vascular resistance, a sustained drop in plasma volume,[125a] and a favorable effect on renal hemodynamics[126] in those patients who respond to chronic thiazide therapy. The importance of sustained plasma volume reduction is emphasized by the finding that liberalization of dietary salt intake can overcome the antihypertensive effects of thiazide therapy. Patients who do not respond to thiazides alone are then placed on one ormore peripheral vasodilators, beta blockers, or centrally acting agents. Salt and water retention is a predictable consequence of vasodilator therapy, hence continued diuretic therapy is indicated.

Early studies suggested that diuretic therapy may reduce peripheral vascular resistance by a direct effect on vascular smooth muscle. These effects can be demonstrated most convincingly with parenteral administration of diuretics, but are not necessarily related to the antihypertensive effect of chronic thiazide therapy. A recent study demonstrated an antihypertensive effect of oral chlorothiazide in patients with severe renal failure.[27] This finding was attributed to a direct vasodilatory effect of the diuretic because there was no increase in potassium and sodium excretion. However, there was a decrease in plasma K^+ levels and an increase in serum uric acid and urea levels, suggesting that there was intravascular volume contraction in these patients presumably secondary to intracellular ion shifts or perhaps an effect of the diuretic on the gastrointestinal system. In another study of stable dialysis patients treated with thiazides, it was concluded that natriuresis was necessary for the antihypertensive action of diuretics.[127] A direct effect of thiazides on peripheral vascular resistance could not be demonstrated in these patients. The issue of a primary effect of diuretics on intravascular volume versus peripheral resistance will not be resolved until the cause for increase peripheral vascular resistance in essential hypertension is more clearly understood.

It is worth reemphasizing the sustained reduction of the plasma volume that occurs in response to chronic thiazide therapy.[125a] It is not practical to measure plasma volumes in all hypertensive patients. However, it is useful to evaluate dietary salt intake and compliance in patients with hypertension.[128] Dietary history and urinary sodium excretion rates may serve to distinguish those patients who overcome the antihypertensive effects of thiazides by increasing salt intake.[29,125,128] Patient compliance may be enhanced by once-a-day dosing with a thiazide that has a 12- to 18-hour duration of action (e.g., hydrochlorothiazide). This approach matches the diuretic effect with the normal pattern of dietary salt intake.

It should also be remembered that blood pressure in both hypertensive and normotensive individuals displays a circadian pattern. Blood pressures are lowest between midnight and 6 o'clock AM and rapidly reach peak levels between 9 o'clock AM and 1 o'clock PM.[129] This pattern coincides with the clinical observation that intracerebral hemorrhage and lacunar infarcts occur during waking hours. Furthermore, rigorous control of the blood pressure during waking hours may result in frank hypotension during the night.

RENAL K^+ WASTING

Increased levels of aldosterone secretion will cause marked renal K^+ secretion as distal Na^+ delivery is increased by diuretics and/or by high dietary salt intake. Increased distal H^+ secretion with generation of a metabolic alkalosis occurs in the same setting. Recent studies suggest that total-body K^+ depletion and hypokalemia may provoke serious cardiovascular consequences due to left ventricular irritability.[103] There is considerable controversy over the long-term effects of diuretic-induced K^+ depletion in patients who are not taking digitalis derivatives. Although benign forms of ventricular ectopy are increased during hypokalemia, evidence is lacking that demonstrates an increased propensity for fatal ventricular arrhythmias or decreased theshold for malignant arrhythmias in the setting of an acute myocardial infarction.[130] K^+ depletion does cause a reduction in the number of Na^+–K^+-ATPase sites in skeletal muscle and may therefore alter the disposition of cardioactive glycosides.[131] In any case, it is well recognized that diuretic-induced K^+ depletion can worsen the clinical toxicity of digitalis derivatives.

Dietary K^+ supplementation is one approach to managing diuretic-induced K^+ depletion. Unfortunately, this approach is relatively expensive, requires steady compliance, and, in the case of oral KCl administration, may not be met with widespread patient approval.

Another approach has recently emphasized the importance of dietary Na^+ intake.[29,125,128] In the steady state, dietary Na^+ intake will be reflected in the urinary excretion of Na^+. This relationship also pertains to patients who are chronically taking thiazides or loop diuretics. Once the initial diuresis is completed, the patient should then maintain normal salt balance. Therefore, even in the setting of chronic diuretic therapy, the daily excretion of Na^+ is an accurate index of intake. If dietary salt intake is excessive, then distal delivery of Na^+ and urinary excretion of Na^+ will be high, and distal K^+ (and H^+) excretion will be stimulated. Moderate restriction of dietary Na^+ intake (60 to 100 mEq/day) has been shown to potentiate the effects of diuretics in essential hypertension and to lessen renal K^+ wasting.[128] Dietary Na^+ restriction is also indicated in states associated with avid renal Na^+ retention (e.g., congestive heart failure, cirrhosis, advanced diabetic nephropathy).

K^+-sparing diuretics are indicated for the patient who has failed to respond to or comply with dietary Na^+ restriction or K^+ supplementation. It is worth emphasizing the beneficial effects of dietary counseling before resorting to additional diuretic intervention.

Fixed-dosage combinations of K^+-sparing diuretics with thiazide agents are currently widely prescribed. The combinations offer the virtue of synergistic effects of Na^+ handling as well as the counteracting side effects. The combination of thiazide plus aldosterone antagonist will inhibit Na^+ reabsorption in the distal convoluted tubule (thiazides) and in the collecting tubule (aldosterone antagonist). This approach is especially useful if secondary aldosteronism has stimulated Na^+ transport in the collecting tubule.

TYPE IV RENAL TUBULAR ACIDOSIS

The hallmark of this group of disorders is hyperkalemia in the presence of normal or moderately reduced glomerular filtration rate (>20 ml/min). It is usually, but not invariably, accompanied by a hyperchloremic metabolic acidosis.[132,133] Hyporeninemic hypoaldosteronism, frequently secondary to diabetes mellitus, is the most common cause of type IV renal tubular acidosis.[132] Other possible pathogenetic mechanisms include (1) impairment in the renin–angiotensin–aldosterone system not due to functional hyporeninemia, such as Addison's disease,[132] primary hypoaldosteronism,[132,] chronic heparin-induced hypoaldosteronism,[132,] pseudohypoaldosteronism types I (end-organ resistance), and II (chloride shunt),[134] a primary renal tubular secretory defect (e.g., sickle cell disease,[135] systemic lupus erythematous,[136] postrenal transplant,[137,138] amyloid,[132] familial,[132] obstructive uropathy,[139]) and (2) inhibition of tubular secretion (e.g. spironolactone, amiloride, triamterene[132]).

The mainstays of treatment include a low-potassium diet; thiazide and loop diuretics; mineralocorticoids, sodium bicarbonate, and cationic exchange resins.[132] The therapeutic modalities prescribed depend upon the nature of the underlying disorder and the status of the patient. For example, patients with a K^+ secretory defect[132,135–137,139] are best treated with diet and a cationic exchange resin. Patients with primary hyporeninemia or hypoaldosteronism are effectively treated with replacement doses of mineralocorticoids. Postrenal transplant hyperkalemia is an example of a disorder that can result from two different mechanisms, impaired secretion of K^+ that is (1) sensitive to thiazide but not necessarily loop diuretics,[140] and (2) hyporeninemia.[137,138] Furosemide and sodium bicarbonate are efficacious in the subgroups with diabetes mellitus. Mineralocorticoid is often ineffective, necessitating supraphysiologic dosages with resultant circulatory overload.[132]

The efficacy of furosemide can result from some combination of augmentation of aldosterone secretion, increased distal Na^+ delivery, and tubular fluid flow. When administered with a nonreabsorbable anion, such as sodium bicarbonate, all the conditions necessary for K^+ secretion are fulfilled.

A chloride shunt has recently been postulated to exist in some patients with hypertension and hyperkalemia.[134] In this uncommon disorder, dietary salt restriction and thiazides constitute the cornerstone of therapy. The proposed pathogenic mechanism involves enhanced chloride reabsorption in the distal nephron. This shunt results in a decreased driving force for K^+ secretion by (1) decreased renin–aldosterone production, and (2) a relative diminution in the intraluminal negative potential difference. The observed superiority of thiazides over loop agents suggests that the location of this shunt is between the sites of action of these two classes of diuretics.

ACUTE RENAL FAILURE

The value of mannitol and loop agents remains uncertain in the treatment and prophylaxis of established or imminent acute renal failure. Loop agents have been used in oliguric acute renal failure with the intent of producing a nonoliguric state. The rationale is to permit better management of fluids, nutritional requirements, and electrolytes, notably potassium and phosphorus. Whether outcome is favorably altered, as it is in patients with established nonoliguric renal failure, is not yet known.

Furosemide can increase urine flow and glomerular filtration in certain experimental models of acute renal failure.[141] Controversy persists in humans as to whether high-dose furosemide can convert an oliguric to a nonoliguric state.[142–144] The direct renal artery injection of furosemide in patients with acute renal failure has had no discernible effects on urine flow or clinical course.[145] In those instances in which furosemide has produced an increase in urine output (necessitating doses of 3.0 g/day), no beneficial effect has been uniformly noted on overall outcome, mortality, dialytic requirements, or duration of acute renal failure.[142–144,146] The prophylactic use of furosemide has not been adequately assessed. Mannitol has been shown to improve renal blood flow and glomerular filtration during and after renal artery hypoperfusion in the experimental setting.[147,148] However, reports in the surgical literature fail to demonstrate convincingly any prophylactic benefit or any substantial effects in established early acute renal failure resulting from noncardiovascular surgery that cannot be otherwise achieved with crystalloid infusion.[146,149–151]

Renal dysfunction that occurs after cardiac surgery with cardiopulmonary bypass is characterized by a nonoliguric state with a fractional excretion of sodium of less than 1 percent. The pathophysiology of this phenomenon is not clear, but the ability of the kidney to abstract sodium requires intact tubular function. Pretreatment with volume expansion and mannitol infusion at the beginning of cardiopulmonary bypass and hourly thereafter may serve to attenuate the severity of renal injury that results from ischemia. The ultimate development of acute renal failure (nonoliguric but with fractional excretion of sodium > 1 percent) is associated with persistent and severe hemodynamic compromise.[152,153]

The manner in which these agents are postulated to work includes the following:

1. An amelioration by mannitol of smooth muscle and tubular cell swelling[107]
2. Maintenance of high luminal flow rates and pressure, thereby minimizing tubular obstruction from cellular and proteinaceous debris (An additional effect would be a minimization of vasoconstriction and decreased glomerular filtration that attends tubular obstruction.)
3. A direct vasodilatory effect to counteract the vasoconstriction seen in acute renal failure
4. Extracellular and intravascular volume expansion by mannitol that could result in decreased blood viscosity and improved renal blood flow
5. Furosemide inhibition of tubuloglomerular feedback

In a clinical setting that predisposes to acute renal failure (e.g., acute intravascular hemolysis with hemoglobinuria due to incompatible blood transfusions or drug-induced hemolysis, acute hyperuricemia, rhabdomyolysis with myoglobinuria), an initial trial of mannitol and/or furosemide is reasonable. Baseline laboratory data, including urinary osmolarity and electrolytes and serum electrolytes, calcium, phosphorus, uric acid, and magnesium, should be obtained before the initiation of therapy. The patient's volume status must be critically assessed before and during treatment to detect volume depletion (and therefore a potentially reversible cause of renal failure) and to avoid cardiovascular compromise that can result from mannitol infusion.

A low urinary sodium concentration during pigment nephropathy may be predictive of reversible acute renal failure.[154] An approach to the oliguric, azotemic patient with pigment nephropathy involves the infusion over 4 hours of 25 g mannitol and 100 mEq sodium bicarbonate added to 1 liter dextrose and water.[155] If a diuretic response ensues, this Cocktail can be repeated. If hypocalcemia is present, then the bicarbonate should be deleted to avoid possible tetanic complications. If a diuretic response does not occur after the initial infusion, then 250 mg intravenous furosemide can be tried.

Severe acute hyperuricemia in lymphoma and leukemia patients treated with chemotherapy has become a rare occurrence since the introduction of allopurinol. The use of diuretics along with a large intake of fluids induces high tubular flow rates and lessens the likelihood of acute uric acid nephropathy. Alkalinization of the urine has been shown to have little protective effect when compared with forced diuresis.[4] However, it would appear prudent, at the onset of treatment, for malignancy to alkalinize the urine so as to increase the solubility of uric acid and xanthine.

The use of cis-platinum, a heavy metal, can result in renal insufficiency and electrolyte disorders, notably magnesium wasting. Cis-platinum nephrotoxicity correlates with both the total dose and the duration of treatment and is probably irreversible. Distal nephron tubular necrosis has been observed in cis-platinum-associated nephrotoxicity. Adequate hydration with high urine flow rates and the constant infusion of 10 g mannitol per hour at the time of cis-platinum infusion and for 6 hours thereafter reduces the incidence and severity of nephrotoxicity.[156]

High-dose methotrexate (>1 g/m^2) can result in tubular necrosis independent of the development of acute uric acid nephropathy. Methotrexate is not appreciably metabolized and requires both glomerular filtration and tubular secretion for excretion. Precipitation within the tubule lumen and disruption of renal transport mechanisms are believed to be the factors responsible for the development of tubular necrosis.[157] Methotrexate is poorly soluble in acid urine. Therefore, to minimize nephrotoxicity, a brisk diuresis and alkalinization of the urine with sodium bicarbonate is employed.

In those patients who are unable to maintain a diuresis and develop intravascular overload, mannitol is the preferred diuretic. Furosemide has the theoretical disadvantage of competing with methotrexate for active tubular secretion and could, therefore, result in intracellular accumulation of methotrexate to nephrotoxic levels.

Radiographic contrast media can result in a nonoliguric acute renal failure, which occurs principally in individuals with preexisting renal insufficiency, (serum creatinine above 2 mg/dl). The azotemic type I diabetic is at an even greater risk. Furthermore, if the preexisting creatinine clearance is less than 20 ml/min, approximately 50 percent of diabetics will not recover renal function.[158] The infusion of 250 ml of 20 percent mannitol in a well-hydrated patient within 1 hour after the injection of contrast dye has been shown to be more effective in reducing the frequency of acute renal failure than hydration alone. More than 90 percent of well-hydrated diabetic patients and 60 percent of nondiabetic patients (mean serum creatinine 3.8 mg/dl) has a reduction in creatinine clearance of at least 25 percent. When a similar group of patients (mean serum creatinine 4.6 mg/dl) received mannitol in addition to hydration, the incidence of acute renal failure was reduced to 35 percent in the diabetic patients and 15 percent in the nondiabetic patients.[159]

Diuretic administration in certain disorders has been temporally related to the development of acute renal failure. The administration of triamterene to healthy individuals being treated with indomethacin has resulted in reversible acute renal failure. Acute tubular necrosis has been reported in furosemide-treated patients with the nephrotic syndrome secondary to minimal change disease. Furosemide and thiazide diuretics are rarely associated with allergic interstitial nephritis.

Renal failure develops in a variable percentage of patients with progressive systemic sclerosis and may present in one of two general patterns. Progressive acute oliguric renal failure, usually associated with severe hypertension, is the classic and best recognized presentation of renal failure. The second and more recently recognized group of patients are those with mild and gradually progressive renal insufficiency, moderate hypertension, and mild proteinuria.[160] These patients appear to be predisposed to developing a superimposed acute renal failure during treatment for congestive heart failure and during episodes of abdominal surgery, pericardial effusion, or volume depletion.[161]

CONCLUSION

Diuretics constitute one of the most important pharmacologic agents prescribed by physicians. The clinical usefulness of these agents has expanded beyond their initial employment as natriuretics. Diuretics have proved efficacious in states of altered Ca^{2+} and H_2O balance, the renal tubular acidoses, and toxic nephropathies, and in the amelioration of the severity of acute tubular necrosis associated with cardiovascular surgery. It is also well recognized that serious and life-threatening complications occur with diuretics. As in all aspects of medicine, the underlying disorder has to be correctly identified and defined and a rational approach constructed. Therapy is initiated and adjusted as dictated by the observed effects of treatment. Through an understanding of their mechanisms of action, diuretics can be effectively and judiciously applied. Because the ability of the body to adjust to acute changes induced by pharmacologic intervention is often compromised in the diseased state, it is important to place into perspective the duration and severity of the disorder and the time course necessary to effect proper treatment. Understanding the sites of diuretic action within the nephron is as important as an appreciation of the time course of the therapeutic response. With these factors in mind, diuretic therapy can be instituted with maximal therapeutic benefit.

REFERENCES

1. Schrier RW, Lehman D, Zacherle B, et al: Effects of furosemide on free water excretion in edematous patients with hyponatremia. Kidney Int 3:30, 1973
2. Warnock DG, Rector FC Jr: Renal acidification mechanism. p. 440. In Brenner BM, Rector FC Jr (eds): The Kidney. 2nd Ed. WB Saunders, Philadelphia, 1981
3. Campbell DA: Effect of Neptazane on intraocular pressure in relation to its systemic action and its clinical application. Br J Ophthalmol 44:415, 1960
4. Conger JD, Falk SA: Intrarenal dynamics in the pathogenesis and prevention of acute urate nephropathy. J Clin Invest 59:786, 1977
5. Bear R, Goldstein M, Phillipson E, et al: Effect of metabolic alkalosis on respiratory function in patients with chronic obstructive lung disease. Can Med Assoc J 117:900, 1977
6. Miller PD, Berns AS: Acute metabolic alkalosis perpetuating hypercarbia: A role for acetazolamide in chronic obstructive pulmonary disease. JAMA 238:2400, 1977
7. Greene MK, Kerr AM, McIntosh IB, et al: Acetazolamide in prevention of acute mountain sickness: A double-blind controlled cross-over study. Br Med J 283:811, 1981
8. Beck LM, Goldberg M: Effects of acetazolamide and parathyroidectomy on renal transport of sodium, calcium and phosphate. Am J Physiol 224:1136, 1973
9. Agus ZS, Goldfarb S, Wasserstein A: Disorders of calcium and phosphate metabolism. p. 985. In Brenner BM, Rector FC Jr (eds): The Kidney. 2nd Ed. WB Saunders, Philadelphia, 1981
10. Sinha TK, Allen DO, Queener SF, et al: Effects of acetazolamide on the renal excretion of phosphate in hypoparathyroidism and pseudohypoparathyroidism. J Lab Clin Med 89:1188, 1977
11. Mudge GH: Drugs affecting renal function and electrolyte metabolism. p. 896. In Gilman AG, Goodman LS, Gilman A (eds): 6th Ed. The Pharmacological Basis of Therapeutics. Macmillan, New York, 1980
12. Streeten DHP, Dalakos TG, Fellerman H: Studies on hyperkalemic periodic paralysis. Evidence of changes in plasma Na and Cl and induction of paralysis by adrenal glucocorticoids. J Clin Invest 50:142, 1971
13. Griggs RC, Engel WK, Resnick JS: Acetazolamide treatment of hypokalemic periodic paralysis. Prevention of attacks and improvement of persistent weakness. Ann Intern Med 73:39, 1970

14. Lemann J Jr, Litzow JR, Lennon JR: Studies of the mechanism by which metabolic acidosis augments urinary calcium excretion in man. J Clin Invest 46:1318, 1967
15. Parfitt AM: Acetazolamide and sodium bicarbonate induced nephrocalcinosis and nephrolithiasis. Arch Intern med 124:736, 1969
16. Krivoy N, Ben-Arien Y, Carter A, et al: Methazolamide-induced hepatitis and pure RBC aplasia. Arch Intern med 141:1229, 1981
17. Webster LT Jr, Davidson CS: Production of impending hepatic coma by a carbonic anhydrase inhibitor. Diamox. Proc Soc Exp Biol Med 91:27, 1956
18. Earley LE, Kahn M, Orloff J: The effects of infusion of chlorothiazide on urinary dilution and concentration in the dog. J Clin Invest 40:857, 1961
19. Burg MB: Renal handling of sodium, chloride, water, amino acids and glucose. p. 328. In Brenner BM, Rector FC Jr (eds): The Kidney. 2nd Ed. WB Saunders, Philadelphia, 1981
20. Kunau RT Jr, Weller DR, Webb HL: Clarification of the site of action of chlorothiazide in the rat nephron. J Clin Invest 56:401, 1975
21. Suki WN, Dawoud F, Eknoyan G, et al: Effects of metolazone on renal function in normal man. J Pharmacol Exp. Ther 180:6, 1972
22. Ross CR, Cafruny EJ: Blockade of the diuretic action of benzothiadiazines. J Pharmacol Exp Ther 140:125, 1963
23. Constanzo LS, Windhager EE: Calcium and sodium transport by the distal convoluted tubule of the rat. Renal Fluid Electrolyte Physiology Suppl 4.) Am J Physiol 235:F492, 1978
24. Taylor A, Windhager EE: Possible role of cytosolic calcium and Na–Ca exchange in regulation of transepithelial sodium transport. Am J Physiol 236(6):F505, 1979
25. Suki WN: Effects of diuretics on calcium metabolism. Mineral Electrolyte Metab 2:125, 1981
26. Porter RH, Cox BG, Heaney D, et al: Treatment of hypoparathyroid patients with chlorthalidone. N Engl J Med 298:577, 1978
27. Jones B, Nanra RS: Double-blind trial of antihypertensive effect of chlorothiazide in severe renal failure. Lancet 2:1258, 1979
28. Ezra D, Iaina A, Kapular S, et al: Evidence for an extra-renal action of chlorothiazide on serum potassium. Mineral Electrolyte Metab 7:285, 1982
29. Fries E: Salt in hypertension and the effects of diuretics. Annu Rev Pharmacol Toxicol 19:13, 1979
30. Coe FL: Clinical stone disease. p. 1. In Brenner BM, Stein JH (eds): Nephrolithiasis. Contemporary Issues in Nephrology. Churchill Livingstone, New York, 1980
31. Coe, FL, Kavalach AG: Hypercalciuria and hyperuricosuria in patients with calcium nephrolithiasis. N Engl J Med 291:1344, 1974
32. Coe, FL: Prevention of kidney stones. Am J Med 71:514, 1981
33. Yendt ER, Cohanim M: Prevention of calcium stones with thiazides. Kidney Int 13:397, 1978
34. Weber DV, Coe FL, Parks JH, et al: Urinary saturation measurements in calcium nephrolithiasis. Ann Intern med 90:180, 1979
35. Crawford JD, Kennedy GC, Hill LE: Clinical results of treatment of diabetes insipidus with drugs of the chlorothiazide series. N Engl J Med 262:737, 1960
36. Earley LE, Orloff J: The mechanism of antidiuresis associated with the administration of hydrochlorothiazide to patients with vasopressin-resistant diabetes insipidus. J Clin Invest 41:1988, 1962
37. Batlle D, Gaviria M, Grupp M, et al: Distal nephron function in patients receiving chronic lithium therapy. Kidney Int 21:477, 1982
38. Singer I: Lithium and the kidney. Kidney Int 19:374, 1981
39. Levy ST, Forrest JN Jr, Heninger GR: Lithium-induced diabetes insipidus: Manic symptoms, brain and electrolyte correlates, and chlorothiazide treatment. Am J Psychiatry 130:1014, 1973
40. Rampini S, Fanconi A, Illig R, et al: Effect of hydrochlorothiazide on proximal renal tubular acidosis in a patient with idiopathic "de Toni–Delore–Fanconi syndrome." Helv Paediatr Acta 23:13, 1968

41. Donckerwolcke RA, Vanstekelenburg J Tilddburg J, et al: Therapy of bicarbonate losing tubular renal acidosis. Arch Child Dis 45:774, 1970
42. Report of Medical Research Council Working Party on Mild to Moderate Hypertension: Adverse reactions to benzflurazide and propranolol for the treatment of mild hypertension. Lancet 2:539, 1981
43. Samaan N, Dollery CT, Fraser R: Diabetogenic action of benzothiadiazines. lancet 2:1244, 1963
44. Hoskins B, Jackson CM: The mechanism of chlorothiazide-induced carbohydrate intolerance. J Pharmacol Exp Ther 206:423, 1978
45. Manuel MA, Steele TH: Changes in renal urate handling after prolonged thiazide administration. Am J Med 57:741, 1974
46. Helgeland A, Hjermann I, Holme I, et al: Serum triglycerides and serum uric acid in untreated and thiazide-treated patients with mild hypertension. The Oslo Study. Am J Med 64:34, 1978
47. Ashraf N, Locksley R, Arieff AI: Thiazide-induced hyponatremia associated with death or neurologic damage in outpatients. Am J Med 70:1163, 1981
48. Kennedy RM, Earley LE: Profound hyponatremia resulting from a thiazide-induced decrease in urinary diluting capacity in a patient with primary polydypsia. N Engl J Med 282:1185, 1970
49. Fichman MP, Vorherr H, Kleeman CR, et al: Diuretic induced hyponatremia. Ann Intern Med 75:853, 1971
50. Popovtzer MM, Subryan VL, Alfrey AC, et al: The actue effect of chlorothiazide on serum-ionized calcium. Evidence for a parathyroid hormone-dependent mechanism. J Clin Invest 55:1295, 1975
51. Agus ZS, Wasserstein A, Goldfarb S: Disorders of calcium and magnesium homeostasis. Am J Med 72:473, 1982
52. Bell RT, Lippman M: Hydrochlorothiazide induced pulmonary edema. Arch Intern Med 139:817, 1979
53. Linton AL, Clark WF, Driedger AA, et al: Acute interstitial nephritis due to drugs: Review of the literature with a report of nine cases. Ann Intern Med 93:735, 1980
54. Rane A, Villeneuve JP, Stone WJ, et al: Plasma binding and disposition of furosemide in the nephrotic syndrome and in uremia. Clin Pharmacol Ther 24:199, 1978
55. Koechel DA: Ethacrynic acid and related diuretics: Relationship of structure to beneficial and detrimental actions. Annu Rev Pharmacol Toxicol 21:265, 1981
56. Warnock DG, Eveloff J: NaCl entry mechanisms across the luminal membrane of the renal tubule. (Editorial review.) (Renal Fluid Electrolyte Physiology 11.) Am J Physiol 242:F561, 1982
57. Dirks JH: Mechanism of action and clinical use of diuretics. Hosp Pract p 99, 1979
58. Dikshit K, Vyden JK, Forrester JS, et al: Renal and extrarenal hemodynamic effects of furosemide in congestive heart failure after acute myocardial infarction. N Engl J Med 288:1087, 1973
59. Lesch M, Caranasos GJ, Mulholland JH: Controlled study comparing ethacrynic acid to mercaptomerin in the treatment of acute pulmonary edema. N Engl J Med 279:115, 1968
60. Martinex-Maldonado M, Eknoyan G, Suki WN: Diuretics in nonedematous states. Physiologic basis for clinical use. Arch Intern Med 131:797, 1973

60b. Tobert JA, Cirillo VJ, Hitzenberger G, et al: Enhancement of uricosuric properties of indacrinone by manipulation of the enantiomer ratio. Clin Pharmacol Ther 29:344, 1981

61. Bennett WM, Van Zee BE: Aucte renal failure from ticrynafen. N Engl J Med 301:1179, 1979
62. Cohen LH, Norby LH, Champion C, et al: Acute renal failure from ticrynafen. N Engl J Med 301:1180, 1979
63. Martinez-Maldonado M: Inappropriate antidiuretic hormone secretion of unknown origin. Kidney Int 17:554, 1980
64. Forrest JN Jr, Cox M, Hong C, et al: Superiority of demeclocycline over lithium in the treatment of chronic syndrome of inappropriate secretion of antidiuretic hormone. N Engl J Med 298:173, 1978
65. Miller PD Linas SL, Schrier RW: Plasma demeclocycline levels and nephrotoxicity: Correlation in hyponatremic cirrhotic patients. JAMA 243:2513, 1980
66. Decaux G, Waterlot Y, Genette F, et al: Treatment of the syndrome of inappropriate

secretion of antidiuretic hormone with furosemide. N Engl J Med 304:329, 1981
67. DeFronzo RA, Braine H, Calvin DM, et al: Water intoxication in man after cyclophosphamide therapy. Ann Intern Med 78:861, 1973
68. Green TP, Mirkin BL: Prevention of cyclophosphamide-induced antidiuresis by furosemide infusion. Clin Pharmacol Ther 29:634, 1981
69. Goldberg M: Hyponatremia. Med Clin North Am 65:251, 1981
69a. Dubois GD, Arieff AI: Symptomatic hyponatremia: The case for rapid correction. In Narins R (Ed): Controversies in Nephrology and Hypertension. Churchill Livingstone, New York, 1984, p 377
70. Hantman D, Rossier B, Zohlman R, et al: Rapid correction of hyponatremia in the syndrome of inappropriate secretion of antidiuretic hormone. Ann Intern Med 78:870, 1973
71. Ayus JC, Olivero JJ, Frommer JP: Rapid correction of severe hyponatremia with intravenous hypertonic saline solution. Am J Med 72:43, 1982
72. Massry SG: Disorders of magnesium metabolism. p. 1639. In Earley LE, Gottshalk CW (eds): Strauss and Welt's Diseases of the Kidney. 3rd Ed. Little, Brown, Boston, 1979
73. Gabow PA, Hanson TJ, Poportzer MM et al: Furosemide-induced reduction in ionized calcium in hypoparathyroid patients. Ann Intern Med 86:579, 1977
74. Gallagher KL, Jones JK: Furosemide-induced ototoxicity. Ann Intern Med 91:744, 1979
75. Vargish T, Benjamin R, Shenkman L: Deafness from furosemide. Ann Intern Med 72:761, 1970
76. Cooperman LB, Rubin IL: Toxicity of ethacrynic acid and furosemide. Am Heart J 85:831, 1973
77. Fernandez PC, Puschett JB: Proximal tubular actions of metolazone and chlorothiazide. Am J Physiol 225:954, 1973
78. Lucci MS, Warnock DG: Effects of anion transport inhibitors on NaCl reabsorption in the rat superficial proximal convoluted tubule. J Clin Invest 64:570, 1979
79. Wollam GL, Tarazi RC, Bravo EL, et al: Diuretic potency of combined hydrochlorothiazide and furosemide therapy in patients with azotemia. Am J Med 72:929, 1982
80. Epstein M, Lepp BA, Hoffman DS, et al: Potentiation of furosemide by metolazone in refractory edema. Curr Ther Res 21:656, 1977
81. Ghose RR, Gupta SK: Synergistic action of metolazone with "loop" diuretics. Br Med J 282:1432, 1981
82. Black WD, Shiner PT, Roman J: Severe electrolyte disturbances associated with metolazone and furosemide. South Med J 71:380, 1978
83. Giebisch G, Stanton B: Potassium transport in the nephron. Annu Rev Physiol 41:241, 1979
84. Sebastian A, Hulter HN, Kurtz I, et al: Disorders of distal nephron function. Am J Med 72:289, 1982
85. Petty KJ, Kokko JP, Marver D: Secondary effect of aldosterone on Na-K ATPase activity in the rabbit cortical collecting tubule. J Clin Invest 68:1514, 1981
86. Tannen RL: Relationship of renal ammonia production and potassium homeostasis. Kidney Int 11:453, 1977
87. Corvol P, Claire M, oblin ME, et al: Mechanism of the antimeralocorticoid effect of spirolactones. Kidney Int 20:1, 1981
88. Stoner LC, Burg MB, Orloff J: Ion transport in cortical collecting tubules: Effect of amiloride. Am J Physiol 227:453, 1974
89. Schambelan M, Sebastian A, Biglieri EG, et al: Amelioration of hypokalemia by amiloride in diverse syndromes associated with renal potassium wasting. Kidney Int 21:157a, 1982
90. Gabow PA, Moore S, Schrier RW: Spironolactone-induced hyperchloremic acidosis in cirrhosis. Ann Intern Med 90:338, 1979
91. Tannenbaum PJ, Rosen E, Flanagan T, et al: The influence of dosage form on the activity of a diuretic agent. Clin Pharmacol Ther 9:598, 1968
92. Mueller A, Steinmetz PR: Spironolactone, an aldosterone agonist in the stimulation of H^+ secretion by turtle urinary bladder. J Clin Invest 61:1660, 1978
93. Ettinger B, Oldroys NO, Sorgel F: Triamterene nephrolithiasis. JAMA 244:2443, 1980
94. Ettinger B, Weil E, Mandel NS, et al: Triam-

terene-induced nephrolithiasis. Ann Intern Med 91:745, 1979
95. Favre L, Glasson P, Vallotton MB: Reversible acute renal failure from combined triamterene and indomethacin. Ann Intern Med 96:317, 1982
96. Shuck J, Shen S, Omensky L et al: Spironolactone hepatitis in primary hyperaldosteronism. Ann Intern Med 95:708, 1981
97. Warren SE, Blantz RC: Mannitol. Arch Intern Med 141:493, 1981
98. Gennari FJ, Kassirer JP: Osmotic diuresis. N Engl J Med 291:714, 1974
99. Arieff AI: Dialysis dysequilibrium syndrome: Current concepts on pathogenesis. p. 367. In Schriener GE, Winchester JF (eds): Controversies in Nephrology. Vol. 4. Georgetown University Press, 1982
100. DeTroyer A: Demeclocycline: Treatment for syndrome of inappropriate antidiuretic hormone secretion. JAMA 237:2723, 1981
101. Chou T-C, Van Der Bel-Kahn J, Allen J, et al: Electrocardiographic diagnosis of right ventricular infarction. Am J Med 70:1175, 1981
102. Cohn JN: Right ventricular infarction revisited. Am J Cardiol 43:666, 1979
103. Holland OB, Nixon JV, Kohnert L: Diuretic-induced ventricular ectopy activity. Am J Med 70:762, 1981
104. Levy M, Seeley JF: Pathophysiology of edema formation. p. 150. In Brenner BM, Rector FC Jr (eds): The Kidney. 2nd Ed. WB Saunders, Philadelphia, 1981
105. Wilkinson SP, Williams R: Renal failure in cirrhosis: Current views and speculations. Adv Nephrol 7:15, 1977
106. Shear L, Ching S, Gabuzda GJ: Compartmentalization of ascites and edema in patients with hepatic cirrhosis. N Engl J Med 282:1391, 1970
107. Earley LE, Martino JA: Influence of sodium balance on the ability of diuretics to inhibit tubular reabsorption. Circulation 42:323, 1970
108. Grausz H, Lieberman R, Earley LE: Effect of plasma albumin on sodium reabsorption in patients with nephrotic syndrome. Kidney Int 1:47, 1972
109. Perez-Ayuso RM, Arroyo V, Planas R, et al: Randomized comparative study of efficacy of furosemide versus spironolactone in non-azotemic cirrhosis with ascites. Gastroenterology 84:978, 1983
110. Gregory PB, Broekelschen PH, Hill MD et al: Complications of diuresis in the alcoholic patient with ascites: A controlled trial. Gastroenterology 73:534, 1977
111. Boyer TD, Warnock DW: Diuretic use and effects in hepatic cirrhosis. Gastroenterology 84:1051, 1983
112. Glassock RJ, Cohen AH, Bennett CM et al: Primary glomerular diseases. p. 1407. In Brenner BM, Rector FC Jr (eds): The Kidney. 2nd Ed. WB Saunders, Philadelphia, 1981
113. Meltzer JI, Keim HJ, Laragh JH, et al: Nephrotic syndrome: Vasoconstriction and hypervolemic types indicated by renin-sodium profiling. Ann Intern Med 91:688, 1979
114. Lowenstein J, Schacht RG, Baldwin D: Renal failure in minimal change nephrotic syndrome. Am J Med 70:227, 1981
115. Bernard DB: Case records of the Massachusetts General Hospital. N Engl J Med 306:221, 1982
116. Chamberlain MJ, Pringle A, Wrong OM: Oliguric renal failure in the nephrotic syndrome. Q J Med 35:215, 1966
117. Connolly ME, Wrong OM, Jones, NF: Reversible renal failure in idiopathic nephrotic syndrome with minimal glomerular changes. Lancet 1:665, 1968
118. Rose BD: Case records of the Massachusetts General Hospital. N Engl J Med 299:136, 1978
119. Yamauchi H, Hopper J Jr: Hypovolemic shock and hypotension as a complication in the nephrotic syndrome: Report of ten cases. Ann Intern Med 60:242, 1964
120. DeWardener HE: Idiopathic edema: Role of diuretic abuse. Kidney Int 19:881, 1981
121. MacGregor GA, Roulston JE, Markandu ND, et al: Is idiopathic oedema idiopathic? Lancet 1:397, 1979
122. MacGregor GA, Tasker PRW, DeWardener HE: Diuretic-induced oedema. Lancet 1:489, 1975
123. Stinebaugh BJ, Schloeder FX: Glucose-induced alkalosis in fasting subjects. J Clin Invest 51:1326, 1972
124. Landsberg L, Young JB: Fasting, feeding and regulation of the sympathetic nervous system. N Engl J Med 298:1295, 1978

125. MacGregor GA, Best FE, Cam JM, et al: Double-blind randomized crossover trial of moderate sodium restriction in essential hypertension. Lancet 1:351, 1982

125a. deCarvalho JGR, Dunn FG, Lohmöller G, et al: Hemodynamic corelates of prolonged thiazide therapy: Comparison of responders and nonresponders. Clin Pharmol Ther 22:875, 1977

126. Van Brummelen P, Woerlee M, Schalekamp MADH: Long-term versus short-term effects on hydrochlorothiazide on renal haemodynamics in essential hypertension. Clin Sci 56:453, 1979

127. Bennett WM, McDonald WJ, Kuehnel E, et al: Commentary: Do diuretics have antihypertensive properties independent of natriuresis? Clin Pharmacol Ther 22:499, 1977

128. Ram CVS, Garrett B, Kaplan NM: Moderate sodium restriction and various diuretics in the treatment of hypertension: Effects on potassium wastage and blood pressure control. Arch Intern Med 141:1015, 1981

129. Millar-Craig MW, Bishop CN, Raftery EB: Circadian variation of blood pressure. Lancet 1:795, 1978

130. Harrington JT, Ishner JM, Kassirer JP: Our national obsession with potassium. Am J Med 73:155, 1982

131. Norgaard AA, Kjeldsen K, Clausen T: Potassium depletion decreases the number of ^{3}H-ouabain binding sites and the active Na^{+}–K^{+} transport in skeletal muscle. Nature 293:739, 1981

132. DeFronzo RA: Hyperkalemia and hyporeninemic hypoaldosteronism. Kidney Int 17: 118, 1980

133. Schambelan M, Sebastian A, Biglieri EG: Prevalence, pathogenesis, and functional significance of aldosterone deficiency in hyperkalemic patients with chronic renal insufficiency. Kidney Int 17:89, 1981

134. Schambelan M, Sebastian A, Rector FC Jr: Mineralocorticoid-resistant renal hyperkalemia without salt wasting (type II pseudohypoaldosteronism): Role of increased chloride reabsorption. Kidney Int 19:716, 1981

135. DeFronzo RA, Taufield PA, Block H, et al: Impaired renal tubular potassium secretion in sickle cell disease. Ann Intern Med 90:310, 1979

136. DeFronzo RA, Cooke CR, Goldberg M, et al: Impaired renal tubular potassium secretion in systemic lupus erythematosus. Ann Intern Med 86:268, 1977

137. Better OS: Nonazotemic hyperkalemia following kidney transplantation. Mineral Electrolyte Metab 3:167, 1980

138. Perez GO, Oster JR: Hyporeninemic hypoaldosteronism after renal transplantation. South Med J 70:363, 1977

139. Batlle DC, Arruda JAL, Kurtzman NA: Hyperkalemic distal renal tubular acidosis associated with obstructive uropathy. N Engl J Med 304:373, 1981

140. DeFronzo RA, Goldberg M, Cooke CR, et al: Investigations into the mechanisms of hyperkalemia following renal transplantation. Kidney Int 11:357, 1977

141. deTorrente A, Miller PD, Cronin RE, et al: Effects of furosemide and acetylcholine in norepinephrine-induced acute renal failure. Am J Physiol 235:F131, 1978

142. Brown CB, Ogg CS, Cameron JS: High dose furosemide in acute renal failure: A controlled trial. Clin Nephrol 13:90, 1981

143. Cantarovich F, Galli C, Benedatti L, et al: High dose furosemide in established acute renal failure. Br Med J 4:449, 1973

144. Kleinknecht D, Ganeval D, Gonzalez-Duque LA, et al: Furosemide in acute oliguric renal failure: A controlled trial. Nephron 17:51, 1976

145. Epstein M, Schneider NS, Befeler B: Effect of intrarenal furosemide on renal function and intrarenal hemodynamics in acute renal failure. Am J Med 58:510, 1975

146. Levinsky NG, Bernard DB, Johnston PA: Enhancement of recovery of acute renal failure: Effects of mannitol and diuretics. p. 163. In Brenner BM, Stein JH (eds): Acute Renal Failure, Contemporary Issues in Nephrology. Churchill Livingstone, New York, 1980

147. Flores J, Dibona DR, Beck CH, et al: The role of cell swelling in ischemic renal damage and the protective effect of hypertonic solute. J Clin Invest 51:118, 1972

148. Morris CR, Alexander EA, Bruns FJ, et al: Restoration and maintenance of glomerular filtration by mannitol during hypoperfusion of the kidney. J Clin Invest 51:1555, 1972

149. Atik M: Prevention of acute renal failure. Am J Surg 108:384, 1964

150. Beall AC, Jr, Holman MR, Morris GC Jr,

et al: Mannitol-induced osmotic diuresis during vascular surgery. Arch Surg 86:34, 1963
151. Yeboah ED, Petrie A, Pead JL: Acute renal failure and open heart surgery. Br Med J 1:415, 1972
152. Hilberman M, Derby GC, Spencer RJ, et al: Sequential pathophysiological changes characterizing the progression from renal dysfunction to acute renal failure following cardiac operation. J Thorac Cardiovasc Surg 79:838, 1980
153. Hilberman M, Myers BD, Carrie BJ, et al: Acute renal failure following cardiac surgery. J Thorac Cardiovasc Surg 77:880, 1979
154. Knochel JP: Rhabdomyolysis and myoglobinuria. Semin Nephrol 1:75, 1981
155. Eneas JF, Schoenfeld PY, Humphreys MH: The effect of infusion of mannitol-sodium bicarbonate on the clinical course of myoglobinuria. Arch Intern Med 139:801, 1979
156. Blachley JD, Hill JB: Renal and electrolyte disturbances associated with cisplatin. Ann Intern Med 95:628, 1981
157. Stoller RG, Jacobs SA, Drake JC, et al: Pharmacokinetics of high-dose methotrexate (NSC-740). Part 3. Ca Chemother Pharmacol 6:19, 1975
158. Harkonen S, Kjellstrand C: Contrast nephropathy. Am J Nephrol 1:69, 1981
159. Anto HR, Chou S-Y, Porush JG, et al: Mannitol prevention of acute renal failure associated with infusion intravenous pyelography. Clin Res 27:407A, 1979
160. Dichoso CC: The kidney in progressive systemic sclerosis. p. 104. In Suki WN, Eknoyan G (eds): The Kidney in Systemic Disease. 2nd Ed. Wiley, New York, 1981
161. Cannon PJ, Hassar M, Case DB, et al: The relationship of hypertension and renal failure in scleroderma to structural and functional abnormalities of the renal cortical circulation. Medicine (Baltimore) 53:1, 1974

26

Total Parenteral Nutrition

Khursheed N. Jeejeebhoy
Mitchell L. Halperin
David Z. Levine

The intake of nutrients is often an accepted event in the day-to-day life of an individual. We eat at regular intervals throughout the day, and any restriction on the intake of food is rarely, if ever, a voluntary act willingly undertaken. Unfortunately, until recently the same view was not taken about persons unable to eat or nourish themselves because of gastrointestinal or systemic disease. In such persons, our ability to maintain life through the use of intravenous fluid and electrolyte replacement often resulted in prolonged starvation, until improvement of gastrointestinal function and/or the patient's condition permitted resumption of an oral diet. Thus in these patients, malnutrition often compromised recovery or even survival, despite control or cure of other morbid conditions.

The availability of techniques for bypassing bowel and giving nourishment intravenously has, in theory, completely eliminated the specter of starvation in patients who have had temporary or permanent damage to the gastrointestinal tract, and has allowed the infusion of supplementary nutrients to those patients who have increased requirements. The ability to nourish persons parenterally has permitted the use of bowel rest to treat patients with various active gastrointestinal diseases, such as Crohn's disease, pancreatitis, and malabsorptive syndromes.

Finally, the ability to give patients defined nutrients has expanded our understanding of requirements of specific ones.

INDICATIONS FOR TOTAL PARENTERAL NUTRITION

While it is technically easy to give total parenteral nutrition, it is undesirable nevertheless to use the parenteral route when nutrients can be given as effectively via the gastrointestinal tract. There are two main reasons: (1) parenteral feeding is more expensive; and (2) it may lead to a greater number of complications. On the basis of these general principles, the indications for parenteral nutrition are as follows.

1. *Gut failure:* The prime indication is functional "gut failure." When the gastrointestinal tract cannot be effectively used to take and/or absorb nutrients, the parenteral route must be used. This problem may be either of a temporary of permanent nature.

2. *Oral route disability:* In the event that the gastrointestinal tract is not functionally capable of nourishing the individual, the decision to give parenteral nutrition has to be based on a prediction of how long this disability will last. In circumstances wherein the oral

route cannot be used for a few days, e.g., after an elective operation in an otherwise healthy individual, it is our arbitrary practice not to give parenteral nutrition as there is no evidence that total parenteral nutrition aids outcome in these circumstances. The difficult cases involve patients who are malnourished and who need surgical procedures of a nature that is unlikely to result in prolonged loss of gastrointestinal function. In such cases, individualized decisions have to be taken.

3. *Bowel rest:* In certain conditions it has been recognized that orally ingested food may result in discomfort and increased disease activity. Under these circumstances avoidance of orally fed nutrients for some weeks may benefit the patient, at least symptomatically, and perhaps may even induce a remission of disease. Conditions treated in this way include Crohn's disease and pancreatitis.

NUTRIENT REQUIREMENTS

Nutrient requirements in patients on total parenteral nutrition are different from those given a normal diet for several reasons. First, by-passing the bowel results in complete systemic delivery of nutrients, while in contrast the proportion of nutrients reaching the systemic circulation after oral ingestion is modified by the bowel and liver. For example, only 20 percent of orally ingested zinc is absorbed, and ingested glutamate is transaminated to aspartate. Second, patients on total parenteral nutrition are often those with serious medical illness, such as sepsis, traumatic injury or tumor, all of which modify requirements. Third, certain metabolic requirements for so-called regrowth of the malnourished patient are not applicable in the stable individual.

The main objective of nutritional therapy is to restore or maintain normal body composition and function. This initially involves restoration or maintenance of lean tissue, followed by repletion of energy stores in the form of adipose tissue. In considering the requirements of restoring versus maintaining lean tissue, it is important to recognize that lean tissue is composed of individual cells with an electrically balanced ionic content. In addition, the cell has a membrane and endoplasmic reticulum. Restoration of all these elements requires the input of a number of nutrients. These include protein as amino acids, as well as intracellular electrolytes such as potassium, calcium, magnesium, phosphorus, and zinc. In addition, the cell membranes require the availability of lipid and carbohydrate moieties. Among the lipid components, certain fatty acids cannot be synthesized from carbohydrates and are thus called essential fatty acids. In the human, the main essential fatty acid is linoleic acid and, less importantly, linolenic acid. Thus it is evident that nutrient requirements are interrelated and require the simultaneous input of amino acids, lipids, electrolytes, and trace elements. The removal of any one element may often prevent the utilization of several others. For example, the absence of nitrogen results in negative potassium and phosphorus balance and vice versa.[1] With these general remarks, let us consider the requirements of specific components.

Amino Acids

Amino acids are the basis of all body proteins. Both the individual components of an amino acid mixture and the total nitrogen input are important.

AMINO ACID COMPOSITION OF THE INFUSED MIXTURE

Animal experiments showed that the growth of an animal depended not only on the amount of protein fed, but on the source of protein as well.[2] Some protein, such as egg, induced rapid growth even when fed in small quantities. In contrast, other protein such as gluten from wheat did not induce the same growth rates, even when given in large quantities. This difference was found to be due to the fact that optimal growth depended on providing a certain amount of each of a variety of amino acids. Rose defined the mixture for the normal human adult,[3] and subsequently a number of amino acid mixtures devised for intravenous infusion have tried to mimic the essential amino acid balance of this formula.

Most mixtures are not as yet ideal in terms of the nonessential amino acid components. This difficulty is partly due to the fact that certain amino acids such as glutamate may have potential central nervous system toxicity when given intravenously,[4] thus precluding their incorporation in a mixture, and partly because most mixtures have glycine and alanine added in excess to make up nonessential nitrogen. Such an excess results in increased levels of these amino acids in plasma during infusion, associated with increased catabolism and urinary losses. In addition, the composition of the mixtures currently available is based on balance studies derived from normal adults, who need only maintenance of tissue protein. The needs of malnourished individuals who are repleting tissue, as well as those who are septic and/or injured are as yet unresolved.

TOTAL NITROGEN INTAKE

While the protein requirements in terms of the amino acid mixture remains in dispute, the need for total nitrogen intake is better defined. Calloway and Spector showed that in normal volunteers, the amount of nitrogen retained, based on nitrogen balance, was dependent on both nitrogen and calorie intake.[5] In normal subjects, they showed that a positive nitrogen balance was only achieved when about 15 g nitrogen was fed with about 3000 kcal/day. However, it should be recognized that these were nongrowing normal adult volunteers in whom there was little potential for tissue repletion. What of the depleted sick patient? To answer this question it is desirable to look at nitrogen balance in depleted subjects given a hypocaloric infusion with varied amounts of protein. Blackburn et al.[6] showed that 1 g/kg amino acid, infused alone without added nonprotein calories, resulted in a better nitrogen balance than did equicaloric amounts of 280 mM (5 percent) dextrose. Later Greenberg et al.[7] showed that the protein-sparing action of amino acids was based on the amount of amino acids given, and did not depend on the substrate-hormone profile. In later studies, Greenberg and Jeejeebhoy[8] showed that, unlike data in normal volunteer studies, the provision of 2 g/kg amino acids to surgical patients as the sole caloric source resulted in a positive nitrogen balance even when caloric utilization exceeded intake, i.e., a negative energy balance. Subsequent studies by Bozetti[9] and Elwyn et al.[10] have supported this finding.

Body composition studies done by Collins et al.[11] showed that body nitrogen was maintained as well by amino acid infusions as by glucose plus amino acids. These findings indicate that in depleted patients the intake of amino acids is of prime importance in defining the occurrence and extent of nitrogen retention.[7]

The above studies have been carried out in the depleted patient. What of patients who are injured and septic and those with tumors? Roulet et al.[12] showed that in septic subjects the provision of about 1.5 g of amino acids/kg body weight resulted in an equilibrium between protein synthesis and catabolism and also a zero or positive nitrogen balance. In patients with small cell cancer of the lung, a similar intake of amino acids maintained total body nitrogen but did not result in its rise.[13] However other studies with graded input need to be done in such patients.

Energy Requirements

Harris and Benedict showed that energy needs in normal subjects were a function of age, sex, and body size.[13a] These workers derived a formula for the needs of these subjects. It is also possible to derive the actual energy requirements by indirect calorimetery. Using these techniques we have found that in normals the two correlate within a ±10 percent error. In depleted subjects, the actual energy expenditure is below normal but appropriate for their reduced body size. In such subjects, an intake of about 30 kcal/kg will meet requirements; anything in excess will result in weight gain.

In contrast, patients who are septic and injured are traditionally believed to need additional calories. Several previous estimates have suggested that caloric requirements are increased by 40 to 60 percent for injury and sepsis and by 100 percent for burns.[14] These estimates have been questioned recently; indeed, it has become apparent that infusing calories in excess of requirements only serves to increase the incidence of both pulmonary and hepatic complications.

In two separate studies, the energy requirements for injured septic patients have been found to exceed by only 13 to 14 percent the predicted value based on their age, sex, and body size.[12,15] However, in patients with oat cell cancer of the lung, the increase in metabolic rate appeared to be more substantial and was 30 percent above the predicted value.[16] In any case, both these estimates are much below previously derived requirements and suggest that even in injured-septic subjects or those with cancer, provision of about 40 kcals/kg per day would result in meeting requirements. If computed on ideal body weight, 40 kcals/kg per day would result in surfeit calories sufficient to induce weight gain. Thus, more than 2400 kcals/day for a 60 kg person is rarely indicated.

SOURCE OF CALORIES: CARBOHYDRATE OR FAT?

In controlled cross-over studies, Jeejeebhoy et al.[17] showed that nitrogen balance was the same when patients were given 1 g/kg amino acids per day in addition to 40 kcal/kg/day nonprotein calories either as glucose alone or as 83 percent fat and 17 percent glucose. This equivalence of fat and carbohydrate in maintaining nitrogen balance has been confirmed in similar patients by a variety of other studies.[18-20] In contrast, it has been claimed by some investigators[21,22] that patients with increased metabolic requirements retain nitrogen better when glucose is the major source of nonprotein calories. Recent evidence does not support these findings. Roulet et al.[12] showed that in septic patients on ventilators, those who received 50 percent of their calories as fat had a better ratio of protein synthesis to catabolism than those receiving glucose alone. MacFie et al.[23] showed that postoperative patients gained total body nitrogen only when at least 60 percent of their nonprotein calories was given as fat.

ESSENTIAL FATTY ACID REQUIREMENTS

In addition to providing energy, lipid emulsions contain linoleic and linolenic acids, neither of which can be synthesized from carbohydrates. These fatty acids are essential for normal membrane structure and function. In their absence, dermatitis, hypermetabolism, increased incidence of infection, and erythrocyte abnormalities occur. Linoleic acid, which is the main essential fatty acid in the human, is converted to a longer-chain fatty acid, which has four double bonds (tetraene), arachidonic acid, which is a precursor for prostaglandin synthesis. In the absence of linoleic acid, oleic acid is converted to a similar long-chain fatty acid with three double bonds (triene) called eicosatrienoic acid. Thus the ratio of triene:tetraene has been used as an index of essential fatty acid deficiency. Collins et al.[24] showed that the infusion of fat-free total parenteral nutrition resulted in an abnormal triene:tetraene ratio that was corrected by giving lipid emulsions.

COMPLICATIONS OF INFUSING CARBOHYDRATES

Two major problems may occur when carbohydrates are the main source of calories. First, the infusion of carbohydrates can result in increased CO_2 production.[15] The increased production of CO_2 may pose a stress for the respiratory system and, in selected patients with preexisting compromised ventilatory function, the condition may be worsened. In addition, injured-septic patients receiving carbohydrate infusions may require increased oxygen consumption,[15] which may also stress a compromised respiratory system. Furthermore, carbohydrate infusions may contribute to the development of a fatty liver.[25]

Both processes appear to be attributable to the fact that carbohydrate infused in excess of 4 mg/kg-min is not completely oxidized.[26] The excess is converted to fat, resulting in increased CO_2 production. The newly synthesized fat is esterified to triglyceride and exported from the liver. When hepatic fat synthesis exceeds the ability of the liver to export the fat, a fatty liver may develop.

WHAT IS THE IDEAL CALORIC SOURCE DURING TOTAL PARENTERAL NUTRITION

Since carbohydrate is inexpensive, and has been used traditionally in IV solutions in North America, it is still often used as an exclusive source of energy. However, from the evidence noted previously, it is best to give a mixture of carbohydrate and fat as a caloric source. This is so for several reasons. First, Wolfe et al.[26] have shown that there is a limit to the proportion of total energy which can be derived from carbohydrate oxidation. Second, in injured-septic patients, fat oxidation continues preferentially, and provision of nonprotein calories as fat enhances protein balance and total body nitrogen. Third, pulmonary and hepatic complications can be caused by carbohydrate infusion. Finally, essential fatty acids can only be provided by infusing fat.

It is thus not logical to employ a fat-free infusion as the sole energy source. Infusing 50 percent of calories as fat and 50 percent as carbohydrate results in a substrate-hormone profile comparable to that seen in persons eating a normal diet, minimizes excess CO_2 production, decreases the tendency to form a fatty liver and prevents essential fatty acid deficiency.

ACID–BASE BALANCE AND ELECTROLYTES

General Considerations

PRODUCTION OF HYDROGEN IONS IN INTERMEDIARY METABOLISM

Although several methods have been used to analyze the acid or base load in the diet, we have chosen to approach this subject based upon a theoretical analysis. Therefore, all major biochemical reactions related to hydrogen ion production, and removal will be taken into account to calculate acid loads from either a typical North American diet or in a sample solution used in total parenteral nutrition. We shall also highlight some of the acid–base disorders encountered in patients receiving total parenteral nutrition.

Hydrogen ions are produced in metabolism when a nutrient is converted into a carbon product that contains a greater net anionic charge than the original nutrient. In general, the reaction is as follows: a neutral substance (glucose) is converted to an anion (lactate$^-$) plus a H^+. Alternatively, a cation (lysine$^+$) is converted into neutral products (urea plus exhaled carbon dioxide) plus a H^+. With this in mind, let us analyze net hydrogen ion production from various foodstuffs.

CARBOHYDRATE. Dietary carbohydrates are ingested in the form of uncharged hexoses or their polymers. These are converted to glycogen, neutral lipid or exhaled carbon dioxide, all of which are also electroneutral. Hence, under normal circumstances, metabolism of these compounds does not lead to net acid production. An exception to the rule that "metabolism of carbohydrates will not produce protons" can occur if these pathways do not go to completion: for example, during hypoxic

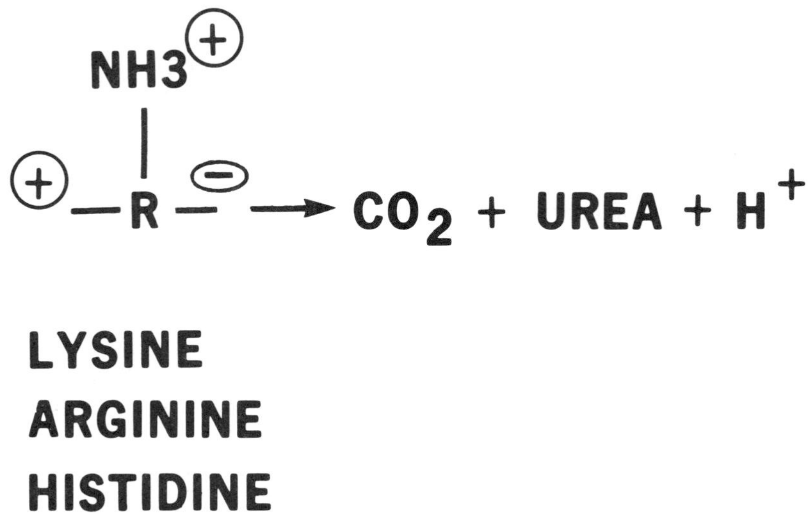

Fig. 26–1. Effect of cationic amino acids on net acid production. For details, see text.

states lactic acid is produced and can accumulate, resulting in a higher hydrogen ion concentration (for review, see refs. 27 and 28).

FAT. The intake of fat is largely in the form of neutral triglyceride; the products are also electroneutral. Thus, metabolism of these compounds will also not contribute to acid–base imbalance. However, during states of relative insulin deficiency, incomplete oxidation of fat results in the production of ketoacids (for review, see refs. 29 and 30).

PROTEIN. Acid production as a result of intermediary metabolism is predominantly due to amino acid oxidation. Since most proteins are ingested at a pH close to neutral, hydrogen ions can be either produced or removed as a result of amino acid oxidation. It is helpful to subdivide these reactions as follows:

1. *Neutral amino acids:* Since these represent most amino acids, and both have no net charge and are converted to neutral products,

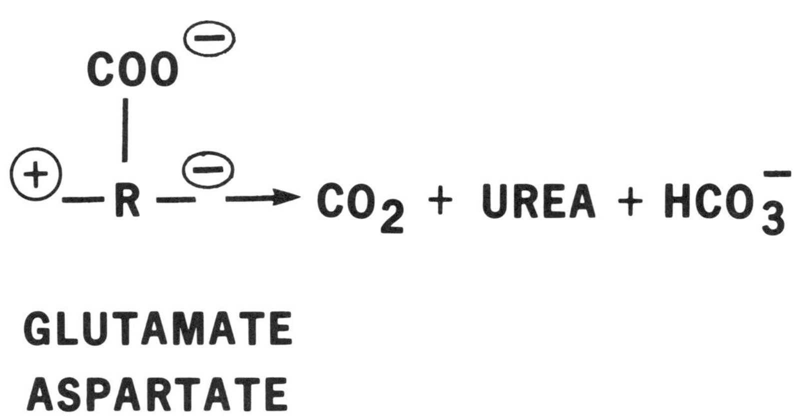

Fig. 26–2. Effect of anionic amino acids on net acid production. For details, see text.

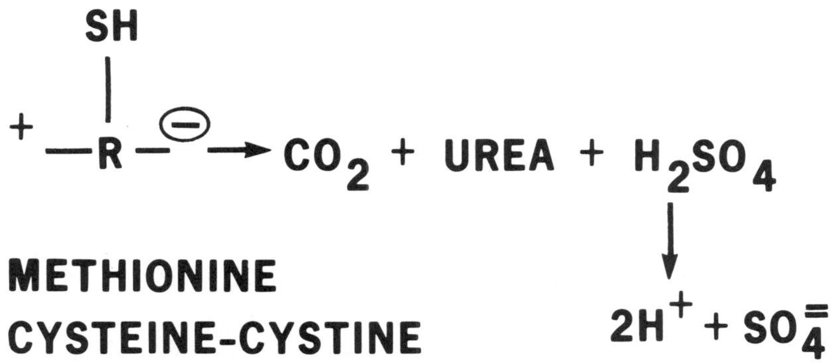

Fig. 26–3. Effect of sulfur-containing amino acids on net acid production. For details, see text.

including urea, exhaled CO_2, neutral lipid, or glucose (glycogen), oxidation of these compounds does not alter acid–base balance.

2. *Cationic amino acids:* oxidation of lysine and arginine produces neutral end products plus hydrogen ions (Fig. 26–1). Hence, 1 mole of protons will be produced per mole cationic amino acid oxidized. Histidine will also carry a net positive charge at neutral pH (~0.5 mole/mole amino acid); hence its oxidation also contributes to hydrogen ion production, but to a lesser degree than other compounds with a higher pK.

3. *Anionic amino acids:* glutamate and aspartate, when metabolized to neutral end products, require that one mole of hydrogen ion be consumed per mole of anionic amino acid metabolized (Fig. 26–2).

4. *Sulfur-containing amino acids:* The oxidation of methionine, cysteine, and cystine results in the production of sulfuric acid plus neutral end products (Fig. 26–3). Hence, two moles of hydrogen ion are produced per mole of sulfur-containing amino acid which is oxidized.[31]

5. *Quantitative analysis of the acid load due to protein oxidation:* In a diet containing 2500 kcal (40 percent as fat, 45 percent as carbohydrate, and 15 percent as protein, 15 percent of 2500 kcal is ~400 kcal) the diet would also contain 100 g protein because proteins have 4 kcal usable energy per gram. If the average molecular weight of amino acids is taken as 100 for convenience, then 1000 mmol amino acids would be consumed and metabolized daily in the nongrowing adult. As shown in Table 26–1, a typical blend of proteins should yield ~120 mmol cationic amino acids, 100 mmol glutamate plus aspartate (consuming 100 mmol protons) and 30 mmol methionine plus cystine/cysteine (producing 60 mmol protons). Thus, the net acid load in this calcu-

Table 26–1. Examples of the Acid Load in a Diet and Intravenous Solutions

	2500-kcal Mixed Diet (mmol H^+)	Travasol 5 percent (mmol H^+)	Hydrolysates: Fibrin (mmol H^+/liter)	Hydrolysates: Casein (mmol H^+/liter)
Cationic amino acids	120	57	20	30
Anionic amino acids	100	0	10	25
Sulfur-containing amino acids	60	43	11	15
Organic anions	?	100	—	—
Titratable acid	?	11	50	32
Total free H^+ load	80[a]	11	71	52

[a] From protein.

lation is 80 mmol hydrogen ion per day from protein oxidation.

If a subject were given intravenous amino acids, a similar analysis could be performed. If the pH of this fluid were far from the neutral range, one would then have to titrate it to determine the additional acid or base load. In practice, this is not a problem as the titratable acid of synthetic amino acid preparations is relatively low (i.e., ~10 to 15 mmol/liter; however, protein hydrolysates can have a titratable acid value that is four times greater).[32,33]

ORGANIC ANIONS. For simplicity, we can divide organic anions into two types with respect to acid–base balance: those that are metabolized to neutral end products and those that are not. Only the former are converted to bicarbonate, whereas the latter play no major role in acid–base balance (see Table 26–2). Because of this fact, one cannot reliably determine the net acid load of foodstuffs by analyzing the mineral ash content of the diet (see section of the conversion of foodstuffs to organic acid in the GI tract for a more detailed discussion).

1. *Metabolized organic anions:* The metabolism of an anion to a neutral end product results in the removal of a hydrogen ion, for example, the oxidation of sodium or potassium lactate or β-hydroxybutyrate to exhaled CO_2 results in the removal of a proton (Fig 26–4). Other examples of anions which are metabolized in humans include acetate, citrate, malate, gluconate, etc. and these have been called "potential bicarbonate." Each mmole metabolized yields 1 mmole of bicarbonate after metabolism to a neutral end product. One should also remember that intestinal bacteria rather than parenchymal cells may metabolize the organic anions and thereby produce the bicarbonate.[34] Should the bacterial flora change in quantity or in species, the rate of bicarbonate production could change considerably.

Finally, some organic anions such as acetoacetate undergo spontaneous, nonenzymatic, decarboxylation to produce the neutral volatile compounds acetone and CO_2. Should acetoacetate be converted to β-hydroxybutyrate, this pathway for proton removal would no longer be available (for review, see ref. 30).

2. *Nonmetabolized organic anions:* Most of the ingested tartrate or oxalate anions which are absorbed from the gastrointestinal tract are excreted in the urine without biochemical modifications.[35] If the compound was either absorbed and excreted with a cation other than hydrogen (or ammonium), or if both absorbed and excreted with these latter cations, it would have no direct influence on acid–base balance. However, if either ingestion or excretion of the compounds (but not both) were coupled with a proton, then these compounds might lead to alterations in acid-base balance. It is the quantity of the latter compounds ingested that creates problems with determining the acid load ingested in the form of the ash of the diet.

METABOLIZABLE CATIONS. The oxidation of a cation to a neutral end product will pro-

Table 26–2. Contribution of Nutrients to Acid–Base Balance

Nutrient	Mechanism	Result
Carbohydrate	Hypoxia	Lactic acid
	Rare causes	Lactic acid
Fat	Insulin deficiency	Ketoacidosis
Protein	$S \rightarrow H_2SO_4$	2 H^+/sulfur aa
	$R—NH_3^+ \rightarrow H^+$	1 H^+/dibasic aa
	$R—COO^- \rightarrow HCO_3^-$	1 HCO_3^-/dicarboxylic aa
Organic anions	$OA^- \rightarrow HCO_3^-$	1 HCO_3^-/OA^-
	OA^- not metabolized	0 HCO_3^-/OA^-

Abbreviations: aa, amino acid; R, organic acid side chain; OA, organic acid anion.

Fig. 26–4. Conversion of an organic anion to bicarbonate via intermediary metabolism. Org A^- = organic anion; $HA°$ = organic acid.

1. $\text{Org } A^- + H^+ ===> HA° ===>$ neutral end product

2. $CO_2 + H_2O ===> H^+ + HCO_3^-$

sum 1 + 2 $\quad \text{Org } A^- ===> HCO_3^-$

duce a proton. For example, ingestion of a mole of ammonium will yield a mole of hydrogen ion plus, in this case, one-half mole of urea. Hence, these compounds must also be considered in the acid–base analysis with respect to dietary intake.

ORGANIC PHOSPHATES. Phosphate diesters (phospholipids, nucleic acids), when metabolized, produce equivalent quantities of dibasic phosphates and hydrogen ions.[36] In contrast, dihydrogenphosphates are added as food preservatives and, as such, also add equivalent quantities of dibasic phosphate plus hydrogen ions to body fluids. Since both the hydrogen ions and their buffer anions are added and excreted together in the urine, these compounds will not result in acidemia unless there is a reduction in GFR or hydrogen ion secretion by the kidney (Fig. 26–5). In contrast, the ingestion of phosphoproteins or dibasic phosphate will provide a buffer anion without the proton and, after excretion as dihydrogen phosphate in the urine, will lead to a true bicarbonate gain.

OXIDATION OF PURINES TO URIC ACID. The normal adult produces only a few mmoles of uric acid per day. These protons make only a small contribution to the overall acid load.

CONVERSION OF NEUTRAL FOODSTUFFS TO ORGANIC ACIDS IN THE GI TRACT. Intestinal bacteria can convert neutral foodstuffs to organic acids. If the protons are absorbed, an acid load is presented to the body. Unless the accompanying anion is metabolized to a neutral end-product or excreted in the urine along with a hydrogen ion (or ammonium ion), acidosis will ensue. The quantitative as-

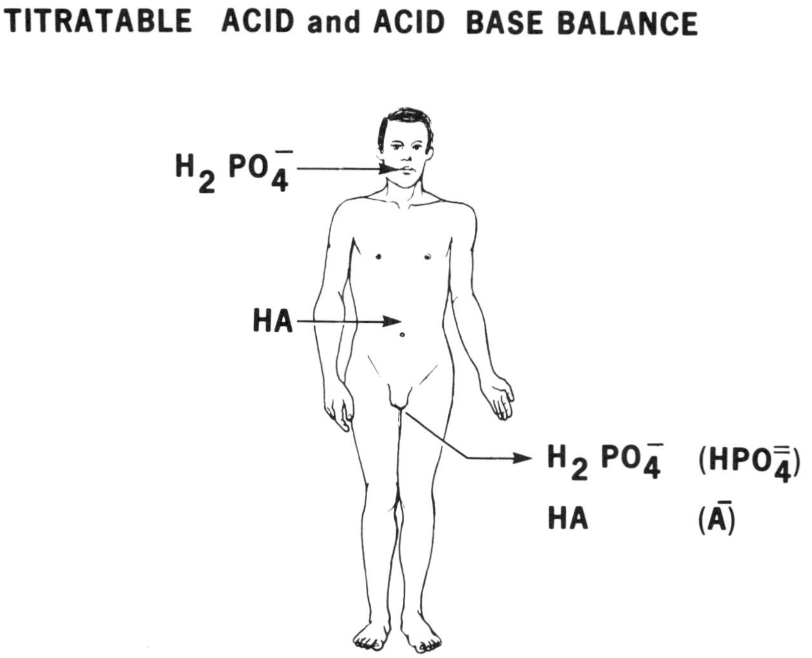

Fig. 26–5. Phosphate and acid–base balance. For details, see text.

pects of this pathway are difficult to evaluate, but probably they vary depending largely on the dietary intake and the composition of the intestinal flora.

MISCELLANEOUS COMPOUNDS. The ingestion of calcium salts of inorganic anions such as calcium chloride results in an acid load for the following reason. In the small intestine, ionic calcium reacts with secreted bicarbonate to produce insoluble calcium carbonate plus hydrogen ions, and the net result is an acid load:

$$Ca^{2+} + HCO_3^- ==> CaCO_3\downarrow + H^+$$

It should also be recognized that the deposition of calcium salts in bone will result in a hydrogen ion load:

$$10\ Ca^{2+} + 4.8\ HPO_4^{2-} + 1.2\ H_2PO_4^- + 2\ H_2O ====> (Ca_3(PO_4)_2)_3 \cdot Ca(OH_2) + 9.2\ H^+ \quad (1)$$

This will make a major contribution during active bone growth.[37] Conversely, an acute removal of hydrogen ions (or generation of bicarbonate) will occur when bone salts are dissolved (reversal of the above reaction).

Should magnesium or calcium hydroxide be ingested together with a cation exchange resin (not in the hydrogen ion form), the resin will bind the divalent cation and prevent the precipitation of the insoluble carbonate in the intestinal tract. As a result, the subject will now have the net intake of an alkali load from the metabolism of the anion portion of the salt but no hydrogen ions produced in equation (1).[38] Therefore, not only must the diet be analyzed, but reactions which produce or remove hydrogen ions in the gastrointestinal tract must be taken into consideration.

Finally, the ingestion of nonresorbable anions in the protonated form, such as exchange resins in the hydrogen ion form, could conceivably cause a proton load if other cations such as potassium were to bind to those anions that must remain in the gastrointestinal tract.

SUMMARY. In the absence of hypoxia and relative insulin deficiency, hydrogen ions are produced from the metabolism of sulfur-containing and cationic amino acids and organic bases, whereas they are removed by metabolism of anionic amino acids and ingested metabolizable organic anions. Small contributions can be made from the metabolism of phospholipids and purines. Should inorganic acids, calcium chloride, or exchange resins be ingested, these could also result in an acid load. These must be included in calculating the acid load of diet or parenteral alimentation solutions. Special metabolic reactions such as bone accretion or dissolution may also alter the daily net acid load.

INDIRECT ANALYSIS

ASHING THE DIET. The acid–base properties of food have also been defined in terms of the potential acidity or alkalinity of the ash remaining after complete combustion, a process whereby organic matter is removed.[39–41] Foods containing an excess of inorganic, or fixed, cations (sodium, potassium, calcium, magnesium) over inorganic or fixed anions (chloride, phosphate, sulfate) are said to have an alkaline ash; the converse is also true. An excess of inorganic cations over inorganic anions implies the presence in the food of organic anions, which, upon metabolism in the body to neutral end products, yield bicarbonate. Similarly, an excess of inorganic anions implies the presence of organic cations, which, upon metabolism, yield hydrogen ions. In order to complete this analysis, one must add the other sources of hydrogen ions from the diet. These sources of hydrogen ions produced from food are the oxidation of sulfur to sulfuric acid, the hydrolysis of phosphate diesters to dihydrogenphosphates, and the oxidation of neutral compounds to organic acids.

There is one major drawback to this form of analysis. Human beings can metabolize only certain of the ingested organic anions (to produce bicarbonate), whereas the ashing procedure removes all the organic anions. Thus, although certain organic anions such as tartrate or oxalate would be ashed, they cannot be quantitatively converted into bicarbonate in humans[35] (or by the bacteria harbored in their gastrointestinal tracts). Therefore, without knowing whether all organic anions will produce bicarbonate in vivo or not, significant errors may result from the ash analysis in the calculation of the potential acid load of the diet. Finally, one cannot be certain that absorption of dietary anions and cations from the gastrointestinal tract will be quantitative. Therefore, without an analysis of the feces, and/or the urine, again large errors in the estimated acid load might result from a simple consideration of the inorganic composition of the ashed diet (this latter criticism also applies to the theoretical analysis presented above).

If neutral organic compounds are ingested and converted to organic acids by the intestinal flora, this would not be apparent from the ashing technique. Furthermore, if the proton and organic anion were absorbed, an acid load would be presented to the host. Should this organic anion be metabolized, the acid load would be removed. In contrast, if this anion were excreted unchanged, an acid load would have to be dealt with. It follows that the ashing procedure is not sufficient for a complete acid–base analysis.

NET ACID EXCRETION. It is also possible to estimate the daily acid load (diet, gastrointestinal tract, and endogenous acid productions) by assuming that the subject is in acid–base balance and that this is achieved by the excretion of net acid in the urine.[42] The net acid is the sum of titratable acid plus ammonium minus bicarbonate in urine.

DISORDERS UNIQUE TO TOTAL PARENTERAL NUTRITION ACID–BASE DISORDERS

Metabolic Acidosis

Since the normal kidney can excrete about 300 mmol ammonium per day when a chronic acid load is given (for review, see ref. 43), exceedingly high protein intakes would be required to be the sole cause of metabolic acidosis. In fact, this will probably never occur during total parenteral nutrition. One can therefore conclude that, should metabolic acidosis be present, other etiologies should be suspected (e.g., see ref. 44).

With respect to renal function, the most likely cause of metabolic acidosis attributable to total parenteral nutrition appears to be a defect in ammonium excretion.[45] While the cause of the defect is not known, there is no evidence to suggest any of the common causes of impaired secretion of ammonia, such as a decrease in circulating glutamine; hyperkalemia; or renal cortical necrosis. Rather, the cause may be an interstitial nephritis which can compromise ammonium short circuiting via the loop of Henle to the medullary collecting duct.[46] However, the cause of the acidosis has not been thoroughly investigated.

Although the infusion of hypertonic dextrose is associated with a modest rise in blood lactate levels, this rarely if ever results in significant clinical acidosis unless an underlying defect in intermediary metabolism is present.[47,48] In addition, high dextrose loads increase blood lactate levels and may further increase any existing high lactate levels in septic patients. Recently, five pediatric oncology patients who were receiving intravenous 4 percent Freamine and 25 percent glucose developed lactic acidosis. In two of these patients, the lactic acidosis responded to a reduction in the rate of glucose infusion, but in the other three it seemed to be an integral part of the disease.[48]

Metabolic acidosis may be caused by the infusion of the glucose substitutes, fructose or sorbitol. Exogenous fructose and fructose derived by the dehydrogenation of sorbitol are rapidly metabolized to lactate. This process may cause lactic acidosis with fructose infusions,[49-53] especially in patients with inborn errors of metabolism. In adults, total parenteral nutrition, providing about 25 percent of nonprotein calories as fructose, has not caused clinical acidosis[54] but may have decreased the adenosine triphosphate content of the liver.[55]

In contrast, serious acidosis and hyperlactatemia have been observed in infants given total parenteral nutrition solutions containing fructose and/or sorbitol.[49-53]

Infusion of hypocaloric (i.e., containing fewer calories than required for metabolic needs) amino acid solutions for so-called protein-sparing therapy is associated with a rise in levels of blood free fatty acids and ketones[7,8] resulting in a situation that is even less marked than that seen in starvation. More serious degrees of ketoacidosis require an explanation other than hypocaloric intake.

Oxidation of amino acids can influence the acid load. The oxidation of most proteins results in an acid load. This acid load can in theory be diminished by adding glutamate to the amino acid mixture, because oxidation of this anionic amino acid results in the removal of a proton. However, intravenously infused glutamate potentially can injure the neonatal brain.[4] Therefore, the addition of glutamate to total parenteral nutrition solutions is not recommended.

In addition, the acid load from protein oxidation during total parenteral nutrition is now avoided by adding the organic anion acetate to the nutrient mixture. The oxidation of acetate produces bicarbonate, which neutralizes the acid load.

All amino acid mixtures have free ammonium and titratable acid. However, in practice they do not seem to result in a significant hydrogen ion load during total parenteral nutrition.[32,33] In fact, the titratable acidity of a synthetic amino acid mixture which can cause acidosis has been found to be only 10 to 15 mEq/liter. The concentration of free ammonium is high in certain protein and amino acid preparations, and this could lead to hyperammonemia in certain vulnerable subjects.[32,33,56,57] It should be emphasized that this hyperammonemia can be toxic for reasons other than the contribution to a systemic acid load.

In infants receiving hypertonic glucose and protein hydrolysate solutions, metabolic acidosis may be produced; hyperosmolality has been implicated in this disorder.[58] In adults, total parenteral nutrition does not cause hyperosmolality because of the enormous capacity of the adult to utilize the infused glucose and amino acids. In contrast, the immature low birth weight infant has a limited capacity to dispose of nutrients. If these are infused rapidly, hyperglycemia, hyperammonemia, acidemia and hypertonicity may ensue.

Metabolic Alkalosis

This disorder should be very rare in total parenteral nutrition. When it occurs, it will most likely be due to some combination of chloride deficiency, ECF volume contraction, potassium deficiency, or more rarely, adrenal cortical hormone administration. Should the total parenteral nutrition solution administered result in a net base load, bicarbonate must be excreted by the kidney to maintain acid–base balance. A problem could occur if renal failure was present as well. Persistent metabolic alkalosis has been reported in dialysis patients awaiting renal transplantation in whom thoracic duct lymph drainage is replaced by protein fractions. Fractions such as proteinate and plasmatein have low chloride concentrations and high concentrations of organic anions which, upon metabolism to neutral end products, generate bicarbonate. Thus, if renal function were impaired to such an extent that it did not permit sufficient bicarbonaturia,[59] metabolic alkalosis might ensue.

Respiratory Acidosis or Alkalosis

In septic-injured patients and those with markedly impaired pulmonary function, high carbohydrate loads might increase CO_2 generation and possibly lead to a raised P_{CO_2}.[15]

FLUID AND ELECTROLYTE DISORDERS

SODIUM. Sodium intake during total parenteral nutrition is usually ~120 mmol/day, but this can be reduced to 20 to 40 mmol/day when salt restriction is desired. In general, severely malnourished patients, when refed with a system rich in carbohydrate, quickly become edematous and may even develop pulmonary edema. It has been shown that feeding carbohydrate tends to induce sodium retention,[60] and this process is exaggerated in malnourished individuals who already have an excess of total body water. In such patients, refeeding (including vitamin and mineral replacements) should be undertaken cautiously, initially restricting both sodium and fluid.

POTASSIUM. During total parenteral nutrition, there is retention of potassium with nitrogen for the restoration of the lean body mass.[1] In addition, the infusion of glucose plus amino acids seems to be associated with a disproportionate rise in body potassium as compared with the infusion of amino acids alone.[11] Hence, total parenteral nutrition solutions should provide at least 90 to 120 mmol potassium per day to aid positive nitrogen balance and avoid hypokalemia. This intake has to be modified in patients with renal failure.

WATER. Nutrients for intravenous use must be dissolved in water; to avoid fluid overload, these solutions must have a caloric density of ~1 kcal/ml, so that the usual energy requirements can be given in ~2000 to 3000 ml fluid. Accordingly, subjects must be able to excrete the administered water load. Water excretion can be compromised if there is either a low rate of delivery of sodium chloride to the ascending limb of the loop of Henle (i.e., during states in which the effective extracellular fluid volume is reduced); if sodium chloride transport in this nephron segment is inhibited (i.e., if loop diuretics such as furosemide were given) or if elevated levels of antidiuretic hormone are present (e.g., high osmolality, extracellular fluid volume contraction, drug intake). Among the most effective ways of evaluating total body water balance is monitoring of the plasma sodium concentration (assuming that hyperglycemia or hyperlipidemia are not complicating the interpretation).

The fluid load administered can be reduced by replacing part of the calories with 20 percent lipid emulsions (calorie density should increase about twofold) or by adding 70 percent dextrose to the solution in a pharmacy. Such solutions are difficult to infuse because of their viscosity.

MAGNESIUM. This is another intracellular cation retained during total parenteral nutrition, especially during the phase of positive nitrogen balance. In fact, to induce a positive nitrogen balance, magnesium administration is required.[61] In practice about 12 to 15 mmol magnesium should be given per day to avoid hypomagnesemia and to maintain magnesium balance.

CALCIUM. Hypercalcemia may complicate total parenteral nutrition therapy and may even result in pancreatitis.[62] The precise cause of this phenomenon is not known, but it is not due to the continued infusion of total parenteral nutrition solutions, as it may continue for a few weeks even when total parenteral nutrition has been discontinued.[63] The process tends to occur when vitamin D is added to total parenteral nutrition solutions[64,65] and may result in metabolic bone disease indistinguishable from osteomalacia. The hypercalcemia is associated with hypercalciuria and marked negative calcium balance.[64] This hypercalcemia, hypercalciuria, and metabolic bone disease can be relieved by withdrawal of vitamin D.[65] On the other hand, these patients have low blood levels of parathormone and 1,25-dihydroxyvitamin D and normal levels of 25-hydroxyvitamin D. Hence, this hypercalcemia is not due to hypervitaminosis of vitamin D, nor is it due to hyperparathyroidism.

It is recommended that vitamin D not be added to total parenteral nutrition solutions, at least in patients receiving total parenteral nutrition for only a few months' duration. The amount of supplemental calcium required to maintain calcium balance does not need to exceed 10 mmol/day.

PHOSPHORUS. Phosphate deficiency was a frequent and severe problem early in the history of total parenteral nutrition, but the addition of phosphate to the administered fluids has largely eliminated this problem. Phosphorus is necessary for positive nitrogen balance.[1] In association with potassium and magnesium, phosphorus is an intracellular ion necessary for repleting the cell mass. In the absence of added inorganic phosphorus during total parenteral nutrition, hypophosphatemia occurs and can result in serious neurologic symptoms.[66] The central nervous system manifestations are described in Chapter 21. The amount of phosphorus required during total parenteral nutrition varies between 10 and 20 mmol phosphate ion per day.

TRACE ELEMENTS

It has been recognized for years that certain trace elements are essential nutrients for animals. In the human, recognition that trace elements are essential for nutrition was slow to come. With the increasing popularity of total parenteral nutrition several syndromes of trace element deficiency have dramatically demonstrated their need. Among trace elements, zinc, copper, chromium, iron, iodine, selenium, and cobalt (as vitamin B_{12}) are clearly essential.

ZINC. Zinc is an essential trace element for a number of metabolic systems. It is essential for DNA synthesis, and its deficiency depresses cell-mediated immunity. It is also important for insulin secretion and for nitrogen retention. If zinc is not added to total parenteral nutrition solutions, then plasma zinc levels fall. Eventually, a syndrome of scaly pustular rash, erythema of palms and soles, and resistant skin infections may occur. There can be loss of hair and an altered sense of taste. Supplementation with zinc can reverse this clinical syndrome and also improves nitrogen balance and insulin secretion. Zinc requirements during total parenteral nutrition were found to be determined by the losses both in urine and from the gastrointestinal tract.[67] The major source of zinc loss was determined to be the gastrointestinal tract in patients with diarrhea and stomas. In such patients losses may vary between 3 and 20 mg zinc per liter of diarrhea or stomal fluid. Urinary losses are increased by increased catabolism.

The requirements for zinc were found to be 2.5 to 3.0 mg/day in patients who were not hypercatabolic and who did not have diarrhea or stomal losses. The needs increased to 6 to 20 mg/day, or even more in hypercatabolic patients with diarrhea.

COPPER. Copper deficiency is less frequent than zinc deficiency in the unsupplemented patient on total parenteral nutrition. It results in a hypochromic anemia, leucopenia and skeletal abnormalities. In patients without diarrhea, the gastrointestinal losses are small, and copper balance can be maintained by the small amounts (0.3 mg/day) present as contaminants in many total parenteral nutrition solutions.[68] In patients with diarrhea, the losses increase, and ~0.5 mg copper is required per day to maintain balance. In contrast, patients with liver disease and jaundice do not excrete copper and they do not require copper supplementation.

CHROMIUM. This trace element is required for glucose homeostasis and insulin action, and deficiency can cause glucose intolerance and peripheral neuropathy.[69] About 20 μg/day is required.

VITAMINS. The vitamin requirements during total parenteral nutrition have not been studied in detail, with a few exceptions. Requirements have been poorly characterized and most current recommendations are based on an extrapolation from Recommended Dietary Allowances for orally administered vitamins. However, recent research in parenterally fed patients has helped clarify this area.

It has been demonstrated that regular use of a well-known multivitamin infusion (MVI) maintained adequate blood levels of many water soluble vitamins including thiamine (B_1), riboflavin (B_2), pyridoxine (B_6), niacin, pantothenic acid, and ascorbic acid (C) in six long-term total parenteral nutrition patients,[25] again demonstrating that adequate levels of water-soluble vitamins can be provided by routine multivitamin preparations.

Vitamin B_{12} and folic acid are not provided in many multivitamin preparations. However, use of vitamin B_{12} in the treatment of pernicious anemia has determined the daily maintenance dose to be 3 to 5 μg. For folic acid, although much larger doses are often given, as little as 0.7 mg/day is sufficient.

The fat-soluble vitamins are supplied in many multivitamin preparations. Vitamin A intoxication and hypercalcemia are rare when patients are given 1500 to 2000 IU/day vitamin A. Interestingly, complete withdrawal of vitamin A in home total parenteral nutrition patients did not cause low serum levels in 11 patients after 6 months. Thus it appears that the margin for error in vitamin A administration is wide.

About 50 IU vitamin E (d,1 alpha-tocopherol) is required daily. Since the polyunsaturated fatty acids in lipid infusions contain some vitamin E (0.4 IU/g fatty acids), most of the vitamin E requirements may be supplied in the lipid infusions, with the rest as additional vitamin.

Vitamin K is normally derived from the diet through the activity of gut bacteria. During total parenteral nutrition, this latter source alone may suffice. However, if changes in gut flora occur, such as alterations following treatment with antibiotics, vitamin K production may no longer be adequate. In this case, supplementation with 10 mg/day Synkavite (sodium menadiol diphosphate) appears sufficient.

Caution is required with vitamin D. Even on a modest intake (by oral standards) of 250 IU/day, metabolic bone disease characterized by hypercalciuria, intermittent hypercalcemia, osteomalacia, and bone pain with fractures has been seen.[65] This responded to the complete withdrawal of vitamin D. On this basis, no intravenous vitamin D is recommended either short or long term, but patients are encouraged to expose themselves to sunlight to maintain normal vitamin D levels from natural sources.

The need for biotin supplementation is not entirely clear. Despite low plasma biotin levels in 6 home total parenteral nutrition patients,[25] there was no demonstrable clinical effect. However, a recent case of biotin-responsive rash and organic acidosis with reduced plasma, blood and urinary biotin concentrations, has been described.[70] Although it appears that this was indeed an acquired defect, the need for routine biotin supplementation is still not resolved.

PROTOCOLS FOR TOTAL PARENTERAL NUTRITION

Parenteral nutrition can be given via the central venous route or through peripheral veins. The former method allows the use of hypertonic solutions while the maximum osmolality of solutions entering a peripheral vein should not exceed 600 mOsm/liter. Hence, the latter route can only be used if lipid emulsions (which are isotonic, see Table 26–3) are used as a major source of nonprotein calories.

Central Venous Administration

INSERTION

Hypertonic total parenteral nutrition solutions will damage the intima of veins and cause thrombosis unless the infusate is rendered isotonic by rapid blood flow. To achieve such a rapid rate of flow it is necessary to infuse these solutions directly into the vena cava, via a catheter advanced to this location after insertion into a central vein. The most successful route of insertion is by infraclavicular puncture of the subclavian vein. The success of this route in part depends on the ease with which the catheter can be anchored and the puncture site can be kept clean and sterile. The catheter insertion should be done aseptically and catheter care performed meticulously to avoid sepsis.[71]

TECHNIQUE OF INFUSION

The amino acid–dextrose–electrolyte–trace element mixture is prepared in a pharmacy under aseptic conditions and stored in plastic liter bags. Vitamins are added just prior to use. The lipid emulsion is available in 10 or 20 percent concentrations in bottles.

The infusion of the amino acid–dextrose mixture and the lipid is undertaken simultaneously via a "Y" connector. The amino acid–dextrose mixture is infused through a drip chamber and tubing to one arm of the Y, and the lipid through the other. These solutions then mix at the common stem of the "Y" and the mixture flows through a tube into the central venous catheter.

TYPICAL NUTRIENT PRESCRIPTION

This prescription is outlined in Table 26–3.

Table 26–3. Protocols for Infusions

Protocols for TPN for Central Venous Infusion	
Glucose as the only source of nonprotein calories.	
8 AM to 8 PM	
2–4 percent amino acids[a] with 25 percent dextrose	1500 ml
Electrolyte additives, as needed[b]	30 ml (approx)
MVI[c] OR	5 ml
Soluzyme plus vitamin C[d]	10 ml
8 PM to 8 AM	
2–4 percent amino acids[a] with 25 percent dextrose	1500 ml
Electrolyte additives, as needed[b]	30 ml (approx)
Trace element mix (1) to (4)[e]	1 ml (each)
Nutrient composition of above regimen	
Amino acids (60 g)	240 kcal
Glucose monohydrate (750 g)	2550 kcal
Total nonprotein energy	2550 kcal
Total volume	3000 ml (approx)
Electrolytes	
Na	130 mmol
K	90–120 mmol
Ca	10 mmol
Mg	12–15 mmol
P	10–20 mmol
Glucose and Lipid nonprotein calories.	
8 AM to 8 PM	
4 percent amino acids[a] with 25 percent dextrose	750 ml
Electrolyte additives, as needed[b]	30 ml (approx)
MVI[c] OR	5 ml
Soluzyme plus vitamin C[d]	10 ml
Intralipid 10 percent[f,g]	500 ml
8 PM to 8 AM	
4 percent amino acids[a] with 25 percent dextrose	750 ml
Electrolyte additives, as needed[b]	30 ml (approx)
Trace element mix (1) to (4)[e]	1 ml (each)
Intralipid 10 percent[f,g]	500 ml
Nutrient composition of the above regimen	
Amino acids (60 g)	240 kcal
Glucose monohydrate (375 g)	1275 kcal
Lipid (100 g)	1100 kcal
Total nonprotein energy	2375 kcal
Total volume	2600 ml (approx)

Peripheral Venous Administration

This system depends on the fact that the lipid emulsion dilutes the hypertonic amino acid–dextrose mixture just prior to its entry into the peripheral vein. Hence, it is critical that the lipid emulsion be infused simultaneously in constant proportion to the amino acid–dextrose mixture through the Y connector, in the same way as the central system. The main difference is the lower dextrose concentration and larger volume of lipid used in order to render the final mixture tolerable to a peripheral vein.

INSERTION

For successful infusion, it is important to select a large vein with good blood flow. To avoid phlebitis and infection, the venipuncture must be done with aseptic precautions and the puncture site carefully dressed and kept aseptic.[71]

TECHNIQUE OF INFUSION

The principle of infusion is the same as for the central system, but it is more critical to ensure careful and continuous mixing of the

Table 26–3 ***Continued***

Protocol for Peripheral Venous Infusion	
8 AM to 8 PM	
6 percent amino acids with 12 percent dextrose	500 ml
Electrolyte additives, as needed[b]	30 ml (approx)
MVI[c] OR	5 ml
Soluzyme plus vitamin C[d]	10 ml
Intralipid 10 percent[g,h]	1000 ml
8 PM to 8 AM	
6 percent amino acids with 12 percent dextrose	500 ml
Electrolyte additives, as needed[b]	10 ml (approx)
Trace element mix (1) to (4)[e]	1 ml (each)
Intralipid 10 percent[g,h]	1000 ml
Nutrient composition of above mixture	
Amino acids (60 g)	240 kcal
Glucose monohydrate (120 g)	408 kcal
Lipid (200 g)	2200 kcal
Total nonprotein energy	2608 kcal

[a] Amino acid concentrations can be increased to give a higher nitrogen intake if desired.

[b] Total electrolytes have been calculated on the assumption that the amino acid mixture used is electrolyte free. If another amino acid source is used, the values will be different. The total input of electrolytes given in this table has been found to be capable of maintaining balance in patients without abnormal losses of gastrointestinal secretions. However, in patients with such losses, appropriate replacement has to be made.

[c] MVI injection (USV Pharmaceutical Corp.).

[d] Soluzyme plus vitamin C (Upjohn).

[e] Trace element mix: 1 ml each of (1) 0.3 mg/ml elemental Cu as cupric chloride ($CuCl_2 2H_2O$), 20 μg/ml elemental Cr as chromic nitrate [$Cr(NO_3)_3$], and 120 μg/ml elemental Se as selenious acid, (H_2SeO_3); (2), 120 μg/ml elemental I as potassium iodide (KI); (3) 3 mg/ml elemental Zn as zinc sulfate ($ZnSO_4 7H_2O$); and (4) 0.7 mg/ml elemental Mn as manganous chloride ($MnCl_3 4H_2O$).

[f] The triglyceride emulsion and dextrose–amino acid mixture are infused concurrently through a central venous line using a Y connector for continuous mixing.

[g] Intralipid 10 percent (Cutter Laboratories).

[h] It is very important in this system that the amino acid–dextrose solution and Intralipid be infused in correct proportions through the Y connector. The concentration of the former must be diluted adequately by constant mixing with the Intralipid to make the dextrose noninjurious to the peripheral vein. An infusion pump is advisable.

acid–dextrose mixture in the Y connector. To achieve this, a dual-channel Holter pump should be used.

TYPICAL NUTRIENT PRESCRIPTION

For general use, mixing 1 liter of a 10 percent amino acid mixture with 1 liter of 25 percent dextrose yields a final mixture of 5 percent amino acid and 12.5 dextrose. By infusing 1.5 liter of this mixture with 1.5 liter of 10 percent lipid emulsion, one can provide 75 g amino acids and 2285 kcal nonprotein energy per day. Electrolytes, trace elements, and vitamins are added as with the protocol for central venous infusion.

REFERENCES

1. Rudman D, Millikan WJ, Richardson TJ, et al: Elemental balances during intravenous hyperalimentation of underweight adult subjects. J Clin Invest 55:94, 1975
2. Munro HN: General aspects of the regulation of protein metabolism by diet and by hormones. p. 381. In Munro HN, Allison JB (eds): Mammalian Protein Metabolism. Vol. 1. Academic Press, New York, 1964
3. Rose WC: Nutritive significance of amino acids. Physiol Rev 18:109, 1938
4. Olney JW, Ho OL, Rhee V: Brain-damaging potential of protein hydrolysates. N Engl J Med 289:391, 1973
5. Calloway DH, Spector H: Nitrogen balance as related to calorie and protein intake in active young men. Am J Clin Nutr 2:405, 1954
6. Blackburn GL, Flatt JP, Clowes GHA, et al: Peripheral intravenous feeding with isotonic amino acid solutions. Am J Surg 125:447, 1973
7. Greenberg GR, Marliss EB, Anderson GH, et al: Protein-sparing therapy in postoperative patients: Effects of added hypocaloric glucose or lipid. N Engl J Med 294:1411, 1976
8. Greenberg GR, Jeejeebhoy KN: Intravenous protein-sparing therapy in patients with gastrointestinal disease. JPEN 3:427, 1979
9. Bozetti F: Parenteral nutrition in surgical patients. Surg Gynecol Obstet 142:1, 1976
10. Elwyn DH: Nutritional requirements of adult surgical patients. Crit Care Med 8:19, 1980
11. Collins JT, Oxby CB, Hill GL: Intravenous amino acids and intravenous hyperalimentation as protein sparing therapy after major surgery: A controlled clinical trial. Lancet 1:788, 1978
12. Roulet M, Jeejeebhoy KN, Shike M, et al: Energy and protein metabolism in critically ill, malnourished and septic patients. (Abst.) JPEN 4:582, 1980
13. Shike M, Feld R, Evans WK, et al: Long-term effect of TPN on body composition of patients with lung carcinoma. (Abst.) JPEN 5:564, 1981

13a. Harris JA, Benedict FG: Standard basal metabolism constants for physiologists and clinicians. p. 223. In A Biometric Study of Basal Metabolism in Man. Carnegie Institution of Washington. Publ. No. 279. JB Lippincott, Philadelphia, 1919

14. Kinney JM, Long CL, Duke JH: Carbohydrate and nitrogen metabolism after injury. p. 103. In Porter R, Knight K (eds): Energy Metabolism in Trauma. (Ciba Foundation Symposium.) Churchill, London, 1970
15. Askanazi J, Carpentier YA, Elwyn DH, et al: Influence of total parenteral nutrition on fuel utilization in injury and sepsis. Ann Surg 191:40, 1980
16. Shike M, Feld R, Evans WK, et al: Energy expenditure in relation to caloric intake in patients with lung carcinoma. JPEN 5:562, 1981 (Abst.)
17. Jeejeebhoy KN, Anderson GH, Nakhooda AF, et al: Metabolic studies in total parenteral nutrition with lipid in man: Comparison with glucose. J Clin Invest 57:125, 1976
18. Bark S, Holm I, Hakansson I, et al: Nitrogen sparing effect of fat emulsion compared with glucose in the post-operative period. Acta Chir Scand 142:423, 1976
19. Gazzaniga AB, Bartlett RH, Shobe JB: Nitrogen balance in patients receiving either fat or carbohydrate for total intravenous nutrition. Ann Surg 182:163, 1975
20. Wannemacher RW, Kaminski MU, Dinter-

man RE, et al: Protein-sparing therapy during pneumococcal infection in rhesus monkeys. JPEN 2:507, 1980
21. Long JM, Wilmore DW, Mason AD Jr, et al: Fat carbohydrate interaction: Nitrogen sparing effect of varying caloric sources for total intravenous feeding. Surg Forum 25:61, 1974
22. Woolfson AMJ, Heatley RV, Allison SP: Insulin to inhibit protein catabolism after injury. N Engl J Med 300:14, 1979
23. MacFie J, Smith RC, Hill GL: Glucose or fat as a nonprotein energy source? A controlled clinical trial. Gastroenterology 80: 103, 1981
24. Collins FD, Sinclair AJ, Royale JP, et al: Plasma lipids in human linoleic acid deficiencies. Nutr Metab 13:150, 1971
25. Jeejeebhoy KN, Langer B, Tsallas G, et al: Total parenteral nutrition at home: Studies in patients surviving 4 months to 5 years. Gastroenterology 71:943, 1976
26. Wolfe RR, Durkot MJ, Allsop JR, et al: Glucose metabolism in the severely burned patient. Metabolism 20:1031, 1979
27. Cohen RD, Woods HF: Clinical and Biochemical Aspects of Lactic Acidosis. Blackwell, Oxford, 1976
28. Park R, Arieff AI: Lactic acidosis. Adv Int Med 25:33, 1980
29. Cahill GH Jr: Ketosis. Kidney Int 20:416, 1981
30. Halperin ML, Goldstein MB, Bear RA, Josse RG: Diabetic comas. Chap. 20. In Arieff AI, DeFronzo R (eds): Fluid, Electrolyte and Acid–Base Disorders. Churchill Livingstone, New York, 1985
31. Hunt JN: The influence of dietary sulphur on the urinary output of acid in man. Clin Sci 15:119, 1956
32. Chan JCM, Malekzadeh M, Hurley J: pH and titratable acidity of amino acid mixtures used in hyperalimentation. JAMA 220:1119, 1972
33. Heird WC, Dell RB, Driscoll Jr, et al: Metabolic acidosis resulting from intravenous alimentation mixtures containing synthetic amino acids. N Engl J Med 287:943, 1972
34. Richardson RMA, Goldstein MB, Stinebaugh BJ, et al: Influence of diet and metabolism on urinary acid excretion in the rat and the rabbit. J Lab Clin Med 94:510, 1979
35. Chadwick VS, Vince A, Killingley M, et al: The metabolism of tartrate in man and the rat. Clin Sci Mol Med 54:273, 1978
36. Lennon EJ, Lemann J Jr, Relman AS: The effects of phosphoproteins on acid balance in normal subjects. J Clin Invest 41:637, 1962
37. Biltz RM, Pellegrino ED, Letteri JM. Skeletal carbonates and acid–base regulation. Min Elect Metab 5:1, 1981
38. Fernendez PC, Kovnat PJ: Metabolic acidosis reversed by the combination of magnesium hydroxide and a cation-exchange resin. N Engl J Med 286:23, 1972
39. Sherman HC, Sinclair JE: The balance of acid-forming and base-forming elements in food. J Biol Chem 3:307, 1907
40. Gonick HC, Goldberg G, Mulcare D: Reexamination of the acid-ash content of several diets. Am J Clin Nutr 21:898, 1968
41. Teree TM, Connerton S: Quantitation of potential metabolic acid in infant food and excreta. Pediatrics 47:239, 1971
42. Relman AS, Lennon EJ, Lemann J Jr. Endogenous production of fixed acid and the measurement of the net balance of acid in normal subjects. J Clin Invest 40:1621, 1961
43. Halperin ML, Goldstein MB, Stinebaugh BJ: Biochemistry and physiology of ammonium excretion. In Seldin DW, Giebisch G (eds): Physiology and Pathology of Electrolyte Metabolism. Raven Press, New York (in press)
44. Chan JCM: The influence of synthetic amino acid and casein hydrolysate on the endogenous production and urinary excretion of acid in total intravenous alimentation. Pediatr Res 6:789, 1972
45. Fraley DS, Adler S, Bruns F, et al: Metabolic acidosis after hyperalimentation with casein hydrolysate. Ann Intern Med 88:352, 1978
46. Sajo IM, Goldstein MB, Sonnenberg H, et al: Sites of ammonia addition to tubular fluid in rats with chronic metabolic acidosis. Kidney Int 20:353, 1981
47. Goldman HI, Karelitz S, Seifter E, et al: Acidosis in premature infants due to lactic acid. Pediatrics 27:921, 1961
48. Merritt RJ, Ennis CE, Thomas DW, et al: Lactic acidosis in pediatric patients with cancer receiving total parenteral nutrition. J Pediatr 99:247, 1981
49. Sahebjami H, Scalettar R: Effects of fructose

infusion on lactate and uric acid metabolism. Lancet 1:366, 1971
50. Bergstrom J, Hultman E, Roch-Norlund AE: Lactic acid accumulation in connection with fructose infusion. Acta Med Scand 184:359, 1968
51. Helmuth WV, Adam PAJ, Sweet AY: The effects of protein hydrolysate-monosaccharide infusion on low birth-weight infants. J Pediatr 81:129, 1972
52. Harries JT: Metabolic acidosis during intravenous feeding of infants. p. 266. In Wilkinson AW (ed): Parenteral Nutrition. (An International Symposium in London, April 30–May 1, 1971.) Churchill Livingstone, London, 1972
53. Aynsley-Green A, Baum JD, Alberti KGMM, et al: Hyperlactataemia during intravenous feeding in childhood. Arch Dis Child 49:647, 1974
54. Vinay P, Bourbeau D, Duranceau A, et al: Metabolic effects of total parenteral nutrition with or without fructose with special reference to the liver adenine nucleotide content. Clin Invest Med 4:87, 1981
55. Bode JC, Zelder O, Rumpelt HJ, et al: Depletion of liver adenosine phosphates and metabolic effects of intravenous infusion of fructose or sorbitol in man and in the rat. Eur J Clin Invest 3:436, 1973
56. Heird WC, Nicholson JF, Driscoll JM Jr, et al: Hyperammonemia resulting from intravenous alimentation using a mixture of synthetic L-amino acids: A preliminary report. J Pediatr 81:162, 1972
57. Johnson JD, Albritto WL, Sunshine P: Hyperammonemia accompanying parenteral nutrition in newborn infants. J Pediatr 81: 154, 1972
58. Sotos JF, Dodge PR, Talbot NB: Studies in experimental hypertonicity. II. Hypertonicity of body fluids as a cause of acidosis. Pediatrics 30:180, 1962
59. Rahilly GT, Berl T: Severe metabolic alkalosis caused by the administration of plasma protein fraction in end-stage renal failure. N Engl J Med 301:824, 1979
60. DeFronzo RA: The effect of insulin on renal sodium metabolism: A review with clinical implications. Diabetologia 21:165, 1981
61. Freeman JB: Magnesium requirements during parenteral nutrition. p. 43. In Hill GL, Jeejeebhoy KN, Kinney JM (eds): Parenteral Nutrition/Canada. Present Status and Newer Developments (Proc. of a Can. Symp.). Communications Media for Education, Princeton, NJ, 1981
62. Izsak EM, Shike M, Roulet M, et al: Pancreatitis in association with hypercalcemia in patients receiving total parenteral nutrition. Gastroenterology 79:555, 1980
63. Manson RR: Acute pancreatitis secondary to iatrogenic hypercalcemia. Arch Surg 108:213, 1974
64. Shike M, Harrison JE, Sturtridge WC, et al: Metabolic bone disease in patients receiving long-term total parenteral nutrition. Ann Intern Med 92:343, 1980
65. Shike M, Sturtridge WC, Tam CS, et al: A possible role of vitamin D in the genesis of parenteral-nutrition-induced metabolic bone disease. Ann Intern Med 95:560, 1981
66. Silvas SE, Paragas PD: Paresthesias, weakness, seizures, and hypophosphatemia in patients receiving hyperalimentation. Gastroenterology 62:513, 1972
67. Wolman SL, Anderson GH, Marliss EB, et al: Zinc in total parenteral nutrition: Requirements and metabolic effects. Gastroenterology 73:458, 1979
68. Shike M, Roulet M, Kurian R, et al: Copper metabolism and requirements in total parenteral nutrition. Gastroenterology 81:290, 1981
69. Jeejeebhoy KN, Chu RC, Marliss EB, et al: Chromium deficiency, glucose intolerance and neuropathy reversed by chromium supplementation, in a patient receiving long-term total parenteral nutrition. Am J Clin Nutr 30:531, 1977
70. Innis SM, Allardyce DB: Possible biotin deficiency in adults receiving long-term total parenteral nutrition. Am J Clin Nutr 37:185, 1983
71. Kennedy G, Jeejeebhoy KN: Home parenteral nutrition. p. 92. In Jeejeebhoy KN (ed): Total Parenteral Nutrition in the Hospital and at Home. CRC Press, Boca Raton, FL, 1983

27

Fluid and Electrolyte Therapy in Children

Norman J. Siegel
William E. Lattanzi

HISTORICAL PERSPECTIVE

Ancient writing from the Greeks, including Hippocrates,[1] and from the Talmud[2] elaborate the effects of diarrheal disease and refer to the use of oral rehydration. In the sixteenth century Sanctorius[3] demonstrated insensible water loss. In the mid-1800s several important occurrences are documented—O'Shaughnessy[4] conceptualized parenteral fluid therapy, Schmidt[5] analyzed blood and body fluid samples, Bernard[6] described the *milieu intereur* and Latta[7] attempted replacement therapy in cholera victims. By the twentieth century, pediatricians had assumed a leading role in the field of electrolyte physiology and parenteral fluid therapy, as recently reviewed by Finberg et al.[8] Acidosis occurring as a consequence of dehydration was described by Howland and Marriot[9] and by Schloss and Stetson.[10] Gamble[11] conceived the compartmentalization of body fluids, and Darrow and co-workers[12,13] emphasized that the metabolic turnover of water differs strikingly in infants, as compared with that in older children and adults, and described the importance of potassium losses in diarrheal states. Grover Powers,[14] professor of pediatrics at Yale and a recognized clinician, suggested a comprehensive approach to fluid and electrolyte therapy in 1926. Although our understanding of the physiology of fluid and electrolytes is better delineated and additional contributions have been made by pediatricians such as Harrison,[15] Holliday and Segar,[16] Weil and Wallace,[17] Winters,[18] and others, our current approach to fluid and electrolyte therapy in children is only a little more sophisticated and complex than that proposed by Dr. Powers.

Parenteral fluid therapy in infants and children must be given careful consideration and special attention. Accordingly, many systems and approaches for the administration of fluids and electrolytes to infants and children have been devised. In large part, these systems are empiric, based on clinical experience, and interchangeable. In this regard, several important factors should be remembered: (1) therapy must be individualized for every patient, as a cookbook approach will only lead to errors and confusion; (2) the patient's condition and response to therapy are the final determinants of the accuracy of all calculations, which are at best only estimates of the patient's needs; and (3) simplicity in the design and execution of parenteral fluid therapy is not only highly desirable, but essential for effective utilization. With these prerequisites in mind, we describe in this chapter a simplified approach to each aspect of parenteral fluid therapy in infants and children as well as the special considerations for fluid administration in newborns and postoperative children.

MAINTENANCE THERAPY

The aim of this aspect of parenteral fluid therapy is to replace water and electrolytes lost under ordinary conditions.[18] Maintenance fluids are designed to maintain water and electrolyte homeostasis with minimal renal compensation. In addition, maintenance fluids should provide 20 percent of caloric needs as protein-sparing calories.

The volume of fluid needed for maintenance therapy is determined from the metabolic rate. Holliday and Segar[16] have provided normal values for energy expenditures by hospitalized infants and children. It is usually assumed that 120 ml water is required for every 100 kcal metabolized. However, endogenous water is provided from the oxidation of carbohydrate, fat, and protein, as well as from intracellular water released during cellular degeneration. If one takes into account these two endogenous sources of water, water of oxidation (17 ml/100 kcal), and performed water (3 ml/100 kcal), it becomes apparent that 100 ml exogenous water must be supplied for each 100 kcal metabolized. Thus, estimates of both caloric expenditure and total maintenance fluid requirement can be made from Table 27–1. For example, a child who weighs 15 kg would have an estimated maintenance fluid requirement of 1250 ml/day, that is, 1000 ml for first 10 kg + 50 ml/kg for next 5 kg = 1000 ml + 250 ml = 1250 ml. Note that for patients weighing more than 80 kg, the proportionate distribution of body water is altered, so that calculations from Table 27–1 may be a significant overestimate of fluid requirement.

Table 27–1. Estimate of Total Maintenance Fluid Requirement for Infants and Children[a]

Body Weight (kg)	Maintenance Fluids (ml/kg-day)
1–10	100
11–20	1000 + 50 over 10 kg
21–80	1500 + 20 over 20 kg

[a] These values assume that the child is afebrile, hospitalized, and at less than normal activity. Also, this sliding scale will estimate average caloric expenditure under these conditions.

In order to maintain normal electrolyte homeostasis, ~2 to 3 mEq Na^+ and Cl^- and 2 to 2.5 mEq K^+ will be required for each 100 kcal expended, or 100 ml of maintenance fluid. In addition, 20 percent of the caloric need should be provided by glucose to minimize protein catabolism and prevent ketosis. If the full volume of estimated maintenance requirement can be administered, sufficient glucose for a protein-sparing effect will be achieved with a 5 percent dextrose solution, that is, 5 g glucose/100 ml fluid. With a little arithmetic, it becomes apparent that a parenteral solution containing 25 to 30 mEq/liter Na^+ and Cl^-, 20 mEq/liter K^+, and 5 percent dextrose will meet the objectives of maintenance fluid therapy when administered at a rate calculated from Table 27–1. A number of such solutions are commonly available commercially.

The quantity of fluids and electrolytes estimated from these calculations of maintenance fluid requirements will provide for losses from two sources: (1) evaporative (insensible) losses, and (2) urinary losses. Evaporative or insensible losses are composed of solute-free water lost through the skin and lungs. This water is used for thermal regulation and to humidify the inspired air. Under ordinary conditions, these losses are approximately 30 to 35 percent of total maintenance volume. Sweat is not included in evaporative fluid losses. Because insensible losses are evaporative, the ambient humidity and temperature will have profound effects on the magnitude of these losses. Infants or children receiving humidified air via an endotracheal tube or dwelling in a mist tent will have a considerable reduction in insensible losses that must be taken into account in calculating maintenance needs. Similarly children with hyperthermia or tachypnea or under a radiant warmer will have exaggerated evaporative losses. A temperature greater than 38°C will increase water requirements by 12.5 percent per degree of fever. Under ordinary circumstances, 33 percent of evaporative losses occur through the lungs and 66 percent from the skin, while total evaporative losses are one-third of maintenance requirements. The volume of fluid calculated to replace evaporative losses should be given as an electrolyte-free solution.

The adequacy of fluid therapy in children who are receiving only fluids to replace evaporative losses is judged best by changes in body weight and serum sodium concentration. If an appropriate volume and composition of fluid have been administered, the weight of the patient should decrease by 0.5 to 1 percent per day because of deficient caloric intake, and the serum sodium should remain stable between 130 to 140 mEq/liter. A more rapid loss of weight or increase in serum sodium would suggest that inadequate fluids have been given, while a gain in weight combined with a fall in serum sodium would imply overhydration. If hydration has been inadequate, one should assess those factors that would increase insensible fluid losses, such as hyperthermia, increased activity, tachypnea, or a dry ambient environment as produced by radiant warmers. If excessive fluids have been given, one should reevaluate insensible fluid requirement in terms of a factor that would reduce evaporative fluid losses, such as humidified air from a respirator, hypothermia, sedation, or reduced activity.

In a hospitalized child, the volume or rate of urine excretion is often used as an index of cardiovascular stability, cardiac output, and peripheral perfusion. In fact, in some instances the adequacy of parenteral fluid therapy is assessed and adjusted according to urine output. Such assumptions concerning urine output and judgments about fluid therapy are not only an oversimplification of complex renal physiology, but are also hazardous for patient management. Under homeostatic conditions, 20 to 25 percent of cardiac output is distributed to the kidneys, 500 ml/min in an adult. Approximately 20 percent of this volume is filtered by the glomerulus (100 ml/min) and, over 24 hours, the proximal tubule is presented with 144 liters glomerular filtrate (i.e., potential urine) and 20,160 mEq (460 g) sodium. The tubules and collecting ducts reabsorb 98 to 99 percent of this filtrate (i.e., 142 liters fluid and 456 g sodium), which results in a final urine output of 2 liters/day containing 4 g sodium. In most circumstances, the kidney will react to maintain intravascular volume and plasma tonicity by balancing the processes of filtration, reabsorption, and secretion.

During maintenance fluid therapy, urinary losses are expected to occur as 280 to 300 mOsm/liter with urine specific gravity 1.010. Caution must be taken that the patient can achieve an isosthenuric urine. In some circumstances (e.g., diabetes insipidus, premature infant), the patient is obligated to produce a more dilute urine, and appropriate increases in the volume of maintenance fluids must be made. On other occasions (e.g., excessive or inappropriate antidiuretic hormone secretion), the patient may not be able to decrease urine osmolarity to 300 mOsm/liter, and the volume of maintenance fluids must be decreased. Under homeostatic conditions, urinary losses account for two-thirds of the total maintenance fluid requirement. Thus, in a stable euvolemic state, a child or adolescent with normal renal function and intact kidneys will generally excrete 1.5 to 3 ml/kg-hr urine, and a urine volume of <0.8 ml/kg-hr can be defined as oliguria.

Maintenance Fluid Therapy in Surgical Patients

Maintenance fluid therapy in pediatric surgical patients requires special considerations. In most hospitals more children are admitted for surgical procedures than for medical problems. By far most of these children will require parenteral fluid therapy during hospitalization. Elective operations in basically well children do not pose major fluid therapy problems. These children should be kept hydrated and euvolemic before surgery, so that deficit losses do not occur. Because evaporative fluid losses from the skin and lungs are relatively high in small infants and young children and because urinary concentrating ability is limited, these patients should not be deprived of fluids for a prolonged period before undergoing surgery. After approximately 4 hours in infants and 6 hours in older children, parenteral fluids should be administered if the patient is to remain without oral fluids before surgery. During the perioperative period, the estimated maintenance fluid requirement (see Table 27–1) is usually reduced by 25 percent in anticipation of antidiuretic hormone release in response to fright, pain, and anesthesia.

Extensive surgical procedures complicate fluid therapy considerably. Opening the abdomen or thorax for an extended period increases evaporative losses. It must be emphasized that the surface area of these spaces is a larger proportion of total body surface area in infants and children, hence the magnitude of these losses may be considerable. In complex circumstances, intravascular monitoring of extracellular fluid volume will be required. The assessment of the state of hydration in postoperative children may be difficult. If a child is voiding at a rate of 2 to 3 ml/kg-hr with a specific gravity of 1.010 or urinary osmolarity of 280 to 300 mOsm/kg, it is likely that the patient has replete intravascular volume. After surgery, most children will have a urine flow rate of 1 to 2 ml/kg-hr because of postoperative antidiuretic hormone release, and additional fluids should not be administered in an attempt to increase urine volume as long as the child is stable and without clinical symptoms of volume depletion. However, if a child is oliguric (i.e., urine volume <0.8 ml/kg-hr) during the postoperative period, one must determine whether the patient has diminished renal perfusion from intravascular volume depletion, acute renal failure, or excessive nonphysiologic antidiuretic hormone release. In many cases, the administration of an isotonic fluid (normal saline or Ringer's lactate) at 1 percent of body weight (10 ml/kg) over 1 hour will result in an increase in urine volume that is sustained. However, if the patient remains oliguric, then an assessment of urinary osmolarity and sodium concentration may be helpful (Table 27–2).

Maintenance Fluid Therapy in Newborn Infants

Many factors influence the amount of water and electrolyte necessary for maintenance fluid therapy in newborn infants. The observa-

Table 27–2. Urinary Sodium and Osmolarity in Evaluation of Oligoanuria

	Decreased Intravascular Volume or Diminished Renal Perfusion	Established Acute Renal Failure	Nonphysiologic ADH Secretion[a]
Urinary Na (mEq/liter)	<10	>50	>50
Fractional Na excretion (FE_{Na})	<1%	>2%	>2%
Urinary osmolarity (mOsm/liter)	>500	~300	>500
$\frac{\text{Urine}}{\text{Plasma}}$ Osmolarity	>1.5	0.8–1.2	>2.0
BUN/serum creatinine	>20	Progressive increase in both	<20

$$\text{Fractional sodium excretion} = \frac{\text{urine}}{\text{plasma}}\ \text{Na} \div \frac{\text{urine}}{\text{plasma}}\ \text{Creatinine}$$

[a] ADH, antidiuretic hormone.

tion that the smaller the baby the larger the percentage of body water has been appreciated for some time.[19] Since fat is virtually absent in babies weighing less than 1500 g, a high percentage of body weight is contributed by water. Widdowson[20] demonstrated that a premature infant weighing 1000 g has total body water of 86 percent, which falls to 68 percent in a 3500-g full-term infant. Water and electrolyte losses vary considerably between babies of even the same weight as a function of many environmental factors. Insensible water loss is influenced by amount of surface area exposed, the velocity of air movement over this surface, and the vapor pressure of water both on the skin and in the air. The evaporative losses from the respiratory tract depend on the differences in absolute humidity of inspired and expired air. Variations in nursery environment, which include the use of single-walled or double-walled incubators, humidified incubator or room air, radiant warmers and/or phototherapy, and respirators, all contribute to the complexity of estimating maintenance fluid requirements of the neonate. The difficulty in deciding how much fluid to give an infant rests in large part with an assessment of the contribution of each of these factors. Wu and Hodgman[21] have shown that evaporative fluid losses are inversely correlated to birth weight and that these losses increase markedly by the use of radiant warmers. Studying infants weighing less than 1500 g, these investigators tested three types of warmers and found that evaporative fluid losses increased from 50 to 100 percent depending on the type of warmer. In infants weighing more than 1500 gs, fluid losses increased from 82 to 190 percent, again varying with the type of warmer. These workers also demonstrated that phototherapy increased evaporative fluid losses and that such losses could be minimized by careful temperature control. Oh and Karechi[22] confirmed that increases in evaporative fluid losses, stool water, and urine losses all contributed to the need for more water in mature infants receiving phototherapy.

The practical aspects of parenteral fluid therapy in newborn infants are complicated by the low margin of reserve in these patients. Inadequate fluids result in rapid dehydration because of increased insensible fluid losses and diminished renal concentrating ability. Excessive fluid administration results in hyponatremia and volume expansion because of a low glomerular filtration rate and limited ability to excrete a volume load. Persistent volume expansion in these small infants can lead to cardiac decompensation and has been associated with increased risk of necrotizing enterocolitis[23] and patent ductus arteriosus.[24] Table 27–3 provides guidelines for maintenance fluid therapy in newborn infants according to the recommendations of Baumgart and associates.[25] Careful and frequent assessment of the state of hydration is essential in the care of these infants.

DEFICIT THERAPY

This aspect of parenteral fluid therapy is designed to evaluate and repair the losses of fluids and electrolytes that occurred before the patient's presentation. As such, there are three essential components to this aspect of fluid therapy: (1) to estimate the degree or severity of dehydration; (2) to determine the type of deficit that has occurred, that is, isotonic, hypertonic, or hypotonic; and (3) to plan an approach to repair the deficit.

Degree or Severity of Dehydration

The degree or severity of dehydration is estimated from the patient's history and clinical condition at the time of initial presentation. No piece of laboratory data other than a documented change in body weight can predict the degree or severity of dehydration. This estimation must be made on the basis of clinical observations and experience. As shown in Table 27–4, the percentage loss of body weight can be correlated with clinical signs and symp-

Table 27–3. Guidelines for Maintenance Fluid Therapy in Newborn Infants[a,b]

	Weight (g)			
Type of Warmer	600–800	801–1000	1001–1500	1501–2000
Radiant warmer				
Volume (ml/kg-day)	120	90	75	65
Dextrose (g/100 ml)	5	10	10	12.5
Saline (%)	0.1	0.2	0.2	0.2
Incubator				
Volume (ml/kg-day)	90	75	65	55
Dextrose (g/100 ml)	7.5	10	10	12.5
Saline (%)	0.1	0.2	0.2	0.2
Either, with shield				
Volume (ml/kg-day)	70	55	50	45
Dextrose (g/100 ml)	7.5	10	12.5	12.5
Saline (%)	0.1	0.2	0.2	0.2

[a] Source: Based on the recommendations of Baumgart S, Langman CB, Sasulshi R, et al: Fluid, electrolytes and glucose maintenance in the very low birth weight infant. Clin Pediatr 21:302, 1982.

[b] The volume of fluid should be increased by 30 percent with phototherapy. Salt-containing solutions are usually not given on the first day of life.

toms. In children with mild (1 to 5 percent) dehydration, the findings are largely historical, that is, history of 12 to 24 hours of vomiting/diarrhea, and so forth, with minimal findings on physical examination. Children with moderate (6 to 10 percent) dehydration have a history of abnormal fluid and electrolyte losses plus physical findings that include tenting skin, sunken eyes and fontanel, slight lethargy, and dry lips and mouth. With severe (11 to 15 percent) dehydration, the patient will usually develop findings of cardiovascular instability (mottling of skin, tachycardia, hypotension) and neurologic involvement (extreme irritability, coma). Dehydration, which occurs over a protracted period, may be more severe than clinically evident. It must be remembered that the findings provide only an index as to the severity of the dehydration and not a precise determination. In fact, the specific degree of volume depletion estimated by several skilled observers in the same patient may vary greatly. Nonetheless, the assessment of the percentage dehydration is an integral part of planning a strategy for treating the patient and, as such, should be done carefully and conscientiously in all children with a history of excess fluid losses.

Table 27–4. Assessment of Degree and Severity of Dehydration in Infants and Children

Degree of Dehydration	Percent Loss of Body Weight (%)	Clinical Finding
Mild	3–5	History of fluid losses, minimal signs, decreased urination
Moderate	6–10	Tenting of skin, lethargy, sunken eyes
Severe	11–15	Hypotension, tachypnea, tachycardia, oliguria, sensorium changes

Type of Deficit

The type of deficit that has occurred can best be estimated from the patient's electrolyte values at presentation. In fact, the tonicity of the fluid that the patient has lost will be the mirror image of the tonicity of the patient's plasma. In practice, the type of dehydration is defined by the osmolarity of the patient's serum at presentation—not by the type of deficit that has occurred. On this basis, states of dehydration are commonly referred to as isotonic (serum osmolarity 270 to 300 mOsm/liter; serum Na^+ 130 to 150 mEq/liter); hypotonic (serum osmolarity <270; serum Na^+

<130); and hypertonic (serum osmolarity >310; serum Na^+ >150). It may be useful to recall that

$$\text{Serum osmolarity} = 2\,(Na^+ + K^+) + \frac{\text{BUN}}{2.8} + \frac{\text{glucose}}{18}$$

Therefore, if blood urea nitrogen (BUN) and glucose are in normal ranges, the serum osmolarity may be estimated by 2(Na^+). Patients with hypertonic dehydration must be given very special attention because of frequent and serious central nervous system complications (e.g., seizures, coma) that occur during rehydration. (See Chapter 21.)

Plan of Approach

There are many approaches to the correction of fluid deficits. Each approach has a number of proponents, and most plans have been extensively evaluated. Most of these programs are interchangeable and share a number of similar principles:

1. Restoration and preservation of cardiovascular function and perfusion of the brain and kidneys are a primary initial concern. Thus, in all forms of dehydration, especially in the child with severe dehydration, therapy should be initiated with a volume expander. This initial rapid rehydration gives the physician time to analyze laboratory data and to reevaluate the patient.
2. Total body repair will require a considerable period of time in all types of dehydration.
3. Half-normal saline (77 mEq/liter sodium and chloride) is a readily available solution well suited as a replacement fluid in most forms of dehydration in children. This fluid is used to replace the bulk of the estimated deficit in most cases.
4. Total body potassium losses cannot be replaced immediately, since potassium is predominantly an intracellular ion. After the child has voided, usually twice, potassium may be added to the parenteral fluids. The concentration of potassium should not ordinarily exceed 40 mEq/liter or a rate of infusion of 0.5 mEq/kg-hr. Potassium is usually added as 20 mEq/liter as either KCl or K_2HPO_4.
5. The adequacy of the corrected volume deficit must be determined on the basis of changes in the patient's appearance, clearing of the signs of dehydration, and increase in weight. Continuous monitoring of the volume and concentration of the patient's urine may be helpful. If the urine contains no protein or glucose, one may assume that extracellular fluid deficits have been corrected when the urine specific gravity reaches 1.010. If available, urine osmolarity may be more helpful in assessing the adequacy of rehydration. Nevertheless, the efficacy of the fluid therapy regimen should not be judged by any one parameter, but must rely on a frequent reassessment of the patient by a skilled observer. One should never be content with the original estimate of dehydration unless the patient is responding appropriately and is showing signs of progressive improvement.

CORRECTION OF FLUID DEFICITS DUE TO HYPOTONIC OR ISOTONIC DEHYDRATION

Plan I makes no provision for maintenance fluid requirements during the period of deficit therapy, and all of the estimated deficit is replaced within 6 to 8 hours. This plan has the advantage of enabling the therapist to concentrate on one aspect (i.e., deficit therapy) of the patient's need at one time and to consider other aspects of fluid therapy separately. The disadvantage of this approach is the relatively rapid infusion of large volumes of fluid, especially in older children. In large part, this approach is generally feasible for younger children with mild to moderate dehydration and no evidence of preexisting renal or cardiac disease. This plan is not generally used for adolescents with diabetic ketoacidosis or for older children with more than 10 percent dehydration.

Plan I

Rapid or initial phase: restore intravascular volume
- *Rate:* 1 to 2 percent of the body weight/hr or 10 to 20 ml/kg-hr
- *Fluid:* Ringer's lactate or normal saline
- *Duration:* 1 to 2 hours, depending on patient's condition [If patient is hypotensive or shocky, give 3 to 5 percent body wt/hr (30 to 50 ml/kg-hr) of plasma or albumin. If shock persists after initial hydration, whole blood may be required.]

Second phase: replacement of deficit
- *Rate:* Calculated and adjusted to replace all of estimated deficit in 6 to 8 hours
- *Fluid:* D5 0.5 NS plus K^+ (20 mEq/liter) after patient has voided twice
- *Duration:* 6 to 8 hours (When urine specific gravity decreases to 1.010, switch to maintenance rate if patient's condition is improved.)

Third phase: reequilibration and stabilization
- *Rate:* Maintenance and ongoing losses
- *Fluid:* 280 mM glucose/77 mM NaCl plus K^+ (20 mEq/liter) after patient has voided twice
- *Duration:* Depends on clinical problems as long as parenteral fluids are required

Plan II provides a slower and more prolonged repair of the deficit. This program provides for estimated maintenance needs during the period of deficit correction. Although this approach requires slightly more complex calculations, it is particularly applicable for older patients with moderate to severe dehydration or patients with known cardiac disease, renal disease, or hypertonic states (i.e., diabetic ketoacidosis, poisoning).

Plan II

Rapid or initial phase: restore intravascular volume
- *Rate:* 1 to 2 percent of the body weight/hr or 10 to 20 ml/kg-hr
- *Fluid:* Ringer's lactate or normal saline
- *Duration:* 1 to 2 hours or less if urine specific gravity <1.015 [If patient is hypotensive or shocky, then give 3 to 5 percent BW/hr (30 to 50 ml/kg-hr) of plasma, albumin.]

Second phase: replacement of extracellular losses
- *Rate:* Calculated to provide one-third of total maintenance fluids plus one-half estimated deficit and replace ongoing losses over 8 hours
- *Fluid:* Usually D5 0.5 NS plus K^+ (20 to 30 mEq/liter) added after patient has voided twice
- *Duration:* 8 hours

Third phase: reequilibration and stabilization
- *Rate:* Maintenance and ongoing losses plus remaining deficit (if necessary, i.e., if urine specific gravity >1.015)
- *Fluid:* Usually D5 0.2 NS + 20 mEq/liter K^+
- *Duration:* Dependent on clinical situation and ongoing losses

CORRECTION OF FLUID DEFICITS DUE TO HYPERTONIC DEHYDRATION

In infants and young children, hypertonic dehydration (see Chapter 21) presents a more complex diagnostic and therapeutic problem.[17,26] In these children, the degree of volume deficit is frequently underestimated. In patients with isotonic or hypotonic dehydration, the clinical signs and symptoms of mild to moderate dehydration occur because of a disproportionate loss of extracellular fluid and preservation of intracellular fluid. With hypertonic dehydration, a greater degree of intracellular fluid loss occurs, and the severity of the volume contraction is more difficult to estimate on the basis of the common clinical signs (Table 27–4). Intracellular volume contraction followed by cell swelling has been proposed as an explanation for the high incidence of seizures and cerebral edema that occurs during the period of rehydration in infants and children with hypertonic dehydration. It is postulated that the osmotic behavior of the brain cell is similar to that of the erythrocyte. When red cells are placed in a hypertonic medium, the cell contracts as water moves from the intracellular to extracellular space and osmotic equilibrium is achieved. If these erythrocytes are then placed in an isotonic solution, they accumulate an excess of water and swell beyond their normal size, developing intracellular edema. To prevent or minimize this phenomenon as it affects the brain cells of children with hypertonic dehydration, fluids should be administered slowly and the estimated deficit should be replaced over 24 to 48 hours.[26] The probability of neurologic complications will be increased (1) in infants and young children, (2) with prolonged dehydration of more than 4 days, (3) when associated with severe hypertonicity (serum Na >170 mEq/liter), and (4) with rapid correction of extracellular osmolarity. Although the sodium deficit in these children is less than that in other types of dehydration, some sodium should be included in the rehydration fluids. Although a variety of special solutions have been devised for use in hypertonic dehydration, in reality it is the rate of infusion rather than the contents of the solution that is the critical factor in minimizing central nervous system complications. We prefer a solution similar to that used for maintenance therapy, that is, 25 to 30 mEq/liter sodium. Using this solution, one-half the estimated deficit should be replaced over 24 to 38 hours, during which time full maintenance fluids should be administered as well. Because the hypertonicity of the plasma will provide a continuous stimulus for antidiuretic hormone release, the volume and concentration of urine will not be as accurate a reflection of repletion of extracellular volume as in the other forms of dehydration. Thus, careful reevaluation of the patient and monitoring of serum sodium concentration will be required. If rehydration is proceeding on schedule, the serum sodium should fall by 0.4 to 0.8 mEq/liter-hr, or 10 to 12 mEq/liter-day. A more rapid fall in serum would suggest overzealous replacement, in which case the rate of rehydration should be slowed, while an increase in serum sodium would suggest inadequate rehydration, in which case the rate of fluid administration should be increased. Hyperglycemia is often evident at presentation and usually disappears during the first few hours of rehydration. However, one must remember that when hyperglycemia is present, effective serum sodium is actually higher than measured, and an initial rise in serum sodium during the first 2 to 3 hours of rehydration may reflect correction of the hyperglycemia and resultant shift of water into cells rather than underhydration. Hypocalcemia also occurs in children with hypertonic dehydration, may complicate the assessment of neurologic signs, and can be corrected by the administration of calcium (4 mg/kg-hr). A plan for deficits repair in patients with hypertonic dehydration might be as follows:

Plan III

Rapid or initial phase: restore intravascular volume
- *Rate:* 1 to 2 percent of the body weight/hr or 10 to 20 ml/kg-hr
- *Fluid:* Ringer's lactate or normal saline
- *Duration:* 1 to 2 hours if patient not hypotensive (Since these fluids contain a high sodium concentration, this rate of infusion will not produce a significant fall in serum sodium but will permit a stabilization of intravascular volume.)

Second phase: slow rehydration and maintenance fluids
- *Rate:* Calculated to provide one-half deficit plus standard maintenance fluids and replace ongoing losses
- *Fluid:* Usually 280 mM glucose/30 mM NaCl with K^+ (20 mEq/liter) added after patient voids twice
- *Duration:* 24 to 48 hours and adjusted so that serum sodium falls by 10 to 12 mEq/liter-day

In each of the three plans for correction of deficits, we have indicated that either Ringer's lactate or normal saline could be administered during the initial phase of therapy, which is designed to restore intravascular volume. In two situations, small infants and patients with metabolic alkalosis, Ringer's lactate should not be used. In small babies, particularly premature infants, lactate may not be readily metabolized, and the administration of this anion would only produce or worsen the development of metabolic acidosis. In children with dehydration secondary predominantly to vomiting, such as infants with pyloric stenosis, the metabolism of lactate to bicarbonate will worsen the metabolic alkalosis. In these two clinical settings the administration of normal saline rather than Ringer's lactate would be preferred during the initial phase of rehydration.

REPLACEMENT THERAPY

This aspect of parenteral fluid therapy is designed to replace ongoing fluid and electrolyte losses from sources other than evaporative (insensible) or urinary fluids. These fluid volumes are not accounted for in the calculation of deficit or maintenance requirements and must be added to maintenance therapy. Since the constituents of these losses are frequently quite different from the composition of maintenance fluids, it may be hazardous to simply increase the volume of maintenance fluids in an attempt to compensate for these losses. Numerous tables estimating the volume and constituents of fluids from various sites are available. However, in most circumstances it is preferable to measure the electrolyte content of these fluids and replace them milliequivalent per milliequivalent and milliliter per milliliter.

The most commonly encountered type of ongoing loss is nasogastric suction. This fluid usually contains a high concentration of chloride and requires replacement with normal saline. Inadequate replacement of chloride losses will result in a hypochloremic–hypokalemic alkalosis. It should also be remembered that excessive urinary losses are not accounted for in the calculation of maintenance fluids. Thus, the child with congenital or acquired diabetes insipidus or the infant with a post-obstructive diuresis after relief of posterior uretheral valves will require additional replacement therapy to cover urinary losses.

In small infants, the magnitude of third-space losses from an ileus, ascites, burn, or wound may be quite difficult to estimate. In such cases, central volume should be monitored to provide a more accurate estimate of the magnitude of these losses.

In children receiving parenteral nutrition, there is a tendency to replace ongoing losses by increasing the volume of the intravenous alimentation solution. Such a procedure may actually produce the paradoxical result of increased volume depletion, particularly in small infants and young children. These patients have a concentrating ability limited to ~400 to 600 mOsm/liter. Thus, for each milliosmole of renal solute load, these patients must excrete 2 ml of urine. The use of intravenous alimentation solutions to replace ongoing losses may present an increased renal solute load without sufficient free water to cover the urine volume that must be excreted. The additional water required for excretion of the solute load will be taken from the intravascular volume and thereby result in volume depletion and hypertonic dehydration. Thus, it is best to replace ongoing losses with a fluid similar in content and volume to that being lost.

ASSESSMENT OF OLIGURIA IN CHILDREN

In children requiring parental fluid therapy, the rate of urine formation is an important index of their clinical condition. On the basis of the expected urine volume, a child or adolescent excreting <0.8 ml/kg-hr urine should be assessed for oliguria. Classically, the causes of oligoanuria have been categorized as prerenal, renal, and postrenal. However, such a classification is neither physiologically based nor accurate. Accordingly, we prefer to evaluate patients for anatomic and pathophysiologic causes of oliguria.

Anatomic Causes

First consideration should be given to the obstruction or occlusion of the major anatomic components of the renal system: artery, vein, ureter, and bladder. It should be emphasized that oliguria will not result from the occlusion of the artery, vein, or ureter to only one kidney, unless the contralateral kidney is absent or nonfunctional. Therefore, one must suspect bilateral renal artery, vein, or ureteral obstruction if these sites are to be implicated as the cause of oliguria. Renal artery thrombosis is rare in children, although it is occasionally encountered in newborn infants as a complication of umbilical artery catheterization.[27-29] The usual clinical presentation for this problem is acute hypertension in a young infant. Likewise, renal vein thrombosis occurs almost exclusively in newborn infants. This diagnosis should be suspected when a patient develops an enlarging flank mass associated with the onset of hematuria, proteinuria, thrombocytopenia, and intravascular coagulopathy.[27-29] The diagnosis of renal vein thrombosis may be difficult to establish and may require arteriography for confirmation. Bilateral ureteral obstruction should be considered in all children who develop oliguria, because this is a potentially acutely correctable situation. Because partial ureteral obstruction produces polyuria and because most children with hydronephrosis present with an abdominal mass or urinary tract infection, ureteral obstruction is an uncommon cause of oliguria. Nonetheless, this possibility should be evaluated using noninvasive imaging techniques such as renal ultrasound.[30,31] The demonstration of two kidneys and the lack of a dilated renal pelvis in at least one kidney will essentially eliminate this diagnosis as the cause of oliguria. Several prospective studies have shown renal ultrasound to be reliable in assessing ureteral obstruction in adults.[30,31] Unless this diagnosis is highly suspected on the basis of the clinical situation, potentially risky or invasive procedures such as an intravenous or retrograde pyelogram should not be done routinely. Finally, bladder outlet obstruction must be evaluated in all children with oliguria, particularly male infants. In this condition, the bladder can often be palpated in children, especially in boys with posterior urethral valves. Even if the bladder cannot be palpated, a catheter may have to be inserted into the bladder to rule out this potentially correctable cause of oliguria. Each of these anatomic sites should be considered before evaluation of the pathophysiologic causes of oliguria.

Pathophysiologic Causes

There are three pathophysiologic conditions in which oliguria occurs: (1) decreased intravascular volume or impaired renal perfusion, (2) acute renal failure, and (3) nonphysiologic antidiuretic hormone secretion. The renal response in each of these clinical settings is highly reproducible and well defined. Although each of these conditions will cause a fall in urine volume below expected levels, the urinary constituents, especially sodium and osmolarity, are characteristic and can be used diagnostically when the kidney has not been manipulated pharmacologically with vasodilators or diuretics (Table 27–2).

A decrease in intravascular volume results in a decrease in cardiac output and renal hypoperfusion, while the glomerular filtration rate is relatively well maintained. Thus, the renal response to either decreased intravascular volume or a primary fall in renal perfusion is similar. In this situation, the renal tubules remain intact, and a marked increase in the reabsorption of solutes and water occurs throughout the nephron. An increase in filtration fraction (GFR/renal plasma flow) produces an increase in peritubular oncotic pressure and results in enhanced reabsorption of tubular fluid in proximal tubular segments. The decrease in renal perfusion stimulates the secretion of renin by the juxtaglomerular apparatus, leading to increased aldosterone production and inducing sodium reabsorption from the distal tubule. Release of antidiuretic hormone in response to decreased intravascular volume increases water reabsorption in the collecting duct. Thus, the urinary sodium concentration is quite low (<10 mEq/liter) and the urinary osmolarity is high (>500 mOsm/liter). In premature infants and in children less than 1 year of age, urinary sodium <20 mEq/liter and osmolarity >400 mOsm/liter would be acceptable values.[32] If the patient is hyponatremic (serum sodium <130 mEq/liter), then fractional sodium excretion (FE_{Na}) is a better index of renal sodium handling. Fractional sodium excretion is the amount of sodium excreted ($U_{Na} \times V$) expressed as a ratio of the amount of sodium filtered (GFR $\times$ P_{Na}). If one substitutes creatinine clearance ($U_{Cr} \times V/P_{Cr}$) for GFR, the FE_{Na} can be expressed as U/P Na $\div$ U/P Cr. Similarly, urine to plasma ratio of osmolarity is a better reflection of water reabsorption in the hyponatremic patient. For example, if a patient had a serum sodium of 120 mEq/liter, the estimated plasma osmolarity would be 240 mOsm/liter, and a urine osmolarity of 360 mOsm/liter would be a urine:plasma osmolar ratio of 1.5 and would represent significant water reabsorption. The increased solute reabsorption that occurs in this condition pertains to constituents other than just sodium, such as urea. Normally, 30 percent of filtered urea is reabsorbed and an increased proportion is reabsorbed when renal perfusion falls. Since creatinine is not reabsorbed to any major extent by the tubule, the enhanced urea reabsorption results in a BUN:creatinine ratio of >20, often referred to as prerenal azotemia, but actually due to the pathophysiologic response of the kidney to diminished perfusion. Renal perfusion may be reduced to the extent of impairing the glomerular filtration rate at which time serum creatinine will rise. In contrast to patients with an established acute renal failure, in whom the serum creatinine increases by 0.5 to 1.5 mg/dl each day, patients with impaired renal perfusion usually have a slower rise in serum creatinine such that the values tend to remain at the same level for several days at a time and to increase in a stepwise fashion rather than a linear pattern.

The renal response to a fixed or established acute renal insult is complex.[33,34] Although the specific mechanisms involved may vary accordingly to the type and intensity of the acute renal injury, an acute loss of glomerular filtration rate and paralysis of tubular function are the characteristic features of acute renal failure. An increase in renal vascular resistance,[28,35] combined with backleak of tubular fluid[36,37] and intratubular obstruction,[38] result in a nearly complete cessation of glomerular filtration rate. Clinically, this is reflected in an increase in both BUN and serum creatinine on a daily basis. It is important to remember that although glomerular filtration rate is virtually nonexistent early in acute renal failure, the absolute value of serum creatinine will not reflect the profound loss of glomerular filtration rate because this value increases only 0.5 to 1.5 mg/dl-day. Thus, in patients with acute renal failure the rate of change in serum creatinine, rather than the actual value itself, is the best index of the level of glomerular filtration rate; a progressive increase in BUN and creatinine is a characteristic feature of this syndrome. Changes in BUN will be affected by a variety of factors, such as catabolic rate, protein load, and medications, including steroids and antibiotics. Consequently, the rate of change in BUN is not a specific index of the level of glomerular filtration rate. The second feature characteristic of acute enal failure is diminished tubular function. Ironically, the term acute tubular necrosis is a better description of tubular function than of anatomic morphology in acute renal failure.[39] Thus, the small volume of urine produced by these patients has a high sodium concentration (>50 mEq/liter) and elevated FE_{Na} (>2 percent). Since both the concentration and dilution of tubular fluid require intact tubular function, the urine of these patients is isotonic to plasma (i.e., urinary osmolarity of 280 to 300 mOsm/liter and urine to plasma osmolar ratio of 0.8 to 1.0). In acute renal failure, a dilute urine would be as unexpected as a concentrated urine, and an isotonic urine is the most consistent feature of this syndrome. In fact, a low urinary sodium concentration and FE_{Na} have been reported in some patients with acute renal failure induced by contrast media.

A variety of clinical conditions have been associated with nonphysiologic release of antidiuretic hormone[40-43] (see Chapter 18) and with a persistently concentrated urine, even though intravascular volume is normal or increased and plasma osmolarity is normal or decreased.[40,44,45] Continual release of antidiuretic hormone results in increased water reabsorption from the collecting duct into the plasma. Consequently, these patients have a concentrated urine (urine osmolarity >500 mOsm/kg, urine:plasma osmolar ratio >2.0) and a diluted plasma (plasma osmolarity <280 mOsm/liter, serum sodium <140 mEq/liter, BUN <15 mg/dl, and uric acid <2 mg/dl). The reabsorption of water from the collecting duct into the plasma also results in intravascular volume expansion, causing a depression of proximal tubular sodium reabsorption and a natriuresis (urinary sodium >50 mEq/liter, FE_{Na} >2 percent).

The urinary sodium concentration and osmolarity are a valid index of the pathophysiologic cause of oliguria only if the urine sample is obtained before the patient has been given: (1) a significant fluid challenge (20 ml/kg-hr) or (2) diuretic agents (mannitol, furosemide, ethacrinic acid). In some situations in which one may not be able to differentiate the cause for the oliguria, two manipulations can be attempted. First, assuming that the patient does not have overt evidence of fluid overload such as pulmonary or peripheral edema, a significant volume challenge (20 to 30 ml/kg-hr) of isotonic fluid can be administered. Since the fluid is isotonic, the potential hyponatremia associated with a fixed renal injury or nonphysiologic antidiuretic hormone secretion should not be exacerbated, and the patient with oliguria secondary to volume depletion or diminished renal perfusion should manifest an increase in urine output. Similarly, the administration of furosemide (4 mg/kg IV) would be expected to result in a diuresis in patients with volume depletion, but would have little or no effect for patients with acute renal failure. It must be remembered that both maneuvers will invalidate the use of urinary sodium concentration, FE_{Na}, or osmolarity in differentiating the cause of oliguria. Moreover, the administration of a potent diuretic may result in severe volume depletion in a postoperative patient with ongoing fluid losses; care must be taken to monitor urine volume and replace fluids carefully in such patients to avoid hypotension or shock.

ORAL FLUID AND ELECTROLYTE THERAPY

Because most episodes of viral gastroenteritis are self-limited and of short duration, pediatricians have traditionally prescribed the use of a number of common commercial products (Table 27–5). These solutions, usually referred to as clear fluids, may vary considerably in electrolyte content, depending on the locality in which they are manufactured; however, within a given community each product is reasonably consistent (Table 27–5). Since 1950, a series of commercial products specifically formulated for rehydration purposes have been approved (Table 27–6). Recently, considerable controversy concerning the optimum electrolyte and glucose concentration that these solutions should contain has arisen.

The interest in oral fluid and electrolyte therapy for dehydration has increased since reports of successful outcomes with this method have been published. Cases of cholera as well as bacterial, viral, and nonspecific diarrhea have been rehydrated using oral therapy.[40,46-48] The solutions used in most of these studies had a sodium concentration of

Table 27–5. Sodium and Potassium Concentration in Commonly Used Clear Fluids[a]

Product Name	October 1971		August 1981	
	Na^+	K^+	Na^+	K^+
	(mEq/liter)	(mEq/liter)	(mEq/liter)	(mEq/liter)
Pepsi Cola	2.75	1.3	2.0	1.2
Coca Cola	1.93	0.8	1.0	0.8
Ginger ale (Canada Dry)	0.99	0.10	2	0.6
Draft-style root beer (Barrel-head)	0.98	0.10	6	0.6
Apple juice (Lincoln)	—	—	2	17.6
Tea (Salada, brewed 1 minute)	0.86	0.22	1	3.3
Chamomile tea			3	6
Jell-O (raspberry)	15.18	0.22	25	0

[a] All values were determined for products purchased from a local grocery store and measured on a standard laboratory flame photometer.

90 mEq/liter and contained 2 to 4 g glucose/100 ml. On the basis of these and other studies, the World Health Organization (WHO) has recommended an oral rehydration solution that has sodium concentration of 90 mEq/liter, potassium concentration of 20 mEq/liter, and 2 g glucose/100 ml.[49] This recommendation has been received with some skepticism because of experience in the 1950s which suggested that a solution containing only 50 mEq/liter of sodium was responsible for increasing the incidence of hypernatremic dehydration. Since this product was prepared by the use of a measuring scoop, errors in dilution may have contributed to the observation that more children with hypertonic dehydration had taken this product as compared with children with isotonic dehydration.[50] It was also believed that 50 mEq/liter sodium would be excessive if this quantity met stool losses only and did not provide adequate free water to replace evaporative fluid losses. In addition to these initial studies by Colle et al.,[50] Franz and Segar[51] found an increase in hypernatremic dehydration in children who had taken a commercial product containing 50 mEq/liter sodium. However, when they fed solutions containing sodium at either 50 or 25 mEq/liter to children with diarrhea, these workers were unable to find a difference in serum sodium between the two groups. The fluid intake for all children in the study averaged 137 ml/kg-day, and this high volume of fluid was probably more important than the differences in sodium content. These studies emphasized the fact that inaccurate preparation of these solutions at home may have been a significant factor in the early experience with oral rehydration and pointed out that with the use of ordinary kitchen utensils the concentration of electrolytes in these solutions may vary greatly. A teaspoon is not a precise measurement, as powders can be heaped or leveled and thus are difficult to measure accurately. Even with a liquid, volumes may range from 3 to 7 ml. Because of the inherent diffi-

Table 27–6. Electrolyte and Carbohydrate Content of Commercially Available Oral Rehydration Solutions[a]

	Electrolyte			
	Na^+ (mEg/liter)	K^+ mEg/liter)	Cl^- (mEg/liter)	Carbohydrate (g/100 ml)
Pedialyte	30	20	30	5
Lytren	30	25	25	7.2
Gatorade	23	3	17	5.9
Hydra-Lyte	84	10	59	2.4
Infalyte	50	20	40	2
Pedialyte RS	60	20	50	2.5

[a] All values based on manufacturer's data.

culty in obtaining reproducible measurements, additional oral hydration solutions were provided to the public as a ready-to-use product in 1967; since that time, most commercial oral electrolyte solutions in this country have been provided as premixed formulations. Although no specific cause-and-effect relationship between the sodium concentration of 50 mEq/liter and the occurrence of hypernatremic dehydration was ever established, the sodium concentration of most commercial products was lowered to 30 mEq/liter (Table 27–6).

Bart and Finberg[52] believe that the sodium concentration of the solution recommended by WHO is too high, especially in children under 2 years of age because of their relatively immature renal function and insensible fluid losses. These investigators also question the advisability of comparing children of the third world, who have been the subject of most large-scale oral therapy studies, with children from developing countries in terms of fluid needs. On this basis, Finberg[53] has proposed that three solutions of varying sodium concentration—75, 40 to 50, and 20 to 25 mEq/liter—be available for oral use. The fluid prescribed would depend on the tonicity of the serum and whether deficit or maintenance therapy was intended. Walker[54] believes that solutions containing 80 to 90 mEq/liter sodium are dangerous if used without supervision and therefore should be available only by prescription and administered under supervision to ensure a high-volume intake. Nalin and Cash,[55] Steinhoff,[56] Woodward,[57] and Sack[58] all defend the use of oral hydration solutions containing 90 mEq/liter Na as safe on the basis of (1) their studies of successful rehydration with this concentration, (2) the principle of replacing losses with similar solutions, and (3) the impracticality of using three different solutions, especially in underdeveloped countries.

Two explanations seem most probable to resolve this apparent discrepancy between past experience, the well-documented observation that losses of electrolyte in patients with diarrhea (other than cholera) are hypotonic, and the current WHO recommendations. The first explanation is that higher concentrations of carbohydrate were used in the past, hence malabsorption of carbohydrate may have occurred and resulted in further water losses and prolonged diarrhea. Rapid transit, bacterial overgrowth in the small intestines, and disaccharidase deficiency may all lead to carbohydrate malabsorption in diarrheal states. Early oral rehydration products contained ~8 g/100 ml carbohydrate from glucose as compared with the 2 to 3 g/100 ml used in the recent formulations (Table 27–6). Sladen and Dawson[59] showed that maximum absorption of isotonic mixtures of glucose and saline were best absorbed when the concentration of glucose was between 56 and 140 mM/liter (1 to 2.5 g/100 ml). Studies have also compared glucose to sucrose as the carbohydrate source, most of which have shown that sucrose is an effective substitute, although one study showed it to be less effective.[60] Another study by Nalin's group on infants confirmed his opinion that glucose is preferable because sucrose produced both a slower correction of electrolyte abnormalities and a higher percentage of patients who needed more than 24 hours for recovery.[61]

The second explanation has to do with the total amount of water ingested as a critical factor in oral rehydration therapy. Since hypotonic fluid is being lost during diarrhea, and the other usual body water losses are either free water (evaporative losses) or hypotonic fluid (sweat losses), the patient's serum would tend to become more hypertonic if inadequate volume of fluid were given. The problem then is to be certain that the patient will take an adequate volume of fluid to prevent hypernatremia. Walker and colleagues[62] showed that the amount of fluid given was the major determinant in the rise or fall of serum sodium in a group of patients with diarrhea. These workers found that serum sodium rose when their patients were given a solution containing 30 mEq/liter sodium at 60 ml/kg-day but that the level fell when the same solution was given at 120 to 150 ml/kg-day. It is known that hypernatremia may develop even if the administered sodium is less than overall losses when sodium absorption exceeds the rate in which the extracellular fluid can be diluted by water from the cells or when sufficient exogenous water is not provided. A case in point is the report of an exclusively breast-fed baby who presented at the age of 2 weeks with moderate-to-severe dehydration and a serum sodium of 178 mEq/liter.[63] No other foods or liquids had been fed, and the infant recovered without evidence of renal disease. She recovered after rehydration with 200 ml/kg of Ringer's lactate for 48 hours, at which time her serum sodium fell to 154 mEq/liter. Although the sodium concentration of Ringer's lactate (130 mEq/liter) is much higher than the usual recommendation for the treatment of hypernatremic dehydration, this case illustrates the primary role of adequate provision of volume for the prevention of hypertonic dehydration.

The success rates of oral rehydration vary in published reports. Pizarro et al.[64] reported 40 neonates with a mean degree of dehydration of 6.7 percent, with five patients being 10 percent dehydrated. Ten patients required admission because of recurrence of dehydration, five of whom required parenteral fluids while the other five were again orally hydrated. These investigators found no complications in this group, including an infant whose initial serum sodium of 168 mEq/liter fell to 140 mEq/liter in 12 hours. Although this paper reported success with oral hydration, the five patients who required parenteral fluid therapy and the five whose condition necessitated rehydration orally actually represent a 25 percent failure rate. Sack et al.[65] reported 89 children, 57 with rotovirus infection, successfully hydrated orally, but the average estimated degree of dehydration was 5 percent. Pizarro et al.[66] reported oral rehydration in 100 children in an emergency room setting. Their degree of dehydration varied between 1 and 10 percent. Parenteral fluids were instituted in eight patients because of persistent vomiting or refusal to take fluids and, more importantly, 13 returned because of failure to maintain hydration at home. The mean emergency room stay was 15.6 ± 8.1 hours.

RECOMMENDATIONS CONCERNING THE USE OF ORAL FLUID AND ELECTROLYTE THERAPY

1. The prescribing of oral hydrating solutions should be taken as seriously as the ordering of parenteral fluids.
2. Health care providers advising the intake of any oral rehydrating solution should specify the volume, concentration, and frequency of the solution to be given. For children under 2 years of age, an intake of at least 120 to 150 ml/kg-day is essential.
3. Any solution containing more than 30 mEq/liter sodium should be administered under medical supervision with careful follow-up evaluation and reassessment of adequacy of rehydration.
4. The carbohydrate concentration in oral rehydration solutions should be ~2 g/100 ml to maximize sodium and water absorption.
5. Clear fluids are justified during the first 24 to 48 hours of a diarrheal episode, since many of the intercurrent diarrheas last a short time.
6. Home-brewed solutions mixed with the usual household utensils are fraught with danger in such cases and should be discouraged.

Ironically, in developed countries we may have more difficulty providing the personnel to administer and closely monitor oral therapy than occurs in third-world nations. Keeping children and parents in busy emergency rooms for long periods of time is also impractical and difficult for both patients and health care providers. Thus, the cost–benefit of this approach is not fully established, but careful attempts at oral rehydration in children with mild degrees of dehydration appear warranted and feasible.

SUMMARY

This chapter provides an overview of the special considerations regarding fluid and electrolyte therapy in infants, children, and adolescents. In most cases, the basic pathophysiologic perturbation that must be considered is similar to that in adults, but a clear recognition of the limitations in adaptation and restricted margin of error in providing fluids and electrolytes to infants and children must be recognized. To this end, the materials in this chapter should provide the basis for an assessment of the clinical situation and at least the initiation of a rational program of fluid and electrolyte therapy in children.

ACKNOWLEDGMENTS

The authors wish to acknowledge the long and dedicated tradition of investigation and innovation in fluid and electrolyte therapy for infants and children that has existed at our institution for the past decade. Clearly, the simplified approach to parenteral fluid therapy presented in this chapter has evolved over a number of years and has benefited from the critique of our colleagues and the experience of our patients. We are also indebted to Ester Nichols, Marie Campbell, and Marilyn Modzelewski, who provided secretarial services.

REFERENCES

1. Adams F: The Genuine Works of Hippocrates, Vols I, and II. William Wood, New York, 1886
2. Kramer B, Kanof A: Diarrhea in children. A historical review. J Pediatr 57:769, 1960
3. Pratt EL: Presidential address, Society for Pediatric Research. Am J Dis Child 96:419, 1958
4. O'Shaughnessy WB: Experiments on blood in cholera. Lancet 1:490, 1831–1832
5. Schmidt C: Charakteristik der epidemischen cholera gegenuber verwandten transsudationsanomialiee. GA Rehyer, Leipzig, 1850
6. Bernard C: Introduction to the Study of Experimental Medicine (1859), Green HC (transl). Harry Shuman, New York, 1949
7. Latta T: Letter to Secretary of Central Board of Health, London, Affording view of rationale and results of his practice in treatment of cholera and saline injections. Lancet 2:274, 1831–1832
8. Finberg L, Kravath R, Fleischman A: Water and Electrolytes in Pediatrics. WB Saunders, Philadelphia. 1982
9. Howland J, Marriot WM: Acidosis occurring with diarrhea. Am J Dis Child, 11:309, 1916
10. Schloss OM, Stetson, RE: Occurrence of acidosis with diarrhea. Am J Dis Child 13:218, 1917
11. Gamble JL: Chemical Anatomy, Physiology and Radiology of Extracellular Fluid. 6th Ed. A Lecture Syllabus. Harvard University Press, Cambridge, Ma, 1954
12. Darrow DC: The significance of body size. Am J Dis Child 98:416, 1959
13. Darrow DC, Pratt EL, Flett J, et al: Disturbances of water and electrolytes in infantile diarrhea. Pediatrics 3:129, 1949
14. Powers GF: A comprehensive plan of treatment for the so-called intestinal intoxication of infants. Am J Dis Child 32:232, 1926
15. Harrison HE: The treatment of diarrhea in infancy. Pediatr Clin North Am 1:335, 1954
16. Holliday MA, Segar WE: Maintenance need for water in parenteral fluid therapy. Pediatrics 19:823, 1957
17. Weil WB, Wallace WM: Hypertonic dehydration in infancy. Pediatrics 17:171, 1956
18. Winters RW: The Body Fluids in Pediatrics. Little, Brown, Boston, Ma, 1973
19. Friis-Hansen B: Body water compartments in children: Changes during growth and related changes in body composition. Pediatrics 28:169, 1951
20. Widdowson EM: Growth and composition of the fetus and newborn. In Assali NS (ed): Biology of Gestation. Vol. II: The Fetus and Neonate. Academic Press, New York, 1978
21. Wu PYK, Hodgman JE: Insensible water loss in preterm infants—Changes with postnatal development and non-ionizing radiant energy. Pediatrics 54:704, 1974

22. Oh W, Karechi H: Phototherapy and insensible water loss in the newborn infant. Am J Dis Child 124:230, 1972
23. Bell E, Warburton D, Stonestreet BS, et al: High volume fluid intake predisposes premature infants to necrotizing enterocolitis. Lancet 2:90, 1979
24. Bell E, Warburton D, Stonestreet BS, et al: Effect of fluid administration on the development of symptomatic patent ductus arteriosus and congestive heart failure in premature infants. N Engl J Med 302:598, 1980
25. Baumgart S, Langman CB, Sasulshi R, et al: Fluid, electrolytes and glucose maintenance in the very low birth weight infant. Clin Pediatr 21:302, 1982
26. Finberg L: Current concepts: Hypernatremic (hypertonic) dehydration in infants. N Engl J Med 289:196, 1973
27. Gordillo-Paniagua G, Velasquez-Jones L: Acute renal failure. Pediatr Clin North Am 23:817, 1976
28. Gianantonio, CA, Vitacco, M., Mendilaharza J, et al: Acute renal failure in infancy and childhood. J Pediatr 61:660, 1962
29. Reimold EL, Don TD, Worthen HG: Renal failure during the first year of life. Pediatrics 59:987, 1977
30. Ellenbogen PH, Scheible FW, Talner LB, et al: Sensitivity of gray scale ultrasound in detecting urinary tract obstruction. AJR 130:721, 1978
31. Sander RC, Jeck DL: B-scan ultrasound in the evaluation of renal failure. Radiology 119:199, 1976
32. Norman ME, Asadi FK: A prospective study of acute renal failure in the newborn infant. Pediatrics 63:475, 1979.
33. Kashgarian M: Acute renal failure. Pathol Annu 15:335, 1980
34. Stein JH, Lifschitz MD, Barnes LD: Current concepts on the pathophysiology of acute renal failure. Am J Physiol 234:F171, 1978
35. Hollenberg NK, Epstein M, Rosen SM, et al: Acute oliguric renal failure in man: Evidence for preferential renal cortical ischemia. Medicine (Baltimore) 47:455, 1968
36. Donohoe JF, Venkatachalam MA, Bernard DB, et al: Tubular leakage and obstruction after renal ischemia: Structural–functional correlations. Kidney Int 13:208, 1978
37. Myers BD, Chui F, Hilberman M, et al: Transtubular leakage of glomerular filtrate in human acute renal failure. Am J Physiol 237:319, 1979
38. Tanner GA, Sophasen S: Kidney pressure after temporary renal artery occlusion in the rat. Am J Physiol 230:1173, 1976
39. Solez K, Morel-Maroger L, Sraer JD: The morphology of "acute tubular necrosis" in man: Analysis of 57 renal biopsies and a comparison with the glycerol model. Medicine (Baltimore) 58:362, 1979
40. Hirschhorn N, McCarthy BJ, Ranney B, et al: Adlibitum oral glucose–electrolyte therapy for acute diarrhea in Apache children. J Pediatr 83:562, 1973
41. Mor J, Ben-Galim E, Abrahamov A: Inappropriate antidiuretic hormone secretion in an infant with severe pneumonia. Am J Dis Child 129:133, 1975
42. Friedman AL, Segar WE: Medical Progress. Antidiuretic hormone excess. J Pediatr 94:521, 1979
43. Kaplan A, Feigin R: Inappropriate secretion of antidiuretic hormone in meningitis. J Pediatr 92:758, 1978
44. Bartter FC, Schwartz WB: The syndrome of inappropriate secretion of antidiuretic hormone. Am J Med 42:790, 1967
45. Verney EB: The antidiuretic hormone and the factors which determine its release. Proc R Soc Lond [Biol] 135:25, 1947
46. Cash DR, Islam RA, Molla M, et al: Oral maintenance therapy for cholera in adults. Lancet 2:370, 1968
47. Sack DA, Eusof A, Merson MH, et al: Oral hydration in rotovirus diarrhea: A double blind comparison of sucrose with glucose electrolyte solution. Lancet 2:280, 1978
48. Sack DA, Islam S, Brown KH, et al: Oral therapy in children with cholera: A comparison of sucrose and glucose electrolyte solution. J Pediatr 96:20, 1980
49. WHO: Treatment and Prevention of Dehydration in Diarrheal Diseases Guide for Use of Primary Health Care Personnel. Scientific Publication No. 336. World Health Organization, Washington DC, 1977
50. Colle E, Ayoub E, Raille R: Hypertonic dehydration (hypernatremia): The role of feedings high in solutes. Pediatrics 22:5, 1958
51. Franz MN, Segar WE: The association of various factors in hypernatremic diarrheal

dehydration. Am J Dis Child 97:298, 1959
52. Bart KJ, Finberg L: Single solution for oral therapy of diarrhea. (Letter.) Lancet 2:633, 1976
53. Finberg L: The role of oral electrolyte–glucose solutions in hydration for children—international and domestic aspects. J Pediatr 96:51, 1980
54. Walker SH: (Letter.) N Engl J Med 304:1238, 1981
55. Nalin DR, Cash, RA: (Letter.) Lancet 2:957, 1976
56. Steinhoff MC: (Letter.) J Pediatr 97:515, 1980
57. Woodward WE: (Letter.) J Pediatr 97:516, 1980
58. Sack DA: (Letter.) J Pediatr 97:517, 1980
59. Sladen GE, Dawson AN: Interrelationships between the absorptions of glucose, sodium and water by the normal human jejunum. Clin Sci 36:119, 1969
60. Nalin DR: Sucrose and oral therapy for cholera and related diarrheas. Lancet 1:1400, 1975
61. Nalin DR, Mata L, Vargus W, et al: Comparison of sucrose and glucose in oral therapy of an infant diarrhea. Lancet 2:77, 1978
62. Walker, SH, Gayhall, VP, Wuintero BA: Sodium and water content of feedings for use of infants with diarrhea. Clin Pediatr 20:101, 1981
63. Clarke A, Markarian M, Griswold W, et al: Hypernatremic dehydration resulting from inadequate breast feeding. Pediatrics 63:931, 1979
64. Pizarro D, Mata L, Posada, G, et al: Oral rehydration in neonates with dehydrating diarrheas. Lancet 2:1209, 1979
65. Sack RB, Pierce NF, Hirschhorn N: Oral therapy in acute diarrhea. Am J Clin Nutr 31:2252, 1978
66. Pizarro D, Posada G, Mohs E, et al: Evaluation of oral therapy for infant diarrhea in emergency room setting: The acute episode as an opportunity for instructing mothers in home therapy. Bull WHO 57:983, 1979

28

Aging and Renal Function

John W. Rowe

This chapter provides an overview of the changes in renal function that occur in adult life, including a discussion of adaptive mechanisms responsible for the regulation of volume and composition of the extracellular fluid. The term aging, as used here, refers to renal changes that occur after attainment of maturity, and in the absence of disease states. Changes before maturity—during childhood and adolescence—are more properly included in the area of growth and development rather than senescence and will not be discussed. An attempt has been made to emphasize only those gerontologic studies in which the study population has been carefully screened to exclude coexisting medical diseases.

RENAL ANATOMY

Advancing age is associated with progressive loss of renal mass in humans, with renal weight decreasing from 250 to 270 g in young adulthood to 180 to 200 g by the eighth decade.[1,2] In the absence of hypertension or marked vascular disease, the senescent kidney maintains its relatively smooth contour. The loss of renal mass is primarily cortical, with relative sparing of the renal medulla. The total number of identifiable glomeruli falls with age, roughly in accord with the changes of renal weight.[3-5] The number of hyalinized or sclerotic glomeruli identified on light microscopy increases from 1 to 2 percent during the third to fifth decade, to as high as 30 percent in some apparently healthy 80-year-olds, with a mean prevalence after age 70 of approximately 10 to 12 percent.[5-7] Of interest is the finding that neither McLachlan and coworkers[5] nor Kaplan and associates[7] could relate the number of absolescent glomeruli at postmortem to coincident vascular abnormalities.

Aging is associated with a loss of lobulation of the glomerular tuft, thus decreasing effective filtering surface. Although the total number of nuclei per glomerulus is unchanged with age, the filtering surface is further diminished by progressive increase in the number of mesangial cells after age 40 years, and a reciprocal decrease in the number and percentage of epithelial cells. The mesangium, which accounts for roughly 8 percent of total glomerular volume at age 45 years, increases to nearly 12 percent by age 70 years.[8] Although the glomerular basement membrane thickens with age, studies of glomerular filtration characteristics, as estimated by dextran clearance, show no change in permeability between ages 20 and 61.[9,10]

Several changes have been documented in the renal tubule with age. As with the glomerulus, the tubular basement membrane thickens.[11,12] In microdissections Oliver[13] observed a lack of relationship between the glomerular and tubular size in kidneys from elderly nonhypertensive patients and noted the presence of intact tubules after the glomeruli had become hyalinized. Conversely, Darmady and co-workers,[11] employing a similar methodology, were unable to identify aglomerular nephrons and found a strong relation between the glomerular and tubular dimensions. Of particular interest is the observation by Darmady and co-workers[11] that diverticuli of the distal nephron, which are essentially absent in kidneys from young individuals, become increasingly prevalent with advancing age, reaching a frequency of three diverticuli per tubule at age 90 years. It has been suggested that these diverticuli represent the origin of the simple retention cysts commonly seen in the elderly.[14,15]

Changes in the intrarenal vasculature with age, independent of hypertension or other renal disease, have been the focus of several excellent studies. It is generally agreed from histologic studies that normal aging is associated with variable sclerotic changes in the walls of the larger renal vessels. These sclerotic changes do not encroach on the lumen and are augmented in the presence of hypertension.[2,11,13,14,16,17] Smaller vessels appear to be spared, with fewer than 20 percent of senescent kidneys from nonhypertensive subjects displaying arteriolar changes.[16,18]

Radiographic studies of the renal vasculature in normotensive subjects from across the adult age range demonstrate an increasing prevalence after the seventh decade of abnormalities similar to those seen in hypertension.[19] The changes observed include abnor-

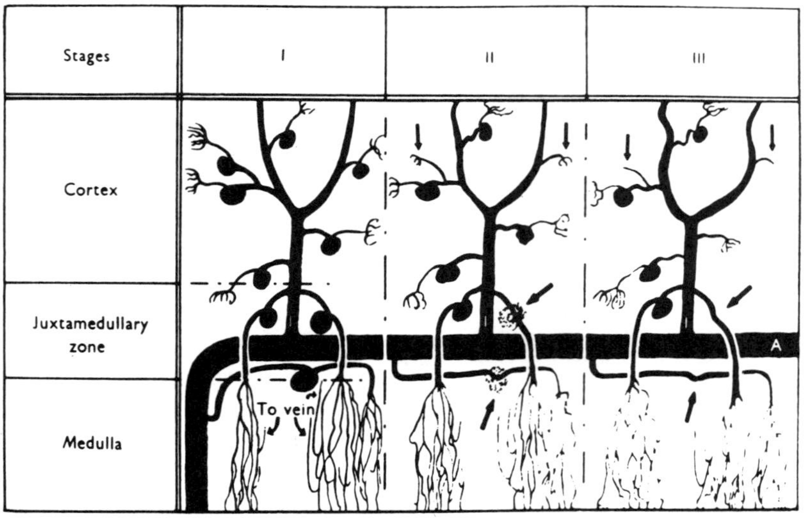

Fig. 28–1. Diagram showing changes in the intrarenal arterial pattern with age (A, arcuate artery; 1, interlobular artery). Stage I, basic adult pattern showing glomerular arterioles. Stage II, partial degeneration of some glomeruli. Two cortical afferent arterioles ramify into remnants of glomerular tufts (small arrows). Two juxtamedullary arterioles pass through partially degenerated glomeruli (large arrows). Note slight spiraling of interlobular arteries and afferent arterioles. Stage III, two cortical afferent arterioles now end blindly (small arrows), and two juxtamedullary arterioles are aglomerular (large arrows). The corresponding glomerular tufts have degenerated completely. The spiraling of interlobular arteries and afferent arterioles is now more pronounced. (From Ljungqvist A, Lagergren C: Normal intrarenal arterial pattern in adult and aging human kidney. J Anat 96:285, 1962. Reprinted with permission of Cambridge University Press.)

mal tapering of interlobular arteries, abnormal arcuate arteries, increased tortuosity of intralobular arteries, and a predilection for age-related vascular abnormalities to occur in the polar region.[19,20]

Combined microangiographic and histologic studies have identified two very distinctive patterns of change in arteriolar–glomerular units with senescence[21,22] (see Figs. 28–1 and 28–2). In one type, hyalinization and collapse of the glomerular tuft are associated with obliteration of the lumen of the preglomerular arteriole and a resultant loss in blood flow. This type of change is seen primarily in the cortical area. The second pattern, seen primarily in the juxtamedullary area, is characterized by the development of anatomic continuity between the afferent and efferent arterioles during glomerular sclerosis. The end point is thus loss of the glomerulus and shunting of blood flow from afferent to efferent arterioles. Blood flow is maintained to the arteriolar rectae verae, the primary vascular supply of the medulla, which are not decreased in number with age.

RENAL PHYSIOLOGY

Renal Blood Flow

A progressive reduction in renal plasma flow of approximately 10 percent per decade from 600 ml/min in young adulthood to 300 ml/min by 80 years is well established.[23] While early studies identified age-related declines in cardiac output that may contribute to this reduction in renal blood flow,[24,25] more recent studies have failed to show a diminution in cardiac output with age.[26,27] Thus the dominant, if not sole, determinant of reduced renal blood flow with age would appear to be the changes in the renal vasculature outlined above. Hollenberg et al.,[28] who employed the

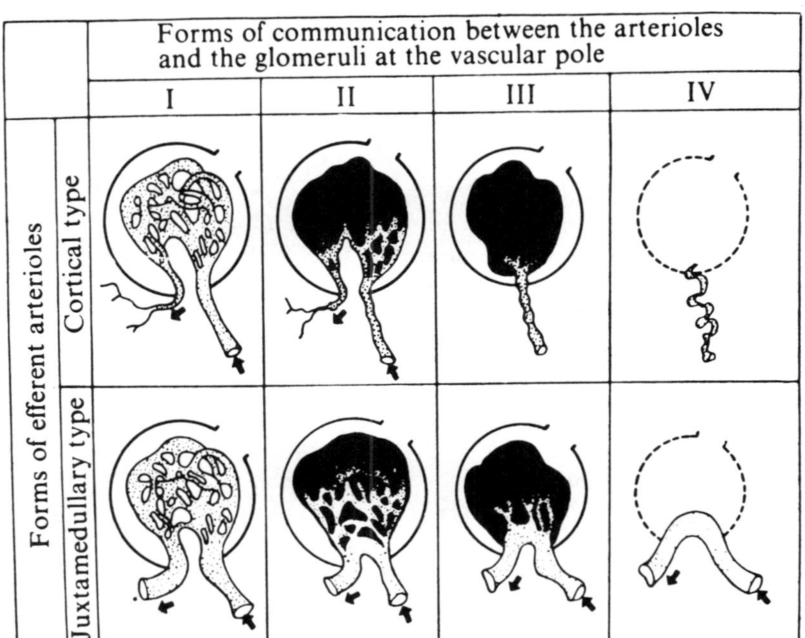

Fig. 28–2. Diagram of the degenerative process in the cortical and juxtamedullary nephrons. (From Takazakura E, Sawabu N, Handu A, et al: Intrarenal vascular changes with age and disease. Kidney Int 2:224, 1972. Reprinted from Kidney International with permission.)

xenon washout technique in a study of 207 healthy potential renal donors ranging in age from 17 to 76 years, reported a highly significant decrease with advancing age in the rapid (cortical) component of blood flow, a finding consistent with the histologic studies showing selective loss of cortical vasculature and preservation of medullary flow. These cortical vascular changes probably account for the patchy cortical defects commonly seen on renal scans in healthy old adults.[29] This histologic and functional demonstration of selective decrease in cortical flow may explain the observation that filtration fraction (glomerular filtration rate divided by renal plasma flow) actually increases with advancing age,[23,30] since outer cortical nephrons have a lower filtration fraction than do juxtamedullary nephrons.

In order to clarify the relative contribution of functional "spasm" to the observed changes in blood flow, Hollenberg et al.[28] studied young and old subjects before and during intraarterial administration of acetylcholine and angiotensin. If age-related functional spasm was present, maximal renal blood flow after acetylcholine-induced vasodilation might be expected to be normal or close to normal in elderly subjects. To the contrary, however, renal blood flow after acetylcholine was markedly decreased with advancing age. The slope of the line relating renal blood flow and age was similar in old and young subjects after acetylcholine, indicating a fixed or structural etiology for the observed decrease in flow with increasing age. Consistent with these findings, the vasoconstrictor response to angiotensin was not influenced by age.

Glomerular Filtration Rate

The major clinically relevant renal functional defect arising from the histologic and physiologic changes described in the preceding sections is a progressive decline in the glomerular filtration rate. Several studies, the results of which have been compiled and standardized by Wesson,[23] have shown that glomerular filtration rate (estimated by inulin clearance) falls progressively throughout the adult age span in men and women. In order to exclude an age-dependent effect on the renal handling of creatinine and to establish the utility of creatinine clearance in gerontological studies, Rowe et al.[31] performed simultaneous inulin and creatinine clearances on 55 healthy men ranging in age from 17 to 93 years. They found no effect of age on the ratio of true creatinine clearance to inulin clearance. Age-adjusted normative standards for creatinine clearance have recently been established employing 24-hour urinary creatinine clearance values on a large community-dwelling male population spanning the adult age range.[31,32] (Fig. 28–3).

In order to obtain a healthy group of elderly subjects, all volunteers were screened with a battery of tests including thorough history and physical examination, resting and postexercise electrocardiograms, glucose tolerance test, and urinalysis. Individuals found to have any evidence of renal disease, urinary tract infection, congestive heart failure, coronary artery disease, cerebrovascular disease, diabetes mellitus, gout, or a history of prostatic surgery were excluded from the study population. Subjects were also excluded if they were taking diuretics or antihypertensive medications. Results in 584 "normal" subjects showed that true creatinine clearance is stable until the middle of the fourth decade, at which time a linear decrease of ~8.0 ml/min/1.73 m^2/decade is observed (Fig. 28–3).

The argument that entire nephrons drop out with advancing age is supported by the rather striking parallel decline in glomerular filtration rate and several proximal tubular functions including maximum excretion of p-aminohipurate[33] and diodrast[34] and maximal absorption of glucose.[35] In addition, it has been shown that the renal threshold for glucosuria, which relates inversely to the degree of "splay" in reabsorptive capacity of individual nephrons, increases with age. A practical clinical correlate of this observation is that a healthy older individual is less likely than his

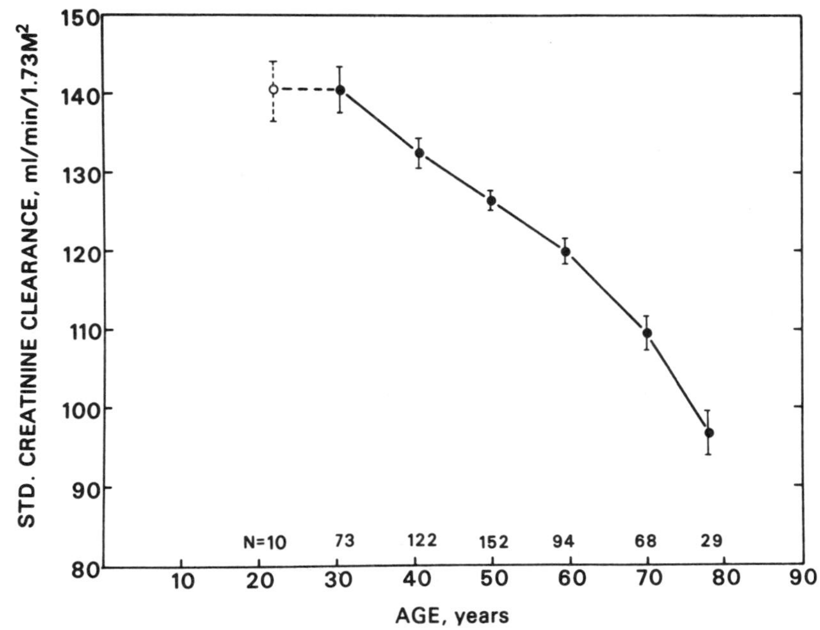

Fig. 28–3. Cross-sectional differences in standard creatinine clearance with age. The number of subjects in each age group is indicated above the abcissa. Values plotted indicate mean ± SEM. (From Rowe JW, Andres RA, Tobin J, et al: The effect of age on creatinine clearance in man: A cross-sectional and longitudinal study. J Gerontol 31:155, 1976. Reprinted by permission of The Gerontologist/The Journal of Gerontology.)

younger counterpart to show a false-positive urinary glucose test in post-prandial screening for diabetes.[36] Likewise, glucose will appear in the urine of a young diabetic patient at a lower blood glucose concentration than in an elderly diabetic.

Despite the highly significant decrease in glomerular filtration rate that occurs with age, there is no elevation in serum creatinine concentration (Table 28–1). Since muscle mass, from which creatinine is derived, falls with age at roughly the same rate as glomerular filtration rate, the rather drastic age-related loss of renal function is not reflected by an increase in the serum creatinine. Thus, serum creatinine will tend to underestimate the decline in glomerular filtration rate in the elderly. From the clinical standpoint, it is important to emphasize that the normal age-related decline in glomerular filtration rate will rarely cause an elevation of serum creatinine above 1.5 mg/dl. Serum creatinine values in excess of 1.5 mg/dl should suggest the presence of intrinsic renal disease or some other associated medical or surgical problem that has adversely affected renal function.

FLUID AND ELECTROLYTE BALANCE

Under normal circumstances, age has no effect on the plasma sodium or potassium concentrations, on the blood pH or on ability to maintain normal extracellular fluid volume. However, the adaptive reserve mechanisms responsible for maintaining constancy of the extracellular fluid volume and composition in response to stress are impaired in the elderly. Consequently acute illness in geriatric patients is often complicated by the development of derangements in fluid and electrolyte balance that delay recovery and prolong hospitalization.

Table 28–1. Cross-Sectional Age Differences in Creatinine Clearance, Serum Creatinine, and 24-Hour Creatinine Excretion

Age (years)	No. of Subjects	Creatinine Clearance (ml/min/1.73 m²)[a]	Serum Creatinine Concentration (mg/100 ml)	Creatinine Excretion (mg/24 hr)
17–24	10	140.2 ±3.7	0.808 ±0.026	1790 ±52
25–34	73	140.1 ±2.5	0.808 ±0.010	1862 ±31
35–44	122	132.6 ±1.8	0.813 ±0.009	1746 ±24
45–54	152	126.8 ±1.4	0.829 ±0.008	1689 ±18
55–64	94	119.9 ±1.7	0.837 ±0.012	1580 ±22
65–74	68	109.5 ±2.0	0.825 ±0.012	1409 ±25
75–84	29	96.9 ±2.9	0.843 ±0.019	1259 ±45

[a] Values indicate mean ± 1 SEM.

Extracellular Volume Depletion

The ability of the aged kidney to conserve sodium in response to sodium deprivation is impaired. When salt intake is acutely reduced (from 100 to 10 mEq/day sodium diet), elderly subjects are capable of maximally decreasing urinary sodium excretion, but their sodium conservation response is sluggish when compared with that of younger adults. In the studies of Epstein and Hollenberg,[37] the half-time for reduction of urinary sodium after salt restriction was 17.6 hours in the young compared with 30.9 hours in old subjects (Fig. 28–4). The cumulative sodium deficit before daily renal loss became equal to intake is thus greater in the elderly. Since old patients are more likely to experience confusion, loss of thirst, and disorientation when acutely ill, this "salt-losing" tendency may be aggravated by failure of adequate salt intake. This will lead to further depletion of the extracellular fluid volume and impaired cardiac, renal, and mental function. This vicious circle is too often continued after hospitalization when physicians, dreading pulmonary edema, are reluctant to administer substantial amounts of sodium-containing fluids intravenously to the acutely ill volume-depleted geriatric patients. This salt-losing tendency of the senescent kidney results from reduced nephron mass, with increased osmotic load per nephron and resultant mild osmotic diuresis, as well as to the important age-related alterations that occur in the renin–aldosterone system.

Basal renin, whether estimated by plasma renin concentration or renin activity, is diminished by 30 to 50 percent in elderly individuals in the face of normal levels of renin substrate. This basal difference between young and old is magnified by maneuvers designed to augment renin secretion such as salt restriction, diuretic administration, or upright posture.[38–40] The lowered renin levels are associated with a 30 to 50 percent reduction in plasma aldosterone concentration as well as a significant reduction in the secretion and metabolic clearance rate of aldosterone.[41] The aldosterone deficiency appears to be related to the coexisting renin deficiency, and not to intrinsic adrenal changes since both the plasma aldosterone and cortisol responses to adrenal corticotropic hormone (ACTH) stimulation are not impaired with advancing age.[39]

The impact of normal aging on plasma renin must be considered when assigning hyper-

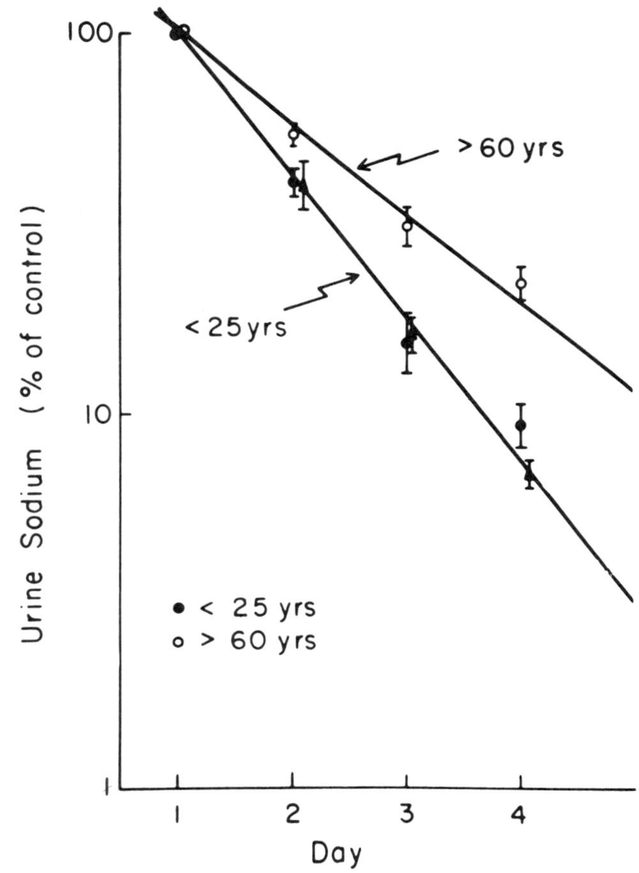

Fig. 28–4. Response of urinary sodium excretion to restriction of sodium intake in man. The mean half-time for eight subjects over 60 years of age was -30.9 ± 2.8 hours, exceeding the mean half-time of -17.6 ± 0.7 hours for subjects under 25 years of age ($p < 0.01$). (From Epstein M, Hollenberg NK: Age as a determinant of renal sodium concentration in normal man. J Lab Clin Med 87:411, 1976.)

tensive patients to specific pathophysiologic groups based on renin level. A geriatric hypertensive patient, or occasionally a normotensive patient with the normal elevation in systolic blood pressure seen with advancing age, may be labeled as having low renin hypertension when actually the renin level is not low but normal for the patient's age. This can lead to confusing or inappropriate conclusions in clinical studies, since the relationship between the normal reduction in renin with aging and the low renin levels seen in some young hypertensive patients is unknown.

The management of sodium depletion and its resultant deleterious effects on cardiac, central nervous system, renal, and intestinal function includes the prompt administration of sodium chloride. If the extracellular depletion is mild, oral administration of fluids and high-sodium-content foods over several days is often sufficient. If volume depletion is more marked, as reflected by decreased blood pressure or tissue turgor or orthostatic hypotension, intravenous administration of isotonic saline is indicated. The administration of hypotonic fluids, such as 5 percent glucose in water or half-normal 0.45 percent saline solutions, will lead to hyponatremia, while failing to correct the salt depletion, and may aggravate the patient's overall condition.

Extracellular Volume Expansion

Excessive sodium retention and volume overload is a commonly encountered problem in older patients. Primarily because of its lower glomerular filtration rate, the senescent kidney is less able to excrete an acute salt load than that of younger individuals. Geriatric patients, with or without preexisting myocardial disease, are thus at risk for expansion of the extracellular fluid volume when faced with the necessity to excrete an acute salt load (from inappropriate intravenous fluids, dietary indiscretion, or as commonly happens, after the administration of sodium-rich radiographic contrast agents such as those used in intravenous pyelography).

The mainstay of management of acute volume expansion with pulmonary congestion remains the intravenous administration of potent diuretics such as furosemide or ethacrynic acid. However, in the absence of preexisting cardiomegaly, administration of excess fluid generally does not result in the precipitation of acute congestive heart failure, but rather in modest weight gain and the appearance of mild peripheral edema. Over the course of several days, this excess salt is generally excreted. The administration of oral diuretics is indicated if the volume expansion aggravates preexisting heart failure or hypertension.

IMPACT OF NORMAL AGING ON WATER ECONOMY

Renal Concentrating Ability

Aging in man is associated with many and varied alterations in endocrine physiology, including changes in hormone synthesis, secretion and end-organ responsiveness. With regard to the hypothalamic–neurohypophyseal–renal axis and its role in regulating water balance, renal concentrating ability declines with age in man. As with any age-related physiologic alteration, it is important to discern whether this represents normal aging or is the consequence of a pathologic change or disease state which is more prevalent in the older subjects. In a large group of community-dwelling self-recruited men (age range 18 to 96 years), who were screened to exclude central nervous system or renal disease, Rowe et al.[42] found a significant age-related reduction in urine concentrating ability in response to water deprivation. These findings support the results of previous smaller studies with less strict patient selection and a more narrow age spectrum.[43,44]

The effect of age on renal response to exogenous vasopressin with age has been studied in two ways. Lindeman et al.[45] showed no age-related difference in response to submaximal Pitressin infusion. Shock and Miller,[46] in infusing vasopressin to achieve maximally effective levels, were able to show an age-related decline in urinary concentrating ability, suggesting that a non-vasopressin-dependent renal mechanism was responsible. One plausible explanation for the age differences seen in these studies is decreased function of the counter current multiplier system. The progressive decline in nephron population with age is associated with a decrease in cortical, but relative sparing of medullary, blood flow. This could result in a relative increase in medullary blood flow per nephron and "washout" of the medullary osmotic gradient which is necessary for the maintenance of the counter current multiplier system and normal urinary concentration.

Vasopressin Secretion

Conclusions regarding the function of the hypothalamoneurohypophyseal tract and water regulation in aging have largely been based on experimental studies conducted on Wistar rats. In these studies, a decrease in hypothalamic neurosecretory material has been seen with age,[47] and an age-related blunting of the antidiuretic response to hypertonic saline has been demonstrated.[48] The presence of a mild form of diabetes insipidus in the senescent Wistar rat,[49] however, makes extrapolation of these findings to human aging hazardous. In addition, opposite findings (increased neurosecretory granules with age) have been seen in other rat species.[50]

Morphologic studies in human subjects

show no evidence of age-related degenerative changes in the supraoptic and paraventricular nuclei, the sites of vasopressin production.[51] To the contrary, in a study of 64 human brains, Buttlar-Brentano found that these nuclei in the elderly are characterized by giant cells (8 to 10 times the size of those seen in youth), many of which are multinucleate and contain several (up to 6) nucleoli, as compared with the single nucleus and nucleolus characteristic of younger subjects.[51]

Helderman et al. described the influence of age on the plasma vasopressin response to infusions of hypertonic saline and ethanol.[52] Studies were performed on healthy young and old men screened extensively to exclude cardiac, renal, endocrine, hepatic, or central nervous system disease by appropriate examination and laboratory tests. All subjects were taking no medications, and subjects for the alcohol experiments refrained from all alcoholic beverages for at least 3 weeks prior to study.

In the hypertonic saline infusions, young (22 to 48 years) and old (52 to 66 years) subjects were administered a continuous intravenous infusion of hypertonic saline for 2 hours. Basal values of osmolality and vasopressin were the same in the two groups. As osmolality rose during the infusion from 290 to 306 mOsm/kg, both groups responded with increases in plasma vasopressin. In the young men, vasopressin increased to 2½ times basal values while the older subjects increased their vasopressin levels to 4½ times basal despite a similar osmotic stimulus (Fig. 28–5). The slope of the curve relating each individual's plasma vasopressin response to the plasma osmolality is a measure of his osmoreceptor sensitivity. When the individual slopes are plotted versus age, it can be seen that older subjects manifest enhanced osmoreceptor sensitivity

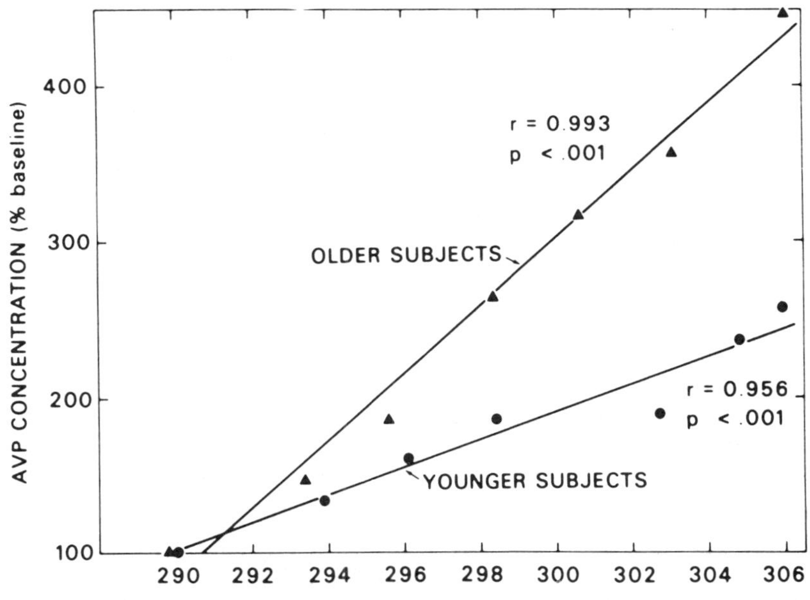

Fig. 28–5. Correlation between serum osmolality and arginine vasopressin (AVP) concentration in younger and older subjects during a 2-hour intravenous infusion of 3 percent NaCl at the rate of 0.1 ml/kg-min. The points represent mean values of osmolality and AVP at successive 20-minute intervals in each age group. (From Helderman JH, Vestal RE, Rowe JW, et al: The response of arginine vasopressin to intravenous ethanol and hypertonic saline in man: The impact of age. J Gerontol 33:39, 1978. Reprinted by permission of The Gerontologist/The Journal of Gerontology.)

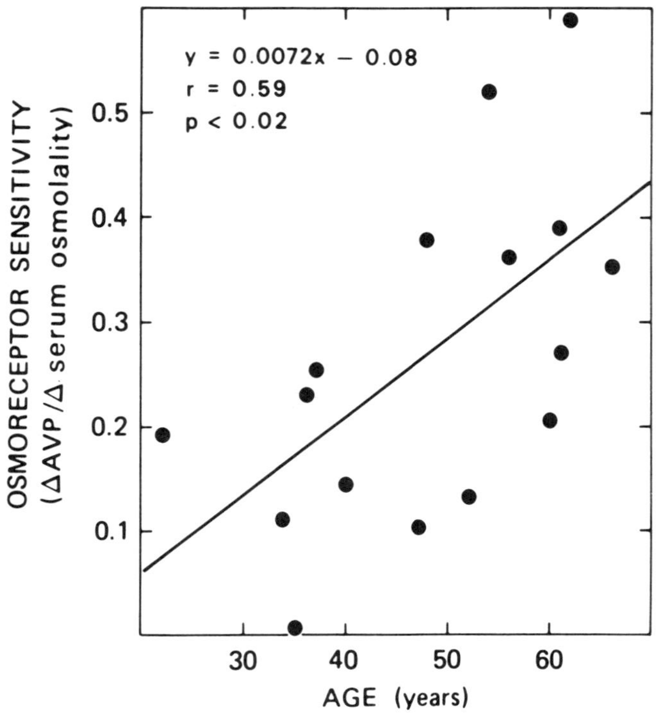

Fig. 28–6. Relationship between age and osmoreceptor sensitivity shown by the slope of plasma arginine vasopressin (AVP) concentration in pg/ml on serum osmolality in mOsm/kg. (From Helderman JH, Vestal RE, Rowe JW, et al: The response of arginine vasopressin to intravenous ethanol and hypertonic saline in man: The impact of age. J Gerontol 33:39, 1978. Reprinted by permission of The Gerontologist/ The Journal of Gerontology.)

with advancing age (Fig. 28–6) ($r = 0.52$; $p < 0.02$).

When alcohol was infused in young and old subjects, vasopressin levels fell promptly, and during the first 30 minutes the rate of fall was similar in both groups. During the second half hour of infusion, vasopressin continued to fall in the young subjects, returning to baseline after the infusion was discontinued. In contrast, in the older men, the suppressive effect of alcohol on arginine vasopressin secretion began to wave after 30 minutes and plasma vasopressin levels returned toward basal values. Thus, there was an escape from the inhibitory effects of ethanol on arginine vasopressin secretion in the older subjects. This may be explained, at least in part, by the increased osmoreceptor sensitivity of elderly subjects shown in the hypertonic saline experiments. Since during the ethanol infusion serum osmolality (corrected for the effect of ethanol on freezing point depression) rose in all subjects, the older group, more sensitive to this stimulus, may have increased arginine vasopressin secretion in spite of ethanol levels which inhibited arginine vasopressin secretion in the young subjects.

In order to investigate whether the increase in osmoreceptor sensitivity with age was a reflection of a generalized age-related increase in vasopressin release or is specific for osmolar stimuli, Rowe et al. evaluated the plasma vasopressin response to upright posture in 12 young (19 to 31 years) and 15 old (68 to 83 years) healthy subjects.[53] Plasma vasopressin rose at least 3.0 pg/ml in 11 of the 12 young subjects. In the old group, plasma vasopressin failed to rise in 7 of the 15 subjects ($p < 0.03$ compared with young group) despite the development of symptomatic hypotension in two of these individuals.

Of particular interest was the finding that plasma norepinephrine rose to similar levels after standing in the elderly and young subjects. The intact norepinephrine response in the elderly indicates that the afferent limb of baroreflex is intact and that the defect causing the age-related failure to release vasopressin upon standing is distal to the medullary vasomotor center. Since elderly subjects readily secrete vasopressin in response to an osmotic challenge, the defect must be proximal to the posterior pituitary and can be tentatively located at a site between the vasomotor center and the posterior pituitary.

The contrasting effects of osmolar and volume pressure stimuli on arginine vasopressin secretion in elderly subjects may be related to impaired baroreflex input to the supraoptic nucleus. Volume–pressure stimuli alter the sensitivity of the osmoreceptor in rats[54] and humans.[55] Volume depletion increases osmoreceptor sensitivity and volume expansion decreases it. Hypertonic saline infusion results in volume expansion and increases in blood pressure, dampening the response of vasopressin secretion to the osmolar stimulus. With an age-related defect in baroreflex-mediated input to the hypothalamus, the dampening effect would be removed, permitting an unrestrained response of the supraoptic nucleus to changes in osmolality.

Hypernatremia

The clinical impact of the aged kidney's inability to regulate salt balance properly under stress is compounded by similar abnormalities in water metabolism. The capacity of elderly individuals to conserve water and elaborate a concentrated urine under conditions of either water deprivation or infusion of anti-diuretic hormone is moderately impaired.[42,46] The cause of the decreased concentrating capacity of the aged kidney probably relates to the concomitant decline in glomerular filtration rate and an age-related decrease in renal response to antidiuretic hormone.

Although the decline in water-conserving capacity with age is not so severe as to have clinical significance under conditions of free access to water, it may become important when fluid intake is limited in the presence of exaggerated insensible losses such as with fever. Under such conditions elevations of the serum sodium concentrations to levels which impair mental function (>160 mEq/liter) is commonly seen in the geriatric age group. Both the salt- and water-losing tendencies of the senescent kidneys contribute to the common clinical presentation of acutely or subacutely ill elderly patients with hypertonic volume depletion.

In the initial management of the patient with severe hypertonic volume depletion, it is important to focus on volume repletion as potentially life saving and to treat such patients with rapid intravenous infusion of isotonic saline until cardiovascular stability is attained. In the presence of marked hypernatremia, these isotonic fluids are actually hypotonic relative to the patient's plasma and serum sodium will begin to fall as volume is expanded. Once blood pressure and intravascular volume are corrected, hypotonic fluids should be administered until the serum sodium is below 150 mEq/liter. Severe hypertonic dehydration in the elderly is uniformly associated with marked alterations in consciousness. Although the volume and the composition of the extracellular fluid may be normalized within 72 hours of admission, mental state alterations commonly persist for some time and slow recovery over 2 weeks is not infrequent. Thus persisting confusion despite normal electrolytes should not necessarily precipitate invasive clinical evaluation. Patience is often rewarded in such cases and the complications of lumbar punctures and invasive radiologic procedures avoided.

Hyponatremia

Perhaps the most serious and least well-recognized electrolyte disorder in geriatric patients is their tendency to develop water intoxication. One survey at a chronic disease facility found serum sodium values below 135 mEq/liter in more than 20 percent of the residents and values below 120 mEq/liter in 10 percent.[56] The clinical presentation of hyponatremia is nonspecific with depression, confusion, lethargy, anorexia, and weakness the most common findings. When hyponatremia is severe (serum sodium concentrations below 110 mEq/liter), seizures and stupor may be seen and central nervous system damage may be irreversible (see Chapter 21). It is not unusual for geriatric patients to become hyponatremic in the setting of any stress, including surgery, fever, or acute viral illness.

Clinical evaluation of the elderly hyponatremic patient usually reveals one of three general causes. One general cause is decreased renal capacity to excrete water as a consequence of acute or chronic reductions in renal blood flow (see Chapter 5). This is seen in patients with extracellular volume depletion, congestive heart failure, hypoalbuminemia associated with cirrhosis or nephrosis or drug-induced hypotension. In addition to the evidence on history and physical examination of the possible presence of any of these disorders, a laboratory examination often reveals prerenal azotemia with BUN elevations out of proportion to the elevations in serum creatinine. A second group of hyponatremic patients are those who develop water intoxication in association with the administration of diuretics (see Chapter 21). The most frequent offenders are the thiazides, which interfere with urinary diluting capacity and the more potent loop diuretics (furosemide and ethacrynic acid), which blunt both dilution and concentration (see Chapter 25). Hyponatremia may be rapid in onset and is generally easily corrected with discontinuation of the diuretic and short-term water restriction.

A third group of patients displays a constellation of findings consistent with oversecretion of antidiuretic hormone as a cause of the water retention (see Chapter 18). These include low serum sodium, evidence of normal renal function (low BUN), normal extracellular fluid volume as determined by clinical examination, and evidence of inappropriate renal water retention (urine osmolality greater than maximally dilute and in most cases more concentrated than serum). In addition, excess antidiuretic hormone secretion, because of the slight ECF expansion and subsequent reduction in aldosterone secretion and elevation of glomerular filtration rate, is associated with the presence of modest to large amounts of sodium in the urine. The relationship between the normal age-related changes in vasopressin physiology discussed above and the apparently high presence of excess antidiuretic hormone secretion in the elderly is not known.

Excess antidiuretic hormone secretion is commonly associated with pneumonia, tuberculosis, stroke, meningitis, subdural hematoma, a variety of pulmonary and central nervous system disorders, and other stresses such as surgery. Although all age groups may develop hyponatremia in these settings, the elderly seem particularly susceptible to this complication.[57] This may also hold true for drug-induced antidiuretic hormone excess. In one study, elderly patients accounted for most cases of hyponatremia developing from use of chlorpropamide.[58]

One must maintain a high degree of suspicion for hyponatremia in geriatric patients, particularly in view of the slow, insidious nature of the development of water intoxication and its nonspecific clinical presentation. Physicians caring for the elderly should be cautious when prescribing medications known to increase antidiuretic hormone secretion, such as chlorpropamide and barbiturates, as well as in the administration of hypotonic fluids in the setting of recent surgery or any acute illness.

Management of water intoxication is dictated by the level and rate of fall of the serum sodium, the clinical manifestations and the cause. In all cases, strict water restriction is appropriate. Medications possibly associated with water intoxication, such as diuretics or agents that increase the effect of antidiuretic hormone (Table 28–2), should be promptly withheld (see Chapter 24). In cases in which hyponatremia is associated with reduced renal

Table 28–2. Drugs Known to Impair Water Excretion and Induce Hyponatremia

Vasopressin	Carbamazepine
Oxytocin	Amitriptyline
Chlorpropamide	Thiothixene
Vincristine	Aspirin
Cyclophosphamide	Acetaminophen
Fluphenazine	Narcotics
Clofibrate	Barbiturates

blood flow, therapy should be aimed at maximizing renal function by either correction of congestive heart failure, volume repletion of patients with extracellular fluid depletion or restoration of blood pressure in hypotensive patients.

Severe hyponatremia (<110 mEq/liter) is associated with seizures or major central nervous system abnormalities and requires prompt correction. The most effective approach is the administration of hypertonic saline; 500 ml of 3 percent sodium chloride safely can be administered intravenously to most patients such that serum sodium is increased at a rate of about 2 mEq/liter per hour until a level of 125–130 mEq/liter is reached. The details and methods of calculation are described in Chapter 21. This will be sufficient to offset the immediate danger while other therapeutic modalities are initiated.

In cases of chronic excess antidiuretic hormone secretion, fluid restriction alone will generally result in a slow return of plasma osmolality toward normal levels. In cases in which fluid restriction is impractical, the water retaining effects of antidiuretic hormone can be inhibited by oral administration of dimethylchlortetracycline in doses of 300 mg bid to tid. This agent induces a state of partial nephrogenic diabetes insipidus and predictably results in correction of hyponatremia over the course of several days. Since it is a potential nephrotoxic agent, the serum creatinine and BUN levels should be followed closely.

POTASSIUM BALANCE

Hyperkalemia

The age-related decreases in renin and aldosterone may contribute to the elderly patient's increased risk of developing hyperkalemia in a variety of clinical settings. Aldosterone represents one of the major protective mechanisms in the prevention of hyperkalemia during periods of potassium challenge. Since tubular mass decreases in old patients, they may be prone to the development of elevated plasma potassium levels, especially in the presence of gastrointestinal bleeding or when given potassium salts intravenously. This tendency toward hyperkalemia is further aggravated in any clinical setting associated with acidosis, since the senescent kidney is sluggish in its response to acid loading, resulting in prolonged depression of blood pH, which can result in a shift of potassium from the intracellular to extracellular fluid compartment. Similarly, diuretics such as spironolactone or triamterene, which impair renal potassium excretion, should be administered with caution to the elderly, and concomitant administration of these agents and potassium should be avoided.

The initial management of hyperkalemia includes discontinuation of any excessive sources of potassium in diet, discontinuation of potassium-sparing diuretics, and the prompt maximization of renal function in patients with volume depletion or heart failure. Severe hyperkalemia, which is reflected by electrocardiographic abnormalities including symmetrically peaked T waves and widened QRS complexes, requires prompt treatment (see Chapter 23) with intravenous calcium salts (calcium chloride or calcium gluconate) which directly antagonize the effect of hyperkalemia on the myocardium and often normalizes the ECG. Also indicated are sodium bicarbonate, glucose and insulin. Such emergency treatment is of only temporary benefit in controlling serum potassium and has no effect on total body potassium. Therefore, simultaneous with these emergency efforts should be the initiation of efforts designed to remove potassium from the body. These include the oral or rectal administration of sodium–potassium exchange resins (Kayexelate), and intravenous diuretic (furosemide or ethacrynic acid) administration, or dialysis.

Hypokalemia

While most generally fit ambulatory elders do not require potassium supplementation when administered diuretics, hypokalemia is a common accompaniment of diuretic therapy in residents of long-term care facilities. This may be due to the more severe hypertension and/or congestive heart failure in such patients, thus leading to the requirement of larger doses of diuretics. Poor dietary potassium intake may also be a contributing factor. Symptoms of hypokalemia, especially muscle weakness, often go unrecognized in institutionalized patients in whom chronic weakness, anorexia and lethargy may be associated with other associated medical illnesses. Potassium administration should be undertaken cautiously in hypochloremic elderly patients, particularly those with evidence of impaired renal function. The serum potassium concentration should be measured at regular intervals, especially in patients on digitalis.

Acid–Base Balance

The normal senescent kidney has a reduced capacity to excrete an acid load, thus aggravating the severity and rapidity of onset of metabolic acidosis from any cause.[59] The etiology spectrum and management of metabolic acidosis is not influenced by age and is discussed in Chapter 7.

Metabolic alkalosis is common in the elderly, especially in acutely ill patients with marked volume depletion or in the setting of chronic diuretic administration. Treatment is the same as for younger adults and generally includes administration of sodium chloride infusions and oral potassium chloride as indicated (see Chapters 7 and 25).

REFERENCES

1. Roessie R, Roulet F: Mass and Zahl in der Pathologie. Berlin J Spungen, 1932
2. Tauchi H, Tsuboi K, Okutomi J: Age changes in the human kidney of the different races. Gerontolica 17:87, 1971
3. Moore RA: Total number of glomeruli in the normal human kidney. Anat Rec 48:153, 1931
4. Dunnill MS, Halley W: Some observations on the quantitative anatomy of the kidney. J Pathol Bacteriol 110:113, 1973
5. McLachan MSF, Guthrie JC, Anderson CK, et al: Vascular and glomerular changes in the aging kidney. J Pathol 121:65, 1977
6. Sworn MJ, Fox M: Donor kidney selection for transplantation. Br J Urol 44:377, 1972
7. Kaplan C, Pasternack B, Shah H, et al: Age-related incidence of sclerotic glomeruli in human kidneys. Am J Pathol 80:227, 1975
8. Sorenson F: Quantitative studies of the renal corpuscles. Acta Pathol Microbiol Scand 85:356, 1977
9. Artursen G, Groth T, Grotte G: Human glomerular membrane porosity and filtration pressure: Dextran clearance data analyzed by theoretical models. Clin Sci 40:137, 1971
10. Morgensen CE: The glomerular permeability determined by dextran clearance using sephadex gel filtration. Scand J Clin Lab Invest 21:77, 1968
11. Darmady EM, Offer J, Woodhouse MS: The parameters of the aging kidney. J Pathol 109:195, 1973
12. Scott EB: Modification of the basal architecture of renal tubule cells in aged rats. Proc Soc Exp Biol Med 117:586, 1964
13. Oliver JR: Urinary system. p. 257. In Cowdry EV (ed): Problems of Aging: Biological and Medical Aspects. Williams & Wilkins, Baltimore, 1939
14. McLachlan MSF: The aging kidney. Lancet 2:143, 1978

15. Baert L, Steg A: Is the diverticulum of the distal and collecting tubules a preliminary stage of the simple cyst in the adult? J Urol 118:707, 1977
16. Williams RN, Harrison TR: A study of the renal arteries in relation to age and to hypertension. Am Heart J 14:645, 1937
17. Yamaguchi T, Omae T, Katsuki S: Quantitative determination of renal vascular changes related to age and hypertension. Jpn Heart J 10:248, 1969
18. Moritz AR, Oldt MR: Arteriolar sclerosis in hypertensive and non-hypertensive individuals. Am J Pathol 13:679, 1973
19. Davidson AT, Talner LB, Downs WM: A study of the radiographic appearance of the kidney in an aging normotensive population. Radiology 92:975, 1969
20. Griffiths GJ, Cartwright GO, McLachlan MSF: Loss of renal tissue in the elderly. Clin Radiol 26:249, 1975
21. Ljungqvist A, Lagergren C: Normal intrarenal arterial pattern in adult and aging human kidney. J Anat 96:285, 1962
22. Takazakura E, Sawabu N, Handu A, et al: Intrarenal vascular changes with age and disease. Kidney Int 2:224, 1972
23. Wesson LG: Physiology of the Human Kidney. Grune & Stratton, New York, 1969
24. Brandfonbrener M, Landsdowne M, Shock NW: Changes in cardiac output with age. Circulation 12:557, 1955
25. Lammerant J, Veall N, DeVisscher M: Observations on cardiac output and "pulmonary blood volume" in normal man by internal recording of the intracardiac flows of 123I labelled albumin. Nucl Med 1:353, 1961
26. Strandell T: Circulatory studies on healthy old men. Acta Med Scand 175 (Suppl): 414, 1964
27. Manyasi DE, Patterson C, Johnson DE, et al: An echocardiographic study of resting left ventricular function in healthy elderly subjects. J Clin Exp Gerontol (in press)
28. Hollenberg NK, Adams DF, Solomon HS, et al: Senescence and the renal vasculature in normal man. Circ Res 34:309, 1974
29. Friedman SA, Raizner AE, Rosen H, et al: Functional defects in the aging kidney. Ann Intern Med 76:41, 1972
30. McDonald RK, Solomon DH, Shock NW: Aging as a factor in the renal hemodynamic changes induced by a standardized pyrogen. J Clin Invest 30:457, 1951
31. Rowe JW, Andres RA, Tobin J, et al: The effect of age on creatinine clearance in man: A cross sectional and longitudinal study. J Gerontol 31:155, 1976
32. Rowe JW, Andres RA, Tobin JD, et al: Age-adjusted normal standards for creatinine clearance in man. Ann Intern Med 84:567, 1976
33. Watkin DM, Shock NW: Agewise standard value for C_{IN}, CpAH and TmpAH in adult males. J Clin Invest 34:969, 1955
34. Davies DF, Shock NW: Age changes in glomerular filtration rate, effective renal plasma flow and tubular excretory capacity in adult males. J Clin Invest 29:496, 1950
35. Miller JH, McDonald RK, Shock NW: Age changes in the maximal rate of renal tubular reabsorption of glucose. J Gerontol 7:196, 1952
36. Butterfield WJ, Keen H, Whechelow MJ: Renal glucose threshold variations with age. Br Med J 4:505, 1967
37. Epstein M, Hollenberg NK: Age as a determinant of renal sodium conservation in normal man. J Lab Clin Med 87:411, 1976
38. Samblin MP, Crane MG, Genest J: Essential hypertension, newer concepts about mechanisms. Ann Intern Med 79:411, 1973
39. Weidmann P, DeMyttenare-Burzstein S, Maxwell M, et al: Effect of aging on plasma serum and aldosterone in normal man. Kidney Int 8:325, 1975
40. Crane MG, Harris JJ: Effect of aging on renon activity and aldosterone excretion. J Lab Clin Med 87:947, 1976
41. Flood C, Gherondache C, Picus G, et al: The metabolism and secretion of aldosterone in elderly subjects. J Clin Invest 46:960, 1967
42. Rowe JW, Shock NW, DeFronzo R: The influence of age on urine concentrating ability in man. Nephron 17:279, 1976
43. Dontas AS, Marketos S, Papanayiouton P: Mechanisms of renal tubular defects in old age. Postgrad Med J 48:295, 1972
44. Lindeman RD, VanBuren HC, Raisz LG: Osmolar renal concentrating ability in young men and hospitalized patients without renal disease. N Engl J Med 262:1396, 1960
45. Lindeman RD, Lee TD, Yienjst MJ, et al: Influence of age, renal disease, hypertension,

diuretics and calcium on the anti-diuretic response to suboptimal infusion of vasopressin. J Lab Clin Med 68:206, 1966
46. Miller JH, Shock NW: Age differences in the renal tubular response to antidiuretic hormone. J Gerontol 8:446, 1953
47. Dunihue FW: Reduced juxtaglomerular cell granularity, pituitary secretory material and width of the zone glomerulosa in aging rats. Endocrinology 77:948, 1965
48. Friedman SM, Hinke JAM, Friedman CL: Neurohypophyseal responsiveness in the normal and senescent rat. J Gerontol 11:288, 1956
49. Friedman SM, Friedman CL, Nakashima M: Effect of pitressin on old-age changes of salt and water metabolism in the rat. Am J Physiol 199(1):35, 1960
50. Frolkis VV, Bezinkov W, Duplinko YK, et al: The hypothalamus in aging. Exp Gerontol 7:169, 1972
51. Buttlar-Brentano, Von L: Zur lebensgesuchte des nucleus basalis tuberomamillaris, supraopticus und paraventricularis unter nomden und pathogenes bedingungen. J Hurforsch 1:337, 1954
52. Helderman JH, Vestal RE, Rowe JW, et al: The response of arginine vasopressin to intravenous ethanol and hypertonic saline in man: The impact of age. J Gerontol 33:39, 1978
53. Rowe JW, Kilgore A, Robertson GL: Age related failure in vasopressin response to volume-pressure stimuli in man. Kidney Int 14:660, 1978
54. Dunn FJ, Brennan TJ, Nelson AE, et al: The role of blood osmolality and blood volume in regulating plasma vasopressin in man. J Clin Invest 52:3212, 1973
55. Robertson GL, Athar S: The interaction of blood osmolality and blood volume in regulating plasma vasopressin in man. J Clin Endocrinol Metab 42:613, 1976
56. Kleinfeld M, et al: Hyponatremia as observed in a chronic disease facility. J Am Geriatr Soc 27:156, 1979
57. Deutsch S, Goldberg M, Dripps RD: Postoperative hyponatremia with the inappropriate release of antidiuretic hormone. Anesthesiology 27:250, 1966
58. Weissman PN, Shenkman L, Gregerman RI: Chlorpropamide hyponatremia. N Engl J Med 284:65, 1971
59. Adler S, Lindeman RD, Yiengst MJ, et al: Effect of acute acid loading on urinary acid excretion by the aging human kidney. J Lab Clin Med 72:278, 1968

Index

The letter t following a page number indicates tabular material

Abdominal pain, in electrolyte disorders, 1130
Absorptagogues, intestinal, 836
Absorption, intestinal, 827
  cAMP affecting, 835
  of calcium, 512
    malabsorption, 544
  calcium affecting, 835
  in colon, 834
  cGMP affecting, 835
  in ileum, 832–833
  in jejunum, 830–832
  of magnesium, 576–579
  malabsorption. *See* Malabsorption
  neurohumoral agents affecting, 836
  of phosphate, 628, 633–635
Acetaldehyde levels, in paraldehyde acidosis, 317
Acetate
  and dialysis hypotension, 786–787
  in hemodialysis, 794–797
    and hypoxemia, 793
  metabolism of, 1198
  in peritoneal dialysis, 798
  pK_A value for, 227t
Acetazolamide, 1160–1162
  and bicarbonate reabsorption, 232
  bicarbonaturia from, 346
  and calcium excretion, 515
  in diuretic-induced alkalosis, 350
  in hyperkalemic periodic paralysis, 449
  hypomagnesemia from, 605
  in mountain sickness, 398
  in salicylate intoxication, 312
Acetoacetate
  coma from, 1017
  decarboxylation of, 1198
  plasma levels in diabetic ketoacidosis, 942t
Acetylcholine
  and magnesium excretion, 590
  receptors on gastric parietal cells, 830
  release in alkalosis, 343
Acetylsalicylic acid. *See* Salicylates
Acid(s), 221–222
  in buffering system, 224–227
  dissociation constant for, and pK_A, 222
  gastric secretion of, 336–337, 352, 830
    in electrolyte disorders, 1130–1131
  normal pK_A values for, 227
  overproduction or administration of, acidosis from, 282–283
  titratable, 232–233, 324
    in peritoneal dialysate, 798
    in respiratory acidosis, 241–242
  urinary excretion of, 231–235
    and daily acid production, 338–339
    in diuretic-induced alkalosis, 346–348
    failure of, and metabolic acidosis, 283–284
    in hypercapnia, 392
    in hypoaldosteronism, 324
    net acid excretion, 233, 323–324, 1201
      in distal renal tubular acidosis, 326
    in pregnancy, 1064–1065
    regulation of, 234
Acid-base balance, 230–257
  in aging, 1244
  and anion gap, 277–280
  in brain and cerebrospinal fluid, 971–972
  buffering in, 224–227, 270–277
    cellular, 236–240
  dialysis affecting
    continuous, 813–814
    hemodialysis, 791–797
    peritoneal, 798–800
  disorders of. *See also* Acidosis; Alkalosis
    in diabetic coma, 941–948
    in hypercalcemia, 530
    hypomagnesemia in, 602
    magnesium excretion in, 595
    mixed disturbances, 406–408
      anion gap in, 279–280
      in diarrhea, 320, 321
      in lung disease, 1161
    neurologic disorders in, 1095–1097
    in pulmonary medicine, 385–409
  and effects of pH in body, 252–257. *See also* pH
  hormones affecting, 244–245
  intracellular, 245–252
  and potassium metabolism, 419
  renal mechanisms in, 231–235, 322–324
  respiratory system in, 240–244
  in total parenteral nutrition, 1195–1201
Acidemia, hyperkalemia in, 421–424, 456, 458–459
Acidifying agents, 355t
Acidity
  definition of, 269
  of solutions, 222–224
Acidosis
  hyperchloremic, 318–335
    in diabetes mellitus, 945
    in diarrhea, 842
    from carbonic anhydrase inhibitors, 1161
    in hypercalcemia, 530
    in renal tubular acidosis, 1181
  hyperkalemic, 422–423, 924–925
  hypokalemic/hyperchloremic, 318–335

Acidosis (*Cont.*)
metabolic, 281–335
ACTH secretion in, 244–245
in aging, 1244
aldosterone levels in, 244, 293
alkalosis with
metabolic, 280, 282
respiratory, 286, 399, 406–408
anion gap in
in chronic renal failure, 714, 790
increased, 278, 296–317
normal, 317–335
anorexia in, 1128
arrhythmias in, 254, 295–296, 1126t, 1127
arterial effects of, 296
bicarbonate loss in, 282
bicarbonate therapy in, 947–948
dangers of, 948
in biliary and pancreatic drainage procedures, 321
bone buffering as defense mechanism in, 237–238
calcium excretion in, 238, 239
calcium metabolism in, 290–293
cardiovascular system in, 254–255, 295–296, 1113–1114
catecholamine secretion in, 293
causes of, 296–335
cellular buffering in, 237–240
coma in, 1096
in diabetic ketoacidosis, 945–948, 956, 1018
in diarrhea, 318–321
and effects of digitalis, 1128
electrolyte metabolism in, 288–293
in ethylene glycol poisoning, 313–314
and failure of renal acid excretion, 283–284
in fasting, 293
from potassium-sparing diuretics, 1172–1173
gastrointestinal effects of, 295
hyperventilation in, 1107
in hypoaldosteronism, fludrocortisone affecting, 919
hypomagnesemia in, 608
hypophosphatemia in, 639
increased acid burden in, 282–283
and insulin binding to adipocytes, 244, 256
insulin resistance in, 1134
lactic acidosis, 301–309. *See also* Lactic acidosis
lethargy and stupor in, 1096
and magnesium transport in kidney, 585, 595
manifestations of, 288–296
metabolism in, 253–254, 293
in methanol poisoning, 314–316
myocardial performance in, 254, 295, 1117–1118
neurologic disorders in, 1026
in nonketotic coma, 952
overcompensated, 399
oxygen-hemoglobin affinity in, 1133
in paraldehyde toxicity, 316–317
pathophysiology of, 281–284
potassium metabolism in, 288–290, 417
pulmonary effects of, 293–295
pulmonary vascular resistance in, 254, 294
renal effects of, 295
in renal failure, acute, 296–297, 676–678
respiratory acidosis with, 406
respiratory compensation in, 284–288, 395–396
pathophysiology of, 286–288
in salicylate intoxication, 309–313
in total parenteral nutrition, 1201–1202
in ureterosigmoidostomy patients, 321–322
vasoconstriction in, venous, 296
vasodilatation in, 296
renal tubular, 322–335
clinical features of, 332–333
combined proximal/distal disease, 333
contrasting features of, 332t
diagnostic studies in, 333–335
distal, 326–331
hyperkalemic, 444–446
incomplete, 331
diuretics in, 1164, 1181
hypokalemia in, 470
hypophosphatemia in, 639, 645
proximal, bicarbonate-wasting, 324–326
in pseudohypoaldosteronism, 922
reduced buffer excretion in, 331–332
treatment of, 335
respiratory, 240–242
acute, treatment of, 400
alkalosis with, metabolic, 406–408, 1161
arrhythmias in, 1127
bicarbonate levels in, 241–242, 396
cardiovascular system in, 1113
causes of, 400t
cerebrospinal fluid in, 972
chronic, treatment of, 402
clinical features of, 400–405
cognitive function in, 1111
coma in, 1095
electrocardiography in, 1123
hallucinations in, 1112
headache in, 1104
hypomagnesemia in, 602
in hypothyroidism, 402
in idiopathic alveolar hypoventilation, 402
lethargy and stupor in, 1095
in lung disease, 405
magnesium excretion in, 595
metabolic acidosis with, 406–408
myocardial performance in, 1117–1118
myoclonus in, 1098
neurologic disorders in, 1024–1025

in neuromuscular disorders, 403–404
overcompensated, 405
in oxygen therapy, 402–403
and posthypercapnic alkalosis, 351, 405
psychiatric manifestations of, 1109
renin secretion in, 245
in total parenteral nutrition, 1202
uremic, 297–301, 677–678, 713–716, 790
bone disease with, 791
Acromegaly
calcium excretion in, 515
hypercalcemia in, 520
hyperphosphatemia in, 651
magnesium absorption in, 579
ACTH
and renal hypertrophy, compensatory, 697
secretion in acidosis, 244–245
as therapy in Addison's disease, 431
Addison's disease, 909–910
clinical and laboratory features of, 430t
etiology of, 429t
hypercalcemia in, 521
hyperkalemia in, 424–425, 429–432
hyponatremia in, 211, 878–880
urinary dilution in, 155–156
Adenohypophyseal disease
hypokalemia in, 883
hyponatremia in, 877–883
Adenoma, parathyroid, 518
Adenomatosis, multiple endocrine, 519
Adenosine monophosphate, cyclic. *See* cAMP
Adenosine triphosphate. *See* ATP
Adipocytes, insulin binding to, in acidosis, 244, 256
Adipsia, 126, 127, 131
in diabetes insipidus, 858
and hypernatremia, 858
Adrenal glands
enzyme defects
mineralocorticoid deficiency in, 910–914
mineralocorticoid excess in, 900–901
hyperplasia, congenital, 910–914
insufficiency, 909–910. *See also* Addison's disease
mineralocorticoid hormones, 893–925. *See also* Mineralocorticoid hormones
β-Adrenergic agents
polydipsia from, 138
and potassium metabolism, 418
β-Adrenergic blockers, hyperkalemia from, 440, 447–448
Adrenergic receptors, and renal sodium excretion, 61
Age
and acid-base disorders from salicylates, 310
and renal function, 1231–1244. *See also* Kidney, aging affecting
and renal hypertrophy, compensatory, 697
and urinary acid excretion, 235
Albright's hereditary osteodystrophy, 541, 550, 551
Albumin
binding to magnesium, 575
calcium binding to, 511
in dialysate water, 811t
hypoalbuminemia
in cirrhosis, 93–94
hypocalcemia from, 540
in nephrotic syndrome, 99–100
solutions used in preeclampsia, 1073
Alcohol
interaction with paraldehyde, 317
lactic acidosis from, 307
and magnesium excretion, 591–592
and osmolality of extracellular fluid, 187
therapy with
in ethylene glycol poisoning, 313, 314
in methanol poisoning, 316
and urinary concentration, 164
and vasopressin levels in aging, 1239–1240
and water metabolism, 1153
withdrawal from
hypomagnesemia in, 602
seizures in, 1092
Alcohol dehydrogenase inhibitors
in ethylene glycol poisoning, 314
in methanol poisoning, 316
Alcoholism
ataxia in, 1107
hallucinations in, 1111
hypocalcemia in, 543
hypomagnesemia in, 592, 600, 606–607
hyponatremia in, 1002–1003
phosphate depletion in, 640, 1015
Aldosterone
and abnormal salt and water processing in cirrhosis, 97–98
antagonists of, 1172–1173, 1180–1181
deficiency of, 906–909. *See also* Hypoaldosteronism
hyperaldosteronism. *See* Aldosteronism
and magnesium absorption, 579
metabolism in uremia, 426–428
and potassium metabolism, 418–419
and potassium secretion, 416
pseudoaldosteronism, 366–367, 479
pseudohypoaldosteronism, 444
secretion of
in acidosis, 244, 293
in diabetes mellitus, 440
evaluation of, 452
in 21-hydroxylase deficiency, 912–913
in pregnancy, 1047–1051
and sodium excretion in nephrotic syndrome, 104
and sodium reabsorption, 26, 49–52
in uremia, 704
and sodium retention in heart failure, 86–88
and urinary acid secretion, 235
Aldosteronism
and alkalosis from loss of gastric juice, 844
in Bartter's syndrome, 360, 904
clinical features and diagnosis of, 366

Aldosteronism (*Cont.*)
and hypertension with hypokalemia and decreased plasma renin, 477
hypomagnesemia in, 608–609
magnesium absorption in, 579
magnesium excretion in, 594
pathogenesis of, 363–366
polydipsia in, 137
potassium-sparing diuretics in, 1172
primary, 363–366, 900
pseudohyperaldosteronism, 366–367, 479
and renal alkalosis, 338
secondary, 366, 902–903
treatment of, 366
Alka-Seltzer, alkali in, 359
Alkalemia, hypokalemia with, 461–462, 481
Alkali therapy. *See also* Bicarbonate, therapy with
alkalosis from, 357–359
in chronic renal failure, 301, 718
hypercalcemia from, 522
in salicylate intoxication, 312
Alkaline phosphatase levels, in chronic renal failure, 749–750
Alkalinity, definition of, 270
Alkalinization
mechanisms in, 230
of urine, carbonic anhydrase inhibitors in, 1160
Alkalosis
metabolic, 335–367
acidosis with
metabolic, 282
respiratory, 406–408, 1161
in aging, 1244
in aldosteronism, 363
anion gap in, 279, 344
arrhythmias in, 254, 1126t
in Bartter's syndrome, 359–362
calcium metabolism in, 344
in calcium metabolism disorders, 363
carbonic anhydrase inhibitors in, 1160–1161
cardiovascular effects of, 342–343, 1114
causes of, 345–367
chloriduric
hypertensive, 363–367
normotensive, 359–363
clinical features of, 342–345
contraction, 335–336
in diarrhea, 336, 842–843
chloride diarrhea, congenital, 356–357
diuretic-induced, 346–350, 1164
acid excretion in, 346–348
clinical features and diagnosis of, 348–350
pathogenesis of, 346–348
treatment of, 350
and effects of digitalis, 1128
from alkali administration, 336, 357–359
from antacids, 358–359
from antibiotics, 350
from bicarbonate added to extracellular fluid, 336–338
from loss of chloride-rich fluid, 335–336
from sodium sulfate, 350
gastric, 336–337, 351–356
clinical features and diagnosis of, 354
correctional phase in, 354
developmental phase in, 353
pathogenesis of, 351–354
steady-state phase in, 353–354
treatment of, 354–356
in gastric juice losses, 844
generation of, 335–338
in 11β-hydroxylase deficiency, 366
in 17α-hydroxylase deficiency, 366
in hypercalcemia, 530
in hyperreninism, 366
hypokalemia in, 340, 341, 344, 362, 461–462, 481
hypomagnesemia in, 602
hypophosphatemia in, 344–345
hypoventilation in, 1107
intestinal, 356–357
ketonuria in, 244
lethargy and stupor in, 1096
magnesium excretion in, 585, 595
maintenance of, 338–342
metabolic effects of, 253–254, 344–345
neurologic disorders in, 1026–1027
neuromuscular effects of, 343–344
oxygen-hemoglobin affinity in, 1133
in peritoneal dialysis, 798–799
posthypercapnic, 350–351, 405
treatment of, 351
potassium secretion in, 417
in pseudohyperaldosteronism, 901–902
in refeeding, 362–363
renal, 337–338, 346–351, 365
evolution of, 365
respiratory alkalosis with, 406–408
respiratory compensation in, 342, 395–396
saline-responsive, 345t, 346–359
saline-unresponsive, 345t, 359–367
seizures in, 1088–1089
tetany in, 1106
in total parenteral nutrition, 1202
in villous adenomas of intestines, 357
over-shoot, 280
respiratory, 242, 393–395
acidosis with, metabolic, 286, 406–408
overcompensated, 399
anion gap in, 279
bicarbonate levels in, 396
cardiovascular system in, 1113
causes of, 397t
cerebrospinal fluid in, 971–972
in cirrhosis, 399
clinical features of, 396–400
cognitive function in, 1111
confusion in, 1110
in dialysis
hemodialysis, 792–793
peritoneal, 798

drug-induced, 398–399, 402, 403
and diarrheal acidosis, 320
in fever, 399
hallucinations in, 1112
hypokalemia in, 461–462
hypophosphatemia in, 637
in hypoxemia, 398
in hypoxia, 397
ketonuria in, 244
lethargy and stupor in, 1096
magnesium levels in, 602
metabolic alkalosis with, 406–408
in mountain sickness, 398
neurologic disorders in, 1025–1026
in pregnancy, 399
in pulmonary edema, 397, 398
reflexes in, 1104
seizures in, 1088
in septic shock, 399
tetany in, 1106
in total parenteral nutrition, 1202
treatment of, 397–400
in ventilator mismanagement, 399–400
Aluminum
accumulation of
and bone disease in renal failure, 729, 730, 755
in osteomalacia, 737–740, 755
management of, 760
in dialysate
dementia from, 806–807, 989–991
and osteomalacia, 807–808
Aluminum hydroxide
in hyperphosphatemia, 754–755
and intestinal absorption of aluminum, 805
and Kayexalate, alkalosis from, 358
Alveolar-capillary diffusion block, 386–387
Amiloride, 1172–1173
acidifying effect of, 346
and calcium excretion, 616
inhibiting potassium secretion, 446, 459, 484
and kallikrein activity, 895
and magnesium excretion, 590–591, 605
in pseudohyperaldosteronism, 902
Amino acids
in brain, 970
in hypernatremia, 1012
oxidation of, 1196–1198
in total parenteral nutrition, 1192–1193
Aminoaciduria, in hypercalcemia, 531
γ-Aminobutyric acid metabolism, in nonketotic coma, 1021
Aminoglycosides
hypomagnesemia from, 607
and magnesium excretion, 592
3-Amino-1-hydroxypropane-1,1-diphosphonate, in hypercalcemia, 537
Amitriptyline, and inappropriate secretion of antidiuretic hormone, 1151
Ammonia
as base combined with hydrogen ion, 221, 233
fecal excretion in diarrhea, 842
production in chronic renal failure, 299–301
urinary excretion of
in chronic renal failure, 715
in hypercalcemia, 530
in hypoaldosteronism, fludrocortisone affecting, 916–917, 919–920
in renal tubular acidosis, 332
Ammonium chloride, as acidifying agent, 355t
cAMP
excretion in pseudohypoparathyroidism, 541
generation inhibition in potassium deficiency, 166
and hydroosmotic response to antidiuretic hormone, 162
and intestinal electrolyte transport, 835
nephrogenous, in hypercalcemia, 534
and phosphaturic effect of parathyroid hormone, 630
production by bone, in acidosis, 239
Amphoteric behavior of substances, 222
Amphotericin B
hypokalemia from, 475
and urinary acidification, 328, 330
and urinary concentration, 164
Ampicillin
alkalosis from, 350
hypokalemia from, 475
Androgens
hypophosphatemia from, 637
and renal hypertrophy, compensatory, 697
Anemia, hemolytic
in electrolyte disorders, 1131
from copper in dialysate, 810
Angiotensin I converting enzyme inhibitor. *See* Captopril
Angiotensin II
and abnormal salt and water processing in cirrhosis, 97–98
as dipsogenic agent, 136, 137
interaction with prostaglandins, 88
plasma levels of
in diabetes insipidus, 133
in polydipsia, 133, 136, 137
in preeclampsia, 1069
in pregnancy, 1054–1055
and sodium excretion, 26, 55–56
in nephrotic syndrome, 104
and sodium retention in heart failure, 86–88
and thirst regulation, 122
Anion gap, 277–280
in ethylene glycol poisoning, 313
in lactic acidosis, 305
in metabolic acidosis
in chronic renal failure, 714, 790
increased, 278, 296–317
normal, 317–335
in metabolic alkalosis, 279, 344
in methanol poisoning, 315
in paraldehyde toxicity, 317
in respiratory alkalosis, 279
in salicylate intoxication, 310
Anorexia, 1128
Anoxemia and encephalopathy, diabetes insipidus with, 857

Antacids
  alkalosis from, 358–359
  hypophosphatemia from, 638
Antibiotics
  alkalosis from, 350
  aminoglycoside
    hypomagnesemia from, 607
    and magnesium excretion, 592
  anion gap increase from, 278–279
Antibodies to glomerular basement membrane, 691
Anticonvulsant therapy, hypocalcemia from, 544
Antidepressants, tricyclic, and inappropriate secretion of antidiuretic hormone, 1151
Antidiuretic hormone, 1173–1174
  antagonists of, 1175
    complications from, 1176
  cellular action of, 162
    in hypercalcemia, 167
  chlorpropamide affecting, 1145–1147
  deficiency of, and central diabetes insipidus, 160, 204
  dipsogenic effect of, 122
  hydroosmotic response to
    cAMP affecting, 162
    lithium affecting, 163
    in potassium depletion, 165–166
  and hypertonic urine production, 152–153
  inappropriate secretion of, 13, 14, 872–877, 993
    chlorpropamide-induced, 1148
    clinical features and pathophysiology of, 872–874
    cyclophosphamide-induced, 1168
    demeclocycline in, 164, 1168, 1176
    diagnosis of, 874–875
      criteria for, 210t
    drug-induced, 874
    etiology of, 157t, 873–874
    from tricyclic antidepressants, 1151
    furosemide in, 1168
    glipizide-induced, 1149
    hyponatremia in, 210–211, 873, 874–875, 995
    in hypothyroidism, 882
    lithium therapy in, 1168, 1175–1176
    in lung diseases, 873
    in neurologic disorders, 873–874
    and osmolality of plasma and urine, 872, 875
    polydipsia in, 135–136
    sodium excretion in, 30
    symptoms of, 874
    treatment of, 210–211, 875–877
    in tumors, 873
    two regions of, 130
    urinary dilution in, 156
  interaction with mineralocorticoids, 897
  and magnesium reabsorption, 585
  and osmolality of urine, 149
  osmotic threshold for, 860–862
    in pregnancy, 1060
  preparations of. *See* Desmopressin; Pitressin
  secretion and release of
    in aging, 1238–1241, 1242
    in Bartter's syndrome, 905–906
    defects with hypodipsia, 129
    in diabetes insipidus, 851
    drugs affecting, 138
    in polydipsia, 133–134
    in pregnancy, 1061–1062
    relation to thirst, 124–125
    stimuli for, 15, 120, 121
  and sodium excretion in pregnancy, 1046
  and urea reabsorption, 150
  and water excretion in glucocorticoid deficiency, 155–156
Antigravity suits, in nephrotic syndrome, 107
Antimetabolite therapy, water metabolism in, 1151–1152
Apathy, in electrolyte disorders, 1108
Apnea, in sleep, 402
Aqueous humor, electrolytes in, 1015t
Arachidonic acid, 1194
  metabolites in inflammatory bowel disease, 839
Areflexia, 1103
Arginine hydrochloride
  as acidifying agent, 355t
  hyperkalemia from, 450
Arousal states, in electrolyte disorders, 1109t, 1110
Arrhythmias, 1125–1128
  in acidosis, 254, 295–296
  in alkalosis, 254
  atrial, 1125–1126
  bradycardia, 1125
  and digitalis, 1127–1128
  and myocardial infarction, 1127
  pH changes in, 254
  ventricular, 1126–1127
Arsenic, in dialysate water, 811t
Arterial conditions. *See* Vasculature
Ascites with cirrhosis. *See also* Cirrhosis
  diuretics in, 1177–1178
  edema and sodium retention in, 89–99
Ash content of diet, 1200–1201
Aspirin. See Salicylates
Asterixis, 1105
Asthma
  bicarbonate therapy in, 254
  respiratory acidosis in, 404
  respiratory alkalosis in, 398
Ataxia, 1107
ATP
  in brain, in uremia, 978
  and cellular pH regulation, 250
  generation from glycolysis, 303
  red cell levels in hypophosphatemia, 1131
ATPase
  calcium, and intestinal electrolyte transport, 828
  calcium-magnesium, and renal calcium transport, 513
  potassium-hydrogen, and intestinal electrolyte transport, 829
  sodium-potassium, 11
    aldosterone affecting, 52
    in brain, in uremia, 978
    deficiency of, and pseudohypoaldosteronism, 923–924
    and intestinal electrolyte transport, 828
Auditory acuity, in electrolyte disorders, 1104

Auditory hallucinations, in electrolyte disorders, 1111–1112
Autonomic nervous system, in dialysis hypotension, 789–790
Azotemia, prerenal, 662–663

Bacterial enterotoxins, diarrhea from, 837, 838
Balance, concept of, 686
Barium
in dialysate water, 811t
poisoning from, hypokalemia in, 462–463
Bartter's syndrome, 359–362, 472–475, 903–906
aldosterone secretion in, 904
amiloride in, 1172
antidiuretic hormone secretion in, 905–906
clinical features and diagnosis of, 361–362, 472t
differential diagnosis of, 467, 469, 475
etiology of, 473–475
hypokalemia in, 473
magnesium depletion in, 906
pathophysiology of, 360–361
sodium chloride reabsorption in, 904–905
treatment of, 362
urinary dilution in, 156
Base(s) and acids, 221–222
Basement membrane, glomerular, antibodies to, 691
Behavioral disorders, 1107–1112
apathy, lassitude and depression in, 1108–1109
arousal states in, 1109t, 1110
cognitive functions in, 1110–1111
confusion, delirium and psychosis in, 1109–1110
in hypocalcemia, 549
polydipsia in, 133, 209
Berylliosis, hypercalcemia in, 521
Bicarbonate
biliary, 321
in body fluids, 4t, 1015t
in brain, 970
in respiratory acidosis, 1025
in respiratory alkalosis, 1026
and carbonic acid buffer system, 227–230, 272–274
in cerebrospinal fluid, 971
in hypercapnia, 1024–1025
in hypocapnia, 1026
colonic handling of, 319
in dialysate, 794, 797
and hypoxemia, 793
exchange for chloride, 386
extracellular, 4t, 275–277
generation from carbon dioxide, 386
hyperbicarbonatemia. *See also* Alkalosis, metabolic
generation of, 335–338
maintenance of, 338–342
intestinal absorption of, in jejunum, 832
intracellular, 4t, 275, 276t
and intracellular electrolyte content, 11
losses of
in chronic renal failure, 298–299
in diabetic ketoacidosis, 945–947
in diarrhea, 842
and metabolic acidosis, 282
in pancreatic fluid, 321, 336, 352, 830
plasma levels of
in acidosis in chronic renal failure, 714
in diabetic ketoacidosis, 942t, 958
in pregnancy, 1064–1065
in respiratory acidosis, 241–242
in respiratory alkalosis, 242
and potassium levels, 423
production from organic anions, 1198
and regulation of cellular pH, 250
renal tubular reabsorption of, 231, 322–324
in acidosis of hyperparathyroidism, 530
in alkalosis, 339
carbon dioxide tension affecting, 389
in chronic renal failure, 298–299, 716
in hyperparathyroidism, 292, 530
parathyroid hormone affecting, 716
secretion in duodenum, 832
secretion in ileum, 833
synthesis of, 336
therapy with, 191t
in acidosis, 947–948
in renal failure, 791
renal tubular, 335
alkalosis from, 336, 357–358
respiratory, 399
in asthma, 254
dangers of, 948, 963
in diabetic ketoacidosis, 963, 965
in diarrhea, 842
in hyperkalemia, 456, 458–459, 674
in renal failure, 803
hypernatremia from, 1007
in lactic acidosis, 308, 400
in methanol poisoning, 316
in renal failure
acute, 674, 678
chronic, 301
in salicylate intoxication, 312
Bile, 830
electrolytes in, 1015t
pH of, 227t
potassium in, 467t
Bile acids, as intestinal secretagogues, 838–839
Biliary drainage, hyperchloremic acidosis from, 321
Bilirubin levels, elevated, affecting renal function, 93
Biotin, in total parenteral nutrition, 1205
Blood, pH of, 227t. *See also* pH, of blood
Blood-brain barrier, 973–974
anatomy of, 974
Blood flow
autoregulation of, 1112–1113
cerebral
in alkalosis, 343
hypercarbia correction affecting, 1089
pH affecting, 256
potassium affecting, 1113
coronary
in alkalosis, 342
in electrolyte disorders, 1115–1116
regional, pH affecting, 256
renal
in acute renal failure, 666–667
aging affecting, 1233–1234
loop diuretics affecting, 1166

Blood flow (*Cont.*)
pH affecting, 256
in remnant kidney, 689–690
Blood pressure. *See also* Hypertension; Hypotension
in electrolyte disorders, 1112–1116
in pregnancy, 1066–1067
Blood volume
decreased. *See* Hypovolemia
in dialysis hypotension, 785–786
in nephrotic syndrome, 100–101
Blue diaper syndrome, 526
Body fluid compartments, 185
Bohr effect, 255
Bone
acidosis affecting, 291
aseptic necrosis in renal transplant patients, 764–765
as buffer source, 237–238, 326–327, 516
in chronic renal failure, 714–715, 790–791
disorders in distal renal tubular acidosis, 327, 333
growth in chronic renal failure, 301
hungry bone syndrome, 547, 601, 637
in hypocalcemia, 550
in hypophosphatemia, 643–644
magnesium in, 600
metastases to, and hypercalcemia, 517
in nephrotic syndrome, 761
pain in renal osteodystrophy, 741
phosphorus in, 626
in renal osteodystrophy, 545, 729–765
resistance to calcemic action of parathyroid hormone, 734
Bradycardia, in electrolyte disorders, 1125
Bradykinin
and intestinal electrolyte transport, 836
and magnesium excretion, 590
plasma levels in cirrhosis with impaired renal function, 98
Brain
acid-base balance in, 971–972
adaptation to hyperglycemia, 1021–1024
amino acids in, 970
in hypernatremia, 1012
bicarbonate in, 970
biochemical changes in uremia, 978–980
blood flow in
in alkalosis, 343
hypercarbia correction affecting, 1089
pH affecting, 256
potassium affecting, 1113
buffering by, 238
in respiratory acidosis, 1025
in respiratory alkalosis, 1026
calcium in, 970
in uremia, 978, 979, 981–982
chloride in, 970
in hypernatremia, 1011–1012
in hyponatremia, 997
dehydration of, hypotonicity in, 193
edema of
in diabetic ketoacidosis, 963–964
in dialysis disequilibrium, 984, 986
in hyponatremia, 996–999
hypotonicity in, 193, 213
extracellular space of, 973–974
glucose levels in hyperglycemia, 1023
glucose oxidation in, 934
hypercalcemia affecting, 1094
hypercarbia affecting, 1095–1096
hypernatremia affecting, 1010–1011
hypoxia in ketoacidosis, 1018
idiogenic osmoles in, 193, 938, 970
in hyperglycemia, 964, 1021–1023, 1090
in hypernatremia, 1012, 1090
in uremia, 979
intravascular coagulation in diabetic ketoacidosis, 1019
lesions with salt wasting, 993–994
magnesium in, 970
natriuretic hormone in, 27. *See also* Natriuretic hormone
osmotically active solutes in, 970–971
pathologic studies of
in hyponatremia, 995–996
in uremia, 980–981
plasma osmolality affecting, 12
potassium in, 970
in hypernatremia, 1011–1012
in hyponatremia, 997
in respiratory acidosis, 1025
in respiratory alkalosis, 1026
sodium in, 970
in hypernatremia, 1011–1012
in hyponatremia, 997
volume regulation in
in hyperosmolality, 17
in hypoosmolality, 16
volume receptors in, 24
water content
in hyperglycemia, 1021
in hypernatremia, 1011–1012
in hyponatremia, 996–999
water deficits affecting, 938
Brattleboro rats, diabetes insipidus in, 859–860
Bromocriptine, and water metabolism, 1153
Buffering, 225–227, 270–277
bone in, 237–238, 326–327, 516
in chronic renal failure, 714–715, 790–791
by brain, 238
in respiratory acidosis, 1025
in respiratory alkalosis, 1026
carbon dioxide-bicarbonate system in, 227–230, 272–274
cellular mechanisms in, 236–240, 249–251
isohydric principle in, 274–275
and reduced buffer excretion in chronic renal failure, 299–301
in respiratory acidosis, 241–242
Burkitt's lymphoma, hyperphosphatemia in, 648
Burns
hyperosmolar syndrome in, 950
hypophosphatemia in, 639

phosphorus, hyperphosphatemia from, 648
potassium loss in, 466
Bursitis, olecranon, in dialysis patients, 744
Butorphanol, diuretic action of, 1152

Cadmium, in dialysate water, 811t
Calcifediol
in chronic renal failure, 758
in vitamin D deficiency, 554
Calcific periarthritis, in uremia, 744, 745
Calcification
of basal ganglia, in hypocalcemia, 549
of soft tissue
in chronic renal failure, 744–746
in eye, 746
periarticular, 745
in skin, 746
vascular, 746
visceral, 745–746
in hypercalcemia, 531–532
hyperphosphatemia with, 650, 651
radiographic features of, 753
Calciphylaxis, inchronic renal failure, 746–748
Calcitonin
and acid-base balance, 245
and calcium excretion, 515
and magnesium absorption, 579
and magnesium excretion, 593
and magnesium reabsorption, 584–585
therapy with
in hypercalcemia, 536–537
hypocalcemia from, 547
Calcitriol
in chronic renal failure, 757–758
parenteral administration of, 759
in vitamin D deficiency, 554
Calcium, 511–554
in brain, 970
in uremia, 978, 979, 981–982
in cerebrospinal fluid, 972–973
channel blockers, coronary vasodilation from, 1116
dietary, in chronic renal failure, 718
extracellular, 4t
hypercalcemia, 516–539. *See also* Hypercalcemia
hypercalciuria in distal renal tubular acidosis, 327
hypocalcemia, 539–554. *See also* Hypocalcemia
interaction with digitalis, 455
intestinal absorption of, 512
in gastrointestinal diseases, 843
malabsorption, 544
in nephrotic syndrome, 761
phosphate depletion affecting, 644
and intestinal electrolyte transport, 835
intracellular, 4t
and magnesium absorption, 577
and magnesium excretion, 591
metabolism of
in acidosis, 290–293
in acute renal failure, 761–763
in alkalosis, 344
in nephrotic syndrome, 760–761
plasma levels of
in alkalosis, 343
in chronic renal failure, 712–713, 749, 755–756
in renal transplant patients, 763–764
protein-bound, 511
renal transport of, 513–515
factors affecting, 514–515
mechanisms in, 513
sites of, 513–514
storage during pregnancy, 1045t
therapy with
in chronic renal failure, 755–756
in hyperkalemia, 454–455
in hypocalcemia, 552, 553
in total parenteral nutrition, 1203
urinary excretion of, 512–513
in acidosis, 238, 239
factors affecting, 514–515
in hypocalciuric hypercalcemia, familial, 519–520
loop diuretics affecting, 1166, 1169
in phosphate depletion, 645
thiazides affecting, 1163
Calcium carbonate therapy, in chronic renal failure, 301, 718
Calcium chloride
as acidifying agent, 355t
in acute hyperkalemia in renal failure, 803
Calcium gluconate, in hyperkalemia, 673–674
Calcium oxalate crystalluria, in ethylene glycol poisoning, 313, 314
Calculi, renal
in diarrheal diseases, 843–844
in distal renal tubular acidosis, 327
from carbonic anhydrase inhibitors, 1162
in hypercalcemia, 528
thiazides in, 1163–1164
triamterene-induced, 1173
Caloric requirements
in pediatric fluid therapy, 1212
in total parenteral nutrition, 1193–1195
Candidiasis
and hypercalcemia, 521, 522
and hypocalcemia, 550
Capillaries
filtration rate in, 19
and lymphatic drainage rate, 28–29, 78
fluid exchange in, 17–18, 52–53, 77–78
Captopril, 1172
effects in heart failure, 86-87
hyperkalemia from, 440, 459
polydipsia from, 137–138
and renal blood flow, 106
Carbamazepine
antidiuretic action of, 1149–1151
in diabetes insipidus, 872
Carbenicillin
alkalosis from, 350
anion gap increase from, 278
hypokalemia from, 475
Carbenoxolone
hypokalemia from, 478
pseudohyperaldosteronism from, 367

Carbohydrates
  malabsorption of, diarrhea in, 840–842
  metabolism of, 1195–1196
  in oral rehydration solutions, 1224t
  in total parenteral nutrition, 1194
    complications from, 1194–1195
Carbon dioxide
  bound to hemoglobin, 386
  conversion to bicarbonate, 228, 386
  excretion through lungs, 386–387
  glucose oxidation to, 934
  hypercapnia, 241–242. *See also* Hypercapnia
  hypocapnia, 242. *See also* Hypocapnia
  partial pressure of, 228
    in acidosis, 284–286
    in alkalosis, 342
    and bicarbonate reabsorption, 389
    and cellular pH, 387–389
    increased, 241–242, 387–389
    reduced, 242
    urinary minus blood gradient
      in acute hypercapnia, 391
      in chronic hypercapnia, 393
      in hypocapnia, 395
    and ventilation regulation, 240–244
  plasma levels in acidosis, in chronic renal failure, 714
  production of, 385
    carbohydrate infusions affecting, 1195
  transport of, 385–386
Carbonic acid
  as buffer with bicarbonate, 227–230, 272–274
  dehydration of, 229
    in renal tubules, 231
  pK_A value for, 227t
Carbonic anhydrase
  and carbon dioxide conversion to bicarbonate, 386
  inhibitors of, 1160–1166
    acetazolamide, 1160–1162. *See also* Acetazolamide
    in alkalinization of urine, 1160
    in alkalosis, 1160–1161
    contraindications to, 1162
    in epilepsy, 1161
    in glaucoma, 1160
    in hyperphosphatemia, 1161
    in mountain sickness, 1161
    in periodic paralysis, 1161
    thiazides, 1162–1166. *See also* Thiazide diuretics
    toxicities of, 1161–1162
  renal, 232, 322–323, 337
Carcinoid syndrome, diarrhea in, 838
Cardiovascular syndrome
  in acid-base disorders, 1113–1114
  calcium levels affecting, 1114
  in electrolyte disorders, 1112–1118
    arrhythmias in, 1125–1128
    coronary circulation in, 1115–1116
    electrocardiography in, 1119–1125
    myocardial performance in, 1116–1119
    vascular tone and blood pressure in, 1112–1115
  in hyperphosphatemia, 1115
  in hypochloremia, 1115
  magnesium levels affecting, 1114–1115
  sodium levels affecting, 1115
Carotid body chemoreceptor for ventilation, 240, 287
Carotid sinus baroreceptors, 23, 43, 81
Carpal tunnel syndrome, in uremia, 744
Castor oil, as intestinal secretagogue, 839
Catecholamines. *See also* Epinephrine; Norepinephrine
  and renal sodium reabsorption, 26, 60–61
  secretion in acidosis, 293
Cation-exchange resin. *See* Kayexalate
Cecal fluid, electrolytes in, 1015t
Cells
  action on mineralocorticoid hormones, 894–897
  dehydration of, 13
    correction of, 14
  in electrolyte disorders, 1131–1132
  hypophosphatemia affecting, 641–643
  pH in
    measurements of, 245–249
    regulation of, 249–251
    relation to extracellular pH, 251–252
  swelling of
    correction of, 14
    in hypoosmolality, 12
  volume of, tonicity affecting, 193–197
  water in, 1. *See also* Intracellular fluid
Cerebral conditions. *See* Brain
Cerebrospinal fluid
  acid-base balance in, 971–972
  calcium in, 972–973
  electrolytes in, 1015t
  glucose in, in cerebral edema, 964
  in hypercapnia, 1024–1025
  magnesium in, 973
  pH of, 227t, 971
    dialysis affecting, 985–986
    and ventilatory control, 240, 287–288
  potassium in, 972
  sink action of, 973
  sodium in, 972
    and renal sodium excretion, 25, 45
    and thirst regulation, 120, 122
Chemoreceptors for ventilation, 240, 287, 288
  alkalosis affecting, 342
Chemotherapy
  hyperphosphatemia from, 648
  hyperuricemia from, 1182–1183
  water metabolism in, 1151–1152
Chewing tobacco
  hypokalemia from, 478
  pseudohyperaldosteronism from, 367
Children, fluid and electrolyte therapy for, 1211–1227. *See also* Pediatric fluid and electrolyte therapy
Chloride
  in body fluids, 4t, 1015t

in brain, 970
in hypernatremia, 1011–1012
in hyponatremia, 997
deficiency of, acid excretion in, 235
extracellular, 4t
in gastric fluid, 352
hyperchloremic acidosis, 318–335. *See also* Acidosis, hyperchloremic
intestinal absorption of
in colon, 834
in ileum, 832–833
in jejunum, 832
intracellular, 4t
losses of, and hyperbicarbonatemia, 335–336
in oral rehydration solutions, 1224t
in pancreatic fluid, 830
in pediatric fluid therapy, 1212
plasma levels
in acidosis in chronic renal failure, 714
in hypercapnia, 243
in hypocapnia, 243
ratio to phosphate in serum, in hypercalcemia, 535
and regulation of cellular pH, 250
renal reabsorption of
in Bartter's syndrome, 474–475, 905
hyperabsorption in distal nephron, 924–925
in hypertension and hyperkalemia, 1181
role in metabolic alkalosis, 340–341
secretion of
in colon, 834
in ileum, 833–834
in jejunum, 832
urinary excretion of
in aldosteronism, 363
in Bartter's syndrome, 361–362
in chronic hypercapnia, 392
in mineralocorticoid excess, 898–899
Chloridorrhea, congenital, 842–843
Chloriduric alkalosis
hypertensive, 363–367
normotensive, 359–363
Chlorothiazide. *See* Thiazide diuretics
Chlorpropamide
in diabetes insipidus, 871
in hypodipsia, 132
hyponatremia from, in aging, 1242
and water metabolism, 1145–1148
Chlorthalidone, and urinary dilution, 154
Cholinergic agonists, and intestinal electrolyte transport, 835, 836
Chorea, 1107
Chromium
in dialysate water, 811t
in total parenteral nutrition, 1204
Chvostek sign
in alkalosis, 343
in tetany, 548
Cimetidine
in alkalosis from nasogastric suction, 844
in gastric alkalosis, 354
Cirrhosis
and abnormal salt and water processing by nephrons, 95–99
mediators of, 97–99
edema in, 89–99. *See also* Edema, in cirrhosis with ascites
hepatic venous outflow obstruction in, 89–92
hypoalbuminemia in, 93–94
hypocalcemia in, 544
LeVeen shunt in, 107
affecting renal function, 91
portal hypertension in, 92
respiratory alkalosis in, 399
single nephron function in, 95–96
sodium retention in, 89–99
Cisplatin
hypomagnesemia from, 607
and magnesium excretion, 592
nephrotoxicity of, 1183
and urinary concentration, 164
and water metabolism, 1151
Citrate
alkalosis from, 359
excretion in distal renal tubular acidosis, 327
pK_A value for, 227t
Clofibrate, in diabetes insipidus, 871–872
Clonidine
polydipsia from, 138
and urinary concentration, 164
and water metabolism, 1152–1153
Clostridium botulinum toxin, respiratory muscle paralysis from, 403
Coagulation, disseminated intravascular, in diabetic ketoacidosis, 1019
Coccidioidomycosis, hypercalcemia in, 521
Cognitive function, in electrolyte disorders, 1110–1111
Colchicine
hypocalcemia from, 547
and urinary concentration, 164
Colitis, ulcerative
hypomagnesemia in, 604
nephrolithiasis in, 843
Colloid osmotic pressure, capillary and interstitial, 17–18
Colon
absorption in, 834
secretions of, 834–835
Colorimetry, for intracellular pH measurements, 248
Coma
in acidosis
metabolic, 1096
respiratory, 1095
diabetic, 933–966
acid-base disorders with, 941–948
and glucose excretion in urine, 935–937
glucose oxidation in, 934
hyperglycemia in, 933–937
and ketoacidosis, 956–966
neurologic disorders in, 1017–1024
nonketotic coma, 948–956
potassium metabolism in, 940–941
water metabolism in, 937–939
electroencephalography in, 1097
in electrolyte disorders, 1092–1097
etiology of, 1093t
in hyponatremia, 1093–1094
in hypophosphatemia, 1097

Coma (*Cont.*)
  in metabolic encephalopathy, 969
  nonketotic hyperosmolar, 948–956
    and absence of ketoacidosis, 942–943
    clinical features of, 948–949
    diagnosis of, 950–951
    etiology of, 949–950
    fever in, 1106
    fluid replacement in, 953–954
    glucose therapy in, 955
    insulin in, 954–955
    laboratory evaluation of, 951–952
    myoclonus in, 1098
    neurologic disorders in, 1020
    potassium therapy in, 954
    preventive nursing care in, 955–956
    saline solutions in, 953
    seizures in, 1090
    sensorium in, 1096
    treatment of, 952–956
    underlying disorders with, 955–956
Concentration of urine, 145–151. *See also* Urine, concentration of abnormal, 156–169
Confusion, in electrolyte disorders, 1108t, 1109–1110
Conn's syndrome. *See* Aldosteronism
Consciousness alterations, in electrolyte disorders, 1092–1097
Constipation, 1129
Contraceptives, oral, and hyperreninemia with hypertension and hypokalemia, 477
Contractility, myocardial, in electrolyte disorders, 1116–1119
Contrast media, radiographic
  renal failure from, 1183
  and urinary concentration, 158
Convulsions. *See* Seizures
Copper
  in dialysate water, 811t
    hemolysis from, 810
  in total parenteral nutrition, 1204
Cor pulmonale, oxygen in, 106
Coronary arteries, in electrolyte disorders, 1115–1116
Coronary blood flow, in alkalosis, 342
Corticosteroids. *See* Glucocorticoids
Corticosterone methyloxidase deficiency, 433, 913–914
Cortisol
  deficiency of, 909–910
    sodium excretion in, 879
    water excretion in, 878–879
  hypercorticolism, hypokalemia in, 883
  plasma levels in pregnancy, 1054
Cortisone
  suppression test in hypercalcemia, 535
  as therapy in Addison's disease, 432
Countercurrent exchanger and multiplier, renal, 147, 150
  aging affecting, 1238
Cramps, muscular, 1099
  etiology of, 1098t
Creatinine in serum
  aging affecting, 1235
  in chronic renal failure, 709–710
  in diabetic ketoacidosis, 958
  and glomerular filtration rate, 684, 694
Crisis
  hypercalcemic, 526–527
    fever in, 1106
    hallucinations in, 1111
  myasthenic, respiratory acidosis in, 403
Crohn's disease
  hypomagnesemia in, 604
  nephrolithiasis in, 843
Crystalluria, in ethylene glycol poisoning, 313, 314
Cushing's syndrome, 901
  hypokalemia in, 479, 883
  nonketotic coma in, 950
Cyclophosphamide
  inappropriate antidiuresis from, 1168
  and water metabolism, 1151

Dehydration
  anion gap in, 278
  cellular, 13
    correction of, 14
    in diabetes mellitus, 937–938
  cerebral, hypotonicity with, 193
  in childhood, fluid therapy in, 1215–1220
  in diabetes insipidus, 852
  hypernatremia in, 1007
    and seizures during therapy, 1089–1090
  hypertonic, 31, 203–204
  hypotonic, 31
  nonketotic coma in, 1020
  in test for diabetes insipidus, 862–866
  in test for thirst deficit, 126
  water intake after, 125, 204
Delirium, in electrolyte disorders, 1108t, 1109–1110
Demeclocycline, 1175
  in inappropriate antidiuretic hormone secretion, 210, 876–877, 1168, 1176
  and urinary concentration, 164
Dementia, in dialysis patients, 806–807, 975, 988–992
Deoxycorticosterone. *See* Desoxycorticosterone
Depression, in electrolyte disorders, 1108–1109
Desferrioxamine, in aluminum-associated osteomalacia, 760
Desipramine, and inappropriate secretion of antidiuretic hormone, 1151
Desmopressin
  chlorpropamide interaction with, 1145
  in diabetes insipidus, 858, 869–870
Desoxycorticosterone
  activity in enzyme disorders, 478
  mineralocorticoid potency of, 900–901
  and potassium excretion in pregnancy, 1058
  serum levels
    in preeclampsia, 1071
    in pregnancy, 1052–1054
  and sodium excretion in pregnancy, 1050
Dexamethasone, in Addison's disease, 431
Dextran therapy, in preeclampsia, 1073
Dextrose monohydrate, 191t

Dextrose solution, in pediatric fluid therapy, 1212
Diabetes insipidus, 203–204
- central or neurogenic, 204, 851–871
  - abnormalities with, 854t
  - animal models of, 859–860
  - in anoxemic encephalopathy, 857
  - in brain tumors, 854
  - carbamazepine in, 872
  - causes of, 161t, 853–854
  - chlorpropamide in, 871
  - clinical features and pathophysiology of, 851–859
  - clofibrate in, 871–872
  - compared to primary polydipsia, 133, 869
  - dehydration studies in, 862–866
  - desmopressin in, 858, 869–870
  - differentiation from nephrogenic diabetes insipidus, 867–869
  - in head trauma, 855–856
  - in histiocytosis X, 854
  - hypernatremia in, 203, 204, 857–858, 1007
  - hypodipsia in, 127, 128, 129
  - idiopathic, 854–855
  - laboratory features of, 860–869
  - lysine vasopressin in, 870
  - in metastatic malignancies, 857
  - osmolality of plasma and urine in, 852–853, 866–868
  - osmotic threshold studies in, 860–862
  - Pitressin tannate in, 870–871
  - polydipsia in, 135
  - in pregnancy, 1062–1063
  - protriptyline in, 1161
  - in sarcoidosis, 857
  - traumatic, 855–856
    - anterior pituitary function in, 856–857
  - treatment of, 869–872
  - two regions of, 130
  - and urinary concentration, 160
- nephrogenic, 204
  - chlorpropamide in, 1145–1147
  - compared to primary polydipsia, 133
  - differentiation from central diabetes insipidus, 867–869
  - etiology of, 161t
  - familial, 161–163
  - lithium-induced, 163–164
  - thiazides in, 1164
  - urinary concentration in, 160–161

Diabetes mellitus
- chlorpropamide in, hyponatremia from, 1147–1148
- comas in, 933–966. *See also* Coma, diabetic
- diarrhea in, 838
- hyperchloremic acidosis in, 945
- hyperglycemia in. *See* Hyperglycemia
- and hyperkalemia in insulin deficiency, 447
- and hypertonicity with hyperglycemia, 190, 198–200
- and hyporeninemic hypoaldosteronism, 433–441, 941
- ketoacidosis in, 941–945, 956–966, 1017–1020
  - bicarbonate levels in, and anion gap, 958
  - bicarbonate losses in, 945–948
  - bicarbonate therapy in, 963, 965
  - blood pH, P_{CO_2} and P_{O_2} in, 958
  - cerebral edema in, 963–964
  - cerebral hypoxia in, 1018
  - clinical features of, 956–957
  - and complications during therapy, 963–965
  - creatinine and BUN levels in, 958
  - and effects of ketonemia, 1017–1018
  - erythrocyte 2,3-DPG levels in, 959, 961
  - fluid and electrolyte replacement in, 960–961, 965
  - hydrogen ion concentration in, 942–943
  - hyperglycemia in, 957
  - hyperosmolality in, 1018–1019
  - hypophosphatemia in, 639
  - insulin resistance in, 244
  - insulin therapy in, 961–963, 965–966
  - ketoacid anion concentration in, 943–945
  - ketone bodies in, 957
  - laboratory evaluation in, 957–959
  - lethargy and stupor in, 1096
  - magnesium deficiency in, 606
  - metabolic acidosis with, 1018
  - neurologic disorders in, 1017
  - phosphorus deficiency in, 958–959, 961
  - potassium levels in, 423, 957–958, 960–961
  - potassium therapy in, 961, 965
  - sodium deficiency in, 957
  - thromboses in, 964–965
  - treatment of, 959–966
- lactic acidosis in, 306
- metabolic acidosis in, 945–948
  - bicarbonate therapy in, 947–948
- sodium metabolism in, 939–940
- water deficiency in, 937–938

Dialysance, and clearance rate
- in hemodialysis, 779
- in peritoneal dialysis, 781

Dialysis, 777–814
- in acute renal failure, 670, 674, 679
- aluminum levels in, 805–808
  - and dementia, 806–807, 989–991
  - and osteomalacia, 739, 740, 755, 807–808
- bone changes from. *See* Osteodystrophy, renal
- copper levels in, 810
- and deionization of water for dialysate, 990–991
- dementia from, 806–807, 975, 988–992
  - aluminum role in, 806–807, 989–991
  - etiology of, 989–991
  - treatment of, 991–992
- disequilibrium syndrome from, 975, 983–988
  - cerebral edema in, 984, 986

Dialysis (*Cont.*)
clinical features of, 984, 987
differential diagnosis of, 988t
management of, 987–988
mannitol in, 1175
pathogenesis of, 984
pH of cerebrospinal fluid in, 985–986
reverse urea hypothesis of, 984–985
and electroencephalographic findings, 976, 977
in ethylene glycol poisoning, 314
fluoridated water in, 810–811
following ultrafiltration procedures, 988
hemodialysis, 777–780
acetate in, 794–797
and acid-base balance, 791–797
bicarbonate in, 794, 797
dementia from, 988–992
disequilibrium syndrome from, 975, 983–988
fluid removal and sodium balance in, 784
hemofiltration in, 780, 786
hypotension from, 784, 785–790, 1175
hypoxemia from, 793
potassium removal in, 801–802, 804
respiratory alkalosis from, 792–793
solute flux in
by convection, 780
by diffusion, 778–779
ultrafiltration in, 780, 786
sequential, 780, 786
water flux in, 779–780
in hypercalcemia, 538
hypercapnia from, 385
in hyperkalemia, 457, 674
hypermagnesemia from, 598
in hypermagnesemia, 599
in methanol poisoning, 316
neurologic disorders from, 975, 983–992
peritoneal, 780–783
and acid-base balance, 798–800
continuous ambulatory, 811–814, 988
acid-base homeostasis in, 813–814
fluid and solute removal in, 812–813
glucose metabolism in, 814
nutrition in, 814
potassium removal in, 813
sodium removal in, 813
trace metal metabolism in, 814
fluid removal and sodium balance in, 784
hypernatremia from, 784
hyperosmolar syndrome from, 950
hypertonic fluid in, effects of, 206
lactic acidosis in, 799–800
and mass transfer coefficient, 782
metabolic alkalosis in, 798–799
potassium removal in, 802–803, 804
respiratory alkalosis in, 798
sieving coefficient in, 782–783
solute flux in
by convection, 782
by diffusion, 781, 782
ultrafiltration in, 782
in salicylate intoxication, 312
and standards for dialysate water, 811t
and sulfate in dialysate, 811
and zinc deficiency, 808–810
Diarrhea, 318–321, 836–844, 1130
acidosis in
hyperchloremic, 318–321, 842
metabolic, 842
acute, 840
alkalosis in
metabolic, 337, 842
respiratory, 320
ammonium excretion in, 842
bicarbonate loss in, 320, 842
calcium absorption in, 843
chloride, congenital, 356–357
chronic, 840
clinical features of, 320, 840t
definition of, 836
etiology of, 838–839
evaluation of, 840
from bacterial enterotoxins, 837, 838
from inflammation of bowel, 839
from ingestion of poorly absorbed solutes, 839
from laxatives, 838–839
from loss of absorptive cells, 839
from neurohumoral agents, 838
hypomagnesemia in, 604
laboratory features of, 320
magnesium absorption in, 843
mechanism of, 836–838
and nephrolithiasis, 843–844
osmotic, 837, 840–842
pathophysiology of, 318–320
potassium loss in, 468–469, 843
secretory, 837, 842–843
sodium loss in, 939
systemic effects of, 840–844
treatment of, 320–321
Dichloroacetate, in lactic acidosis, 308–309
Dichloromethylene diphosphonate, in hypercalcemia, 537
Diet. *See* Nutrition
Diffusion, nonionic, 233
Diffusion block, alveolar-capillary, 386–387
DiGeorge syndrome, 540
Digitalis
effects in electrolyte disorders, 1119, 1127–1128
hyperkalemia from, 446, 450
hypomagnesemia from, 607–608
interaction with calcium, 455
toxicity of
in alkalosis, 342
hypokalemia affecting, 482
Digoxin, potassium depletion from, without hypokalemia, 479
Dihydrogen phosphate, 222
Dihydroxytachisterol, in chronic renal failure, 758
24,25-Dihydroxyvitamin D_3, in chronic renal failure, 758–759
Dilution of urine, 144–145. *See also* Urine, dilution of abnormal, 152–156
Dioctyl sodium sulfosuccinate, as intestinal secretagogue, 839

Diphenylhydantoin
in inappropriate antidiuretic hormone secretion, 211, 876
and urinary concentration, 164
and water metabolism, 1153
2,3-Diphosphoglycerate in red cells
in diabetic ketoacidosis, 959, 961
in hypophosphatemia, 642, 1131
in metabolic acidosis, 294–295
and oxygen affinity for hemoglobin, 1133
pH affecting, 255–256
in phosphate depletion, 1016
Diphosphonate therapy, in hypercalcemia, 537
Disodium etidronate, in hypercalcemia, 537
Dissociation constant for acids, and pK_A, 222
Diuretics, 1159–1184
abuse of, 362
detection of, 470, 475
chloride excretion in, 467
acetazolamide, 1160–1162. *See also* Acetazolamide
adverse effects of, 108
alkalosis from, 346–350
antidiuretic hormone antagonists, 1175
and calcium excretion, 515
carbonic anhydrase inhibitors, 1160–1166
clinical uses of, 1176–1184
in diabetes mellitus
potassium loss from, 941
water loss from, 938
water retention from, 939
edema from, 1179
in hyperkalemia, 456
in hypertension, 1179–1180
hypocalcemia from, 548
hypokalemia from, 469–470, 482
hypomagnesemia from, 605–606
hyponatremia from, in aging, 1242
hypotonic urinary loss from, and hypernatremia, 206
loop agents, 1166–1170. *See also* Ethacrynic acid; Furosemide
contraindications to, 1170
therapeutic uses of, 1167–1169
thiazides with, 1170–1171
toxicities of, 1169–1170
and magnesium reabsorption and excretion, 585, 590–591
osmotic, 1174
polydipsia from, 137
potassium-sparing, 1171–1173, 1180–1181
in preeclampsia, 1074
in renal failure, acute, 669, 1181–1184
in renal potassium wasting, 1180–1181
in renal tubular acidosis, 335, 1181
salt intake with, 107–108
thiazide, 1162–1166. *See also* Thiazide diuretics
loop agents with, 1170–1171
and urinary concentration, 157–160
and urinary dilution, 154
Donnan equilibrium, 3, 4–6
Dopamine
and intestinal electrolyte transport, 835, 836
and magnesium excretion, 590
and renal sodium excretion, 26, 62
urinary, in pregnancy, 1054
and water metabolism, 1153
Doxapram, respiratory alkalosis from, 398
Drinking behavior, thirst in. *See* Thirst
Drug-induced conditions
hyperkalemia, 440–441, 446, 450, 459
hyperosmolar syndrome, 950
hypocalcemia, 547–548
hypokalemia, 464
hypomagnesemia, 606–608
hyponatremia, 999
inappropriate antidiuretic hormone secretion, 157t, 874
magnesium excretion changes, 591–592
nephrotoxic acute renal failure, 664
osteomalacia, 737
polydipsia, 133, 137–138
renin-aldosterone axis impairment, 440–441
respiratory acidosis, 402, 403
respiratory alkalosis, 398–399
Drugs affecting water metabolism, 1145–1153
antimetabolites, 1151–1152
bromocriptine, 1153
clofibrate, 1149
clonidine, 1152–1153
diphenylhydantoin, 1153
dopamine, 1153
ethanol, 1153
narcotic agents, 1152
sulfonylureas, 1145–1149
tricyclic compounds, 1149–1151
Duodenum, bicarbonate secretion in, 832
Dysphagia, 1129

Eclampsia of pregnancy, 1067
Edema, 77–108
cerebral. *See* Brain, edema of
in cirrhosis with ascites, 89–99
diuretics in, 1177–1178
and hepatic venous outflow obstruction, 89–92
and portal hypertension, 92
and portasystemic shunting, 92–93
treatment of, 106–107
urinary dilution in, 153
diuretic-induced, 1179
diuretics in, 1176–1179
in heart failure, congestive, 78–89
effector mechanisms in, 82–89
hormones affecting, 86–89
peritubular factors in, 82–85
prostaglandins affecting, 88–89
renal nerves affecting, 89
renin-angiotensin-aldosterone system in, 86–88
sensing mechanisms in, 78–82
urinary dilution in, 153
and hyponatremia, 213
and mechanisms in interstitial fluid volume accumulation, 77–78
in nephrotic syndrome, 99–106
treatment of, 107
in preeclampsia, 1070

Edema (*Cont.*)
prevention by local regulatory mechanisms, 19–31
pulmonary
from saline solutions in hyponatremia, 213
from water intake in hypernatremia, 207
loop diuretics in, 1167
paraldehyde-induced, 317
and respiratory alkalosis, 397, 398
refractory, loop diuretics in, 1167
treatment of, factors affecting, 106–108
urinary dilution in, 153
Effective solutes, 187
Eicosatrienoic acid, 1194
Electrocardiography, in electrolyte disorders, 1119–1125
P wave in, 1119
P-R interval in, 1119–1120
QRS complex in, 1120–1121
Q-T interval in, 1122–1123
S-T segment in, 1123
T wave in, 1124–1125
U wave in, 1125
Electroencephalography
in coma, 1097
in dialysis dementia, 989
in electrolyte disorders, 1097
in hypernatremia, 1009–1010
in hyperparathyroidism, 982
in hyponatremia, 995
in renal failure
acute, 976
chronic, 977–978
Electrolytes in body fluids, 3–4
Embolism, renal arterial, 663–664
Emotional disorders, in electrolyte disorders, 1110
Encephalopathy. *See also* Neurologic disorders
anoxemic, diabetes insipidus from, 857
dialysis. *See* Dialysis, dementia from
metabolic, 969
uremic, 975–976
Endocrine disorders
hypocalcemia in, 550–551
hypomagnesemia in, 608–609
β-Endorphin, and vasopressin release, 1152
Endotoxemia, and respiratory alkalosis, 320
Enemas, phosphate, hyperphosphatemia from, 647
Energy requirements
in pediatric fluid therapy, 1212
in total parenteral nutrition, 1193–1195
Enkephalins
and intestinal electrolyte transport, 836
and thirst regulation, 122
Enteritis
regional
hypomagnesemia in, 604
nephrolithiasis in, 843
viral, 839
Enterotoxins, bacterial, diarrhea from, 837, 838
Enuresis, in diabetes insipidus, 851
Epilepsy. *See also* Seizures
and seizures in alkalosis, 1088
Epinephrine
hyperkalemia from, 447
hypokalemia from, 464
and potassium metabolism, 418
serum levels in pregnancy, 1054
Erythrocytes
2,4-DPG in. *See* 2,3-Diphosphoglycerate in red cells
hypophosphatemia affecting, 641–642
metabolism in electrolyte disorders, 1131
volume regulation in
in hyperosmolality, 16–17
in hypoosmolality, 15
Estrogen
hypocalcemia from, 547
and phosphate metabolism, 651
serum levels in pregnancy, 1054
Ethacrynic acid, 1166–1170
alkalosis from, 346–350
and calcium excretion, 515
in cirrhosis with ascites, 1177
in hyperkalemia, 456
hypotonic urinary loss from, and hypernatremia, 206
in nephrotic syndrome, 1178
in renal failure, acute, 669
toxicities of, 1169–1170
uricosuric congeners of, 1167–1168
and urinary concentration, 157
and urinary dilution, 154
Ethamivan, respiratory alkalosis from, 398
Ethanol. *See* Alcohol
Ethylene diamine tetraacetate, in hypercalcemia, 537
Ethylene glycol
acidosis from, 313–314
treatment of, 314
metabolism of, 313
and osmolality of extracellular fluid, 187
poisoning from, hypocalcemia in, 548
Euphemia, 270
in metabolic acidosis, 281–282
Exercise, hyperkalemia from, 448–449
Extracellular fluid, 1, 185. *See also* Interstitial fluid; Plasma
bicarbonate in, 275–277
electrolytes in, 4t
osmolality of, 186–187
volume of, 2–3
aging affecting, 1236–1238
in chronic renal failure, 699–700
contraction of
in alkalosis, 335–336
in diabetes, 939
decreased. *See* Hypovolemia
in hypernatremia, 203–207
in hyponatremia, 209–213
and magnesium excretion, 590
in pregnancy, 1042–1044
receptors for. *See* Volume receptors
regulation of, 17–18, 686–687
and sodium excretion. *See* Sodium, urinary excretion of
and thirst regulation, 121–122
and vascular volume maintenance, 20–21, 28–31
Extracellular space of brain, 973–974
Extrapyramidal disorders, 1107

Eyes
calcification in chronic renal failure, 746
in electrolyte disorders, 1104, 1105
in hypocalcemia, 549

Fanconi syndrome
hypophosphatemia in, 639
and renal tubular acidosis, 325, 333
Fasciculations, 1098
etiology of, 1098t
Fasting, acidosis in, 293
Fat
metabolism of, 1196
in total parenteral nutrition, 1194, 1195
Fatty acids
as intestinal secretagogues, 839
malabsorption of, 837
in total parenteral nutrition, 1184, 1194
Feces. See Stool
Fever, 1106
oxygen-hemoglobin affinity in, 1133
respiratory alkalosis from, 399
Fibrin deposition, cerebral intravascular, in diabetic ketoacidosis, 1019
Fludrocortisone
in Addison's disease, 432
in hyperkalemia, 459, 460
in hyporeninemic hypoaldosteronism, 916–921
Fluid
compartments of body, 1, 185. *See also* Extracellular fluid; Intracellular fluid
losses of. *See also* Dehydration
cutaneous, 203, 205
in diabetes
decreased, 939
increased, 938
gastrointestinal, 119
and hypernatremia or hypertonicity, 203–204
hypotonic, 204–206
insensible, 119, 203
in children, 1212–1213
and fluid replacement, 671
pulmonary, 203
replacement of
in childhood, 1211–1227
in diabetic ketoacidosis, 960–961, 965
in diarrhea, 841
in hypernatremia, 204, 206, 1013–1014
in insensible fluid losses, 671
in nonketotic coma, 953–954
Fluorescent probes, for intracellular pH measurements, 248
Fluoride
in dialysate water, 811t
osteomalacia from, 740, 810–811
9α-Fluoroprednisone in nasal spray, hypokalemia from, 478
Fluphenazine, and inappropriate secretion of antidiuretic hormone, 1151
Folic acid
deficiency of, methanol poisoning in, 315
as therapy in chronic renal failure, 718
in total parenteral nutrition, 1205
Food intake. *See* Nutrition
Formic acidosis, methanol-induced, 315
Fructose, intracellular phosphate shifts from, 637
Furosemide, 1166–1170
alkalosis from, 346–350
and calcium excretion, 515
in cirrhosis with ascites, 1177–1178
in hypercalcemia, 762, 1167
in hyperkalemia, 456
hypomagnesemia from, 605–606
in hyponatremia, 1168–1169
in hyporeninemic hypoaldosteronism, 921
hypotonic urinary loss from, and hypernatremia, 206
in inappropriate antidiuretic hormone secretion, 211, 876, 1168
and magnesium reabsorption, 585
in renal failure, acute, 669, 1181–1183
in symptomatic hypotonicity, 214
thiazides with, 1170–1171
toxicities of, 1169–1170
tubular necrosis from, 1183
and urinary concentration, 157
and urinary dilution, 154

Gastrectomy, vitamin D deficiency from, 544
Gastric alkalosis, 351–356
Gastric juice, 830
acid in, 336–337, 352, 830
in electrolyte disorders, 1130–1131
composition of, 352
electrolytes in, 1015t
loss of, systemic effects of, 844
pH of, 227t
potassium in, 466, 467t
Gastrin
hypercalcemia affecting levels of, 1130
receptors on gastric parietal cells, 830
Gastroenteritis, viral, 839
Gastrointestinal tract
absorption in, 827. *See also* Absorption, intestinal
as bicarbonate source, 336–337
colonic bicarbonate handling, 319
diarrhea, 836–844
disorders of
hypokalemia in, 466–469
hypomagnesemia in, 603–605
hypophosphatemia in, 644
total parenteral nutrition in, 1191–1192
in electrolyte disorders, 1128–1131
electrolyte transport in, 828–829
calcium pump in, 828
carrier-mediated, 829
channels or pores in, 829
extracellular, 829
potassium-hydrogen pump in, 829
sodium-potassium pump in, 828
fluid loss from, 119
hypernatremia in, 205
intestinal alkalosis, 356–357
intestinal transport, 830–836
in colon, 834–835
in ileum, 832–834

Gastrointestinal tract (*Cont.*)
intracellular mediators of, 835
in jejunum, 830–832
neurohumoral control of, 835–836, 838
in metabolic acidosis, 295
pH of intestinal juice, 227t
secretions of, 827
biliary, 830
in colon, 834–835
gastric, 830
in ileum, 833–834
in jejunum, 832
neurohumoral agents affecting, 836, 838
pancreatic, 830
salivary gland, 829–830
small bowel fluid electrolytes, 1015t
water transport in, 828
Gentamicin
and magnesium excretion, 592
respiratory muscle paralysis from, 403
and urinary concentration, 164
Geophagia, hypokalemia in, 465
Glaucoma, carbonic anhydrase inhibitors in, 1160
Glipizide, diuretic action of, 1149
Glomerular filtrate
normal amounts of, 144
reabsorption of, 144–145
Glomerular filtration
in acute renal failure, 667
aging affecting, 1234–1235
in chronic renal failure, 683–684
evaluation of, 694–695
in cirrhosis, 95
and creatinine in serum, 684, 694
diuretics affecting, 1159
and glucose excretion, 936–937
and hyperbicarbonatemia maintenance, 338–339
in hypercalcemia, 166, 167, 528–529
hyperfiltration, 439
in lithium-induced polyuria, 163
of magnesium, 579–580
in nephrotic syndrome, 101
phosphate ultrafiltration, 629
in potassium depletion, 165
in preeclampsia, 1070
in pregnancy, 1044–1046
in protein malnutrition, 157
in remnant kidney, 690
single-nephron, in glomerular disease, 691
and tubuloglomerular feedback, 339
Glomerulosclerosis
in chronic renal failure, 692
diabetic, 694
in reflux nephropathy, 694
Glomerulus, renal
aging affecting, 1231
antibodies to basement membrane, 691
diseases of, renal function in, 690–695
Glucagon, and magnesium reabsorption and excretion, 585, 593
Glucocorticoids
compared to mineralocorticoids, 897–898
deficiency of, 909–910
compared to mineralocorticoid deficiency, 155
hyponatremia in, 211, 878–880
and distribution of body sodium and water, 879–880
and intestinal electrolyte transport, 836
and magnesium excretion, 594
therapy with
and aseptic necrosis of bone in renal transplant patients, 764–765
in hypercalcemia, 536
Gluconeogenesis, 934
pH affecting, 253
Glucose
in brain, in hyperglycemia, 1023
and calcium excretion, 515
in cerebrospinal fluid, in cerebral edema, 964
dietary precursors of, 934
as effective solute, 187
hyperglycemia. *See* Hyperglycemia
hypoglycemic agents, oral, lactic acidosis from, 306–307
intestinal absorption of, in jejunum, 831
intracellular phosphate shifts from, 636–637
and magnesium absorption, 577
and magnesium excretion, 593, 607
metabolism of, 303
in continuous ambulatory peritoneal dialysis, 814
osmotic diuresis from, and hypotonic fluid loss and hypernatremia, 205–206
oxidation of, obligatory, 934
production from endogenous sources, 934
renal reabsorption of, in hypercalcemia, 531
removal systems for, 934–937
therapy with
in hyperkalemia, 456, 674
in renal failure, 803
hyperosmolar syndrome from, 950
in nonketotic coma, 955
in pediatric fluid therapy, 1212
in renal failure, acute, 674, 679
in total parenteral nutrition, 1194
and tubuloglomerular feedback activity, 439–440
and urinary concentration, 158, 159
urinary excretion of, 935–937
Glyburide, diuretic action of, 1148–1149
Glycerol, 191t
as effective solute, 187
and osmolality of extracellular fluid, 187
Glycogen, conversion to glucose, 934
Glycolysis
and ATP generation, 303
pH affecting, 253
Glycosuria, thiazide-induced, 1165
Glycyrrhizic acid
hypokalemia from, 478
pseudohyperaldosteronism from, 366–367
cGMP, and intestinal electrolyte transport, 835
Gout
hypophosphatemia in, 639
thiazide-induced, 1165

Granulomatous diseases, hypercalcemia in, 521–522
Gravity, specific, 8
Growth in childhood, after renal transplantation, 765
Growth hormone
  and acid-base balance, 245
  and hypercalcemia in acromegaly, 520
  and magnesium absorption, 579
  and magnesium excretion, 593
  and phosphate metabolism, 651
  and renal hypertrophy, compensatory, 697
Guanabenz, and urinary concentration, 164
Guanosine monophosphate, cyclic, and intestinal electrolyte transport, 835
Guillain-Barré syndrome
  and inappropriate antidiuretic hormone secretion, 874
  respiratory acidosis in, 403

Hallucinations, in electrolyte disorders, 1111–1112
Halophenate, antidiuretic action of, 1149
Hamburger shift, and bicarbonate exchange for chloride, 386
Head trauma, diabetes insipidus from, 855–856
Headache, 1104–1105
Hearing changes
  in electrolyte disorders, 1104
  from loop diuretics, 1170
Heart
  in acidosis, 254–255, 295–296
  in alkalosis, 342–343
  calcification in chronic renal failure, 746
  in dialysis hypotension, 785
  in hypercalcemia, 527
  in hyperkalemia, 453–454, 673, 1113
  in hypocalcemia, 550
  in hypokalemia, 481
  in hypophosphatemia, 643
  infarction with arrhythmias, in electrolyte disorders, 1127
  pH affecting, 254–255
  volume receptors in, 22–23, 40–42, 79–80
Heart failure, congestive
  diuretics in, 1176–1177
  edema and renal sodium retention in, 78–89. *See also* Edema, in heart failure
  and respiratory alkalosis, 397
  treatment of, 106
Hematocrit, and renal sodium excretion, 27, 46
Hematologic effects of electrolyte disorders, 1131–1133
Hemodialysis, 777–780. *See also* Dialysis
Hemoglobin
  carbon dioxide bound to, 386
  and cell volume regulation, 16
  oxygen dissociation from
    in acidosis, 294–295
    in alkalosis, 345
    in electrolyte disorders, 1132–1133
    pH affecting, 255
Hemolytic anemia
  in electrolyte disorders, 1131
  from copper in dialysate, 810
Henderson-Hasselbalch equation, 224, 273
Henle's loop, as countercurrent multiplier, 147
Heparin, hyperkalemia from, 440–441, 459
Heparinoid administration, and aldosterone excretion in pregnancy, 1049, 1050–1051
Hepatorenal syndrome, LeVeen shunt in, 107
Histamine receptors, on gastric parietal cells, 830
Histiocytosis X, diabetes insipidus from, 854
Histoplasmosis, hypercalcemia in, 521
Homeostasis, 686
  in chronic renal failure, 688–689
  extrarenal control of, 686–687
  intrinsic renal control of, 687–688
Hormones
  and acid-base balance, 244–245
  in electrolyte disorders, 1133–1134
  role in excretory processes, 687
Hungry bone syndrome, 547
  hypomagnesemia in, 601
  hypophosphatemia in, 637
Hydrochloric acid
  as acidifying agent, 355t
  gastric secretion of, 336–337, 352, 830
    in electrolyte disorders, 1130–1131
  as therapy in gastric alkalosis, 355–356
Hydrocortisone, in hypercalcemia, 536
Hydrogen ions, 221–222
  and acidity of solutions, 222–224
  in brain, in dialysis disequilibrium, 986–987
  combined with ammonia, 221, 233
  concentrations related to pH, 269–270
  in diabetic ketoacidosis, 942–943
  gastric secretion of, 351–352
  mineralocorticoids affecting secretion of, 895–897
  production from foodstuffs, 1195–1201
  renal secretion of, 231, 323
Hydropenia, renal response to, 140–141
5-Hydroperoxyeicosatetraenoic acid (HPETE), as intestinal secretagogue, 836, 839
Hydrostatic pressure, capillary and interstitial, 17–18, 52–53
β-Hydroxybutyrate
  deaths from infusions of, 1017
  oxidation of, 1198
  plasma levels in diabetic ketoacidosis, 942t, 957
β-Hydroxybutyric acidosis, in paraldehyde toxicity, 317
18-Hydroxycorticosterone
  plasma levels of
    in hypoaldosteronism, 436–437
    in type 1 corticosterone deficiency, 433
  urinary, in pregnancy, 1054
5-Hydroxyeicosatetetraenoic acid (HETE), as intestinal secretagogue, 836, 839
11β-Hydroxylase deficiency, 366, 432, 477–478
  mineralocorticoid excess in, 900–901

17α-Hydroxylase deficiency, 366, 433, 477–478
  mineralocorticoid excess in, 900–901
21-Hydroxylase deficiency, 432, 911–913
Hyperaldosteronism. *See* Aldosteronism
Hypercalcemia, 516–539
  abdominal pain in, 1130
  acid-base disorders in, 530
  acid-base metabolism in, 292–293
  acid secretion in, 1130
  in acromegaly, 520
  in adrenal insufficiency, 521
  alkalosis in, 363
  anorexia in, 1128
  arrhythmias in, 1126t
  ataxia in, 1107
  auditory acuity in, 1104
  and calcification of soft tissue, 531–532
  cardiovascular system in, 527, 1114
  catheterization of thyroid veins in, 535
  causes of, 516–526
  and chloride:phosphate ratio in serum, 535
  cognitive function in, 1111
  constipation in, 1129
  cortisone suppression test in, 535
  crisis in, 526–527
    fever in, 1106
    hallucinations in, 1111
  depression in, 1109
  diagnostic approach to, 532–533
  differential diagnosis of, 532–535
  documentation of, 532
  electrocardiography in, 1119, 1120, 1121, 1122, 1125
  eye changes in, 1104
  gastrointestinal manifestations of, 527–528
  in granulomatous diseases, 521–522
  headache in, 1104, 1105
  in hyperparathyroidism
    primary, 513–519
    tertiary, 525
  hypertension with, 527
  in hyperthyroidism, 520
  in hypervitaminosis A, 523
  hypocalciuric, familial, 519–520
  hypokalemia with, 530–531
  hypomagnesemia with, 608
  hypoparathyroidism with, 341
  idiopathic, of infancy, 525
  in immobilization, 522
  lethargy and stupor in, 1094
  loop diuretics in, 1166, 1167
  magnesium excretion in, 591
  in malignancies, 517–518
  in milk-alkali syndrome, 522–523
  miscellaneous causes of, 525–526
  in multiple endocrine syndromes, 519
  nausea and vomiting in, 1129
  nephrogenous cAMP in, 534
  in Paget's disease, 522
  pancreatitis in, 1131
  paresthesias in, 1104
  in pheochromocytoma, 520–521
  phosphate excretion in, 535
  psychiatric manifestations of, 1109
  radioimmunoassay of parathyroid hormone in, 533–534
  reflexes in, 1104
  in renal failure
    acute, 525, 676, 762
    chronic, 749, 756
  renal manifestations of, 528–531
  in renal transplant patients, 524–525, 763–764
  in sarcoidosis, 521
  seizures in, 1091–1092
  signs and symptoms of, 526–532
  thiazide-induced, 523–524, 1165–1166
  treatment of, 535–539
    in acute disease, 538
    agents in, 536–538
    in chronic symptomatic disease, 538–539
    in mild disease, 539
    in moderate disease, 538
  urinary concentration in, 166–168
  in vitamin D intoxication, 523
  vitamin D metabolite levels in, 534
  weakness in, 1102–1103
Hypercalciuria, idiopathic, thiazides in, 1163–1164
Hypercapnia, 387–394
  acid excretion in, 234
  acute, 387–389
    renal response to, 389–393
  in alkalosis, 335, 341, 342
  apathy and lassitude in, 1108
  asterixis in, 1105
  brain changes in, 1025
  cardiovascular system in, 1113
  cerebrospinal fluid in, 1024–1025
  chronic, 391–393
  correction of, and cerebral blood flow decrease, 1089
  papilledema in, 1105
  and posthypercapnic alkalosis, 350–351
  reflexes in, 1103, 1104
  and respiratory acidosis. *See* Acidosis, respiratory
  seizures in, 1088–1089
Hypercarbia. *See* Hypercapnia
Hyperglycemia
  in diabetic comas, 933–937
  in diabetic ketoacidosis, 957
  glomerular filtration rate in, 936–937
  and glucose excretion in urine, 935–937
  glucose oxidation in, 934
  hypertonicity with, 190, 198–200
  and idiogenic osmoles in brain, 964, 1021–1023, 1090
  lethargy and stupor in, 1093
  and nonketotic coma, 948–956, 1020
    seizures in, 1090
  sodium levels in, 199–200
  thiazide-induced, 1165
  water metabolism in, 937–939
Hyperkalemia, 419–460
  in abnormal potassium distribution, 446–450
  and acid excretion in urine, 234
  acidemia in, 421–424, 456, 458–459
  in acidosis, 288–290, 422–423
  in acute renal failure, 672–674
  in Addison's disease, 424–425, 429–432
  in aging, 1243–1244
  aldosterone secretion in, 447, 452

arrhythmias in, 1126t
bicarbonate therapy in, 456, 458–459
calcium infusions in, 454–455
clinical features of, 453–454
in decreased distal sodium delivery, 424–425
in diabetes mellitus, 941
diagnostic tests in, 450–453
dialysis in, 457
diet in, 457–458
in digitalis overdose, 446, 450
diuretics in, 456
drug-induced, 440–441, 446, 450, 459
and effects of digitalis, 1119, 1128
electrocardiography in, 1119, 1120, 1121, 1122, 1123, 1124
in enzyme deficiencies, 432–433
etiology of, 421t
exercise-induced, 448–449
fasciculations in, 1098
from increased potassium input, 424
from potassium-sparing diuretics, 1172–1173
heart in, 453–454, 673, 1113
hormones released in, 1134
hypertension with, chloride shunt in, 1181
hypertonic saline in, 455–456
in hypoaldosteronism
  hyporeninemic, 433–441, 914–916
  selective, 443–444
in insulin deficiency, 447
insulin and glucose in, 456
Kayexalate in, 456–457, 460
in lupus erythematosus, 442–443
neuromuscular manifestations of, 454
in obstructive uropathy, 443
in periodic paralysis, 449, 1100–1101
pseudohyperkalemia, 420–421
in pseudohypoaldosteronism, 444, 922
reflexes in, 1103, 1104
in renal failure
  acute, 425–429
  end-stage, 800–801
    treatment of, 803–804
in renal transplant patients, 443, 1181
in renal tubular acidosis, 444–446, 924–925, 1181
renin secretion in, 451–452
in sickle cell disease, 441–442
  pregnancy with, 1059
in tissue damage, 449–450
treatment of, 453–460
  in acute disease, 454–457
  in chronic disease, 457–460
weakness and paralysis in, 1100
Hyperlipidemia, thiazide-induced, 1165
Hypermagnesemia, 596–599
  arrhythmias in, 1126t
  cardiovascular system in, 1114–1115
  in chronic renal failure, 597, 749, 756
  clinical features of, 598–599
  electrocardiography in, 1119, 1120, 1121, 1122, 1124
  etiology of, 596–598
  from magnesium therapy, 598
  magnesium excretion in, 591, 597–598
  myocardial performance in, 1118–1119
  nausea and vomiting in, 1129
  neurologic disorders in, 1094–1095
  paralytic ileus in, 1129
  reflexes in, 1103, 1104
  sensory changes in, 1104
  treatment of, 599
  weakness and paralysis in, 1101
Hypernatremia, 200–207, 1007–1014
  acute, 1009
  adipsic, 858
  in aging, 1241
  brain damage in, anatomic, 1010–1011
  brain water and electrolyte content in, 1011–1012
  cardiovascular system in, 1115
  chorea in, 1107
  classification of, 200–203
  cognitive function in, 1111
  confusion in, 1110
  in diabetes insipidus, 203, 204, 857–858, 1007
  in diabetes mellitus, 940
  differential diagnosis of, 202t
  and effects of hyperosmolality, 1009, 1010
  electroencephalography in, 1009–1010
  essential, 203
    asymptomatic, 858, 867
    definition of, 131
    hypodipsia in, 127–128, 129–132
    symptomatic, 132
  etiology of, 1007t
  extracellular fluid volume in
    decreased, 204–206
    increased, 206–207
    normal, 203–204
  fever in, 1106
  from peritoneal dialysis, 784
  hyperosmolality and cell dehydration with, 13
  hypotension with, 204
  and idiogenic osmoles in brain, 1090
  lethargy and stupor in, 1093
  mortality in, 1008, 1012–1013
  muscle cramps in, 1099
  muscle rigidity in, 1107
  myoclonus in, 1098
  in myotonic dystrophy, 868
  nausea and vomiting in, 1128
  neurologic disorders in, 1008–1009
  physiologic responses to, 14
  reflexes in, 1104
  in renal failure, acute, 672
  in salt poisoning of infants, 1009, 1090
    chorea in, 1107
    fever in, 1106
  seizures in, 1089–1090
  symptoms of, 1008–1009
  thirst in, 203
  treatment of, 204, 1013–1014
Hyperosmolality, 10
  brain adaptation in, 970, 1012
  and hypernatremia, 1009, 1010
  hypotonicity with, 200
  in ketoacidosis, 1018–1019
  and myoclonus, 1098
  in nonketotic coma, 950, 1020
  physiologic responses to, 14–15
  seizures in, 1089–1090
  signs and symptoms of, 13
  volume regulatory increase in, 16–17

Hyperparathyroidism, 518–519
acid-base disorders in, 530
anorexia in, 1128
and aseptic necrosis of bone, 765
bicarbonate reabsorption in, 292, 716
dysphagia in, 1129
familial, 519
headache in, 1105
hypertension in, 527
hypophosphatemia in, 638–639
magnesium absorption in, 578
magnesium deficiency in, 600, 608
magnesium excretion in, 592–593
nausea and vomiting in, 1129
neurologic disorders in, 982
normocalcemic, 532
pancreatitis in, 528, 1131
peptic ulcers with, 527–528, 1130
primary, 518–519
radiation-induced, 518–519
renal calculi in, 528
in renal failure
acute, 674–676
chronic, 710–712, 731–736
tertiary, 525
weakness in, 1102–1103
Hyperphosphatemia, 646–652
and calcification of soft tissues, 650, 651
carbonic anhydrase inhibitors in, 1161
cardiovascular system in, 1115
causes of, 647–651
evaluation of, 647
from phosphate enemas, 647
in hyperthyroidism, 650–651
hypocalcemia with, 546, 651
in hypoparathyroidism, 649
in increased phosphate load, 647–649
endogenous sources of, 648–649
exogenous sources of, 647–648
in lactic acidosis, 305
in pseudohypoparathyroidism, 649–650
in renal failure
acute, 651, 675, 676, 761
chronic, 651, 748
control of, 754–755
signs and symptoms of, 651–652
treatment of, 652
in vitamin D intoxication, 647
Hyperreflexia, 1103, 1104
Hypertension
in aldosteronism, 363, 900
in chloriduric alkalosis, 363–367
in Cushing's syndrome, 901
diuretics in, 1179–1180
hypercalcemia with, 527, 1114
hyperkalemia with, chloride shunt in, 1181
hypokalemia with, 476–479, 1113
hypomagnesemia with, 1114
intracranial, mannitol in, 1175
malignant, and hyperreninemia with hypokalemia, 476
polydipsia from, 136
portal, in cirrhosis, 92
in pregnancy, 1066–1070
classification of, 1067–1068
and preeclampsia, 1068–1070
in pseudohyperaldosteronism, 366, 901–902
Hyperthermia, malignant, hyperphosphatemia in, 649
Hyperthyroidism
acid-base balance in, 245
calcium excretion in, 515
hypercalcemia in, 520
hyperphosphatemia in, 650–651
hypomagnesemia in, 608
magnesium absorption in, 579
magnesium excretion in, 593
nonketotic coma in, 950
polydipsia in, 136
Hypertonia, and muscle rigidity, 1107
Hypertonic solutions, 191t
Hypertonicity, 7, 190, 195
hyperglycemia with, 190, 198–200
and hyponatremia, 207
and intracranial hemorrhage, 193
treatment of, 204
Hyperuricemia
in chemotherapy, 1182–1183
ethacrynic acid congeners in, 1167–1168
in lactic acidosis, 305
in metabolic acidosis, 295
in preeclampsia, 1070
thiazide-induced, 1165
Hyperventilation, 1107
bicarbonate levels in, 242
phosphorus levels in, 243
psychogenic, 398
and respiratory alkalosis, 396
in salicylate intoxication, 310
Hypoalbuminemia. *See* Albumin, hypoalbuminemia
Hypoaldosteronism, 906–909
acid excretion in, 324, 906
and distal renal tubular acidosis, 331
in enzymatic defects, 432–433
hyperkalemia in, 447
hyporeninemic, 433–441, 914–921
aldosterone levels in, 434–437
clinical features of, 433–434
in diabetes mellitus, 941
fludrocortisone in, 916–921
hyperkalemia in, 914–916
and hypertension with hypokalemia, 477–479
and renal tubular acidosis, 1181
renin secretion in, 437–440
pseudohypoaldosteronism, 444, 921–924
selective, hyperkalemia in, 443–444
Hypocalcemia, 539–554
anorexia in, 1128
arrhythmias in, 1126t
cardiovascular system in, 550, 1114
causes of, 539–548
chorea in, 1107
cognitive function in, 1111
dental changes in, 550
depression in, 1109
diagnostic approach to, 551–552
in diarrhea, 843, 1130
drug-induced, 547
and effects of digitalis, 1128
electrocardiography in, 1120, 1122, 1124

endocrine manifestations of, 550–551
fasciculations in, 1098
from postgastric surgery, 544
hallucinations in, 1111
in hepatobiliary disease, 544
in hungry bone syndrome, 547
and hyperparathyroidism, 731
in hyperphosphatemia, 546, 641
hypoalbuminemia with, 540
in hypomagnesemia, 542–543, 610
in hypoparathyroidism, 540–542
lethargy and stupor in, 1094
mental retardation in, 549
miscellaneous causes of, 547–548
movement disorders in, 549
muscle rigidity in, 1107
myocardial performance in, 1116–1117
myopathy in, 549–550
neonatal, 547
in nephrotic syndrome, 545, 760
ocular manifestations of, 549
in pancreatitis, 546–547
papilledema in, 1105
paresthesias in, 1104
in pseudohypoparathyroidism, 541–542
psychiatric disorders in, 549, 1109
reflexes in, 1104
in renal failure
acute, 674–676, 762
chronic, 545, 749
prevention of, 755–756
renal manifestations of, 551
in renal transplant patients, 764
seizures in, 549, 1091–1092
signs and symptoms of, 548–552
skeletal manifestations of, 550
tetany in, 548–549, 1106
treatment of, 552–554
in acute disease, 552–553
in chronic disease, 553
in vitamin D deficiency, 553–554
in vitamin D deficiency, 543–546
in anticonvulsant therapy, 544–545
in hepatobiliary disease, 544
and nutritional rickets, 543–544
postoperative, 544
in vitamin D-dependent rickets, 545–546
weakness in, 1102
Hypocapnia
acid excretion in, 234
in acidosis, 284–286
brain changes in, 1026
cardiovascular system in, 1113
in diabetic ketoacidosis, 958
in hemodialysis, 792
renal response to, 393–395
and respiratory alkalosis. *See* Alkalosis, respiratory
Hypocarbia. *See* Hypocapnia
Hypochloremia, cardiovascular system in, 1115
Hypodipsia, 126–132, 203
and defects in antidiuretic hormone release, 129
in diabetes insipidus, 127, 128, 129, 858
in essential hypernatremia, 127–128, 129–132
in hypothalamic damage, 129
osmoregulatory defects with, 129
primary, 126–132
pure, 128–129
symptoms of, 126
tests in, 126
and threshold for thirst, 127
treatment of, 132
Hypoglycemic agents, oral, lactic acidosis from, 306–307
Hypokalemia, 460–484
abdominal pain in, 1130
and acid excretion in urine, 234
in acidosis
hyperchloremic, 318–335
renal tubular, 333, 470
in adenohypophyseal disease, 883
in aging, 1244
in aldosteronism, 363, 900
and alkalemia, 461–462
in alkalosis, 340, 341, 344, 461–462, 481
arrhythmias in, 1126t
in barium poisoning, 462–463
in Bartter's syndrome, 360, 472–475, 903
clinical features of, 480–481
confusion and delirium in, 1110
constipation in, 1129
in Cushing's syndrome, 901
in diarrhea, 321, 468–469, 843
in dietary deficiency, 465
diuretic-induced, 469–470
drug-induced, 464, 475–476
and effects of digitalis, 1128
electrocardiography in, 1119, 1121, 1122, 1123, 1124, 1125
estimation of potassium deficit in, 479–480
etiology of, 460t, 481–482
in extrarenal potassium wasting, 466–469
fasciculations in, 1098
from transfusions of frozen erythrocytes, 464–465
in gastrointestinal disorders, 466–469
hallucinations in, 1112
heart in, 481
in hypercalcemia, 530–531
hypertension with, 476–479, 1113
and decreased plasma renin, 477–479
decreased aldosterone with, 477–479
increased aldosterone with, 477
and hyperreninemia, 476–477
and normal plasma renin, 479
lethargy in, 1094
in leukemia, 464
in loss of gastric juice, 844
in magnesium deficiency, 471–472
neuromuscular disorders in, 481
paralytic ileus in, 1129
paresthesias in, 1104
in periodic paralysis, 463–464, 100–1101
polydipsia in, 137
potassium-sparing diuretics in, 1172

Hypokalemia (*Cont.*)
in pseudohyperaldosteronism, 901–902
reflexes in, 1103, 1104
renal effects of, 481
severe depletion in, 362
treatment of, 479–484
vascular tone in, 1112–1113
in vomiting, 466–467
weakness and paralysis in, 1099–1100
Hypomagnesemia, 599–612
in acid-base disorders, 602
in acidosis, 608
in alcohol withdrawal, 602
in alcoholism, 606–607
in aldosteronism, 608–609
in aminoglycoside therapy, 607
anion gap in, 279
apathy and lassitude in, 1108
arrhythmias in, 1126t
ataxia in, 1107
cardiovascular system in, 1114
clinical features of, 609–610
confusion and delirium in, 1110
definition of, 599–601
in diabetes mellitus, 607, 611
diagnosis of, 600t
in diarrhea, 843
dilutional, 603
diuretics causing, 605–606, 1166, 1169
drug-induced, 606–608
in endocrine disorders, 608–609
etiology of, 601–609
fasciculations in, 1098
in gastrointestinal disorders, 603–605
hallucinations in, 1111
in hungry bone syndrome, 601
in hypercalcemia, 531, 608
in hyperthyroidism, 608
hypocalcemia in, 542–543, 551, 610
hypokalemia in, 471–472
insulin-induced, 602–603
in malabsorption syndromes, 603–604
in metabolic disorders, 608
myoclonus in, 1098
nausea and vomiting in, 1129
neurologic disorders in, 1094
nystagmus in, 1105
in pancreatitis, acute hemorrhagic, 601
paralytic ileus in, 1129
in parathyroid disorders, 608
paresthesias in, 1104
in phosphate depletion, 608
postoperative, 603
prophylaxis of, 611
in protein-calorie malnutrition, 602, 603
reflexes in, 1104
renal causes of, 605–609
in renal failure, chronic, 756
in renal tubular defects, 609
seizures in, 1092
tetany in, 1106
treatment of, 610–612
in mild or asymptomatic disease, 611–612
in severe or symptomatic disease, 612
weakness and paralysis in, 1102
Hyponatremia, 207–214, 992–1007
acute, 994
in Addison's disease, 910
in adenohypophyseal disease, 877–883
in aging, 1241–1243
anorexia in, 1128
apathy and lassitude in, 1108
ataxia in, 1107
brain water and electrolyte content in, 996–999
carbamazepine-induced, 1151
cardiovascular system in, 1115
causes of, 992t
and central pontine myelinolysis, 1000–1002
cerebral, 993–994
chronic, 994–995
classification of, 207–209
cognitive function in, 1110–1111
coma in, 1093–1094
in diabetes mellitus, 940
from chlorpropamide, 1147–1148
in diabetic ketoacidosis, 957
differential diagnosis of, 208t
diuretic-induced, 211, 212, 994, 1165
drug-induced, 999
electroencephalography in, 995
in endocrinopathies, 211
extracellular fluid volume in
decreased, 211–212
increased, 212–213
normal, 209–211
factitious, 197–198
fasciculations in, 1098
in glucocorticoid deficiency, 878–880
hallucinations in, 1112
headache in, 1104
and hypertonicity, 207
in hypothyroidism, 880–883
hypotonic, 209
in inappropriate antidiuretic hormone secretion, 164, 210–211, 872–873, 874–875
lethargy and stupor in, 1093–1094
loop diuretics in, 1168–1169
mortality in, 1002–1004
muscle rigidity in, 1107
myoclonus in, 1098
nausea and vomiting in, 1128
neurologic disorders in, 994, 995
papilledema in, 1105
pathology in, 995–996
physiologic responses to, 14
potassium depletion with, from diuretics, 154
in polydipsia, primary, 209–210
in pseudohypoaldosteronism, 922
pseudohyponatremia, 207
psychiatric manifestations of, 1109
reflexes in, 1103, 1104
in renal failure, acute, 672
in reset osmostat syndrome, 209–210, 211
in salt-wasting syndromes, 993–994
cerebral, 993–994
diuretic-induced, 994
renal, 993
seizures in, 1090–1091
signs and symptoms of, 12–13, 994–995
taste loss in, 1104
thiazide-induced, 1165
treatment of, 999–1007
rapid, 1004–1005
slow, 1005–1006
in symptomatic hypotonicity, 213–214

weakness and paralysis in, 1102
Hypoosmolality, 10
physiologic responses to, 14
signs and symptoms of, 12–13
volume regulatory decrease in, 15–16
Hypoparathyroidism, 540–542
acid production in, 1130
cataracts in, 1104
chorea in, 1107
hypercalcemia with, 341
hyperphosphatemia in, 649
hypomagnesemia in, 608
idiopathic, 540–541
partial, 540
postoperative, 540
pseudohypoparathyroidism, 541–542
pseudoidiopathic, 542
weakness in, 1102
Hypophosphatemia, 635–646
in acidosis, 639
in alcoholism, 640
in alkalosis
metabolic, 344–345
respiratory, 637
in androgen therapy, 637
animal studies of, 1016
antacids causing, 638
ataxia in, 1107
biochemical features of, 641–645
in burns, 639
in carbohydrate load, 636–637
causes of, 635–641
clinical studies of, 641–645, 1015–1016
coma in, 1097
confusion and delirium in, 1110
definition of, 635
in diabetic ketoacidosis, 639, 958–959, 961
in dietary phosphate deficiency, 637–638
fasciculations in, 1098
from intracellular phosphate shifts, 636–637
gastrointestinal tract in, 644
in gout, 639
hallucinations in, 1112
hematologic effects of, 641–643
hemolytic anemia in, 1131
in hungry bone syndrome, 637
hyperalimentation-induced
leukocytes in, 1132
platelets in, 1131–1132
in hypercalcemia, 531
in hyperparathyroidism, 638–639
lactate infusions causing, 639
lethargy and stupor in, 1097
in malabsorption syndromes, 638
muscular system in, 643
myocardial performance in, 1117
nausea and vomiting in, 1129
neurologic disorders in, 645, 1014–1017
in osteomalacia, 737
oxygen-hemoglobin affinity in, 1133
paresthesias in, 1104
red cell metabolism in, 1131
in refeeding, 637
reflexes in, 1103, 1104
renal responses to, 644–645
in renal transport patients, 641, 764
in rickets, 639, 640, 643
skeletal system in, 643–644
treatment of, 645–646
in vitamin D deficiency, 639, 640
vomiting causing, 638
weakness and paralysis in, 1101
Hyporeflexia, 1103–1104
Hypotension
in hemodialysis, 784, 785–790
acetate role in, 786–787
autonomic dysfunction in, 789–790
intravascular volume and cardiovascular dynamics in, 785–786
hypoxemia in, 787
mannitol in, 1175
osmolarity of plasma in, 787–788
in hypermagnesemia, 1114–1115
hypernatremia with, 204
in hypocalcemia, 1114
Hypothalamus
disorders of
hypodipsia in, 129
polydipsia in, 858
osmoreceptor in, 119. *See also* Osmoreceptors
Hypothermia
in diabetic ketoacidosis, 957, 958
oxygen-hemoglobin affinity in, 1133
Hypothyroidism
hyponatremia in, 211, 880–883
magnesium absorption in, 579
magnesium excretion in, 593
and renal hypertrophy, compensatory, 697
respiratory acidosis in, 402
urinary dilution in, 153–154
water retention in, 881–883
Hypotonic fluid loss, 204–206
Hypotonicity, 7, 190, 196
in cerebral dehydration, 193
in cerebral edema, 193
hyperosmolality with, 200
and hyponatremia, 209
in inappropriate antidiuretic hormone secretion, 210
symptomatic, 213–214
Hypoventilation, 1106–1107
idiopathic alveolar, 402
in metabolic alkalosis, 342
and respiratory acidosis, 400
Hypovolemia
in Addison's disease, 910
in hyperaldosteronism, secondary, 902–903
hypernatremia in, 204–206
and hyponatremia, 211–212
in preeclampsia, 1071–1074
in prerenal azotemia, 662
urinary dilution in, 152–153
Hypoxemia
and dialysis hypotension, 787
in hemodialysis, 793
and respiratory alkalosis, 398
Hypoxia
cerebral, in ketoacidosis, 1018
and respiratory alkalosis, 397

Ibuprofen
in Bartter's syndrome, 361, 362
hyperkalemia from, 438
Idiogenic osmoles. *See* Brain, idiogenic osmoles in
Ileal fluid, electrolytes in, 1015t
Ileum
absorption in, 832–833
secretions of, 833–834

Ileus, paralytic, 1129–1130
Immobilization, hypercalcemia from, 522
Immune-complex nephritis, 690–691
  glomerulotubular balance in, 103
Immune mechanisms, pH affecting, 256
Indacrinone, uricosuric effects of, 1167
Indomethacin
  in Bartter's syndrome, 361, 362
  hyperkalemia from, 441, 459
    in hyporeninemic hypoaldosteronism, 438
Infants, maintenance fluid therapy for, 1214–1215
Insulin
  binding to adipocytes, in acidosis, 244, 256
  and calcium excretion, 515
  deficiency of, hyperkalemia in, 447
  and magnesium excretion, 593–594
  output affected by extracellular pH, 244
  and potassium metabolism, 417–418, 437
  and sodium reabsorption, 26
  therapy with
    in diabetic ketoacidosis, 961–963, 965–966
    in hyperkalemia, 456, 674
      in renal failure, 803
    hypokalemia from, 464, 481
    hypomagnesemia from, 602–603, 607
    in lactic acidosis, 309
    in nonketotic coma, 954–955
Interstitial fluid, 1, 185
  characteristics of, 3–4
  electrolyte concentrations in, 4t
  exchange with plasma, 17–18
  volume of
    accumulation in edema. *See* Edema
    regulation of, 19
Intestinal conditions. *See* Gastrointestinal tract
Intracellular fluid, 1, 185
  bicarbonate in, 275–277
  deficiency in diabetes mellitus, 937–938
  electrolyte concentrations in, 4t
  volume of, 2–3
    abnormalities in, 11–13
    in chronic renal failure, 700
    regulation of, 10–17
    regulatory decrease in, 15–16
    regulatory increase in, 16–17
    and vascular volume regulation, 28–31
Intravascular fluid, 185
  volume regulation, 20–31
Iodine, radioactive, hypoparathyroidism from, 540
Ischemia, renal, 664
Isohydric principle, in buffer pairs, 274–275
Isophosphamide, and urinary concentration, 164
Isoproterenol
  hypokalemia from, 464
  polydipsia from, 138
Isotonic fluid, loss or gain of, 194

Jaundice, renal function in, 93
Jejunoileal bypass for obesity, and nephrolithiasis, 843
Jejunum
  absorption in, 830–832
  secretions of, 832

Kallikrein
  and abnormal salt and water processing in cirrhosis, 98
  and sodium transport, 895
Kayexalate
  aluminum hydroxide with
    alkalosis from, 358
    in chronic renal failure, 301
  in hyperkalemia, 456–457, 460, 674
    in renal failure, 804
Kernicterus, renal function in, 93
Ketoacidosis
  diabetic, 941–945, 956–966, 1017–1020. *See also* Diabetes mellitus, ketoacidosis in
  in fasting, 293
Ketone bodies, in diabetic ketoacidosis, 943–945, 957
Ketonemia, and coma in diabetic ketoacidosis, 1017–1018
Ketonuria
  in alkalosis, 244
  in starvation, 293
Kidney
  abnormal salt and water processing in cirrhosis, 95–99
    mediators of, 97–99
  and acid-base balance, 231–235
  in acidosis, 292, 295
  acute failure of, 661–680
    acidosis in, 283–284, 296–297, 676–678
    bicarbonate therapy in, 674, 678
    calcium metabolism in, 674–676, 761–763
    diagnosis by exclusion, 662–666
    dialysis in, 670, 674, 679
    diuretics in, 669, 1181–1184
    etiology of, 664
    fluid replacement in, 671
    from radiographic contrast media, 1183
    glomerular filtration rate in, 667
    glucose infusions in, 674, 679
    hypercalcemia in, 525
    hyperkalemia in, 425–429
    hypermagnesemia in, 597
  hyperparathyroidism in, 674–676
    hyperphosphatemia in, 651
    initiation phase of, 662
      acidosis in, 677
      hyperparathyroidism and hypocalcemia in, 675–676
      nutrition in, 678–679
      potassium homeostasis in, 673
      sodium chloride and water balance in, 670
    insulin therapy in, 674
    ischemic, 664
    Kayexalate in, 674
    maintenance phase of, 662
      acidosis in, 677–678
      hyperphosphatemia and hypocalcemia in, 676
      nutrition in, 679
      potassium homeostasis in, 673–674

sodium chloride and water balance in, 670–672
nephrotoxic, 664
neurologic disorders in, 976
nonoliguric, 661
nutrition in, 678–679
oliguric, 661
pathophysiology of, 666–669
phosphate levels in, 674–676
physiologic abnormalities in, 669–679
and pigment nephropathy, 664
potassium homeostasis in, 672–674
prevention of, 669
recovery phase of, 662
acidosis in, 678
hypercalcemia in, 676
nutrition in, 679
potassium homeostasis in, 674
sodium chloride and water balance in, 672
renal blood flow in, 666–667
rhabdomyolysis in, 648, 676
in scleroderma, 1183
sodium chloride and water balance in, 670–672
triamterene-induced, 1173, 1183
tubular function abnormalities in, 667–668
vitamin D metabolism in, 675–676, 762
aging affecting, 1231–1244
and acid-base balance, 1244
anatomy in, 1231–1233
blood flow in, 1233–1234
and extracellular fluid volume, 1236–1238
glomerular filtration rate in, 1234–1235
and hyperkalemia, 1243–1244
and hypernatremia, 1241
and hypokalemia, 1244
physiology in, 1233–1235
urinary concentration in, 1238
and vasopressin secretion, 1238–1241
in alkalosis, 346–351
in Bartter's syndrome, 360
bicarbonate reabsorption in, 231–232
as bicarbonate source, 337–338
blood flow in. *See* Blood flow, renal
calcium transport in, 513–515
chronic failure of, 683–719
acidosis in, 283–284, 297–301, 713–716, 790
bone disease with, 791
aldosterone metabolism in, 426–428
and alkaline phosphatase activity, 749–750
ammonium excretion in, 715
bicarbonate reabsorption in, 298–299, 716
buffer excretion in, 299–301
calcifications of soft tissue in, 744–746
calcium intake in, 755–756
calcium metabolism in, 712–713, 749
and compensatory renal hypertrophy, 695–699
creatinine appearance in, 709–710
effects of nephron loss in, 683–686
extracellular fluid volume in, 699–700
glomerular filtration rate in, 683–684
evaluation of, 694–695
glomerular function in, 690–695
glomerulosclerosis and proteinuria in, 692
homeostasis in, 688–689
augmented signal for excretion in, 688
enhanced end-organ response in, 689
prolonged signal for excretion in, 688–689
in hypercalcemia, 528–529
hyperkalemia in, 425–429
hypermagnesemia in, 597
hyperparathyroidism in, 731–736
hyperphosphatemia in, 651
hypocalcemia in, 545
hyponatremia in, 213
intracellular fluid space in, 700
lactic acidosis in, 307
magnesium levels in, 713, 749, 756
neurologic disorders in, 977–978
nitrogen metabolism in, 709–710
nocturia in, 708–709
in nonglomerular disease, 689–690
nutritional requirements in, 717–718
and parathyroid hormone as uremic toxin, 748
phosphate excretion in, 715–716
phosphate retention in, 732–733
phosphorus metabolism in, 710–712, 748–749
polydipsia in, 136
potassium homeostasis in, 705–707
progressive course of, 692–694
prevention of, 718–719
renal blood flow in, 689–690
and renal osteodystrophy, 729–765
reversible causes of, 717t
sodium homeostasis in, 299, 699–705
solute balance in, 688–689
treatment of, 301, 716–719
tubular function in, 684–685
tubular handling of sodium in, 701–705
in animals, 702–703
in glomerular disease, 703–704
in humans, 701–702
in nonglomerular disease, 702–703
mediators of, 704–705
urea accumulation in, 709
uric acid levels in, 710
urinary concentration in, 168–169, 707–709
urinary dilution in, 154–155, 707–709
vitamin D metabolism in, 735–736
vitamin D sterols in, 756–759
parenteral, 759
concentration of urine in, 145–151
dilution of urine in, 144–145

Kidney (*Cont.*)
gluconeogenesis in, 934
in hypercalcemia, 528–531
in hypercapnia
acute, 389–393
chronic, 392–394
hypertrophy of, compensatory, 695–699
conditioning factors in, 697
humoral regulation of, 697–698
and kidney cell growth in culture, 698
and loss of mass versus loss of function, 696–697
and new nephron formation, 695–696
and renotropin activity, 697–698
sites of, 696
stimuli for, 696–698
work hypothesis of, 698–699
in hypocalcemia, 551
in hypocapnia, 393–395
in hypophosphatemia, 644–645
in jaundice, 93
magnesium reabsorption in, 580–596
mineralocorticoid hormones affecting, 893–894
minimal-change lesions, sodium retention in, 101, 104
natriuretic hormone in, 27. *See also* Natriuretic hormone
nephrocalcinosis, 166
neural system in. *See* Renal nerves
parenchymal diseases, 663
phosphate transport in, 629–633
potassium excretion regulation, 414–417
potassium secretion in tubules
defect in, 441–446
evaluation of, 452
inhibition of, 446
preeclampsia affecting, 1070–1071
in pregnancy, 1044–1065
salt-wasting syndromes, 993
in diabetes mellitus, 939–940
single nephron function in cirrhosis, 95–96
sodium retention sites in nephron
in cirrhosis, 95–99
in nephrotic syndrome, 101–104
sodium excretion. *See* Sodium, urinary excretion and solute homeostasis, 139–140, 687–688
transplantation of
and aseptic necrosis of bone, 764–765
and calciphylaxis, 746–748
calcium levels after, 524–525, 763–764
and growth in children, 765
hyperkalemia from, 443, 1181
phosphorus levels after, 641, 764
tubular acidosis, 322–335. *See also* Acidosis, renal tubular
tubular reabsorption of glomerular filtrate, 144–145. *See also specific reabsorbed substances*
tubuloglomerular feedback
glucose affecting, 439–440
and renin-angiotensin activation, 667
volume receptors in, 24, 43–44
and water balance regulation, 139
water deprivation and water ingestion affecting, 140–141
water excretion
abnormal, 151–169
normal, 139–151
and solute-free water clearance, 141–144
Kinin, and abnormal salt and water processing in cirrhosis, 98
Krebs cycle, pH affecting, 253
Kussmaul respiration, in acidosis, 294
Kyphoscoliosis, respiratory acidosis in, 404

Lactate
in blood
in diabetic ketoacidosis, 942t
in hypocapnia, 242–243
in brain, in respiratory alkalosis, 1026
daily turnover of, 304
oxidation of, 1198
in peritoneal dialysis, 798
pK_A value for, 226, 227t
therapy with, hypophosphatemia from, 639
urinary excretion of, 304
Lactate dehydrogenase reaction, 302
Lactic acidosis, 301–309
anion gap in, 305
bicarbonate therapy in, 400
blood sample collections in, 305
clinical features of, 305–308
in diabetes mellitus, 306
ethanol-induced, 307
hyperphosphatemia in, 649
laboratory findings in, 305
in liver failure, 307
in methanol poisoning, 316
pathogenesis of, 302–305
in peritoneal dialysis, 799–800
phenformin-induced, 306–307
potassium levels in, 423
in renal failure, 307
in seizures, 307
in shock, 305
in total parenteral nutrition, 1201
treatment of, 308–309
in tumor patients, 307
type A, 305, 306
type B, 305, 306
Lactose
intolerance to, 836–837
and magnesium absorption, 577
Lactulose, diarrhea from, 839
Lassitude, in electrolyte disorders, 1108
Laxative abuse
diarrhea from, 838–839
and hyperphosphatemia, 647
hypokalemia from, 469
hypomagnesemia from, 604
phosphate levels in, 546
Lead, in dialysate water, 811t
Lethargy and stupor, 1092–1097
in acidosis
metabolic, 1096
respiratory, 1095
in alkalosis, 1096–1097
in diabetic ketoacidosis, 1096

etiology of, 1093t
in hypercalcemia, 1094
in hyperglycemia, 1093
in hypernatremia, 1093
in hypocalcemia, 1094
in hypokalemia, 1094
in hyponatremia, 1093–1094
in hypophosphatemia, 1097
Leukemia
acute myeloid, hypokalemia in, 464
diabetes insipidus in, 857
hyperphosphatemia in, 648
Leukocytes, in electrolyte disorders, 1132
Leukocytosis, in lactic acidosis, 305
LeVeen shunt, in cirrhosis, 107
renal function after, 91
Licorice
hypokalemia from, 478
pseudohyperaldosteronism from, 366–367
Liddle's syndrome, 366–367, 479, 901–902
Linoleic acid, 1194
Lipid
emulsions of, 1194
in serum, and factitious hyponatremia, 197
thiazide-induced hyperlipidemia, 1165
Lithium
as antidiuretic hormone antagonist, 1175
hypercalcemia from, 526
in inappropriate antidiuretic hormone secretion, 211, 876, 1168, 1175–1176
polydipsia from, 137
polyuria from, 163–164
side effects of, 1176
Liver
as buffer source, 238
cirrhosis of. *See* Cirrhosis
failure of, lactic acidosis in, 307
gluconeogenesis in, 934
volume receptors in, 24–25, 45–46, 90
Lungs
calcification in chronic renal failure, 746
carbon dioxide excretion through, 386–387
diseases of
acid-base disorders in, 385–409
acidosis in, respiratory, 404–405
alkalosis in, respiratory, 398
and inappropriate antidiuretic hormone secretion, 157t, 873
function in metabolic acidosis, 293–295
pH affecting, 254
Lupus erythematosus
and inappropriate antidiuretic hormone secretion, 874
renal potassium secretion in, 442–443
Lydia Pinkham's Compound, pseudohyperaldosteronism from, 367
Lymphatic drainage rate, 19
and capillary filtration, 28–29, 78
Lymphectasia, intestinal, hypomagnesemia in, 604
Lymphocytes, volume regulation in, 16
Lymphomas, hyperphosphatemia in, 648
Lysine hydrochloride, as acidifying agent, 355t
Lysine-vasopressin, in diabetes insipidus, 870

Magnesium, 575–612
in brain, 970
in cerebrospinal fluid, 973
depletion of
anorexia in, 1128
in Bartter's syndrome, 906
cognitive function in, 1111
dysphagia in, 1129
and effects of digitalis, 1128
electrocardiography in, 1120, 1121, 1122, 1123, 1124–1125
hormones released in, 1134
hypokalemia in, 471–472
diarrhea from, 839
dietary, 576
and urinary magnesium excretion, 594–595
distribution of, 575
extracellular, 4t
gastrointestinal losses of, 603–605
glomerular filtration of, 579–580
hypermagnesemia, 596–599. *See also* Hypermagnesemia
hypomagnesemia, 599–612. *See also* Hypomagnesemia
intestinal transport of, 576–579
characteristics of, 579
defects in, 605
endocrine factors in, 578–579
factors affecting, 577–579
in gastrointestinal diseases, 843
phosphate depletion affecting, 644
physicochemical factors in, 577
intracellular, 4t
metabolism in chronic renal failure, 713
in plasma, 575–576
in chronic renal failure, 749, 756
protein-bound, 575
renal handling of, 579–596
in ascending limb of Henle's loop, 583–586
changes in, 590–596
in collecting tubule and collecting duct, 587
defects in, 609
in distal tubule, 586–587
in pars recta and descending limb of Henle's loop, 583
in proximal convoluted tubule, 580–583
therapy with
and effects of digitalis, 1128
hypermagnesemia from, 598
in hypocalcemia, 552
in total parenteral nutrition, 1203
urinary excretion of, 588–596
in acid-base disorders, 595
adrenal steroids affecting, 594
alcohol affecting, 591–592
aminoglycosides affecting, 592
calcitonin affecting, 593
calcium affecting, 591
cisplatin affecting, 592
coupled with potassium excretion, 588

Magnesium (*Cont.*)
dietary magnesium affecting, 594–595
diurnal variation in, 596
extracellular fluid volume affecting, 590
filtered load affecting, 589–590
glucagon affecting, 593
growth hormone affecting, 593
in hypermagnesemia, 591, 597–598
in hypophosphatemia, 645
insulin and glucose affecting, 593–594
loop diuretics affecting, 1166, 1169
measurements of, 601
parathyroid hormone affecting, 592–593
in phosphate depletion, 591
renal vasodilatation affecting, 590
thyroid hormone affecting, 593
vitamin D affecting, 595–596
Malabsorption
of calcium, 512
of carbohydrate, diarrhea in, 840–842
of fatty acids, 837
and hypocalcemia, 1130
and hypophosphatemia, 638
Malignancies. *See* Tumors
Malnutrition
hypomagnesemia in, 602, 603
hyponatremia in, 1002–1003
nystagmus in, 1105
urinary concentration in, 156–157
Mannitol, 191t, 1174
in dialysate, 1175
diarrhea from, 839
as effective solute, 187
in hypotension from hemodialysis, 1175
hypotonic urinary loss from, and hypernatremia, 206
in intracranial hypertension, 1175
and magnesium reabsorption, 582–583, 585
in oliguria, 1175
and osmolality of extracellular fluid, 187
in renal failure, acute, 669, 1181–1183
and salt and water excretion in cirrhosis, 95
toxicity of, 1176
and urinary concentration, 158–159
and urinary dilution in heart failure, 153
Medulla oblongata, respiratory control center in, 240, 287, 288
Mental changes. *See also* Behavioral disorders
in electrolyte disorders, 1107–1112
in inappropriate antidiuretic hormone secretion, 874
in nonketotic coma, 950–951
Mental retardation, in hypocalcemia, 549
Mercurial diuretics
alkalosis from, 346
and urinary concentration, 157
and urinary dilution, 154
Mercury, in dialysate water, 811t
Metabolism
acidosis affecting, 293
alkalosis affecting, 344–345
in electrolyte disorders, 1133–1134
pH affecting, 253–254
Methanol
and osmolality of extracellular fluid, 187
poisoning from, 314–316
diagnosis of, 315–316
treatment of, 316
Methotrexate, tubular necrosis from, 1183
Methoxyflurane, and urinary concentration, 164
4-Methylpyrazole
in ethylene glycol poisoning, 314
in methanol poisoning, 316
Metolazone
alkalosis from, 346–350
hypotonic urinary loss from, and hypernatremia, 206
and urinary dilution, 154
Microelectrodes, for intracellular pH measurements, 246–247
Micropuncture studies, renal
of calcium reabsorption, 513, 514
of chloride reabsorption in potassium depletion, 363
in cirrhosis, 96
in hyperbicarbonatemia, 339
of magnesium reabsorption, 580, 582, 583, 584, 586
in nephrotic syndrome, 102–104
of potassium excretion, 414, 415, 416
by remnant kidney, 705
of potassium secretion in acidosis, 461
Milk
hyperphosphatemia from, 647
phosphate in, 646
Milk-alkali syndrome, 359, 515
hypercalcemia in, 522–523
Mineralocorticoid hormones, 893–925
cellular action of, 894–897
compared to glucocorticoids, 897–898
deficiency of, 906–925
in Addison's disease, 909–910
in adrenal enzyme defects, 910–914
compared to glucocorticoid deficiency, 155
and corticosterone methyl oxidase deficiency, 913–914
in experimental states, 906–909
in hyporeninemic hypoaldosteronism, 914–921
in pseudohypoaldosteronism, 921–924
in renal hyperkalemia and acidosis, 924–925
excess of, 898–906
in adrenal enzyme defects, 900–901
in aldosteronism
primary, 900
secondary, 902–903
in Bartter's syndrome, 903–906
in Cushing's syndrome, 901
in experimental states, 898–900
in pseudohyperaldosteronism, 901–902

and hydrogen ion transport, 895–897
interaction with antidiuretic hormone, 897
and potassium transport, 897
renal responses to, 893–894
and sodium transport, 894–895
Mithramycin
in hypercalcemia, 536, 762
hypocalcemia from, 547
Moniliasis
and hypercalcemia, 521, 522
and hypocalcemia, 550
Monohydrogen phosphate, 222
Morphine, and water metabolism, 1152
Mountain sickness
carbonic anhydrase inhibitors in, 1161
respiratory alkalosis in, 398
Movement disorders, in hypocalcemia, 549
Muscle
as buffer source, 238
electrolytes in, 4
Muscular disorders, 1097–1104
in hyperkalemia, 454
in hypocalcemia, 549–550
in hypokalemia, 481
in hypophosphatemia, 643
myoclonus in, 1097–1098
in renal osteodystrophy, 742–743, 758
respiratory acidosis in, 403–404
stretch reflexes in, 1103–1104
weakness and paralysis in, 1099–1103
Myasthenic crisis, respiratory acidosis in, 403
Myelinolysis, central pontine, and hyponatremia, 1000–1002
Myeloma, multiple, hypercalcemia in, 526
Myocardial infarction, and renal sodium excretion, 80
Myocardial performance. *See also* Heart
in acidosis, 254, 295, 1117–1118
in hypermagnesemia, 1118–1119
in hypocalcemia, 1116–1117
in hypophosphatemia, 1117
in potassium depletion, 1119
Myoclonus, 1097–1098
etiology of, 1098t
Myopathy. *See* Muscular disorders
Myotonic dystrophy, hypernatremia in, 858
Myxedema. *See* Hypothyroidism

Nafcillin, hypokalemia from, 475
Naproxen, hyperkalemia from, 438
Narcotics
respiratory acidosis from, 402
and water metabolism, 1152
Nasogastric suction
and fluid loss in children, 1220
loss of gastric juice in, 844
Natriuretic hormone, 24, 26–27, 64–65, 705
and abnormal salt and water processing in cirrhosis, 98–99
in brain, 27
in kidney, 27
in pregnancy, 1046–1047
and sodium retention in nephrotic syndrome, 104–105
Nausea and vomiting, 1128–1129. *See also* Vomiting
Neoplasia. *See* Tumors
Nephritis
antiglomerular basement membrane, 691
immune-complex, 690–691
Nephrocalcinosis, 166
in distal renal tubular acidosis, 327
in hypercalcemia, 529
Nephrolithiasis. *See* Calculi, renal
Nephrotic syndrome
calcium metabolism in, 760–761
diuretics in, 1178
hypocalcemia in, 545
puromycin, 692
sodium retention and edema in, 99–106
mediators of, 104–105
nephron sites of, 101–104
treatment of, 107
and urinary dilution, 153
steroid-resistant, 101
vitamin D metabolism in, 760–761
volume regulation in, 101
Nervous system, central. *See* Neurologic disorders
Neurologic disorders, 1087–1097
in acidosis
metabolic, 1026–1027
respiratory, 1024–1026
in alkalosis
metabolic, 343–344, 1026–1027
respiratory, 1024–1026
coma in, 1092–1097. *See also* Coma
in diabetic coma, 1017–1024
in dialysis, 975, 983–992
electroencephalography in, 1097
in hypermagnesemia, 1094–1095
in hypernatremia, 1008–1009
in hyperparathyroidism, 982
in hypomagnesemia, 1094
in hyponatremia, 994, 995
inappropriate antidiuretic hormone secretion in, 157t, 873–874
lethargy and stupor in, 1092–1097
in nonketotic hyperosmolar coma, 951, 1020
in phosphate depletion, 645, 1014–1017
seizures in, 1087–1092
in uremia, 974, 992
in acute renal failure, 976
and biochemical changes in brain, 978–980
in chronic renal failure, 977–978
encephalopathy in, 975–976
parathyroid hormone role in, 981–983
pathology of brain in, 980–981
in water intoxication, 994
Neuropsychiatric disorders. *See* Behavioral disorders
Neurotoxins, uremic, 979, 981–983
Newborn infants, maintenance fluid therapy for, 1214–1215
Nicotine, and urinary concentration, 164
Nifedipine, and intestinal electrolyte transport, 835
Nikethemide, respiratory alkalosis from, 398

Nitrogen
intake in total parenteral nutrition, 1193
metabolism in uremia, 709–710
Nocturia, in chronic renal failure, 708–709
Norepinephrine
and renal tubular reabsorption, 60
respiratory effects of, 398
serum levels of
and dialysis hypotension, 789
in pregnancy, 1054
Nuclear magnetic resonance, for intracellular pH measurements, 248–249
Nutrition
and dietary deficiency of potassium, 465
glucose intake and hepatic gluconeogenesis, 934
in hyperkalemia, 457–458
magnesium in foods, 576
malnutrition
hypomagnesemia in, 602, 603
hyponatremia in, 1002–1003
nystagmus in, 1105
urinary concentration in, 156–157
in peritoneal dialysis, continuous ambulatory, 814
phosphate intake, 628, 633
in renal failure
acute, 678–679
chronic, 717–718
total parenteral, 1191–1208
acid-base balance and electrolytes in, 1195–1201
acidosis in
metabolic, 1201–1202
respiratory, 1202
alkalosis in
metabolic, 1202
respiratory, 1202
amino acids in, 1192–1193
calcium in, 1203
carbohydrates in, 1194
complications from, 1194–1195
central venous administration of, 1205–1206
in children, 1220. *See also* Pediatric fluid and electrolyte therapy
chromium in, 1204
copper in, 1204
energy requirements in, 1193–1195
fat in, 1194, 1195
fatty acids in, 1194
fluid and electrolyte disorders in, 1202–1204
hypophosphatemia from, 1016
leukocytes in, 1132
platelets in, 1131–1132
indications for, 1191–1192
magnesium in, 1203
nitrogen intake in, 1193
nutrient requirements in, 1192–1195
peripheral venous administration of, 1207–1208
phosphorus in, 1204
potassium in, 1203
sodium in, 1202–1203
trace elements in, 1204–1205
vitamins in, 1203, 1204–1205
water in, 1203
zinc in, 1204
and vitamin D deficiency, 543–544
Nystagmus, 1105

Obesity jejunoileal bypass for, and nephrolithiasis development, 843
Obstructive uropathy, 663
hyperkalemia in, 443
Olecranon bursitis, in dialysis patients, 744
Oleic acid, 1194
Oliguria
in children, 1220–1223
mannitol in, 1175
Oncotic pressure of plasma, 6
Osmolality, 185–187
of brain, in uremia, 978–979
and distribution of salt and water, 8–9
effective, 6, 187
of extracellular fluid, 10
hyperosmolality. *See* Hyperosmolality
hypoosmolality, 12–16
of plasma, 6–7
alterations in, effects of, 12
and brain tissue changes, 970–971
in cirrhosis, 95
in dehydration, 1216–1217
in diabetes insipidus, 852–853, 866–868
and dialysis hypotension, 787–788
in ethylene glycol poisoning, 314
in inappropriate antidiuretic hormone secretion, 872, 875
normal range of, 119
in pregnancy, 1059–1061
relation to urine osmolality, 141
and thirst sensation, 120–121
and specific gravity, 8
of stool, 837
and thirst mechanisms, 14–15, 120–121
and tonicity, 7–8
total, 6
of urine
antidiuretic hormone affecting, 149
in diabetes insipidus, 852–853, 866–868
in inappropriate antidiuretic hormone secretion, 872, 875
water deprivation and water ingestion affecting, 140–141
Osmoles, idiogenic. *See* Brain, idiogenic osmoles in
Osmoreceptors, 119
aging affecting, 1239–1240
defective, in diabetes insipidus, 852–853
high-set, 853
and asymptomatic hypernatremia, 858, 867
and reset osmostat syndrome, 130, 209–210, 211
Osmoregulation in pregnancy, 1060
Osmotic diuresis, hypotonic fluid loss in, and hypernatremia, 205–206
Osmotic diuretics, 1174. *See also* Mannitol
and urinary concentration, 158–160
Osmotic gradient, renal corticopapillary, and urinary concentration, 145–150

Osmotic pressure, colloid, capillary and interstitial, 17–18
Osmotic threshold studies, in diabetes insipidus, 860–862
Osteitis fibrosa, 729, 730
  clinical features of, 741
  radiographic features of, 750–753
Osteoclast activating factor, hypercalcemia from, 518
Osteodystrophy, renal, 545, 729–765
  acidosis affecting, 791
  Albright's hereditary, 541, 550, 551
  alkaline phosphatase activity in, 749–750
  biochemical features of, 748–749
  bone pain in, 741
  and calciphylaxis, 746–748
  calcium intake in, 755–756
  calcium levels in, 749
  clinical features of, 741–743
  and extraskeletal calcifications, 744–746
  and hyperparathyroidism, 731–736
  magnesium levels in, 749, 756
  management of, 754–760
  mixed, 729
    factors in, 740–741
  myopathy in, 742–743, 758
  osteitis fibrosa in, 729, 730
  osteomalacia in, 729, 730–731
  parathyroid surgery in, 759–760
  phosphorus levels in, 748–749
    and control of hyperphosphatemia, 754–755
  pseudogout in, 743–744
  radiographic features of, 750–753
  skeletal pathology in, 729, 730–731
  vitamin D sterols in, 756–759
    parenteral, 759
Osteolysis, and hypercalcemia in malignancies, 517
Osteomalacia, 729, 730–731
  aluminum accumulation in, 737–740, 755
  aluminum-induced, 807–808
    management of, 760
  in anticonvulsant therapy, 544–545
  aplastic, 729, 731
  clinical features of, 742
  drug-induced, 737
  fluoride-induced, 810–811
  from gastric surgery, 544
  in hypophosphatemia, 643
  isolated, 729, 730
  phosphate depletion in, 737
  radiographic features of, 753
  in vitamin D deficiency, 543, 550
  vitamin D metabolism in, 736–737
  weakness in, 1102
Osteosclerosis, in chronic renal failure, 752–753
Ototoxicity of loop diuretics, 1170
Oxalate
  excretion in ethylene glycol poisoning, 313, 314
  pK_A value for, 227t
Oxilorphan
  diuretic action of, 1152
  in inappropriate antidiuretic hormone secretion, 876
Oxygen
  anoxemia and encephalopathy, diabetes insipidus with, 857
  delivery to tissues
    acidosis affecting, 293–295
    pH affecting, 254–256
  dissociation from hemoglobin
    in acidosis, 294
    in alkalosis, 345
    in electrolyte disorders, 1132–1133
    pH affecting, 255
  hypoxemia
    and dialysis hypotension, 787
    in hemodialysis, 793
    and respiratory alkalosis, 398
  hypoxia
    cerebral, in ketoacidosis, 1018
    and respiratory alkalosis, 397
  partial pressure of, and ventilation regulation, 240–244
  therapy with
    in cor pulmonale, 106
    in dialysis hypotension prevention, 787
    respiratory acidosis from, 402–403
Paget's disease of bone, hypercalcemia in, 522
Pain
  abdominal, in electrolyte disorders, 1130
  and inappropriate antidiuretic hormone secretion, 874
Pancreatic juice, 830
  bicarbonate in, 336, 352
  drainage of, hyperchloremic acidosis from, 321
  electrolytes in, 1015t
  loss of, systemic effects of, 845
  pH of, 227t
  potassium in, 467t
Pancreatitis, 1131
  acute hemorrhagic, hypomagnesemia in, 601
  and hypercalcemia, 528
  hypocalcemia in, 546–547
Papilledema, 1105
  in hypocalcemia, 549
Paraldehyde toxicity, 316–317
Paralysis, 1099–1103. *See also* Weakness and paralysis
  periodic
    carbonic anhydrase inhibitors in, 1161
    familial, 1100–1101
    hyperkalemic, 449
    hypokalemic, 463–464
  of respiratory muscles, 403
Paralytic ileus, 1129–1130
Paraproteinemia
  hypercalcemia with, 526
  sodium levels in, 197
Parathyroid gland
  hyperparathyroidism. *See* Hyperparathyroidism
  hypoparathyroidism. *See* Hypoparathyroidism
  surgery of
    hypoparathyroidism from, 540
    in osteodystrophy, 759–760
Parathyroid hormone
  and bicarbonate reabsorption, 716
    in renal acidosis, 298–299
  and bicarbonate wasting in hyperparathyroidism, 530
  calcemic action of, bone resistance to, 734
    in acute renal failure, 762
  and calcium excretion, 514
  and cellular buffering of acid, 238–239

Parathyroid hormone (*Cont.*)
immunoreactive, in chronic renal failure, 731, 750
and magnesium absorption, 578–579
and magnesium reabsorption and excretion, 582, 584, 591–593
and neurologic disorders in uremia, 981–983
and phosphate reabsorption, 630–631
phosphate retention affecting, 732–733
plasma levels of
in acidosis, 291, 292
in acromegaly, 520
in hyperthyroidism, 520
in hypocalciuric hypercalcemia, familial, 520
in pheochromocytoma, 521
in renal failure, acute, 675–676
in renal transplant patients, 524
radioimmunoassay of, 533–534
shift of set-point for, 732, 757
tumor production of, 517
as uremic toxin, 748
Paresthesias, in electrolyte disorders, 1104
Parietal cells, gastric, 830
Parotid glands, secretions of, 829–830
Pediatric fluid and electrolyte therapy, 1211–1227
in dehydration, 1215–1220
assessment of severity of, 1215–1216
hypertonic, 1217, 1218–1220
hypotonic, 1216, 1217–1218
isotonic, 1216, 1217–1218
historical aspects of, 1211–1212
maintenance fluids in, 1212–1215
in newborn infants, 1214, 1215
in surgical patients, 1213–1214
and oliguria assessment, 1220–1223
oral fluids in, 1223–1226
parenteral fluids in, 1212–1220
replacement fluids in, 1220
Penicillin
alkalosis from, 350
anion gap increase from, 278
Peritoneovenous shunting in cirrhosis, 107
renal function after, 91
Perspiration. *See* Sweat
pH
and acid excretion in urine, 234
of bile, 227t
of blood, 227t
in diabetic ketoacidosis, 942t, 958
and myocardial contractility, 1118
and oxygen-hemoglobin affinity, 1133
and potassium levels in serum, 422–423
in pregnancy, 1064
of brain
in acidosis, respiratory, 1025
in alkalosis, respiratory, 1026
in diabetic ketoacidosis, 1018
dialysis affecting, 986
in hypercarbia, 1095
mitochondrial, in uremia, 979
in uremia, 979
of cerebrospinal fluid, 227t, 971
dialysis affecting, 985–986
in hypercapnia, 1024
and ventilatory control, 240, 287–288
compared to hydrogen ion concentration, 223–224
and electrolyte content of cells, 11
fecal, 227t
of gastric juice, 227t
of intestinal juice, 227t
intracellular, 227t
carbon dioxide tension affecting, 387–389
measurements of, 245–249
chemical equilibria in, 247
colorimetry and fluorescent probes in, 248
distribution of weak acids or bases in, 246
microelectrodes in, 246–247
nuclear magnetic resonance in, 248–249
tissue homogenates and lysates in, 247
in muscle, 238
regulation of, 249–251
relation to extracellular pH, 251–252
in various tissues, 249
metabolic effects of, 253–254
of pancreatic juice, 227t
and regional blood flow, 256
relation to hydrogen ion concentration, 269–270
relation to pK_A, 224–227
of saliva, 227t
and tissue oxygen delivery, 254–256
of urine, 227t
in hypoaldosteronism, fludrocortisone affecting, 919–920
in renal tubular acidosis, 334
Phagocytosis, in hypophosphatemia, 643
Phenformin, lactic acidosis from, 306–307
Phenothiazines, polydipsia from, 133, 138
Phentolamine, and renal blood flow in cirrhosis, 99
Phenytoin. *See* Diphenylhydantoin
Pheochromocytoma
hypercalcemia in, 520–521
thyroid carcinoma with, 519
Phosphates. *See* Phosphorus and phosphates
Phosphofructokinase
inhibition by ATP, 303
pH action on, 253
Phospholipids, and acid-base balance, 1199
Phosphoproteins, and acid-base balance, 1199
Phosphoric acid, pK_A value for, 227t
Phosphorus and phosphates, 625–652
in bone, 626
and calcium excretion, 515

depletion of
anorexia in, 1128
cognitive function in, 1111
hypomagnesemia in, 608
neurologic disorders in, 1014–1017
dietary, 628–633
in chronic renal failure, 718
increases in, 647
restriction of, 635, 637–638, 641, 644
in uremia, 710
and urinary phosphate excretion, 631
distribution of, 625–626
extracellular, 4t
as filtered buffer, 232
hyperphosphatemia, 646–652. *See also* Hyperphosphatemia
hypophosphatemia, 635–646. *See also* Hypophosphatemia
intestinal absorption of, 628, 633–635
in chronic renal failure, 748
mechanisms of, 634–635
intracellular, 4t
shifts in, 636–637
and magnesium absorption, 577
and magnesium reabsorption and excretion, 586, 591
metabolism in chronic renal failure, 710–712
organic, metabolism of, 1199
plasma levels of
in chronic renal failure, 748–749
and prevention of hyperphosphatemia, 754–755
composition of, 626–627
hyperventilation affecting, 243
in hypocalcemia, 551
regulation of, 628–629
in renal transplant patients, 764
protein-bound, 629
ratio to chloride in serum, in hypercalcemia, 535
renal handling of, 629–633
assessment of, 631–633
factors affecting, 630t
retention of, and parathyroid hormone secretion, 732–733
therapy with
in hypercalcemia, 537
hyperphosphatemia from, 648
preparations in, 646t
in total parenteral nutrition, 1204
ultrafiltration of, 629
urinary excretion of, 628
in chronic renal failure, 715–716
in hypercalcemia, 535
phosphate deprivation affecting, 644–645
in renal tubular acidosis, 331–332
Phototherapy, and fluid losses in infants, 1215
Phrenic nerve palsy, respiratory acidosis in, 403
Phytic acid, and magnesium absorption, 577
Pigment nephropathy, 664
mannitol in, 1182
Pitressin
in diabetes insipidus, 858, 870–871
renal response to, in aging, 1238
Pituitary
adenohypophyseal disease
hypokalemia in, 883
hyponatremia in, 877–883
hypopituitarism, anterior, hyponatremia in, 211
renotropic factor in, 697
in traumatic diabetes insipidus, 856–857
p*K* values for acids, 227t
and acid strength, 271–272
Plasma, 1
electrolytes in, 4t, 1015t
exchange with interstitial fluid, 17–18
oncotic pressure of, 6
osmolality of, 6–7
volume of
decreased. *See* Hypovolemia
in dialysis hypotension, 785–786
in nephrotic syndrome, 100–101
Platelets
in Bartter's syndrome, 361
in electrolyte disorders, 1131–1132
in hypophosphatemia, 643
pH affecting, 257
Pneumothorax, respiratory acidosis in, 404
Polydipsia
in diabetes insipidus, 851
drugs causing, 133, 137–138
in hypercalcemia, 166–167
primary, 132–139, 858
in aldosteronism, 137
clinical features of, 132–133
compared to central diabetes insipidus, 133, 869
in hypertension, 136
hyponatremia in, 209–210
osmoregulatory defects with, 135–136
in potassium depletion, 137
pure, 134
in renal failure, 136
tests in, 133–134
in thyrotoxicosis, 136
treatment of, 138–139
psychogenic, 858
treatment of, 872
urinary concentration in, 160
Polystyrene sulfonate. *See* Kayexalate
Polyuria
in diabetes insipidus, 851
in hypercalcemia, 166–167
lithium-induced, 163
Pontine myelinolysis, central, and hyponatremia, 1000–1002
Porphyria, acute intermittent
hypomagnesemia in, 603
and inappropriate antidiuretic hormone secretion, 874
Portal hypertension, in cirrhosis, 92
Portal vein, volume receptors in, 24–25
Portasystemic shunts, as therapeutic procedure, 92–93
and renal function in cirrhosis, 92–93
Posture
and plasma volume in nephrotic syndrome, 101
in pregnancy
and plasma volume, 1044
and sodium excretion, 1055–1057, 1071
and urinary concentration, 1063–1064

Posture (*Cont.*)
and water excretion, 1060–1061
and renin secretion, 451
Potassium
and blood flow autoregulation, 1112–1113
in body fluids, 4t, 1015t
in brain, 970
in hypernatremia, 1011–1012
in hyponatremia, 997
in cerebrospinal fluid, 972
depletion of
apathy and lassitude in, 1108
cognitive function in, 1111
electrocardiography in, 1120, 1121, 1123
hyponatremia with, from diuretics, 154
hypotonicity from, 190
myocardial performance in, 1119
paralytic ileus in, 1129
tetany in, 1106
thiazide-induced, 1164
urinary concentration in, 164–166
without hypokalemia, 479
dietary
in chronic renal failure, 718
deficiency of, 465
distribution of, 413–414
in diabetic ketoacidosis, 957–958, 960–961
in hyperkalemia, 446–450
in hypokalemia, 461
as effective solute, 187
extracellular, 3, 4t, 413
homeostasis of
in acute renal failure, 672–674
in chronic renal failure, 705–707
extrarenal, 417–419
regulation of, 687
hyperkalemia, 419–460. *See also* Hyperkalemia
hypokalemia, 460–484. *See also* Hypokalemia
increased input of, 424
intestinal absorption of
in colon, 834
in jejunum, 832
intracellular, 3, 4t, 413
losses of
in diabetes mellitus, 941
in gastric juice, 844
in nonketotic coma, 951
metabolism of
in acidosis, 288–290
aldosterone affecting, 418–419
in diabetic coma, 940–941
epinephrine affecting, 418
insulin affecting, 417–418, 437
plasma levels of
blood pH affecting, 422–423
in hyperchloremic acidosis, 318
and renal sidum excretion, 27
removal by dialysis
in hemodialysis, 801–802, 804
in peritoneal dialysis, 802–803, 804
renal reabsorption of, 415–417
mineralocorticoids affecting, 897
renal tubular secretion of
defect in, 441–446
evaluation of, 452
inhibition of, 446, 459, 484
renal wasting syndromes, 903–906
diuretics in, 1180–1181
from carbonic anhydrase inhibitors, 1162
replacement therapy
in diabetic ketoacidosis, 961, 965
in diarrhea, 841, 842
intravenous solutions in, 483–484
in nonketotic coma, 954
oral rehydration solutions in, 483, 1224t
pediatric fluid therapy in, 1212
in total parenteral nutrition, 1203
secretion by colon, 834
sodium-potassium pump, 11
in stool, 413, 843
storage during pregnancy, 1045t
uptake by extrerenal tissues, 452–453
urinary excretion of, 414
coupled with magnesium excretion, 588
in dialysis patients, 800–801
in gastric alkalosis, 353
in hypercapnia, 392
in mineralocorticoid excess, 899
in pregnancy, 1058–1059
renal regulation of, 414–417
Potassium chloride therapy
in diuretic-induced alkalosis, 350
in gastric alkalosis, 354
Potassium-sparing diuretics, 1171–1173, 1180–1181
Preeclampsia, 1067
diuretics in, 1074–1075
edema in, 1070
hypertension in, 1068–1070
kidney in, 1070–1071
salt restriction in, effects of, 1072
salt tolerance test in, 1071
sodium retention in, 1070–1071
volume loading in, 1071–1074
Pregnancy, 1041–1075
abnormal, alterations in, 1064
acid excretion in, 1064–1065
aldosterone levels in, 1047–1051
alkalosis in, respiratory, 399
bicarbonate levels in, 1064–1065
desoxycorticosterone levels in, 1052–1054
diabetes insipidus in, 852, 1062–1063, 1064
estrogen levels in, 1054
fluid volume alterations in, 1042–1044
glomerular filtration rate in, 1044–1046
hypertension in, 1066–1070
classification of, 1067–1068
and preeclampsia, 1068–1070
natriuretic hormone levels in, 1046–1047
posture in
and plasma volume, 1044
and sodium excretion, 1055–1057, 1071
and urinary concentration, 1063–1064
and water excretion, 1060–1061
potassium homeostasis in, 1058–1059

renin-angiotensin system in, 1054–1055
salt restriction in, effects of, 1041, 1057, 1075
in preeclampsia, 1072
in sickle cell disease, hyperkalemia in, 1059
sodium excretion in, 1044–1047
sodium reabsorption in, 1047–1057
urinary concentration and dilution in, 1063–1064
vasopressin secretion in, 1061–1062
water handling in, 1059–1063
weight gain in, 1041–1042
Progesterone
and aldosterone excretion in pregnancy, 1047, 1048–1049
and potassium excretion in pregnancy, 1058–1059
respiratory alkalosis from, 398
and salt retention in preeclampsia, 1071
and sodium excretion in pregnancy, 1046
Prolactin
and renal sodium retention, 26
serum levels in preeclampsia, 1071
Propoxyphene, and urinary concentration, 164
Propranolol, hyperkalemia from, 440, 447–448
Prorenone, 1172
Prostaglandins
and abnormal salt and water processing in cirrhosis, 98
and hypercalcemia, 518
and inflammatory bowel disease, 839
inhibitors of
in Bartter's syndrome, 361, 362, 474
hyperkalemia from, 441, 459
in hyporeninemic hypoaldosteronism, 438
and intestinal electrolyte transport, 835, 836
plasma levels in preeclampsia, 1069–1070
renal synthesis of
in Bartter's syndrome, 473–474
in hypercalcemia, 168
in potassium deficiency, 166
and renin release, 438
and sodium excretion, 26, 61, 62–64
and sodium retention
in heart failure, 88–89
in nephrotic syndrome, 105
and thirst regulation, 122
urinary excretion of, in uremia, 705
uterine synthesis of, in pregnancy, 1055
Protein
calcium binding to, 511
in cerebrospinal fluid, 971
dietary, in chronic renal failure, 717–718
extracellular, 4t
fractions for volume expansion, alkalosis from, 359
intracellular, 4t
magnesium binding to, 575
metabolism to glucose, 934
oxidation of, 1196–1198
phosphate bound to, 629
plasma levels of, and renal sodium excretion, 27, 46
Protein-calorie malnutrition
hypomagnesemia in, 602, 603
urinary concentration in, 156–157
Proteinuria
in chronic renal failure, 692
in nephrotic syndrome, 99–100
in preeclampsia, 1070
Protriptyline, in diabetes insipidus, 1151
Pseudoaldosteronism, 366–367, 479, 901–902
Pseudogout, and renal osteodystrophy, 743–744
Pseudohyperaldosteronism, 366–367, 479, 901–902
Pseudohyperhypoparathyroidism, 650
Pseudohyperkalemia, 420–421
Pseudohypoaldosteronism, 444, 921–924
types 1 and 2, 924–925
Pseudohyponatremia, 197–198, 207
Pseudohypoparathyroidism, 541–542
hyperphosphatemia in, 649–650
Pseudoketosis, in paraldehyde acidosis, 317
Pseudotetany, 1106
Psychiatric disorders, 1107–1112. *See also* Behavioral disorders
Psychogenic conditions
hyperventilation, 398
polydipsia, 858
Psychosis
in electrolyte disorders, 1108t, 1109–1110
and inappropriate antidiuretic hormone secretion, 874
Purines, oxidation of, 1199
Puromycin nephrosis, 692
Pyelonephritis
glomerular filtration in, 690
renal concentrating defect in, 708
in ureterosigmoidostomy patients, 322
Pyridoxine, in chronic renal failure, 718
Pyruvate dehydrogenase, 303
Pyruvic acid metabolism, 302–304

Radiation therapy, hyperparathyroidism from, 518–519
Radiography
contrast media in
renal failure from, 1183
and urinary concentration, 158
in renal diseases, 666
in renal osteodystrophy, 750–753
Radioimmunoassay of parathyroid hormone, 533–534
Radioiodine, hypoparathyroidism from, 540
Receptors
chemoreceptors for ventilation, 240, 287, 288
alkalosis affecting, 342
and osmoregulation. *See* Osmoreceptors
volume. *See* Volume receptors
Refeeding
alkalosis in, 362–363
hypophosphatemia from, 637

Reflexes, in electrolyte disorders, 1103–1104
Rehydration solutions, oral, 1223–1226
Renal artery stenosis, and hyperreninemia with hypertension and hypokalemia, 476–477
Renal nerves
  and abnormal salt and water processing in cirrhosis, 99
  affecting sodium excretion, 25–26, 56–62, 81
    in nephrotic syndrome, 104
  and sodium retention in heart failure, 89
Renin
  and abnormal salt and water processing in cirrhosis, 97–98
  and aldosterone secretion regulation, 435
  hyperreninemia
    in Bartter's syndrome, 360
    in hypertension with hypokalemia, 476–477
    primary, 366
  hyporeninemic hypoaldosteronism, 433–441, 914–921
  plasma levels of
    aging affecting, 1236–1237
    decreased, in hypertension with hypokalemia, 477–479
    in diabetes insipidus, 133
    in polydipsia, 133, 136
    in preeclampsia, 1069
    in pregnancy, 1054–1055
  secretion of
    in diabetes mellitus, 440
    evaluation of, 451–452
    in hypercapnic acidosis, 245
    by tumors, 477
  and sodium excretion in nephrotic syndrome, 104
  and sodium retention in heart failure, 86–87
Renotropin, 697–698
Renovascular disease, 663–664
Resins, cation-exchange. *See* Kayexalate
Respiration
  hyperventilation in, 1107
  hypoventilation in, 1106–1107
  in metabolic acidosis, 294
  and regulation of carbon dioxide tension, 229–230
Respiratory acidosis, 240–242
Respiratory alkalosis, 242, 393–395
Respiratory distress
  adult, pulmonary function in, 254
  in infants, bicarbonate affecting, 230
Respiratory system. *See also* Lungs
  and acid-base balance, 240–244
  in metabolic acidosis, 284–288, 294
  in metabolic alkalosis, 342
Rhabdomyolysis
  and acute renal failure, 648, 676
    calcium metabolism in, 762
  in hot climates, 466
  and hypercalcemia, 525, 1102
  hyperkalemia in, 449–450
  and hyperphosphatemia, 546, 648
  in hypophosphatemia, 643, 1101
Ricinoleic acid, as intestinal secretagogue, 839
Rickets
  hypophosphatemia in, 639, 640, 643
  nutritional, 543–544
  vitamin D-dependent, 545–546
  vitamin D-resistant, 546
  weakness in, 1102
Rigidity, muscular, 1107
Ringer's lactate, in pediatric fluid therapy, 1220
Rolaids, alkali in, 359

Salbutamol
  in hyperkalemic periodic paralysis, 449
  hypokalemia from, 464
Salicylates, 309–313
  acid-base changes from, 310
  alkalosis from, respiratory, 398–399
  intoxication from
    clinical features of, 310–311
    diagnosis of, 311
    treatment of, 311–313
  metabolic effects of, 309–310
Saline solutions
  in diabetic ketoacidosis, 960, 965
  in diarrhea, 841, 842
  in gastric alkalosis, 354
  in hypercalcemia, 536, 762
  in hyperkalemia, 455–456
  hypernatremia from, 1007
  hypertonic, 191t, 206–207
  in hyponatremia, 213, 1005–1006
  in hypotonicity, symptomatic, 213–214
  in inappropriate antidiuretic hormone secretion, 876
  isotonic, in hypernatremic volume depletion, 206
  in nonketotic coma, 953
  in pediatric fluid therapy, 1218–1220
  and vasopressin levels in aging, 1239–1240
Saliva, 829–830
  electrolytes in, 1015t
  pH of, 227t
  potassium in, 467t
Salivary glands, secretions of, 829–830
Salt intake. *See* Sodium, dietary
Saralasin
  and blood pressure in pregnancy, 1055
  and renal plasma flow in puromycin nephrosis, 692
Sarcoidosis
  bicarbonate levels in, 363
  diabetes insipidus in, 857
  hypercalcemia in, 521
Scintiscans of bone, in renal osteodystrophy, 753–754
Scleroderma, renal failure in, 1183
Secretagogues, intestinal, 836, 838
Seizures, 1087–1092
  in acidosis, 1089
  in alcohol withdrawal, 1092
  in alkalosis, 1088–1089
  carbonic anhydrase inhibitors in, 1161
  in hypercalcemia, 1091–1092
  in hypernatremia, 1089–1090
  in hyperosmolality, 1090
  in hypocalcemia, 549, 1091–1092
  in hypomagnesemia, 1092
  in hyponatremia, 1090–1091
  lactic acidosis in, 307
  in nonketotic hyperglycemia, 1021, 1090

Selenium, in dialysate water, 811t
Senokot, as intestinal secretagogue, 839
Sensory changes, in electrolyte disorders, 1104
Serotonin, and intestinal electrolyte transport, 835, 836
Shock
  lactic acidosis in, 305
  septic, respiratory alkalosis in, 399
Shohl's solution
  in acidosis with renal failure, 791
  in chronic renal failure, 301, 718
  in renal tubular acidosis, 335
Sickle cell disease
  in pregnancy, hyperkalemia in, 1059
  renal potassium secretion in, 441–442
Silver, in dialysate water, 811t
Sipple's syndrome, 519
Skeletal conditions. *See* Bone
Skin
  calcification in chronic renal failure, 746
  disorders in hypocalcemia, 550
Sleep apnea, 402
Sodium
  in body fluids, 4t, 1015t
  in brain, 970
    in hypernatremia, 1011–1012
    in hyponatremia, 997
  cerebral salt wasting, 872
  in cerebrospinal fluid, 972
    and renal sodium excretion, 25, 45
    and thirst regulation, 120, 122
  decreased distal delivery of
    and dilution of urine, 152–153
    and hyperkalemia, 424–425
  deficiency of, in diabetes, 939–940
  dietary
    in chronic renal failure, 718
    and diuretic use, 107–108
    in pseudohypoaldosteronism, 922, 924
    restriction of
      in Bartter's syndrome, 905
      in diuretic-induced alkalosis, 350
      effects in aging, 1236
      in preeclampsia, 1072
      in pregnancy, effects of, 1041, 1057, 1075
      in renal potassium wasting, 1180
  distribution of, glucocorticoids affecting, 879–880
  as effective solute, 187
  electrogenic transport of
    in distal renal tubular acidosis, 330
    mineralocorticoids affecting, 894–895
    and potassium secretion, 1172
    thiazides affecting, 1162–1163
  excess of, in diabetes mellitus, 940
  extracellular, 3, 4t, 39
  in gastric fluid, 352
  homeostasis in renal failure
    acute, 670–672
    chronic, 699–705
  hypernatremia, 200–207, 1007–1014. *See also* Hypernatremia
  hyponatremia, 207–214. *See also* Hyponatremia
  intestinal absorption of
    in colon, 834
    in ileum, 832–833
    in jejunum, 831
  intracellular, 3, 4t
  loading studies
    in preeclampsia, 1071
    in pregnancy, 1057
  losses of
    gastrointestinal, 939
    in sweat, 939
  and magnesium absorption, 577
  metabolism in diabetes mellitus, 939–940
  in oral rehydration solutions, 1224t
  and osmolality of extracellular fluid, 186–187
  in pediatric fluid therapy, 1212
  plasma levels of
    in diabetes insipidus, 852
    in hyperglycemia, 199–200
    in nonketotic coma, 951
    and renal sodium excretion, 27
    and tonicity of body fluids, 197–198
  and regulation of cellular pH, 250
  renal reabsorption of
    in alkalosis, 338, 341
    in Bartter's syndrome, 905
    in heart failure, peritubular factors in, 82–85
    in pregnancy, 1047–1057
    in uremia, 701–705
  renal retention of
    in aging, 1237–1238
    in cirrhosis with ascites, 89–99
      nephron sites of, 95–96
    edema in. *See* Edema
    in heart failure, 78–89
    in nephrotic syndrome, 99–106
    in preeclampsia, 1070–1071
    therapy affecting, 106–108
  renal wasting of, 993
    in diabetes mellitus, 939–940
  storage during pregnancy, 1045t
  in total parenteral nutrition, 1202–1203
  urinary excretion of
    afferent mechanisms in, 21–25, 39–47
    aldosterone affecting, 26, 49–52
    angiotensin affecting, 26, 55–56
    blood composition affecting, 27, 46
    in cortisol deficiency, 879
    dietary sodium affecting, 39
    efferent mechanisms in, 25–27, 47–67
    glomerular filtration rate affecting, 28, 47–48
    and glomerular-tubular balance, 48–49
    humoral factors in, 26–27
    in hypercalcemia, 530
    in mineralocorticoid excess, 898–899
    natriuretic hormone affecting. *See* Natriuretic hormone

Sodium (*Cont.*)
physical factors affecting, 52–55
in pregnancy, 1044–1047
posture affecting, 1055–1057, 1071
prostaglandins affecting, 26, 61, 62–64
in renal failure
acute, 672
chronic, 299
renal medullary tonicity affecting, 62
renal nerves affecting, 25–26, 56–62, 81
renal perfusion pressure affecting, 27, 43–44, 54–55, 81
tubular reabsorption affecting, 28, 48
volume receptors affecting, 21–27
water immersion affecting, 40, 79, 91
Sodium-potassium pump, 11. *See also* ATPase, sodium-potassium
Sodium salts of acids, and anion gap increase, 278
Sodium sulfate
alkalosis from, 350
in hypercalcemia, 536
Solutes
balance of, kidney role in, 139–140
effective, 187
Somatostatin, and intestinal electrolyte transport, 836
Sorbitol
in cerebrospinal fluid, in hyperglycemia, 1024
diarrhea from, 839
as effective solute, 187
as therapy in hyperkalemia, 457
Soy-protein formula diet, alkalosis from, 359
Specific gravity, 8
Spinal cord injury, respiratory acidosis in, 403
Spironolactone, 1172–1173
acidifying effect of, 346
action in cirrhotic patients, after water immersion, 95
in cirrhosis with ascites, 1177–1178
effects in pseudohypoaldosteronism, 924
in hypertension with aldosteronism, 900
inhibiting potassium secretion, 446, 459, 484
and magnesium excretion, 590, 605
Sprue, nontropical, 839
hypomagnesemia in, 603–604
Starling forces, and capillary fluid exchange, 17–18, 52–53, 78
Starvation, acidosis in, 293
Steatorrhea, 1130
Stomach. See Gastric juice
Stool
normal weight of, 836
osmolality of, 837
pH of, 227t
potassium in, 843
Stress, and inappropriate antidiuretic hormone secretion, 874
Stretch reflexes, in electrolyte disorders, 1103–1104
Stupor. *See* Lethargy and stupor
Succinylcholine
hyperkalemia from, 450
respiratory muscle paralysis from, 403
Sulfasalazine, in inflammatory bowel disease, 839
Sulfate
in dialysate, 811t
diarrhea from, 839
extracellular, 4t
intracellular, 4t
Sulfonylureas
and antidiuretic hormone release, 138
and urinary concentration, 164
and water metabolism, 1145–1149
Surgery
parathyroid, in osteodystrophy, 759–760
and pediatric fluid therapy, 1213–1214
and postoperative conditions
hyperphosphatemia, 649
hypomagnesemia, 603
hypoparathyroidism, 540
vitamin D deficiency, 544
Sweat
electrolytes in, 1015t
fluid loss in, 203, 205
potassium loss in, 466
sodium loss in, 939

Tamoxifen, hypercalcemia from, 526
Taste sensation
loss of, in hyponatremia, 1104
and polydipsia, 137
Temperature
and fever, 1106
respiratory alkalosis from, 399
hypothermia in diabetic ketoacidosis, 957, 958
malignant hyperthermia, hyperphosphatemia in, 649
and oxygen-hemoglobin affinity, 1133
Tendon rupture, in uremia, 744
Terbutaline, hypokalemia from, 464
Testosterone, and compensatory renal hypertrophy, 697
Tetany, 1105–1106
in hypocalcemia, 548–549, 1091
paresthesias in, 1104
Theophylline, respiratory alkalosis from, 398
Thiamine, in lactic acidosis, 309
Thiazide diuretics, 1162–1166
alkalosis from, 346–350
and calcium excretion, 515
in cirrhosis with ascites, 1177
contraindications to, 1166
in extracellular fluid volume reduction, 1163
extrarenal action of, 1163
hypercalcemia from, 523–524
in hypercalciuria, 1163–1164
in hyperkalemic periodic paralysis, 449
in hypertension, 1179–1180
hypomagnesemia from, 605
hyponatremia from, 211, 212, 994
hypotonic urinary loss from, and hypernatremia, 206
loop agents with, 1170–1171
and magnesium excretion, 590
in nephrogenic diabetes insipidus, 1164
in nephrotic syndrome, 1178
in preeclampsia, 1074

in renal tubular acidosis, 335, 1164
toxicities of, 1164–1165
and urinary dilution, 154
Thioridazine
polydipsia from, 138
water intoxication from, 1151
Thiothixene, and inappropriate secretion of antidiuretic hormone, 1151
Thirst, 119–139
adipsia, 126, 127, 131
and antidiuretic hormone release, 124–125
clinical studies of, 123–125
in diabetes insipidus, 851
in hypernatremia, 203
hypodipsia, 126–132, 203. *See also* Hypodipsia
osmolality affecting, 14–15
polydipsia, primary, 132–139, 858. *See also* Polydipsia
regulation of
abnormal, 125–139
neuroanatomy of, 122–123
normal, 120–125
stimuli for, 120–122
osmolal, 120–121
volumetric, 121–122
threshold for, 124–125, 127
Thrombosis
in diabetic ketoacidosis, 964–965
renal vein, 664
Thyrocalcitonin. *See* Calcitonin
Thyroid gland
hyperthyroidism. *See* Hyperthyroidism
hypothyroidism. *See* Hypothyroidism
medullary carcinoma of
diarrhea in, 838
pheochromocytomas with, 519
surgery of, hypoparathyroidism from, 540
Thyroid hormone
and magnesium absorption, 579
and magnesium excretion, 593
Thyroid vein catheterization, in hyperparathyroidism, 535
Ticarcillin, hypokalemia from, 475
Ticrynafen, uricosuric effects of, 1167–1168
Tienilic acid, uricosuric effects of, 1167–1168
Titrable acids, 232–233, 324
in peritoneal dialysate, 798
in respiratory acidosis, 241–242
Tobacco chewing
hypokalemia from, 478
pseudohyperaldosteronism from, 367
Tolazamide
diuretic action of, 1147
and water excretion, 1148
Tolbutamide, hyponatremia from, 1148
Tonicity, 7–8, 119, 187
and cell volume, 193–197
in dehydration, 1216–1217
disorders of, 190–214
effective solutes affecting, 187–190
hypertonicity, 7, 190, 195. *See also* Hypertonicity
hypotonicity, 7, 190, 196. *See also* Hypotonicity
in isolated alterations of solutes or body water, 190–193
medullary, and renal sodium excretion, 62
and potassium metabolism, 419
sodium levels affecting, 197–198
Tooth disorders, in hypocalcemia, 550
Transfusions of frozen erythrocytes, hypokalemia from, 464–465
Transplantation of kidney. *See* Kidney, transplantation of
Trauma
diabetes insipidus from, 855–856
and inappropriate antidiuretic hormone secretion, 873
Triamterene, 1172–1173
acidifying effect of, 346
inhibiting potassium secretion, 446, 459, 484
and magnesium excretion, 590, 605
in pseudohyperaldosteronism, 902
nephrolithiasis from, 1173
renal failure from, 1173, 1183
Tricyclic compounds, and water metabolism, 1149–1151
Trousseau sign
in alkalosis, 343
in tetany, 549
Tuberculosis
hypercalcemia in, 521
and inappropriate antidiuretic hormone secretion, 873
Tumors
of brain, diabetes insipidus in, 854
cancer cell growth in, pH affecting, 257
hypercalcemia in, 517–518
hypophosphatemia in, 640
inappropriate antidiuretic hormone secretion in, 157t, 873
lactic acidosis in, 307
metastatic, diabetes insipidus from, 857
multiple endocrine neoplasia, 519
type 1, 519
type 2, 519
parathyroid hormone produced by, 517
renin-secreting, 477
thyroid medullary carcinoma
diarrhea in, 838
pheochromocytoma with, 519
villous adenoma, intestinal, 357
Tums, alkali in, 359

Ulcer, peptic, and hyperparathyroidism, 527–528, 1130
Ultrafiltration procedure, and dialysis, 988
in hemodialysis, 780, 786
in peritoneal dialysis, 782
Urea
clearance from brain, in dialysis, 984–985
hypotonic urinary losses from, and hypernatremia, 206
renal reabsorption of, 149–150
as therapy in inappropriate antidiuretic hormone secretion, 211
and urinary concentration, 158
Urea nitrogen levels, in diabetic ketoacidosis, 958

Uremia
  dialysis in. *See* Dialysis
  neurologic disorders in, 974–992
    in acute renal failure, 976
    and biochemical changes in brain, 978–980
    in chronic renal failure, 709, 977–978
    encephalopathy in, 975–976
    parathyroid hormone role in, 981–983
  neurotoxins in, 979, 981–983
Ureterosigmoidostomy, hyperchloremic acidosis from, 321–322
Uric acid
  daily production of, 1199
  hyperuricemia. *See* Hyperuricemia
  plasma levels of
    in chronic renal failure, 710
    in preeclampsia, 1070
Urine
  acid excretion in, 231–235. *See also* Acid, urinary excretion of
  alkalinization of, carbonic anhydrase inhibitors in, 1160
  calcium excretion in, 512–513. *See also* Calcium, urinary excretion of
  composition changes in, 665t
  concentration of, 145–151
    abnormal, 156–169
    in aging, 1238
    and corticopapillary osmotic gradient, 145–150
    demeclocycline affecting, 164
    in diabetes insipidus
      central, 160
      nephrogenic, 160–163
    disorders of, 158t
    diuretics affecting, 157–160, 1174
    in hypercalcemia, 166–168, 529–530
    lithium affecting, 163–164
    in miscellaneous disorders, 168t
    in polydipsia, 160
    in potassium depletion, 164–166
    in pregnancy, 1063–1064
    in protein malnutrition, 156–157
    in renal insufficiency, 168–169
    in uremia, 707–709
  crystalluria in ethylene glycol poisoning, 313, 314
  dilution of, 144–145
    abnormal, 152–156
    in adrenal insufficiency, 155–156
    in Bartter's syndrome, 156
    diuretics affecting, 154, 1174
    in edema, 153
    in inappropriate antidiuretic hormone secretion, 156
    in myxedema, 153–154
    in pregnancy, 1063–1064
    in renal insufficiency, 154–155
    in uremia, 707–709
    in volume depletion, 152–153
  glucose excretion in, 935–937
  magnesium excretion in, 588–596. *See also* Magnesium, urinary excretion of
  pH of, 227t
    in hypoaldosteronism, fludrocortisone affecting, 919–920
    in renal tubular acidosis, 334
  phosphate excretion in, 628. *See also* Phosphorus and phosphate, urinary excretion of
  sediment alterations in, 665t
  specific gravity of, 8
  volume of
    in diabetes insipidus, 851
    oliguria
      in children, 1220–1223
      and hyperkalemia, 424–425
    in pediatric fluid therapy, 1213
    and solute excretion, 139–140

Van't Hoff equation, 5
Vasa recta system, countercurrent arrangement in, 150
Vasculature
  arterial volume receptors, 23, 42–44
  calcification in chronic renal failure, 746
  electrolyte disorders affecting, 1110t, 1112–1116
  filtration rate in capillaries, 19
    and lymphatic drainage rate, 28–29, 78
  fluid exchange in capillaries, 17–18, 52–53, 77–78
  intravascular fluid, 185
  portasystemic shunt formation, 92–93
  renal, aging affecting, 1232–1233
  venous volume receptors, 21–22, 40, 79–80
  volume regulation in, 20–31
    by external balance, 21–28
    by internal redistribution, 28–31
Vasoactive intestinal polypeptide, and intestinal electrolyte transport, 836
Vasoconstriction, venous, in metabolic acidosis, 296
Vasodilatation, in metabolic acidosis, 296
Vasodilators, and renal blood flow, 106
Vasopressin. *See* Antidiuretic hormone
Ventilation
  in metabolic acidosis, 284–288, 293–294
  regulation of, 240–244, 386
    chemoreceptors in, 240, 287, 288
      alkalosis affecting, 342
Ventilation/perfusion mismatch, 386
Ventilator use, respiratory alkalosis from, 399–400
Verapamil, and intestinal electrolyte transport, 835
Vinca alkaloids
  and urinary concentration, 164
  and water metabolism, 1151
Viscosity of serum, and measurements of sodium levels, 197
Visual hallucinations, in electrolyte disorders, 1111–1112
Vitamin A
  intoxication from, hypercalcemia in, 523
  in total parenteral nutrition, 1205

Vitamin B_6, in chronic renal failure, 718
Vitamin B_{12}, in total parenteral nutrition, 1205
Vitamin C, in chronic renal failure, 718
Vitamin D
  activation in metabolic acidosis, 291
  deficiency of
    hypocalcemia in, 543–546
    hypomagnesemia in, 604
    hypophosphatemia in, 639, 640
    and rickets, 545–546
    treatment of, 553–554
    weakness in, 1102
  intoxication from
    bicarbonate levels in, 363
    hypercalcemia in, 523
    hyperphosphatemia in, 647
  and magnesium absorption, 578
  and magnesium excretion, 595–596
  measurements in serum, 551–552
  metabolism of, 512
    in nephrotic syndrome, 760–761
    in osteomalacia, 736–737
    in renal failure
      acute, 675–676, 762
      chronic, 735–736
    in uremic myopathy, 743
  metabolites in hyperparathyroidism, 534
  sensitivity to, in sarcoidosis, 521
  therapy with, 553–554
    in chronic renal failure, 718, 756–759
      parenteral sterols in, 759
    in hypocalcemia, 552–553
  in total parenteral nutrition, 1203, 1205
Vitamin E, in total parenteral nutrition, 1205
Vitamin K, in total parenteral nutrition, 1205
Volume of body fluid, 2–3. *See also* Extracellular fluid; Intracellular fluid
Volume receptors
  arterial, 23, 42–44
  atrial, 22, 41–42, 79–80
  in brain, 24
  carotid sinus, 23, 43, 81
  in central nervous system, 25, 44–45
  in heart, 22–23, 40–42, 79–80
  hepatic, 24–25, 45–46, 90
  in plasma space, 20
  renal, 24, 43–44, 81
  sites of, 21–25, 40–46
  in thoracic low-pressure system, 21–23, 40–42, 79–80
  venous, 21–22, 40, 79–80
Vomiting
  in acidosis, 295
  in electrolyte disorders, 1128–1129
  and gastric alkalosis, 352
  gastric juice loss in, 844
  hypokalemia from, 466–467
  hypophosphatemia from, 638
  sodium loss in, 939
  surreptitious, 362
    and chloride in urine, 467, 475
    clinical features of, 467

Water
  balance of, 185
    kidney role in, 139–140
    regulation of, 119
    in renal failure, acute, 670–672
  brain content of
    in hypernatremia, 1011–1012
    in hyponatremia, 996–999
  content of body, 2
    increase in, 14
    reduction of, 14
  deionization of, for dialysate, 990–991
  distribution of, 187–190
    in diabetes mellitus, 937, 938–939
    glucocorticoids affecting, 879–880
  excess of, in diabetes mellitus, 938–939
  immersion in
    and plasma renin activity in nephrotic syndrome, 101
    and renal sodium excretion, 40, 79
      in cirrhosis, 91, 95
  as therapy
    in cirrhosis with ascites, 107
    in nephrotic syndrome, 107
  intake of
    after dehydration, 125
    in diabetes mellitus
      decreased, 937
      increased, 938
    in hypodipsia, 132
    renal response to, 140–141
    restriction in inappropriate antidiuretic hormone secretion, 210
  intestinal transport of, 828
  intoxication from
    in aging, 1241–1243
    brain pathology in, 996
    confusion and delirium in, 1110
    neurologic disorders in, 994
    in polydipsia, 133
  intracellular deficiency of, in diabetes mellitus, 937–938
  loading test
    in diabetes insipidus, 860–861
    in inappropriate antidiuretic hormone secretion, 875
  losses of. *See* Dehydration; Fluid, losses of
  metabolism of
    in aging, 1238–1243
    drugs affecting, 1145–1153
  renal excretion of, 139–169
    abnormal, 151–169
    agents affecting, 1173–1176
    in cortisol deficiency, 878–879
    in hypothyroidism, 881–883
    normal, 139–151
    in pregnancy, 1060–1061
    and solute-free water clearance, 141–144
  retention in hypothyroidism, 881–883
  in stool, in diarrhea, 836
  total body water, 185
    distribution of, 187–190
    isolated alterations in, 190
    in pregnancy, 1042–1044
  in total parenteral nutrition, 1203

Weakness and paralysis, 1099–1103
  etiology of, 1099t
  in hypercalcemia, 1102–1103
  in hyperkalemia, 1100
  in hypermagnesemia, 1101
  in hypocalcemia, 1102
  in hypokalemia, 1099–1100
  in hypomagnesemia, 1102
  in hyponatremia, 1102
  in hypophosphatemia, 1101
  hypoventilation in, 1107
Weight gain in pregnancy, 1041–1042
Wermer's syndrome, 519
Whipple's disease, hypomagnesemia in, 604
Zinc
  deficiency of, in dialysis patients, 808–810
  in dialysate water, 811t
  in total parenteral nutrition, 1204
Zollinger-Ellison syndrome, 519
  hypercalcemia in, 1130
  hyperparathyroidism with, 528